PEDIATRIC UROLOGY PRACTICE

PEDIATRIC UROLOGY PRACTICE

Edmond T. Gonzales, MD
Texas Children's Hospital
Baylor College of Medicine
Houston, Texas

Stuart B. Bauer
Children's Hospital Medical Center
Boston, Massachusetts

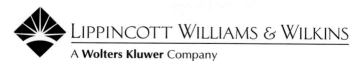

LIPPINCOTT WILLIAMS & WILKINS
A **Wolters Kluwer** Company
Philadelphia · Baltimore · New York · London
Buenos Aires · Hong Kong · Sydney · Tokyo

Editor: Craig Percy
Developmental Editor: Ellen DiFrancesco
Marketing Manager: Melissa Harris
Production Editor: June Choe

Copyright © 1999 Lippincott Williams & Wilkins

351 West Camden Street
Baltimore, Maryland 21201-2436 USA

227 East Washington Square
Philadelphia, PA 19106

The publisher is not responsible (as a matter of product liability, negligence or otherwise) for any injury resulting from any material contained herein. This publication contains information relating to general principles of medical care which should not be construed as specific instructions for individual patients. Manufacturers' product information and package inserts should be reviewed for current information, including contraindications, dosages and precautions.

Printed in the United States of America

Library of Congress Cataloging-in-Publication Data

Pediatric urology practice / [edited by] Edmond T. Gonzales, Stuart B. Bauer.
   p.   cm.
   Includes bibliographical references and index.
   ISBN 0-397-51368-2 (alk. paper)
   1. Pediatric urology. I. Gonzales, Edmond T. II. Bauer, Stuart
B. (Stuart Barry), 1943– .
   [DNLM: 1. Urogenital Abnormalities. 2. Urologic Diseases—Child.
3. Urologic Diseases—Infant. WS 320 P3757 1999]
RJ466.P384 1999
618.92′6—dc21
DNLM/DLC
for Library of Congress   99-13237
                         CIP

The publishers have made every effort to trace the copyright holders for borrowed material. If they have inadvertently overlooked any, they will be pleased to make the necessary arrangements at the first opportunity.

To purchase additional copies of this book, call our customer service department at **(800) 638-3030** or fax orders to **(301) 824-7390.** International customers should call **(301) 714-2324.**

00 01 02 03 04
2 3 4 5 6 7 8 9 10

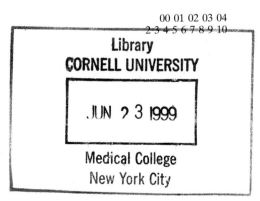

Preface

Over the past few decades, Pediatric Urology has been defined clearly as an area of special interest within the filed of Urology. Every major text in Urology separates Pediatric Urology from all other areas of interest. The major journals in Urology, likewise, give special notation and position to Pediatric Urology. The subspecialty now has accredited fellowship training programs with inservice examinations and numerous research laboratories at major pediatric institutions exploring the causes and effects of pediatric urologic diseases. Today, Pediatric Urology remains the standard by which other disciplines within Urology should be organized and judged.

These special considerations for Pediatric Urology reflect the accepted truism that "children are not just small adults." The time span defined as childhood extends from the newborn period to late adolescence. As a result, Pediatric Urology encompasses a dynamic, rapidly changing environment that demands special knowledge and skills that vary markedly for each age group. To be sure, the management of obstructive uropathy in a three-pound premature infant requires very different responsibilities and expertise compared with the treatment of a similar lesion in a 9-year-old child. The rapid expansion and application of new advances within the parameters of Pediatrics, i.e., neonatology, intensive medical care, nephrology, infectious disease and anesthesiology has broadened the opportunities for the well-trained Pediatric Urologist to provide definitive reconstruction for major urologic anomalies to smaller and sicker infants than was even remotely possible a couple of decades ago. Improved techniques in regional anesthesia and postoperative pain management also allow these procedures to be done with much less postoperative discomfort than was possible just a few short years ago, as well. Early reconstruction of complex urologic anomalies has yielded substantially better results and minimized the long-term sequelae that many children with these conditions experienced in the past. In fact, the safety of pediatric anesthesia for all age groups has allowed Pediatric Urologists to devise new and imaginative ways to correct complicated anomalies and to look beyond not only the technical procedures necessary to manage the physical deformities but also to consider the psychological effects of surgical reconstruction.

This book strives to define the very subspecialty which Pediatric Urology is—an area of medicine that demands delicate, unique surgical expertise, an understanding of the physiology of the maturing urinary tract, an appreciation of the pyschological impact that reconstruction has on the child and his family and a compassion for and willingness to undertake and manage the many nonsurgical urologic conditions that are common to pediatric urologic practice, i.e., dysfunctional voiding and urinary infection. The text begins with a very thorough chapter on the pediatric physical examination. This is positioned first in recognition of the paramount responsibility that all physicians have, who assume the surgical care of an infant or child, in recognizing the possibility of coexistant problems and systemic manifestations of many disease processes. The clinician needs to be aware how to approach the child and learn what he or she can tell us by their physical nature and behavior. The chapters that immediately follow discuss other important issues in pediatric medicine including radiology, nephrology and anesthesia that allow us to diagnose and manage the children comprehensively and efficiently. These were placed towards the beginning of the book to re-emphasize the importance of having a complete understanding of the unique aspects that Pediatrics demands before one focuses on the management of a specific pediatric urologic disorder.

This text should be of interest to practitioners and students of Urology as well as to all physicians interested in Pediatrics. The charge to all authors was to look at what is new and how it applies to Pediatrics. The literature is replete with contributions that describe traditional surgical approaches to various urologic problems, but a consolidation of what is new in molecular biology, smooth muscle physiology, and diagnostic imaging studies relating to Pediatric Urology has not been readily available until now. Also, every effort has been made to keep this text current. These objectives have been admirably met by all of the invited authors.

The editors would like to take this opportunity to thank the authors for their dedication and commitment to excellence. The quality of this work will ultimately be judged by the many individual efforts that went into its formation. The editors would like to express special appreciation to Kellie Poudrier, whose persistence and deadline orientation kept us on a straight and true path; and to Carlyn Schum who assisted in editing all the chapters. Without their help we may never have completed this task.

Edmond T. Gonzales, Jr.
Stuart B. Bauer
March 1, 1999

Contributors

Julia Spencer Barthold, MD   *Children's Hospital of Michigan, Department of Pediatric Urology, Detroit, Michigan, Chapter 32: Intersex States*

Thomas Bartholomew, MD   *Methodist Plaza, San Antonio, Texas, Chapter 31: Other Disorders of the Penis and Scrotum*

Laurence S. Baskin, MD   *Chief, Pediatric Urology, Department of Urology, UCSF Medical Center, San Francisco, California, Chapter 36: Hernia/Hydrocele*

David A. Bloom, MD   *Professor of Surgery, Chief of Pediatric Urology, Section of Urology, The University of Michigan, Ann Arbor, Michigan*

Timothy B. Boone, MD, PhD   *Associate Professor, Scott Department of Urology, Baylor College of Medicine, Houston, Texas, Chapter 22: Neurogenic Bladder: Etiology and Diagnostic Evaluation*

Eileen D. Brewer, MD   *Texas Children's Hospital, Renal Services, Houston, Texas, Chapter 5: Management of Renal Failure in Children*

Robert J. Carpenter, Jr., MD   *Associate Professor of Obstetrics and Gynecology; Associate Professor of Human and Molecular Genetics, Baylor College of Medicine, Houston, Texas, Chapter 6: Management of the High-Risk Fetus: Prenatal Diagnosis and Therapy*

Anthony J. Casale, MD   *Associate Professor, Department of Urology, Indiana University School of Medicine, J.W. Riley Hospital for Children, Pediatric Urology Division, Indianapolis, Indiana, Chapter 13: Posterior Urethral Valves and Other Obstructions of the Urethra*

Robert L. Chevalier, MD   *Benjamin Armistead Shepherd Professor, Chair, Department of Pediatrics, University of Virginia, Department of Pediatrics, Charlottesville, Virginia, Chapter 8: Prenatal and Perinatal Nephrology: Compensatory Renal Growth*

Ross M. Decter, MD   *Associate Professor of Surgery, Director, Pediatric Urology, The Milton S. Hershey Medical Center, Hershey, Pennsylvania, Ch 23: Nonsurgical Management of Neurogenic Bladder*

David A. Diamond, MD   *Associate Professor of Surgery, Harvard Medical School; Division of Urology, Children's Hospital, Boston, Massachusetts, Chapter 27: Vesicoureteral Reflux*

Steven G. Docimo, MD   *Associate Professor of Urology and Pediatrics, Director, Pediatric Endocrinology, The James Buchanan Brady Urological Institute, Johns Hopkins Hospital, Baltimore, Maryland, Chapter 29: Cryptorchidism*

Jan E. Drutz, MD   *Director, Continuity Clinics Teaching Program, Associate Professor of Pediatrics, Baylor College of Medicine, Department of Pediatrics, Houston, Texas, Chapter 1: The Pediatric Physical Examination*

S. Jean Emans, MD   *Associate Professor of Pediatrics, Harvard Medical School; Chief, Division of Adolescent/Young Adult Medicine, Children's Hospital, Adolescent Medicine, Boston, Massachusetts, Chapter 33: Menstrual Problems in the Adolescent*

Scott A. Engum, MD   *Riley Hospital for Children, Indiana University Medical Center, Department of Pediatric Surgery, Indianapolis, Indiana, Chapter 2: Surgery Physiology of the Neonate*

Sandra K. Fernbach, MD   *Professor of Radiology, Northwestern Medical School, Evanston Hospital, Department of*

Radiology, Evanston, Illinois, Chapter 7: Imaging the Urinary Tract in Children

John P. Gearhart, MD   *Professor and Director of Pediatric Urology, Professor of Pediatrics, Brady Urological Institute, Johns Hopkins Hospital, Baltimore, Maryland, Chapter 21: Bladder and Cloacal Exstrophy*

Nancy L. Glass, MD   *Associate Professor of Anesthesiology and Pediatrics, Baylor College of Medicine; Director, Operating Room Clinical Services, Texas Children's Hospital, Department of Anesthesia, Houston, Texas, Chapter 3: Pediatric Anesthesia*

Ricardo González, MD   *Professor of Virology, Wayne State University, Chief, Pediatric Urology, Children's Hospital of Michigan, Department of Pediatric Urology, Detroit, Michigan, Chapter 38: Urogenital Sinus and Cloacal Anomalies*

Saul Greenfield, MD   *Pediatric Urology Associates, Buffalo, New York, Chapter 25: Physiology of Micturition and Dysfunctional Voiding*

John T. Herrin, MBBS, FRACP   *Associate Clinical Professor of Pediatrics, Harvard Medical School, Director of Clinical Services, Division of Nephrology, The Children's Hospital, Boston, Massachusetts, Chapter 4: General Nephrology: Workup of Hematuria, Tubular Disorders*

Douglas Husmann, MD   *Mayo Clinic, Department of Urology, Rochester, Minnesota, Chapter 18: Ureteral Ectopia, Ureteroceles, and Other Anomalies of the Distal Ureter*

David B. Joseph, MD   *Chief of Pediatric Urology, Department of Surgery, The University of Alabama at Birmingham, The Children's Hospital of Alabama, Birmingham, Alabama, Chapter 20: Prune Belly Syndrome and Other Disorders of Abnormal Detrusor Development*

Evan J. Kass, MD   *William Beaumont Hospital, Chief, Pediatric Urology, Royal Oak, Michigan, Chapter 30: Varicoceles*

Michael Keating, MD   *Codirector, Pediatric Urology, The Nemours Children's Clinic, Orlando, Florida, Chapter 14: Effect of Obstruction on the Detrusor: Congenital and Acquired*

Antoine Khoury, MD   *Head of Pediatric Urology and Associate Professor of Surgery, Division of Urology, Hospital for Sick Children, Toronto, Ontario, Canada, Chapter 39: Role of Urinary Diversion in Childhood: Continent, Temporary, or Otherwise*

Harry P. Koo, MD   *Assistant Professor of Surgery, Section of Urology, The University of Michigan, Ann Arbor, Michigan*

Bruce R. Korf, MD   *The Children's Hospital, Department of Genetics, Boston, Massachusetts, Chapter 10: Clinical Genetics and Heritable Disorders in Pediatric Urology*

Leslie Kushner, PhD   *Department of Urology, Long Island Jewish Medical Center, New Hyde Park, New York, Chapter 9: Molecular Basis of Pediatric Urologic Disease*

Charlotte Massad, MD   *Pediatric Urology, Atlanta, Georgia, Chapter 12: Ureterovesical Junction Obstruction and Other Retroperitoneal Obstructions*

Daniel McMahon, MD   *Department of Urology, Children's Hospital Medical Center, Akron; Pediatric Urology, Akron, Ohio, Chapter 19: Anatomic Abnormalities of the Bladder*

Phillip Nasrallah, MD   *Chief of Pediatric Urology, Children's Hospital Medical Center of Akron, Ohio, Associate Professor of Urology, Northeastern Ohio , Universities College of Medicine, Pediatric Urology, Akron, Ohio, Chapter 19: Anatomic Abnormalities of the Bladder*

John C. Pope, IV, MD   *Pediatric Urology, Vanderbilt University Medical Center, Nashville, Tennessee*

Frederick J. Rescorla, MD   *Associate Professor of Surgery, Riley Hospital for Children, Indiana University Medical Center, Department of Pediatric Surgery, Indianapolis, Indiana, Chapter 2: Surgery Physiology of the Neonate*

Mark A. Rich, MD   *Pediatric Urology, Orlando, Florida, Chapter 9: Relevant Molecular Biology: Steroid Receptor Function, Gene Expression, Growth Factors, Oncogenes*

Richard C. Rink, MD *Robert A. Garrett Professor of Pediatric Urology Research, Indiana University School of Medicine, Chief, Pediatric Urology, James Whitcomb Riley Hospital for Children, Urology Division, Indianapolis, Indiana, Chapter 24: Surgical Options in Managing the Neurogenic Bladder*

Michael Ritchey, MD *University of Texas, Health and Science Center, Division of Pediatric Surgery, Houston, Texas, Chapter 35: Pediatric Oncology*

David R. Roth, MD *Associate Professor of Urology, Scott Department of Urology, Baylor College of Medicine, Texas Children's Hospital, Pediatric Urology, Houston, Texas, Chapter 28: Hypospadias*

Richard Schlussel, MD *Assistant Professor of Urology, Mount Sinai Medical Center, Department of Urology, New York, New York, Chapter 17: Disorders of Renal Position and Parenchymal Development*

Linda Shortliffe, MD *Stanford University Medical Center, Department of Urology, Stanford, California, Chapter 15: Diagnostic Maneuvers to Differentiate Obstruction From Nonobstructive Ureteral Dilation*

Lydia A. Shrier, MD, MPH *Instructor of Pediatrics, Harvard Medical School, Assistant in Medicine, Children's Hospital, Department of Adolescent Medicine, Boston, Massachusetts, Chapter 33: Disorders of the Female Genitalia and Menarche*

Richard I. Silver, MD *Assistant Professor of Urology and Pediatrics, Jefferson Medical College, Thomas Jefferson University, Philadelphia, Pennsylvania, Attending*

Pediatric Urologist, Department of Surgery, Alfred I. duPont Hospital for Children, Wilmington, Delaware, Chapter 29: Cryptorchidism

Steve J. Skoog, MD *Professor of Surgery and Pediatrics, Director, Pediatric Urology, Doenbeckers Childrens' Hospital, Oregon Health Sciences University, Division of Urology & Renal Transplantation, Portland, Oregon, Chapter 37: Imperforate Anus and Caudal Regression Syndrome*

F. Bruder Stapleton, MD *Pediatrician-in-Chief, Children's Hospital & Medical Center, Seattle, Washington, Chapter 34: Urolithiasis in Children*

George Steinhardt, MD *Glennon Children's Hospital, Department of Urology, St. Louis, Missouri, Chapter 11: Ureteropelvic Junction Obstruction*

William R. Strand, MD *Center for Pediatric Urology, Dallas, Texas, Chapter 26: UTI: Pathogenesis, Defense Mechanisms, Bacteriologic Virulence*

J. Lynn Teague, MD *University of Missouri, School of Medicine—Columbia, Section of Urology, Columbia, Missouri, Chapter 16: Disorders of the Adrenal Gland*

Julian Wan, MD *Assistant Professor of Urology, State University of New York at Buffalo; Department of Pediatric Urology, Children's Hospital of Buffalo; Pediatric Urology Associates, Buffalo, New York, Chapter 25: Physiology of Micturition and Dysfunctional Voiding*

J. Stuart Wolf, Jr., MD *Assistant Professor of Surgery, Section of Urology, The University of Michigan, Ann Arbor, Michigan*

Dedication

The editors would like to dedicate this book to our wives, Lynn Gonzales and Lee Bauer, who acknowledged and respected the time we spent in bringing this endeavor to fruition, and to all the children, our patients, who will benefit from the dissemination of knowledge this book imparts to the pediatric urologic clinician.

Contents

CHAPTER 1

The Pediatric Physical Examination

Jan E. Drutz

In recent years, sophisticated technological advances in medicine have proved to be remarkably beneficial in the diagnostic process, yet the well-performed history and the physical examination remain the clinician's most important tools. They are venerated elements of the art of medicine; the best series of diagnostic tests we have.[1] A thorough history is generally more valuable than the examination.

Regardless of the reason for a patient's visit, however, a relatively complete physical examination should be carried out each time. Numerous medical anecdotes relate instances in which the examination revealed findings unrelated and unexpected from the patient's chief complaint and major concerns. On occasion, a limited or inadequate examination may miss a significant condition, mass lesion, or potentially life-threatening condition.

GENERAL PRINCIPLES

The Approach

After years of experience, seasoned examiners become aware of and are able to avoid potential pitfalls often encountered on entering a patient's room. The patient's chart should be carefully reviewed, and the identity of the patient and others in the room should be confirmed before entering. Most physicians have experienced the discomfort of walking into a patient's room and greeting the patient, parent, or caregiver by the wrong name or had the correct name but the wrong chart in hand.

To avoid a potentially embarrassing situation, the examiner should always knock on the door and await a response before entering. Small children standing on the other side could be easily injured by the door handle or by the door's impact as it is being opened.

Whether the physician and caregiver have previously met or not, it is appropriate to greet everyone in a cordial manner, maintaining a professional yet friendly demeanor. Infants older than 6 months and anxious toddlers who are leery of strangers are often more comfortable when held by their caregiver. To gain the child's confidence and to avoid an early adversarial relationship, the physician should try using a calm approach, a reassuring smile, and a toy or bright object as a diversion. During the history-taking portion, an appropriate distance should be maintained. Once the physical examination is about to begin, the physician's approach should be cautious and nonthreatening.

Infants younger than 6 months who have no stranger anxiety and children older than 30 to 36 months who are familiar with the examining physician and/or who possess a trusting demeanor generally cooperate during the examination without being held. Physical examination of 5- to 12-year-old children is usually easy to perform, because these children are generally not apprehensive and tend to be cooperative.

The History

For patients in the neonatal age range through early childhood, historical information almost strictly depends on the caregiver. To obtain pertinent information regarding a 5- to 12-year-old child, the physician must still rely primarily on the caregiver, although attention should be given to the relevant and often honest comments made by the patient.

Key elements in the history-taking process include establishing a warm, caring atmosphere and asking questions in a nonconfrontational, seemingly unhurried manner. The terminology and language used by the examiner should be appropriate for the educational level of the caregiver and the age and educational level of the patient. Good eye contact and a sense of undivided attention should be maintained. The physician should sit opposite the caregiver and/or patient at a comfortable distance, unencumbered by large objects such as desks or tables. Outside interruption by the medical staff and by telephone calls should be kept to a minimum. An effort should be made to maintain an uninterrupted dialogue, to write few notes, and to refer to written data as little as possible.

The Physical Examination

Before beginning and again after completing the examination, the examiner should wash his or her hands thoroughly, preferably with an antiseptic soap and warm water. When appropriate, protective gloves should be worn. Patients and caregivers alike are well aware when the examiner fails to carry out this seemingly routine procedure.

Skilled clinicians employ different techniques to gain pediatric patient cooperation. The use of toys, distracting objects, and pictures help in the examination of young children, infants, and toddlers. Engaging the 2- to 4-year-old in stories or a discussion of imaginary animals frequently creates an effective diversion. Food, in the form of chewable snacks, or liquid refreshments are generally used as a means of pacification, depending on the stage of the examination.

When an otherwise normal-acting child older than 4 years fails to cooperate for an examination, even in the presence of a familiar caregiver, it may be an indication of either an earlier traumatic encounter between the patient and another examiner or a failure on the part of the current examining physician to use the correct approach. Consideration should be given to the possibility of an underlying psychosocial problem or personality defect in an otherwise normal-appearing child who is older than 4 years and who proves to be totally combative or extremely uncooperative.

For patients old enough to understand but who appear apprehensive, the examiner should explain what is going to be done during the examination and allow them to look at and touch any of the instruments to be used. If there is potential for pain or discomfort, patients old enough to understand should be told in advance.

For the most part, physical examination of the adolescent patient is performed in the absence of caregivers. Pertinent historical information, anticipatory guidance, and preventive health care issues are discussed more openly between doctor and adolescent in the absence of an accompanying adult. When examining an adolescent of the opposite sex, the physician should make certain an appropriate chaperone is present.

If a patient has a complaint, sign, or symptom that appears to involve a particular part of the anatomy, that part of the examination should be last. An example is a patient complaining of right lower quadrant abdominal pain, thought to be the result of appendicitis. By not examining that part of the body first, the physician may be able to divert the patient's attention away from the involved area and rule out other possible causes of the pain.

Patient privacy should be respected. If a patient objects to being unclothed or to wearing an examination gown, allow him or her to remain clothed until a specific part of the anatomy must be checked. When an area needs to be examined, the patient should be asked to remove or pull free the garments that are hindering visualization, palpation, or auscultation.

The order in which the physical examination is conducted is often age specific and depends on examiner preference. For an infant and younger child, the physician may prefer to begin by examining the eyes—noting the red-light reflex, extraocular eye muscle movements, and visual tracking—and then move to other parts of the body or organ systems before finally examining the ears, which are sensitive. For the older, more cooperative child, the examination might begin at the head and progress down the body; the neurologic examination would be performed last.

STANDARD MEASUREMENTS

Height, Weight, Head and Chest Circumference

Measurement of the standard growth parameters throughout childhood and adolescence is essential in helping assess normal development[2]. Data obtained should be plotted on standard growth curves to determine progress (Figs. 1.1–1.8). With each periodic well child visit, height (length) and weight should be measured. Frontal-occipital head circumference should be recorded routinely until the patient is 2 or 3 years old. Thereafter, only height and weight need to be routinely obtained. In the child younger than 2 years, measuring body length when the child is in the supine position is preferable to trying to obtain an accurate measurement while the child is standing. In older children, the height measurement should always be done with the patient standing.

Because infants dislike having their head circumference measured, the procedure should be attempted only at the conclusion of the physical examination. To obtain an accurate head circumference measurement, the measuring tape should encircle the head and include an area 1 to 2 cm above the glabella anteriorly and the most prominent portion of the occiput posteriorly. Chest circumference is measured at the time of the newborn examination, but it is not a part of the routine examination for well child visits. Measure the chest circumference at the nipple line. In the majority of newborns and in children 12 to 18 months old, head circumference is 1 to 2 cm larger than the chest circumference. An exception is the normal rapidly growing head of the premature infant. When not explained by other factors, a disproportionately large head may be indicative of hydrocephalus or macrocephaly. A smaller than normal head circumference constitutes microcephaly and suggests

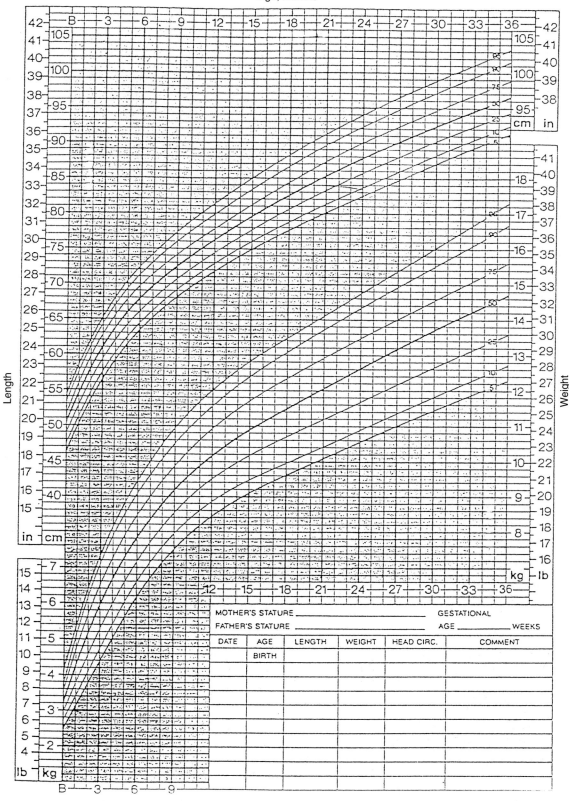

FIG. 1.1. National Center for Health Statistics (NCHS) percentiles of physical growth in boys—birth to 36 months of age. Reprinted with permission from Ross Laboratories, Columbus, OH, and modified from Hamill PW, Drizd TA, Johnson CL, et al. Physical growth: National Center for Health Statistics percentiles. Am J Clin Nutr 1979;32:607–629.

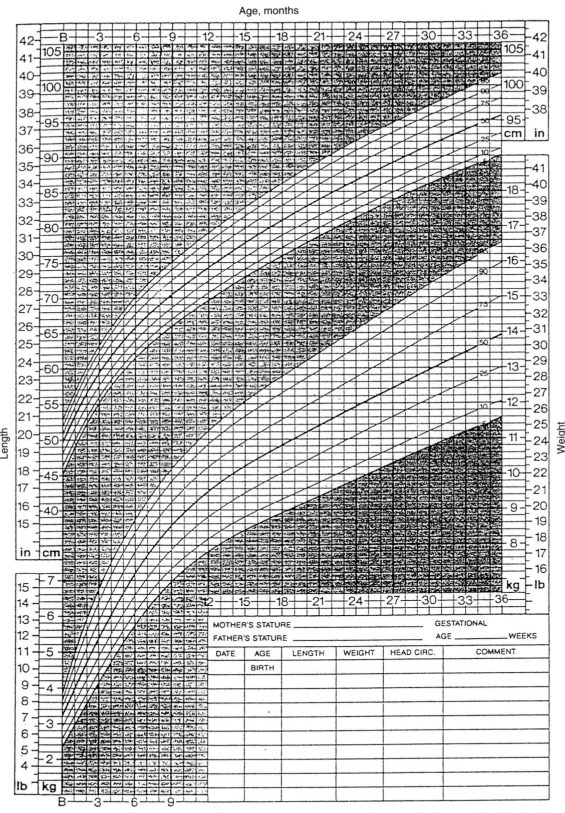

FIG. 1.2. NCHS percentiles of physical growth in girls—birth to 36 months of age. Reprinted with permission from Ross Laboratories, Columbus, OH, and modified from Hamill PW, Drizd TA, Johnson CL, et al. Physical growth: National Center for Health Statistics percentiles. Am J Clin Nutr 1979;32:607–629.

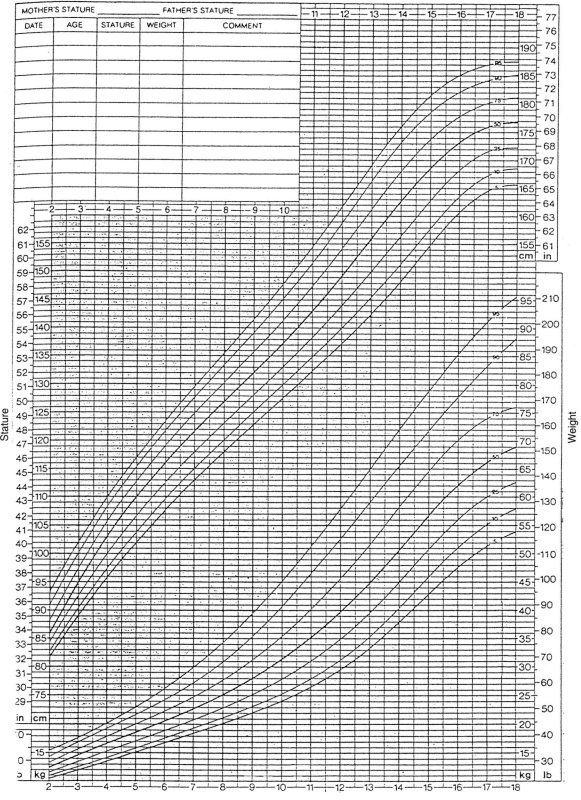

FIG. 1.3. NCHS percentiles of physical growth in boys—2 to 18 years of age. Reprinted with permission from Ross Laboratories, Columbus, OH, and modified from Hamill PW, Drizd TA, Johnson CL, et al. Physical growth: National Center for Health Statistics percentiles. Am J Clin Nutr 1979;32:607–629.

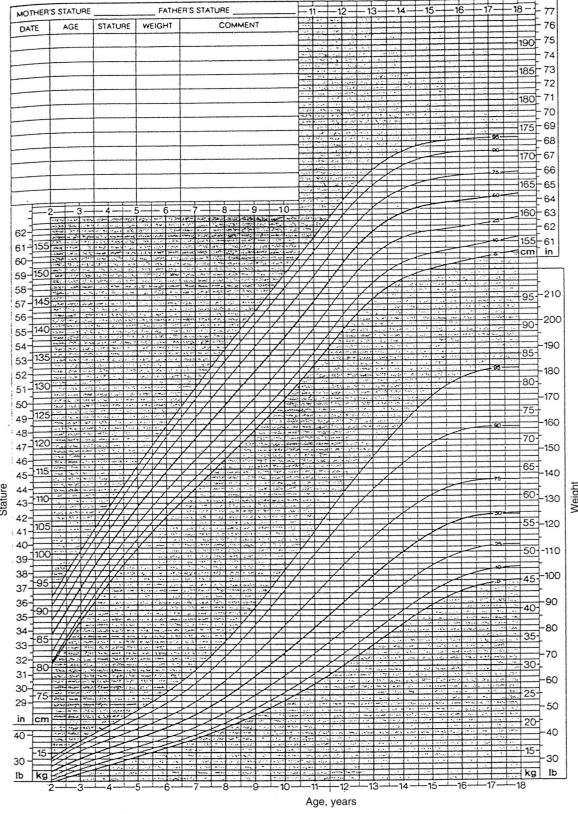

FIG. 1.4. NCHS percentiles of physical growth in girls—2 to 18 years of age. Reprinted with permission from Ross Laboratories, Columbus, OH, and modified from Hamill PW, Drizd TA, Johnson CL, et al. Physical growth: National Center for Health Statistics percentiles. Am J Clin Nutr 1979;32:607–629.

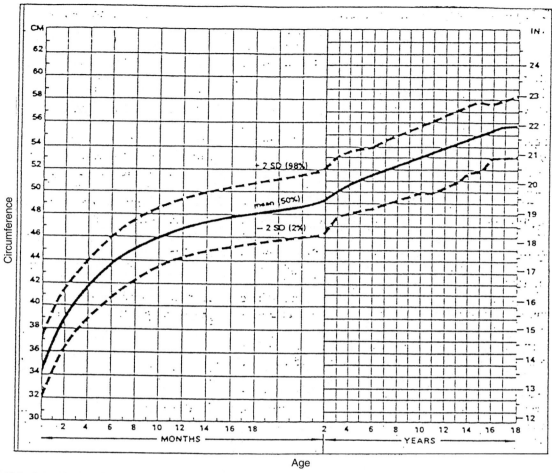

FIG. 1.5. Head circumference in boys. Reprinted with permission from Nelhaus G. Composite international and interracial graphs. Pediatrics 1968;41:106–114.

potential underlying neurologic deficits. In some children, however, small head size may be normal.

Temperature

The routine measurement of a patient's temperature at the time of an examination is not always necessary. When a temperature measurement is needed, the technique and appropriate site for measurement are age dependent. Rectal temperature recordings in infants and young children are preferred, although axillary recordings (about 2° below rectal temperatures) are acceptable. Rectal temperature measurements should be done with the patient in the prone position with the legs slightly flexed at the hips and knees; the thermometer is directed anteriorly at an angle of approximately 20° to the surface of the examination table.[3,4]

Oral temperature readings (about 1° below rectal temperatures) should not be obtained until the child is old enough to understand how to hold and retain an oral thermometer under the tongue. Battery-operated and electronic thermometers for recording oral or rectal temperatures are generally reliable and fast. Compared to rectal thermometers, infrared tympanic thermometers, which are inserted into the external auditory canal, give inconsistent readings.[5]

Respiratory Rate

The normal range for the respiratory rate depends on the age of the child. In 1- to 2-month-old infants, there is a wide range of normal readings, from 30 to 80 breaths per minute; however, a resting breathing rate higher than 30 breaths/min in infants older than 6 months should be considered abnormal. For children older than 4 years, including adolescent patients, normal rates range from 15 to 22 breaths/min.[6] Accurate determination of the respiratory rate should be attempted only when the patient is asleep or at rest. It can be obtained by auscultation, palpation, or direct observation. A sustained breathing rate in excess of the upper limit of normal generally indicates primary respiratory

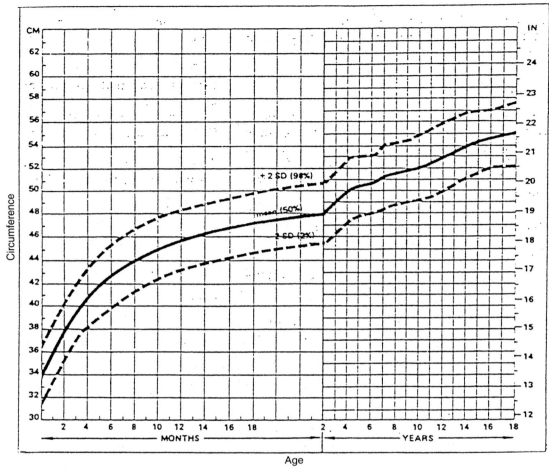

FIG. 1.6. Head circumference in girls. Reprinted with permission from Nelhaus G. Composite international and interracial graphs. Pediatrics 1968;41:106–114.

tract disease; it may also occur secondary to a metabolic disorder, infectious disease, high fever, or underlying heart disease.

Pulse

According to Ti,[7] "Those who wish to know the inner body feel the pulse and thus have the fundamentals for diagnosis." Like the respiratory rate, the normal heart rate varies with age. Up to 3 months of age, the range is 90 to 210 beats/min; from 3 months to 2 years of age, 100 to 190 beats/min; from 2 to 10 years of age, 60 to 140 beats/min; and above 10 years of age, 60 to 100 beats/min.[8,9] The heart rate can be obtained by direct auscultation or palpation of the heart or by palpation of peripheral arteries (carotids, femorals, brachials, or radials). A heart rate above the upper limits of normal may indicate primary cardiac disease; it may also occur secondary to an underlying systemic or metabolic disorder, infectious disease, or high fever.

Blood Pressure

It is often difficult to obtain an accurate blood pressure reading in children. Falsely elevated blood pressures frequently occur in the agitated child. In most circumstances, routine blood pressure measurements should not be attempted until the patient is at least 3 years old.[2,10] The examining area should be quiet, and the child should be in a relative resting state before the physician should make any attempt at measurement. Although infants may be measured while in a supine position, children should be sitting. The right arm, resting on a supportive surface at heart level, is the extremity of choice for measurement.[11,12]

Patients old enough to understand should be shown the blood pressure device before the examiner attempts to take a measurement. To gain his or her cooperation, the patient should be allowed to play with the device or feel the cuff inflate. Blood pressure devices include the standard extremity cuff and mercury bulb sphygmomanometer, the hand-held aneroid manometer, and the

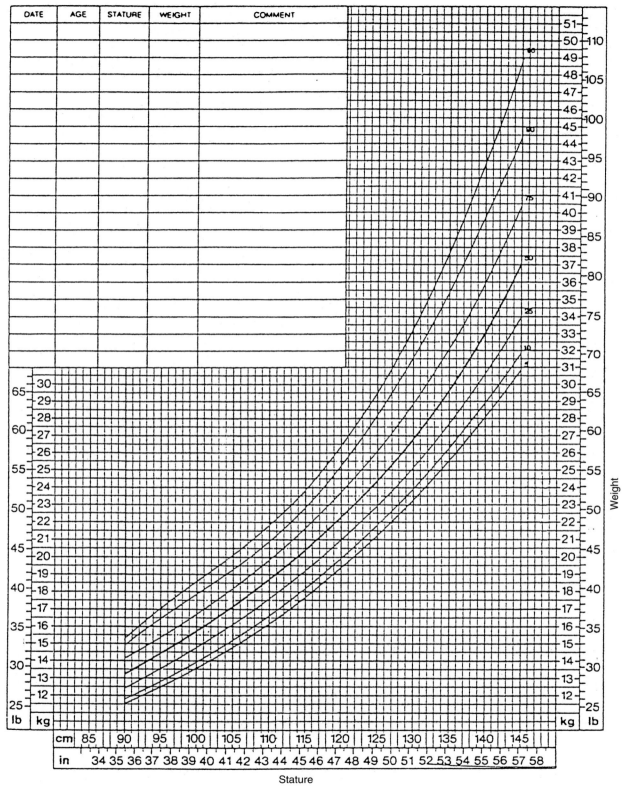

FIG. 1.7. NCHS percentiles of prepubescent physical growth in boys. Reprinted with permission from Ross Laboratories, Columbus, OH, and modified from Hamill PW, Drizd TA, Johnson CL, et al. Physical growth: National Center for Health Statistics percentiles. Am J Clin Nutr 1979;32:607–629.

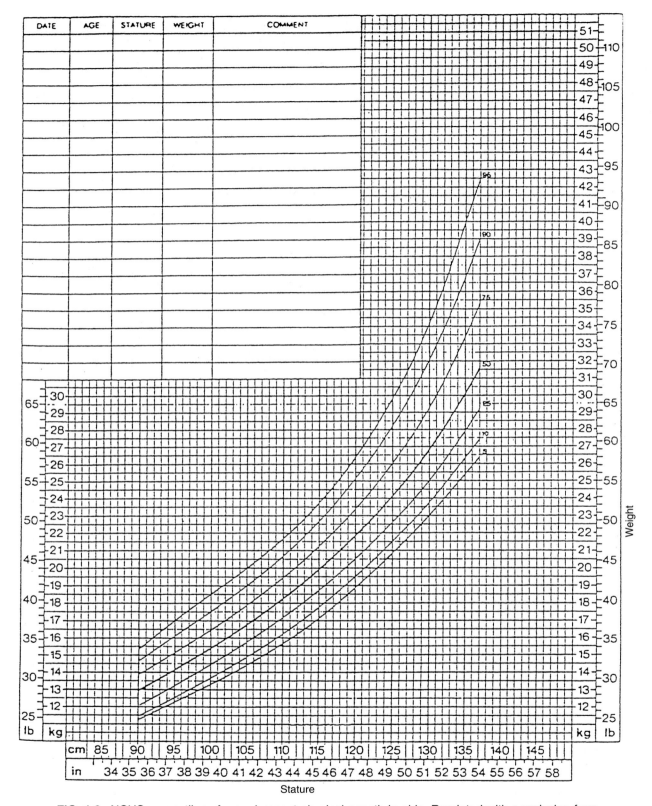

FIG. 1.8. NCHS percentiles of prepubescent physical growth in girls. Reprinted with permission from Ross Laboratories, Columbus, OH, and modified from Hamill PW, Drizd TA, Johnson CL, et al. Physical growth: National Center for Health Statistics percentiles. Am J Clin Nutr 1979;32:607–629.

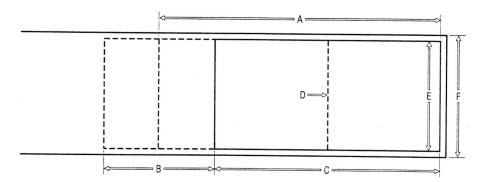

FIG. 1.9. Dimensions of the bladder and cuff in relation to arm circumference. **A,** Ideal arm circumference; **B,** range of acceptable arm circumferences; **C,** bladder length; **D,** midline of bladder; **E,** bladder width; **F,** cuff width. Reprinted with permission from Perloff D, Grim C, Flack J, et al. Human blood pressure determination by sphygmomanometry. Circulation 1993;88: 2450–2467.

relatively new Doppler and oscillometric devices. Cuff size should be appropriate to the size of the child's upper right arm; the bladder width of the cuff should be approximately 40% of the upper arm circumference, measured midway between the olecranon and the acromion. The bladder width will usually cover 80 to 100% of the circumference of the arm[12] (Figs. 1.9–1.12). The systolic pressure measured in the lower extremity is generally about 20 mm Hg higher than that measured in the upper extremity.

Blood pressure measurements for children younger than 3 years are indicated when there is evidence of underlying renal disease, such as a tumor, nephrotic syndrome, glomerulonephritis, pyelonephritis, or renal artery stenosis. Another reason for measuring the blood

pressure in this age group is the finding or suspicion of underlying cardiovascular disease, such as coarctation of the aorta or patent ductus arteriosus (PDA).

For all age groups, in addition to the disorders mentioned above, elevated blood pressures are associated with neuroblastomas, pheochromocytomas, thyroid disease, neurofibromatosis, Cushing disease, intoxication from or ingestion of various substances, increased intracranial pressure, and myriad other disorders. It is wise to keep in mind that elevated systolic pressures alone are frequently noted in patients after vigorous exercise, excessive agitation, or during febrile illnesses.

Abnormally low blood pressure recordings are noted in patients with heart failure from a number of causes and in patients in a shock-like state, such as sepsis or hypovolemia. A rapid change in the patient's position

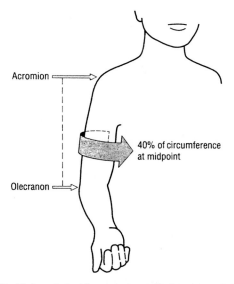

FIG. 1.10. Determining the proper cuff size: step 1. The cuff bladder width should be approximately 40% of the circumference of the arm, measured at a point midway between the acromion and olecranon. Reprinted with permission from National High Blood Pressure Education Program Working Group on Hypertension Control in Children and Adolescents. Update on the 1987 task force report on high blood pressure in children and adolescents: a working group report from the National High Blood Pressure Education Program. Pediatrics 1996;98:649–658.

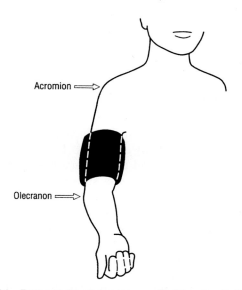

FIG. 1.11. Determining the proper cuff size: step 2. The cuff bladder should cover 80 to 100% of the circumference of the arm. Reprinted with permission from the National High Blood Pressure Education Program Working Group on Hypertension Control in Children and Adolescents. Update on the 1987 task force report on high blood pressure in children and adolescents: a working group report from the National High Blood Pressure Education Program. Pediatrics 1996;98: 649–658.

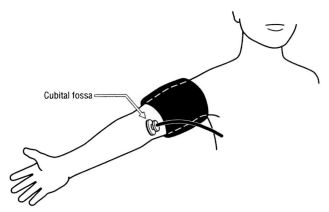

Cubital fossa

FIG. 1.12. Blood pressure should be measured with the cubital fossa at heart level, and the arm should be supported. The stethoscope bell is placed over the brachial artery pulse, proximal and medial to the cubital fossa, below the bottom edge of the cuff. Reprinted with permission from the National High Blood Pressure Education Program Working Group on Hypertension Control in Children and Adolescents. Update on the 1987 task force report on high blood pressure in children and adolescents: a working group report from the National High Blood Pressure Education Program. Pediatrics 1996;98:649–658.

from supine to standing or sitting may result in orthostatic hypotension. Widened pulse pressures may be seen in patients with aortic regurgitation, arteriovenous fistulas, PDA, or hyperthyroidism; narrowed pulse pressures are found in patients with subaortic or aortic valve stenosis and occasionally in those with hypothyroidism.

As with pulse and respiratory rates in children, blood pressure varies with age. Standard reference charts that give the ranges of normality should be consulted[12] (Tables 1.1 and 1.2).

GENERAL APPEARANCE

Upon entering a patient's room, the examiner, by observation alone, may gain significant insight into important social and family dynamics. Terms used to describe a patient's general appearance may include degree of comfort (calm, nervous, shy), state of well-being (normal, ill appearing, distressed), activity level (sedate, alert, active, fidgety), physical appearance (neat, disheveled, unkempt), behavior and attitude (happy, sad, irritable, combative), body habitus (overweight, underweight, short, tall), and nutritional status (malnourished, normal, corpulent). If the infant, toddler, or child to be examined is not in close proximity to the caregiver and there is no eye contact between them and/or the patient lacks animation and has no social smile, the possibility of neglect should be considered. Psychosocial intervention may be warranted.

If a child appears ill, particular attention should be paid to the way the patient has positioned himself or herself. A child who lies completely still on the examina-

tion table, is verbally responsive, but noticeably winces when an attempt is made to change position may have an acute abdomen; a patient who is sitting upright, is bent slightly forward at the waist with the arms extended and hands resting on the knees and is breathing with some degree of difficulty might be experiencing an exacerbation of asthma.

If an infant who is about to be examined is crying when the physician enters the examination room, the pitch and intensity of the cry should be noted. A boisterous hardy cry may be somewhat reassuring, whereas a weak and listless cry may indicate a seriously ill infant. In contrast, a high-pitched screeching cry could indicate increased intracranial pressure, reaction to a painful injury, toxic reaction, strangulated inguinal hernia, or another serious disorder.

Note the patient's breathing pattern and skin color. If the patient has rapid, shallow respiration yet appears to be in no acute distress, the underlying cause could be primary pulmonary disease or respiratory compensation for metabolic acidosis.

Before touching the patient, the examiner should evaluate the child's developmental status. The patient's motor function, interaction with surrounding objects and people, response to sounds, and speech pattern give clues about whether the patient is normal or is in need of extensive developmental assessment.

SKIN

Examination of the skin requires careful inspection and palpation. When describing individual skin abnormalities, the examiner should describe color and size and whether the lesions, tumors, rashes, or defects are raised or flat, coalescent or isolated, well localized or diffuse, pruritic or nonpruritic. Terms such as *papule, macule, pustule, vesicle, bullae,* and *nodule* describe the appearance of rashes and have meaning for most health professionals. Because skin lesions from different causes can have the same appearance, however, the physician must be careful to make the correct diagnoses and recommend the correct treatment. A carefully taken history and good physical examination can be of significant benefit in helping to differentiate among various disorders.

Essentially all lesions originating in the skin of children are benign. Lesions without an altered appearance of the epidermis, however, may not be easy to categorize. A mass that moves freely over the underlying fascia is most likely to be present in the subcutaneous tissue and should be considered benign. If the lesion is fixed to the underlying fascia or the examiner is unsure of what is being felt, malignancy is a possibility and an appropriate referral should be made.[13]

Palpation of the skin may reveal rough, coarse, or dry areas in the region of the neck, knee, or elbow,

TABLE 1.1. *Blood pressure levels for the 90th and 95th percentiles of blood pressure for boys aged 1 to 17 years by percentiles of height*

Age, years	Blood pressure percentile[a]	Systolic blood pressure by percentile of height, mm Hg[b]							Diastolic blood pressure by percentile of height, mm Hg[b]						
		5%	10%	25%	50%	75%	90%	95%	5%	10%	25%	50%	75%	90%	95%
1	90th	94	95	97	98	100	102	102	50	51	52	53	54	54	55
	95th	98	99	101	102	104	106	106	55	55	56	57	58	59	59
2	90th	98	99	100	102	104	105	106	55	55	56	57	58	59	59
	95th	101	102	104	106	108	109	110	59	59	60	61	62	63	63
3	90th	100	101	103	105	107	108	109	59	59	60	61	62	63	63
	95th	104	105	107	109	111	112	113	63	63	64	65	66	67	67
4	90th	102	103	105	107	109	110	111	62	62	63	64	65	66	66
	95th	106	107	109	111	113	114	115	66	67	67	68	69	70	71
5	90th	104	105	106	108	110	112	112	65	65	66	67	68	69	69
	95th	108	109	110	112	114	115	116	69	70	70	71	72	73	74
6	90th	105	106	108	110	111	113	114	67	68	69	70	70	71	72
	95th	109	110	112	114	115	117	117	72	72	73	74	75	76	76
7	90th	106	107	109	111	113	114	115	69	70	71	72	72	73	74
	95th	110	111	113	115	116	118	119	74	74	75	76	77	78	78
8	90th	107	108	110	112	114	115	116	71	71	72	73	74	75	75
	95th	111	112	114	116	118	119	120	75	76	76	77	78	79	80
9	90th	109	110	112	113	115	117	117	72	73	73	74	75	76	77
	95th	113	114	116	117	119	121	121	76	77	78	79	80	80	81
10	90th	110	112	113	115	117	118	119	73	74	74	75	76	77	78
	95th	114	115	117	119	121	122	123	77	78	79	80	80	81	82
11	90th	112	113	115	117	119	120	121	74	74	75	76	77	78	78
	95th	116	117	119	121	123	124	125	78	79	79	80	81	82	83
12	90th	115	116	117	119	121	123	123	75	75	76	77	78	78	79
	95th	119	120	121	123	125	126	127	79	79	80	81	82	83	83
13	90th	117	118	120	122	124	125	126	75	76	76	77	78	79	80
	95th	121	122	124	126	128	129	130	79	80	81	82	83	83	84
14	90th	120	121	123	125	126	128	128	76	76	77	78	79	80	80
	95th	124	125	127	128	130	132	132	80	81	81	82	83	84	85
15	90th	123	124	125	127	129	131	131	77	77	78	79	80	81	81
	95th	127	128	129	131	133	134	135	81	82	83	83	84	85	86
16	90th	125	126	128	130	132	133	134	79	79	80	81	82	82	83
	95th	129	130	132	134	136	137	138	83	83	84	85	86	87	87
17	90th	128	129	131	133	134	136	136	81	81	82	83	84	85	85
	95th	132	133	135	136	138	140	140	85	85	86	87	88	89	89

[a]Blood pressure percentile was determined by a single measurement.
[b]Height percentile was determined by standard growth curves.
(From the 1987 Task Force Report on High Blood Pressure in Children and Adolescents: A Working Group Report from the National High Blood Pressure Education Program. Pediatrics 1996;98:649–658.)

which are often found in patients with atopic dermatitis. Large patches of coarse papular lesions palpable over the dorsal surfaces of the upper arms and thighs of an older child or adolescent may be compatible with hyperkeratosis pilaris. An elongated or patchy area of moist, erythematous, denuded, pruritic skin may be seen in patients with contact dermatitis caused by poison ivy. Pink, raised, pruritic, lesions of various sizes and shapes, diffusely scattered over the body are found in patients with urticaria.

Skin Color

Variations from normal skin color could indicate a previously undiagnosed disorder. A yellow tint to the skin may be compatible with jaundice (hyperbilirubinemia) or carotenemia. The latter condition can be found in infants and toddlers whose diets consist of large amounts of strained yellow vegetables, particularly carrots. Unlike jaundice, the skin color is characteristically more yellow-orange and more noticeable over the palms and soles, sparing mucosal tissue and the sclerae. Although the diet is a major cause of carotenemia in childhood, some diseases, such as nephrosis, diabetes mellitus, anorexia nervosa, liver disease, and hypothyroidism, can also produce the condition.[14]

Jaundice can be differentiated from carotenemia by the yellow-green skin color, yellow sclerae and mucous membranes, and the darkly colored urine and lightly colored stools. Collection of bile pigment accounts for the change in tissue color. Disorders giving rise to hyperbilirubinemia include neonatal (physiologic) jaundice, hemolytic anemias, hepatitis, enzyme defects, and biliary tree obstruction.[15]

TABLE 1.2. *Blood pressure levels for the 90th and 95th percentiles of blood pressure for girls aged 1 to 17 years by percentiles of height*

Age, years	Blood pressure percentile[a]	Systolic blood pressure by percentile of height, mm Hg[b]							Diastolic blood pressure by percentile of height, mm Hg[b]						
		5%	10%	25%	50%	75%	90%	95%	5%	10%	25%	50%	75%	90%	95%
1	90th	97	98	99	100	102	103	104	53	53	53	54	55	56	56
	95th	101	102	103	104	105	107	107	57	57	57	58	59	60	60
2	90th	99	99	100	102	103	104	105	57	57	58	58	59	60	61
	95th	102	103	104	105	107	108	109	61	61	62	62	63	64	65
3	90th	100	100	102	103	104	105	106	61	61	61	62	63	63	64
	95th	104	104	105	107	108	109	110	65	65	65	66	67	67	68
4	90th	101	102	103	104	106	107	108	63	63	64	65	65	66	67
	95th	105	106	107	108	109	111	111	67	67	68	69	69	70	71
5	90th	103	103	104	106	107	108	109	65	66	66	67	68	68	69
	95th	107	107	108	110	111	112	113	69	70	70	71	72	72	73
6	90th	104	105	106	107	109	110	111	67	67	68	69	69	70	71
	95th	108	109	110	111	112	114	114	71	71	72	73	73	74	75
7	90th	106	107	108	109	110	112	112	69	69	69	70	71	72	72
	95th	110	110	112	113	114	115	116	73	73	73	74	75	76	76
8	90th	108	109	110	111	112	113	114	70	70	71	71	72	73	74
	95th	112	112	113	115	116	117	118	74	74	75	75	76	77	78
9	90th	110	110	112	113	114	115	116	71	72	72	73	74	74	75
	95th	114	114	115	117	118	119	120	75	76	76	77	78	78	79
10	90th	112	112	114	115	116	117	118	73	73	73	74	75	76	76
	95th	116	116	117	119	120	121	122	77	77	77	78	79	80	80
11	90th	114	114	116	117	118	119	120	74	74	75	75	76	77	77
	95th	118	118	119	121	122	123	124	78	78	79	79	80	81	81
12	90th	116	116	118	119	120	121	122	75	75	76	76	77	78	78
	95th	120	120	121	123	124	125	126	79	79	80	80	81	82	82
13	90th	118	118	119	121	122	123	124	76	76	77	78	78	79	80
	95th	121	122	123	125	126	127	128	80	80	81	82	82	83	84
14	90th	119	120	121	122	124	125	126	77	77	78	79	79	80	81
	95th	123	124	125	126	128	129	130	81	81	82	83	83	84	85
15	90th	121	121	122	124	125	126	127	78	78	79	79	80	81	82
	95th	124	125	126	128	129	130	131	82	82	83	83	84	85	86
16	90th	122	122	123	125	126	127	128	79	79	79	80	81	82	82
	95th	125	126	127	128	130	131	132	83	83	83	84	85	86	86
17	90th	122	123	124	125	126	128	128	79	79	79	80	81	82	82
	95th	126	126	127	129	130	131	132	83	83	83	84	85	86	86

[a]Blood pressure percentile was determined by a single reading.
[b]Height percentile was determined by standard growth curves.
(From Update on the 1987 Task Force Report on High Blood Pressure in Children and Adolescents: A Working Group Report from the National High Blood Pressure Education Program. Pediatrics 1996;98:649–658.)

A bluish gray discoloration of the skin may be a side effect of a drug or caused by the ingestion of a toxic substance. The parts of the body most often involved are the face, neck, and extremities.[16]

Pigmentation

Hyperpigmented or hypopigmented skin lesions may have clinical significance. Hypopigmented areas are often benign but may be compatible with various disease states.[17] Small hypopigmented or depigmented areas may be the result of postinflammatory lesions, pityriasis alba, or tinea versicolor. Patients with neuroectodermal disorders, such as tuberous sclerosis, often have hypopigmented ash leaf spots. Streaked areas of hypopigmentation are characteristically seen in hypomelanosis of Ito. Vitiligo, an autosomal trait of variable penetrance, is a patterned loss of pigmentation

secondary to the destruction of melanocytes. Albinism is an entity with total or nearly complete absence of pigmentation.

A rare autosomal recessive immunologic disorder with diffuse oculocutaneous hypopigmentation, leukocyte dysfunction, and recurrent infections is Chediak-Higashi syndrome. Patients with this disorder have fair skin; light blond hair; translucent irises; and renal, hematologic, and neurologic abnormalities.[18]

Increased skin pigmentation owing to an excess of melanin may be localized or diffuse. Between one and four light brown macular lesions (café au lait spots) no greater than 0.5 to 1.0 cm at their largest diameter (depending on the patient's age) is a normal finding in many patients. Larger and more numerous café au lait spots may be seen in neurofibromatosis, Bloom syndrome, ataxia telangiectasia, and several other syndromes.[19]

More darkly pigmented cutaneous tumors that appear anywhere on the body may be present at birth or appear years later. Congenital and dysplastic nevi (usually developing during the second decade of life) often become melanoma. Melanoma lesions, though rarely found in infants and children, have an irregular border with deeply pigmented or varied colored areas, may have ulcerations or satellite lesions, and have a tendency to grow.[13, 16]

Acquired nevi (not present at birth) are less than 1 cm in diameter, may be flat or slightly raised, are light brown to black in color, and have discrete regular borders. They develop during the first several decades of life and often eventually disappear. Though the vast majority of acquired nevi are harmless, certain changes indicate a need for biopsy and histologic evaluation, including rapid darkening, changes in size or borders, ulceration, itching, pain, or bleeding.[13]

Vascular Lesions

Vascular lesions commonly seen in children may have clinical significance. The most common vascular lesion seen in infants is a pink macular stain (salmon patch, stork bite, angel's kiss) most often found on the nape of the neck, glabella, upper eyelids, forehead, and nasolabial folds. These require no treatment, and the vast majority clear within the first year of life.[20]

Strawberry hemangiomas—benign neoplasms composed of proliferating vascular endothelium—are seen in 2.6% of newborns. Approximately 90% of these neoplasms undergo spontaneous involution by the time the patient is 9 years old. When these hemangiomas affect the visual pathway or respiratory tract or result in platelet trapping (Kasabach–Merritt syndrome), interventional therapy with steroids, laser therapy, or α interferon-2a should be considered. Rapidly growing facial hemangiomas may require systemic steroids and injections of α interferon-2a.[21]

A potentially more serious situation may arise if the patient has a disorder known as diffuse neonatal hemangiomatosis. This condition is associated with multiple disseminated hemangiomas involving the skin and viscera, which may lead to high-output cardiac failure, portal hypertension, neurologic abnormalities, and gastrointestinal or urinary tract bleeding.[22]

Vascular lesions that neither proliferate nor involute and are caused by inborn errors of vascular morphogenesis are termed venous malformations.[23] They grow in proportion to the growth of the child and may require treatment. The facial port wine stain, the most frequently occurring example of this condition, is often associated with a neurocutaneous disorder (Sturge–Weber syndrome). Port wine staining of one of the extremities may be associated with soft tissue hypertrophy and overgrowth of the underlying bone (Klippel–Trenaunay syndrome or Parkes–Weber syndrome).[16, 23]

For the cosmetic and psychological treatment of this vascular lesion, a tunable pulsed dye laser may be used.[24]

Other Lesions

Among the more common skin lesions seen in childhood are warts, pyogenic granulomata, and sebaceous cysts. Though cosmetically unattractive, warts on the hands and feet do not always require treatment, and most regress spontaneously. Warts in the genital or perianal areas should alert the examiner as to the possibility of sexual abuse. Pyogenic granulomata are benign, generally small, raised papules appearing anywhere on the skin.[13] They bleed easily and are best treated with silver nitrate or electrocautery. Sebaceous cysts occur at anatomical sites where hair is present. If unsightly or bothersome, they should be surgically removed. Whenever a pigmented lesion (with or without a tuft of hair), a vascular lesion, a soft tissue mass, or a skin defect is found over the midline of the head, neck, or back, the examiner should be suspicious of a potential underlying neurologic defect.

Lymph Nodes

The appropriate examination of the lymph nodes requires careful inspection and palpation. The approach should be symmetrical and sequential, e.g., beginning with simultaneous palpation of the occipital and posterior cervical nodes, followed by palpation of the anterior cervical nodes, preauricular and postauricular nodes, submental nodes, supraclavicular nodes, axillary nodes, and inguinal nodes.

In normal children between 2 years of age and early adolescence, superficial, enlarged, freely movable, nontender lymph nodes are easily palpable, particularly in the anterior cervical chain. Cervical and inguinal nodes 1 to 1.5 cm in diameter are frequently found but generally remain enlarged only for a short period of time.[25] Nodes up to 3 mm in diameter in the axilla and submandibular areas are often found in the otherwise normal child. Palpable posterior auricular, occipital, submental, supraclavicular, epitrochlear, and popliteal nodes are uncommon.[26] Any node larger than 3 mm in the neonate and in children older than 12 years should be considered as possibly abnormal.[27]

Routine examination of the lymph nodes includes attention to size, mobility, tenderness, and adhesion to adjacent tissues as well as to the temperature and condition of the overlying skin.[28] Nodes that grow slowly are generally benign, whereas those that grow rapidly and are rubbery hard, nontender, and matted tend to be malignant. Enlarged tender nodes with increased warmth to the overlying skin are usually infected.

Supraclavicular nodes are normally not palpable. When they are, early biopsy is recommended, particularly in children who have been ill with a fever for more than 1 week or who have experienced weight loss and when the node is fixed to the overlying skin without evidence of inflammation.[13] Such nodal enlargement may be compatible with malignancy. Supraclavicular nodes on the right drain the lung and esophagus while those on the left drain the lung, stomach, small intestine, kidney, and pancreas.[27]

Lymph node enlargement elsewhere can be cautiously observed; however, careful follow-up and accurate measurement are required. Nodes that drain an extremity may become enlarged as a result of a primary infection or lymphoma or an inflammatory reaction in the distal extremity. Lymphadenopathy in the inguinal area may suggest a sexually transmitted disease.

HEAD

Visualization of the head for shape and the presence of hair, scalp defects, unusual lesions or protuberances, lacerations, and abrasions or contusions should constitute the initial part of the examination. In the newborn infant, asymmetrical head shape may be the result of molding, caput succedaneum, cephalhematoma, or overlapping or premature closure of sutures.

Throughout the first 24 to 36 months of life, a child's head circumference should be measured at each regularly scheduled well child visit. Measurements should be plotted on a standard head circumference growth chart to determine percentile for age and rate of growth. Percentile growth curves from birth to 36 months of age are included on most growth charts (Figs. 1.5 and 1.6). Approximately 75% of adult head size is reached by 2 years of age.[29]

Palpation of the head of a child of any age may reveal unusual masses, lesions, or scalp defects. Firm or hard masses include exostoses or calcified hematomas. Soft tissue masses include hemangiomas, dermoid cysts, encephaloceles, and infected scalp lesions. Palpation of the anterior and posterior fontanelles should be fairly easy during the first several weeks of the child's life. The posterior fontanelle, located at the juncture of the sagittal and lambdoid sutures, usually closes at 2 to 4 months of age. The anterior fontanelle, located at the juncture of the metopic, sagittal, and coronal sutures, generally closes between 10 and 24 months of age. The normal time of closure depends somewhat on the patient's gestational age at birth.

Palpation of the fontanelles should be done with the patient in the upright position. Although early closure of either fontanelle should alert the examiner to the possibility of developing microcephaly, it is not unusual for this to occur in an otherwise normal child. Early closure may actually represent the growth of fibrous tissue, which precedes bony closure by several months. The posterior fontanelle is usually no greater than 1 to 1.5 cm in diameter. Through the first 6 months of life,

the anterior fontanel is generally 3 to 6 cm in diameter. Both fontanelles are normally soft and relatively flat.

Visible or palpable pulsations of the anterior fontanelle are common, especially in the crying or agitated infant. Bounding pulsations or persistent tenseness of the fontanelle may indicate increased intracranial pressure. A depressed or sunken anterior fontanelle may be compatible with dehydration or malnutrition. Palpation of the parietal area of the skull, particularly in a premature infant, may elicit an unusual spring-like bony compressability (craniotabes), similar to the sensation of pushing in the side of a Ping-Pong™ ball. Persistent craniotabes beyond the age of 6 to 9 months may be found in children with several disorders, including syphilis and rickets.[3]

Auscultation of the skull for a bruit is occasionally helpful in detecting an arteriovenous malformation. The presence of an audible bruit in a child during the first several years of life may not be abnormal. As the child gets older, systolic bruits take on more significance, although their presence is not necessarily pathologic. A transmitted cardiac murmur may give rise to an audible cranial bruit, eliminated readily by gentle pressure over the ipsilateral carotid artery.

Intracranial defects, such as hydranencephaly and hydrocephaly, can be transilluminated with a Chun gun or flashlight fitted circumferentially with a rubber or sponge cup. Unlike the skull of the normal child, light will be transmitted far beyond the circumferential rim of the instrument being used if the patient has either of these defects or anencephaly.

Attention to the texture, pattern, and abundance or absence of scalp hair can help determine an underlying problem. Dry scaling areas of the scalp may be caused by psoriasis or seborrheic dermatitis. A bald spot over the occipital area is frequently found in infants placed in the supine position for sleeping and developmentally delayed children who fail to change head position. A white forelock, associated with congenital deafness, may be found in patients with Waardenburg syndrome.[30] Twisted, short, fragile hair can be associated with Menkes syndrome.[31] Coarse, dry hair is a finding in patients with hypothyroidism. Patches of alopecia may be found in patients with tinea capitus, trichotillomania, ectodermal dysplasia, and alopecia areata and at the site of a scalp probe or intravenous insertion.

FACE

The clinician should pay close attention to the patient's anatomical facial structures. The size of the mouth; the shape of the lips; the length of the philtrum; the size and shape of the nose; the distance between the eyes; the width of the palpebral fissures; and the size, shape, and position of the pinnae are all important. Atypical facial features may reveal a phenotypic pattern compatible with a particular syndrome attributable to maternal drug ingestion or a specific genetic or chromosomal abnormality.

Periorbital or facial edema may occur as part of a systemic allergic reaction or be the first indication of nephrotic syndrome. Unilateral orbital or facial edema may occur as a result of an insect bite or periorbital or orbital cellulitis. Unilateral or bilateral facial swelling not caused by edema may be secondary to an infectious process or, in the case of mumps, parotid gland swelling. Submandibular soft tissue swelling may be the result of lymphadenopathy or salivary gland pathology.

Unilateral facial paralysis secondary to a peripheral or central facial nerve defect may be attributable to a traumatic injury, viral or bacterial infection, or other abnormality. Tense rigid facial muscles are seen in patients with hypocalcemia, tetanus, and other infections. Asymmetry of the eyes may be the result of prominent epicanthal folds, a difference in the size of the globes, or ptosis.

EYES

Patient cooperation and compliance are essential to a good eye examination. Infants and younger children are best examined if held upright in the comforting arms of their caregiver with their attention drawn to a toy or bright object. Infants tend to be easier to examine than 18-month to 3-year-old children, who can be uncooperative. By age 6 to 8 years, children are usually able to sit alone facing the examiner and to follow directions.

Before using the ophthalmoscope or touching the child, the examiner should note the position and spacing of the eyes, width of palpebral fissures, eye color, appearance of the sclera and conjunctiva, condition of the eyelids, pupillary size, and eye movement. Widened or narrow palpebral fissures may be the norm for some patients but be part of a syndrome complex in others. Examination of eyelids should include the lashes, color, presence of ptosis, and skin defects. Erythematous or violaceous eyelids may be the result of hemangiomas or vascular malformations or may appear secondary to trauma, infection, metastasis, or connective tissue disorders.

Small linear creases involving the lower eyelid (Dennie lines or Morgan folds) are seen in patients with allergies.[32] Edematous eyelids may be the result of hypoproteinemia as part of the nephrotic syndrome. A mild degree of unilateral or bilateral congenital ptosis, often of undetermined cause, is commonly seen. Acquired causes of ptosis, e.g., myasthenia gravis, third cranial nerve palsy, and ophthalmoplegic migraine, need to be determined.

Flaking, erythema, and mild swelling of the eyelid margins are seen in patients with blepharitis, which is often attributable to seborrheic dermatitis of the scalp or face. A stye (external hordeolum) presents as a painful inflammation of the hair follicles or accessory glands along the lid margin; infection generally owing to *Staphylococcus aureus*. A chalazion (internal hordeolum) is a nontender nodular lesion located deeper in the eyelid, caused by chronic inflammation of a meibomian gland.

Eye discharge or excessive tearing from one or both eyes may indicate a pathologic condition. Purulent discharge can occur as a result of bacterial infection (e.g., *Neisseria gonorrhea*) or chemical irritant (e.g., silver nitrate). Abundant tearing may result from a blocked tear duct, presence of a foreign body, allergic reaction, infection, or glaucoma. Inflammation of the conjunctivae (conjunctivitis) may be caused by an infectious process, irritants, toxins, emotional problems, crying, or systemic disorders (e.g., Kawasaki disease). Subconjunctival hemorrhages owing to injury or inflammation are generally benign and self-limiting. Epithelial hyperplasia that gives rise to a mildly uncomfortable yellowwhite lesion involving the bulbar conjunctiva (pinguecula) should be differentiated from a pterygium, a similar-appearing painless lesion that may grow over the cornea.[33]

To assess extraocular muscle movement, a penlight, finger, or other object should be used. Symmetrical movement of the eyes should be noted as the patient's eyes follow the finger or object as it tracts superiorly, inferiorly, laterally, medially, and obliquely. Any evidence of nystagmus should be noted.

The corneal light reflex should be tested to determine eye alignment (Fig. 1.13). When a light source is held directly in front of a patient who is staring straight ahead, normal eye alignment will reveal a symmetric reflex in the center of each pupil. If the light reflex in one eye is inwardly displaced, that eye is exotropic; if outwardly displaced, it is esotropic; and if superiorly or inferiorly displaced, it is hypertropic.[33]

In the cooperative patient, the cover-uncover eye test is a more accurate test for ocular alignment (Fig. 1.14). Testing should be done with the patient looking first at a near object and then at a far object As the patient fixates on the object, one eye is rapidly covered with a hand or occluder and the other eye is observed for movement. Normally there should be no movement of either eye as they are alternately tested.

Strabismic gaze or lack of parallel visual axes can be normal during the first several months of life. Persistent strabismus, regardless of age, should be referred to an ophthalmologist for further evaluation. A number of factors could interfere with the normal visual axis, including eye muscle weakness, cranial nerve involvement, cataract, chorioretinitis, and retinoblastoma. In young infants and children, pseudostrabismus can be seen in the presence of unilateral or bilateral epicanthal folds.

An infant's interest and attentiveness to bright light and the accompanying pupillary response indicate his or her ability to see. Visual fixation can be assessed in

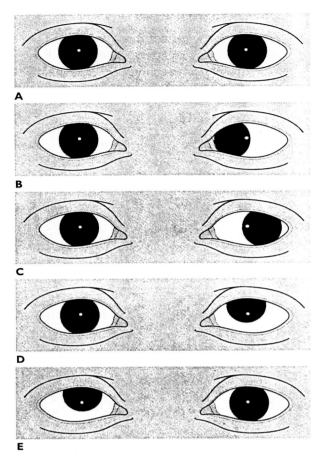

FIG. 1.13. A, Normal alignment as revealed by the corneal light reflection test. The light reflections are centered on both corneas. **B,** In left esotropia, the light reflection is outwardly displaced on the left cornea. **C,** In left exotropia, the light reflection is inwardly displaced on the left cornea. **D,** In left hypertropia, the light reflection is downwardly displaced on the left cornea. **E,** In right hypertropia, the light reflection is downwardly displaced on the right cornea. Reprinted with permission from Trobe JD. The physician's guide to eye care. San Francisco: American Academy of Ophthalmology, 1983.

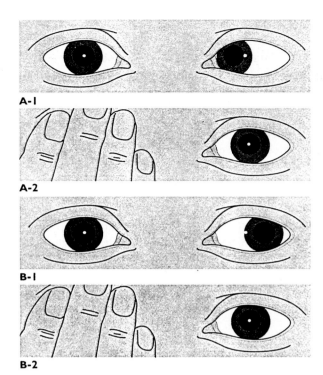

FIG. 1.14. A-1, With the patient's gaze directed straight ahead, the corneal reflections noted during the cover–uncover test indicate left esotropia. **A-2,** When the right eye is occluded, the left eye moves outward to pick up the fixation. **B-1,** With the patient's gaze directed straight ahead, the corneal reflections indicate left exotropia. **B-2,** When the right eye is occluded, the left eye moves inward to pick up the fixation. Reprinted with permission from Trobe JD. The physician's guide to eye care. San Francisco: American Academy of Ophthalmology, 1983.

infants by observing their ability to focus on an object or, more often, on their parent's face. The use of a rotating multicolored drum also helps determine the presence of sight. The patient with an intact visual pathway will have nystagmus when the drum is turned, whereas the eyes of a visually impaired patient will not move.

Ophthalmoscopic examination of the eyes should begin at a distance with the beam of light projected onto the upper facial area. The lens setting should be at zero. From a distance of several feet, visualization of each fundus is confirmed by the presence of the bilateral normal red reflex. In more darkly pigmented individuals, the reflex may be more gray than red.[34] Any opacities involving anatomic structures through which the light must pass will create a dull or abnormal color. Occasion-

ally, visualization of this reflex through the ophthalmoscope is difficult. Alternatively, a hand-held otoscope with the magnifying lens moved out of the examiner's field of vision may be used. While the examiner looks through the otoscopic aperture, the beam of light can be directed onto each eye separately or onto both eyes simultaneously, allowing for better visualization of the red reflex.

Examination of the cornea should reveal a clear transparent membrane. Adequate visualization entails use of an ophthalmoscope set at +8 to +6 diopters. Any corneal opacity is abnormal, including that owing to haziness or ulceration. A hazy cornea may be seen in a number of disorders, such as metabolic disease, glaucoma, and vitamin deficiency. Ulcerations may appear as a result of infection, foreign body, connective tissue disease, or trauma. Traumatic lacerations and acute ulcerations are extremely painful and are accompanied by photophobia, conjunctivitis, and pupillary constriction.

After visualization of the cornea, the anterior chamber should be examined with the ophthalmoscopic lens set at about +6 diopters. It should be completely free of opacities. Blood in the anterior chamber is a result of trauma. Turbidity and cellular debris in the chamber are caused by inflammation of the iris and ciliary muscle secondary to an autoimmune reaction.

To examine the iris and lens, the ophthalmoscopic setting should be +4 to +2 diopters. Cataracts, noted as a white pupillary reflex (leukocoria), can be seen without use of an ophthalmoscope. In a well-lit room or in natural sunlight, cataracts appear white or gray; and through the ophthalmoscope, they are dark or almost black. They can be congenital or acquired and may be the result of infection, metabolic disease, drugs, toxins, traumatic injury, glaucoma, or retinoblastoma. Visual impairment generally develops. If the cataract remains small, however, no visual difficulty may occur. Certain dermatologic abnormalities and several musculoskeletal, central nervous system, and craniofacial syndromes can give rise to cataracts. Two renal syndromes, Lowe and Alport, have cataracts as a major component, as does a primary hepatic condition, Zellweger (cerebrohepatorenal) syndrome.[34]

Examination of the retina and optic disk require ophthalmoscopic lens settings of 0 to −2 diopters. When close to the patient, the examiner can clearly visualize the optic disk; blood vessels; and more laterally, the macula. The fundus should be pink to red; in anemic patients and in darkly pigmented individuals, it may be gray-white. If an almost completely white and somewhat opaque light reflex is noted, impairing the examiner's ability to identify the optic disk, blood vessels, and macula, consideration should be given to the possibility of cloudy cornea, lens opacity, retinoblastoma, retinopathy of prematurity, or retinal detachment.[35]

Visual acuity in the infant and younger child can be tested by having them look at and follow the expression and movement of their caregiver's (or other person's) face. The physician should also note their response to optokinetic testing with a rotating multicolored drum and determine fixation with the cover–uncover test. For children older than 3 to 4 years, Allen cards (pictures of familiar objects, such as a car, cake, horse, and bird), and the HOTV test can be used to assess acuity. For the child 4 to 6 years old, the tumbling *E* test can be used; and for children who have mastered the alphabet, the standard Snellen eye chart can be considered.

For a child old enough to cooperate, visual field assessment can be conducted by having the child sit opposite the examiner at a distance of only a few feet and telling him or her to look at a particular part of the examiner's face, e.g., the nose. With both arms fully extended in opposite directions, the examiner begins wiggling a toy or the fingers of one hand and asks the patient to indicate (verbally or by pointing) when the movement comes into the child's visual field. Assuming the examiner has normal visual fields, assessment of any significant loss or deficiency in the patient can be determined. All four visual field quadrants should be tested. For the older patient, the examiner may choose to carry out the test by holding up a certain number of fingers and having the patient identify them when they come into range.

EARS

The examiner should note the relationship of the ears to the rest of the face, particularly the shape and position of the pinnae. If the superior rim of the pinnae is below a line drawn posteriorly from the superior orbital rim, the possible association with a renal anomaly should be considered; e.g., the absence of kidneys as seen in Potter syndrome. Malformation of the pinnae may be found in syndromes that affect mandibulofacial structures (e.g., Treacher Collins or Goldenhar syndrome).

Protruding, anteriorly placed pinnae can be a normal anatomical variant. If the external ear is displaced outward and anteriorly, consideration should be given to a diagnosis of mastoiditis, external otitis, cellulitis, or another disease process. Preauricular skin tags, although occasionally associated with hearing loss, generally have no clinical significance. Ear pits involving the pinnae and preauricular skin pits are also unlikely to be associated with a hearing loss, except in branchio-oto-renal syndrome.[36] Occasionally, a pit located just in front of the tragus may extend into a subcutaneous cyst and become infected.

Palpation of the tragus or pinnae may elicit significant pain in the patient with external auditory canal irritation. The canal can become swollen, erythematous, and painful as a result of a foreign body, external otitis, insect bite, or furuncle. In such situations, discomfort and swelling may become so significant that visualization of the tympanic membrane becomes difficult.

To complete the examination of the ear, the clinician should have an appropriate otoscope containing an excellent light source (preferably a halogen light). The diameter of the external auditory canal varies considerably among children; thus a range of specula should be available. To thoroughly visualize the external auditory canal and tympanic membrane, the examiner must clear the canal of excessive cerumen and foreign material. A flexible cerumen spoon or firm curette with a smooth, rounded edge can be used to gently remove cerumen with minimal trauma. When the cerumen is firm, thick, or dry and crusting, an ear wax softener (e.g., ℞Murine, ℞Cerumenex, or ℞Debrox) can be beneficial. A ™Water-Pik may be used to direct a stream of water into the canal under low pressure to pulverize and flush out difficult-to-remove cerumen. Foreign bodies in the canal should be removed under direct visualization using an operating microscope and appropriate forceps or suction equipment.

Once the anatomical structures are clearly visible, otoscopic examination should proceed as painlessly as possible. Visualization can be achieved best when the patient is sitting either in an upright position or lying supine with head appropriately tilted. The examiner should insert the otoscopic speculum into the external auditory canal as gently as possible; and to steady the position of the instrument to prevent discomfort, the ulnar aspect of the hand holding the instrument should be comfortably braced against the patient's face or forehead. At the same time, the thumb and index finger of the opposite hand should be used to pull the respective pinnae superiorly and posteriorly, allowing for maximal visualization of the external auditory canal.

For the patient who is difficult to examine, the caregiver should be instructed to hold the child firmly on his or her lap, holding the child's flailing legs between his or her own legs. The patient's head should be turned to the side and securely positioned to rest on the caregiver's shoulder or chest. Alternatively, the child should be placed in a supine position with extended arms and elbows firmly pinioned at the sides and extended legs gently immobilized by the weight of the accompanying adult's body lying over the thighs, knees, and lower legs. If available, the use of a papoose-like device to secure the patient is even more beneficial.

The smooth pink external auditory canal is normally short and straight in the infant and younger child and somewhat longer and more angulated in the older patient. Tympanic membranes are generally translucent, occasionally allowing for visualization of several middle ear structures (umbo, manubrium of the malleus, round window niche, pars flaccid, and chorda tympani nerve). The normal tympanic membrane can vary slightly in color and appearance; inexperienced examiners should not misinterpret what they are seeing.

Despite otoscopic evidence or a normal light reflex from the tympanic membrane, little information is gleaned regarding middle ear function. The degree of mobility of the tympanic membrane, using pneumatic otoscopy or tympanometry, however, can provide helpful information. Both techniques require a tight seal between the speculum or rubber ear piece and the external auditory canal. Movement is best visualized in the posterosuperior quadrant of the ear drum.

In the patient with normal middle ear pressure, the tympanic membrane moves inward with slight positive pressure and outward with slight negative pressure. If positive pressure produces no movement and negative pressure produces exaggerated movement, the middle ear has significant negative pressure. A full ear drum accompanied by fluid and air in the middle ear will move with positive pressure but will have no movement with negative pressure. A bulging ear drum caused by excessive middle ear effusion and little to no air will exhibit nearly complete or total absence of mobility.[37]

Erythema alone is not indicative of otitis media; but dull appearance, loss of normal mobility, and absence of distinctive landmarks are helpful diagnostic criteria. Fullness or bulging of the drum may or may not be present. Occasionally, a patient may have acute otitis media but no obvious middle ear fluid or loss of mobility. When a bulging ear drum is present without other signs or symptoms of otitis media, consideration should be given to retained middle ear effusion after an episode of otitis media or blood in the middle ear space after trauma. Water retention alone rarely if ever accounts for a distended ear drum.

The most common bacterial pathogens accounting for otitis media in childhood are *Streptococcus pneumoniae*, nontypable *Haemophilus influenzae*, and *Moraxella catarrhalis*. If the drum is perforated, purulent discharge may be found in the external auditory canal. In the presence of an intact tympanic membrane after an episode of otitis media, 40% of patients will have a middle ear effusion 1 month later; 2 and 3 months later, 20 and 10% of patients, respectively, still will have middle ear effusion.

With chronic middle ear effusion, patients are frequently found to have retracted tympanic membranes. The finding of a perforated ear drum alone is indicative of traumatic injury as a result of a foreign body, increased barometric pressure, iatrogenic injury, or previous surgical incision for ventilating tubes.

Several techniques are available for assessing hearing in children.[37] Gross hearing can be assessed by observing an infant's physical response to sound. A startle response, eye blinking, and turning toward the sound are normal reactions. In the older more cooperative child, crude testing can be carried out by standing close to the patient and mouthing relatively inaudible words into the child's ear or whispering words at a distance of 1 to 2 feet from one ear while occluding the external auditory canal of the opposite ear. The child can then be asked to repeat what was said. More formal testing can be done in the relatively uncooperative child using acoustic impedance measurements or an auditory brainstem response. For the more cooperative younger patient, various behavioral tests are available; the older child can undergo standardized audiometric testing.

A hearing deficit may result from an infectious disease, may be associated with a hereditary renal disorder, may be congenital and idiopathic, may be drug related, or may be a component of numerous syndromes. There may be a conductive or neurosensory problem or a combination of both. If the patient is old enough to cooperate, the Rinne and Weber tests should be employed to determine which type of problem is involved.

To test for conductive loss (the Rinne test), the examiner should place the flat end of a vibrating tuning fork handle (preferably 512 dB) over the mastoid process (bone conduction) and ask the patient to indicate when sound is no longer heard. The vibrating fork should then be held 1 to 2 inches from the meatus of the external auditory canal (air conduction). Patients with normal hearing will be able to hear sound longer by air conduction. Both ears should be tested. The vibrating fork should then be placed in the center of the patient's forehead to determine if there is unilateral bone conduction (neurosensory) or air conduction hearing loss (the Weber test). Ordinarily, the patient should be able to hear the sound equally well in both ears. If the patient has air conduction hearing loss in one ear, the sound will be heard better in that ear. If there is unilateral neurosensory loss, the sound will be better heard on the opposite side.[3]

NOSE

Examination of the nose should be conducted with the patient's head tilted back in a sniffing position and the physician sitting directly opposite the patient. The shape, size, and position of the nose should be noted. Inspection of internal structures should be done using a bright light source and nasal speculum or, for the smaller child, an ear speculum. To reduce patient discomfort and to steady the head, the examiner should position the outer ulnar aspect of the hand not holding an instrument against the patient's forehead; the thumb of that hand is used to elevate the tip of the nose. This allows for optimal visualization of each vestibule, the nasal turbinates, septum, and mucosal surfaces.

Normally, the mucosal surfaces are pink and the vestibules are patent and easily visible to the level of the middle turbinates. The septum should be in the midline, although a slight deviation is acceptable. Transient septal deformity secondary to in utero positioning may be noted in the newborn. When septal perforation is present, the differential diagnosis should include infectious diseases, inhaled drugs (particularly cocaine), and traumatic injury.

Swelling, bleeding, abnormal lesions, and types of secretions should be noted. Thin serous or watery nasal discharge may be seen in patients with allergic rhinitis or in those with a viral upper respiratory tract infection (URI). An almost crystal clear nasal discharge may occur as a result of leaking cerebral spinal fluid, diagnosable by a glucose dipstick. A more viscous nasal discharge may be noted in patients during the latter stages of a viral URI. Thick purulent nasal discharge may be seen in patients with either a viral or bacterial infection involving the nasopharynx or sinuses. In a patient with unilateral, malodorous, purulent nasal discharge, an impacted foreign body should be suspected.

Although epistaxis is not unusual in childhood, the examiner should always inquire about the frequency, amount of blood, time of day, duration of the incident, and whether the bleeding was from one or both nasal passageways. For most children, nose bleeds are infrequent, of short duration, occur primarily in the winter months, involve either or both sides of the nose, and emanate from the small blood vessels in the anterior nasal septum (Kiesselbach's plexus).[38] Prolonged bleeding may be the result of a bleeding dyscrasia or traumatic injury. An angiofibroma, seen primarily in teenage males, is occasionally a cause for recurrent, prolonged, unilateral epistaxis.

If there is apparent nasal obstruction in a newborn, the examiner should rule out the possibility of choanal atresia by attempting to pass a small-gauge feeding tube or French catheter through each nasal passageway. Occluded nasal passageways caused by boggy nasal mucosa may develop as a result of allergies, vasomotor rhinitis, or overuse of nasal decongestants. Nasal polyps caused by allergies or associated with cystic fibrosis may cause unilateral or bilateral nasal obstruction. Adenoidal enlargement may obstruct the nasopharynx, making nasal breathing difficult and creating the typical open-mouth adenoid facies.

MOUTH AND THROAT

Examination of the mouth should begin with visual inspection of the lips for color, texture, and anatomical defects. The width of the vermilion border and the shape and size of the orifice should be noted. Abnormal findings may be compatible with multisystem disorders such as Williams syndrome or those resulting from maternal substance abuse as seen in the fetal alcohol syndrome.

Mouth examination should include the gingiva, teeth, buccal mucosa, salivary ducts, tongue, palate, tonsils, and uvula. Ulcerations of the lips, gingiva, and/or mucosal surfaces may be compatible with herpetic stomatitis, aphthous ulcers, metabolic disorders, drug reactions, or secondary complications from underlying immunosuppressive disease. Extensive inflammation and erosion of surfaces may be the result of primary infection or poor oral hygiene with secondary infection. Obstructed salivary ducts may be caused by concretions, leading to the development of a cyst-like structure in the floor of the mouth (ranula) or by inflammation leading to painful swelling in the area of the parotid gland. Fissuring or cracking of the tongue may be a normal variant but can occur with poor hydration and vitamin deficiency. Defects in the hard and/or soft palate should be noted, particularly midline cleft palate defects. Dimpling of the soft palate and/or the presence of a bifid uvula may be found with a submucosal cleft.[39]

The development and continued good health of dentition in childhood is extremely important. Deciduous tooth eruption generally begins at 6 months of age with the appearance of upper and/or lower central incisors, followed over the next 18 months by the eruption of lateral incisors, canines, and molars. By the age of 2, the majority of toddlers should have the full complement of 20 teeth.[29] Misshapen or absent teeth or significant delay in the development of these teeth may be found in patients with underlying metabolic disorders, infectious diseases, or various syndromes.

Visualization of the palatine tonsils generally does not occur until the child is 6 to 9 months old. Once fully developed, the tonsils remain enlarged throughout childhood. Unless they become a nidus of significant recurrent infection or are enlarged enough to obstruct normal breathing, removal is not necessary. Bacterial infection of the throat and tonsils with group A β-hemolytic *Streptococcus* may be indicated by the classic appearance of tonsillar enlargement with erythema and exudate, a "strawberry" tongue, petechiae of the soft palate and uvula, and enlarged tender anterior cervical nodes. Frequently, however, the patient with a streptococcal infection will have few if any of these findings. Enlarged tonsils with exudate may be caused by other infectious organisms, such as diphtheria and Epstein–Barr virus.

Examination of the pharynx usually requires visualization only. Pharyngitis may be indicated by erythema and/or pharyngeal adenopathy (cobblestoning). It can be caused by viral, bacterial, or fungal disease, by a chemical irritant or as a complication of some other condition. Soft tissue lesions and foreign body injuries should be noted.

NECK

Examination of the neck is accomplished best with the patient either sitting or standing. The head should be in the midline position comfortably held in extension. The size and position of anatomical neck structures should be noted. A webbed-shape neck may be associated with Turner syndrome and redundant posterior neck folds can be seen in patients with Down syndrome. A short neck with a low hairline and limited range of motion may be the result of bony anomalies of the cervical spine associated with Klippel–Feil syndrome. Klippel–Feil syndrome patients frequently have accompanying genitourinary abnormalities. A short neck also occurs with congenital hypothyroidism and with one of the mucopolysaccharidoses (e.g., Hurler or Morquio).

Distended or pulsating neck veins may indicate obstruction to right heart return (e.g., mediastinal masses) or impaired cardiac function (e.g., pericarditis or poor myocardial contractility). Distended pulsating carotid arteries are normally seen in patients who are emotionally upset and after vigorous exercise. If the finding persists, significant disorders such as aortic insufficiency, patent ductus arteriosus (PDA), hypertension, and severe anemia must be considered.[27]

A head tilt can result from several different conditions. In the infant, torticollis may be the result of sternocleidomastoid muscle fibrosis secondary to in utero pressure or trauma during delivery, myopathy, denervation, or venous occlusion.[40] Head tilt may occur in patients with a visual defect and in those with a posterior fossa tumor or neuroblastoma. Patients with severe gastroesophageal reflux may exhibit a head tilt as a compensatory maneuver to help reduce the discomfort of reflux esophagitis (Sandifer syndrome).[41]

A soft tissue, freely movable, cystic mass in the midline of the neck superior to the upper border of the thyroid cartilage is most compatible with a thyroglossal duct cyst. Other midline lesions of the neck include sebaceous cysts, small abscesses, lipomas, and dermoids.

Below the thyroid cartilage, the thyroid gland separates into two symmetrical lobes and curves posteriorly around the sides of the trachea and esophagus. Palpation of the thyroid is accomplished best with the examiner positioned behind the standing or sitting patient. The fingers of the examiner's hands should be gently positioned over the respective lobes, which are normally soft, smooth, and not enlarged. When the patient swallows, the thyroid gland can be felt to move upward. Only repetitive palpation of the thyroid of many patients will give the examiner the feel for normal size, shape, and contour.

Moving the hands from the midline to lateral structures of the neck, the examiner should feel for abnormal masses. Within the sternocleidomastoid muscle, a firm mass could be caused by fibrosis or a benign or malignant tumor. Branchial cleft cysts palpable in the upper portion of the neck are soft and smooth. Cystic hygromas and lymphangiomas of the neck, which generally transilluminate easily, may vary in size and shape and are not tender. Additional detectable soft tissue structures include hemangiomas, dermoid cysts, lipomas, and neurofibromas.[42]

A few shotty, freely movable, nontender lymph nodes in the anterior and posterior cervical chain are palpable in a large number of young children and are considered normal. Enlarged, firm, nontender, freely movable or fixed neck nodes can be found in patients with lymphoma, Hodgkin's disease, and other metastatic disease. Enlarged nodes that are tender, warm, and painful to movement are compatible with lymphadenitis. The most common bacterial organism causing lymphadenitis is *Staphylococcus aureus*. Other bacterial causes include group A β-hemolytic *Streptococcus, Mycobacterium tuberculosis,* atypical mycobacterium, and *Bartonella henselae.* Common viral causes for lymphadenitis include Epstein–Barr virus, cytomegalovirus, measles, rubella, and varicella viruses. Numerous infectious and noninfectious causes for lymphadenopathy and lymphadenitis must be considered for a complete differential diagnosis.[28]

CHEST

Chest Wall

Before auscultating or percussing the heart or lungs and before palpating the chest wall and breast tissue, the examiner should observe and inspect the chest wall carefully. Normally, the chest is symmetrical; and in the infant or young child, it is almost round. With aging, the transverse diameter increases. When a persistently round, barrel-shaped chest is seen in an older child, the examiner should consider the possibility of an underlying chronic pulmonary disease, such as cystic fibrosis or chronic asthma.

The shoulders should be examined, especially in the newborn, for clavicular fractures and foreshortened or absent clavicles. Nipple alignment and the distance between nipples should be noted. Accessory nipples along the milk line are normal. A shield-like chest with widely spaced nipples can be found in patients with Turner syndrome. The width of the ribs and length of the sternum should be noted.

An asymmetrical chest wall may be present as a result of scoliosis or an underlying cardiac disease that creates a precordial bulge. Poland syndrome, consisting of syndactyly and ipsilateral absence of the sternal head of the pectoralis major muscle, gives rise to an asymmetrical chest wall with an inferiorly placed ipsilateral nipple.[43] A mild degree of pectus excavatum (funnel chest) or pectus carinatum (pigeon breast) is a common finding in an otherwise normal patient. Pectus excavatum frequently becomes accentuated with even mild degrees of airway obstruction. Surgical correction for persistent mild to moderate pectus carinatum or excavatum generally is not indicated.[44]

In the normal child, inspiration results in expansion of the chest wall and depression of the diaphragm. In the patient with unilateral pneumonia, pneumothorax, atelectasis, or a foreign body lodged in one of the mainstem bronchi, inspiration can cause the diaphragm to rise and the chest wall to collapse on the involved side. Bilateral paradoxical breathing can be seen in patients with neuromuscular disease.[27]

Breasts

Like the staging of pubic hair development and genital maturation, breast development staging is based on standards established by Marshall and Tanner[45, 46] (Fig. 1.15). The range is from no evident breast tissue (stage 1) to complete adult development (stage 5). Infants of either sex often have transient breast tissue enlargement secondary to perinatal maternal estrogen stimulation, which may remain for several months before spontaneous regression occurs. There is generally no discernible difference between boys and girls under the age of 8 years in the size and shape of the chest wall.

Sometime in early adolescence, both males and females may experience the development of a firm and often tender-to-touch unilateral or bilateral subareolar nodule. In approximately 66% of normal boys, these nodules occur as part of the developmental pattern of adolescent male gynecomastia. They develop as a result of direct testicular secretion of estrogen and the peripheral conversion of prohormones to estrogen. The size of these nodules decrease over 1 to 2 years, although residual nontender remnants may remain.[47]

True male gynecomastia can occur; and in the majority of cases, the cause is undetermined. Possible causes include drugs (digitalis, isoniazid, cimetidine, phenothiazine, and antidepressants), breast tumors, adrenal and gonadal lesions, gonadal dysgenesis, hyperthyroidism, Klinefelter syndrome, malnutrition, renal disease, and severe liver disease.[48]

In the United States, the mean age for the start of breast development in girls is between 8.5 and 10 years.[49] Precocious breast development in girls can be normal, although attention should be given to other possible explanations. True assessment of breast tissue development and size is best determined with the patient in the supine position. While the breast area is being examined, the patient's head should be in the midline resting on the palm of the ipsilateral hand. The pattern for examination should be in concentric circles proceeding peripherally from the infraclavicular and axillary areas toward the areola.

Obese patients may have pseudoprecocious breast area enlargement, in which the areola is small, the nipple is flat, and the breast tissue is soft. In normal breast development, the areola is large, the nipple is raised, and the surrounding tissue is firm. If the breasts fail to develop by middle to late adolescence, consideration should be given to the possibility of gonadal dysgenesis, adrenal hyperplasia, pituitary dysfunction, or significant malnutrition (anorexia nervosa).[50]

Lungs

Observation of the patient's breathing pattern should be foremost in the examination of the lungs. The rate, rhythm, and depth of breathing should be carefully noted. The occurrence of a periodic sigh is normal in everyone. Shallow rapid breathing can be seen with anatomical defects, pulmonary infection, pleuritic disease, and metabolic disorders. Slow breathing can occur as a result of central nervous system pathology, metabolic disease, and drug effect. Vigorous exercise, a state of anxiety, and metabolic acidosis cause deep rapid breathing. A prolonged expiratory phase occurs in patients with an acute exacerbation of reactive airway disease or true asthma. A sleeping infant may have brief periods of rapid breathing alternating with respiratory pauses.[51]

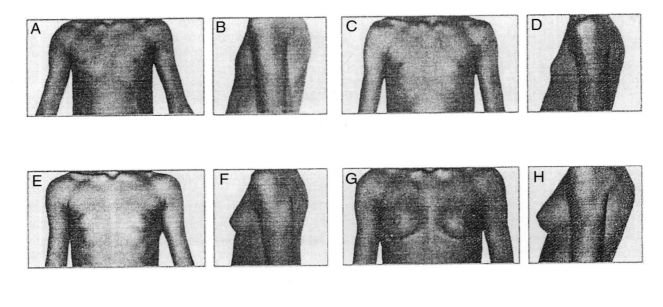

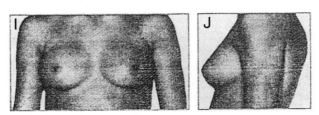

FIG. 1.15. Pubertal development of the size of female breasts. **A and B,** In stage 1, the breasts are preadolescent; there is elevation of the papilla only. **C and D,** In stage 2, the breast buds develop. A small mound is formed by the elevation of the breast and papilla; the areolar diameter enlarges. **E and F,** In stage 3, the breasts and areola continue to enlarge; there is no separation of the contours. **G and H,** In stage 4, there is a projection of the areola and papilla, forming a secondary mound above the level of the breast. **I and J,** In stage 5, the breasts are fully mature; the areola has recessed to the general contour of the breast.

Thorough auscultation of lung fields in children is sometimes difficult, and successful examination frequently depends on the age of the child. Fear of the examiner and discomfort from illness generally account for the patient's uncooperative behavior. An experienced clinician, aware of the difficulty of auscultation of a noncompliant, often screaming, child, concentrates on the inspiratory phase, with the realization that little will be gained by trying to listen during the expiratory phase. Some of the anxiety may be alleviated if a caregiver holds the child.

An organized symmetrical approach to auscultation of the lung fields should be used. Sequential examination should proceed from one side of the chest to the other, comparing breath sounds in anatomically similar areas. Either the bell or the diaphragm of the stethoscope may be used, depending on the size of the child. The diaphragm is more appropriate for listening to the lungs of larger patients.

The sounds produced by breathing may help localize a particular area of involvement or specific pathologic condition. Ordinarily, deep mouth breathing produces clear, soft breath sounds over the lungs. Atypical breath sounds in the form of rales, rhonchi, or wheezes are heard most often in patients with underlying pulmonary disease. Upper airway congestion in small children often produces coarse sounds that, when transmitted through the larger airways, may give the impression of an underlying lung abnormality. Coughing and/or vigorous crying will frequently clear a congested upper airway, helping the clinician distinguish between upper and lower airway sounds.

In small children, an inspiratory high-pitched stridorous sound with or without significant respiratory distress may be the result of narrowing at or near the larynx or anywhere along the trachea. It may be attributable to a croup-like illness, anatomical defect, mass lesion, foreign body, or external obstruction. Patients in severe respiratory distress with stridor may have epiglottitis. When absent or decreased breath sounds are heard over a particular lung area, spoken words may sound muffled or the letter *E* may sound more like an *A*. This is especially true in a child with a segmental or lobar consolidation. Fairly well localized squeaky crackles during respiration may be due to a pleural friction rub.

Heart

Before cardiac auscultation and palpation are initiated, the examining physician should devote particular attention to the patient's general appearance. Central and peripheral color, nutritional status, respiratory rate and effort, presence of sweating, and chest contour should be noted. Jugular venous distention, peripheral edema, and evidence of hepatitic engorgement suggest right ventricular dysfunction.[52]

The clinician may evaluate the heart in older, cooperative patients at any time during the examination; however, it is best to evaluate the heart in infants and younger children early in the examination. Palpation of the cardiovascular system should begin with the peripheral pulses. The pulsatile rate, regularity, and degree of fullness should be noted. Palpation can be used in the diagnosis of valvular lesions, for assessment of ventricular function, and as a source of information about the patient's hemodynamic status.[52]

A rapid pulse may indicate congestive heart failure, an arrhythmia, or an underlying respiratory problem and may occur as a direct result of anxiety or agitation. Bounding pulses suggest aortic insufficiency, PDA, truncus arteriosus, or an arteriovenous malformation. An extremely slow pulse rate could mean heart block, a central nervous system problem, or a metabolic abnormality. Simultaneous palpation of pulses in the upper extremities and then contralateral palpation of pulses in an upper and lower extremity should be done to help determine the presence of an aortic or peripheral artery filling defect, e.g., coarctation of the aorta (COA).

Palpation of the heart through the chest wall determines the apical impulse and the presence of a heave, tap, or thrill. Because the right ventricle remains dominant in the newborn, a palpable lift, better appreciated with the heel of the hand, is best felt in the area of the left lower sternal border. In a patient with left ventricular hypertrophy, a heave can be detected best with the palm and proximal surfaces of the fingers of the right hand.[52] A tap due to pressure overload is felt near the apex as a well-localized sharp impulse.

A thrill is a palpable loud murmur of grade IV to VI. Thrills associated with specific cardiac defects are often well localized. A thrill at the left upper sternal border is usually caused by pulmonary valve or pulmonary artery stenosis (PAS); one at the right upper sternal border is the result of aortic stenosis (AS). A thrill along the left lower sternal border generally is the result of a ventricular septal defect (VSD), and one at the suprasternal notch can be caused by either a PDA, PAS, COA, or AS.

Auscultation of the heart can be achieved using either the bell or the diaphragm of the stethoscope. The bell is designed for listening to low-frequency sounds; and the diaphragm, for high-frequency sounds. Thorough evaluation necessitates auscultation of all areas of the precordium as well as the back, neck, and axillary areas. The process should entail noting the rate and rhythm and listening carefully for the normal first and second heart sounds. Close attention should be given to detecting ejection clicks, systolic and diastolic murmurs, pericardial friction rubs, extra heart sounds, and diastolic rumbles.

The first heart sound is generally a singular sound caused by nearly simultaneous closure of the tricuspid and mitral valves and is best heard at the apex. Splitting of the first heart sound may be detectable in the presence of an Ebstein anomaly or a right bundle branch block pattern. The second heart sound, best heard at the left upper sternal border, is caused by the closure of the pulmonary and aortic valves and is normally split with inspiration, less so with expiration. A third heart sound, although unusual, can be heard in normal children, at the apex or along the lower left sternal border, and is attributed to the turbulence of rapid filling of the left ventricle. A dilated, noncompliant ventricle may create an abnormally loud third heart sound. The rhythm of the first, second, and third heart sounds together should produce a beat similar to the sound of the three syllables in the word *Kentucky*. An abnormal fourth sound, present in patients with decreased ventricular compliance, when heard in sequence with the first and second heart sounds creates a beat similar to the three syllables in the word *Tennessee*. The rapid beat of the first, second, third, and/or fourth sounds, common in congestive heart failure sounds like the rhythm of a horse's gallop.

Murmurs are characterized by the intensity and quality of the sound they create, when they occur in the cardiac cycle, their location, and whether they are transmitted. The intensity of murmurs are graded on a scale of I to VI. Grade I murmurs are nearly inaudible, whereas grade III murmurs are loud but have no palpable thrill. Grade V murmurs can be heard when the stethoscope is barely touching the chest wall, and grade VI murmurs are audible when the stethoscope is not touching the chest wall. High-pitched, blowing murmurs are heard with mitral regurgitation (MR) and VSD. Harsh murmurs are heard in patients with AS or PAS. Murmurs described as having a vibratory or humming sound are generally innocent and of no significance.

Most murmurs occur during systole and are either ejection or regurgitant murmurs. Those heard along the left upper sternal border may be caused by AS or PAS, pulmonary branch stenosis (PBS), tetralogy of Fallot (TOF), COA, or other defect (generally minor). Those heard along the right upper sternal border may be the result of either supravalvular, valvular, or subvalvular

AS. Murmurs along the lower left sternal border may be caused by VSD, tricuspid regurgitation (TR), TOF, idiopathic hypertrophic subaortic stenosis (IHSS), or even an innocent Still's murmur. Murmurs at the apex can be found in patients with MR, mitral valve prolapse, AS, IHSS, or an innocent murmur. Regurgitant murmurs are heard in patients who have VSD, MR, or TR.

Murmurs heard during diastole may occur in early, middle, or late diastole. Those in early diastole are caused by aortic or pulmonary valve incompetence. Those in middle diastole occur secondary to anatomic stenosis of the mitral or tricuspid valve and are generally preceded by a loud third heart sound. Those in late diastole are due to vigorous atrial contraction, resulting in a rapid injection of blood into the ventricle. A continuous murmur is one that begins in systole and lasts throughout most of diastole. Continuous murmurs can be heard in patients with PDA, COA, or venous hum.[53]

A large number of children, sometime during their lifetime, will be found to have an innocent or functional murmur with no anatomical abnormality; for example, the common but transient functional murmur best heard over the left precordium in patients with increased cardiac output secondary to high fever. An innocent grade I to III murmur noted in early infancy is the result of peripheral pulmonary branch stenosis, best heard at the base of the heart and bilaterally in each axilla and over the back. The continuous murmur of a venous hum occurs in the early years of childhood, is most readily audible over the upper thoracic and jugular areas with the patient in an upright position, and disappears when gentle pressure is applied to the jugular vein or when the patient's head is turned fully to the opposite shoulder. A Still's murmur is best heard along the lower left sternal border or apex, occurs in middle systole, has an intensity no greater than grade III, and has a vibratory or musical quality. The innocent pulmonary ejection murmur, detected most often in adolescents, is heard best in middle systole in the second left intercostal space. It has a harsh quality and an intensity no greater than grade III.[54]

ABDOMEN

Visualization of a child's abdomen for contour, symmetry, pulsations, peristalsis, peripheral vascular irregularities, and skin markings is best done in good light with the patient supine and the examiner positioned at the patient's right side. Although often seen after a patient has eaten, abdominal distention noted at other times may indicate abnormal gas-filled loops of bowel, a ruptured viscus, fecal retention, mass lesion, or ascites. A scaphoid abdomen may be found in a patient with upper gastrointestinal obstruction or as a result of starvation. Peristaltic waves may be seen on occasion but vascular pulsations generally are not visualized. The

presence of hyperpigmented or hypopigmented skin lesions may be normal. Vascular lesions other than hemangiomata are usually not present.

Abdominal wall protrusions are frequently seen. In the infant, toddler, and younger child, umbilical hernias are commonly present, particularly among black children. The majority of umbilical hernias are uncomplicated, require no surgery, and resolve spontaneously. Diastasis recti and small epigastric hernias, if not readily visible, can be elicited by having the patient raise his or her head off the examining table while lying supine or by having the child tense the abdominal muscles. These hernias do not require surgical correction.

Abdominal auscultation is often difficult and unrewarding in the active, uncooperative child but may be of significant benefit in the child experiencing abdominal discomfort. Active bowel sounds are often heard in patients with gastroenteritis and are usually decreased or absent in patients with appendicitis or intestinal obstruction. Stenosis involving the aorta or iliac, femoral, or renal arteries may give rise to an audible abdominal bruit. Some examiners have employed an auscultatory technique to determine the inferior margin(s) of the liver and/or spleen by listening with a stethoscope over the patient's abdomen while gently scratching the abdominal skin surface with a blunt instrument. Starting in the ipsilateral lower quadrant of the organ being examined and advancing superiorly, the examiner is able to identify the lower border of the liver or spleen when a change in sound from tympany to dullness is heard.

Percussion helps detect mass lesions and organ size and can often help identify local areas of pain. Solid or fluid-filled structures, such as a urine-filled bladder, produce a dull sound to percussion, whereas gas-filled loops of bowel produce tympany.

When a distended abdomen is thought to be the result of ascites, percussion can be used to help make the diagnosis. The patient should be supine, and percussion should begin peripherally. At first, dullness will be noted; but as percussion advances centrally, the air-filled loops of intestine, forced to the midline by ascitic fluid, will emit a tympanitic sound. When the patient turns to one side or the other, the locations of tympany and dullness shift as the fluid moves into dependent areas. A fluid wave can be produced when the examiner strikes one flank area with the tips of the fingers of one hand and detects gentle pressure with the other hand on the opposite flank.[55] This finding is better demonstrated by employing the aid of an assistant who at the same time has placed the ulnar surfaces of both fully extended hands pointing toward one another along the midline of the abdomen.

Palpation is extremely beneficial for determining liver, kidney, and spleen size and for detecting abdominal masses. An examiner's warm hands and initial gentle, soft touch may go a long way in gaining the cooperation of the patient for deeper, more thorough palpation. The often ticklish younger child may require a calm, reassuring touch, and no initial hand movement by the examiner. After a few moments, these children are instructed to take a deep breath and then exhale slowly while the examiner applies firm steady pressure to the abdomen. By repeating the procedure in all four quadrants, a fairly complete examination can be achieved.

The softer and less tense the abdominal musculature, the more easily organs and mass lesions can be felt. In the obese child, a two-hand technique may have to be used with the fingers of one hand applying pressure on top of the fingers of the other hand. When peritonitis is suspected, rebound tenderness may be elicited by pressing firmly and slowly on the abdomen and then quickly releasing pressure. Subsequent wincing by the patient or other audible or visual sign of pain confirms the examiner's impression.

Because the abdominal wall of children is usually thin, the organs are relatively easy to palpate. When attempting to feel the liver, the examiner should stand on the patient's right side, placing the fingers of the right hand over the right middle to lower quadrant in a somewhat oblique position. Palpation should progress in a superior direction, until the lower edge of the liver is detected. With the left hand under the right flank, the examiner should place gentle cephalad-directed pressure on the liver until the edge of the liver is felt with the right hand. A similar maneuver in the left upper quadrant and posterior flank helps determine the inferior margin of the spleen.

The kidneys can be palpated in much the same way as the liver and spleen. Renal tenderness can be easily determined in a cooperative child with pyelonephritis through percussion of the flank areas. A firm striking blow to the flank area with the ulnar surface of the closed fist will elicit discomfort in the patient with renal infection.

In the child with suspected appendicitis, the presence of several positive physical findings may help make the diagnosis. Early in the inflammatory process, patients may complain of pain in the periumbilical area making the examiner less suspicious of appendiceal involvement. Over time, the pain generally localizes to the right lower quadrant and light palpation may elicit tenderness and guarding. Deeper palpation and quick release of pressure may create rebound tenderness. In advanced cases of appendicitis, significant abdominal muscular rigidity may develop, making palpation difficult.

Other physical findings and observations may help solidify the diagnosis of appendicitis. These patients often will have difficulty climbing onto the examination table. Once on the table, they will remain supine reluctant to make any movement. Internal rotation of the right thigh at the hip, while the knee and hip are flexed, will stretch the obturator muscle and elicit pain if the appendix is inflamed. Psoas muscle irritation from an inflamed appendix can be demonstrated by having the supine patient raise the right thigh while at the same time an examiner applies firm hand pressure just proximal to the knee. Digital examination of the anterior rectal wall may elicit pain. Although such findings may be compatible with appendicitis, other pathologic conditions—psoas muscle abscess, ovarian cyst, pelvic inflammatory disease, and passage of urinary tract stones (particularly in older children)—should be considered in the differential diagnosis.

EXTREMITIES

The approach to the examination of the extremities of the older child and adolescent is similar to that of the adult, but examination of the extremities of infants and younger children requires an understanding of anatomical limitations and acceptable variations in normal alignment. Examination should begin with careful visualization of the upper and lower extremities looking for appropriate alignment, unusual masses or protuberances, joint deformities, missing or fused digits, and/or integument abnormalities. Attention should be paid to muscle mass. Adverse effects from maternal drugs, congenital defects, and chromosomal/genetic abnormalities may cause limb deformities and limb length discrepancies.

Physical examination of the extremities should include determining the range of motion of all joints. Normal, full-term newborn infants have significant flexion contractures of the upper and lower extremities, limiting the range of motion. Within normal anatomical limits of a particular joint, flexion, extension, abduction, adduction, supination, pronation, eversion, and inversion should be demonstrated. Variation from normal between paired joints and extremities should also be noted. For older children, the clinician should evaluate the gait as well as the sitting and standing postures.

Palpation of the extremities should be done to determine areas of tenderness, swelling, and increased or decreased temperature. Any one or all of these findings may be noted at sites of fracture, bone or joint disease, infection, and sprain. Clavicular fractures in the newborn may be undetected in the immediate neonatal period; on subsequent examination of the clavicles, these patients may have unilateral or bilateral swelling (callous formation) and tenderness. The tone and strength of the muscles should be examined. Patients with Duchenne muscular dystrophy, who have pseudohypertrophy of muscle groups, will (deceptively) appear to have adequate muscle mass, despite having decreased muscle tone and strength.

In infants and toddlers, femoral anteversion, tibial torsion, and metatarsus adductus are commonly found. The vast majority of these anatomical variations are present as a result of in utero positioning and tend to correct spontaneously. Minimal intervention, consisting of passive range of motion exercises, may help enhance the correction. Prolonged malalignment of the feet and/or legs may occur as a result of poor postural positioning, for example, if the child habitually sits in the reversed tailor position or sleeps in the prone knee–chest position with the feet crossed beneath the pelvis.

In the early months of walking, infants have a normal, wide-based gait; the legs are often rotated externally, and the feet are flat. The more normal gait of childhood develops with anatomical and neurologic maturity. Toe walking, found in patients with cerebral palsy, may be a transient finding in some normal infants. Passive range of motion of the foot will help distinguish a tight heel cord that is limiting normal dorsiflexion from the full range of motion seen in the otherwise normal toe walker. Toeing in and toeing out, seen frequently in early childhood, generally correct over time. In the majority of cases, corrective shoes, splints, and braces provide little if any benefit and are not recommended.

Developmental Dysplasia of the Hip

Thorough examination of the hips for evidence of joint laxity or dislocation should be performed on every infant from shortly after birth until several months after independent walking. Findings compatible with developmental dysplasia of the hip may be detected in the newborn period, and abnormal signs present at that time may disappear. Until an infant is approximately 2 months old, two diagnostic maneuvers with the patient in the supine position may help make an early diagnosis. The Barlow maneuver reveals dislocation and is carried out by flexing the leg at the hip and adducting the thigh while applying pressure in a posterior direction along the long axis of the femur. The Ortolani maneuver reveals reduction and is demonstrated by hip flexion and abduction of the thigh while replacing the femoral head into the acetabulum with a lift of the leg in an anterior direction.[56]

In the supine infant with unilateral hip dislocation, subtle physical findings may include asymmetric abduction of the hips, loss of hip and knee flexion contractures, and asymmetric skin folds with the legs held in extension. A sign of unilateral dislocation demonstrable at any age is seen in the supine position with both hips flexed to 90°, knees flexed, and feet flat on a level surface (Allis, Perkins, or Galeazzi sign). In this position, the knees are normally at the same level. With unilateral dislocation, the head of one femur will be displaced posteriorly and the knee on that side will lower than the other knee. In the patient with bilateral dislocated hips, no asymmetry may be seen. An abnormal gait, limp, or waddle may be the only sign of dislocation in the older child. Bilateral dislocation in this age group may be suspected by visualization of a widened perineum.

Child with a Limp

Possible causes of a limp include infection; neuromuscular or neurologic problems; primary bone, cartilage, ligament, and/or joint abnormalities; allergic and/or inflammatory processes; oncologic diseases; mass lesions; and foreign bodies. Examination of a septic joint will reveal warmth, pain, and tenderness at the site with limited range of motion. Osteomyelitis is indicated by localized erythema and edema; the child may refuse to move the involved extremity. Patients with avascular necrosis of the femoral head (Legg–Calvé–Perthes disease) have a gait abnormality, loss of hip rotation and abduction, pain in the hip or anterior thigh, and eventually wasting of the thigh and gluteal muscles.

Toxic synovitis, generally seen in very young children, is manifest by a limp, hip or thigh pain, limited range of hip motion, and exquisite discomfort and guarding when the flexed hip is gently abducted or adducted while the patient is supine. The patient with slipped capital femoral epiphysis may present with sudden onset of uncomfortable weight bearing and pain involving the groin, thigh, and/or knee.[57] When the involved hip is flexed, a pathognomic finding of slipped epiphysis is simultaneous external rotation and abduction of the hip.[40]

In the preadolescent or adolescent, unique problems involving the lower extremity may account for pain and/or limitation of motion. Among these are knee problems owing to either Osgood–Schlatter disease or chondromalacia patella.

GENITOURINARY SYSTEM

The physical findings and approach to examination of the genitourinary system are age dependent. The neonatal examination should focus particularly on congenital anomalies. In the male, attention should be paid to penile length, foreskin anatomy, location of the urethral meatus, scrotal anatomy (including rugae), the presence and location of the testes, and the presence of abnormal scrotal or inguinal masses.

The tightly adherent foreskin should be gently retracted to reveal the urethral meatus in its normal anatomical position at the tip of the glans penis. Forceful retraction is never indicated, particularly in the infant. If the urethral meatus is found on the ventral surface proximal to the glans (hypospadias), a hooded foreskin and chordae are generally present. Epispadius is diagnosed when the urethral meatus is found on the dorsal surface of the penis. Appropriate imaging studies to rule out additional genitourinary abnormalities are warranted if either hypospadias or epispadius is present.

Attention to the development of scrotal rugae helps determine the gestational age of male neonates. Poorly developed shallow rugae are found in significantly preterm infants. Fully developed deep rugae are evident in the term infant. The physician's hands and fingers must be in the proper position for an appropriate examination of the scrotum for testes and other normal and abnormal masses. Ideally, the index finger and/or middle finger of the examining hand should be placed over the posterior aspect of the scrotum, and the thumb of that hand should be positioned over the anterior aspect of the scrotum.

If the scrotal sack is empty, each inguinal canal should be carefully examined for retained testicular tissue. The infant or young child should be in a supine position. With the index and middle finger of the examining hand positioned over the inguinal canal, the examiner should palpate the length of the canal and attempt to gently express any retained testicular tissue into the scrotum. At the same time, the middle finger, index finger, and thumb of the opposite hand should be properly positioned to palpate the ipsilateral proximal scrotum for any testicular tissue entering from the inguinal canal.

Even if previous examinations have revealed the presence of scrotal testes, it is important to re-examine the scrotum at each subsequent well child visit. Some boys have palpable testes in the scrotum on one visit; but months to years later, a subsequent examination reveals that the testes have spontaneously ascended into the inguinal canal or into an intra-abdominal position.[58] The persistence of an undescended testis beyond 1 year of age warrants surgical exploration.

Occasionally, palpation of the scrotum reveals unilateral or bilateral fullness in addition to the normally palpable testis(es). Transillumination of the area using a narrow-beam, bright light source will frequently reveal either a fluid-filled hydrocele or an indirect inguinal hernia. Hydroceles generally spontaneously regress during the first 12 to 18 months of life. Occassionally, they are accompanied by hernias, sometimes making it difficult to distinguish between the two. Hernias usually fill the inguinal area and the upper two-thirds of the scrotum, whereas hydroceles may be confined to the scrotal area alone.

Although genitourinary examination of the older infant and toddler requires the same meticulous evaluation as in the neonate, the findings may be somewhat different. If the examiner has difficulty palpating scrotal testes, the patient should be placed in a sitting knee–chest position to help force the testes into a dependent position. Testicular palpation may be enhanced further by having the patient assume that same position in a warm tub of water.

The foreskin of an uncircumcised penis may be difficult to retract. Fusion of the inner epithelium of the prepuce and the epithelium of the glans account for the nonretractability. After the first few years of life, squamous cells eventually keratinize, and the prepuce separates from the glans, allowing for normal retraction.[59] In 90% of boys, the process is complete by age 5.[60] Occasionally, the glans becomes traumatized or infected, producing erythema and swelling (balanitis). Foreskin that has been forcibly retracted and not returned to its normal anatomical position may create a ligature around the penile shaft (paraphimosis) that requires immediate medicosurgical intervention.

Genitourinary examination of female neonates requires careful inspection of anatomical structures. Proper visualization should be done with the infant in a supine position, legs flexed and abducted at the hips. There is normally no visible distinction between the labia majora and labia minora in the young girl. Gentle separation of the labia will reveal the clitoris, vaginal introitus, and urethral meatus. If the clitoris is large and posterior labial fusion is noted, virilization secondary to congenital adrenal hyperplasia should be ruled out.

Inferior to the clitoris is the urethral meatus and inferior to it, the vaginal introitus. Patency of the vaginal introitus should be established. Many infants have vaginal tags, which are of no significance and eventually spontaneously regress. In the first few days after birth, a transient, blood-tinged, mucoid vaginal discharge may be seen secondary to maternal estrogen withdrawal. A unilateral soft tissue mass in the inguinal or labial areas may represent a direct inguinal hernia.

Female infants and toddlers are best examined in the supine position with the legs abducted at the hips. Gentle posteriolateral retraction of the skin surrounding the inferior vulvar rim provides optimal visualization. Anatomically and physiologically, there is generally little change in this area from the time of birth. Occasionally, a thin tissue membrane adherent to labial skin, but not impeding urethral flow, will obscure visualization of the underlying vulvar anatomy. This membrane may develop as a result of poor hygiene. Management of this condition consists of instructions to the caregivers regarding appropriate cleansing of the area and/or daily application of a thin layer of estrogen cream for 2 to 3 weeks.

The physician must understand individual sensitivity issues regarding the genitourinary examination of the older child. The admonition from parents, teachers, and guardians that a child should not allow anyone to see or touch their private areas without their permission causes some children to become apprehensive and uncooperative. Recognizing this, the physician who is about to begin an examination of the genitalia should explain to the patient why there is need for examination of the area and how the examination will be performed, including what instruments, if any, will be used. Appropriate gowning and/or covering should be provided, and careful attention should be given to making sure the procedure is painless.

As the male approaches adolescence, at an average age of 11 to 12 years, the first sign of pubertal onset is testicular enlargement (Tanner stage 2). Testicular length before puberty is normally 1.5 to 2 cm. As the patient advances into puberty, testicular length can be determined using a measuring tape or calipers; alternatively, testicular size and volume can be determined with the use of orchidometer beads. When testicular growth is questionable, ultrasound measurements should be made.[61] Although somewhat smaller than the right testicle, the left testicle tends to be positioned lower in the scrotum. Most varicoceles collapse when the patient assumes a supine position.

In addition to testicular growth at this stage, pubic hair becomes evident, at first long and straight and later curling. With advancement through puberty, penile enlargement begins in stage 2 and continues through stage 5. Accurate measurement of penile length is best achieved by using a ruler, retracting the pubic fat away from the proximal shaft, and stretching the penis to its full length. By Tanner stage 4, pubic hair becomes more abundant spreading to involve the symphysis pubis and eventually the thighs. Prolonged onset of male puberty is generally attributable to constitutional delay and warrants close follow-up.

Genital examination of the preadolescent female is best conducted either with the patient in the supine position with legs in a frog-like position, flexed and abducted at knees and hips, or with the patient prone in a knee–chest position. Vaginal mucosa in the preadolescent is thin, moist, and somewhat red. The examiner should look for any signs of trauma, irritation, or discharge. In early puberty, a normal watery, non-foul-smelling vaginal discharge may be present. The presence of blood, purulent discharge, or foul odor requires investigation. Evidence of trauma or blood should raise the possibility of sexual abuse. In the younger child with genital blood or foul odor, the examiner should consider the possibility of a vaginal foreign body.

Clitoral size should be determined by the clitoral index, a measurement expressed in square millimeters and calculated from the product of the length and width of the clitoris; charts indicating the normal clitoral index by age are available. When measurements indicate clitoral enlargement for age, causes for androgen stimulation should be sought, including congenital adrenal hyperplasia and abnormal karyotype.[62]

In preadolescent females, unusual soft tissue masses may be seen in the vulvar area. An edematous, violaceous, nontender, donut-shaped mass may be noted surrounding the urethral meatus, particularly in black females younger than age 10 years. This abnormality is the result of urethral prolapse with eversion of the mucosa through the external meatus. Bleeding from this area may be the presenting complaint. A lesion found predominantly in white preadolescent girls is a prolapsed ectopic ureterocele, which protrudes through the urethral meatus. Other vulvar lesions include paraurethral cyst, imperforate hymen (leading to hydrocolpos or hydrometrocolpos), and rarely a grapelike cluster (caused by sarcoma botryoides).[63, 64]

Generally, the first sign of puberty (Tanner stage 2) for girls is breast development, followed shortly thereafter by the growth of pubic hair (Fig. 1.16). Delayed onset of puberty beyond age 14 years requires a thorough investigation to rule out significant organic causes. In females, unlike males, this delay cannot be explained on constitutional grounds. Rapid growth in girls begins during Tanner stage 2 and slows considerably after the onset of menses (usually in Tanner stage 4); females usually grow only 1 to 2 inches thereafter.

Examination of the adolescent male should include visualization of the urethral meatus for any discharge and the penile and scrotal skin for unusual lesions. The clinician should also palpate the scrotum for testicular position, hernias, and abnormal masses (such as a varicocele). The normal testicular surface feels smooth, whereas an adjacent varicocele feels like a clump of worms

Adolescent varicoceles (dilatation of spermatic cord veins) can be detected more frequently if the patient

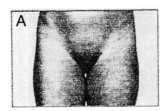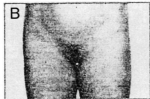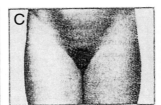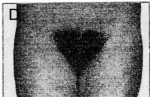

FIG. 1.16. Pubertal development of female pubic hair. In stage 1, there is no pubic hair. **A,** In stage 2, there is sparse growth of long, slightly pigmented downy hair, straight or only slightly curled, primarily along the labia. **B,** In stage 3, the hair is considerably darker, coarser, and more curled. The hair spreads sparsely over the junction of the pubes. **C,** In stage 4, the hair, now adult in type, covers a smaller area than in an adult and does not extend onto the thighs. **D,** In stage 5, the hair is adult in quantity and type; there is extension onto the thighs.

is examined while standing. Accurate adolescent Tanner staging is determined by assessing penile and testicular size and the extent of pubic hair development.

In addition to examining the genitalia, the physician should inspect the perianal area for fissures, hemorrhoids, or abnormal lesions. If there are any abnormal findings, the adolescent should be appropriately informed and counseled. Normal findings also should be communicated to the patient, particularly to those who have been somewhat apprehensive during the examination. The examiner should routinely teach Tanner stage 4 and 5 males the appropriate technique for performing testicular self-examination.[65, 66]

An adolescent female should be examined in the same position as described for the preadolescent. Tanner staging should be assessed, and attention should be given to looking for abnormal vaginal discharge and vaginal or vulvar lesions. Estrogen stimulation of the vaginal mucosa produces a thickened, dull pink mucoid surface. A thin, white, non-foul-smelling liquid discharge (leukorrhea) is normally present in the otherwise asymptomatic patient.

Evidence of trauma, ulcerative or inflammatory lesions, and abnormal vaginal discharge warrants appropriate speculum examination along with specific laboratory studies and cultures when indicated. Bimanual examination of the uterus in a supine preadolescent or adolescent female can be accomplished by palpating the anterior rectal wall with the gloved index finger of one hand while palpating and applying pressure to the lower midline abdominal area with the other hand. If not indicated for other reasons, vaginal examination is recommended for all sexually active females.[2]

ANUS AND RECTUM

Examination of the anus and rectum is relatively standard for all age groups. Inspection of the perianal area under normal circumstances should reveal an intact, symmetrically wrinkled, area of pigmented skin. Aside from the rare finding of an imperforate anus or an anteriorly placed anus, anatomical abnormalities in the pediatric age group are unusual. External hemorrhoids and prolapsed internal hemorrhoids are found primarily in older patients. Perianal fissures caused by straining during defecation and passage of hard stools or by dry irritated skin are seen in all age groups, particularly infants. Careful attention should be noted regarding bruises, tears, and lacerations in patients suspected of having been sexually abused.

Digital rectal exams are not routinely carried out as part of the regular physical examination of children. When digital examination becomes necessary, the examiner should remain sensitive to the potential embarrassment and discomfort for the patient. The patient and/or guardian should be given an easily understandable explanation of why the examination is being done and what discomfort might be involved. The examination is performed best with the patient lying on his or her left side and legs flexed at the hips and knees. Gloves and an appropriate lubricant should be used.

In the child with a lower abdominal mass and/or history of constipation or infrequent passage of stools, a rectal examination may help make the diagnosis. A smooth-walled rectal vault with soft stool in the rectal ampulla is the normal finding. A palpable abnormal mass or blood-tinged stool on a gloved finger requires more extensive investigation.

BACK

The back examination is relatively standard for all ages. Spinal alignment, structural asymmetry, soft tissue masses, skin lesions, and points of tenderness should be noted. The vertebral column should be straight with alignment along an imaginary vertical line from the midpoint of the occiput to the gluteal cleft. The level of the shoulders, scapulae, and pelvic rims should be symmetrical. Any midline soft tissue lesion overlying the spine should raise suspicion of the possibility of an underlying neurologic defect.

Infants born with midline skin, underlying soft tissue, or bony defects of the spine may have any of several lesions, including a meningocele, myelomeningocele, lipomeningocele, diastematomyelia, abscess, or tumor. With many of these lesions, the neurologic deficits may be severe enough to lead to genitourinary tract, gastrointestinal tract, and/or lower extremity impairment. The presence of scoliosis in the neonate has great significance because it produces cosmetic problems and potential underlying visceral and/or neurologic dysfunction. Nearly 33% of children with congenital scoliosis may have associated urinary tract anomalies.[67] Flattened buttocks and shortening of the cephalad extent of the gluteal cleft is the classic sign of sacral agenesis. To confirm the diagnosis, the physician must ask the caregiver about maternal insulin-dependent diabetes and must order a lateral radiologic image of the lower spine.

Darkly pigmented neonates and infants through at least the first year of life, may have one or a number of bluish macular skin lesions over the back. These lesions, termed Mongolian spots, are benign accumulations of elliptical melanocytes and regress spontaneously after 1 to 2 years. Midline dimples in the skin overlying the coccyx generally have a visible intact base and are of no significance. Dimples above that level require further examination, including imaging, to rule out underlying neural tube involvement.

All patients should undergo examination of the spine for scoliosis, particularly children in the preadolescent years. Proper examination necessitates complete unobstructed visualization of the back. The patient should be standing straight, but not rigid, with feet together and arms at the sides. Asymmetry of the back structures should be noted. For the second phase of the examination, the patient should be asked to bend over at the waist with legs straight, feet together, arms in a dependent position with the tips of the thumbs apposed, and head directed toward the floor in a relaxed position. The presence of a rib hump or abnormal curvature should be noted.

In addition to inspection for scoliosis, the spine should be examined for kyphosis and lordosis. A normal lumbar lordotic curvature, giving rise to a pot-bellied appearance, is found in the majority of toddlers. In almost all of them, spontaneous resolution of the curvature occurs as the patient advances into early childhood. Mild lumbar lordosis and/or thoracic kyphosis, found in many patients, requires no intervention. More prominent forms of either deformity warrant thorough evaluation.

NEUROLOGIC EXAMINATION

Aside from the sequence in which it is performed, the neurologic examination of a child varies little from that for an adult. Neurologic assessment of older children and adolescents begins with determining the mental status; next the cranial nerves, muscle tone and strength, deep tendon reflexes, cerebellar function, and sensory responses are tested.

Adequate examination of the infant and younger child usually requires the protective security provided by the caregiver's lap and the use of toys and bright objects to provide diversion or visual attention. The method of determining mental status depends on the age of the patient. For the infant and younger child, mental status is based on language and motor skills as well as on social interaction. For infants and young children, the sensory, motor, and cerebellar examinations might begin with the lower extremities; whereas for school-aged children, the examinations begin with the head, neck, and/or upper extremities. With the exception of the first cranial nerve (not often or easily tested in infants and small children), cranial nerve function can be tested in much the same way as in adults.

Assessing cerebellar and motor function and strength in the infant or toddler requires close observation. While the patient is engaged in normal activity, the examiner should look for appropriate alternate or symmetric movement of the trunk, head, and extremities. Upper extremity muscle tone and strength can be assessed in various ways. For the infant as young as 4 months, an examiner can make the determination based on the ability of the patient to pull to a sitting position while holding onto the examiner's fingers. Alternatively, assessment can be judged by noting an infant's upper trunk resistance against the examiner's hands held under the

patient's axillae as he or she is being lifted into the air. Lower extremity tone and strength can be assessed by noting an infant's ability to bear weight while standing supported.

Deep tendon reflexes can be elicited at any age, but in infants younger than 33 weeks gestation, reflex responses are diminished. In preterm and near-term infants, an examiner's finger placed over the tendon to be tested can be lightly struck with a percussion hammer to elicit a reflex. Complete absence of deep tendon reflexes may be attributable to anterior horn cell disease or peripheral neuropathy. Deep tendon reflexes with an exaggerated response may occur as a result of upper motor neuron pathology.

Many developmental reflexes present in the newborn disappear within the first year of life. The rooting, palmar grasp, and Moro reflexes are gone by 2 to 4 months of age; and the tonic neck response disappears by 3 to 6 months of age.[27, 68] Plantar flexion of the toes, elicited by firm finger pressure at the plantar metatarsal-phalangeal joint area, may be present for the first several months of life. Dorsiflexion of the great toe and fanning of the smaller toes (Babinski reflex), elicited by stroking the lateral aspect of the plantar surface of the foot in a posterior to anterior direction, is a normal finding up to about 18 months of age. For older patients, the normal Babinski reflex is characterized by plantar flexion of the great toe with no movement of the other toes.

In males, the cremasteric reflex can be demonstrated by stroking the inner thigh area in an anterior to posterior direction and noting ipsilateral scrotal retraction and testicular rise. The lack of response or an asymmetrical response is compatible with a corticospinal tract abnormality. Occasionally, the response will be absent in otherwise normal boys younger than 6 months and older than 12 years.[27]

Except in an unusual situation, a thorough neurologic examination of every patient is not necessary. Patients who present with or who are found to have neurologic or neuromuscular abnormalities on examination should undergo a complete neurologic assessment.

REFERENCES

1. Sackett DL, Rennie D. The science of the art of the clinical examination. JAMA 1992;267:2650–2652.
2. Committee on Psychosocial Aspects of Child and Family Health, 1995–1996. Guidelines for health supervision III. Elk Grove Village, IL: American Academy of Pediatrics, 1997.
3. Bates B. A guide to physical examination and history taking. 6th ed. Philadelphia: Lippincott, 1995.
4. Rowe PC. Pediatric procedures. In: Oski FA, DeAngelis CD, Feigin RD, Warshaw JB, eds. Principles and practice of pediatrics. Philadelphia: Lippincott, 1990:2010–2023.
5. Yaron M, Lowenstein SR, Koziol-McLain J. Measuring the inaccuracy of the infrared tympanic thermometer: correlation does not signify agreement. J Emerg Med 1995;13:617–621.
6. Gillette PC, Garson A Jr., Crawford F, et al. Dysrhythmias. In: Adams FH, Emmanouilides GC, eds. Moss' heart disease in in-

fants, children, and adolescents. 4th ed. Baltimore: Williams & Wilkins, 1983:925–939.

7. Ti H. Nei ching su wen [The yellow emperor's classic of internal medicine; Keith I, trans.] Berkeley: University of California Press, 1966.

8. Ziegler RF. Electrocardiographic studies in normal infants and children. Springfield, IL: Thomas, 1951.

9. Tudbury PB, Atkinson DW. Electrocardiograms of 100 normal infants and young children. J Pediatr 1950;36:466–481.

10. Sinaiko AR. Hypertension in children. N Engl J Med 1996; 335:1968–1973.

11. Task Force on Blood Pressure Control in Children, National Heart, Lung, and Blood Institute. Report of the Second task force on blood pressure control in children—1987. Pediatrics 1987;79:1–25.

12. National High Blood Pressure Education Program Working Group on Hypertension Control in Children and Adolescents. Update on the 1987 task force report on high blood pressure in children and adolescents: a working group report from the National High Blood Pressure Education Program. Pediatrics 1996;98:649–658.

13. Putnam TC. Lumps and bumps in children. Pediatr Rev 1992;13:371–378.

14. Leung AK. Carotenemia. Adv Pediatr 1987;34:223–248.

15. Gollan JL, Knapp AB. Bilirubin metabolism and congenital jaundice. Hosp Pract 1985;20:83–106.

16. Hurwitz S. Clinical pediatric dermatology. 2nd ed. Philadelphia: Saunders, 1993.

17. Vanderhooft SL, Francis JS, Pagon RA, et al. Prevalence of hypopigmented macules in a healthy population. J Pediatr 1996; 129:355–361.

18. Amichai B, Zeharia A, Mimouni M, et al. Picture of the month. Arch Pediatr Adolesc Med 1997;151:425–426.

19. Korf BR. Diagnostic outcome in children with multiple café au lait spots. Pediatrics 1992;90:924–927.

20. Burns AJ, Kaplan LC, Mulliken JB. Is there an association between hemangioma and syndromes with dysmorphic features? Pediatrics 1991;88:1257–1267.

21. Eskowitz RAB, Mulliken JB, Folkman J. Interferon α-2a therapy for life-threatening hemangiomas of infancy. N Engl J Med 1992;326:1456–1463.

22. Hurwitz S. Vascular skin lesions: accentuate the positive. Contemp Pediatr 1992;9:92–109.

23. Mulliken JB, Young AE. Vascular birthmarks: hemangiomas and malformations. Philadelphia. Saunders, 1988.

24. Garden JM, Polla LL, Tan OT. The treatment of port-wine stains by the pulsed dye laser. Arch Dermatol 1988;124:889–896.

25. Margileth AM. Cervical adenitis. Pediatr Rev 1985;7:13–24.

26. Chesney PJ. Cervical adenopathy. Pediatr Rev 1994;15:276–285.

27. Barness LA. Manual of pediatric physical diagnosis. 6th ed. St. Louis: Mosby Year Book, 1991.

28. Carpentieri U, Smith LR Jr, Daeschner CW III. Approach to a child with enlarged lymph nodes. Tx Med 1983;79:58–60.

29. Athreya BH, Silverman BK. Pediatric physical diagnosis. Norwalk, CT: Appleton-Century-Crofts, 1985.

30. Waardenburg PJ. A new syndrome combining developmental anomalies of the eyelids, eyebrows, and nose root with pigmentary defects of the iris and head hair and with congenital deafness. Am J Hum Genet 1951;3:195–253.

31. Hart DB. Menkes' syndrome: an updated review. J Am Acad Dermatol 1983;9:145–152.

32. Morgan DB. A suggestive sign of allergy. Arch Dermatol Syph 1948;57:1050.

33. Trobe JD. The physician's guide to eye care. San Francisco: American Academy of Ophthalmology, 1993.

34. Walton DS. Eye evaluation in the newborn. In: Oski FA, DeAngelis CD, Feigin RD, Warshaw JB, eds. Principles and practice of pediatrics. Philadelphia: Lippincott, 1990:468–470.

35. Nelson LB, Calhoun JH, Harley RD, eds. Pediatric ophthalmology. 3rd ed. Philadelphia: Saunders, 1991.

36. Eavey RD. Management strategies for congenital ear malformations. Pediatr Clin North Am 1989;36:1521–1534.

37. Bluestone CD, Klein JO. Otitis media in infants and children. Philadelphia: Saunders, 1988.

38. Henretig FM. Epistaxis. In: Fleischer G, Ludwig S, eds. Textbook of pediatric emergency medicine. Baltimore: Williams & Wilkins, 1993:175–177.

39. Gray SD, Parkin JL. Congenital malformations of the mouth and pharynx. In: Bluestone CD, Stool SE, Kenna MA, eds. Pediatric otolaryngology. 3rd ed. Philadelphia: Saunders, 1996: 985–998.

40. Renshaw TS. Pediatric orthopedics. Philadelphia: Saunders, 1986.

41. Murphy WJ Jr, Gellis SS. Torticollis with hiatus hernia in infancy: Sandifer syndrome. Am J Dis Child 1977;131:564–565.

42. Zitelli BJ. Evaluating the child with a neck mass. Contemp Pediatr 1990;7:90–112.

43. Lord MJ, Laurenzano KR, Hartmann RW Jr. Poland's syndrome. Clin Pediatr 1990;29:606–609.

44. Haller JA, Colombani PM, Humphries CT, et al. Chest wall constriction after too extensive and too early operations for pectus excavatum. Ann Thorac Surg 1996;61:1618–1625.

45. Marshall WA, Tanner JM. Variations in pattern of pubertal changes in girls. Arch Dis Child 1969;44:291–303.

46. Marshall WA, Tanner JM. Variations in pattern of pubertal changes in boys. Arch Dis Child. 1970;45:13–23.

47. Kulin HE, Muller J. The biologic aspects of puberty. Pediatr Rev 1996;17:75–86.

48. Eraunstein GD. Diagnosis and treatment of gynecomastia. Hosp Pract 1993;28:37–46.

49. Herman-Giddens ME, Slora EJ, Wasserman RC, et al. Secondary sexual characteristics and menses in young girls seen in office practice: a study from the pediatric research in office settings network. Pediatrics 1997;99:505–512.

50. Copeland KC. Variations in normal sexual development. Pediatr Rev 1986;8:47–55.

51. Guilleminault C. State of sleep and apnea in infants (near miss for SIDS and controls). Breathing in the fetus and newborn. Paper presented at the 12th Mead Johnson Symposium on Perinatal and Developmental Medicine, Marco Island, FL, Dec 4–8, 1977.

52. Parrino TA. Hands on the heart: palpation of the cardiovascular system. Hosp Pract 1989;4A:103–115.

53. Lehrer S. Understanding pediatric heart sounds. Philadelphia: Saunders, 1992.

54. Perloff JK. The clinical recognition of congenital heart disease. 3rd ed. Philadelphia: Saunders, 1987.

55. AH Robins Co. Physical examination of the abdomen [GI series]. Richmond, VA: Robins, 1974

56. Mooney JF III, Emans JB. Developmental dislocation of the hip: a clinical overview. Pediatr Rev 1995;16:299–303.

57. Crawford AH. Slipped capital femoral epiphysis. J Bone Joint Surg Am 1988;70:1422–1427.

58. Garcia J, Navarro E, Guirado F, et al. Spontaneous ascent of the testis. Brit J Urol 1997;79:113–115.

59. Snyder HM III. To circumcise or not. Hosp Pract 1991;26: 201–207.

60. Cooper GG. Therapeutic retraction of the foreskin in childhood. Brit Med J 1983;286:186–187.

61. Walc L, Bass J, Rubin S, Walton M. Testicular fate after incarcerated hernia repair and/or orchiopexy performed in patients under 6 months of age. J Pediatr Surg 1995;30:1195–1197.

62. Sane K, Peskovitz OH. The clitoral index: a determination of clitoral size in normal girls with abnormal sexual development. Pediatrics 1992;120:264–266.

63. Lowe FC, Hill GS, Jeffs RD, Brendler CB. Urethral prolapse in children: insights into etiology and management. J Urol 1986;135:100–103.

64. Nussbaum AR, Lebowitz RL. Interlabial masses in little girls: review and imaging recommendations. Am J Roentgenol 1983; 141:65–71.

65. Equal time for men: teaching testicular self-examination [Editorial]. J Adolesc Health Care 1986;7:273–274.

66. Goldenring JM. A lifesaving exam for young men. Contemp Pediatr 1992;9:63–85.

67. Keim HA, Hensinger RN. Spinal deformities. Clin Symp 1989; 41:10–13.

68. Fishman MA. Pediatric neurology. Orlando, FL: Grune & Stratton, 1986.

CHAPTER 2

Surgical Physiology of the Neonate

Scott A. Engum and Frederick J. Rescorla

Infants with surgically correctable disorders often have other conditions that threaten survival, requiring surgeons to understand general neonatal physiology. During the neonatal period, the infant possesses distinctive and rapidly changing physiologic characteristics secondary to adaptation to the extrauterine environment, organ maturation, and rapid growth and development. Low birth weight is a major determinant of neonatal mortality and has been recognized since 1930, when Yllpo argued that newborn infants weighing ≤2500 g had a substantially increased risk of death.[1]

Advances in the care of the premature newborn have resulted in improved survival (Table 2.1); however, birth weight, especially for very low birth weight infants, still accounts for a substantial amount of the variation in neonatal mortality within and between countries.[2, 3] Neonatal survival rates for very low birth weight (<1500 g) infants increased during the 1980s, especially among the extremely low birth weight (<1000 g) subgroup.[4-8] The reported 20 to 30% reduction in neonatal mortality[9-11] has been attributed to a number of factors, including (a) a greater number of high-risk pregnant women enrolled in prenatal care programs,[12] (b) the expanded availability of neonatal intensive care units,[13] (c) advances in ventilator technology,[14] (d) an increased use of artificial surfactant,[15] and (e) the option of therapeutic abortion.[16]

The effects of the severity of illness appear to be completely independent of birth weight with two exceptions. First, the effects of an extremely low birth weight (<1000 g) are so powerful that the mildness of the illness is not protective. Second, the effects of marginal increases in an already extremely severe illness—score for neonatal acute physiology (SNAP) >20 to 25—do not seem to increase mortality risk.[3] Care of critically ill newborns requires trained personnel and specialized equipment. The care of such babies is best accomplished in designated regional medical centers that are capable of providing pediatric surgical and neonatal intensive care.

TRANSPORTING THE NEWBORN SURGICAL PATIENT

The transfer of sick and premature neonates, whether within the hospital or to a tertiary center, requires specialized personnel, equipment, and management. Regionalization of perinatal care has been recognized as a potential means of reducing perinatal mortality and morbidity.[17-20] It involves designating a regional perinatal center, assessing care levels at all perinatal facilities in the region, and establishing a network of perinatal services. Although antenatal referral is the goal, in certain situations, such as advanced labor, intrapartum complications, or undiagnosed prenatal conditions, postnatal transport is necessary. In these cases, anticipation of potential neonatal problems is critical. Optimal neonatal stabilization requires skills in oxygen administration and monitoring, airway management (laryngoscopy, tracheal intubation, suctioning, assisted ventilation, chest compressions), emergency administration of drugs and fluids, and maintenance of thermal stability. In addition, the ability to recognize and decompress a tension pneumothorax by aspiration may be required.

Efficient pretransport and intratransport stabilization are associated with decreased transport-related mortality and improved outcome of these neonates.[21] Neonatal stabilization may take as long as 1.5 h because of the complexity of these patients' problems.[22] The once-popular concept of "grab and run" or "swoop and scoop" was thought be the optimal way to move patients to the facility in which definitive care would take place; however, this approach is justified only in rare situations. In the current era of air transport (by which speed can save lives), physicians must remember not only the spectacular benefits of this technology but also the disadvantages and challenges it brings to the caregiver. During air transport, the predominant factor affecting human physiology is altitude and its associated hypoxemic hypoxia, stagnant hypoxia, and alterations in gas expansion. Other factors may also produce negative physiologic

TABLE 2.1. *Mortality risk by birth weight group*

Mortality rate, %	Birth weight, g
31	<750
20	750–999
8	1000–1499
1	1500–2499
2	>2499

Data from Stevens SM, Richardson DK, Gray JE, et al. Estimating neonatal mortality risk: an analysis of clinicians' judgments. Pediatrics 1994;93:945–950.

responses or stresses, including noise, vibration, motion, temperature fluctuations, and humidity changes. When transporting the neonatal surgical patient in all environments (in hospital or via ground ambulance or air transport), the physician must observe the following precautions: maintain normal body temperature with the use of an incubator, maintain meticulous airway management by using a bulb syringe or suction device, maintain gastric decompression (to minimize the risk of aspiration) by either fasting or using an oral gastric tube, and protect the patient by transporting with the proper identification and copies of the medical history.

DETERMINING GESTATIONAL AGE AND NEWBORN CLASSIFICATION

Newborn infants can be classified into four groups, based on the level of maturation and physical development: *(a)* term infant, gestational age >38 weeks and body weight >2500 g; *(b)* preterm infant, gestational age <38 weeks and body weight appropriate for age; *(c)* small for gestational age (SGA), gestational age >38 weeks and body weight <2500 g; and *(d)* large for gestational age (LGA), gestational age >38 weeks and body weight >4000g (or >90th percentile for age).

Infants with surgically treatable lesions frequently weigh <2500 g. It is important to distinguish premature infants from those born with intrauterine growth retardation (IUGR). Preterm infants are born before 38 weeks of gestation, regardless of the birth weight. Some of the characteristics of a preterm infant include thin and transparent skin, absence of plantar creases, soft and malleable fingers, poor ear cartilage development, males with undescended testicles and underdeveloped scrotum, and females with enlarged labia minora and small labia majora. Preterm infants are at risk for developing hyaline membrane disease, intraventricular hemorrhage, hypothermia, and patent ductus arteriosus and may have a poor suck reflex and inadequate gastrointestinal absorption. In preterm infants, especially infants <34 weeks of gestation, both classification as SGA and the presence of maternal risk factors predict a poor

neonatal outcome. This is consistent with the theory that suggests a strong relationship between preterm delivery and IUGR and considers SGA preterm infants to be at increased risk for morbidity and mortality.[23, 24]

SGA newborns are thought to suffer from IUGR as a result of placental, maternal, or fetal factors. The understanding, diagnosis, and evaluation of suspected IUGR are hampered by the heterogeneous nature of the condition and its imprecise definition. The most commonly used definition of IUGR equates it with the small for gestational age infant, i.e., an infant whose birth weight is less than a specific level based on his or her gestational age (usually the 10th or 5th percentile).[25, 26] But IUGR actually implies a pathologic process that affects normal fetal growth, resulting in an infant whose size is less than his or her inherent potential, not simply an infant who is SGA; thus the terms are not truly synonymous.[27] SGA infants may weigh the same as some preterm newborns; however, the two groups have different physiologic characteristics.

NEONATAL INTENSIVE CARE MONITORING

Continuous monitoring of the neonate in the neonatal intensive care unit reveals trends that can assist the surgeon and neonatologist in assessing responses to therapy and provides early warning of potential catastrophes, so they may be avoided with intervention. Many episodes of sudden deterioration in the neonate are preceded by more gradual changes in the clinical condition. Noninvasive monitoring of many parameters, including oxygen saturation levels, has become standard practice in the neonatal patient population.

Transcutaneous Monitors

The use of transcutaneous (skin) oxygen and carbon dioxide monitoring in critically ill neonates provides information regarding oxygenation and ventilation that may not otherwise be readily available. Control of oxygenation levels is important for preventing retrolental fibroplasia and hypoxia; and carbon dioxide levels are valuable for managing multiple forms of mechanical ventilation, especially high-frequency ventilation. Although transcutaneous oxygen and carbon dioxide levels do not equal arterial levels under normal conditions, a transcutaneous monitor is a useful adjunct to blood gases because it provides continuous information.[28, 29] Transcutaneously measured oxygen is less closely associated with arterial levels than is similarly measured carbon dioxide; however, the technique does provide a potentially useful indication of arterial oxygenation in neonates who require intensive care, particularly if relative changes within an individual patient are considered.

Pulse Oximetry

Pulse oximeter monitors have become common place in the newborn intensive care unit. Pulse oximetry was developed in 1974,[30] although it was not initially introduced into clinical practice. It is based on the physical principle that oxygenated (infrared band 850 to 1000 nm) and deoxygenated (infrared band 600 to 750 nm) hemoglobin have different absorption spectra. This oxygen-monitoring technique has some shortfalls; however, in combination with transcutaneous oxygen monitoring, it can alert clinicians to dangerously high Pa_{O_2} levels and potential hyperoxemia. In patients in whom neither movement artifact nor hyperoxemia is a problem, the use of a pulse oximeter alone will usually be sufficient. Even the most sophisticated noninvasive oxygen-monitoring system cannot replace the gold standard of directly measuring arterial blood gases; however, pulse oximetry allows the physician to increase the intervals between arterial blood gas determinations.

Arterial Blood Gas

Although arterial blood gases are extremely useful, their measure involves an invasive procedure, requiring an arterial puncture or intra-arterial catheter. Capillary blood samples are frequently used in the neonatal intensive care unit as an alternative to arterial blood gases. Capillary blood is "arterialized" by topical vasodilators or heat, which increases blood flow to the sample site, allowing the clinician to obtain a freely flowing sample and minimizing exposure to the atmosphere (which falsely raises Pa_{O_2}).[31] Capillary blood pH and carbon dioxide tension are highly correlated with arterial samples; Pa_{O_2} is less reliable. Venous blood monitoring allows the evaluation of carbon dioxide levels in patients who have a central venous catheter. Peripheral venous samples are strongly affected by the local circulatory or metabolic environment and have limited usefulness. Although there can be a significant discrepancy between arterial and venous values, the correlation is generally best when the venous measurements are within the normal physiologic range (Table 2.2). Basing management decisions on abnormal venous measurements is not advised.

TABLE 2.2. *Average blood gas values by site*

Site	pH	Pa_{O_2}	Pa_{CO_2}
Artery	7.35–7.45	55–65	35–45
Vein	7.25–7.30	30–45	45–55
Capillary	7.30–7.35	40–60	40–45

Central Venous Access and Monitoring

The use of central venous catheters has increased along with the complexity of neonatal intensive care units. There have been a few reports of the successful use of the intraosseous route in the resuscitation of neonates in whom central venous access was not possible.[32] Besides the inability to maintain peripheral intravenous access, indications for central venous catheter placement include hemodynamic monitoring and central hyperalimentation as well as the need to infuse medications that cannot be given peripherally. Commonly used sites are the internal and external jugular, subclavian, and femoral veins; the saphenous and antecubital veins are also used, with advancement of the catheter into a central location. Central venous pressure monitoring, which involves serial measurements made with an electronic transducer, is not commonplace for the neonate. Central venous pressure may be altered by positive pressure ventilation, pericardial tamponade, and increased intrathoracic or abdominal pressure.

Neonatal Blood Values

Critical parameters of the pulmonary and cardiovascular systems in humans is the oxygen saturation of hemoglobin contained in the RBCs and the subsequent delivery of oxygen to the tissues to meet the cells' energy demands for function and growth. An inadequate volume of RBCs constitutes the ultimate physiologic cause of anemia in the neonate. Although most neonates receive many blood transfusions during the course of their hospitalization, data regarding transfusion practices for this group are scarce. It has been estimated that 38,000 premature neonates receive more than 300,000 RBC transfusions annually.[33] Surveys have found considerable variation in neonatal transfusion practices.[34]

Hepatitis has always been a concern of homologous blood transfusions, but it was the outbreak of AIDS that stimulated a national evaluation of traditional transfusion practices. The pros and cons of directed donors have been debated. Although the practice is widely available for neonatal transfusions, it accounts for <10% of such transfusions.[35]

THERMOREGULATION

Body temperature is a precisely controlled physiologic variable[36] (Fig. 2.1). Appropriate temperature is critical to bodily functions. Neonates, unfortunately, are prone to temperature instability. At birth, the transition from the uterus to extrauterine life creates a significant challenge to the infant's thermoregulatory system. This problem is accentuated by the physiologic function of infants and their small body size. The cutaneous vasculature is morphologically immature at birth; the disorderly

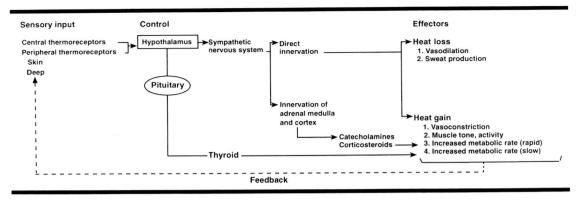

FIG. 2.1. The process of thermoregulation.

capillary network gradually develops into an organized subpapillary plexus and papillary loops during the first weeks of life.[37] The thermoregulation of skin blood flow is considered to be mature and functional in the newborn.[38] Thermoregulatory responses balance heat production and heat loss. Body heat produced through metabolism is precisely balanced against heat loss through conduction, radiation, evaporation. and convection. Unless immediate attention is devoted to heat loss, an infant's body temperature can drop significantly in the first few minutes of life.[39] Neonates have a higher metabolic rate than do children and adults; however, the body heat generated by body mass is lost over the infants' relatively large surface area. This creates a significant imbalance between a small heat-producing body mass and a large surface area for heat loss; thus neonates have a high caloric requirement for supporting temperature regulation and balance. Important factors in thermoregulation include insulation, heat loss and gain, and the thermal response.

Insulation

Insulation reduces heat transfer, and its effectiveness is inversely related to conductivity and directly related to thickness. Insulation may be classified as internal or external. Internal insulation includes the skin, musculoskeletal structures, and subcutaneous body tissues (primarily fat). Fat is a highly effective insulating material owing to its poor heat conductance and relative thickness. The fat layer, which appears at 26 to 29 weeks of gestational age, may be fairly thin in the preterm infant.[40] In addition, internal insulation is more efficient after the ability to decrease cutaneous blood flow through vasomotor control develops.

External insulation primarily modifies the heat transfer at the body's surface. The two main forms of external insulation are clothing and the still-air boundary. Both factors are controlled by the caregiver.

Heat Loss and Gain

Heat is lost or gained by convection, conduction, radiation, and evaporation. When attempting to modify the thermal environment, the clinician must differentiate between application of heat and reduction of heat loss, because the infant is thermally insensitive to the particular route of heat gain or loss.

Convection is the transfer of heat between a solid surface (the infant) and either the air or a liquid environment. Convection loss is affected by the infant's large surface area, air flow velocities and turbulence, temperature gradient, and diameter of the infant's limbs. Incubators operate on convection principles. Rather than warm the infant, the incubator reduces convective heat loss by decreasing the gradient between the air and skin temperatures. Radiation and evaporation heat losses still occur, however; opening the side ports can increase turbulence and thus increase convection heat losses. Other sources of heat loss are cool rooms, corridors, and outside air; drafts from air vents, windows, and doors; and fans and air-conditioners, all of which can be minimized with the routine use of an incubator.

Conduction is the transfer of heat between two solid surfaces that are in contact. Conduction is affected by the solid surface conductivity coefficient, the size of the surface area in contact, and the temperature gradient between the surfaces. Common sources of conduction heat loss include cool mattresses, blankets, scales, tables, x-ray plates, and clothing. Overheating can occur from heating pads, hot water bottles, and chemical bags. To prevent conductive losses, warm the solid surface before allowing contact with the infant and place some form of insulation between the object and the infant.

Radiation is the transfer of heat by electromagnetic infrared waves between solid surfaces that are not in contact. The factors that affect radiant heat flux include the emissivity of the radiating surfaces, the temperature gradient between the solid surfaces, the surface area of the solids, and the distance between the solid surfaces.

Radiant heating devices, such as heat lamps and photo-therapy units, can cause overheating, because the air temperature in the incubator does not include radiant temperature and thus does not accurately represent the degree of infant heating. In addition, the incubator must not be placed near cold or hot external windows or walls or in direct sunlight.

Evaporation produces heat loss through the energy used in the conversion of water to a gaseous state. Evaporative losses may be insensible or sensible. Evaporation is affected by vapor pressure, air velocity, and the infant's surface area. Evaporative loss increases when the body surface is wet (in the delivery room or from bathing) and when cool lotions, solutions, wet packs, or soaks are applied.

Thermal Responses

Regulation of body temperature depends on vasomotor activity, change in motor tone and activity, and modification of heat production. If the first-line defenses do not conserve heat, then the baby compensates by increasing both cellular metabolism and skeletal muscle tone and activity (shivering) to increase heat production. Shivering is poorly developed in infants, and nonshivering thermogenesis (brown fat metabolism) is the primary heat production mechanism in the neonate. Brown adipose tissue cells can be identified at 26 to 28 weeks of gestation and continue to increase until 3 to 5 weeks postdelivery. Brown fat metabolism and heat production are thus reduced in the preterm infant and may be minimal in the extremely low birth weight neonate.

Infants not only are prone to heat loss but can also overheat owing to their large surface area, limited insulation, and limited sweating ability. These factors, coupled with an increased basal metabolic rate, raise the body temperature, which is difficult for the neonate to reduce. Sweating is the only means of decreasing body heat when the environmental temperature is greater than the core body temperature.

Because of immature motor and cognitive abilities, the neonate has limited and subtle thermoregulatory behaviors. The infant's activity level may be altered by the thermal environment; warm infants sleep or seem lethargic, whereas cool infants are active. Frequently, infants will be flexed when cool and extended when warm.[41, 42] Irritability may suggest an alteration in thermal comfort, alerting the caregiver to change the thermal environment.

Research defining normal infant body temperature is typically conducted under neutral thermal conditions. Current recommendations from the American Academy of Pediatrics and the American College of Obstetrics and Gynecology are to maintain rectal and axillary temperatures between 36.5 and 37.5°C (97.7 to 99.5°F) and abdominal skin temperatures between 36 and 36.5°C (96.8

to 97.9°F) for neonates.[43] Unfortunately, there is little information available about normal temperatures for extremely low birth weight infants. It has been suggested that very small infants be placed in incubators with the air temperature maintained above the body core temperature.[44] Current thought suggests that thermoneutrality is met when central and skin temperatures are within normal limits for healthy very low birthweight infants in week 1 of life (36.7 to 37.3°C; 98.1 to 99.1°F) and change less than 0.2 to 0.3°C (0.36 to 0.54°F) per hour.[45]

FLUID MANAGEMENT

Oral fluid intake is initiated after delivery in all newborn infants. For healthy infants with a mature sucking reflex (older than 32 to 34 weeks of gestational age), bottle or breast feeding is offered within 1 to 2 h postdelivery. The volume of oral nutrition is typically on demand and spontaneously increases over the first couple days of life to 120 to 200 mL/kg/day.

In contrast, infants and neonates who are admitted after delivery to the intensive care unit for observation or intense therapy typically require intravenous fluid management for stabilization. The use of peripheral intravenous cannulas for the provision of neonatal intensive care is a commonly accepted practice and is essential for the administration of fluids, medications, and nutrition; however, it can lead to potentially serious complications. The current incidence of complications in this setting is unknown, although studies have shown that 46% of infants have had at least one complication related to therapy when the intravenous cannula was in place for more than 24 h.

An average of 3.7 sloughs per infant (range: 1 to 26) has been reported.[46] Infiltration may lead to sloughing of the skin, which may be severe enough to mandate grafting and to cause loss of function. Treatments to lessen the severity of intravenous catheter–related sloughs have been anecdotally reported and include gentle massage of the infiltrated area,[47] multiple punctures over the infiltrated area,[48] and medications such as hyaluronidase.[49] Infiltration with vasoactive agents (e.g., epinephrine, norepinephrine, and dopamine) can cause severe local vasoconstriction, which can be treated with the local infiltration of phentolamine (0.1 to 0.2 mg/kg body weight). Intravenous infiltration with aminophylline, calcium solutions (>1%), dextrose solutions (>10%), nafcillin, parenteral nutrition solutions, or potassium solutions (>100mEq/L) may lead to large defects; lesions larger than 2 cm should be treated with hyaluronidase (15 units) injected locally into several areas of the infiltrate. The median half-life of intravenous catheters in infants has been shown in comparative surveys to be shorter (36 h) than that in adults (72 h).[50, 51] Other studies have determined that the mean patency for intravenous catheters in neonates is approximately

26.1 h when hyperalimentation is given through the catheter and is 58.7 h when heparin is added to the total parenteral nutrition (TPN) fluids.[52] Co-infusion of a lipid solution may prolong the survival of infusion catheters possibly by providing a protective lining for the endothelium and by decreasing the sclerogenic effect of the TPN by neutralizing the solution.[53]

To calculate the daily maintenance fluid requirement for a newborn infant, the physician must take into account insensible water loss, renal solute excretion, and any current deficits or excesses. Multiple physiologic factors must be evaluated, including (a) losses by evaporation, third space, or external; (b) metabolic demands; and (c) pre-existing fluid deficits or excesses. In low birth weight, low gestational age infants, insensible water loss (which is difficult to measure) is increased because of the developmental characteristics of the skin, the need for a high ambient air temperature to maintain thermal balance, the presence of a relatively large surface area, and the frequent use of radiant warmers and phototherapy.[54–56] Thus maintenance fluids for small, preterm infants have generally been increased on an empirical basis to three to four times (volumes per kilogram body weight) that given to larger, term infants to compensate for the assumed increase in insensible water loss.

After administering the initial intravenous fluid volume for 4 to 8 h, the newborn should be reassessed by observing urine output and concentration. Fluid management is a dynamic process and requires frequent reassessment. It may also be necessary to evaluate changes in serial serum sodium concentrations, blood urea nitrogen, creatinine concentration, and osmolarity.

Initial fluid management in the neonate involves either 5% or 10% dextrose solution at a rate of 80 to 100 mL/kg/day (4 to 8 mg/kg/min of glucose) to keep the blood sugar levels within a normal range. Infants weighing <1000 g at birth are usually started on 5% dextrose solution until they have proven they can tolerate the glucose concentration without hyperglycemia. Depending on the disease process, some neonates may require large volumes (up to 300 mL/kg/day) of fluid intake to avoid dehydration (Table 2.3). Weighing as frequently as every 8 to 12 h may be necessary to follow neonates and/or to identify neonates who are at increased risk of dehydration. Neonates with respiratory distress syndrome may have improved pulmonary function with increased urine output;[57] however, there has been much debate about the merits of high or low initial fluid intake in the newborn who has respiratory distress syndrome. It is believed that initial fluid intakes of 60 to 80 mL/kg/day for the first few days of life may be associated with fewer occurrences of patent ductus arteriosus (PDA) with cardiac failure and pulmonary edema, intraventricular hemorrhage, and bronchopulmonary dysplasia.[57, 58] It may be extremely difficult to maintain these fluid limits in the neonate in the face of hypoglycemia, hypoxia, acidosis, hypotension, or severe asphyxia, because treatment of these disorders may require the administration of extra fluids.

When assessing fluid needs after surgery, it is important to account for the volume and electrolyte concentration of all intravenous infusions administered during the operation. Frequently, large volumes of Ringer's lactate, normal saline, blood, and plasma are given; and the total sodium content given during this time can be as high as four times that of normal intake. It is important to obtain blood chemistry measurements after surgery to identify any electrolyte abnormality and to determine postoperative fluids. Serial measurements of urine flow and concentration are the most helpful guides to fluid management of the neonate. Typically, if the volume of fluid administered is low, urine output falls and the urine becomes more concentrated; if excess fluid is given, urine output increases and the urine becomes more dilute. There is no off-the-shelf intravenous solution that is ideal for all neonates, and low birth weight and sick neonates must have regular electrolyte profiles to determine the appropriate fluid content and administration rate.

RENAL FUNCTION IN THE NEONATE

Neonatal renal function is different from that of adults and is critical for maintaining body homeostasis. Although structurally complete by 36 weeks of gestational age, the neonatal kidney is still functionally immature. The functions of the neonatal kidney are similar to those of the adult organ and include regulation of water and electrolyte balance, excretion of metabolic waste products and foreign substances, regulation of vitamin D and erythrocyte production, and control of arterial blood pressure.

At 34 to 36 weeks of gestation, neonates have approximately 1 million nephrons (the number found in adults); further maturation and hypertrophy continue into infancy. In infants born at less than 34 weeks of gestational age, nephrons will continue to form at a rate similar to that found for in utero development.[59] Although the neonate may have a full complement of nephrons, the nephrons are smaller and less functional than those of older infants. Maturation of renal function after birth

TABLE 2.3. *Usual maintenance water requirements*

Group	Water, mL/kg/24 h
Baseline	80–100
Moderate surgical conditions (ostomy, atresia)	100
Severe surgical conditions (gastroschisis, volvulus)	150–200
Necrotizing enterocolitis with perforation	125–200

TABLE 2.4. *Normal serum creatinine concentrations*

Group	Serum creatinine, mg/dL	
	Age 1–2 weeks	Age 3–6 months
Preterm neonate	1.0–2.0	0.4–0.8
Full term neonate	0.6–1.0	0.2–0.6

is based on postbirth age rather than gestational age for infants who have the adult number of nephrons. Maturation in premature infants is related to both gestational age and postbirth age. In all neonates, however, glomerular filtration and tubular function are different from those in children and adults (Table 2.4). The glomeruli of newborns are only two-fifths the size of adults' glomeruli, and the tubules are one-tenth as long.[60] The glomerular surface area is approximately 10% of the adult value.[61] Therefore, neonates are not able to concentrate urine and absorb sodium in the same way adults do.

The glomerular filtration rate (GFR) increases rapidly at birth and doubles during the first few weeks of life. This is owing to a redistribution of placental blood, an increase in renal blood flow, and an increase in arterial blood pressure, and a resultant decrease in renal vascular resistance[59, 62] as well as increases in glomerular permeability and filtration surface area.[63] Even with the increase after birth, a neonate's GFR is only 20 to 35% of adult values (20 to 40 mL/min in term infants; 100 to 120 mL/min in adults).[59, 64] The glomerular filtration rate in term infants reaches adult levels (factored for body surface area) by 2 years of age;[63] the GFR in very low birth weight infants catch up term infants after 9 months of age.[65] This finding is primarily explained by the proportionately low renal blood flow and high renal vascular resistance (high renin levels in the first 3 to 6 weeks of life result in high resistance in the afferent arterioles) in the neonate compared to adults.[66, 67] The lower GFR makes it more difficult for neonates to excrete a water load and makes them more susceptible to overhydration and water intoxication. In addition, the lower GFR influences drug clearance by increasing the drug's half-life.[68, 69] The ability to clear drugs is also related to postbirth age, because renal function matures rapidly after birth.[69]

The tubular portions of the neonate kidney are smaller than those of the adult and are functionally immature; thus the neonate is unable to transport sodium, urea, chloride, and glucose owing to reduced renal thresholds. Because the integrity of the tubular lumen is also altered, reabsorbed substances can leak back into the tubule, increasing the likelihood that the infant will lose solute in the urine.

The renal handling of sodium in all infants is different from that in adults but is most pronounced in premature infants. This difference is related to the fact that a greater proportion of the renal blood flow is medullary (more sodium conservation than excretion) in neonates and to the degree of maturation of the proximal and distal tubules.[70] In newborns, the medullary nephrons are larger and more functionally mature than the cortical nephrons.[71, 72] In term neonates, the longest proximal tubule is 11 times larger than the smallest tubule, yielding a wide range of available surface area for reabsorption. Newborns also have shortened loops of Henle.[73] Generally, most infants are in a positive sodium balance. At term, the neonatal nephrons are biased toward the reabsorption of filtered sodium for growth. This bias is the result of high aldosterone levels, attributable to a blunted renin feedback response.[74] Very low birth weight infants, however, have the opposite bias. Nearly 100% of infants younger than 30 weeks of gestational age and 40% of infants at 30 weeks of gestation are in negative sodium balance,[75] which puts them at significant risk of sodium imbalance because of the high urinary sodium losses. These losses are the result of a short proximal tubule (the major site of sodium reabsorption) and distal tubules that are relatively less responsive to aldosterone.[74] Thus, until their renal function matures, very low birth weight infants may need higher sodium replacements during the first few weeks of life than do term infants.[75, 76]

Growing infants tend to be in a positive potassium balance, because their kidneys conserve potassium, allowing it to be incorporated into growing tissues. Thus neonatal serum levels are higher than those of adults.[59] Potassium losses may increase in infants experiencing stress, suffering from malnutrition (negative nitrogen balance), or receiving diuretics or parenteral fluid therapy.[70, 77]

Infants are at increased risk for glycosuria because of their lowered transport maximum for glucose (adult average = 350 mg/min/1.73 m^2; neonates = 60 to 80 mg/min/1.73 m^2).[78] Even with this low transport maximum for glucose, few neonates are glycosuric, except for very low birth weight infants, who may have transient glycosuria.[59] The most common cause of glucosuria in hospitalized infants is intravenous infusion of dextrose at rates that exceed the tubular reabsorptive threshold for glucose. The fractional reabsorption of glucose is normally >99%.[79] Very low birth weight infants, however, are unable to excrete a glucose load because of the low GFR and thus are at risk for hyperglycemia.[76]

Compared to adults, neonates have a reduced threshold for proximal tubular bicarbonate reabsorption;[80] the threshold gradually increases with the increase in the GFR. It is important to be aware of the physiologically reduced level of plasma total bicarbonate in neonates to avoid misdiagnosing renal tubular acidosis.[81] In addition, the neonate has a reduced ability to respond to an acid load.[82]

At birth, the neonate has a natural tendency toward hypocalcemia owing to decreased calcium stores, renal immaturity, and relative hypoparathyroidism secondary to suppression by high fetal calcium levels. Newborn calcium levels usually reach their nadir 24 to 48 h after delivery. Preterm infants, newborn surgical patients, and infants from complicated pregnancies (mother is diabetic or received bicarbonate infusions) are at the greatest risk for hypocalcemia. Because of difficulties in estimating ionic calcium levels from total serum levels, most nurseries now measure ionized calcium levels. In addition, parathyroid hormone release is suppressed at birth, resulting in a decrease in serum calcium and a secondary increase in parathyroid hormone production. The same infants at risk for hypocalcemia are also at risk for hypomagnesemia. The most common cause of hypercalciuria in neonates is iatrogenic. Calciuric drugs, such as furosemide and glucocorticoids, increase the risk of nephrocalcinosis or nephrolithiasis.[83] These factors can lead to renal dysfunction in childhood.[84] In contrast, initial tubular reabsorption of phosphate is high in preterm (75%) and term (95%) infants until regular feeding is begun.[85, 86] Because of their normally high phosphate concentration, any neonate with a serum phosphate level <4 mg/dL should be evaluated for phosphate wasting. Following the neonatal period, the tubular reabsorption of phosphate should remain consistently above 85%; lower values should alert the physician to other health disorders.

Oliguria is the most helpful sign of renal impairment in the neonate, and a delay in the first void in a newborn may signal a renal disorder. Preterm neonates generally void earlier than term and post-term neonates.[87] Most infants (66%) void in the first 12 h of life; 23% void in the delivery room. By 24 h of life, 93% of infants have voided; and by 48 h, 98% have voided.[88] Magnesium sulfate given to the mother may cause neuromuscular blockade and a transient urinary tract hypotonia in the neonate, leading to delayed voiding. Any neonate who remains anuric beyond the 1st day of life requires an evaluation for renal insufficiency. Urine output in term

Characteristic	Effects
TABLE 2.5. *Effects of neonatal renal function*	
Decreased GFR	• Difficulty excreting water loads with risk of overhydration and water intoxication • Narrow margin of safety for fluid management • Tendency for water retention and edema (especially pulmonary edema) • Increased half-life of drugs (e.g., antibiotics) • Altered drug doses and dosing intervals • Risk of hyperglycemia in VLBW infants
Tubular function Sodium	• Increased loss in urine (especially in VLBW infants) • Changes in other electrolytes, with risk of acidosis, hyperkalemia, and hypoglycemia • Limited ability to excrete excess sodium
Glucose	• Inability to handle exogenous load, with risk of hyperglycemia • Risk of hyponatremia and dehydration
Bicarbonate	• Decreased ability to compensate for acid–base abnormalities, with risk of acidosis (especially preterm infants)
Decreased concentrating ability	• Risk of dehydration

VLBW, very low body weight.

infants averages 15 to 16 mL/kg/day; output is somewhat higher in preterm infants (24 to 38 mL/kg/day). Minimal urine output in all neonates is 1 to 2 mL/kg/h after the first 48 h of life.[77] Because acute renal failure results in a progressively positive solute balance, a urine flow rate <1 m L/kg/h is an accepted criterion for the definition of oliguria in the neonate.

The newborn infant can produce dilute urine comparable to adult levels owing to the integrity of the loop of Henle and the distal tubule, which matures relatively early.[64] The limitation in GFR, however, still places the neonate at risk for overhydration. Neonates can concentrate urine to only 500 to 700 mOsm/L, whereas adults concentrate urine to 1200 to 1400 mOsm/L (Fig. 2.2).[77, 89] The reduction in concentration is related to the inability of the neonate to produce and maintain a concentration gradient via the countercurrent multiplier system. Limitations in the neonate include relatively short loops of Henle, decreased solute in the interstitial space, and less available urea.[62, 64, 77] Because neonates use their proteins for growth, they do not excrete as much urea as do adults. Receptors in the distal tubule and collecting duct have a limited response to antidiuretic hormone (ADH), which also contributes to the neonate's reduced ability

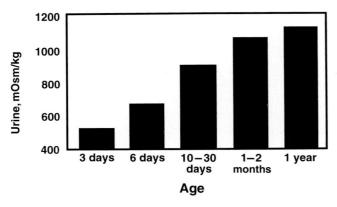

FIG. 2.2. Renal concentrating capacity of a full-term neonate. Adult concentrating capacity is approached within the 1st month of life.

to concentrate urine. Inappropriate ADH secretion occurs in term neonates suffering birth asphyxia, intracerebral hemorrhage, or respiratory distress syndrome.[90, 91] In later childhood, the maximal concentrating ability of very low birth weight infants is not different from that of age-matched peers.[65]

The implications of neonatal renal function are summarized in the Table 2.5.[92] These limitations create a narrow margin for error in the management of neonatal fluid and electrolyte balances. Even healthy neonates are limited in their renal function capabilities and the ability to maintain appropriate fluid and electrolyte homeostases. If the infant is critically ill and experiences further compromise, fluid and electrolyte management becomes a complicated challenge for the caregiver.

NUTRITION

Neonatal Glucose Management

Glucose, a necessary nutrient in maintenance therapy, has important functions. As it is converted into glycogen by the liver, it improves hepatic function. By supplying necessary calories for energy, it spares body protein and minimizes the development of ketosis present with the oxidation of fat stores for essential energy in the absence of added glucose. Carbohydrates provide an indispensable source of calories for the infant who is unable to receive oral sustenance[93] (Table 2.6). When carbohydrates are inadequate, the body uses its fat to supply calories. The by-products of this process are ketones, acidic molecules that neutralize bicarbonate and produce a metabolic acidosis. The only by-products excreted from carbohydrate metabolism are water and carbon dioxide. Carbohydrates, by providing calories for essential energy, also reduce catabolism of protein, which is especially important during the stress response when renal excretion of nitrogen exceeds the intake.

Prompt recognition of hypoglycemia is important to avoid prolonged hypoglycemia its associated neurologic damage.[94, 95] Symptoms of neonatal hypoglycemia are often subtle and include lethargy, apnea, cyanosis, hypothermia, and seizure.[96-98] The working definition of *neonatal hypoglycemia* is a plasma glucose <40 mg/dL in

TABLE 2.6. *Caloric distribution in the preterm infant*

Function	Calories used, %
Maintenance and thermoregulation	42
New tissue components (development)	38
Lost in feces and urine	10
Activity	6
Tissue synthesis	4

Data from Sauer PJ, Dane HJ, Visser HK, et al. Longitudinal studies on metabolic rate, heat loss, and energy cost of growth in low birth weight infants. Pediatr Res 1984;18:254–259.

the first 24 h of life and a level of 40 to 50 mg/dL after the first 24 h of life.[94] Glucose levels in the neonate are determined by glucose reagent strips (which require visual inspection or reflective photometry) and serum glucose tests. Reagent strips provide a value quickly and with minimal blood requirements;[99] however, the readings may be inaccurate because of variations in technique.[94, 99] The most accurate means of measuring blood glucose is through laboratory analysis of serum.[94] Venous sample sites provide a slightly lower value than do arterial sites.[100-102]

Premature infants have lower glycogen stores than do term infants; and very low birth weight infants have almost no glycogen stores,[94, 96] making them more susceptible to hypoglycemia. An increased metabolic rate associated with respiratory distress, hypothermia, sepsis, or other disorders can further compromise these borderline infants.[96] In addition, some infants may be at risk for hypoglycemia secondary to increased glucose use related to hyperinsulinism if they have a diabetic mother. In addition, tocolytic therapy can cause maternal hyperglycemia, resulting in a similar fetal hyperinsulinism and neonatal hypoglycemia.[103]

The mainstay therapy of hypoglycemia is anticipation and prevention. At risk infants (tocolytic use or diabetic mother) should receive early enteral feedings or an intravenous dextrose infusion. A neutral thermal environment and periods of uninterrupted rest are important for minimizing metabolic demands and conserving energy.[97] The treatment for acute hypoglycemia is intravenous dextrose—2 mL/kg $D_{10}W$ (200 mg/kg glucose)[104]— followed by a constant infusion of 6 to 8 mg glucose/kg/min, which may require titration to as high as 15 mg/kg/min. If a central line is present, the clinician may use hypertonic infusion up to $D_{25}W$. Blood glucose monitoring should be performed every 30 to 60 min during the acute phase of therapy. An infusion of 100 mL $D_{10}W$/kg/day provides 6.67 mg/kg/min of dextrose, which is usually adequate to maintain normal serum glucose levels.

Premature neonates receiving intravenous glucose solution may be prone to hyperglycemia because of their relatively immature metabolic regulatory process, which results in an inability to stop producing endogenous glucose, and their ineffective insulin response, which leads to a general insensitivity to glucose.[105, 106] In addition, theophylline, caffeine, lipids, and steroids administered during the newborn period;[107, 108] increased circulating catecholamines related to stress;[105, 106] and depression of insulin secretion and end organ receptor response present with sepsis[103] may cause increased blood glucose levels. Generally, a serum level >150 mg/dL indicates hyperglycemia. Hyperglycemia can cause an osmotic diuresis, leading to dehydration and fluid shifts, which may increase the risk for intraventricular hemorrhage.[103, 105, 106] The majority of neonates with hyperglycemia can be treated by decreasing the amount of glucose in their intravenous fluids. Hypotonic solutions less than $D_{2.5}W$ should be avoided to minimize complications related to hypo-osmolarity.[107, 109] The use of insulin to treat severe hyperglycemia may be considered;[106, 107, 109] however, there is disagreement regarding the level of glucose at which therapy should be initiated.[103, 110] Although insulin therapy may allow the infant to receive larger infusions of glucose (increased calories for growth), the role of this practice remains controversial.[106]

Protein Metabolism

Protein is another important nutrient for maintenance therapy. Although a neonate may be adequately maintained on glucose, water, vitamins, and electrolytes for a limited time, over the long run, protein losses must be replaced. Protein is necessary for cellular repair, healing of wounds, and synthesis of vitamins and some enzymes.

In contrast to healthy adults who exist in a state of neutral nitrogen balance, infants need to be in a positive nitrogen balance to achieve satisfactory growth and development. Infants can retain up to two-thirds of the metabolized protein intake when on both oral and intravenous diets.[111, 112] In contrast to adults, infants may remain in positive nitrogen balance despite suboptimal energy intake.[113, 114] Studies of the dynamic protein response to feeding support the view that both protein and calories are necessary to achieve the positive nitrogen balance. A total of 24 amino acids have been identified, of which 9 are essential in infants. Arginine, cystine, and taurine are essential for low-birthweight infants. New tissue cannot be formed unless all the essential amino acids are present in the diet simultaneously; the absence of only one essential amino acid will result in a negative nitrogen and protein balance. Protein requirements vary with the age of the patient, and neonates have the highest requirements. Healthy, growing term infants who drink 150 to 200 mL human milk/kg/day ingest between 2.0 and 2.8 g protein/kg/day; the same infants fed the same volume of commercial formula receive between 2.2 and 3.0 g protein/kg/day.[115] The protein requirements of premature infants are estimated to be 1.2 to 2.9 g/kg/day as birth weight increases from 700 to 2500 g.[116] Premature infants should not receive excessive protein, however, because lower IQ scores have been identified with infants who were fed a formula containing >3.5 g/kg/day protein.[117] Glutamine is a major energy source for intestinal mucosal cells and other rapidly proliferating cells. Most commercially available amino acid solutions do not include glutamine, although that may soon change.

Fat Metabolism

Fats are a major source of nonprotein calories for the body. Simple lipids, such as triglycerides, are the most abundant fat in the body and food sources. Triglycerides are hydrolyzed in the blood stream to free fatty acids. If triglycerides are not hydrolyzed, they accumulate and are removed by the reticuloendothelial tissue.[118] This overload can lead to decreased pulmonary diffusion, resulting in hypoxia,[119] pathologic deposition of exogenous triglycerides in tissues,[120] and hyperphospholipidemia and hypercholesterolemia.[121] Intravenous lipids delivered early in the neonatal period can displace plasma albumin–bound bilirubin with fatty acids, increasing the risk of kernicterus if the neonate has hyperbilirubinemia.[122]

Humans do not synthesize linoleic acid; therefore, it must be supplied in the diet (1 to 2% of calories) and is considered an essential fatty acid. Deficiencies of essential fatty acids may lead to skin dryness, thickening, and desquamation as well as a rash. The inclusion of approximately 0.5 g lipid/kg/day in the intravenous diet, along with protein and glucose, eliminates deficiencies in essential fatty acids.[123] Continuous infusions of 1 to 3 g lipids/kg/day, as recommended, should be monitored by periodically measuring serum triglyceride levels.[118]

Vitamins

Vitamins, although not nutrients, are necessary for the use of nutrients. Vitamin C and the various B complex vitamins are the most frequently used in parenteral therapy. These water-soluble vitamins are not retained by the body and are lost through urinary excretion. Because of this loss, parenteral therapy requires larger doses for adequate maintenance than does oral therapy. The B complex vitamins play an important role in the metabolism of carbohydrates and in maintaining gastrointestinal function. Vitamin C promotes wound healing and is frequently used for the surgical patient. Vitamins A and D are fat-soluble vitamins; they can be stored in the body and are not generally required by the patient on maintenance therapy.

THERAPEUTIC DRUG MONITORING IN NEONATES

Although therapeutic drug monitoring is well developed in adults, the practice in neonates is based on extrapolation from adult models. There are several reasons to perform therapeutic drug monitoring in neonates. Drug effects are often not easily measurable because of the absence of verbal skills, and subtle signs of toxicity or lack of effect may go unnoticed.[124] Furthermore, neonates undergo maturation of both renal and hepatic functions, not seen in adults;[125–128] and neonates have a rapidly changing physiologic status related to weight and body compartments.[129] In light of these variables, drug monitoring is perhaps more crucial in the neonatal period than in any other age group.

TABLE 2.7. *Factors that affect drug metabolism and monitoring*

Tubular secretion
GFR
Conjugation and glucuronidation
Cytochrome P450
Pancreatic enzymes
Enterohepatic circulation
Bilirubin level
Albumin binding
Total body weight
Fat content

TABLE 2.8. *Drugs commonly monitored in neonates*

Drug	Half-life, h
Antibiotics	
Amikacin	5–7
Gentamicin	3–7
Tobramycin	4–9
Vancomycin	3–6
Antiepileptics	
Phenobarbital	60–120
Phenytoin	20
Miscellaneous	
Caffeine	40–200
Theophylline	20–40

A number of factors affect the unique deposition of drugs in the neonate, including *(a)* volume of distribution, *(b)* metabolism, *(c)* renal excretion, *(d)* circulating total protein and albumin levels, *(e)* changes in regional blood flow of extremities, *(f)* impaired enteral absorption, and *(g)* the infusion pump method. Neonates have volume of distribution differences and a higher water volume (80 to 90%), particularly in younger gestational age groups, compared to adults. Neonates metabolize drugs at a slower rate than do older babies, because of the immaturity of a number of their hepatic enzyme systems (cytochrome P450), which changes the half-life of drugs.[124] Renal excretion, which involves glomerular filtration and tubular secretion, alters the effects of drugs, because neonatal GFR can be as low as 30% of adult levels.[127] Although renal elimination can be estimated from the creatinine clearance value, the changing GFR and tubular secretion rates in neonates make the method somewhat impractical for this age group. A particular drug's solubility may dramatically influence the effect.[129]

Neonates have less circulating total protein and albumin than do adults, and fetal albumin has a lower affinity for most drugs than does adult albumin. Blood pH, bilirubin levels, and free fatty acid concentration affect the amount of displaced drug and can cause an abnormal concentration for a given dose of a drug.[125, 126, 128, 130] Numerous other factors may influence the distribution of a drug in the neonate, including decreased regional blood flow in the extremities, which changes the uptake for intramuscular or subcutaneous sites;[126] impaired enteral absorption; and the effects of pancreatic secretions, all of which influence the bioavailability of medications given orally or parenterally[131] (Table 2.7).

Although assays are available for many medications, drug monitoring is necessary only in certain circumstances. Drugs with known toxicity or chronically used drugs should be considered for monitoring, and drugs that are influenced by changes in body function should be monitored at the steady state and as bodily functions mature or deteriorate. Drugs that are commonly monitored in the neonate are listed in Table 2.8.

RESPIRATORY FAILURE IN THE NEONATE

The treatment of respiratory failure in neonates, infants, and children has advanced significantly since the advent of mechanical ventilators.[132] Despite improvement, long-term ventilation use is still associated with mortality and morbidity related to chronic lung disease and developmental delay.[133, 134] No single modality for the treatment of respiratory failure has become the magic bullet, and newer therapies are being explored to improve outcomes. The goal of mechanical ventilation is to provide adequate alveolar oxygen and carbon dioxide exchange while avoiding lung damage and depression of cardiovascular function. This section reviews some of the most common methods of ventilation and therapy for the neonate with respiratory distress.

Exogenous surfactant therapy has had a significant impact on the care of premature infants. Endogenous pulmonary surfactant stabilizes alveoli by reducing surface tension. Both natural (human or animal derived) and synthetic surfactant reduce mortality risk by 35 to 40%, whether given prophylactically at the time of delivery to high-risk infants or given after the onset of clinical respiratory distress syndrome. As a result of extensive testing, exogenous surfactant therapy has become the standard of care in the prophylaxis and treatment of respiratory distress syndrome in premature infants.

Conventional mechanical ventilators are the main vehicle for the delivery of ventilatory assistance and are classified by the method used to change from inspiration to expiration. The termination of inspiratory flow may be triggered when a preset pressure is reached (pressure cycled), a preset time has elapsed (time cycled), or a preset volume has been delivered (volume cycled). Neonates are most commonly ventilated with time-cycled, pressure-limited ventilators (Table 2.9). Compared to other ventilators, time-cycled ventilators are less expensive, more reliable, and easier to operate. Because of their increased mechanical complexity, however, volume-cycled ventilators are often capable of additional modes of ventilation.

TABLE 2.9. *Initial ventilator settings*

Setting	Level
Volume ventilator	
Mode	Synchronized intermittent mandatory ventilation
F_{IO_2}, %	100
Rate, bpm	
Older children	12–15
Younger children	15–20
Infants	20–30
Tidal volume, mL/kg	12–15
PEEP, torr	3–5
Pressure ventilator	
Mode	Intermittent mandatory ventilation
F_{IO_2}, %	100
Rate, bpm	20–30
PIP, torr	20–30
PEEP, torr	3–5
I:E ratio	1:2

PEEP, positive end-expiratory pressure; *PIP,* peak inspiratory pressure; *I:E,* inspiratory:expiratory.

High-frequency ventilation (HFV) is designed to improve gas exchange by use of high respiratory rates (up to 2400 bpm) and a low tidal volume that is close to the anatomical dead space in an effort to reduce the adverse effects of assisted ventilation.[135] This method of ventilation theoretically decreases barotrauma to the lungs; however, the mean airway pressure remains the same. The ventilator delivers gas in a high-velocity stream (high-frequency jet ventilation) or through oscillations created by a piston or diaphragm (high-frequency oscillatory ventilation).[136] Some authors have noted a lower rate of air leak syndrome with the use of high-frequency ventilation, but a higher incidence of intracranial hemorrhage has also been noted.[137] Other authors have noted no differences in mortality, intracranial hemorrhage, or air leaks between HFV and conventional ventilation.[138]

Liquid ventilation is a relatively new therapy for acute respiratory failure, with theoretical advantages over conventional mechanical ventilation for safe, effective gas exchange in the surfactant-deficient lung. Liquid perflurocarbons have low surface tension, have a high solubility coefficient for oxygen and carbon dioxide, and lack of toxicity, which allows for gas exchange in the lungs through a liquid medium. Some centers are currently investigating this method of ventilation.

Nitric oxide, an endogenous vasodilator otherwise known as endothelium-derived relaxing factor, is a selective pulmonary vasodilator when administered as a gas. Inhaled nitric oxide activates guanylate cyclase, which increases intracellular cGMP, thus reducing intracellular calcium and causing vasodilatation. With this method of delivery, nitric oxide is delivered specifically to the pulmonary vasculature. There are two potential side effects of inhalational nitric oxide therapy: methe-

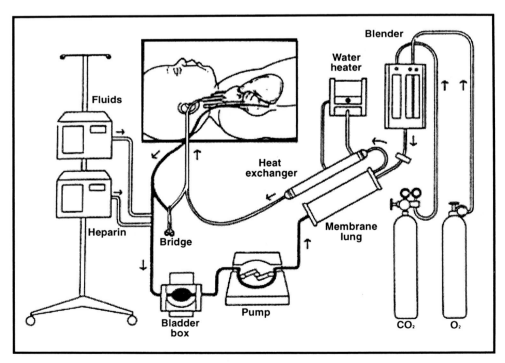

FIG. 2.3. Extracorporeal membrane circuit used for both venoarterial and venovenous bypass. Blood is drained by gravity from the patient and then pumped to the membrane lung where it is oxygenated, heated, and returned to the patient.

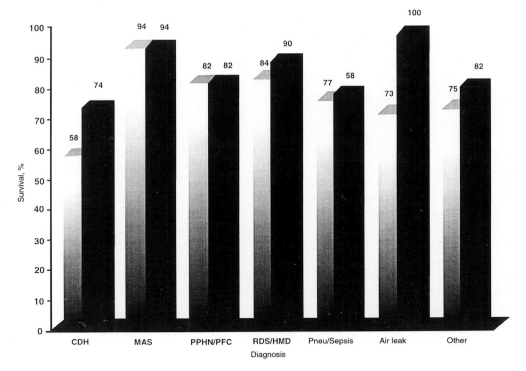

FIG. 2.4. Neonatal ECMO survival rates by diagnosis. *CDH,* congenital diaphragmatic hernia; *MAS,* meconium aspiration; *PPHN/PFC,* persistent pulmonary hypertension/persistent fetal circulation; *RDS/ HMD,* respiratory distress syndrome/hyaline membrane diseases; *PNEU/SEPSIS,* pneumonia/sepsis; *AIR LEAK,* air leak syndrome. □, data from Extracorporeal Life Support Organization. Extracorporeal membrane oxygenation registry report. International summary. July 1996; ■, data from Extracorporeal Life Support Organization. Extracorporeal membrane oxygenation registry report. James Whitcomb Riley Hospital, Indianapolis, IN. July 1996.

moglobinemia and lung injury (nitric oxide is a free radical that can elicit a local response). This modality has improved persistent pulmonary hypertension of the neonate, improved oxygenation, and minimized ventilation-perfusion mismatches.

Extracorporeal membrane oxygenation (ECMO), no longer considered an innovative therapy for infants with severe respiratory failure, is the standard mode of therapy. Bartlett's initial studies have been followed in the treatment of >10,000 infants and children treated with ECMO.[139] ECMO is a technique of prolonged nonpulsatile extracorporeal cardiopulmonary bypass that is achieved through extrathoracic vascular cannulation (venovenous, venoarterial). In simplest terms, ECMO involves draining venous blood (internal jugular or atrial catheter), circulating it through an artificial lung in which oxygen is added and carbon dioxide is removed, and returning it by a vein (venovenous bypass) or artery (venoarterial bypass) (Fig. 2.3) ECMO is quite invasive and expensive and carries associated pulmonary and neurologic morbidity.[140] It should be reserved for infants and children with severe respiratory failure who have failed conventional modes of ventilation (Fig. 2.4).[141, 142]

IMMUNE SYSTEM OF THE NEONATE

Neonates are at high risk time for infectious diseases,[143, 144] particularly with entry sites at the mucosal surfaces of the gastrointestinal tract and the respiratory tract. This implies that cellular mechanisms associated with the induction and/or expression of adaptive immunity are not fully functional at birth, an idea that has been supported by a wide body of data from humans and experimental studies.[145] At birth, the term infant is immunologically competent but suffers from several problems that may increase the risk of sepsis. Newborns have very thin and permeable skin that can be easily injured, allowing entry of bacteria. The neonatal ileum may also absorb macromolecules (bacteria).

Maternal IgG crosses the placenta beginning at approximately 30 weeks of gestation. At term, fetal IgG levels approximate maternal levels. At birth, the neonate quickly develops his or her own IgM and IgA; however, the premature infant may have delayed production of these immunoglobulins, increasing the risk of sepsis. The preterm infant has profound and prolonged physiologic hypogammaglobulinemia; and very low birthweight infants are still hypogammaglobulinemic at 9 months old, compared to term infants. Deficiencies in any of the components of the immune system (cell-mediated or humoral immunity, complement, and neutrophil function) may lead to dramatic clinical presentations with multiple or unusual infections. Such premature infants are able to mount protective specific antibody responses to common vaccines or pathogens as early as 3 months after birth.[146] After birth, serum IgG levels fall (half-life = 3 weeks) at a rate similar to that seen in agammaglobulinemic patients after IgG infusion. The nadir serum IgG level is reached at 4 to 6 months (physiologic trough), increasing the risk of infection at that time. Serum IgG levels then rise, approaching adult levels at 2 to 6 years of age.[147]

IgM, on the other hand, does not cross the placenta; and newborn levels are about 10% of adult levels. IgM rises during infancy and can be elevated in response to congenital infections or a hyper-IgM syndrome. Adult levels of IgM are reached at 1 to 2 years of age. Serum IgA also does not cross the placenta; neonates levels are approximately 1% of adults levels. Levels rise gradually, reaching adult levels in adolescence. Secretory IgA is virtually absent from newborn secretions but can be found in colostrum and breast milk. Production of secretory IgA occurs earlier than serum IgA and can approach adult levels by 2 years of age. Little serum IgE crosses the placenta, and the implications in the neonate are unknown.

Premature infants have lower complement levels than do term infants and adults,[148] and compromised opsonic activity makes them susceptible to infection. In addition, neutrophil counts are lower in premature neonates,[149] and such infants are particularly likely to deplete their granulocyte stores during sepsis. Because neutrophil phagocytosis and killing partly depends on serum opsonization, the low levels of two major opsonins (IgG and complement) in preterm infants render them especially vulnerable to invasive organisms.[150]

Infections at young gestational ages are important clinical problems, often associated with high mortality. The number of infections at extremely young ages is likely to increase in the future owing to better survival rates for premature babies. In addition, AIDS and HIV-related infections will probably affect an increasing number of patients. Immunization of these neonates is important. Infants born to mothers who are HBsAg positive are at risk of perinatally acquired infections. This risk ranges from <10% (anti-HBe positive mother) to 70 to 90% (HBeAg positive mother).[151] Infants infected by perinatal transmission have a 90% risk of chronic infection, and up to 25% of such infants will die of chronic liver disease as adults.[152] Hepatitis B vaccine should be administered at birth to all babies if possible (in an effort to eliminate hepatitis B), and all babies born to carrier mothers should receive further doses at 1 and 6 months.[153] If the mother is either HBe-Ag positive or has an unknown hepatitis status, the neonate should also receive hepatitis B immune globulin (HBIG) within 24 h of birth. Other infant immunizations begin at 2 months of age.

SUMMARY

The development of neonatal intensive care units has led to a dramatic decline in the mortality of sick newborns. Infants managed in high-volume (>15 patients/day) level III intensive care units have a significantly lower risk-adjusted mortality than do infants in all other units.[154] In addition, the costs for the birth of infants at high-volume level III nurseries are no higher than those at other hospitals with neonatal intensive care units. This is sobering data, and each health care provider should re-evaluate the practice of allowing high-risk mothers to deliver in facilities without level III capabilities.

REFERENCES

1. Rooth G. Low birthweight revised. Lancet 1980;1:639–641.
2. Guyer B, Wallach LA, Rosen SL. Birth-weight standardized neonatal mortality rates and the prevention of low birth weight: how does Massachusetts compare with Sweden? New Engl J Med 1982;306:1230–1233.
3. Stevens S M, Richardson D K, Gray J E, et al. Estimating neonatal mortality risk: an analysis of clinicians' judgments. Pediatrics 1994;93:945–950.
4. Luke B, Williams C, Minogue J, Keith L. The changing pattern of infant mortality in the US: the role of prenatal factors and their obstetrical implications. Int J Gynaecol Obstet 1993;40:199–212.
5. Overpeck MD, Hoffman HJ, Prager K. The lowest birth weight infants and the US infant mortality rate: NCHS 1983 linked birth/infant death data. Am J Public Health 1992;82:441–444.
6. Phelps DL, Brown DR, Tung B, et al. Twenty-eight-day survival rates of 6676 neonates with birth weights of 1250 g or less. Pediatrics 1991;87:7–17.
7. Kilbride HW, Daily DK, Claflin K, et al. Improved survival and neurodevelopmental outcome for infants less than 801 g birth weight. Am J Perinatol 1990;7:160–165.
8. Hack M, Fanaroff AA. Outcomes of extremely low birth weight infants between 1982 and 1988. New Engl J Med 1989;321:1642–1647.
9. Victorian Infant Collaborative Study Group. Improving the quality of survival for infants of birth weight <1000 g born in non-level-III centers in Victoria. Med J Aust 1993;158:24–27.
10. Ens Dokkum MH, Schreuder AM, Veen S, et al. Evaluation of care for the preterm infant: review of literature on follow-up of preterm and low birth weight infants. Report from the collaborative Project on Preterm and Small for Gestational Age Infants (POPS) in the Netherlands. Paediatr Perinat Epidemiol 1992; 6:434–459.
11. Heinonen K, Hakulinen A, Jokela V. Survival of the smallest. Time trends and determinants of mortality in a very preterm population during the 1980s. Lancet 1988;2:204–207.
12. Hakala TH, Ylikorkala O. Effective prenatal care decreases the incidence of low birth weight. Am J Perinatol 1989;6:222–225.
13. Hack M, Horbar JD, Malloy MH, et al. Very low birth weight outcomes of the National Institute of Child Health and Human Development Neonatal Network. Pediatrics 1991;87:587–597.
14. Desmond MM. A review of newborn medicine in America: European past and guiding ideology. Am J Perinatol 1991;8:308–322.
15. Schwartz RM, Luby AM, Scanlon JW, Kellogg RJ. Effect of

surfactant on morbidity, mortality, and resource use in newborn infants weighing 500 to 1500 g. New Engl J Med 1994;330:1476–1480.

16. Puffer RR. Family planning issues relating to maternal and infant mortality in the United States. Bull Pan Am Health Organ 1993;27:120–134.

17. Johnson KG. The promise of regional perinatal care as a national strategy for improved maternal and infant care. Public Health Rep 1992;97:134–139.

18. Killam AP, Barrett JM, Cotton RB. The impact of a tertiary perinatal center on survival of the very low birth weight infant. J Tenn Med Assoc 1981;74:870–872.

19. Lucey JF. Why we should regionalize perinatal care. Pediatrics 1973;52:488–491.

20. McCormick MC, Shapiro S, Starfield BH. The regionalization of perinatal services. Summary of the evaluation of a national demonstration program. JAMA 1985;253:799–804.

21. Shenai JP, Major CW, Gaylord MS, et al. A successful decade of regionalized perinatal care in Tennessee: the neonatal experience. J Perinatol 1991;11:137–143.

22. Whitfield JM, Buser MK. Transport stabilization times for neonatal and pediatric patients prior to interfacility transfer. Pediatr Emerg Care 1993;9:69–71.

23. Ott WJ. Intrauterine growth retardation and preterm delivery. Am J Obstet Gynecol 1993;168:1710–1717.

24. Wolf EJ, Vintzileos AM, Rosenkrantz TS, et al. Do survival and morbidity of very low-birth-weight infants vary according to the primary pregnancy complication that results in preterm delivery? Am J Obstet Gynecol 1993;169:1233–1239.

25. Ott WJ. The diagnosis of altered fetal growth. Obstet Gynecol Clin North Am 1988;5:237–263.

26. Ott WJ .Defining altered fetal growth by second-trimester sonography. Obstet Gynecol 1990;75:1053–1059.

27. Seeds JW. Impaired fetal growth: definition and clinical diagnosis. Obstet Gynecol 1984;64:303–310.

28. Vyas H, Helms P, Cheriyan G. Transcutaneous oxygen monitoring beyond the neonatal period. Crit Care Med 1988;16:844–847.

29. Task Force on Transcutaneous Oxygen Monitors. Report of consensus meeting. Pediatrics 1989;83:122–125.

30. Aoyagi T, Kishi M, Yamaguchi K, Watanabe S. Improvement of the earpiece oximeter (in Japanese). Abstract of 13th Conference of Japan Society of Medical Electronics and Biological Engineering, Osaka, Japan, 1974:90–91.

31. Garg AK. "Arterialized" capillary blood [Letter]. Can Med Assoc J 1972;104:16.

32. Alba RM, Lopez MJR, Flores JC. Use of the intraosseous route in resuscitation in a neonate. Int Care Med 1994;20:529–533.

33. Strauss RG. Transfusion therapy in neonates. Am J Dis Child 1991;145:904–911.

34. Sacher RA, Strauss RG, Luban NLC, et al. Blood component therapy during the neonatal period: a national survey of red cell transfusion practices, 1985. Transfusion 1990;30:271–276.

35. Levy GJ, Strauss RG, Hume H, et al. National survey of neonatal transfusion practices: I. Red blood cell therapy. Pediatrics 1993;91:523–529.

36. Thomas K. Thermoregulation in neonates. Neonatal Netw 1994;13:15–22.

37. Perera P, Kurban AK, Ryan TJ. The development of the cutaneous microvascular system in the newborn. Br J Dermatol 1970;82:86–91.

38. Bruck K, Bruck M, Lemtis H. Temperature regulation in the newborn infant. Biol Neonate 1961;3:65–119.

39. Mann TP. Observations on temperatures of mothers and babies in the perinatal period. J Obstet Gynecol Br Commonwealth 1968;75:316–321.

40. Jakubovic HR, Ackerman AB. Structure and function of skin: development, morphology, and physiology. In: Moschella SL, Jurley HJ, eds., Dermatology. 3rd ed. Philadelphia: Saunders 1992:3–87.

41. Rutter N, Hull D. Response of term babies to a warm environment. Arch Dis Child 1979;54:178–183.

42. Harpin VA, Chellappah G, Rutter N. Responses of the newborn infant to overheating. Biol Neonate 1983;44:65–75.

43. American Academy of Pediatrics and American College of Obstetrics and Gynecology. Thermal regulation. In: Brann AW, Cefalo RC, eds., Guidelines for perinatal care. 1983;225–231.

44. Wheldon AE, Hull D. Incubation for very immature infants. Arch Dis Child 1983;58:504–508.

45. Sauer PJJ, Dane HJ, Visser HKA, New standards for neutral thermal environment of healthy very low birth weight infants in week one of life. Arch Dis Child 1984;59:18–22.

46. Collinge JM, Aranda JV. Nonmetabolic complications of neonatal intravenous therapy: epidemiologic considerations. Am J Perinatol 1984;1:185–189.

47. Davidson DC, Gilbert J Severe extravasation injury. Br Med J 1985;291:217.

48. Chandavasu O, Garrow E, Valda V, et al. A new method for the prevention of skin sloughs and necrosis secondary to intravenous infiltration. Am J Perinatol 1986;3:4–5.

49. Zenk KE, Dungy CI, Greene GR, Nafcillin extravasation injury: use of hyaluronidase as an antidote. Am J Dis Child 1981; 135:1113–1114.

50. Wright A, Hecker JF, Lewis GBH. Use of transdermal glyceryl trinitrate to reduce failure of intravenous infusions due to phlebitis and extravasation. Lancet 1985;2:1148–1150.

51. Hecker JF. Failure of infusions from extravasation and phlebitis. Anesth Intens Care 1989;17:433–439.

52. Alpan G, Eyal F, Springer C, et al. Heparinization of alimentation solutions administered through peripheral veins in premature infants: a controlled study. Pediatrics 1984;744:375–378.

53. Pineault M, Chessex P, Piedboeuf B, Bisaillon S. Beneficial effect of confusing a lipid emulsion on venous patency. J Parenter Enteral Nutr 1989;13:637–640.

54. Wu PKY, Hodgman JE. Insensible water loss in preterm infants: changes with postnatal development and non-ionizing radiant energy. Pediatrics 1974;54:704–712.

55. Fanaroff AA, Wald M, Gruber HS, Klaus MH. Insensible water loss in low birthweight infants. Pediatrics 1972;50:236–245.

56. Oh W, Karecki H. Phototherapy and insensible water loss in the newborn infant. Am J Dis Child 1972;124:230–232.

57. Coulter DM. Postnatal fluid and electrolyte changes and clinical implications. In: Brace RA, Ross MG, Robillard JE, eds., Fetal and neonatal body fluids: the scientific basis for clinical practice [Reproductive and perinatal medicine]. Ithaca, NY: Perinatology Press, 1989;11:319–367.

58. Costarino A, Baumgart S. Modern fluid and electrolyte management of the critically ill premature infant. Pediatr Clin North Am 1986;33:153–178.

59. Brion L P, Satlin LM, Edelmann CM. Renal disease. In: Avery GB, Fletcher MA, MacDonald MC, eds., Neonatology: pathophysiology and management of the newborn. 4th ed. Philadelphia: Lippincott, 1994;792–886.

60. Fetterman GH, Shuplock NA, Phillipp FJ, Gregg HS. The growth and maturation of human glomeruli and proximal convolutions from term to adulthood: studies in microdissection. Pediatrics 1965;35:601–619.

61. Jose PA, Fildes RD. Postnatal development of renal function. The tiny baby [Mead Johnson symposium on perinatal and developmental medicine, No. 33]. Evansville, IN: Mead Johnson, 1990.

62. Aperia A, Braberger O, Herin P, Zetterstrom R, Postnatal development of renal function in pre-term and full-term infants. Acta Paediatr Scand 1981;70:183–187.

63. Rubin MI, Bruck E, Rapaport M. Maturation of renal function in childhood: clearance studies. J Clin Invest 1949;28:1144–1162.

64. Yared A, Barakat AY, Ichikawa I. Fetal nephrology. In: Eden RD, Boehm FH, eds., Assessment and care of the fetus. Norwalk, CT: Appleton & Lange, 1990;69–91.

65. Vanpee M, Blennow M, Linne T, et al. Renal function in very low birth weight infants: normal maturity reached during early childhood. J Pediatr 1992;121:784–788.

66. Spitzer A. Factors underlying the increase in glomerular filtration rate during postnatal development. In: Spitzer A, ed., The kidney during development: morphology and function. New York: Masson, 1982:121–134.

67. Green R, Hatton TM. Renal tubular function in gestation. Am J Kidney Dis 1987;9:265–269.

68. Guignard JP. Drugs and the neonatal kidney. Dev Pharmacol Ther 1982;4(Suppl 1):19–27.
69. Yaffe SJ. Antimicrobial therapy and the neonate. Obstet Gynecol 1981;58(Suppl):85S–94S.
70. Siegel SR. Hormonal and renal interaction in body fluid regulation in the newborn infant. Clin Perinatol 1982;9:535–557.
71. Linshaw MA. Concentration and dilution of urine. In: Polin RA, Fox WW, eds., Fetal and neonatal physiology. Philadelphia: Saunders, 1992:1239–1257.
72. Anand SK. Maturation of renal function. In: Taeusch HW, Ballard RA, Avery ME, eds., Diseases of the newborn, 6th ed. Philadelphia: Saunders, 1991:841–849.
73. Seaman SL. Renal physiology part II: fluid and electrolyte regulation. Neonatal Netw 1995;14:5–11.
74. Costarino AT, Baumgart S. Controversies in fluid and electrolyte therapy for the premature infant. Clin Perinatol 1988;15:863–878.
75. Al-Dahhan J, Haycock GB, Nichol B, et al. Sodium homeostasis in term and preterm infants. I. Renal aspects. Arch Dis Child 1983;58:335–342.
76. Blackburn ST, Loper DL. Maternal, fetal and neonatal physiology: a clinical perspective. Philadelphia: Saunders, 1992.
77. Guignard JP, John, EG. Renal function in the tiny, premature infant. Clin Perinatol 1986;13:377–401.
78. Robillard JE, Sessions C, Kennedy RL, Smith FG. Maturation of the glucose transport processes by the fetal kidney. Pediatr Res 1978;12:680–684.
79. Rossi R, Danzebrink S, Linnenburger K, et al. Assessment of tubular reabsorption of sodium, glucose, phosphate and amino acids based on spot urine samples. Acta Paediatr 1994;83:1282–1286.
80. Svenningsen NW. Renal acid-base titration studies in infants with and without metabolic acidosis in the postnatal period. Pediatr Res 1974;8:659–672.
81. Schwartz GJ, Haycock GB, Chir B, et al. Late metabolic acidosis: a reassessment of the definition. J Pediatr 1979;95:102–107.
82. Kerpel-Fronius E, Heim T, Sulyok E. The development of the renal acidifying processes and their relation to acidosis in low-birth-weight infants. Biol Neonate 1970;15:156–168.
83. Jacinto JS, Modanlou HD, Crade M. Renal calcification incidence in very low birth weight infants. Pediatrics 1988;81:31–35.
84. Downing GJ, Egelhoff JC, Daily DK, et al. Kidney function in very low birth weight infants with furosemide-related renal calcifications at ages 1 to 2 years. J Pediatr 1992;120:599–604.
85. Karlen J, Aperia A, Zetterstrom R. Renal excretion of calcium and phosphate in preterm and term infants. J Pediatr 1985; 106:814–819.
86. Arant BS Jr. Developmental patterns of renal functional maturation compared in the human neonate. J Pediatr 1978;92:705–712.
87. Clark DA. Times of first void and first stool in 500 newborns. Pediatrics 1977;60:457–459.
88. Sherry SN, Kramer JC. The time of passage of first stool and first urine. J Pediatr 1955;46:158–159.
89. Sujov P. Plasma and urine osmolality in full-term and pre-term infants. Acta Paedtr Scand 1984;73:722–726.
90. Kaplan SL, Feigin RD. Inappropriate secretion of antidiuretic hormone complicating neonatal hypoxic ischemic encephalopathy. J Pediatr 1978;92:431–433.
91. Stern P, LaRochette FT Jr, Little GA. Role of vasopressin in water imbalance in the sick newborn. Kidney Int 1979;6:956.
92. Tucker Blackburn S. Renal function in the neonate. J Perinat Neonatal Nurs 1994;8:37–47.
93. Sauer PJ, Dane HJ, Visser HK, et al. Longitudinal studies on metabolic rate, heat loss, and energy cost of growth in low birth weight infants. Pediatr Res 1984;18:254–259.
94. Cornblath M, Schwartz R. Hypoglycemia in the neonate. J Pediatr Endocrinol 1993;6:113–129.
95. Pildes RS, Lilien LD. Metabolic and endocrine disorders. In: Fanaroff AA, Martin JM, eds., Neonatal-perinatal medicine: diseases of the fetus and infant. 5th ed., St. Louis: Mosby Year Book 1992:1152–1292.
96. Cole MD. New factors associated with the incidence of hypoglycemia: a research study. Neonatal Netw 1991;10:47–50.
97. Fantazia D. Neonatal hypoglycemia. J Obstet Gyencol Neonatal Nurs 1984;13:297–301.
98. Stokowski LC, Metabolic disorder. In: Beachy P, Deacon J, eds., Care curriculum for neonatal intensive care nursing. Philadelphia: Saunders, 1992:281–286.
99. Conrad PD, Sparks JW, Osberg I, et al. Clinical application of a new glucose analyzer in the neonatal intensive care unit: comparisons with other methods. J Pediatrics 1989;114:281–287.
100. Butler LA, Karp T, McCance KL, Ward RM. Neonatal glucose determinations obtained from an umbilical artery catheter: evaluation for accuracy using an in vitro model. Neonatal Netw 1993;12:31–35.
101. Brown MS, Nelson S, Stewart BJ. Detection of neonatal hypoglycemia: a comparison of three reagent strips. Nurse Pract 1988;13:15–24.
102. Jacob J, Davis RF. Differences in serum glucose determinations in infants with umbilical artery catheters. J Perinatol 1988;8:40–42.
103. Pildes RS, Pyati SP. Hypoglycemia and hyperglycemia in tiny infants. Clin Perinatol 1986;13:351–375.
104. Karp TB, Scardino C, Butler LA. Glucose metabolism in the neonate: the short and sweet of it. Neonatal Netw 1995;14:17–23.
105. Simeon PS. The premature infant with hyperglycemia: use of continuous insulin infusion. J Perinat Neonatal Nurs 1992; 6:52–60.
106. Grasmick L. Continuous insulin infusion for the treatment of hyperglycemia in premature infants. Neonatal Pharmacol Q 1992;1:47–54.
107. Stiles AD, Cloherty JP. Metabolic problems. In: Cloherty JP, Stark AR, eds., Manual of neonatal care. 3rd ed. Boston: Little, Brown, 1991:339–343.
108. Amspacher KA. Meeting the challenge of neonatal hypoglycemia. J Perinat Neonatal Nurs 1992;6:43–51.
109. Gomella TL. Hyperglycemia. In: Gomella GL, Cunningham M, Eval F, eds., Neonatology: management, procedures, on-call problems, diseases, drugs. Norwalk, CT: Appleton & Lange, 1992:210–213.
110. Cowett RM. Hypoglycemia and hyperglycemia in the newborn. In: Polin RA, Fox WW, eds., Fetal and neonatal physiology. Philadelphia: Saunders, 1993:406–418.
111. Zlotkin SH, Bryan MH, Anderson GH. Intravenous nitrogen and energy intakes required to duplicate in-utero nitrogen accretion in prematurely born infants. J Pediatr 1981;99:115–120.
112. Catzeflis C, Schutz Y, Micheli JL, et al. Whole body protein synthesis and energy expenditure in very low birth weight infants. Pediatr Res 1985;19:679–687.
113. Pierro A, Carnielli V, Filler RM, et al. Characteristics of protein sparing effect of total parenteral nutrition in the surgical infant. J Pediatr Surg 1988;23:538–542.
114. Winthrop AL, Filler RM, Smith J, et al. Analysis of energy and macronutrient balance in the postoperative infant. J Pediatr Surg 1989;24:686–689.
115. Gross SJ, David RJ, Bauman L, et al. Nutritional composition of milk produced by mothers delivering preterm. J Pediatr 1980;96:641–644.
116. Ziegler EE, O'Donnell AM, Nelson SE, et al. Body composition of the reference fetus. Growth 1976;40:329–341.
117. Menkes JH, Welcher DW, Levi HS, et al. Relationship of elevated blood tyrosine to the ultimate intellectual performance of premature infants. Pediatrics 1972;49:218–224.
118. Bryan MH, Shennan A, Griffin E, et al. Commentary: intralipid—its rational use in parenteral nutrition of the newborn. Pediatrics 1976;58:787–790.
119. Perreira GR, Fox WW, Stanley CA, et al. Decreased oxygenation and hyperlipidemia during intravenous fat infusions in premature infants. Pediatrics 1980;66:26–30.
120. Friedman Z, Marks KH, Maisels MJ, et al. Effect of parenteral fat emulsion on the pulmonary and reticuloendothelial system in the newborn infant. Pediatrics 1978;61:694–698.
121. Griffin E, Breckenridge WC, Kuksis A, et al. Appearance and characterization of lipoprotein X during continuous intralipid infusions in the neonate. J Clin Invest 1979;64:1703–1712.
122. Odell GB, Cukier JO, Osterea EM Jr, et al. The influence of fatty acids on the binding of bilirubin to albumin. J Lab Clin Med 1977;89:295–307.
123. Friedman Z, Danonn A, Stahlman, MT, et al. Rapid onset of

essential fatty acid deficiency in the newborn. Pediatrics 1976; 58:640–649.

124. Gilman JT. Therapeutic drug monitoring in the neonate and pediatric age group. Clin Parmacokinet 1990;19:1–10.

125. Reed MD, Besunder JB. Developmental pharmacology: ontogenic basis of drug disposition. Pediatr Clin North Am 1989; 36:1053–1074.

126. Morselli PL. Clinical pharmacology of the perinatal period and early infancy. Clin Parmacokinet 1989;17(Suppl 1):13–28.

127. Gilman JT. Neonatal drug therapy. Int Pediatr 1990;5:311–317.

128. Besunder JB, Reed MD, Blumer JL. Principles of drug biodisposition in the neonate, part 1. Clin Parmacokinet 1988;14: 189–216.

129. Polin RA, Fox WW. Fetal and neonatal physiology. Philadelphia: Saunders 1992:107–178.

130. Besunder JB, Reed MD, Blumer JL. Principles of drug biodisposition in the neonate, part 2. Clin Parmacokinet 1988;14: 261–286.

131. Kearns GL, Reed MD. Clinical pharmacokinetics in infants and children: a reappraisal. Clin Parmacokinet 1989;17(Suppl 1): 29–67.

132. Daily WJ, Smith PC, Mechanical ventilation of the newborn infant. Curr Prob Pediatr 1971;1:3–14.

133. Schwendeman CA, Clark RH, Yoder BA, et al. Frequency of chronic lung disease in infants with severe respiratory failure treated with high-frequency ventilation and/or extracorporeal membrane oxygenation. Crit Care Med 1992;20:372–377.

134. Adolph V, Ekelund C, Smith C, et al. Developmental outcome of neonates treated with extracorporeal membrane oxygenation. J Pediatr Surg 1990;25:43–46.

135. Cornish JD, Clark RH. Alternative therapies for respiratory failure. In Arensman RM, Cornish, JD, eds., Extracorporeal life support. Boston: Blackwell Scientific, 1993:68–88.

136. Clark RH. High-frequency ventilation. J Pediatr 1994;124: 661–670.

137. HiFo Study Group. Randomized study of high-frequency oscillatory ventilation in infants with severe respiratory distress syndrome. J Pediatr 1993;122:609–619.

138. Clark RH, Yoder BA, Sell MS. Prospective randomized comparison of high-frequency oscillation and conventional ventilation in candidates for extracorporeal membrane oxygenation. J Pediatr 1994;124:447–454.

139. Bartlett RH, Gazzaniga AB, Jefferies MR, et al. Extracorporeal membrane oxygenation (ECMO) cardiopulmonary support in infancy. Trans Am Soc Int Organs 1976;22:80–93.

140. Towne GH, Lott IT, Hicks DA, et al. Long-term follow-up of infants and children treated with extracorporeal membrane oxygenation (ECMO): a preliminary report. J Pediatr Surg 1985; 20:410–414.

141. Extracorporeal Life Support Organization. Extracorporeal membrane oxygenation registry report. International summary. July 1996.

142. Extracorporeal Life Support Organization. Extracorporeal membrane oxygenation registry report. James Whitcomb Riley Hospital, Indianapolis, IN. July 1996.

143. Holt PG. Postnatal maturation of immune competence during infancy and early childhood. Pediatr Allergy Immunol 1995; 6:59–70.

144. Holt PG. Immunoprophylaxis of atopy: light at the end of the tunnel? Immunol Today 1994;15:484–489.

145. Holt PG. Environmental factors and primary T-cell sensitization to inhalant allergies in infancy: reappraisal of the role of infectious and air pollution. Pediatr Allergy Immunol 1995;6:1–10.

146. Whitelaw A, Parkin J. Development of immunity. Br Med Bull 1988;44:1037–1051.

147. Wedgwood JF, Palmer R, Weinberger B. Development of the ability to make IgG and IgA in newborns and infants. Mt. Sinai J Med 1994;61:409–415.

148. Hill HR. Host defenses in the neonate: prospects for enhancement. Semin Perinatol 1985;9:2–11.

149. McIntosh N, Kempson C, Tyler RM. Blood counts in extremely low birth weight infants. Arch Dis Child 1988;63:74–76.

150. Fleer A, Gerrards LJ, Aerts P, et al. Opsonic defense to *Staphylococcus epidermidis* in the premature neonate. J Infect Dis 1985;152:930–937.

151. Stevens CE, Neurath RA, Beasley RP, Szmuness W. HBeAg and anti-Hbe detection by radioimmunoassay: correlation with vertical transmission of hepatitis B virus in Taiwan. J Med Virol 1979;3:237–241.

152. Begg NT. Immunoprophylaxis at extremes of age. J Antimicrob Chemother 1994;34:121–128.

153. Expanded Programme on Immunization. EPI for the 1990s. Weekly Epidemiol Rec 1992;67:11–15.

154. Phibbs CS, Bronstein JM, Buxton E, Phibbs RH. The effects of patient volume and level of care at the hospital of birth on neonatal mortality. JAMA 1996;276:1054–1059.

CHAPTER 3

Pediatric Anesthesia

Nancy L. Glass

Many advances in anesthesia have accompanied new initiatives in pediatric surgery. New agents and techniques have been developed that allow for rapid onset and offset of unconsciousness, better analgesia, and fewer side effects during the recovery period. These advances have paralleled other changes in medicine, including the pressure to provide more and more care to patients who will go home early in the postoperative period. Busy operative suites require efficient turnover along with rapid discharge after most routine procedures. Smaller, sicker children arrive on the day of surgery to be cared for by a surgeon who has had little time to prepare and who may have seen the patients only once before, as a result of new pressures and referral patterns from managed care organizations. The child's first contact with the anesthesiologist may be immediately before surgery. Effective care of children under these circumstances depends on good communication among surgeons and anesthesiologists.

New inhalational agents both speed the loss of consciousness and, because of their low solubility in blood, are associated with a quicker recovery. Intravenous drugs with similar recovery properties have also been developed. A greater reliance on regional anesthesia and analgesia, especially in genitourinary surgery, has decreased the requirements for opiate agents, the use of which is frequently accompanied by nausea and vomiting. Improved treatments for pain and postoperative nausea and vomiting facilitate smooth recovery and discharge after surgery.

This chapter focuses on the preparation of children for surgery and on common anesthetic techniques used in genitourinary surgery. For additional information on specific medications, indications, limitations, and dosages, the practitioner should refer to the hospital formulary guide or pediatric drug handbook.[1]

PREOPERATIVE PREPARATION OF THE PATIENT

Preoperative evaluation of the pediatric surgical patient involves a review of the medical history, a physical examination, any indicated laboratory studies, and an assessment of the child's psychological and emotional state. For healthy children, the majority of the preoperative visit is focused on explaining the anesthetic plan to the parents and on securing the child's cooperation and understanding. Instructions for the day of surgery, including fasting (nothing by mouth; NPO) guidelines, are reviewed, and an assessment is made about the need for preoperative sedation. Parental consent for anesthesia care is obtained.

Preoperative laboratory evaluations are limited to the studies indicated for the individual patient. In many facilities, there are no required studies; in others, studies are frequently recommended for specific groups of patients. For example, hemoglobin and hematocrit measures may be advised for children <1 year old in an attempt to ascertain unrecognized nutritional anemias.[2] In some facilities, urine pregnancy tests are required for all menstruating females, regardless of the menstrual history; however, Malviya et al.[3] demonstrated in a prospective study of 525 procedures that the menstrual history was in agreement with the pregnancy test results in each adolescent questioned.

Other tests commonly performed include serum electrolytes for patients taking diuretics and urinalysis for children with chronic infections to rule out bacteriuria when the urinary tract is manipulated. Typing and cross matching for a blood transfusion is generally reserved for procedures in which a large blood loss can be reasonably anticipated. Coagulation profiles are not justifiable without either a patient or a family history of perioperative bleeding.

Upper Respiratory Infections and Fever

The onset of acute illness immediately before scheduled surgery frustrates and disappoints families, surgeons, and anesthesiologists and is the major reason for canceled surgery in pediatric facilities. Of these illnesses, upper respiratory infections (URIs), with their attendant secretions, malaise, and reactive airways, are the most common. The presence of a new onset URI, with cough and coryza, is associated with a higher than usual incidence of laryngospasm and intraoperative wheezing and need for supplemental oxygen in the postoperative period.[4]

In one prospective study, children with a URI were 2 to 7 times more likely to experience adverse respiratory events during the perioperative course than children without a URI; for children who are intubated for the procedure, the risk of respiratory complications was increased 11-fold.[5] Based on concerns about possible complications, conventional teaching has dictated that children with early URIs not undergo elective procedures. But for how long should the surgery be postponed? Airway hyperreactivity can be demonstrated for 4 to 6 weeks after onset of a respiratory infection. And practically speaking, because young children have an average of 8 to 10 URIs per year, it would be difficult to schedule surgery in between infections. Some authors have suggested that a minimum of 2 weeks elapse after onset of infection before rescheduling the procedure. Even at that point, some children will still have increased secretions and a nocturnal cough, but constitutional symptoms should have abated.

There continues to be controversy surrounding the necessity of canceling surgery in otherwise healthy children with URIs. Tait and Knight[6] prospectively studied a cohort of nearly 500 children and found no significant difference in the anesthetic course between children with and without URIs. Similarly, Rolf and Coté[7] reported no increase in laryngospasm but an increased incidence of minor desaturation events and bronchospasm in intubated children with URIs. They concluded, however, that these intraoperative events are minor, easily managed, and without long-term sequelae. Tait et al.[8] demonstrated that the use of a laryngeal mask airway instead of an endotracheal tube was associated with a lower incidence of adverse airway events in children with upper respiratory infections. With these and similar data in mind, many anesthesiologists are now willing to anesthetize otherwise healthy children with URIs who are scheduled for superficial surgery. Whether this practice can be extended to children undergoing more invasive procedures is not clear. Careful attention to detail and meticulous airway care should minimize the risk of perioperative complications for children with URIs.

The sudden onset of fever alone may not require the cancellation of surgery but may serve as a warning that the child is developing a respiratory infection or other acute illness. A careful examination should reveal a likely source. The decision to proceed should take into account whether fever in the postoperative period may confuse assessment of the wound or surgical site.

Chronic Medical Conditions

The presence of chronic medical conditions and their impact on anesthetic care are explored in the preoperative assessment. In general, children with significant chronic conditions should be seen by the pediatrician before elective surgery so that any necessary adjustments to ongoing therapy may be instituted.

Infants who were significantly premature represent a special group and may have multiple organ system involvement and ongoing morbidity. Infants born younger than 37 weeks of gestational age are at risk for postoperative apnea after general anesthesia, even if they did not experience apnea in the neonatal period.[9] How long such infants are at risk is a matter of some controversy. Most hospitals admit these infants for 24 h of postoperative cardiorespiratory monitoring until they have achieved a postconceptual age of 52 to 56 weeks, a standard that varies by institution. These infants also experience a higher than usual incidence of reactive airway disease, most often related to the history of neonatal respiratory distress syndrome. Consequently, they may experience bronchospasm or laryngospasm or may require a period of postoperative ventilation before extubation of the trachea. Cardiac conditions, including some degree of right heart failure and/or pulmonary hypertension, are also common in infants with prolonged lung disease.

Congenital heart anomalies are more common in premature infants than in full-term infants and may require ongoing medical therapy. For older children with congenital heart disease, the condition itself and the nature of the proposed surgery determine the type of preoperative assessment required. Children with functional limitations and those with cyanotic heart disease should see their cardiologist before major or invasive surgery to make sure their condition is optimal. For children without functional limitations, a careful history and physical examination should suffice for anesthesia planning purposes. Prophylaxis for subacute bacterial endocarditis is required for most structural heart lesions. Note that prophylaxis for procedures involving incision or biopsy of surgically scrubbed skin or for circumcision is no longer recommended. The practitioner is referred to the most recent American Heart Association guidelines for specific details.[10]

Children with neurologic conditions may require special preparation for surgery. The child with a static or stable lesion, such as spastic cerebral palsy, presents no special challenges, whereas a child with an unstable seizure pattern may require a medication adjustment before surgery. For a child with an indwelling ventriculoperitoneal shunt, that the surgeon communicate with the neurosurgeon who placed the shunt is essential if the peritoneum will be entered. Exteriorization of the shunt may be necessary if there is a likelihood of bacterial contamination.

Congenital anomalies and genetic conditions may not influence the surgical procedure but may significantly affect the anesthetic care. For example, the surgery for repair of an inguinal hernia in a child with Duchenne muscular dystrophy might be straightforward; but because the child would be at an increased risk for malignant hyperthermia and significant cardiomyopathy, the anesthesia must be a special preparation. In general, the clinician should gather as much information as possible about a child with an unusual condition and must share the information with the anesthesiologist well in advance of the procedure.

Children with asthma should be free from an acute attack at the time of elective surgery. Many parents, on the suggestion of their pediatrician, will intensify maintenance therapy before scheduled surgery to minimize the chances of an exacerbation. Continuing medications and respiratory treatments up to the time of surgery is advisable for children with severe asthma.

Children with sickle-cell disease require special mention, because standard perioperative care for these children has changed considerably in recent years. Hemoglobin electrophoresis determination is no longer required, and exchange transfusions are not routine. Decisions about preoperative transfusion is based on hemoglobin level and the invasiveness of the procedure. For superficial surgery, including most genitourinary and laparoscopic surgery, the updated guidelines are used; for major intra-abdominal procedures, consultation with a hematologist is advised. Simple transfusion to a hematocrit of 30 or 32% and adequate perioperative hydration appear to protect children undergoing peripheral surgery who have no history of perioperative sickle-cell-associated complications and no prior history of acute chest syndrome against sickling in the perioperative period.[11] Koshy et al.[12] demonstrated in a cohort of 3765 children and adults with sickle-cell disease that perioperative transfusions decreased the risk for acute chest syndrome and pain crises in the postoperative period. In their series, there were no perioperative deaths in children <14 years of age. Conventional guidelines for anesthetic care, including attention to hydration, body temperature, and humidification and warming of inhaled gases, still apply.

Consent for Anesthesia

One of the most frequently asked questions by parents is, What are the risks of general anesthesia for children? To some extent, the fear of anesthesia has been enflamed by stories in the tabloid press and from investigative television shows. It is unfortunate for the patients' families that we are asked this question just before the beginning of surgery, when anxieties are heightened. In fact, for most healthy children, the risk of having serious problems from anesthesia (death or disability) is less than the risk of injury traveling to the facility for surgery.

Several studies have attempted to look at the risk of perioperative complications. Cohen et al.[13] examined anesthetic outcomes prospectively in 29,200 procedures at a large pediatric facility from 1982 to 1987. Approximately 95% of the children were healthy (physical status I or II), and nearly half were outpatients. Children <1 month of age were at the highest risk for adverse perioperative events or death; these same children were those most likely to be undergoing major cardiac or abdominal surgery. Overall, the incidence of death was 4 per 10,000 anesthetics in this cohort. The authors did not attempt to separate adverse events or deaths related to the surgical procedure.

Tiret et al.[14] studied 40,240 cases of anesthetics given to pediatric patients in 440 general and pediatric hospitals in France between 1978 and 1982. They found that infants <1 year of age had a higher risk of major anesthetic complications (4.3 per 1000) than do older children (0.5 per 1000), although there were no infant deaths in this series. There was a positive correlation between the risk of anesthetic complications and increasing physical status score, number of co-existing diseases, and emergency nature of the procedure; risks were also associated with a preoperative fasting period of <8 h.

Complications from common regional anesthetic techniques are infrequent and difficult to study. Giaufre et al.[15] published a multi-institutional prospective study of 24,409 French children given general anesthetics, including regional blocks; 60% of these were caudal epidural injections. There were 25 minor incidents involving 24 patients; none resulted in lasting sequelae or medicolegal action. The rate of complications from central blocks was 1.5 per 1000. The authors pointed out that all of the complications occurred in the operating room and were easily managed by experienced anesthesiologists. In an accompanying editorial, Berde[16] noted that the Giaufre et al. study may have underrepresented the true complication rate, because few indwelling epidural catheters were included in the sample and few of the regional blocks included opioids; these techniques are expected to be accompanied by a higher rate of complications outside the operating room. Nevertheless, the use of regional anesthesia by trained anesthesiologists seems to have an acceptable safety record.

In light of the low risk of perioperative death in pediatric patients, Kain et al.[17] asked whether parents wished to be told about the risks of anesthesia during the preoperative interview. In their prospective study, the authors found that most parents wanted to know—and believed they had a right to know—about possible anesthetic complications. Kain et al. concluded that it was appropriate to include the risk of death in a discussion with the parents of anesthetic risks and demonstrated that having such a discussion with the anesthesiologist just before surgery did not increase parental anxiety.

Fasting Guidelines

Traditional guidelines mandating that nothing be ingested after midnight on the day of surgery were based on Mendelson's[18] pivotal 1946 paper that described the pathophysiology of aspiration. Features influencing the severity of gastric aspiration include airway obstruction from aspiration of solid material and the volume and pH of the aspirate. Unfortunately, strict adherence to the NPO-after-midnight standard may mean, for example, that a young child who goes to bed at 8 P.M. and has surgery at 12:00 P.M. the following day may have a 16-h fluid deficit. More recent research has demonstrated that the risk of aspiration in healthy children is extremely low and that ingestion of clear liquids up to 2 h before elective surgery does not alter this risk.[19] Gastric volume and pH were unaffected by the ingestion of clear fluids. Welborn et al.,[20] however, showed that some young patients were actually hypoglycemic after a prolonged fast.

Most pediatric facilities have now liberalized the fasting guidelines, although there remains considerable variation. In general, the ingestion of milk and solids is prohibited after midnight of the surgical day. Clear liquids may be taken as desired until 2 to 4 h before surgery. Preoperative instructions may be altered for children with delayed gastric emptying or gastroesophageal reflux.

There is also disagreement regarding the fasting guidelines for infants who are exclusively breast-fed. In some studies, breast milk was found to clear the stomach faster than does infant formula.[21] Litman et al.[22] compared gastric volumes and acidity in infants who either ingested clear liquids or nursed approximately 2 h before surgery. They found no differences between the groups; however, more of the breast-fed group had residual gastric volumes >1 mL/kg. Even so, a correlation between the rate of gastric emptying (or residual volume) after nursing and the risk of aspiration still cannot be drawn. Without conclusive evidence to support clinical practice, some centers allow breast-feeding until 2 h before the procedure, whereas others require cessation of nursing 3 to 4 h before surgery.

The ingestion of chewing gum or hard candy, frequently offered by parents to satisfy hungry children awaiting surgery, is also somewhat controversial. Chewing gum has traditionally been thought to stimulate gastric secretion and elevate residual volume, so its ingestion was strictly prohibited. Newer studies fail to confirm these findings, although most centers continue restrictions against these products.[23]

Regularly scheduled medications may be taken before surgery, with the possible exception of diuretics, nonsteroidal anti-inflammatory drugs (NSAIDs), and aspirin. Management of the morning insulin dose for diabetics on the day of surgery depends on the child's history, the duration of the expected fasting period, and the type of surgery involved.

When children who have just eaten present for urgent or emergent surgery, the anesthesiologist and surgeon must discuss the need for surgery against the increased risk of regurgitation and aspiration. Because gastric emptying is delayed in children who are acutely ill, anxious, and in pain, waiting an arbitrary number of hours before proceeding may give the physicians a false sense of security that the stomach is empty. In an effort to provide adequate protection from aspiration, allowing urgent surgery to proceed, administer agents that hasten gastric motility and raise gastric pH and use a rapid-sequence induction technique with cricoid pressure.

PREOPERATIVE SEDATION

Since the 1950s clinical practice surrounding the premedication of children for surgery has ranged from sedating all children to sedating a select group. There is general acceptance that many children between the ages of 12 months and 5 to 6 years of age require sedation to facilitate separation from parents at the time of surgery. Not all children in this age group, however, require sedation; some go willingly with an anesthesiologist who is relaxed and friendly and who has taken the time to explain to the patient what he or she can expect in the operating room. Creation of a child-friendly environment, with age-appropriate toys and wagons, promotes cooperation and comfort. Some children with previous anesthetic experience, provided that the experience was positive, develop a familiarity with the induction sequence and may be offered the opportunity to demonstrate some control by selecting the candy flavor for the anesthesia mask.

There is considerable individual variation in the response of the child and parents to the operative experience. The child's personality and coping mechanisms determine, in large part, how he or she is likely to respond to the separation from family members and to the induction of anesthesia. Parental anxiety is readily transmitted to the child; sometimes allaying parental concerns will lessen the milieu of anxiety so that sedation becomes unnecessary. It is helpful to ask the parents about the child's responses to other stressful events, including visits to the doctor and separation from parents (e.g., at daycare, with baby-sitters).

Some children will need preoperative sedation. This group might include patients with developmental delay, for whom a strange environment might be threatening, because age-appropriate coping strategies are absent or delayed. Children who are blind or deaf may also need sedation, because of difficulty communicating their needs and fears to the medical team. Allowing these children to wear hearing or visual aids into the operating room until induction is completed may facilitate a smooth induction. Most children who do not speak or understand the language spoken by members of the operating team should be sedated to ensure their comfort and cooperation.

Younger children may need sedation to ease the separation from their parents, but older children and adolescents undergoing life-threatening or mutilating surgery may have realistic fears about the procedure, postoperative pain, loss of function, and survival. These patients should be offered sedation for anxiolysis, because one of the coping styles of older children—stoic nonchalance—is frequently a cover for considerable anxiety, with its attendant tachycardia, sweating, and hypertension.

Routes of Administration and Medications for Sedation

The fastest route for the administration of sedatives is the intravenous route, which may be difficult in the pediatric outpatient who arrives for surgery without vascular access. Establishing an intravenous line can be accomplished with minimal discomfort if an eutectic mixture of local anesthetic (EMLA) cream is applied over the dorsum of the hand, but it takes 1 h to have an effect.[24] It has been demonstrated that the use of an EMLA cream decreases the pain of starting the intravenous catheter but may not diminish the anxiety associated with the procedure, especially in older children.[25, 26] Medications that can be administered intravenously for sedation include benzodiazepines, ketamine, opiates, barbiturates, and a combination these. Which medication is chosen depends on the time of sedation, proximity to the operating room, and the ability to provide appropriate monitoring after administration of agents that can cause respiratory depression. Opioids are most appropriate when preoperative pain is present, because they are otherwise not ideal sedatives.

Because children are usually afraid of being stuck with a needle, the most popular route for administration of sedatives is the oral route. Midazolam is the most commonly used drug (0.5 to 1.0 mg/kg) and is administered 15 to 30 min before the induction of anesthesia.[27] A lower dose per body weight will work well in older children, if sufficient time is allowed for effect and if the preoperative environment is quiet and soothing. The disadvantages of the oral route include the child refusing to ingest an unpalatable substance, the child spitting out or regurgitating part of the dose, and the time required for absorption and effect. Midazolam's bitter taste has been creatively addressed by many clinicians, because this medication is available only in the parenteral form, which is a hydrochloride salt. One popular suggestion is to suspend the midazolam in 10 to 15 mL of a very concentrated powdered drink.[28] Similar onset and duration may be obtained with the administration of oral ketamine (6 mg/kg).[29] Like midazolam, ketamine has a bitter taste that is difficult to mask; and although ketamine, unlike midazolam, provides analgesia, its use may be associated with a slower arousal and readiness for discharge. For older children, the administration of oral diazepam on arrival at the hospital is an inexpensive option that offers considerable anxiolysis without excessive sedation.

Another approach is oral transmucosal fentanyl, which is fentanyl prepared in a hard candy matrix on a small stick; this preparation depends on direct absorption from the oral mucosa rather than on swallowing and gastric absorption.[30] The child is encouraged to suck on a lozenge that administers 10 to 15 μg/kg fentanyl over 10 to 20 min; thus the patient gradually relaxes. One disadvantage is the potential for respiratory depression, which requires monitoring during and after administration. In addition, there is a significant incidence of nausea and vomiting both before and after surgery.[31] Unfortunately, the use of the fentanyl ℞Oralet does not decrease the opiate needs in the perioperative period, as demonstrated in children undergoing tonsillectomies.[32]

Intranasal administration, like oral dosing, eliminates needle fear. Because the dose is directly absorbed into the systemic circulation, onset times are fast and the doses required are small. Disadvantages include irritation of the nasal mucosa and a bitter taste in the posterior pharynx. Intranasal administration has been described for ketamine, midazolam, and sufentanil.[33]

Intramuscular sedation, which was once the standard of care, is now usually reserved for patients who refuse other routes of sedation and who, by virtue of their size or strength, pose a threat to their own safety or to the safety of the operating room personnel. Pentobarbital, midazolam, and ketamine can all be administered intramuscularly. Use of rectal premedication has likewise decreased in popularity, because of issues of comfort and respect for the child's modesty and privacy; methohexital, ketamine, and midazolam have all been given by this route.[34]

It is important to recognize that the administration of sedation in doses high enough to ease anxiety may be accompanied by respiratory depression or loss of airway reflexes. Sedatives should be given by personnel who are trained to monitor for these effects and who understand that sedation is part of a continuum leading to the induction of anesthesia. Considerable individual variation in response is the expected norm.

Disadvantages of Preoperative Sedation

Disadvantages to preoperative sedation include incomplete or inadequate sedation, delay of surgery while waiting for the sedatives to work, and paradoxical effects of sedation. For most commonly used oral sedatives, it is difficult to demonstrate that the use of premedication delays discharge from the postanesthesia care unit (PACU). In a cohort of children younger than 3 years who required myringotomies, I found that premedication with midazolam for this short procedure was related to an increased incidence of postoperative delirium; this effect was exacerbated in the absence of effective analgesia. Use of long-acting sedatives (e.g., such as droperidol, thiopental, and promethazine) may be accompanied by a delayed return to consciousness after short surgery.

Alternatives to Preoperative Sedation

Alternatives to preoperative sedation require preoperative preparation of the child and parents and may include tours of the operating room facility, which can be conducted by nurses, Child Life professionals, or trained hospital volunteers. Familiarity with the environment, equipment, and smells of the operating room may eliminate the need for sedation. Increasingly, hospitals are providing videotapes or books for use with the tours to prepare young children for surgery. Expectations for the anesthetic and surgical experience can be discussed, and the child's questions can be addressed.

Other behavioral approaches to facilitate cooperation include taking the children to the operating room in wagons or on riding toys instead of stretchers and letting the patients enter the operating room in their own clothes. Allowing the child to pick the candy flavor for the mask, playing induction games (such as blowing up the balloon and counting the breaths on the capnograph), and using age-appropriate induction stories are likely to result in a smooth induction. I recommend that a healthy child be allowed to go to sleep while sitting upright on the operating room table or in someone's lap, and I delay placing the monitors until the child begins to get sleepy.

Some facilities allow the parents to be present at the induction of anesthesia as a means of avoiding separation anxiety. Parents may be invited into the operating room itself in cover gowns or scrub attire or into an induction room outside the clean corridor. In general, the parents should not be present for induction of children <1 year of age, of children with difficult airway anatomy, or of children who require a rapid-sequence induction for emergency surgery. Advantages of allowing the parents to be with the patient include eliminating the need for preoperative sedation and providing parental and patient satisfaction. Disadvantages to this practice include excessive parental anxiety that is transmitted to the child, parental distress at watching a young child struggle during induction, and parental syncope. In addition, if the induction is not done in the operating room, extra equipment is needed for maintaining anesthesia and monitoring during transport.

Remember that the purpose of allowing the parents to be present at induction is the comfort of the child. The anesthesiologist should be the only individual charged with the ultimate responsibility for choosing the patient–parent duo who would benefit from this induction option. Parents whose goals include watching the anesthesiologist to make sure he or she is doing the job correctly are poor candidates for the induction room. Parents who are excessively and demonstratively anxious will not be able to help their child, and parental presence may not prevent resistance to the mask or to the odor of the anesthetic. Kain[35] noted that the children benefiting most from parental presence at induction are not the youngest children with separation anxiety but the calm, older child with parents of a similar temperament.

Parental presence at induction cannot be seen as a way of hastening room turnover, because both anesthesiologist and circulating nurse must be present. The operating room must be fully prepared before induction; all appropriate support equipment, including intravenous supplies and airway management tools should be assembled in the induction room, even if their use is not expected in that location. A transport stretcher, monitors, oxygen supply, and volatile anesthetic vaporizer are required.

As expected, there are differences in practice among facilities regarding parental presence at induction. Because of the effort required in this endeavor, it is important to determine whether the benefits of this practice outweigh the disadvantages and potential costs. Several ongoing studies are comparing parental presence with preoperative sedation of children of different ages.

INDUCTION OF ANESTHESIA

The most common induction techniques are inhalation and intravenous induction; preference for one technique over the other for healthy children is based largely on institutional practice and individual habit. Monitoring during induction and maintenance of anesthesia include heart rate and blood pressure, oxygen saturation, temperature, and some measure of adequacy of ventilation (capnography, anesthesiologist's hand on the bag during spontaneous ventilation, precordial stethoscope). Auditory alarms on the anesthesia machine assist but do not replace observation and auscultation.

Inhalation

Inhalation induction with either halothane or sevoflurane and nitrous oxide in oxygen is the most commonly performed induction sequence in the United States. Allowing the nitrous oxide to take effect for 45 to 60 s before adding the more pungent volatile agent minimizes resistance. Another technique is to hold the mask close to the child's face without actually touching it until the anesthetic effect begins. Allow older children to choose the flavor of candy oil the anesthesiologist rubs inside the mask to give them a measure of control during induction and facilitate acceptance of the unfamiliar odors of the mask and anesthetic. Other distraction techniques (e.g., singing, telling stories, and rocking during induction) are practiced by many skilled anesthesiologists. Sevoflurane, the newest anesthetic agent, has an odor that is well accepted by most children and provides a faster induction than does halothane.[36] This property is particularly helpful if the child begins to struggle on induction, as unconsciousness can be rapidly achieved using high concentrations in only a few breaths.

Intravenous

For the child who arrives in the operating room with an intravenous line already in place, induction of anesthesia can be easily accomplished with injection of an agent or combination of agents that might include a barbiturate, propofol, ketamine plus a benzodiazepine, or opioid. Again, the choice of agent is guided by the child's condition, anesthetic requirements for the procedure, and the practitioner's preference. Thiopental, the intravenous induction agent to which all others are compared, provides a rapid onset of sleep with doses of 3 to 5 mg/kg; return to consciousness occurs within 10 to 15 min after a single dose. Thiopental has no analgesic properties, provides no muscle relaxation, and does not suppress airway reflexes adequately for intubation with a single induction dose. Discomfort upon injection is minimal.

Faster awakening with less residual effect is associated with propofol, a newer agent. In addition, propofol has a narcotic-sparing effect, i.e., less opiate is required for a given procedure than if thiopental were the induction agent.[37] Although there may some intrinsic antiemetic effect from propofol, the requirement for less narcotic contributes to less nausea and vomiting and facilitates earlier discharge from day surgery. Unfortunately, the injection of propofol is quite painful, particularly when administered into the small veins of the dorsum of the hand. This effect can be mitigated by administering lidocaine before the injection, adding lidocaine to the mixture, or giving an earlier dose of either ketamine or alfentanil. It should be noted that dose requirements for both induction and maintenance are higher in children than in adults.[38]

Both thiopental and propofol can cause a significant decrease in cardiac output, related to a decrease in venous return; most children respond with tachycardia. For children who are hypovolemic or who have underly-

ing cardiac disease, the resulting hypotension may be poorly tolerated. For these children, ketamine may be the preferred choice, either by itself, or in combination with a benzodiazepine or opiate, because the sympathomimetic effects may support cardiac output during induction. Ketamine is the only induction agent that also provides analgesia.

Intramuscular

Intramuscular induction may be the preferred route for an uncooperative child who arrives in the operating room without an intravenous line and who will not tolerate an inhalation induction. Ketamine, midazolam, and methohexital are all possible choices for an intramuscular induction and may be combined with antisialagogues or muscle relaxants.[34] Faster induction has been accomplished with injection into the deltoid muscle than into the lateral thigh.

Rectal

Induction of anesthesia with the administration of rectal medications is a technique preferred in a few institutions. The smooth transition from sedation to the induction of anesthesia is a reported advantage, and allowing parents to be present during drug administration may be comforting to the child. Methohexital and thiopental are the most commonly used agents. Disadvantages include stooling after administration with loss of drug and effect, and the potential for development of proctitis with methohexital. The use of thiopental may prolong recovery and delay discharge; methohexital does not cause a similar delay.[34] Rectal induction is rarely appropriate after the age of toilet training. This technique will probably become even less common as practitioners accumulate more experience with the newer sedative agents.

MAINTENANCE OF ANESTHESIA

For the majority of children undergoing genitourinary surgery, the maintenance of anesthesia is provided via a balanced technique consisting of volatile anesthetic agents with or without nitrous oxide, neuromuscular blocking agents, and intravenous opiates. Once the trachea has been intubated, maintenance of neuromuscular blockade is seldom required for groin surgery but may facilitate both opening and closing of midline abdominal wounds and costal incisions in the lateral (kidney) position. In many cases, a regional anesthetic block, administered before the incision, is used to supplement intraoperative anesthesia and to provide postoperative analgesia. Another popular technique is the continuous infusion of propofol (50 to 150 μg/kg/min), used alone or to supplement nitrous oxide and a volatile agent;

rapid arousal is an advantage of this technique. Adjunctive agents, including antiemetics, may also be administered.

Airway Management

Choice of airway management technique for a given procedure depends on the patient's underlying condition, whether there will be a surgical requirement for muscle relaxation and controlled ventilation, and to some extent on the expected duration of the procedure. Controlling the airway by placing an endotracheal tube is the standard technique to which all others are compared. Intubation of the trachea protects the patient from regurgitation and aspiration of gastric contents and allows the application of continuous positive airway pressure to for either spontaneous or controlled ventilation. The development of laryngospasm with traction on the spermatic cord is also prevented with intubation, although the patient can still cough and strain unless adequate anesthetic levels and/or muscle relaxation are also given.

Mask ventilation with spontaneous respirations is the simplest technique and is appropriate for many healthy children undergoing common urology procedures, including inguinal hernia repair. It is the least traumatic way to manage the airway and is associated with the lowest incidence of postoperative sore throat.

The laryngeal mask airway (LMA) is a relatively new device; it consists of a cuffed airway that sits in the posterior pharynx.[39,40] The LMA avoids instrumentation of the vocal cords and is associated with a lower incidence of sore throat than is endotracheal intubation. Although it was designed primarily for use in spontaneously breathing patients, controlled ventilation can be done with the LMA if strict attention is given to avoiding excessive pressures and gastric distention. Contraindications to its use include obesity, known gastroesophageal reflux, and a full stomach. One advantage to the LMA in urology patients is that it frees up the hands of the anesthesiologist for performing regional anesthetic blocks.

Fluid Management

After the induction of anesthesia, an intravenous catheter is placed to establish a route for the administration of medications and fluid. For most healthy children, isotonic fluid replacement with lactated Ringer's solution is an acceptable choice. Fluids are administered with the goals of providing hourly maintenance fluids, replacing the fasting deficit, replacing estimated blood loss, and accounting for third space losses. The intravenous line offers a route for the immediate delivery of emergency medications, should those be necessary. Addition of dextrose to the intravenous fluids may be ap-

propriate for the smallest infants, for diabetic patients who are also receiving insulin, and for children receiving parenteral nutrition.

Although many formulas have been recommended for fluid administration, one simple guideline is the 4–2–1 rule: The hourly maintenance rate for a child is 4 mL/kg for the first 10 kg body weight, 2 mL/kg for the second 10 kg, and 1 mL/kg for each kg thereafter. The hourly maintenance rate is then multiplied by the number of hours the child fasted to calculate the fasting deficit. Some practitioners replace all of the fasting deficit before discharging the patient from the hospital, whereas others are more lax as long as the child is awake and tolerating oral fluids. Cardiovascular responses to fluid administration and blood loss guide fluid therapy during more extensive procedures, and placement of a urinary catheter is recommended for long procedures or when considerable dissection and third space fluid losses are anticipated.

REGIONAL ANESTHESIA AS AN ADJUNCT TO GENERAL ANESTHESIA

There has been an explosion of interest in regional anesthetic techniques in pediatric anesthesia practice. Regional techniques provide a continuum of analgesia, extending from the intraoperative to the postoperative period. Only rarely are these techniques used alone in children, who may not tolerate being awake during surgery. One exception is the use of the subarachnoid block (spinal anesthesia) in formerly premature infants still at risk for postoperative apnea in whom common urology procedures may be done without general anesthesia.

It is a far more common practice to perform a regional block after induction but before the incision. It is then easy to demonstrate a decreased requirement for volatile anesthetic after the block is established, particularly for lumbar and caudal epidurals. More limited nerve blocks can be similarly effective if done before the incision. Regional blocks decrease opiate requirements both in the operating room and in the PACU and thus decrease the incidence of postoperative nausea and vomiting. Aside from decreased anesthetic requirements, a combined general and regional technique allows for the rapid recovery of consciousness and ensures patient comfort upon awakening. Epidural and spinal anesthesia have also been shown to blunt the hormonal response to the stress of surgery.

One disadvantage of combining general and regional anesthesia is a slight increase in the time required to prepare the patient for surgery. In most cases, this time is recovered at the conclusion of the procedure because the patient rapidly awakens. The theoretical disadvantage of exposing the patient to the risks of both general and regional anesthesia has not been confirmed in clinical studies. There is, however, the issue of an undesired motor blockade at the end of surgery, a problem that is largely avoidable when dilute concentrations of local anesthetics are used. The time to first void can also be increased by the use of neuraxial blocks, but rarely requires intervention. Because many day surgery units no longer require patients to void before discharge, a slight delay in the first void should not prolong the hospital stay.

SPECIFIC REGIONAL ANESTHETIC AND ANALGESIC TECHNIQUES

For many urology procedures several different regional blocks will provide effective surgical anesthesia and postoperative analgesia. The choice of block may depend on the age of the child, parental expectations, and the preferences of the anesthesiologist and surgeon.

Analgesia for Circumcision

Anesthesia for circumcision can be done with the application of local anesthetic gel, EMLA cream, a ring block of the penis, a dorsal penile nerve block (DPNB), or a caudal epidural block. For either lidocaine gel or EMLA cream to be most effective for circumcision, the foreskin must be retractable. It is important to note that EMLA cream is not approved by the U.S. Food and Drug Administration for application to mucosal surfaces. There is a risk of developing methemoglobinemia from absorption of the prilocaine component, especially in the neonate. In a recent report[41] describing the use of EMLA cream for circumcision in 68 infants, however, this complication was not seen.

The ring block of the penis and the DPNB are both simple and effective blocks for providing distal penile analgesia and can be performed by either the urologist or the anesthesiologist. Injecting a ring of local anesthesia into the skin at the base of the penis provides effective analgesia for circumcision.[42] The classic DPNB, with a midline injection beneath Buck's fascia, provides effective penile analgesia but carries the risk of puncturing the corpus cavernosa, which results in gangrene.[43] The subpubic approach to the DPNB[44] requires two injections into the space below Buck's fascia but carries a lower risk of damaging neurovascular structures. Either lidocaine or bupivacaine can be used; the effects of lidocaine last 1 to 1.5 h, whereas bupivacaine provides 4 to 6 h of pain relief. Epinephrine should not be included in any penile block.

Caudal Epidural Block

The caudal epidural block is the most commonly performed regional block in children. It is used to provide analgesia for procedures below the diaphragm, including circumcision, inguinal hernia repair, hypospadias repair, ureteral reimplantation, and orchidopexy. The caudal block is performed with the child in the lateral position and the hips flexed onto the abdomen. Local anesthetic is injected through the sacral hiatus, which forms where the lowest sacral vertebrae fail to fuse. The sacral hiatus is readily palpated in children from the neonatal period through adolescence.

Needle choice for this block varies. I recommend a blunt, short-bevel needle attached to a syringe; other authors prefer intravenous catheters or butterfly needles. The issues relating to needle choice are identification of the caudal space, stabilization of the needle during injection of local anesthetic, avoidance of puncturing the subarachnoid membrane, and the detection or prevention of an intravascular injection of local anesthetic. For more complex procedures, when a continuous caudal technique is chosen, a standard epidural catheter may be threaded into the caudal space using either a Tuohy or a Crawford epidural needle.

Choice of medication for caudal block depends on the goals for analgesia and the desired duration of the block. For most outpatient procedures, a dilute concentration of bupivacaine, lidocaine, or ropivacaine is selected. The use of lidocaine is associated with a greater degree of motor blockade and a shorter duration of action than is bupivacaine or ropivacaine. Between 4 and 6 h of analgesia can be expected from caudal bupivacaine; the use of concentrations >0.25% may result in significant motor block at the conclusion of the procedure.[45] Ropivacaine, the newest local anesthetic agent, has less potential for cardiac toxicity than does bupivacaine, even in the event of unexpected intravascular injection.[46] The addition of epinephrine to local anesthetics increases the intensity and duration of the block by decreasing systemic absorption.[47] In young infants anesthetized with halothane, however, the addition of epinephrine to bupivacaine has been associated with ventricular tachycardia or bradycardia with ST-T wave changes.[48,49]

The addition of an opiate to caudal epidural analgesia has gained in popularity, especially for the more extensive procedures, such as the complicated hypospadias repair. Fentanyl added to the local anesthetic prolongs the duration of caudal analgesia and permits the use of a more dilute solution of local anesthetic, decreasing the risk of motor blockade and urinary retention.[50] The administration of caudal morphine, with or without local anesthetic, may provide analgesia lasting up to 24 h for abdominal procedures. This duration of effect is only loosely associated with the dose given; but higher doses are accompanied by a higher incidence of respiratory depression, pruritus, and somnolence.

Because the time of greatest risk for respiratory depression from caudal fentanyl occurs with systemic absorption soon after injection, discharge from the hospital following most procedures need not be delayed. Respiratory depression from epidural morphine, however, may be delayed 6 to 12 h after administration; this will necessitate admission of the patient to a special care unit where respiratory monitoring can be accomplished, either with pulse oximetry, respiratory telemetry, or hourly observation and counting of the respiratory rate. Infants younger than 1 year old are more susceptible to respiratory depression with both fentanyl and morphine than are older children.[50] And just as with systemic administration, all epidural opiates have the potential to cause nausea and vomiting, so prophylactic administration of antiemetics should be considered.

Ilioinguinal–Iliohypogastric Block

The ilioinguinal–iliohyppogastric block is less commonly performed than the caudal epidural. This block is appropriate for inguinal hernia repair, varicocele ligation, and orchidopexy but not for surgery on the testis. The nerves can be directly injected by the surgeon at the time of exposure; filling the wound with local anesthetic and allowing the drug to remain there for several minutes also blocks these nerves. These approaches do not provide pre-emptive analgesia and may not completely anesthetize the incision. Another approach is to inject at the point where the nerves are closest to the skin: 0.5 to 1.0 cm medial to and inferior to the anterior superior iliac spine. A blunt needle is inserted perpendicularly to the skin until a fascial pop is felt, indicating that the needle has penetrated the aponeurosis of the external oblique muscle. About two-thirds of the calculated dose of local anesthetic is injected beneath the muscle fascia, and the remainder is injected into the subcutaneous space as the needle is removed. A modification of this block[51] includes a second injection at the level of the external ring to block the peripheral ilioinguinal nerve. If the second injection is done before the procedure for pre-emptive analgesia, it may distort the anatomy during dissection. Other common problems with the ilioinguinal–iliohypogastric block are the need to supplement analgesia in the PACU and a transient weakness in the distribution of the femoral nerve.

The ilioinguinal–iliohypogastric block is ideal for older children and adolescents undergoing a unilateral hernia repair. Absence of motor weakness, which may be seen transiently with caudal blocks, is an advantage in this age group. One additional benefit is not having to move a larger child in the lateral position while anesthetized.

A number of studies have attempted to compare different blocks for postoperative analgesia in children. Several reports show that caudal analgesia and the ilioinguinal–iliohypogastric block are roughly equivalent for pain relief after hernia repair and orchidopexy.[52,53] Tobias et al.,[54] however, reported the caudal block was more efficacious for hernia repairs when laparoscopic inspection of the peritoneum was included in the procedure. Blaise and Roy[55] reported that caudal analgesia was more effective than either penile block or systemic analgesics for boys undergoing hypospadias repair.

Continuous Epidural Anesthesia

Continuous epidural anesthesia is generally limited to patients who will be staying in the hospital after major procedures. Examples of urology procedures for which continuous epidural analgesia would be ideal are ureteral reimplantation, bladder repair, and pyeloplasty. In most children, placement of epidural catheters is done after the induction of anesthesia. One exception to this might be the placement of thoracic epidural catheters; ideally, the practitioner should be able to question the child about paresthesias when inserting this catheter. Because of the risks involved, thoracic catheters should be placed only by experienced physicians.

Commercial epidural kits are widely available and contain an ever-widening variety of needle styles and catheters; personal preference and experience dictate choice. For most children, the larger catheters are easy to place and are associated with a lower incidence of kinking and other difficulties in the postoperative period. Key issues are the integrity of the connection between the catheter and the infusion tubing and the reliability and flexibility of the infusion pump. But most important is the ability of the anesthesiologist to provide 24-h management of epidural analgesia: trouble-shooting, response to emergency situations, patient evaluation, and adjustments to therapy. Despite the advantages of epidural therapy, its use requires an intense professional commitment.

Ideally, the catheter tip will be placed in close proximity to the surgical site. When this can be done, a dilute concentration of local anesthetic, combined with an opioid and infused at a minimal rate, provides excellent analgesia. If the catheter tip cannot be placed close to the surgical site or if the incision is a long vertical one, higher infusion rates will be necessary; motor blockade and urinary retention are more common in this situation.

Surgical anesthesia can be provided with boluses of local anesthesia or by continuous infusion. Doses of local anesthetic required for surgical anesthesia are generally higher than those required for postoperative analgesia. Attention must be paid to maximum total doses, expressed as milligrams per kilogram per hour. Opioids are also commonly administered.

Spinal Anesthesia

There has been a resurgence of interest in spinal anesthesia in children, particularly for the formerly premature infant undergoing surgery. This population is particularly prone to postoperative apnea after general anesthesia, whether or not the infant experienced apnea in the postnatal period.[56] The risk is highest in infants <52 weeks postconceptual age, but isolated reports of apnea following general anesthesia have occurred in infants up to 60 weeks postconceptual age.

Spinal anesthesia allows the surgeon to perform lower abdominal, groin, and lower extremity procedures without administering general anesthesia or manipulating of the airway. One limitation is that the doses of local anesthesia do not last as long in young infants compared with older children or adults. For example, tetracaine (0.4 mg/kg) with glucose and epinephrine will give approximately 90 min of operating time, which may be insufficient for some procedures.[57] The addition of epinephrine prolongs the duration of the block.

Other technical aspects of successful spinal anesthesia in infants include inserting the intravenous line in the lower extremity after the block has been placed. Blood pressure does not fall in infants after spinal anesthesia, so fluid loading is not required.[58] In addition, blood pressure can be measured on a lower extremity to avoid disturbing the infant while the procedure is under way. Although performing the lumbar puncture is generally simple, having a skilled baby holder is crucial; the neck must be supported in the neutral position if the spinal is done while the infant is sitting to prevent airway obstruction. And finally, it is important to minimize the fasting period carefully, offering glucose water up to 2 h before the procedure so that the infant will not be excessively fussy and fidgety.

The hungry, fussy infant may tempt the practitioner to administer a mild sedative. The benefits of spinal anesthesia in this special population of former premature infants at risk for postoperative apnea are eliminated by sedation, as demonstrated in a prospective study that compared general and spinal anesthesia.[59] Because later studies reported apnea after regional anesthesia without sedation, in practice, most facilities still admit infants who are at risk for postoperative apnea for overnight observation, even if a spinal or caudal anesthetic was performed.[60,61]

EMERGENCE FROM ANESTHESIA

When the operative procedure is complete, the anesthetic is discontinued. The stomach and oropharynx are suctioned. Any residual neuromuscular blockade is reversed, if applicable. The endotracheal tube or LMA is removed when the patient has recovered airway reflexes and established a regular breathing pattern. Supplemental doses of pain medication may be administered if necessary.

When it has been determined that the patient's airway is secure, the child may be transported to the PACU. Decisions to transport the patient with oxygen depend on the presence of underlying cardiorespiratory conditions, adequacy of air exchange, and distance from the operating room to the PACU. After vital signs and airway patency have been checked, the anesthesiologist gives to the PACU nurse a report that details the anesthetic course, including pertinent history, induction and anesthetic techniques, untoward intraoperative events, and medications administered.

DISCHARGE FROM THE PACU

Each PACU must establish criteria for discharge to home or transfer to an inpatient unit. The Aldrete and Kroulik[62] recovery score is a simple scoring system that assigns points to each of five criteria: activity level, respirations, circulation (blood pressure), consciousness, and color. The Steward recovery score is similar but is geared toward a simpler evaluation of children.[63] Regardless of which scoring system is used, the criteria for discharge from the PACU to the home setting must require that the child be awake or easily arouseable, be free from pain and nausea, and be able to maintain normal oxygen saturation on room air without airway support. It is notable that neither the Aldrete and Kroulik nor the Steward scoring system identifies children whose oxygen saturation is >95%, because these systems were established before the development of the pulse oximeter.[64] Vital signs need to be within normal range for age and should approximate preadmission vital signs for that child. Ambulation is not necessary for infants and toddlers but is necessary for older children and adolescents.

For patients being admitted to the hospital, recovery parameters are similar, except that patients do not need to be able to ambulate or tolerate oral fluids. Some children who are admitted to the hospital after major abdominal surgery may require the administration of oxygen by mask or nasal cannula for 12 to 24 h postsurgery and monitoring of pulse oximetry until room air saturation is adequate.

POSTOPERATIVE ANALGESIA

For children who are discharged on the day of surgery, awakening from anesthesia pain free is the first step in effective postoperative pain management. This can be accomplished with regional anesthesia, intravenous opiates, intravenous ketorolac, or a combination of these. Rectal acetaminophen (40 mg/kg) at the beginning of the procedure can be a helpful adjunct.[65] Supplemental intravenous opiates may be given as needed in the PACU before discharge, and a discharge prescription for oral pain medication should be provided by the surgeon (Table 3.1).

There are several choices for postoperative analgesia for patients remaining in the hospital after major genitourinary surgery. Often, such therapy is a continuation of intraoperative management and should certainly be part of the presurgery discussion with the patient and parents.

TABLE 3.1. *Postoperative pain management: oral therapy*

Agent	Formulation	Dosage
Acetaminophen	• Liquid: 80, 120, 160, 325 mg/5 mL • Tab: 80, 160, 325, 500, 650 mg	10–15 mg/kg q4h
Ibuprofen	• Liquid: 100 mg/5 mL • Tab: 200, 400, 600, 800 mg	4–10 mg/kg q6–8h
Ketorolac	• Tab: 10 mg	0.1–0.2 mg/kg q6h[a]
Acetaminophen plus codeine	• Liquid: (A 120 mg + C 12 mg)/5 mL • Tab: A 325 mg + C various	1 mg/kg q4h[b]
Acetaminophen plus hydrocodone (℞Vicodin)	• Liquid: (A 120 mg + H 2.5 mg)/5 mL • Tab: A 500 mg + H 2.5 or 5 mg	0.1–0.2 mg/kg q4h[c]
Meperidine	• Liquid: 5 mg/5 mL	1–1.5 mg/kg q4h

[a]Total of 5 days only.
[b]Based on codeine.
[c]Based on hydrocodone.

Following the practice in most pediatric facilities, I discourage the use of intramuscular opiates on an as-needed basis. Children will deny pain and suffer needlessly when pain relief requires an injection. The use of intramuscular agents is associated with a slow onset of analgesia and may be difficult to titrate to the level of pain experienced. Contrary to traditional teaching, the use of intramuscular agents does not protect the patient from excessive sedation or respiratory depression from the opiate.

Intravenous Analgesia

The simplest technique is the use of intermittent doses of intravenous opiate given at scheduled intervals (Table 3.2). For example, intravenous morphine administered every 2 h will maintain patient comfort in most instances, as long as the dose ordered is sufficient. If the patient is excessively sedated, the dose can be decreased, maintaining the 2-h interval. Clearance is prolonged in neonates, so adjustments in dose and interval may be necessary. The success of the scheduled intermittent dosing depends on timely nursing observation and response if the analgesia provided is insufficient. As-needed dosing is likely to result in significant periods of patient discomfort and may negatively affect sleep quality.

Other choices include intermittent doses of meperidine, methadone, or hydromorphone. Meperidine remains a popular choice for postoperative pain; however, meperidine differs from morphine in that intravenous administration may depress cardiac output and result in tachycardia.[66] Continued administration of meperidine over several days may lead to the accumulation of metabolites that cause delirium, tremors, and convulsions.[67] Thus it should be limited to short-term use. Meperidine has a long half-life, provides excellent analgesia, and may be appropriate for severe pain and for chronic or terminal use. Hydromorphone provides similar analgesia to that of morphine, but its use may be associated with fewer side effects. Morphine remains the gold standard for pain relief for most children.

Ketorolac is the only NSAID that is available in parenteral form for use in the perioperative period. In one study of pediatric surgical patients undergoing superficial procedures, ketorolac (0.9 mg/kg) compared favorably with morphine (0.1 mg/kg), with less postoperative emesis.[68] It has also compared favorably with caudal bupivacaine for children undergoing hernia repair. Other studies have confirmed that ketorolac is effective for mild to moderate postoperative pain but may not be sufficient by itself for more invasive procedures. Disadvantages include concerns about intraoperative and postoperative bleeding. Whether ketorolac is appropriate for a given procedure may depend on the surgical site.

In addition, like other NSAIDs, ketorolac may be associated with renal failure, even in the absence of pre-existing renal disease.[69] The manufacturer recommends limiting total (intravenous and oral) ketorolac therapy

TABLE 3.2. *Postoperative pain management: intravenous therapy*

	Intermittent dosing		Patient-controlled analgesia				Maximum dose, mg/kg/h
Agent	Dose, mg/kg	Frequency, h	Concentration	Bolus	Interval, min	Basal infusion, kg/h	
Morphine	0.1	2–3	1 or 5 mg/mL	10–30 µg/kg	6–10	10–30 µg	0.1–0.15
Fentanyl	0.001	1–2	10 µg/mL	0.5–1 µg/kg	6–10	0.5–1 µg	0.002–0.004
Hydromorphone	0.015	3–4	0.5 or 1 mg/mL	3–5 µg/kg	6–10	3–5 µg	0.015–0.02
Meperidine	1.0	2–3	10 mg/mL	0.15–0.25 mg/kg	6–10	0.15–0.25 mg	1.0
Ketorolac	0.5[a]	6					

[a]Up to a maximum of 30 mg; maximum daily dose = 120 mg. Limited to 5 days of therapy.

to 5 days, because of the risk of serious gastrointestinal bleeding. The drug should be discontinued immediately if epigastric pain or dark stools develop. Although ketorolac is not a replacement for potent opioids in the treatment of postoperative pain, it may significantly decrease opiate requirements, thereby minimizing sedation, nausea, and vomiting.

The use of patient-controlled analgesia (PCA) pumps for children has gained wide acceptance. Children over the age of approximately 5 years are able to associate pushing the PCA button with pain relief and can be encouraged to use the button if they are uncomfortable. Younger children who have experience playing video games may be able to understand the relationship between pushing a button and receiving medication for pain; successful PCA use has been described in children as young as 2 and 3 years old. Several institutions have begun to allow parents to administer analgesia when the parents clearly understand the importance of the child being awake before administering the next dose of medication. In situations in which the parents are not judged suitable for this role, the nursing staff can manage the pump. Nurse-controlled analgesia eliminates many of the clerical and nursing barriers to adequate analgesia and saves the time required to prepare an intravenous dose. The need to respond frequently and promptly, however, may limit this option in busy nursing units.

Medications that have been used for PCA pumps include morphine, meperidine, fentanyl, and hydromorphone. Morphine is the most frequently used; for patients who experience severe itching, fentanyl or hydromorphone may be substituted. Meperidine is not recommended for use beyond 3 or 4 days, because of concerns about excitement, delirium, and possible seizures. Hydromorphone is a good alternative to morphine if side effects are troubling.

For older children who have undergone upper abdominal or thoracic procedures or who have extensive incisions, standard PCA regimens may not provide adequate analgesia at night. Such patients awaken in pain when the plasma level of the opiate falls below a threshold level; a number of interval doses will be required, perhaps over more than 1 h, before these patients are comfortable enough to fall asleep again. To solve this problem, it may be necessary to provide a background infusion of opiate in addition to the PCA dosing schedule. A continuous infusion will facilitate nighttime analgesia but may need to be discontinued during the day if the patient remains excessively somnolent.

Epidural Analgesia

Epidural analgesia is commonly used to provide pain relief after abdominal and pelvic procedures, generally as a continuation of intraoperative anesthetic care. Although thoracic epidurals are provided in some centers for upper abdominal or thoracic procedures, this technique should be performed by only practitioners with training and expertise in this area. Standard epidural catheters can be placed either by the caudal or by the lumbar route. Many investigators have reported success in threading caudal catheters up to the thoracic area in young infants, but this practice generally becomes more difficult the older the patient.[70,71] The main disadvantage to the caudal route is the possibility of fecal soiling and contamination of the catheter in young children. Lumbar epidural catheters can be placed without difficulty even in neonates.

The choice of infusion varies among institutions but most commonly consists of both dilute local anesthetic and opiate. Occasionally, only opiate is used. Some degree of motor blockade with a combined technique is not uncommon; and for this reason, many patients with postoperative epidurals require maintenance of the urinary catheter. Children receiving local anesthetics via the epidural route should ambulate only with assistance. To maximize flexibility of the analgesia provided, some pain services offer patient-controlled epidural analgesia (PCEA). The primary advantage of this technique is that it allows the patient the opportunity to self-administer analgesia before uncomfortable procedures or physical therapy.

The most common side effects of epidural therapy are nausea and vomiting, motor blockade, oversedation, and pruritus.[72] Premature (unintended) catheter removal is sometimes necessary for leaking at the skin insertion site, occlusion of the catheter, unilateral analgesia, local erythema or infection, or other catheter-related reason. Backache has commonly been reported in adults after the use of lumbar epidural anesthesia but is less often reported in children.

Weaning from epidural therapy, as from intravenous opiates, generally occurs 1 to 4 days postsurgery, when the child begins to tolerate oral fluids. One practice is to administer oral analgesics after the epidural infusion has been stopped; if analgesia is adequate, the catheter is removed. If the chest has been entered or after a thoracotomy for a Wilms tumor, the physician might leave the epidural in place until the chest tube has been removed.

Oral Analgesia

Oral pain medications are ideal if the patient tolerates oral fluids or if it is time to wean the patient from intravenous or epidural therapy, generally 1 to 3 days after major surgery. Simple analgesics, such as acetaminophen and ibuprofen, can considerably decrease the amount of more potent agents required, either by the intravenous or the oral route. One strategy is to order acetaminophen or ibuprofen on a scheduled basis; then to administer more potent agents for severe or break-through pain. Another strategy is to transfer the patient from intravenous therapy to a combination of an oral opioid and a simple analgesic, such as acetaminophen with codeine or oxycodone. Multiple different preparations are available in liquid, tablet, and capsule form. Tolerance of one agent in preference over another is largely a matter of individual variation. The practitioner should be familiar with several choices and with the equipotent doses of each. Oxycodone may be tolerated better than codeine.

COMMON POSTOPERATIVE PROBLEMS

The administration of opiates, either parenterally or as a part of a regional anesthetic technique, increases the likelihood of postoperative nausea and vomiting. Other contributing factors include the kind of surgery performed, the level of preoperative anxiety, the anesthetic technique, previous history of postoperative emesis, and a history of motion sickness during long automobile trips. Forcing early postoperative oral fluids has also been associated with an increased incidence of postoperative emesis.[73] It should also be recognized that vomiting after hernia repair or orchidopexy may be related to inadequately treated pain.[34] Medications associated with a low incidence of postoperative nausea and vomiting include propofol and ketorolac.

Practitioners are divided between those who provide nausea prophylaxis to all patients and those who administer such medications only if the child complains of nausea or vomits in the early postoperative period. Ondansetron, the newest antiemetic, is effective as a prophylactic agent but less so as a rescue agent. The main disadvantage of its widespread use is cost. Other effective agents include droperidol, metoclopramide, and perphenazine. One major advantage of ondansetron and metoclopramide is that they do not cause sedation, which can make the assessment of respiratory depression associated with epidural therapy or PCA therapy more difficult.

All opiates also have the potential for causing pruritus, which does not by itself indicate an allergic response to the medication. This irritating side effect can be treated with diphenhydramine, which may further potentiate sedation. An alternative treatment is the opiate antagonist naloxone, given either as small boluses or as a continuous infusion. In a dose range of 2 to 4 μg/kg/h, naloxone will reverse pruritus and nausea without reversing analgesia.

A frequent complaint is that of a sore throat from the endotracheal tube or laryngeal mask, which is generally self-limited in nature. Specific therapy may include the use of over-the-counter lozenges, which contain local anesthetics.

More troublesome postoperative respiratory problems include upper airway obstruction, croup, laryngospasm, and bronchospasm. Upper airway obstruction resulting in stridor is often related to residual anesthetic effects on muscle tone; it resolves with positioning maneuvers or with the placement of oral or nasal airways. Suctioning of oropharyngeal secretions may also be helpful. Laryngospasm generally occurs in children who are not completely awake when the endotracheal tube is removed. One common sequence is coughing on secretions that impinge on the vocal cords, followed by vocal cord adduction. Most laryngospasm responds to oxygen delivered with positive pressure to the airway, along with a jaw thrust maneuver. Less frequently, a small dose of succinylcholine will be necessary to relax the vocal cords and allow for effective oxygenation and ventilation. Rarely, pulmonary edema will follow the relief of prolonged laryngospasm.[74]

Croup is reported to occur in about 1% of children who are intubated for general anesthesia; this complication is most common in children aged 1 to 4 years, those with a previous history of intubation, and those whose intubation was traumatic.[75] Current practice of testing for air leak around the endotracheal tube may have decreased this incidence in recent years. Most croup resolves with humidified oxygen, but some children will benefit from inhalation of nebulized racemic epinephrine. Patients who require this treatment should be observed for several hours to make sure the stridor does not recur.

Bronchospasm is an uncommon postoperative event, except in asthmatic children, who may experience bronchospasm in response to the stimulation of the endotracheal tube or LMA. Nebulization of a β-agonist agent with oxygen should promptly treat this difficulty.

Cardiovascular complications after general anesthesia are not common in children without congenital heart disease. Hypotension in PACU usually reflects inadequate replacement of intraoperative fluid losses. Hypertension in the absence of intrinsic renal dysfunction may indicate pain or excessive fluid administration.

SUMMARY

Exciting new techniques have expanded the possibilities for anesthesia care and pain management for children undergoing surgery. Ongoing research is focused on new intravenous medications for the induction and maintenance of anesthesia and is using data on receptor physiology to fashion "on–off" anesthesia. Ultra-short-acting intravenous opiates, such as remifentanil, may begin to play a larger role in pediatric anesthesia as clinical experience accumulates. New delivery systems for local anesthetics may enhance effects and minimize toxicity; the administration of older agents, such as ketamine and clonidine, into the epidural space as adjuncts to local anesthetics may also greatly improve the efficacy of these blocks. Despite these and other advances in anesthetic physiology and pharmacology, the hallmarks of pediatric anesthesia remain vigilance and attention to detail.

REFERENCES

1. Yaster M, Krane EJ, Kaplan RF, et al. Pediatric pain and sedation handbook. St. Louis: Mosby, 1997.
2. Roy WL, Lerman J, McIntyre BG. Is preoperative haemoglobin testing justified in children undergoing minor elective surgery? Can J Anaesth 1991;38:700–703.
3. Malviya S, D'Errico C, Reynolds P, et al. Should pregnancy testing be routine in adolescent patient prior to surgery? Anesth Analg 1996;83:854–858.
4. Betts EK, Cameron C. Controversies in anesthesia: should children with upper respiratory tract infections receive general anesthesia for elective surgical procedures? Anesthesiol Rev 1994;21:139–143.
5. Cohen MM, Cameron CB. Should you cancel the operation when a child has an upper respiratory tract infection? Anesth Analg 1991;72:282–288.
6. Tait AR, Knight PR. The effects of general anesthesia on upper respiratory tract infections in children. Anesthesiology 1987;67:930–935.
7. Rolf N, Coté CJ. Frequency and severity of desaturation events during general anesthesia in children with and without upper respiratory infections. J Clin Anesth 1992;4:200–203.
8. Tait AR, Pandit UA, Voepel-Lewis T, et al. Use of the laryngeal mask airway in children with upper respiratory tract infections: a comparison with endotracheal intubation. Anesthesiology 1998;86:706–711.
9. Coté CJ, Zaslavsky A, Downes JJ, et al. Postoperative apnea in former preterm infants after inguinal herniorrhaphy: a combined analysis. Anesthesiology 1995;82:809–822.
10. Dajani AS, Taubert KA, Wilson W, et al. Prevention of bacterial endocarditis: recommendations by the American Heart Association. JAMA 1997;277:1794–1801.
11. Vichinsky EP, Haberkern CM, Neumayr L, et al. A comparison of conservative and aggressive transfusion regimens in the perioperative management of sickle cell disease. N Engl J Med 1995;333:206–213.
12. Koshy M, Weinar SJ, Miller ST, et al. Surgery and anesthesia in sickle cell disease. Blood 1995;86:3676–3684.
13. Cohen MM, Cameron CB, Duncan, PG. Pediatric anesthesia morbidity and mortality in the perioperative period. Anesth Analg 1990;70:160–167.
14. Tiret L, Nivoche Y, Hatton F, et al. Complications related to anaesthesia in infants and children. A prospective survey of 40,240 anaesthetics. Br J Anaesth 1988;61:263–269.
15. Giaufre E, Dalens B, Gombert A. Epidemiology and morbidity of regional anesthesia in children: a one-year prospective survey of the French language society of pediatric anesthesiologists. Anesth Analg 1996;83:904–912.
16. Berde C. Regional anesthesia in children: what have we learned? [Editorial]. Anesth Analg 1996;83:897–900.
17. Kain ZN, Wang SM, Caramico L, et al. Parental desire for perioperative information and informed consent: a two-phase study. Anesth Analg 1997;84:299–306.
18. Mendelson CL. The aspiration of stomach contents into the lungs during obstetric anesthesia. Am J Obstet Gynecol 1946;52:191–205.
19. Schreiner MS, Triebwasser A, Keon TP. Ingestion of liquids compared with preoperative fasting in pediatric outpatients. Anesthesiology 1990;72:593–597.
20. Welborn LG, McGill WA, Hannallah RS, et al. Perioperative blood glucose concentrations in pediatric outpatients. Anesthesiology 1986;65:543–547.
21. Cavell B. Gastric emptying in infants fed human milk or infant formula. Acta Paediatr Scand 1981;70:639–641.
22. Litman RS, Wu CL, Quinlivan JK. Gastric volume and pH in infants fed clear liquids and breast milk prior to surgery. Anesth Analg 1994;79:482–485.
23. Dubin SA, McCranie JM. Sugarless gum chewing before surgery does not increase gastric fluid volume or acidity. Can J Anaesth 1994;41:603–606.
24. Hallen B, Olsson GL, Uppfeldt A. Pain-free venipuncture. Effect of timing of application of local anaesthetic cream. Anaesthesia 1984;39:969–972.
25. Soliman IE, Broadman LM, Hannallah RS, McGill WA. Comparison of the analgesic effects of EMLA (eutectic mixture of local anesthetics) to intradermal lidocaine infiltration prior to venous cannulation in unpremedicated children. Anesthesiology 1988;68:804–806.
26. Manuksela EL, Korpela R. Double-blind evaluation of a lignocaine-prilocaine cream (EMLA) in children. Effect on the pain associated with venous cannulation. Br J Anaesth 1986;58:1242–1245.
27. Feld LH, Negus JB, White PF. Oral midazolam preanesthetic medication in pediatric outpatients. Anesthesiology 1990;73:831–834.
28. Peterson MD. Making oral midazolam palatable for children [Letter]. Anesthesiology 1990;73:1053.
29. Gutstein HB, Johnson KL, Heard MB, Gregory GA. Oral ketamine preanesthetic medication in children. Anesthesiology 1992;76:28–33.
30. Feld LH, Champeau MW, van Steenis CA, Scott JC. Preanesthetic medication in children: a comparison of oral transmucosal fentanyl citrate versus placebo. Anesthesiology 1989;71:373–377.
31. Epstein RH, Mendel HG, Witkowski TA, et al. The safety and efficacy of oral transmucosal fentanyl citrate for preoperative sedation in young children. Anesth Analg 1996;83:1200–1205.
32. Dsida RM, Wheeler M, Birmingham PK, et al. Premedication of pediatric tonsillectomy patients with oral transmucosal fentanyl citrate. Anesth Analg 1998;86:66–70.
33. Karl HW, Keifer AT, Rosenberger JL, et al. Comparison of the safety and efficacy of intranasal midazolam for preinduction of anesthesia in pediatric patients. Anesthesiology 1992;76:209–215.
34. Cauldwell CB. Induction, maintenance and emergence. In: Gregory GA, ed., Pediatric anesthesia. 3rd ed. New York: Churchill Livingstone, 1994:227–259.
35. Kain ZN. Parental presence during induction of anaesthesia. Pediatr Anaesth 1995;5:209–212.
36. Naito Y, Tamai S, Shingu K, et al. Comparison between sevoflurane and halothane for paediatric ambulatory anaesthesia. Br J Anaesth 1991;67:387–389.
37. Borgeat A, Popovic V, Meier D, Schwander D. Comparison of propofol and thiopental/halothane for short duration ENT surgical procedures in children. Anesth Analg 1990;71:511–515.
38. Smith I, White PF, Nathanson M, Gouldson R. Propofol: an update on its clinical use. Anesthesiology 1994;81:1005–1043.
39. Brain AI. The laryngeal mask—a new concept in airway management. Br J Anaesth 1983:55:801–805.
40. Brain AI, McGhee TD, McAteer EJ, et al. The laryngeal mask airway: development and preliminary trials of a new type of airway. Anaesthesia 1985;40:356–361.
41. Taddio A, Stevens B, Craig K, et al. Efficacy and safety of lidocaine-prilocaine cream for pain during circumcision. N Engl J Med 1997;336:1197–1201.
42. Broadman LM, Hannallah RS, Belman B, et al. Post-circumcision analgesia—a prospective evaluation of subcutaneous ring block of the penis. Anesthesiology 1987;67:399–402.
43. Sara CA, Lowry CJ. A complication of circumcision and dorsal nerve block of the penis. Anaesth Intensive Care 1984;13:79–85.
44. Dalens B, Venneuville G, Dechelotte P. Penile block via the subpubic space in 100 children. Anesth Analg 1989;69:41–45.
45. Wolf AR, Valley RD, Fear DW, et al. Bupivacaine for caudal analgesia in infants and children: the optimal effective concentration. Anesthesiology 1988;69:102–106.
46. Moller R, Covino BG. Cardiac electrophysiologic properties of bupivacaine and lidocaine compared with those of ropivacaine, a new amide local anesthetic. Anesthesiology 1990;72:322–329.
47. Warner MA, Kunkel SE, Offord KO, et al. The effect of age, epinephrine, and operative site on the duration of caudal analgesia in pediatric patients. Anesth Analg 1987;66:995–998.

48. Freid EB, Bailey AG, Valley RD. Electrocardiographic and hemodynamic changes associated with unintentional intravascular injection of bupivacaine with epinephrine in infants. Anesthesiology 1993;79:394–398.

49. Ved SA, Pinosky M, Nicodemus H. Ventricular tachycardia and brief cardiovascular collapse in two infants after caudal anesthesia using a bupivacaine-epinephrine solution. Anesthesiology 1993;79:1121–1123.

50. Murat I. Pharmacology. In: Dalens B, ed., Regional anesthesia in infants, children, and adolescents. Baltimore: Williams & Wilkins, 1995:114–118.

51. Dalens B. Nerve blocks of the trunk. In: Dalens B, ed., Regional anesthesia in infants, children, and adolescents. Baltimore: Williams & Wilkins, 1995:476–479.

52. Hannallah RS, Broadman LM, Belman BA, et al. Comparison of caudal and ilioinguinal/iliohypogastric nerve blocks for control of post-orchiopexy pain in pediatric ambulatory surgery. Anesthesiology 1987;66:832–834.

53. Fisher QA, McComiskey CM, Hill JL, et al. Postoperative voiding interval and duration of analgesia following peripheral or caudal nerve blocks in children. Anesth Analg 1993;76:173–177.

54. Tobias JD, Holcomb GW, Brock JW, et al. Analgesia after inguinal herniorrhaphy with laparoscopic inspection of the peritoneum in children: caudal block versus ilioinguinal/iliohypogastric block. Am J Anesthesiol 1995;22:193–197.

55. Blaise G, Roy WL. Postoperative pain relief after hypospadias repair in pediatric patients; regional analgesia versus systemic analgesics. Anesthesiology 1986;65:84–86.

56. Liu LP, Coté CJ, Goudsouzian NG, et al. Life-threatening apnea in infants recovering from anesthesia. Anesthesiology 1983;59:506–510.

57. Rice LJ, DeMars PD, Whalen TV, et al. Duration of spinal anesthesia in infants less than one year of age. Comparison of three hyperbaric techniques. Reg Anaesth 1994;19:325–329.

58. Dohi S, Naito H, Takahashi T. Age-related changes in blood pressure and duration of motor block in spinal anesthesia. Anesthesiology 1979;50:319–323.

59. Welborn LG, Rice LJ, Hannallah RS, et al. Postoperative apnea in former preterm infants: prospective comparison of spinal and general anesthesia. Anesthesiology 1990;72:838–842.

60. Krane EJ, Haberkern CM, Jacobson LE. Postoperative apnea, bradycardia, and oxygen desaturation in formerly premature infants: prospective comparison of spinal and general anesthesia. Anesth Analg 1995;80:7–13.

61. Watcha MF, Thach BT, Gunter JB. Postoperative apnea after caudal anesthesia in an ex-premature infant. Anesthesiology 1989;71:613–615.

62. Aldrete JA, Kroulik D. A postanesthetic recovery score. Anesth Analg 1970;49:924–934.

63. Steward DJ. A simplified scoring for the post-operative recovery room. Can Anaesth Soc J 1975;22:111–113.

64. Soliman IE, Patel RI, Ehrenpreis MB, et al. Recovery scores do not correlate with postoperative hypoxemia in children. Anesthesiology 1988;67:53–56.

65. Birmingham PK, Tobin MJ, Henthorn TK, et al. Twenty-four hour pharmacokinetics of rectal acetaminophen in children: an old drug with new recommendations. Anesthesiology 1997;87:244–252.

66. Priano LL Vatner SF. Generalized cardiovascular and regional hemodynamic effects of meperidine in conscious dogs. Anesth Anal 1981;53:613–620.

67. Yaster M, Maxwell LG. Opioid agonists and antagonists. In: Schechter NL, Berde CB, Yaster M, eds., Pain in infants, children, and adolescents. Baltimore: Williams & Wilkins, 1993:158–171.

68. Watcha MF, Jones MB, Lagueruela RG, et al. Comparison of ketorolac and morphine as adjuvants during pediatric surgery. Anesthesiology 1992;76:368–372.

69. Buck ML, Norwood VF. Ketorolac-induced acute renal failure in a previously healthy adolescent. Pediatrics 1996;98:294–296.

70. Bösenberg AT, Bland BAR, Schulte-Steinberg O, Downing JW. Thoracic epidural anesthesia via the caudal route in infants. Anesthesiology 1988;69:265–269.

71. Gunter JB, Eng C. Thoracic epidural anesthesia via the caudal approach in children. Anesthesiology 1992;76:935–938.

72. Wood CE, Goresky GV, Klassen KA, et al. Complications of continuous epidural infusions for postoperative analgesia in children. Can J Anaesth 1994;41:613–620.

73. Schreiner MS, Nicolson SC, Martin T, Whitney L. Should children drink before discharge from day surgery? Anesthesiology 1992;76:528–533.

74. Lee KWT, Downes JJ. Pulmonary edema secondary to laryngospasm in children. Anesthesiology 1983;59:347–349.

75. Koka BV, Jeon IS, Andre JM, et al. Postintubation croup in children. Anesth Analg 1977;56:501–505.

CHAPTER 4

General Urology: Workup of Hematuria and Tubular Disorders

John T. Herrin

A number of patients have disorders that overlap the interface between nephrology and urology, making a cooperative approach necessary for optimal care. Included in this group are patients with hematuria and those with primary or secondary disorders of renal tubular function who may present with renal calculi, metabolic abnormalities (e.g., acidosis, alkalosis, or electrolyte disturbances), urinary concentrating defects, urinary tract anomalies, infections, or disturbances of statural growth.

Hematuria is a common manifestation of many renal and nonrenal diseases (e.g., bleeding and coagulation disorders and sepsis). Gross hematuria is a dramatic and worrying, although relatively uncommon, symptom, accounting for 1.3 in 1000 emergency department visits.[1] In pediatric practice, gross hematuria is not necessarily a sign of serious disease; however, microscopic hematuria has become one of the more frequent symptoms seen in patients referred to nephrologic and urologic practice, because of the widespread use of chemical dipstick urine testing. Although convenient, the sensitivity of dipstick testing may cause a number of patients to undergo unnecessary, expensive, and stressful workups, unless strict adherence to the definition of the abnormality is made.[2, 3] Microscopic hematuria occurs in 0.25 to 1.6% of children and is perplexing and confusing to families.[4–7]

In adults with hematuria, the risk of malignancy is high enough that the workup traditionally includes thorough imaging and visual inspection of the upper and lower urinary tract, particularly in males >50 years of age.[8, 9] In children, glomerular lesions and congenital anomalies are present in a relatively high proportion of patients, and tumor risk is low and largely confined to the 2- to 4-year-old age group.[10] Because bleeding may occur at any level in the urinary tract, from the glomerulus to the meatus, the physician must understand the major causes of hematuria to avoid subjecting the patient to unnecessary procedures (Tables 4.1 and 4.2). A nondirected approach is expensive, stressful, and time-consuming. If a cause is not demonstrated on screening, further testing is relatively invasive and has a small yield of significant treatable lesions.

An understanding of the sensitivity of the testing dipstick is necessary, because the readings range from trace to 1+ in normal patients.[2, 3] The test patch absorbs several microliters of urine, hence more erythrocytes react than correspond to 1 μL. Low-grade excretion of both RBCs and protein occurs daily in normal children. Further chemical strip testing does not specifically test for blood and protein, so that false-positive and -negative results occur. Patients with >1+ heme on dipstick testing should also show 3 to 4 RBCs per high power field (HPF) in a centrifuged urine specimen or 6 RBCs/mm^3 before being defined as having hematuria, which requires further investigation. Dodge et al.[7] showed that two of three successive specimens should meet positive criteria for clinical significance; their study also demonstrated that most patients with true hematuria have other symptoms.

PATHOPHYSIOLOGY

Hematuria may be the result of the disruption of the endothelial–epithelial barrier. A physical disruption of the barrier may be caused by trauma, neoplasia, arteriovenous malformation, or vascular accident (infarction). Inflammation of endothelial–epithelial barrier (e.g., glomerulonephritis) leads to cytokine production and damage to the basement membrane, resulting in the loss of RBCs through the glomerulus between capillary endothelial cells or epithelial cells and from the basement membrane itself. Bleeding between tubular epithelial cells is associated with tubulointerstitial disease. When the endothelial–epithelial barrier is disrupted, bleeding from the lower urinary tract can occur between the mucosal cells lining the renal pelvis, ureter, bladder, or urethra.

TABLE 4.1. *Principal causes of hematuria*

Glomerular disease
- IgA nephropathy***
- Hereditary nephritis
- Acute glomerulonephritis syndrome

Infections
- Viral***
- Bacterial
- Other

Anomalies
- Hydronephrosis***
- Cystic disease
- Vascular

Hematologic
- Coagulopathy***
- Thrombocytopenia
- Sickle-cell disease*
- Renal vein thrombosis

Hypercalciuria*** and kidney stones

Exercise
- Primary
- Secondary*

Trauma*

Drugs

Tumors
- Wilms tumor** (especially in 2- to 6-year olds)
- Renal cell carcinoma
  Von Hippel–Lindau disease
  Tuberosclerosis
  Random

Asterisks indicate relative frequency of hematuria.

TABLE 4.2. *Causes of hematuria by age*

Newborn
- Congenital abnormalities
- Renal vascular disorders
  Arterial thrombosis
  Venous thrombosis
- Renal cortical necrosis

Infant (1–24 months)
- Renal venous thrombosis
- Congenital abnormalities
- Urinary tract infection
- Hemolytic uremic syndrome
- Wilms tumor

Child (2–12 years)
- Hemorrhagic cystitis
- Trauma
- Acute glomerulonephritis
- IgA nephropathy
- Hereditary nephritis
  Alport syndrome
  Thin basement membrane disease
- Henoch–Schonlein purpura
- Hypercalciuria

Adolescent (12–18 years)
- Trauma
- Menstruation
- Acute glomerulonephritis
- IgA nephropathy
- Hereditary nephritis
  Alport syndrome
  Thin basement membrane disease
- Hypercalciuria
- Renal calculi

Hematuria in patients with renal calculi or hypercalciuria is associated with intraluminal irritation and mucosal trauma. The irritation may be caused by calcium microcrystals.[11] Bleeding may also be caused by arteriovenous malformation, abnormal blood vessels in polyps, and damage from drugs (e.g., cyclophosphamide).

Transient hematuria in conjunction with fever and hypercatabolic states is likely to be the result of hemodynamic changes, although the exact mechanism is not understood. Exercise-induced hematuria can be caused by traumatic bladder contusion with venous bleeding, which has been observed on cystoscopy in long-distance runners,[12] and glomerular bleeding, which seems to be proportional to the degree of exercise.[13] It has been postulated that glomerular bleeding is secondary to the renal vasoconstriction that occurs during exercise to allow the redistribution of blood to the skeletal muscles. The subsequent relative increase in efferent versus afferent arteriolar constriction is mediated by angiotensin, resulting in nephron hypoxia, increased glomerular permeability, and exudation of RBCs into the urinary space.

INITIAL WORKUP

Figure 4.1 is a flow chart that directs the physician through a cost-efficient, logical, and minimally invasive workup. The aim of testing patients with hematuria is to identify the cause of the bleeding, to discover any potentially serious or progressive conditions, and to develop a rational plan for therapy. The principle is to initiate studies that are likely to determine if additional urologic or nephrologic evaluation is indicated (Table 4.3).

Because the occurrence of hematuria is distressing to the family, particularly with gross hematuria, the optimal time for review is while the hematuria is present. Urinary findings provide a guide to testing and allow the physician to offer support to the patient and family. Urine color, presence of clots or stones, and careful microscopy may suggest the site and cause of bleeding and allow directed urologic, radiologic, or nephrologic studies (Table 4.4). Early evaluation should confirm the hematuria and include a complete urinalysis, which should be performed as soon as practical in patients with gross hematuria.

Patients with asymptomatic hematuria who have no proteinuria or overt renal anomaly have an excellent overall prognosis.[14] Although patients with microscopic hematuria and low-grade proteinuria can have progressive renal disease, most patients without significant proteinuria or hypocomplementemia have stable renal

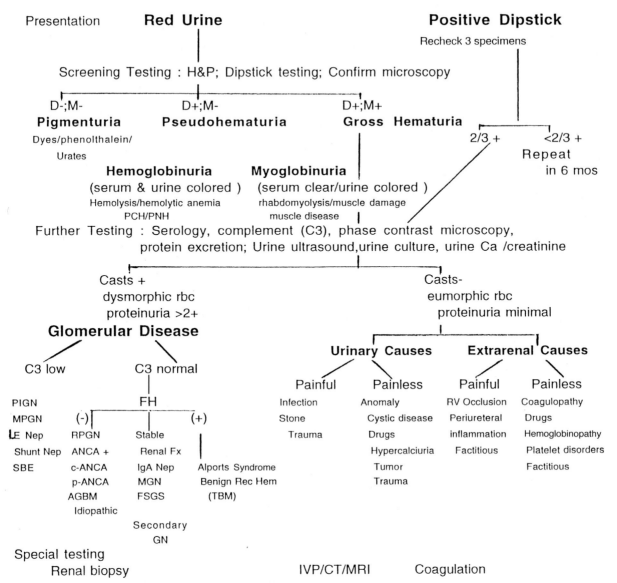

FIG. 4.1. Flow chart for the workup of pediatric hematuria. *H&P,* history and physical examination; *D,* dipstick test (+, positive; −, negative); *M,* microscopy for RBCs (+, >6/HPF; −, ≤6/HPF); *PCH,* paroxysmal cold hemoglobinuria; *PNH,* paroxysmal nocturnal hemoglobinuria; *Ca,* calcium; *Cr,* creatinine; *PIGN,* postinfectious glomerulonephritis; *MPGN,* membranoproliferative glomerulonephritis; *Le nep,* Lupus nephritis; *Shunt nep;* nephritis associated with a ventriculoatrial shunt; *SBE,* nephritis associated with subacute bacterial glomerulonephritis; *FH,* family history; *RPGN,* rapidly progressive glomerulonephritis; *ANCA,* antineutrophil cytoplasmic antibody; *c-ANCA,* Wegener granulomatosis; *p-ANCA,* myeloperoxidase ANCA; *AGBM,* Goodpasture syndrome; *Fx,* fraction; *MGN,* membranous glomerulonephritis; *FSGS,* focal segmental glomerular sclerosis; *GN,* glomerulonephritis; *TBM,* thin basement membrane disease (benign familial hematuria); *RV,* right ventricle; *IVP,* intravenous pyelogram.

function over a prolonged period.[15] Further testing is thus aimed at defining any associated factors in patients with suspected glomerular disease.

Building a Database

The following data will facilitate a directed treatment approach for patients with hematuria. Although a care-

ful history and a physical examination are important in the diagnostic process, determining gross versus microscopic hematuria, assessing the associated pain, and conducting a careful urinalysis are the keys to differentiation in a directed approach to hematuria (Tables 4.4 and 4.5). Furthermore, the clinician should note the color of the urine and place special emphasis on the presence of proteinuria out of proportion to the degree

TABLE 4.3. *Appropriate studies for hematuria*

All patients
- History
  Macroscopic versus microscopic
  Red colored versus tea or coke colored
  Presence of pain
  Presence of clots
  Urinary sediment with casts
  Family history of stones, deafness, keratoconus, renal
    failure, and dialysis
- Physical examination
  Mass
  Local lesion
  Hypertension
  Rash or purpura
  Arthritis or arthralgia
- Other studies
  Urinalysis
    RBC morphology
    Casts
    Urine culture
    CBC (including platelets)
    Complement (C3)
  Ultrasound
    Renal
    Bladder
Selected patients
- Anti-group A and -group B streptococci
- Antineutrophil antibody
- Urine erythrocyte morphology
- Phase contrast
- Coulter counter
- Skin and throat cultures
- Sickle-cell disease screening
- Coagulation and bleeding
- Voiding cystourethrogram
- Audiologic examination
- Ophthalmologic examination
- CT and MRI studies
Invasive procedures (indicated by screening)
- Renal biopsy
- Cystoscopy (adults)
- Angiogram

TABLE 4.4. *Clinical localization of hematuria*

Upper urinary tract bleeding
- Brown (coke or tea) color
- Moderate proteinuria
- Cellular casts
- Dysmorphic red cells
- Renal tubular cells
Lower urinary tract bleeding
- Red color
- Minimal proteinuria
- Terminal bleeding
- Clots and particles
- Normal red cell morphology

to the three-glass test. Protein excretion and microscopy are useful for differentiating glomerular causes (which are diagnosed via serologic testing) from nonglomerular causes (which require definition of anatomy and exclusion of kidney stone disease and hypercalciuria).

Other studies that help determine the site of bleeding in hematuria include phase contrast microscopy, formal cytology analysis of urinary sediment (including cells and casts), Wright staining, and Coulter counter measurement of the urinary RBC size. Among these methods, only the phase contrast review for dysmorphic RBCs has attained a place in the general workup. Early studies, largely on adult populations, identified morphological criteria that define the sites of origin of glomerular and nonglomerular red cells through phase contrast microscopy[16] and Wright staining.[17] Coulter counter Measures of RBC size have also been used. Few reports of such correlations are found in the pediatric literature.[18, 19]

Phase microscopy has the advantage of providing a simple review for the presence of casts and is highly correlated with site of origin of the RBCs. This technique, however, requires experience for accurate interpretation. Mixed populations can occur in disorders in which both glomerular and nonglomerular bleeding coexist (e.g., IgA nephropathy).[16, 20] Furthermore,

of hematuria. Casts indicate glomerular or tubular damage as the cause of the hematuria.

If possible, the parents or caregivers should collect a sample of the first discolored urine (even if it must be retrieved from the toilet bowl) so the physician can test for blood; the red urine may be caused by a dye or pigment. Samples of any subsequent voids made before the examination date should also be provided.

If the hematuria is associated with pain, I ask patients to provide a "three-glass" sample, which reveals a general location of the bleeding site (Table 4.6). If the hematuria is painless, I ask the family to provide urine samples, which are used to create a familial urinalysis profile (Table 4.5; Fig. 4.1). This profile may reveal an inherited nephropathy, or a concurrent family exposure to infection as the cause of the hematuria. Urine color may provide a clue to the site of bleeding and correlates

TABLE 4.5. *Clinical approach to hematuria*

Condition	Macroscopic hematuria	Proteinuria (casts)	Pain
Anomalies	+++	− to +	Present
IgA nephropathy	+++	− to ++	− to +
Infection	++	− to +	Present
Coagulopathy	++	− to +	−
Hypercalciuria or kidney stones	++	−	−
Exercise	++	− to +	− to +
Trauma	++	− to +	− to ++
Drugs	++	− to +	− to ++
Tumor	+ to ++	− to +	−

+, present and relative degree; −, absent.

TABLE 4.6. *The three-glass urine test*

Procedure
- The patient cleans off the urethral meatus.
- The patient voids sequentially into three separate containers so that, if possible, the first 5–10 mL urine is collected in container 1, the majority of the urine is collected in container 2, and the final 2–5 mL is collected in container 3.

Interpretation

Possible bleeding site	Container 1	Container 2	Container 3
Urethra	+	−	−
Bladder	−	−	+
Kidney	+	+	+

Sample does (+) or does not (−) contain blood.

dysmorphic red cells may occur in approximately 10% of cases of nonglomerular bleeding, so interpretation must be used in conjunction with other indicators of the bleeding site.[18]

Clinical Evaluation of the History and Physical Examination

History

When taking the history, the clinician should concentrate on determining the nature of the hematuria. The examiner should note whether the bleeding is the first or a recurrent episode and whether the hematuria is gross or microscopic. The patient should be questioned about any associated pain. (Gross hematuria, particularly when painful, is likely to have a urologic or anatomical cause.) The site and character of the pain and the pattern of its radiation (to the loin, inguinal area, or abdomen) should be determined.

The history should also exclude or assess the possibility of trauma. Direct trauma may produce contusion, rupture, vascular damage, or structural damage to the bladder or urethra; and even minimal trauma may produce hematuria if renal anomalies or hydronephrosis are present.

The clinician should note the amount of bleeding. Spontaneous, heavy bleeding is uncommon, except in renal vascular anomalies, cystic disease, and tumors. In such cases, the blood is usually bright red, and the urine has clots or stringy; fibrinous material. Note that urine can be heavily blood stained by relatively small blood losses; 2.5 to 5 mL blood per 1 L urine will render the urine grossly blood stained. The examiner should obtain an estimate of the hematocrit from a spun urine sample. If the hematocrit is high, a formal urinary hematocrit should be ordered to determine the urgency of finding the bleeding site and gaining control.

The history should include any indication of recent or present infection. Pharyngitis and impetigo in particular

raise the possibility of postinfectious glomerulonephritis (PIGN). It is important to determine whether a streptococci or other culture was obtained, because the prognosis for recovery from poststreptococcal glomerulonephritis (PSGN) is excellent, even if the initial symptoms are severe.[21]

Other acute nephrites can be progressive, e.g., membranoproliferative glomerulonephritis (MPGN).[21] Associated features of secondary nephritic syndromes include *(a)* arthritis, arthralgia, and butterfly distribution facial rash or serositis of lupus erythematosus and *(b)* cough, hemoptysis, and pulmonary hemorrhage seen in pulmonary–renal syndromes (e.g., Wegener granulomatosis, Goodpasture syndrome, Churg–Strauss syndrome, and polyarteritis nodosa). Although rare in childhood, these conditions are signs of true renal emergencies and require urgent diagnosis and therapy.

Hematuria concurrent with an infection is more likely the result of a preexisting mesangial disease or glomerular abnormality (e.g., IgA nephropathy, MPGN, resolving PIGN, and familial nephritis) than the result of a new immune complex related to PIGN.[14, 21] A latent period of 2 to 3 weeks between pharyngeal or skin infection and the onset of hematuria is typical of PIGN, whereas drug-induced acute interstitial nephritis leads to hematuria during the course of treatment.[19]

Exercised-induced hematuria may occur with trauma. It may also be seen in patients with another underlying cause for the bleeding, for example, renal anomalies, glomerular disease, or kidney stone disease. Hematuria may be related to a change in the renal hemodynamics of an otherwise healthy individual; this is the so-called athletic pseudonephritis, in which casts may be present that clear after 24 to 48 h rest. Joggers may experience venous bleeding from the wall or dome of the bladder that is accompanied by small clots or fibrinous material.[12, 13, 22]

The clinician should determine the presence of pain, which is a further clue to the cause of the hematuria (Table 4.5). Bleeding associated with a tumor is usually painless, unless a complication, such as obstruction or infection, occurs. Thus a renal ultrasound should be obtained for patients with painless hematuria, unless a clear alternative diagnosis exists or the family history or uranalysis profile is positive. Furthermore, a renal ultrasound should be conducted for children in the high-risk-for-tumor age group (2 to 5 years), even when another apparent cause for the hematuria is present.

Pain associated with hematuria is common in urologic diseases in which dysuria or colic may be present, but pain is uncommon in most patients with glomerulonephritis. Loin pain may be present in patients with IgA nephropathy, exudative glomerulonephritis, and rapidly progressive glomerulonephritis. The pain in such cases is often bilateral or colicky in character and may represent an increase in intrarenal pressure or surface bleeding. If hematuria is painful, the clinician should obtain a three-glass test, an ultrasound examination, and a screening for a random urine calcium:creatinine (Ca:Cr) ratio (Table 4.6).

Full Family History

When obtaining the full family history, the clinician should pay close attention to the presence of a renal or urologic abnormality, such as hydronephrosis, vesicoureteric reflux, and renal cystic disease (autosomal dominant or recessive polycystic disease, medullary cystic disease, and medullary sponge kidney).[23] Specific review of other family members with renal calculi, including the type and chemical composition of the stone (if analyzed), should be pursued.

The clinician should make a particular effort to identify within the family renal failure, deafness, and keratoconus, which are associated with progressive hereditary nephritis. The family history should be scrutinized for benign microscopic or recurrent gross hematuria. The examiner may need to review the patient's genealogy to differentiate between the X-linked dominant form and the autosomal recessive form of Alport syndrome and to reveal benign familial hematuria (or thin basement membrane disease).

The clinician should also examine the family history for potential bleeding or clotting anomalies and symptoms of an acquired bleeding disorder (e.g., idiopathic thrombocytopenic purpura, Henoch–Schonlein purpura, and hemolytic uremic syndrome), or platelet abnormality (including drug exposure, viral infection, and leukemia).[24–31]

Physical Examination

During the physical examination, the clinician should review the patient's growth parameters (height and weight), which may suggest an underlying chronic condition. The clinician should also perform a full review of the genital and perineal anatomy and a careful examination of the abdomen for masses or tenderness. The skin should be examined for purpura, bruising, rashes, infections, and the characteristic lesions of tuberosclerosis (ash-leaf areas, Shagren patches, adenoma sebaceum); telangiectasia (von Hippel–Lindau disease); and a malar rash (lupus erythematosus). Hematuria may be associated with arthritis and serositis, and tuberosclerosis and von Hippel–Lindau disease may cause profound bleeding. Purpura and bruising suggest vasculitis (Henoch–Schonlein purpura) and the possibility of a bleeding or coagulation disorder.

The clinician should check the patient's blood pressure, which may be elevated with glomerulonephritis, particularly in conjunction with acute nephritic syndromes, vasculitis syndromes, vascular malformations, and arteriovenous fistulae.

A urinary chemistry analysis may help the clinician determine the cause of the hematuria. Urinary calcium and creatinine levels and the urinary protein:creatinine ratio are particularly helpful. Urinary calcium and creatinine should be measured from a random urine sample; their values will be elevated if the hematuria is the result of microcrystallization of calcium. The result of urine calcium/creatinine is compared to a reference value of 0.2 for a random single-void urine sample.

Note that urinary calcium excretion rises after a meal or calcium loading; thus if a random screening reveals a high level of calcium, confirmatory measures of 24-h excretion should be obtained. Urinary calcium excretion >150 mg/m^2/24 h or 4.5 mg/kg/24 h is abnormal and should alert the clinician to investigate further.

The urinary Ca:Cr ratio provides a semiquantitative measure of protein excretion and is useful for assessing the potential of a glomerular disease. A urine culture and a sensitivity test are ordered if the uranalysis suggests a urinary infection and if the diagnosis is not obvious from the screening.

The clinician should obtain an ultrasound examination to define anatomical lesions in patients with painful hematuria who may have potential congenital renal anomalies, a family history of cystic disease, or a renal tumor. Additional testing may be needed, depending on the clinical review.

A Practical Minimal Workup for Hematuria

The first steps are to take a detailed history, perform a physical examination, and order a full urinalysis to build the database (Table 4.4). Some patients may have more than one cause for the hematuria; hence a screening urine culture; renal ultrasound to exclude anomaly, stone, or tumor; and a random urine Ca:Cr ratio are necessary, particularly in patients with macroscopic hematuria. Measurement of the C3 component of complement and at least a semiquantitative estimation of protein excretion (via the urinary protein:Cr ratio) are necessary for patients in whom proteinuria and/or casts suggest glomerulopathy or interstitial disease.

A complete blood examination, including platelet count, is mandatory only in patients for whom the cause cannot be defined on the basis of the initial study. Specialized bleeding and clotting studies may be required if suggested by early screening. Sickle-cell screening should be performed in appropriate patients.

FURTHER INVESTIGATION AND MANAGEMENT BASED ON THE MINIMAL WORKUP

Anomalies

Congenital anomalies predispose the patient to infection and potential deterioration in renal function. It is important that the anomalies be identified and that prompt joint management between the pediatric nephrologist and the pediatric urologist be instituted. A high index of suspicion is indicated when hematuria occurs after minimal trauma.[32]

Renal Calculi

Evaluation for renal calculi includes an assessment for complications (obstruction and infection). Ultrasound, intravenous urogram, and occasionally CT scan or retrograde pyelogram may be needed to demonstrate the anatomy and guide treatment (removal versus the potential for spontaneous passage). Stone analysis is extremely important for establishing a cause: The family and patient should strain the urine to obtain the stone if it is spontaneously passed. When the acute crisis has passed, evaluation of the cause begins.

Further investigation should include appropriate testing to identify whether the patient has hypercalciuria or renal tubular disorders. Examples of such diagnostic tests are the urine Ca : Cr ratio or 24-h calcium excretion (hypercalciuria), urine and serum pH (renal tubular acidosis), cyanide nitroprusside screening and urinary amino acid profile (cystinuria), and oxalate excretion and glycolate : glycerate ratio (hyperoxaluria). The stone analysis may suggest other tests.

Renal Cystic Disease

The differential diagnosis of cystic disease rests on an assessment of the anatomy (by diagnostic imaging and/or biopsy), including an evaluation of both kidneys and the liver along with the detailed family history (Table 4.5). The terminology for cystic disorders of the kidney is confusing, because a number of classification systems exist (e.g., clinical, histologic, radiologic); thus it is essential to use the proper terms when discussing these disorders.

By convention, *multicystic disease* refers to the condition of multicystic dysplasia. The term is usually applied to the unilateral, nonfunctional renal mass (although occasional bilateral lesions do occur). This cystic dysplasia anomaly is usually associated with ureteral atresia. Hematuria is rare with multicystic disease, because the ureter is not patent.

Polycystic disease of the kidney refers to the inherited forms: autosomal recessive polycystic kidney disease (ARPKD) and autosomal dominant polycystic kidney disease (ADPKD). Gross hematuria is common with ADPKD but is rare with other forms of cystic disease (which may, however, include microscopic hematuria).

The differential diagnosis of cystic disease is extensive,[23] and the clinician must distinguish among the different forms of inherited cystic disease, renal dysplasia, and cysts associated with other syndromes (Table 4.7).

TABLE 4.7. *Differential diagnosis of renal cystic disease*

Inherited cystic disease
- ARPKD
- ADPKD
- Nephronophthisis (medullary cystic disease–familial juvenile nephrophthisis complex)
- Glomerulocystic disease

Cystic dysplasia

Renal cysts associated with multiple malformation syndromes
- Meckel syndrome (microcephaly, polydactyly, posterior encephalocele)
- Zellweger cerebrohepatorenal syndrome
- Jeune syndrome (asphyxiating thoracic dystrophy, short limbs)
- Laurence–Moon–Biedel syndrome (obesity, mental retardation, retinal dysplasia, polydactyly)
- Ivemark syndrome (renohepatopancreatic dysplasia)
- Orofacial digital syndrome type 1

Cysts associated with trisomy syndromes
- Trisomy 9, 13, 18, 21 (renal cystic disease, biliary dysgenesis)

Cysts associated with phacomatosis (differential diagnosis: ADPKD)
- Von Hippel–Lindau disease
- Bourneville syndrome (tuberous sclerosis)

Cortical cystic disease
- Glomerulocystic disease
- Diffuse chronic tubulointerstitial nephritis with microcysts
- Pluricystic hypoplasia (neonatal renal failure, hypoplasia, no interstitial fibrosis)
- Congenital nephrotic syndrome Finish type (differential diagnosis: mesangial sclerosis; note relation to Drash syndrome, congenital syphilis)

Medullary cystic disease
- Medullary cystic disease–familial juvenile nephrophthisis complex
- Medullary sponge kidney (canalicular precalyceal tubular ectasia; Cacchi–Ricci disease)

Undefined cystic disease

Urinary Tract Tumor

Tumors of the genitourinary tract can be classified according to both site and specific histopathology. Primary tumors may be subdivided into Wilms tumor and rare tumors (clear cell carcinoma, rhabdoid tumors, mesoblastic nephroma, renal cell carcinoma, sarcoma, and lymphoma).[33] Wilms tumor accounts for almost 95% of tumors in childhood and may be manifest as hematuria, hypertension, or a mass.[34] Other tumors are not generally associated with hematuria. Bladder, prostate, and vaginal rhabdomyosarcoma are more likely to cause urinary retention or a mass; but epithelial carcinoma of the bladder, although rare, may cause hematuria. Cooperative management among the pediatric urologist, pediatric hematologist, and oncologist is required.

Glomerulonephritis

In a patient suspected of having glomerulonephritis as the cause for the hematuria, serologic definition and a knowledge of the natural history are necessary for determining the appropriate therapy and assessing the need for urgent treatment. The cause is defined by reviewing the history and physical examination (latent period, pain, family review) supplemented by serologic and chemical surveys to evaluate renal function and the rate of deterioration.

The serologic review should include antistreptococcal antibodies, antiDNAaseB (ANDB), antistreptolysin-O (ASLO), streptozyme, complement (especially C3), antineutrophil cytoplasmic antibodies (ANCA), and anti–glomerular basement membrane (GBM) (including ELISA and Western blot). Extended lupus testing should include spectrum antinuclear antibody (ANA), anti-dsDNA, anti-sDNA anti-Sjögren syndrome A and B (anti-SS-A, anti-SS-B), lupus anticoagulant, extractable nuclear antibody (ENA), antiribonucleoprotein (anti-RNP), and anti-Smith (anti-Sm). Additional tests are IgA level and hepatitis screening.[35]

Recognition of the clinical syndrome in glomerular disease allows the physician to focus on the appropriate investigation and therapy. Acute nephritis is defined by hematuria with casts, proteinuria, edema, elevated blood pressure, and mild azotemia. Nephrotic syndrome is defined by massive proteinuria with other features of nephritis. Rapidly progressive glomerulonephritis (RPGN) is defined by increasing BUN and creatinine, often with oliguria. Other conditions are chronic, slowly progressive glomerulonephritis; asymptomatic hematuria or proteinuria; secondary glomerulonephritis in which symptoms of the primary disease coexist with the renal symptoms (e.g., Henoch-Schönlein purpura and lupus erythematosus); and pulmonary–renal syndromes (e.g., Wegener granulomatosis and Goodpasture syndrome).

Urinalysis and serum chemistries are used to monitor the progress of pulmonary–renal syndromes, and nonspecific therapy is instituted to control blood pressure and prevent or limit the development of edema (caused by water and salt retention). Dietary restriction of potassium, phosphate, and protein is a prophylaxis against the development of electrolyte abnormality. Renal biopsy is indicated if the natural history of the glomerulonephritis is atypical, e.g., when there is a persisting hypocomplementemia (not corrected in 4 months or the disease is associated with fluctuating levels), an unexplained or steroid-resistant nephrotic syndrome, or a progressive secondary disease. Biopsy should also be performed if a potentially toxic therapy is required.

Urgent therapy is necessary for RPGN, Goodpasture syndrome, Wegener granulomatosis, and ANCA-associated disease. The treatment for these disorders is potentially toxic and consists of pulse-dose steroids, pulse-dose intravenous cyclophosphamide, and plasmapheresis. Urgent serologic review and an early renal biopsy are indicated if the patient is experiencing rapid deterioration of renal function.

IgA nephropathy is the most common cause of recurrent macroscopic hematuria. The hematuria is synpharyngitic rather than latent, as in PIGN. Serum IgA levels are elevated in approximately 40% of patients with an acute infection. Because IgA nephropathy can be a progressive disease (15 to 30% of older patients progress to renal failure),[36, 37] differentiation from benign hematuria syndromes and resolving postinfectious glomerulonephritis is necessary. There is a correlation between proteinuria and renal failure; thus follow-up and consideration of interventional therapy are appropriate if proteinuria develops.

Sickle-Cell Disease

Patients with either sickle-cell disease or sickle-cell trait may present with gross hematuria. Bleeding in this population, however, is relatively uncommon. The series described by Ingelfinger et al.[1] did not include any patients with sickle-cell anemia. Bleeding is more common in patients with sickle-cell trait and more common from the left kidney. Between attacks, the urine is generally clear of microscopic hematuria. Sickle-cell nephropathy usually includes concentrating defects or acidification defects but may include proteinuria, nephrotic syndrome, or progressive nephropathy.[38]

TUBULAR DISORDERS

Primary tubular disorders are uncommon or rare in clinical practice but affect children of all ages (Table 4.8). The importance of primary tubular lesions lies in their propensity to cause growth disturbances, renal calculi, and hypertension.[39] They may present with an abnormal urinalysis or polyuria–polydipsia with high urine output, which may lead to ureteric or bladder dilatation, particularly if minor anatomic anomalies (low-grade obstruction) are present.

Secondary abnormalities of tubular function are more common and occur in patients with urinary tract

TABLE 4.8. *Renal tubular disorders: urologic implications*

Primary disorders
- Proximal
  Fanconi syndrome
  Proximal renal tubular acidosis
- Distal
  Renal tubular acidosis
  Hypercalciuria
  Nephrogenic diabetes insipidus
Secondary disorders
- Obstruction
  Acidosis
  Concentrating defects
- Infection
  Acidosis

obstruction, (particularly with congenital obstruction). They often have a permanent effect on the developing tubules, including persisting concentrating and acidification defects.

Clinical Presentation

Patients with tubular disorders may have a variety of symptoms and conditions, including a dilated urinary tract, enuresis, and polyuria. Urinary-concentrating defects are associated with primary disorders, such as nephrogenic diabetes insipidus and Bartter syndrome; but they are more commonly the result of secondary disorders with obstructive uropathy. An appropriate testing profile is outlined in Table 4.9.

Renal calculi can form as the result of excess excretion of a relatively insoluble solute (secretory hypercalciuria, cystinuria, urate nephropathy) or as nephrocalcinosis or nephrolithiasis secondary to renal tubular acidosis, hypercalciuria, or hyperoxaluria. Tubular disorders are associated with abnormalities in the urinalysis, disorders of growth, hypertension, and Fanconi syndrome.

The chemical analysis of a patient with a tubular disorder may reveal an abnormal electrolyte profile, which suggests Fanconi syndrome (hypophosphatemic, hypokalemic acidosis) or Bartter syndrome (hypokalemic, hypochloremic, alkalosis). Reduced bicarbonate levels may indicate renal tubular acidosis, and elevated levels may indicate Bartter syndrome.

Bony abnormalities and abnormalities of calcium, phosphorus, and alkaline phosphatase are also common with tubular disorders. Reduced serum phosphate levels are typical of Fanconi syndrome and hypophosphatemic

TABLE 4.9. *Evaluation of renal tubular disorders*

Review the genetic background
 • Detailed family history
 • Family urinalysis profile
 • Blood and urine screening
Assess the symptoms
 • Polyuria and polydipsia
 • Renal colic and hematuria
 • Growth retardation
Conduct a physical examination
 • Growth
 • Rickets
Request a laboratory profile
 • GFR
 • Serum and urine pH
 • Potassium, phosphorus, alkaline phosphatase
 • Serum and urine osmolarity
 • Urine amino acids
 • Blood and urine screening
Order radiologic images
 • Long bones (growth, rickets)
 • Bone age
Perform urolithiasis
 • Chemical examination

rickets, whereas concurrent hypocalcemia suggests vitamin D abnormalities. Elevated alkaline phosphatase is associated with tubular hypophosphatemic syndromes and vitamin D abnormalities; and excess phosphaturia is found in Fanconi syndrome, hypophosphatemic rickets, and hyperparathyroidism.

Hypomagnesemia may occur in primary congenital renal tubular wasting disorders and with drug-induced magnesium deficiencies that are secondary to tubular damage (e.g., cis-platinum, aminoglycoside, and loop diuretic administration).[39]

Tools for Evaluation in Renal Tubular Disease

Diagnosis rests on the demonstration of urine solute excretion in excess of normal, expected values (Table 4.9).[39] Comparison of urinary and plasma levels of the substance with the concurrent plasma and urine creatinine concentrations allows the physician to estimate the handling characteristics. The direct ratio of excretion of calcium to creatinine or protein can be used for comparison. Sometimes the characteristics of the excretion pattern of a substance may provide a more sensitive measure. For example, fractional excretion of a substance (FE_x) is used to examine sodium, potassium, and uric acid handling or tubular reabsorption of a substance phosphate (TRP). In practice, the solute : creatinine ratio allows a random urine sample to be used for the evaluation of cystine, oxalate, and citrate excretion and allows the calculation of the risk of symptomatic disease. Solute excretion per milliliter urine (GFR) is used to evaluate uric acid excretion. Using random samples is more convenient than collecting 24-h specimens, although formal loading tests with evaluation of the excretion pattern are still sometimes necessary for demonstrating abnormal physiology or identifying the risk of abnormal tubular function.

If calculi are a recurrent problem or stone analysis suggests the consideration of tubular disorders, then appropriate testing should be instituted as outlined earlier.

REFERENCES

1. Ingelfinger JR, Davis AB, Grupe WE. Frequency and etiology of gross hematuria in a general pediatric setting. Pediatrics 1977;59:557.
2. Freni SC, Heederik GJ, Hol C. Centrifigation techniques and reagent strips in the assessment of microhematuria. J Clin Pathol 1977;30:336.
3. Leonards J. Simple test for hematuria compared with established tests. JAMA 1962;179:807.
4. Vehaskari VM. What is the prevalence of asymptomatic microscopic haematuria and how should such children be managed? Pediatr Nephrol 1989;3:32.
5. Hisano S, Kwano M, Hatae K, et al. Asymptomatic isolated microhaematuria: natural history of 136 children. Pediatr Nephrol 1991;5:578.
6. Murakami M, Yamamoto H, Ueda Y, et al. Urinary screening of

elementary and junior high-school children over a 13-year period in Tokyo. Pediatr Nephrol 1991;5:50.

7. Dodge WF, West EF, Smith EH, et al. Proteinuria and hematuria in school children: epidemiology and early natural history. J Pediatr 1976;88:327–347.

8. Woolhandler S, Pels, et al. Dipstick screening of asymptomatic adults for urinary tract disorders. JAMA 1989;262:1215.

9. Mohr DN, Offord KP, Owen RA, Melton LJ. Asymptomatic microhematuria and urologic disease. JAMA 1986;256:224.

10. Kaplan MP. Hematuria in childhood. Pediatr Rev 1983;5:99.

11. Garcia CD, Miller LA, Stapelton FB. Natural history of hematuria associated with hypercalciuria in children. Am J Dis Child 1991;145:1204.

12. Blacklock NJ. Bladder trauma in the long-distance runner: 10,000 metres hematuria. Br J Urol 1977;49:129.

13. Alyea EP, Parish HH, Durham NC. Renal response to exercise: urinary findings. JAMA 1958;167:807.

14. West CD. Asymptomatic hematuria and proteinuria in children: causes and appropriate diagnostic studies. J Pediatr 1976; 89:173.

15. Hisano S, Ueda K. Asymptomatic haematuria and proteinuria: renal pathology and clinical outcome in 54 children. Pediatr Nephrol 1989;3:229.

16. Fairley KF, Birch DF. Hematuria: a simple method for identifying glomerular bleeding. Kidney Int 1982;21:105.

17. Chang B. Red cell nephrology aid to diagnosis of hematuria. JAMA 1984;252:1747.

18. Stapelton FB. Morphology of urinary red blood cells: a simple guide in localizing the site of hematuria. Pediatr Clin North Am 1987;34:561.

19. Rizzoni G, Braggion F, Zacchello G. Evaluation of glomerular and nonglomerular hematuria by phase-contrast microscopy. J Pediatr 1987;103:370.

20. Hill PA, Davies DJ, Kincaid-Smith P, Ryan GB. Ultrastructural changes in renal tubules associated with glomerular bleeding. Kidney Int 1989;36:992.

21. Couser WG, Johnson RJ. Postinfectious glomerulonephritis. In: Neilson EG, Couser WG, eds., Immunologic renal diseases. Philadelphia: Lippincott-Raven, 1997;915–943.

22. Fassett RG, Owen JE, Fairley J, et al. Urinary red-cell morphology during exercise. Br Med J 1982;285:1455.

23. Bernstein J, Slovis T. Polycystic diseases of the kidney. In: Edelmann CM, ed., Pediatric kidney disease. 2nd ed. Boston: Little, Brown, 1992: 1139–1157.

24. Corrigan JJ. Hemorrhagic and thrombotic disease. In: Behrman RE, Kliegman RM, Arvin AM, eds. Nelson Textbook of Pediatrics, 15th ed. Philadelphia: 1996;1422–1438.

25. Tryggvason K, Zhou J, Hostikka SL, Shows TB. Molecular genetics of Alport syndrome. Kidney 1993;43:38.

26. Gubler M, Levy M, Broyer M, et al. Alport's syndrome: a report of 58 cases and a review of the literature. Am J Med 1981;70:493.

27. Mochizuki T, Lemmink HH, Mariyama M, et al. Identification of mutations in the alpha 3(IV) and alpha 4(IV) collagen genes in autosomal recessive Alport syndrome. Nature Genet 1994;8:77.

28. Barker DF, Hostikka SL, Zhou J, et al. Identification of mutations in the COL4A5 collagen gene in Alport syndrome. Science 1990;248:1224.

29. Lemmink HH, Nillesen WN, Mochizuki T, et al. Benign familial hematuria due to mutation of the type IV collagen alpha 4 gene. J Clin Invest 1996;98:1114.

30. Cosio FG, Falkenhain ME, Sedmak DD. Association of thin glomerular basement membrane with other glomerulopathies. Kidney Int 1994;46:471.

31. Gauthier B, Trachman H, Frank R, et al. Familial thin basement membrane nephropathy in children with asymptomatic microhematuria. Nephron 1989;51:502.

32. Lieu TA, Fleisher GR, Mahboudi S, et al. Hematuria and clinical findings as indications for intravenous pyelography in pediatric blunt trauma. Pediatrics 1988;82:216.

33. LaQuaglia MP. Genitourinary tract cancer in childhood. Semin Pediatr Surg 1996;5:49.

34. Young JL, Miller RW. Incidence of malignant tumours in US children. J Pediatr 1975;86:254.

35. Jennette JC, Falk RJ. Serologic diagnostic techniques in renal disease. In: Narins R, Stein JH, eds., Contempory issues in nephrology. New York: Churchill Livingstone, 1992;25:145–181.

36. Ibels L, Gyory A. IgA nephropathy: analysis of the natural history, important factors in the progression of the renal disease and a review of the literature. Medicine 1994;73:79.

37. Berg UB, Widstam-Attorps UC. Follow up of renal function and urinary protein excretion in childhood IgA nephropathy. Pediatr Nephrol 1993;7:123.

38. Bhathena DB, Sondheimer JH. The glomerulopathy of homozygous sickle cell hemoglobin (SS) disease: morphology and pathogenesis. J Am Soc Nephrol 1991;1:1241.

39. Chesney RW. Clinical study of renal tubular disease. In: Barakat AY, ed., Renal disease in children. New York: Springer-Verlag, 1989:185–206.

CHAPTER 5

Management of Renal Failure in Children

Arundhati S. Kale and Eileen D. Brewer

ACUTE RENAL FAILURE

Acute renal failure (ARF) is defined as an abrupt decrease in glomerular filtration rate (GFR) that is usually reversible. Although ARF may be associated with oliguria (urine output <300 ml/m^2/day) or anuria (no urine output in a 24-h period), neither is necessary to make the diagnosis. There are many causes of ARF in children (Table 5.1). It is important to distinguish prerenal azotemia from intrinsic renal failure and postrenal obstruction to institute appropriate therapy.[1, 2] Although fluid administration is indicated for the first, fluid restriction is more appropriate for the second, and measures to relieve or bypass obstruction are most appropriate for the last. Prolonged prerenal azotemia may result in acute tubular necrosis (ATN), especially if the period of ARF exceeds 24 h. Once the diagnosis is established, identification and management of the metabolic complications are indicated. The clinical and laboratory features of ARF are outlined in Table 5.2. Guidelines for management are discussed below.

Fluid Therapy

Clinical assessment of the patient's hydration status is extremely important in guiding fluid therapy. Signs of dehydration associated with a history of fluid losses from diarrhea and/or vomiting suggest the possibility of prerenal azotemia. The diagnosis is supported by laboratory analyses showing a high urinary specific gravity (>1.020), a low urinary sodium concentration (<20 mEq/L), a low fractional excretion of sodium (<1%), a high urine osmolality (>500 mOsm/kg water), and a serum BUN:creatinine ratio of >20 (Table 5.3).[1] The critical values are different for neonates whose renal tubules are less mature.[1, 3] Appropriate fluid resuscitation should result in correction of azotemia. Prerenal azotemia also occurs in conditions associated with clinical edema and intravascular volume contraction, such as nephrotic syndrome or congestive heart failure. Fluid resuscitation must be done carefully in the presence of congestive heart failure.

Intrinsic ARF is usually associated with fluid overload, which clinically manifests itself as edema and/or hypertension and, if severe enough, with pulmonary edema and congestive heart failure.[1, 2] In the absence of pulmonary edema or heart failure, conservative management with fluid restriction is usually enough. To maintain a euvolemic state in such cases, fluids should be restricted to insensible water losses (400 mL/m^2/day) plus replacement of measured urinary and gastrointestinal losses. When the patient with ARF is moderately to severely overloaded with fluids, fluids should be replaced at less than insensible water loss plus urine and gastrointestinal output to allow for net fluid loss. Fluid status should be assessed closely, including monitoring the patient's weight at least daily in acute situations.

In the case of intrinsic ARF from acute tubular necrosis, anticipation and recognition of the polyuric phase is extremely important, especially in infants and small children, for whom urinary salt and water losses may be quite significant and may lead to prerenal azotemia if fluid restriction is continued. In infants and children with obstructive uropathy associated with ARF, relief of obstruction is followed by increased urinary salt and water losses owing to postobstructive osmotic diuresis and to alterations in tubular transport and tubuloglomerular feedback.[4] Timely replacement of this fluid is critical to avoid hypotension and dehydration.

In the presence of pulmonary edema or congestive heart failure, aggressive diuretic therapy may be indicated. Loop diuretics, such as furosemide, given intravenously in a dose of 1 to 3 mg/kg every 6 h, are most effective.[1, 2] Other diuretics, such as bumetanide and thiazide, offer no added advantages. The combination of a loop diuretic and either oral metolazone or intravenous chlorothiazide may help if the patient becomes refractory to loop diuretics alone. Renal-replacement therapy (RRT) may be required if diuretic therapy fails.

TABLE 5.1. *Causes of acute renal failure*

- Prerenal
  Dehydration
  Hypotension or shock
  Hypovolemia (hemorrhage, burns, trauma)
  Congestive heart failure
  Peripheral vasodilation (septicemia)
  Renal artery thrombosis or embolus
  Drugs (nonsteroidal anti-inflammatories; angiotensin-converting enzyme inhibitors)
- Intrinsic renal
  Acute tubular necrosis
    Ischemic
    Nephrotoxic drugs (aminoglycosides, colistin, amphotericin B, cyclosporine, cisplatin)
    Tumor lysis syndrome
    Rhabdomyolysis (heat stroke, crush injury)
  Acute interstitial nephritis
    Nephrotoxic drugs (methicillin, amoxicillin, sulfa, ciprofloxacin, furosemide, allopurinol, α interferon)
    Poststreptococcal
    Allergic
  Acute glomerulonephritis
  Hemolytic uremic syndrome
- Postrenal obstructive
  Congenital anomalies (posterior urethral valves, neurogenic bladder)
  Tumor (abdominal lymphoma)
  Stones
  Traumatic injury to ureters or bladder
  Blocked urinary catheter

Hypertension with ARF

In oligoanuric ARF, inability of the kidney to excrete salt and water results in fluid overload, which causes hypertension. Fluid and salt restriction and a trial of diuretic therapy is warranted when fluid overload is

TABLE 5.2. *Clinical features of acute renal failure*

- Physical findings
  Edema
  Hypertension
  Pallor
  Respiratory distress if pulmonary edema, congestive heart failure
  Seizures, coma
- Laboratory findings
  Urinalysis
    Proteinuria
    Hematuria
    Active sediment
- Serum analysis
  Increased BUN, creatinine
  Hyponatremia, hypernatremia
  Hyperkalemia
  Metabolic acidosis
  Hypocalcemia
  Hyperphosphatemia
  Hypermagnesemia
  Hyperuricemia
  Anemia

thought to be the cause of hypertension.[1,2] Primary renal or vascular disease, however, may lead to renin-mediated hypertension, which will not respond to this treatment alone. Blood pressure norms vary with the age, sex, and size of the patient.[1,2,5] Hypertension is defined as a sustained elevation of systolic or diastolic pressure >95the percentile for age and sex. Mild hypertension (95th to 99th percentile) is usually not treated, but moderate to severe hypertension (>99the percentile) requires immediate intervention. Commonly used agents are calcium channel blockers (nifedipine), angiotensin-converting enzyme (ACE) inhibitors (captopril, enalapril), and β-blockers (propranolol). Severe hypertension with hypertensive encephalopathy requires the use of rapidly acting agents like diazoxide (3 to 5 mg/kg/dose rapid IV bolus), labetalol (1 to 3 mg/kg/h, continuous IV infusion), and sodium nitroprusside (0.5 to 1.0 μg/kg/min).[1,2] The use of these agents requires close monitoring of the vital signs in an intensive care setting to avoid overshoot hypotension.

Electrolyte Abnormalities

Sodium

Serum sodium concentration may be normal, low, or high in ARF.[1] Hyponatremia, which is defined as a serum sodium level <130 mEq/L, commonly occurs secondary to the dilutional effect of excessive water retention. Mild hyponatremia rarely causes clinical symptoms and is easily corrected with fluid restriction. Severe hyponatremia, defined as a serum sodium level <120 mEq/L, is rare but may cause seizures and other CNS symptoms and requires rapid correction with hypertonic saline. The intravenous use of 3% NaCl, which contains 0.517 mEq/mL sodium, is advocated in symptomatic hyponatremia. The general rule of thumb is that 3% NaCl at 5 mL/kg be given over 1 to 2 h raises the serum sodium concentration by 5 mEq/L. The goal is to raise the level to approximately 120 mEq/L. Rapid correction to normal levels is contraindicated. Hypernatremia, defined as serum sodium concentration >150 mEq/L, most often occurs when large amounts of sodium bicarbonate are administered to correct severe metabolic acidosis.[1] Renal-replacement therapy may be needed to correct severe hypernatremia in the oligoanuric patient.

Potassium

The most serious electrolyte abnormality of ARF is hyperkalemia, which may lead to ECG changes and has the potential to cause arrhythmias and cardiac arrest.[1,2,6] Mild hyperkalemia, although asymptomatic, must be recognized so that preventive measures can be taken to avoid more serious complications. Potassium intake should be restricted. In the presence of metabolic acido-

TABLE 5.3. *Biochemical indices of acute renal failure[a]*

Index	Prerenal	Intrinsic renal	Postrenal obstructive
Urine specific gravity	>1.020	1.010–1.020	<1.020
Urine sodium concentration, mEq/L	<20	>40	>40
Fractional excretion of sodium,[b] %	<1	>2	1–2
Urine osmolality, (mOsm/kg)	>500	<350	<350
BUN : creatinine ratio	>20	10	10

[a]Values for neonates are different from those listed owing to renal tubular immaturity.

[b]Fractional excretion of sodium = [(urine sodium concentration × serum creatinine concentration) ÷ (serum sodium concentration × urine creatinine concentration)] × 100

sis, correction of acidosis with a base supplement is indicated. For persistent mild to moderate hyperkalemia without ECG changes, treatment may be initiated with oral or rectal sodium polystyrene (Kayexalate®; 0.5 to 1 g/kg/dose as often as every 6 h, if needed). Sodium polystyrene is an ion exchange resin that exchanges sodium for potassium, which is eventually removed from the body through the stool. Diuretic therapy, which increases potassium excretion, may be useful, especially if the patient has nonoliguric ARF.

Severe hyperkalemia associated with ECG changes warrants rapid correction. Intravenous administration of 10% calcium gluconate (0.5 to 1 ml/kg over 5 to 10 min with cardiac monitoring), should be given first, especially if the patient is hypocalcemic. Calcium stabilizes the cardiac cell membrane to counteract the effects of hyperkalemia.[1,2] Rapid correction of metabolic acidosis with intravenous sodium bicarbonate (1 to 2 mEq/kg) or administration of concentrated dextrose (25 to 50%; 1 g/kg IV over 30 min) followed by regular insulin (0.1 U/kg IV) results in rapid intracellular movement of the potassium ion and a decrease in the serum potassium concentration.[1,2] Serum glucose must be monitored closely to avoid hypoglycemia after the glucose and insulin infusion. Frequently, all three therapeutic interventions may be necessary to treat hyperkalemia. Dialysis is indicated if the above measures are not successful and the patient is oligoanuric.

Hypokalemia may occur during the polyuric phase of ATN because of urinary losses of potassium in the presence of continued potassium restriction. Serum potassium should be monitored closely as urine output increases. Measurement of the urinary potassium concentration helps guide the appropriate replacement of potassium during the polyuric phase of ATN.

Acidosis

Metabolic acidosis is a common complication of ARF. Maintaining the serum pH > 7.2 is important for preserving cellular functions (e.g., enzyme activity).[1] Although acidosis by itself may be asymptomatic, it can affect the status of other electrolytes, such as potassium and calcium. Acidosis potentiates the effects of hyperka-

lemia but protects against the symptoms of hypocalcemia. Acidosis can be corrected with base supplements, such as intravenous sodium bicarbonate, intravenous acetate, oral sodium bicarbonate, and oral citrate. Hypocalcemia must be corrected before treating acidosis to avoid tetany.[1] Intractable acidosis usually requires dialysis for correction.

Calcium and Phosphorus

Hyperphosphatemia occurs as a result of decreased phosphate excretion owing to lowered GFR. Hyperphosphatemia leads to hypocalcemia and increased parathyroid hormone secretion. Dietary phosphate restriction along with phosphate binders, such as calcium carbonate, are recommended treatment. The use of aluminum salts as phosphate binders has been given up in children because of the dangers of aluminum absorption.[6,7] Excess aluminum can cause bone disease, liver disease, and CNS toxicity. Dementia and seizures are the worst CNS complications and usually occur after long-term use of aluminum salts. Using calcium salts has the added advantage of providing supplemental calcium to correct the hypocalcemia of ARF. Symptomatic hypocalcemia requires the immediate administration of intravenous calcium gluconate.

Other Electrolytes

Hypermagnesemia and hyperuricemia require no specific treatment. Hypermagnesemia rarely causes symptoms, but hypotension and neuromuscular depression can occur if serum magnesium concentration exceeds 5 mg/dL. Attention should be paid to excluding magnesium from the total parenteral nutrition (TPN) fluids in the presence of ARF and a high serum magnesium concentration. Although uric acid levels are elevated with renal failure, the elevation is the result of decreased excretion and not increased production of urate. The chances of developing uric acid nephropathy are low, because the filtration of urate is decreased and the intrarenal precipitation of uric acid is minimized. In hyperuricemia secondary to tumor lysis syndrome, uric acid production is increased, so treatment with allopurinol and alkalinization of urine is important for decreasing the incidence of uric acid nephropathy.[8]

CNS Toxicity

Neurologic symptoms of ARF include irritability, somnolence, seizures, and coma.[2] Uremic coma is extremely rare today, because of early intervention with dialysis. Seizures may occur as a consequence of electrolyte disturbances, such as severe hyponatremia or severe hypertension. Muscle twitching caused by tetany may occur secondary to hypocalcemia. Identification and treatment of the underlying condition are necessary for reversing the neurologic changes.

Hematologic Abnormalities

Anemia associated with ARF is usually dilutional as a result of fluid overload. In some conditions, like the hemolytic uremic syndrome, anemia is largely the result of hemolysis. Packed red blood cell (PRBC) transfusion (5 to 10 ml/kg) is indicated only in the presence of symptomatic anemia, active hemolysis, or bleeding. Elective PRBC transfusion may be needed when hemoglobin falls to low levels (<5 to 6 g/dL). If the patient is receiving hemodialysis, PRBC transfusions are safely given during the hemodialysis treatment to prevent hyperkalemia and fluid overload. Platelet dysfunction secondary to uremia may cause oozing or bleeding at surgical sites, which may respond to intravenous administration of deamino-8-d-arginine vasopressin (DDAVP; 0.2 to 0.4 μg/kg/dose).[2]

Infections

Healing is delayed in the presence of uremia. Surgical wounds should be examined carefully, and prompt antibiotic treatment instituted if infection is suspected. Prolonged use of urinary catheters and drains should be avoided.

Renal-Replacement Therapy

A variety of techniques for RRT are now available for use with ARF, including peritoneal dialysis (PD), hemodialysis (HD), continuous arteriovenous hemofiltration (CAVH) without dialysis, continuous arteriovenous hemofiltration with dialysis (CAVHD), continuous venovenous hemofiltration (CVVH) without dialysis, and continuous venovenous hemofiltration with dialysis (CVVHD).[1,9] The choice of modality for RRT depends on the clinical setting and should be made in consultation with a pediatric nephrologist.

Peritoneal Dialysis

Peritoneal dialysis is the preferred dialysis modality for infants and children, because it is more efficient in children than in adults and because rapid hemodynamic changes can generally be avoided.[1,2,6] A peritoneal dialysis catheter, which may be uncuffed and placed at the bedside or cuffed and inserted surgically, is used for performing the exchanges. Manual exchanges using 10 to 30 ml/kg of commercially available PD solutions containing high-concentration dextrose (1.5 to 4.25%) can be performed even in the smallest infants. Automated programmable cyclers are available for use in larger infants and children. Small volumes are initially used to avoid fluid leaks around the catheter, and the volume is gradually increased to a target of 40 mL/kg/exchange. Fluid and electrolyte status must be monitored closely in all patients receiving PD therapy.

The most serious complication of peritoneal dialysis is peritonitis.[1,2,6] The first sign of peritonitis is usually a cloudy dialysis effluent, followed by clinical symptoms such as fever, abdominal pain, nausea, and vomiting. Diagnosis is made by the presence of >100 WBC/mm^3 in the effluent, >50% of which are neutrophils. After a culture of the effluent is obtained, treatment is begun with intraperitoneal antibiotics for 10 to 14 days. Antibiotic choice is adjusted according to results of the culture. Other complications of PD include hypotension secondary to excess fluid removal, electrolyte disturbances (e.g., hyponatremia or hypokalemia), and mechanical problems with the PD catheter (e.g., kinking, fibrin clots, obstruction by omentum or poor position within the abdomen).

Hemodialysis

Hemodialysis is indicated if there is a need for rapid correction of severe hyperkalemia, intractable metabolic acidosis, severe hyperphosphatemia, and fluid overload. It is also used if the abdomen is unsuitable for PD owing to recent surgery; adhesions; or an acute process, such as intussusception in a patient with hemolytic uremic syndrome. Performance of hemodialysis, especially in infants and small children, requires specifically trained personnel.[1,2,6] It also requires a large double-lumen venous catheter for access. A large single-lumen catheter may be used under special circumstances and with special equipment, but recirculation within the system limits the effectiveness of HD. Appropriate dialyzers are selected according to patient size and dialyzer urea clearance. Rapid urea clearance may lead to a steep fall in serum osmolality and cerebral edema. The patient may then experience headache, nausea, vomiting, or muscle cramps, followed by seizures and coma. This clinical picture is known as the dialysis disequilibrium syndrome[1,2,6] and can be avoided by slow urea clearance and by the administration of an osmotic agent, such as mannitol, early in the dialysis procedure. The rate of fluid removal during HD should also be slow to avoid hypotension. The patient must be continuously monitored by experienced staff during the HD procedure.

CAVH, CAVHD, CVVH, and CVVHD

CAVH and CAVHD require both arterial and venous catheter placement for access.[1] The circuit is driven by the patient's own heart rate and blood pressure and easily clots when the blood pressure falls. Pump-driven CVVH or CVVHD avoids the need for arterial access and the limitations of poor blood flow through the circuit at low blood pressures. Only a single venous dual-lumen catheter or two venous catheters are required for CVVH and CVVHD access.[1,9] Because the circuit is driven by a mechanical blood pump, special equipment and continuous pressure monitoring of the equipment are required. The primary indication for CAVH and CVVH is fluid removal. Fluid removal is achieved at a slow, continuous pace, which results in more hemodynamic stability. Another advantage of slow, continuous fluid removal is the ability to provide nutrient-rich replacement fluids (TPN or enteral tube feedings) to these catabolic patients without worsening their fluid overload. The dialysis component can be added if necessary to improve clearances.

ARF in Neonates

The causes of ARF in neonates are usually related to congenital anomalies of the urinary tract or perinatal events.[1-3] Prerenal azotemia may be secondary to twin-to-twin transfusion, maternal antepartum hemorrhage, or other perinatal events that lead to hypotension in the newborn. The biochemical indices of ARF are different for the neonate than for the older infant or child because of renal tubular immaturity. Prerenal azotemia is associated with a urine osmolality >350 mOsm/kg water and a fractional excretion of sodium <2.5%.[1-3] Urinary sodium concentration, specific gravity, and the serum BUN:creatinine ratio are not reliable indicators for neonates with ARF. Congenital anomalies of the urinary tract associated with ARF include renal hypoplasia or dysplasia, polycystic kidney disease, renal agenesis, bilateral severe vesicoureteral reflux, and obstructive uropathies (e.g., posterior urethral valves, ureteropelvic junction obstruction, ureterovesical junction obstruction, urethral diverticulum, ureterocele, and neurogenic bladder). Intrinsic renal diseases include ATN owing to perinatal asphyxia, and congenital infections, such as syphilis or toxoplasmosis. Use of nephrotoxic antibiotics for the treatment of sepsis may also lead to nonoliguric ARF as in older children and adults.

Prerenal azotemia requires treatment with intravenous fluids. It must be noted that insensible fluid losses are much higher in neonates, largely because of their greater surface area for body weight.[2,3] Use of radiant warmers and concomitant phototherapy significantly increase insensible water losses to as much as 80 to 100 mL/kg/day.

Management of established renal failure in neonates is similar to that in children and includes fluid restriction, prevention of hyperkalemia and hyperphosphatemia by limiting intake, and correction of hypocalcemia and acidosis. Frequent laboratory testing, usually at least daily, is necessary to monitor the appropriateness of the therapy. When dialysis is indicated, PD is the preferred modality.[1,2] Hemodialysis is technically feasible, if needed, but should be done only in centers with specially trained pediatric dialysis staff. CAVH, CAVHD, CVVH, and CVVHD can also be performed successfully in neonates when the appropriate equipment and an experienced staff are available.[9]

CHRONIC RENAL FAILURE AND END-STAGE RENAL DISEASE

The diagnosis of chronic renal failure (CRF) in a child can be quite devastating to the patient and family, especially if end-stage renal failure (ESRD) occurs. ESRD is defined as the point at which the GFR decreases to 10 mL/min/1.73 m^2 or less. In recent years, advances in medical therapy and in dialysis and renal transplantation have made it possible for these patients to have a relatively normal lifestyle. Early medical intervention in the course of patients with CRF may prevent the occurrence of severe complications, such as growth failure and bone disease.[6] Early referral to a pediatric nephrologist is therefore indicated in patients identified with this diagnosis. The incidence, causes, and clinical manifestations of CRF and ESRD are discussed elsewhere in this book; this chapter focuses on the management of these patients. The general categories of medical management are outlined in Table 5.4.

Nutrition

Children with CRF or ESRD easily become malnourished because of poor caloric intake owing to the anorexia associated with uremia and to dietary restrictions in fluid, sodium, potassium, and/or phosphorus.[2,6,10] Every effort should be made to provide at least the recommended dietary allowance (RDA) of calories for age. If height and weight fall below the normal percentiles and if food intake is inadequate, special nutritional supplements may be needed. Supplements designed especially for patients with renal failure have a high caloric density and can be used even when fluid restriction is necessary. In infants and small children, adequate caloric intake can be ensured with the use of nasogastric

TABLE 5.4. *Management of chronic renal failure*

- Nutrition
  Calories: at least 100% RDA
  Protein: 0.5–1.5 g/kg/day
- Edema or fluid overload
  Dietary sodium and fluid restriction
  Diuretics: furosemide, metolazone
- Hypertension
  Dietary sodium restriction
  Drugs: calcium channel blockers, ACE inhibitors,
    β-blockers
- Electrolytes
  Metabolic acidosis: sodium bicarbonate, acetate, or ci-
    trate supplements
  Hyperkalemia: ion exchange resin (Kayexalate®)
- Renal osteodystrophy
  Phosphate binders: calcium carbonate, calcium acetate
  Vitamin D metabolites: calcitriol, dihydrotachysterol
- Anemia
  Iron supplements
  Recombinant erythropoietin
- Growth failure
  Nutritional support
  Control of acidosis and renal osteodystrophy
  Recombinant human growth hormone

tube feeding or gastrostomy feeding. One of the principal causes of retarded growth with CRF is malnutrition, and providing adequate calories has been shown to affect growth favorably.[6, 10]

The issue of protein intake is controversial.[6, 10] In experimental models of renal failure, increased protein intake has been shown to accelerate the progression of renal failure. Protein restriction has been recommended for adults with renal failure, but the degree to which protein must be restricted can interfere with usual dietary preferences and lead to poor intake and calorie malnutrition. In children, protein requirements for growth must be balanced against any potential benefits for retarding disease progression. In general, protein intakes of 1.0 to 1.5 gm/kg/day are recommended. This amount may need be increased for nephrotic children, who have excess protein losses in the urine, or for children undergoing PD, who have excess protein losses in the dialysis effluent.

Metabolic abnormalities that accompany CRF and ESRD include hyperkalemia and metabolic acidosis. Dietary potassium restriction becomes necessary when the child reaches ESRD. When dietary restriction is not effective, oral sodium polystyrene (0.5 to 4 g/kg/day in two to four divided doses) can be used. Correction of metabolic acidosis is achieved with oral alkali supplementation, either sodium citrate or sodium bicarbonate (1 to 4 mEq/kg/day in two to four divided doses). Uncorrected chronic acidosis can contribute to growth retardation and worsen renal osteodystrophy.

Hyperlipidemia occurs frequently with CRF and ESRD.[10] Long-term effects of hyperlipidemia in chil-

dren are unknown, but the potential for early atherosclerosis is a concern.[2] Little is known of the safely and effectiveness of lipid-lowering drugs in children, so they are not routinely recommended. Systematic investigation of lipid-lowering drugs in children with CRF is greatly needed.

Renal Osteodystrophy

Children with CRF and ESRD have secondary hyperparathyroidism and deficient production of 1,25-dihydroxyvitamin D, which can lead to bone disease. Three types of renal osteodystrophy are identified.[11, 12] High-turnover bone disease and osteitis fibrosa occur when excessive parathyroid hormone (PTH) is predominant. Phosphate retention owing to decreased renal excretion from renal failure leads to hypocalcemia, which stimulates excess PTH secretion. Low-turnover bone disease occurs when deficient production of 1,25-dihydroxyvitamin D predominates. Renal damage reduces 1-hydroxylation of 25-hydroxyvitamin D to 1,25-dihydroxyvitamin D, the active form of vitamin D, which is produced in the distal renal tubule. As a result, intestinal calcium absorption is decreased, causing hypocalcemia and poor calcification of bones, which leads to osteomalacia. This form of renal osteodystrophy can be worsened by the use of aluminum salts as phosphate binders. Aluminum is absorbed in the intestine and deposited in tissues, including the bones, where it is turned over slowly compared to calcium, causing severe osteomalacia.[6, 7, 11]

Citrate, like that found in buffered citrate solutions used for the management of acidosis, markedly enhances intestinal absorption of aluminum and should never be used with aluminum salts.[11] To avoid the complications of aluminum toxicity, the use of aluminum salts has been virtually given up in children. Adynamic or aplastic bone disease occurs when both osteoblastic and osteoclastic activities are low. The exact cause is unknown, but aluminum toxicity and the oversuppression of PTH secretion as result of treatment with vitamin D metabolites and high-dose calcium may play important roles in the pathogenesis.[11, 12]

Treatment of renal osteodystrophy requires medications, although dietary restriction of phosphorus may help.[11] Major dietary sources of phosphorus are dairy products and meats. Commonly used infant formulas are cow milk based and have a high phosphate content. In infants with CRF or ESRD, low-phosphate-containing formulas like ™Similac PM 60/40 should be used instead of the usual formulas. Soy formulas are particularly high in phosphorus and should be avoided completely. Protein restriction, as described above, translates into restricted milk and meat intake, which automatically limits phosphate intake in older children. Dietary phosphorus restriction alone is not enough to maintain serum phosphorus in the normal range for age without requiring a diet too restrictive to provide adequate nourishment. Phosphate binding medications, usually in the form of calcium salts such as calcium carbonate and calcium acetate, are needed. Regular laboratory monitoring allows the dose to be adjusted to avoid hypercalcemia. Calcium salts are best taken with meals for maximum effectiveness, but will still be effective if taken regularly at other times if needed to improve patient acceptance and compliance.

The use of vitamin D metabolites and analogues is also important. For infants, the analogue dihydrotachysterol—the only commercial preparation available in liquid form—is widely used. Dihydrotachysterol must be 25-hydroxylated by the liver for activity in the body. In older children and adults, the actual metabolite 1,25-dihydroxyvitamin D_3 (known as calcitriol), which comes in a capsule form, is used in dosages that range from 0.25 to 1.5 μg/day. An injectable form of calcitriol is also available for hemodialysis patients. Routine laboratory monitoring is needed to prevent hypercalcemia, which is the predominant side effect of vitamin D metabolite therapy. Parathyroidectomy is rarely necessary as a form of treatment for secondary hyperparathyroidism in childhood because of the effectiveness of the vitamin D metabolite and phosphate-binder therapies.

Anemia

The anemia of renal failure is typically normocytic and normochromic. Microcytic anemia may, however, be seen in association with iron deficiency, which occurs in CRF and ESRD because of nutritional deficiency or microscopic blood loss in the stools. Correction of iron deficiency with iron supplements is usually the first step in the treatment of anemia associated with CRF and ESRD. The dose is 2 to 6 mg/kg/day of elemental iron given orally. Intravenous iron can also be used, especially for HD patients. The healthy kidney is responsible for the production of erythropoietin, the hormone that stimulates RBC production by the bone marrow. When the kidney is diseased, deficiency of erythropoietin can occur, leading to decreased red blood cell production and anemia. Recombinant human erythropoietin is now commercially available and is used routinely in the management of anemia of both CRF and ESRD.[2,6,10] The starting dose is 50 U/kg/dose subcutaneously twice a week for CRF patients or patients on peritoneal dialysis and intravenously three times a week for patients on hemodialysis. Erythropoietin use minimizes or eliminates the requirement for blood transfusions. Repeated transfusions lead to iron overload and also have the potential to cause HLA sensitization. Correction of anemia with erythropoietin improves exercise tolerance; promotes a general sense of well-being; and improves appetite, which has led to hyperkalemia in some patients from increased intake. Other potential adverse consequences of erythropoietin are hypertension and increased episodes of clotting of arteriovenous access for dialysis.

Hypertension

The association of hypertension with renal disease is well known in children. In CRF and ESRD, hypertension can be caused by salt and water retention or by excessive renin production or by both.[6] Treatment is the same as outlined for ARF.

Growth Failure

Linear growth is adversely affected in CRF and ESRD, because of several factors, including uncorrected metabolic acidosis, poor caloric intake, renal osteodystrophy, and resistance to the action of growth hormone owing to the presence of inhibitory binding proteins in uremic serum.[6,10] Recombinant human growth hormone used in supraphysiologic doses and administered as a daily subcutaneous injection has been shown to improve growth velocity and improve height percentiles in affected children. Final adult height is still below normal for most patients—even with growth hormone treatment—unless treatment is begun early, especially in infants and young children who are most affected by long-term growth failure.

Significant developmental delay may occur in children with CRF and ESRD.[6,10] Poor nutrition, decreased muscle strength, and socioeconomic factors play roles in the developmental delay. Promotion of good nutrition and growth hormone therapy may improve muscle strength and gross motor development. Early intervention programs with physical and occupational therapy services must be used to maximize the developmental potential of these children.

Psychosocial

Disruption of normal lifestyle, stress of dialysis, and retarded physical growth affect the mental well-being of patients and their families.[6,10] Patients may experience poor school performance and disrupted peer relationships. The incidence of divorce in parents of children with chronic illnesses is higher than in the general population. Depression is common in dialysis patients, especially adolescents. Of all renal-replacement therapies that are available, renal transplantation is the most successful, in terms of both medical and psychosocial issues. After successful transplantation, children grow better and return to an almost normal lifestyle.

Dialysis

Most children become symptomatic with anorexia, nausea, lethargy, and poor school performance when

TABLE 5.5. *Advantages and disadvantages of dialysis modalities*

Dialysis	Advantages	Disadvantage
Peritoneal dialysis		
CAPD	Mobility	Labor intensive for patient and family
CCPD and NIPD	Low labor intensity	Need specialize equipment
Hemodialysis	No labor for patient and family; minimal infection risk	Hospital based[a]; requires trained pediatric staff; vascular access difficult in small children

CAPD, chronic ambulatory peritoneal dialysis; *CCPD,* continuous cycling peritoneal dialysis; *NIPD,* nightly intermittent peritoneal dialysis.
[a]In most places.

they reach ESRD; and initiation of dialysis therapy or performance of a renal transplant is indicated at that time. Dialysis modality is chosen based on age, size, psychosocial, and socioeconomic factors. The advantages and disadvantages of the various dialysis modalities are given in Table 5.5.

Hemodialysis

Hemodialysis removes fluid and waste products from the patient's blood, which flows rapidly on one side of a semipermeable dialysis membrane into the dialysis fluid, which flows rapidly in the opposite direction on the other side of the membrane. Clearance of urea, creatinine, potassium, phosphorus, and other small and middle molecules occurs in this fashion. Adequacy of dialysis is currently gauged by the effectiveness of the measured urea clearance. HD in children should be performed in special renal units that are equipped with suitable pediatric equipment and staffed with specially trained pediatric nurses, dieticians, and social workers in addition to a pediatric nephrologist.[2, 6] The HD procedure must be done for 3 to 4 h, three times a week for adequate removal of fluid and waste products. In anuric small infants, hemodialysis often needs to be done four times a week for adequate fluid removal.

A working vascular access is the mainstay of chronic HD.[6] Ideally, a surgically created arteriovenous fistula (AVF) is preferred, because it has the lowest incidence of complications., such as thrombosis, venous stenosis, and infection. An AVF may not be possible in a very small children because their blood vessels may be too small. Surgically placed arteriovenous grafts (AVGs) make of ™Gore-Tex are an alternative to fistulas. Both AVFs and AVGs are typically placed in the nondominant forearm. For the small child, a femoral AVG may be the only alternative for technical reasons. Complications of permanent vascular access include thrombosis, accidental hemorrhage, limb length discrepancy, and infection. For infants and for children weighing <10 kg, both AVF and AVG are technically difficult. In these children, semipermanent access with cuffed dual-lumen catheters may be used for many months. The most common sites of insertion are the internal jugular and the subclavian vein. Complications include infection, catheter thrombosis, central venous stenosis, and thrombosis. Stenosis and thrombosis are more common with subclavian vein catheters but can occur with both.

Children undergoing chronic hemodialysis typically require stringent dietary and fluid restriction. Compliance with this regimen is often difficult, so the incidence of predialysis hypertension and hyperkalemia are high in the pediatric population. Treatment of anemia, renal osteodystrophy, and growth failure as outlined above must be continued, even after starting chronic dialysis.

Peritoneal Dialysis

PD is the preferred modality for children, especially infants. The procedure involves instillation of dialysate fluid through an indwelling catheter into the peritoneal cavity followed by emptying after a desired equilibration time. Each instillation is called an *exchange,* and multiple exchanges are done daily. The peritoneal membrane acts as a semipermeable dialysis membrane; and diffusion of urea, creatinine, potassium, phosphate, and other molecules into the dialysate solution takes place because of a concentration gradient between blood and the dialysis fluid. PD offers several advantages for the pediatric patient:[6] It is technically easier than other forms of dialysis, especially for the small child, and it can be done at home by the patient, parent, or guardian. Because the procedure is performed daily instead of three times a week like HD, diet and fluid restrictions may be less stringent. Protein restriction is not usually necessary, because of obligatory protein losses into the dialysis effluent. Anemia, renal osteodystrophy, and growth failure need to be treated in any dialysis patient, as outlined above.

Performance of chronic PD requires access to the peritoneal cavity with a specialized, cuffed PD catheter. A variety of sizes and designs are available for pediatric patients. Accurate positioning of the PD catheter is critical to successful function. A ™Dacron cuff attached to the catheter is placed at the peritoneal entrance, around which a pursestring suture is applied to create a near watertight seal to hold the catheter in position. The catheter then exits the skin through a tight subcutaneous tunnel, either below or above the belt line. Above the belt line is preferred in infants and non-toilet-trained children, to avoid contamination in the diaper area. Efforts are also made to place the PD catheter exit site away from draining ureterostomies or nephrostomies. A second ™Dacron cuff positioned near the skin exit site, used in adults, is not generally used in children because of the high incidence of erosion of the cuff through the skin.

PD may be done manually or mechanically. When dialysis exchanges are performed manually, the procedure is termed continuous ambulatory peritoneal dialysis (CAPD). Typically, four to five exchanges are done daily. Daytime exchanges are usually done every 3 to 5 h; then a long dwell is left in the peritoneal cavity at night. CAPD requires patient and parental commitment, is labor intensive, and may be associated with frequent infections if aseptic technique is not carried out rigorously with each bag exchange.

Automated programmable cyclers limit the work involved in doing exchanges and the number of times the catheter must be opened, exposing the patient to the risk of infection. When a cycler is used for part of the day or night followed by a long dwell when off the cycler, the procedure is termed continuous cycling peritoneal dialysis (CCPD). When only nighttime exchanges are done, the procedure is termed nightly intermittent peritoneal dialysis (NIPD). For both procedures, 7 to 10 exchanges are performed, usually at night during sleep; the dwell time lasts 45 to 60 min. The child is free during the day to attend school and take part in other activities. Newer cyclers are smaller and more portable, which adds to the patient's independence and the family's ability to travel if desired.

The most important complication of PD is acute bacterial peritonitis. The first sign of peritonitis is usually cloudy dialysis fluid followed by abdominal pain and sometimes fever, vomiting, or diarrhea. Staphylococci are the infecting organisms in the majority of cases. The diagnosis of peritonitis is made when cellular analysis of cloudy effluent reveals >100 WBC/mm^3 with >50% predominance of polymorphonuclear cells. Treatment should be instituted rapidly with intraperitoneal instillation of antibiotics. First-generation cephalosporins are well tolerated and may be effective for most staphylococcal infections, unless the patient lives in an area known to have a high incidence of cephalosporin-resistant staphylococci. Gram negative bacteria require third-generation cephalosporins or aminoglycosides for treatment. Fungal peritonitis is rare but should be considered in patients with persistent cloudy fluid that is culture negative. Most infections respond well to intraperitoneal antibiotics; but for some gram negative bacterial and fungal infections, removal of the PD catheter

may be necessary. These infections are also associated with a high incidence of peritoneal scarring, sometimes requiring a change to hemodialysis because of membrane failure.

Other complications of PD include exit site and tunnel infections, which usually respond to oral antibiotics. Mechanical failure may be attributed to PD catheter kinking, poor positioning, or occlusion by fibrin or omentum. In many centers, partial or complete omentectomy is performed at the time of catheter insertion to avoid this complication.[6] The incidence of inguinal and ventral hernias is high as a result of constant high intra-abdominal pressure. When diagnosed, these require surgical correction.

RENAL TRANSPLANTATION

Renal transplantation is the preferred treatment modality for children and adolescents with ESRD.[13] After successful renal transplantation, patients feel better and have a more normal lifestyle. Recent advances in immunosuppressive therapy have increased success rates. Several other factors, such as congenitally poor bladder function and noncompliance with medications, still limit good outcome after renal transplantation in children and adolescents.

Urologic Considerations

Obstructive uropathy is the cause of ESRD in many children.[14] Careful evaluation of the urinary bladder and upper urinary tracts is extremely important in these patients during pretransplant evaluation. Posterior urethral valves, prune belly syndrome, and spina bifida are associated with poor bladder function and sometimes require augmentation procedures. Clean intermittent catheterization can be continued posttransplant, if necessary. Refluxing ureters or persistent hydronephrosis predispose patients to urinary tract infections after posttransplantation immunosuppression is begun; nephroureterectomy may be warranted in such situations.

Donor Selection

Living related donor (LRD) kidney transplants have the best survival rates.[13, 14] The 1-year graft survival exceeds 90% in LRD transplants, compared to 80 to 85% in cadaveric transplants.[14] HLA matching has also been shown to affect graft survival; an HLA identical donor is best. For children receiving an LRD transplant, parents are the source in >50% cases; siblings are the next most common source. On average, about 45% of children with ESRD receive LRD transplants and 55% receive cadaveric kidneys. Risk factors for poor graft survival after cadaveric renal transplant include donor age

<6 years, recipient age <2 years, HLA-DR (class II) antigen mismatches, cold ischemia time prolonged >24 h, African-American background, prior transfusions, and previous transplants.

Recipient Selection

Active malignancy is the only absolute contraindication to transplantation in pediatric patients. In the case of bilateral Wilms tumor, a patient who remains recurrence- and metastasis-free >1 year is considered an optimal candidate for proceeding with renal transplantation. Other relative contraindications for transplantation in pediatric patients are small recipient size and a history of poor compliance with the medical regimen. For technical reasons, children weighing <10 kg may be considered too small for transplantation in many centers; in these centers, children are treated with dialysis until target growth parameters are met. Compliance with diet and medications must be evaluated and addressed in all patients, especially in the adolescent age group. Noncompliance with immunosuppressive therapy can lead to rejection and graft loss. Donor kidneys are a relatively rare resource and, if possible, should not be wasted in situations in which poor compliance with therapy is already known to be a difficult problem.

A number of underlying renal diseases, especially those with an immunologic basis, can recur in the transplanted kidney.[13-15] Common examples are focal segmental glomerulosclerosis, IgA nephropathy, membranoproliferative glomerulonephritis, membranous nephropathy, and hemolytic uremic syndrome. Even when the incidence of recurrence is fairly high, recurrence may not lead to graft loss.

Immunosuppression

Common drugs used for immunosuppression therapy for renal transplantation are listed in Table 5.6. Prednisone is the most commonly used corticosteroid, both for maintenance therapy and for reversal of acute rejection. Generally, corticosteroids are initiated at a high dose immediately posttransplant, rapidly weaned in the next 4 to 8 weeks to a lower dose, and then tapered to a final maintenance dose. Maintenance doses are usually achieved after 3 to 6 months and vary from 0.1 to 0.3 mg/kg/day to 0.3 to 0.5 mg/kg/day, taken on alternate days.[13] Alternate-day therapy is usually instituted to promote growth. Side effects associated with the chronic use of corticosteroids include facial and truncal weight gain (Cushingoid appearance), poor linear growth, hypertension, hyperlipidemia, aseptic necrosis of the femoral head, diabetes, and cataracts. Short courses of high-dose oral prednisone or intravenous methylprednisolone (steroid pulse) are used to treat acute rejection episodes.[13]

TABLE 5.6. *Drugs Used for Renal Transplant Immunosuppression*

Induction therapy
  Methylprednisolone
  Cyclosporine
  Antibodies: OKT$_3$, Antithymocyte globulin, or Antilymphocyte globulin
Maintenance therapy
  Monotherapy—cyclosporine alone
  Dual therapy—prednisone and cyclosporine
  Triple therapy—prednisone, cyclosporine and azathioprine, or mycophenolate mofetil
  Quadruple therapy—Antibody induction followed by triple therapy
Acute rejection therapy
  Methylprednisolone or prednisone oral pulse
  OKT-3
  Antithymocyte globulin, antilymphocyte globulin
  Mycophenolate mofetil
New agents with limited experience in children with renal transplants
  Tacrolimus
  Mycophenolate mofetil
  Sirolimus
  Monoclonal antibodies: daclizumab, basiliximab

Since the early 1980s, cyclosporine (℞Sandimmune, ℞Neoral) has become the mainstay of transplant immunosuppressive therapy. It is a cyclic polypeptide produced by the fungus *Beauvaria nivea*. Its mechanism of action is suppression of T-lymphocytes, especially T-helper cells, and inhibition of interleukin-2.[13,16] Both T-helper cells and interleukin 2 play important roles in the cascade leading to acute rejection. Dosing of cyclosporine in children is somewhat complicated, because of variable metabolism at different ages. Younger children tend to require higher doses. Dosing interval is generally every 12 h, and trough blood levels are used to guide therapy. Concomitant use of other drugs, like anticonvulsants which increase cyclosporine metabolism, must be carefully monitored and cyclosporine doses adjusted accordingly, usually by frequent measurement of cyclosporine blood levels. The main disadvantage of cyclosporin is its nephrotoxicity. Acute nephrotoxicity associated with high drug levels is generally reversible, but chronic toxicity can lead to irreversible fibrosis and scarring in the transplanted kidney.

Azathioprine (Imuran®; 1 to 2 mg/kg/day PO) is used in many centers along with prednisone and cyclosporine for maintenance therapy.[13,16] Azathioprine is a purine analogue that is incorporated into cellular DNA and inhibits synthesis of RNA, T-lymphocyte activation, and monocyte proliferation. Side effects include hepatotoxicity and bone marrow suppression with an increased risk of infection and anemia. Complete blood cell counts should be followed meticulously when azathioprine is used. Azathioprine does not have a role in the treatment of acute rejection. It is not specific and is likely to be replaced by newer, more specific generations of transplant antirejection drugs.

Tacrolimus (Prograf®; formerly known as FK506) is a macrolide antibiotic compound produced by *Streptomyces tsukubaensis,* which has a similar mechanism of action to cyclosporine by inhibiting interleukin 2 and T-lymphocyte activation.[16] Tacrolimus has been used instead of cyclosporine for maintenance therapy and sometimes for rescue from acute rejection. Experience with pediatric kidney transplants is limited, but growing. Tacrolimus and cyclosporine should not be used together, because of the potential for synergistic toxicities.

Sirolimus (Rapamune®; previously known as rapamycin) is another macrolide antibiotic that is structurally similar to tacrolimus but has a different mechanism of action.[16] It impairs the ability of cytokines to trigger proliferation of T-lymphocytes. Sirolimus interferes with the action of tacrolimus but has synergy with cyclosporine. Combination therapy with sirolimus and cyclosporine may be effective for preventing acute rejection. Clinical trials in adults are in progress.

Mycophenolate mofetil (CellCept®) is a new immunosuppressive drug, and experience with it in children is limited.[17,18] Mycophenolate mofetil inhibits a key enzyme in the de novo synthesis of purine nucleotides in both T- and B-lymphocytes and prevents their proliferation. It has been used instead of azathioprine with prednisone and cyclosporine for induction and maintenance therapy. It has also been used successfully for rescue therapy for acute rejection in adults and children.

Antibodies directed against lymphocytes have been used extensively in the prevention and treatment of rejection. Antithymocyte globulin and antilymphocyte globulin are polyclonal antibodies that have been used for induction and rescue therapy.[13,16] Risks of polyclonal antibody therapy include infection with or reactivation of latent viral diseases, such as cytomegalovirus and Epstein–Barr virus. Acute infection with Epstein–Barr virus has been shown to be a major risk factor predisposing the patient to posttransplant lymphoproliferative disease. Secondary malignancy also occurs to a greater extent in patients who have received polyclonal antibodies. Monoclonal antibodies with greater specificity against T-lymphocytes are also available. OKT$_3$ has been used extensively in children in many centers for induction and rescue from acute rejection, but it has significant side effects.[13,16] Two monoclonal antibodies—daclizumab (Zenapax®)[19,20] and basiliximab (Simulect®)—are now available for induction therapy.[21] Both block the interleukin 2 receptor and have few apparent side effects. Experience with these drugs in children is extremely limited.[19]

Long-Term Prognosis

The overall success rate of renal transplantation in children has shown consistent improvement over the last two decades of the twentieth century. With the development of newer, safer immunosuppressive drugs, graft survival is likely to be more prolonged in the future. Recent analysis of data from the North American Pediatric Transplant Cooperative Study shows a projected 5-year graft survival of about 78% in LRD transplants and 60% for cadaveric transplants in children and adolescents.[14,15] The predominant reasons for hospitalization in the first 6 months after transplant were acute rejection, bacterial or viral infection, and hypertension. Patient mortality rates were low. LRD transplant recipients had a 96% patient survival rate, and cadaveric transplant recipients had a 93% survival rate. Malignancy was reported in 1.2% of cases and was predominantly posttransplant lymphoproliferative disease.[13,14]

REFERENCES

1. Siegel NJ, Van Why SK, Boydstun II, et al. Acute renal failure. In: Holliday MA, Barratt TM, Avner ED, eds., Pediatric nephrology. 3rd ed. Baltimore: Williams & Wilkins, 1994:1176–1203.
2. Mentser M, Mahon J. Renal failure. In: O'Donnell B, Koff SA, eds., Pediatric urology. 3rd ed. Butterworth-Heinemann, 1997: 260–277.
3. Brion LP, Satlin LM. Clinical significance of developmental renal physiology. In: Polin RA, Fox WW, eds., Fetal and neonatal physiology. 2nd ed. Philadelphia: Saunders, 1998:1677–1691.
4. Chevalier RL, Gomez RA. Obstructive uropathy. In: Holliday MA, Barratt TM, Avner ED, eds., Pediatric nephrology. 3rd ed. Baltimore: Williams & Wilkins, 1994:994–1005.
5. National High Blood Pressure Education Program. Update on the 1987 task force report on high blood pressure control in children and adolescents: a working group report from the National High Blood Pressure Education Program. Pediatrics 1996; 98:649–658.
6. Kohaut EC. Chronic renal failure; end stage renal disease. In: Oski FA, DeAngelis CD, Feigin RD, Warshaw JB, eds., Principles and practice of pediatrics. 2nd ed. Philadelphia: Lippincott, 1994:1772–1780.
7. Andreoli SP, Bergstein JM, Sheppard DJ. Aluminum intoxication from aluminum containing phosphate binders in children not undergoing dialysis. N Engl J Med 1984;310:1079–1082.
8. Jones DP, Mahmoud H, Chesney RW. Tumor lysis syndrome: pathogenesis and management. Pediatr Nephrol 1995;9:206–212.
9. Smoyer WE, McAdams C, Kaplan BS, Sherbotie JR. Determinants of survival in pediatric continuous hemofiltration. J Am Soc Nephrol 1995;6:1401–1409.
10. Wassner SJ. Conservative management of chronic renal insufficiency. In: Holliday MA, Barratt TM, Avner ED, eds., Pediatric nephrology. 3rd ed. Baltimore: Williams & Wilkins, 1994:1314–1338.
11. Salusky IB, Ramirez JA, Goodman WG. Disorders of bone and mineral metabolism in chronic renal failure. In: Holliday MA, Barratt TM, Avner ED, eds., Pediatric nephrology. 3rd ed. Baltimore: Williams & Wilkins, 1994:1287–1304.
12. Hruska KA, Teitelbaum SL. Renal osteodystrophy. N Engl J Med 1995;333:166–174.
13. Yadin O, Grimm P, Ettenger R. Renal transplantation in children: clinical aspects. In: Holliday MA, Barratt TM, Avner ED, eds., Pediatric nephrology. 3rd ed. Baltimore: Williams & Wilkins, 1994:1390–1418.
14. Kohaut EC, Tejani A. The 1994 annual report of the North American Pediatric Renal Transplant Cooperative Study. Pediatr Nephrol 1996;10:422–434.
15. Kashtan CE, McEnery PT, Tejani A, Stablein DM. Renal allograft survival according to primary diagnosis: a report of the North

American Pediatric Transplant Cooperative Study. Pediatr Nephrol 1995;9:679–684.

16. Suthanthiran M, Strom TB. Renal transplantation. N Engl J Med 1994;331:365–376.

17. Weber LT, Shipkova M, Lamersdorf T, et al. Pharmacokinetics of mycophenolic acid (MPA) and determinants of MPA free fraction in pediatric and adult renal transplant recipients. German Study Group on Mycophenolate Mofetil Therapy in Pediatric Renal Transplant Recipients. J Am Soc Nephrol 1998;8:1511–1520.

18. Ettenger R, Cohen A, Nast C, et al. Mycophenolate mofetil as maintenance immunosuppression in pediatric renal transplantation. Transplant Proc 1997;29:340–341.

19. Ettenger RB. New immunosuppressive agents in pediatric renal transplantation. Transplant Proc 1998;30:1956–1958.

20. Vincenti F, Kirkman R, Light S, et al. Interleukin-2 receptor blockade with Daclizumab to prevent acute rejection in renal transplantation. New Engl J Med 1998;338:161–165.

21. Nashan B, Moore R, Amiot P. Randomized trial of basiliximab versus placebo for control of acute cellular rejection in renal allograft recipients. Lancet 1997;350:1193–1198.

CHAPTER 6

Management of the High-Risk Fetus: Prenatal Diagnosis and Therapy

Robert J. Carpenter Jr., Edwina J. Popek, and Tom Rowe

The introduction of ultrasound revolutionized the evaluation and management of the fetus in the late twentieth century.[1-8] The ability to see inside the uterus and visualize its contents developed first as brightness-mode-generated amplitude spikes that measured only the distance between two points within the fetus. It is now possible to achieve two-dimensional, real-time, high-resolution imaging by which the clinician can view both normal and abnormal anatomy. Major advancements in transducer technology and the development of multifrequency transducer heads allows the evaluation of fetal behavior and the study of organs and their associated physiologic processes. The enhanced resolution generates differential densities in the organ or tissue being imaged, allowing accurate assessment of the structure. In addition, the rapid increase in microprocessor speed and the substantial decrease in cost of sonographic equipment have brought this equipment into the offices of the generalist obstetrician and family medicine physician. This high-quality ultrasonic scanning equipment makes it possible to identify fetal malformations.

Multipopulation studies of total fetal anomalies and specific genitourinary anomalies have been published. In a study of 11,986 pregnancies in Malmo, Sweden, overall malformation frequency of 0.5%.[5] Fetal uropathy occurred in 0.28% of pregnancies, and urinary tract dilation in 0.18%. A higher frequency of genitourinary malformations (0.48%) was reported by a Finnish study that examined 4,586 pregnancies. Similar findings were noted by other authors.[9-13] Scott and Renwick[9] reported a frequency of 0.3% for urinary tract anomalies, and 57.2% of the anomalies found consisted of hydronephrosis. Moretti et al.[10] noted a substantial increase in urinary tract anomalies from 6.9% in 1978–1982 to 12.4% in 1983–1984 in 103,484 births. Isolated urinary tract lesions accounted for 66 of 91 of the anomalies and obstructive disorders made up 60% of the recognized anomalies. Chitty[14] reviewed multiple series of fetal anomalies. Through postnatal follow-up, 84% of antenatally diagnosed anomalies were confirmed. Many series do not adequately define the anomalies included in the study, especially facial and intracranial anomalies. Furthermore, the cause of the malformations is often not noted, and many authors do not identify chromosomal abnormalities or recognize multiple malformation syndromes.

The increased fluid retention in the genitourinary tract allows for rapid recognition of developmental anomalies. The density differential between the normally placed kidneys and the anteriorly situated liver provides the contrast necessary to assess the common anomalies seen in obstetrical ultrasound studies. When an anomaly of the urinary tract is identified, multiple specialties of medicine are often involved in its assessment and subsequent management; obtaining the necessary information becomes the major focus of the initial management of the abnormality. During the evaluation period, stress and the uncertainty concerning the outcome often have a negative affect on the family. This chapter assesses many issues that help provide comprehensive and continuous care to the family.

EMBRYOLOGY OF THE GENITOURINARY TRACT

Many anomalies affecting the kidney have their origins in the failure of metanephric differentiation and the ingrowth of the primitive ureteric bud into the metanephric blastema and its subsequent differentiation.[15, 16] Failure of renal development and failure of collecting duct formation yield the most common malformations of renal agenesis and multicystic renal dysplasia. The ureteric bud arises from an outpouching of the caudal end of the mesonephric or Wolffian duct, where it curves medially to join the cloaca. It grows posteriorly and cranially into the metanephric blastema. The ampulla of

TABLE 6.1. *Osathanondh and Potter classification*

Type		Description
1		Infantile polycystic disease
2		Multicystic kidney
	2A	Large cysts
	2B	Small cysts
3		Adult polycystic kidneys
4		Obstructive uropathy

Reprinted with permission from Osathanondh V, Potter EL. Pathogenesis of polycystic kidneys: survey of results of microdissection. Arch Pathol 1964;77:510–512.

TABLE 6.2. *Classification of renal cystic diseases*

I. Polycystic disease
  A. ARPKD
    1. Classic infantile polycystic disease
    2. ARPKD and congenital hepatic fibrosis in older individuals
  B. ADPKD
    1. Classic adult polycystic disease
    2. ADKPD in infants (glomerulocystic disease)
II. Glomerular cystic disease
III. Localized cystic disease
IV. Renal cysts associated with syndromes of multiple malformations
V. Medullary cystic disease
  A. Medullary sponge kidney
  B. FN-MCD complex
VI. Multiocular renal cysts
VII. Renal dysplasia with cysts
VIII. Simple renal cysts
IX. Acquired renal cystic disease
X. Miscellaneous extrarenal cysts

Modified from Risdon RA. Development, developmental defects, and cystic diseases of the kidney. In: Heptinstall RH, ed., Pathology of the kidney. 4th ed. Boston: Little, Brown, 1992;1:93.
ARPKD, autosomal recessive polycystic kidney disease; *ADPKD,* autosomal dominant polycystic kidney disease; *FN-MCD,* familial nephronophthisis–medullary cystic disease.

the ureteric bud undergoes multiple branchings, which produce 15 generations of nephron formation. Each new ampullary region develops new branch points, providing additional generations of nephrons. The initial branch points coalesce, creating the renal pelvis and sequentially the calices and papillary collecting ducts. By 10 weeks of gestation, nephron development has begun; urine formation is seen by 13 to 14 weeks of gestation.

Some disorders of renal formation and organization have an underlying genetic basis. Osathanondh and Potter,[17–23] in their classic microdissection studies, elucidated much of the underlying anatomic principles for these structural aberrations. Their classification system is considered to be a pivotal point for more recent attempts at classification (Table 6.1). Because these lesions are frequently recognized during fetal evaluations, it is important to recognize the differences among the Osathanondh and Potter types. Despite the utility of their scheme, more recent classification systems have been proposed that are based on clinopathologic, genetic, and pathoradiologic correlations rather than just morphology.

The difficulties intrinsic to the simple classification system proposed by Osathanondh and Potter have promoted many, more rigorous classification systems. A committee of the Section of Urology of the American Academy of Pediatrics has proposed more precise terminology for the many diseases seen in the developing kidney.[24] A classification system suggested by Risdon[25] is shown in Table 6.2. A review of these systems helps solidify an understanding of the complex and voluminous issues relating to the pathology of the fetal genitourinary system. Excellent sources for such information are available.[26, 27]

Osathanondh and Potter Type 1: Diffuse Autosomal Recessive Cystic Renal Dysplasia

Patients with autosomal recessive polycystic kidney disease (ARPKD) have large kidneys (up to 10 times the expected size) that maintain their reniform shape (Fig. 6.1).[17–19] The relative paucity of nephrons and the apparent excessive duct structures are associated with

rudimentary or normal medullary development. Elongated cysts are found in the cortex, and medullary pyramids are normally formed (Fig. 6.2). The ureter and renal pelvis are patent and small. A hypoplastic bladder completes the lower genitourinary tract, because urine is usually not produced in normal amounts. The basic defect is cyst formation from hyperplasia and dilation of the interstitial portions of the ureteric bud, specifically the collecting tubules.

Sonography of a fetus with ARPKD reveals enlarged, dense kidneys secondary to the increased connective tissue. The kidneys will not appear to contain visible cysts, even with the highest resolution scanners,

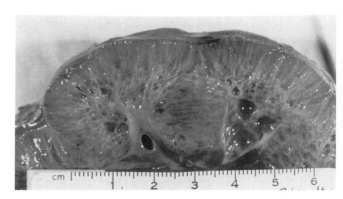

FIG. 6.1. Kidney from a 34-week-old fetus with ARPKD. The cut surface has a spongy appearance. Within the cortex, there are radially oriented, dilated channels that are derived from collecting ducts. There may be large, round cysts within the renal medulla.

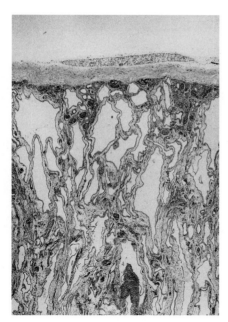

FIG. 6.2. Cysts associated with ARPKD are lined by low cuboidal to columnar epithelium. Interspersed between the cysts are nephrons that are histologically normal and are probably normal in number, which may explain why adequate urine is produced, nearly to term in some cases. There is minimal or no increase in fibrous tissue between the cysts. (Hematoxylin and eosin.)

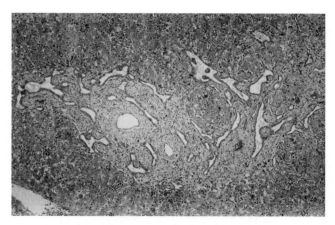

FIG. 6.3. Liver section showing a fine reticular pattern of fibrosis. There is a marked proliferation of bile ducts with abnormal branching. Diffuse portal fibrosis may extend into the lobule, and bile duct cysts are rarely seen. (Hematoxylin and eosin.)

although a few round medullary cysts may be seen. The enlarged kidneys often completely fill the abdomen, significantly increasing the abdominal circumference. The kidneys are seen to kiss one another, owing to their increased size. Although variations in the presentation of different fetuses within a sibship may allow for variable collections of amniotic fluid under most circumstances, by 20 to 24 weeks of gestation a marked reduction in amniotic fluid will be noted.

A number of other autosomal recessive syndromes are associated with enlarged kidneys (Table 6.3). These syndrome can be differentiated from classical ARPKD by underlying histological differences in cyst shape and other clinical findings. A constant characteristic of many of these autosomal recessive syndromes is the co-association of hepatic enlargement, cystic changes, and fibrosis (Fig. 6.3). The exact relationship between

TABLE 6.3. Diffuse renal cystic dysplasia

- Meckel syndrome, Goldston syndrome, Simopoulos syndrome, Miranda syndrome
- Short-rib polydactyly syndromes, Jeune syndrome, Ellis–van Creveld syndrome, Elajalde syndrome
- Robert syndrome
- Zellweger syndrome
- Trisomy 9 and 13
- Glutaric aciduria type 2
- Renal–hepatic–pancreatic dysplasia

ARPKD and congenital hepatic fibrosis (CHF) is unknown. Several other genetic disorders are frequently seen with similar diffuse cystic dysplasia (Fig. 6.4). The gene for ARPKD has been mapped to chromosome 6p21-cen. Linkage analysis is possible if the parents and proband have markers linked to the disease.[28]

Osathanondh and Potter Type 2: Multicystic Renal Dysplasia

Multicystic renal dysplasia is the most common form of renal anomaly seen sonographers that has significant potential for an adverse affect on the fetus. It is most frequently seen as a unilateral condition and has a frequency of 1 in 3000 live births in the United States. From a sonographic perspective, multiple cysts of varying size

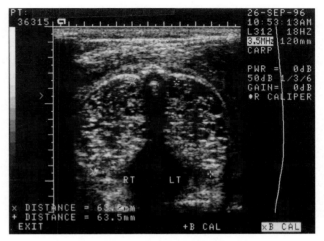

FIG. 6.4. Bilaterally enlarged multicystic dysplastic kidneys with variously sized cysts. The etiology was intravesical obstruction.

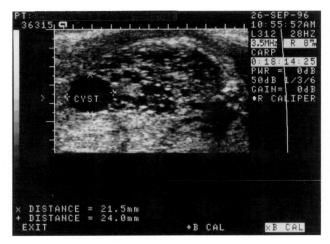

FIG. 6.5. Longitudinal view of a kidney showing variously sized cysts, including one large cyst (21 × 24 mm). Cysts were also seen in other areas of the kidneys.

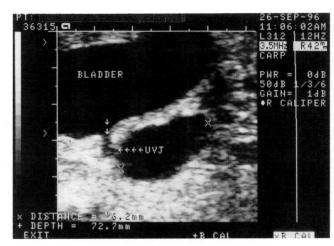

FIG. 6.6. Megacystis with bladder wall thickening. The intravesical cord of the left ureter (*UVJ*) and dilation of the distal ureter (*X–X*) can be seen.

are associated with an enlarged, medially positioned renal pelvic-like structure (Fig. 6.5). Dysplasia is almost always noted when cystic disease is present. An echogenic dense kidney can, however, have severe dysplastic changes without demonstrating cystic disease. The severity of the renal findings and their disturbance of nephron function depend on the completeness of the obstructive process.[20]

Three sites within the genitourinary tract can be obstructed. The most common location of unilateral and bilateral obstruction is where the renal pelvis meets the proximal ureter. The ureteropelvic junction (UPJ) obstruction is often incomplete, resulting in renal pelvis dilation with minimal affect on renal function or complete obstruction with a nonfunctioning fetal organ (see Chapter 11). The second site of ureteric obstruction is at the level of the ureterovesical junction (UVJ) (see Chapter 14). The resultant increase in upper urinary tract pressure can create renal dysfunction, which may range from mild to severe. Severe bilateral disease will most commonly cause oligohydramnios; if no urine production is present, anhydramnios occurs. In the latter situation, Potter's sequence will be seen on examination of the neonate.

The third obstruction is infravesical (Fig. 6.6), which may be partial or complete obstruction of the posterior urethral valves, urethral agenesis, or urethral atresia (see Chapter 13).

In the classical case of multicystic renal dysplasia, the obstruction is always high, at the level of the UPJ or even more proximal, and the ureteral lumen is usually completely obliterated. The increased intrarenal pressure yields pathologic findings that demonstrate cysts of various sizes distributed randomly throughout the kidney (Figs. 6.7 and 6.8). In some cases, the kidney may be small and solid. Adjacent parenchyma may have

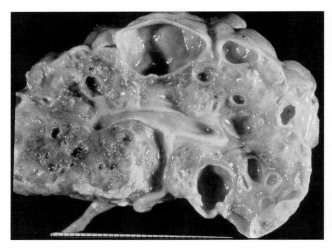

FIG. 6.7. Gross kidney showing cyst formation throughout the cortex and medulla. The calyceal system is normal in this case.

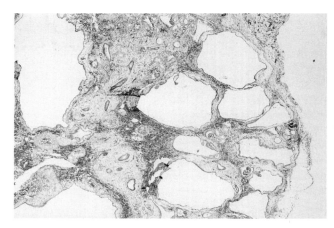

FIG. 6.8. Dysplasia. Note the loss of the corticomedullary relationship. (Hematoxylin and eosin.)

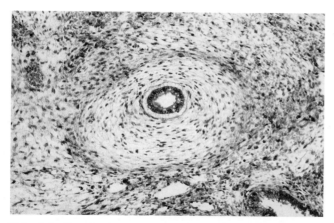

FIG. 6.9. Dysplasia. Note the tubules lined by primitive-appearing epithelium and surrounded by fibromuscular stroma. (Trichrome.)

metaplastic cartilage and blastema. Primitive tubule formation may be seen within the dysplastic kidney (Fig. 6.9) and there is loss of the corticomedullary relationship. Cartilage is seen in <50% of dysplastic kidneys and is more common in kidneys that are smaller than expected for gestational age. Marked dilation of the entire genitourinary tract, with hydroureters and megacystis (Fig. 6.10), can occur in these obstructive states and in other abnormal developmental processes, such as prune belly syndrome (see Chapter 23). The postnatal spectrum of multicystic dysplasia has been described.[29]

Osathanondh and Potter Type 3: Autosomal Dominant Polycystic Kidney Disease

Autosomal dominant polycystic kidney disease (ADPKD) is a common form of renal disease seen in 0.1% of the general population. Although most common in adult patients, ADPKD affects fetuses, infants, and children. The gene responsible for 85% of ADPKD is located in band 16p13.3 (polycystic kidney disease 1). Mutations within the 52-kb unit of genomic DNA making up the gene are responsible for the most severe forms of this disease. Three duplications of the genomic region are present within band 16p13.1. Peral et al.[30, 31] determined additional mutations located within this gene. Furthermore, three other genes sharing substantial homology with the polycystic kidney disease 1 (PKD1) gene are located in this area. In some families, there is no tight linkage with the α-globin gene; this mutation (PKD2) was found in bands (4q13–23).

In some cases, ADPKD can be identified in utero. Cysts, ranging from a few millimeters to several centimeters, are scattered throughout the renal cortex and medulla, often associated with large volumes of normal parenchyma. Ravine et al.[32] suggested the sonographic diagnostic criteria for this disease. When ADPKD is seen in the neonate, the corticomedullary junctions remain relatively well demarcated and the disease is asymmetric. When seen in the fetus or neonate, few, small cysts are noted. In the severely affected infant, multiple discrete cysts of various sizes are seen in both the renal cortex and the medulla.[33] Eventually, molecular tool will be readily available for evaluating the disease in the fetal and neonatal kidney.[34]

THE DUPLEX KIDNEY

The development of a duplex collection system is believed to originate from a second ureteral bud arising from the mesonephric duct distal to the initial ureteric bud and entering the metanephric blastema distal to the initial ureteric bud. The condition is commonly unilateral and creates a bifid system in 70% of cases.[35] The double ureters from a duplex kidney have their entrances into the bladder and are inverted relative to the collecting systems they drain. The orifice of the lower pole ureter enters more cranially and lateral to the upper pole ureter, which enters caudally and more medially. One-third of the renal parenchyma is drained by the upper collecting system, and the remainder is drained by the lower collecting system. Stenosis of the distal orifice of the upper collecting system results in dilation of the ureter and the upper pole pelvis. The ballooning of the submucosal segment of the anterior ureteric wall into the bladder lumen results in an ureterocoele (Fig. 6.11). Ureterocoeles will be present in approximately 50% of bladders when hydronephrosis of the upper pole is seen.[36]

SONOGRAPHY OF THE FETAL GENITOURINARY TRACT

High-resolution transabdominal or transvaginal scanners can recognize fetal kidneys as early as 12 weeks of

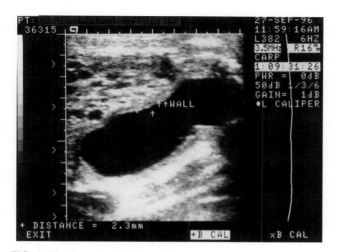

FIG. 6.10. A markedly dilated (80 × 30 mm) with a thickened bladder wall.

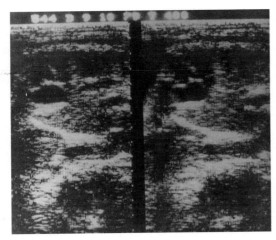

FIG. 6.11. Bilateral ureteroceles divide the fetal bladder into quadrants.

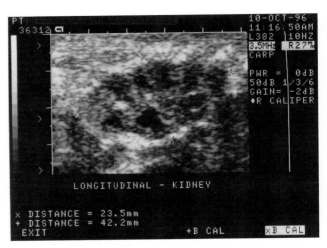

FIG. 6.13. Longitudinal view a third-trimester kidney showing the normal hypoechoic medullary pyramid. Note the hyperechoic rim of the kidney, which represents the deposition of perirenal fat.

gestation.[37] The normal paraspinous location appears as an elliptical mass of tissue when seen in the transverse plane across the fetal abdomen. The so-called glasses on a nose image is easily identifiable as a hypoechoic density, which is distinguished from the liver anteriorly (Fig. 6.12). In the longitudinal paraspinous view, the elongated kidney can be readily seen parallel to the spine (Fig. 6.13) In the medial central pole of the kidney, an echo-free space representing the renal pelvis can be seen in 25% of normal fetuses (Fig. 6.14); an AP measurement of 4 mm is considered normal up to the 27th week of gestation. In the third trimester, an AP diameter up to 7 mm is considered normal.

As pregnancy progresses, an echogenic rim can be noted around the renal fossa, which represents perinephric fat deposits (Figs. 6.15 and 6.16). Concurrently, a change in the appearance of the kidney occurs as the more water filled medullary regions become more hypoechoic than the surrounding renal cortex. The change in medullary density allows the clinician to identify lobulations within the fetal kidney. This normal component of fetal anatomy must be recognized and separated from the more dire critical cystic changes that may occur in the multicystic, dysplastic kidney.

Renal ectopia (which has a reported frequency of 1 in 12,000 clinical and 1 in 900 autopsy cases) can be identified by prenatal sonography. In a series of 22,611 patients examined over 3 years, Meizner et al.[38] identified 26 pelvic kidneys, 13 on each side. Most of the ectopic locations (24 of 26) were recognized after 24 weeks of gestation.

Renal agenesis may occur as a de novo event before the 31st day of fetal development or in association with other anomalies or syndromes (frequency = 0.1 to 0.3

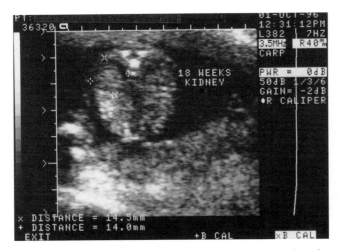

FIG. 6.12. Sonogram of an 18-week-old fetus showing the bilateral low echogenic kidneys. *Callipers,* right kidney.

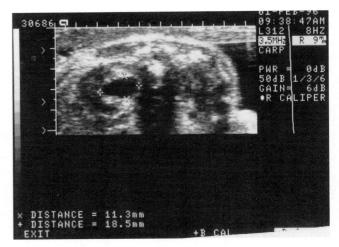

FIG. 6.14. Unilateral UPJ obstruction in an otherwise normal kidney. Note the marked pyelectasis without evidence of hydronephrosis or lower urinary tract abnormality.

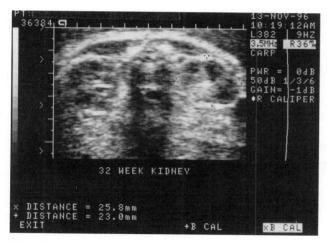

FIG. 6.15. Normal kidneys (*cursors*) in a 32-week-old fetus demonstrating the glasses-on-a-nose appearance.

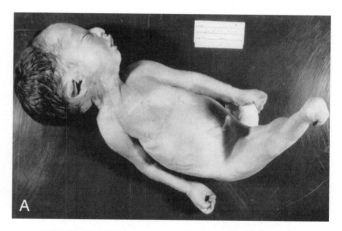

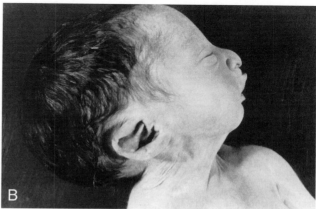

FIG. 6.17. A, Sirenomelia with agenesis of urogenital and anal outflow tracts. **B,** Face of the same fetus showing the beak-like protuberance and flattened ears of Potter syndrome. (Similar findings are found in any child with prolonged anhydramnios, regardless of the underlying cause.)

per 1000 births). Cases reported have possible X-linked, autosomal recessive, and autosomal dominant inheritance. Renal agenesis may be diagnosed as early as 12 weeks of gestation.[39] Sirenomelia (mermaid fetus), a specific malformation complex associated with bilateral renal agenesis and an absent bladder, has been diagnosed in the early second trimester[40] (Fig. 6.17). Both sonography and radiology can demonstrate the presence of two parallel femurs.

Traditionally, the absence of paravertebral reniform masses in both transverse and parasagittal planes is sufficient for diagnosis of renal agenesis, because anhydramnios is universally present. The use of color Doppler sonography can rapidly assess the location and/or presence of the renal arteries as they originate from the aorta. DeVore[41] measured the distance from the aortic bifurcation to the normal point of origin of the renal vessels. If the renal vessels cannot be identified in the

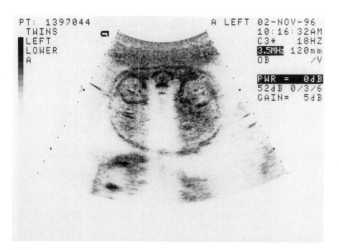

FIG. 6.16. Kidneys of a third-trimester fetus showing midline shadowing.

expected range (±99% prediction interval), then renal agenesis must be considered in the differential diagnosis (Table 6.4). Unilateral renal agenesis occurs, but its precise frequency is not known. Estimates of a 4 to 20 times greater frequency than bilateral agenesis have been made. Unless a contralateral abnormality of renal development is present, the amniotic fluid volume is normal, as is subsequent development in utero. The contralateral kidney is often enlarged (Fig. 6.18); this greater mass suggests the absence of the normal contralateral kidney. Mandell et al.[42] summarized the antenatal ultrasound findings that are seen in children who are subsequently shown to have a unilateral absent or nonfunctioning kidney.

Peters et al.[43] performed surgery on 60-day-old fetal sheep to study the effects of obstruction. In 55 fetal sheep of different gestational ages, renal growth rates had increased. Acceleration of growth was seen before gestational day 95 (term = 135 to 140 days). DNA analysis indicated that the increase in size was not the result of renal water content. The protein:DNA ratios were

TABLE 6.4. *Length from the bifurcation of the iliac arteries to the renal arteries compared to femur length*

Femur, mm	1st prediction interval, mm	Mean, mm	99th prediction interval, mm
10	1.6	6.2	10.8
15	3.1	7.7	12.3
20	4.7	9.3	13.9
25	6.2	10.8	15.4
30	7.7	12.3	16.9
35	9.2	13.8	18.4
40	10.7	15.3	19.9
45	12.2	16.8	21.4
50	13.8	18.4	23.0
55	15.3	19.9	24.5
60	16.8	21.4	26.0
65	18.3	22.9	27.5
70	19.8	24.4	29.0

Modified from DeVore GR. The value of color Doppler sonography in the diagnosis of renal agenesis. J Ultrasound Med 1995;14:443–449.

similar to those seen in a hyperplastic process. The RNA : DNA ratio decreased, indicating a high rate of cellular proliferation. The glomerular number did not increase with the in utero compensatory growth. Subsequently, Mandell et al.[44] measured solitary kidneys and contralateral multicystic dysplastic kidneys in 22 human fetus and compared them to 40 normal fetuses, documenting compensatory hypertrophy in the human fetus. Because the fetal kidney is a dynamically growing organ, an understanding of the normal processes in the human fetus should help clarify the disease states that can occur in utero. The changes in DNA and RNA : DNA ratios found in sheep fetuses are also expected to occur in human fetuses.

Koff and Peller[45] observed growth changes in neonates and young children with unilateral renal disease or agenesis. The increasing size of the unaffected kidney suggests that function is impaired in the contralateral

kidney. Mesrobian et al.[46] documented the existence of unilateral multicystic dysplasia in three fetuses. Later during either fetal or early postnatal life, absence of the abnormal kidney was confirmed. These three fetuses represent the first recognized cases of unilateral renal agenesis owing to a dysplastic process. The authors suggested that the development of a blind ureter without an attached kidney may be the result of this process. Ashley and Mostofi[47] recognized a dysplastic process in 19 of 157 cases of unilateral renal agenesis. They suggested that the process may represent the known autosomal dominant form of renal dysplasia.

The ureter is not visualized in its normal nondistended form. It can, however, be visualized in the absence of intrinsic renal pathology in the form of primary megaureter. This is an uncommon finding seen in the fetus; Deter et al.[48] reported the first in utero diagnosis of primary megaureter. When significant obstructive disease is present, the distended, elongated, and sinusoidal-like ureter appears as an echo-free column running from the medial border of the kidney to the bladder. In some fetuses, the intravesical portion of the ureter is dilated (Fig. 6.6). Occasionally, active peristalsis of the distended hydroureter is seen.

In the fetus, the bladder is a thin-walled sac seen at the level of the pelvic brim as an intra-abdominal structure. The umbilical arteries run parallel to the bladder's lateral walls throughout pregnancy. In some situations (e.g., oligohydramnios; obesity; and shadowing by overlying fetal tissues, especially the skeleton), the umbilical arteries cannot be clearly seen within the umbilical cord proper. The arteries can be identified and counted in their paravesical location.[49] The use of color Doppler ultrasound also allows for rapid visualization as the umbilical arteries course beside the bladder. Nonvisualization of the fetal bladder strongly suggests a significant anatomic or functional abnormality of the genitourinary tract (Table 6.5). Brumfield et al.[50] reviewed 98 patients who were referred between 16 and 24 weeks of pregnancy for oligohydramnios. In 23 of 25 fetuses with nonvisualization of the bladder, a severe anatomic malformation was noted. Megacystis can be identified as early as 10 to 14 weeks of pregnancy. Sebire et al.[51] identified 15 of 24,492 fetuses with megacystis,

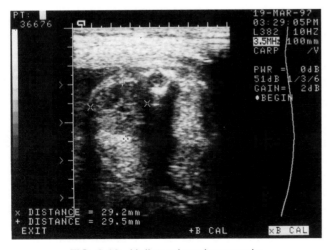

FIG. 6.18. Unilateral nephromegaly.

TABLE 6.5. *Causes for nonvisualization of the fetal urinary bladder*

- Bilateral renal agenesis
- Bilateral multicystic dysplastic kidney
- Severe bilateral UPJ or UVJ obstruction
- Severe infantile ARPKD
- Severe intrauterine growth retardation
- Persistent cloaca
- Bladder or cloacal exstrophy
- Combination of above
- Fetal ADPKD

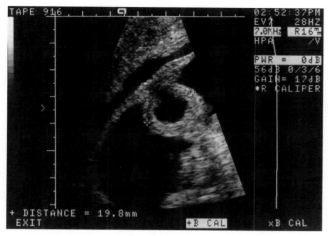

FIG. 6.19. Thickened bladder wall in a 19-week-old fetus with urethral artresia. Note the urinary ascites on each side of the wall, following spontaneous rupture of the bladder.

TABLE 6.7. *Urinary tract abnormalities*

I. Renal agenesis or severe hypoplasia
II. Crossed renal ectopia and pelvic kidneys
III. Obstructive uropathy or urinary tract dilatation
   A. UPJ obstruction
   B. UVJ obstruction and megaureter
   C. Urethral level obstruction or megacystis
IV. Renal cystic disease
   A. Cystic renal dysplasia
   B. Multicystic dysplastic kidney disease
   C. Infantile ARPKD
   D. Adult ADPKD
   E. Syndromes associated with renal cysts
V. Renal tumors
VI. Cloacal anomaly
VII. Bladder exstrophy

based on a minimal longitudinal diameter of 8 mm. In 3 of 15 (20%) fetuses with megacystis, a chromosomal anomaly was noted. In the 12 chromosomally normal fetuses, spontaneous resolution occurred in 7; the remaining 4 progressed to severe obstructive uropathy.

When obstructive uropathies cause bladder distention and hypertrophy of the bladder muscle, the thickened walls of the bladder are readily seen on sonographic studies; the thickness can be measured (Fig. 6.19; Table 6.6). Marked megacystis can lead to failure of the urachus to close; and spontaneous decompression of the distended urinary tract may occur via the patent urachus into the amniotic sac.[52] Decompression of the genitourinary tract may also occur through rupture of the dilated ureter or rupture of a distended renal cyst either into a pararenal, extraperitoneal location, which causes a urinoma,[53] or into the peritoneal cavity, which causes urinary ascites.[54, 55] This decompression may occur in both unilateral and bilateral diseases. In the fetus, decompression does not improve the prognosis of renal function as it does in the infant.[56] A strong selection bias may be present, because fetal disease likely represents an early-onset severe disease process. In some circumstances, a large urinoma may precipitate obstruction of the fetal gastrointestinal tract.[57]

The urethra is not normally seen in antenatal sonographic studies. Rare cases of congenital megalourethra are known.[58] Sepulveda et al.[58] described one 24-week-old fetus with prune belly syndrome who had a dilated scaphoid urethra devoid of a focal portion of the corpus spongiosum. Megalourethra has been associated with other extragenital lesions in about half of both scaphoid and fusiform types. Perinatal mortality is significantly increased when other anomalies are noted. Mortality rates are reported to be as high as 60% and 22.5% for the fusiform and scaphoid types, respectively.

Genital anomalies may be diagnosed antenatally with a high degree of accuracy. Ambiguous genitalia, severe hypospadias, and cryptorchidism have all been identified.[59] The genitourinary tract may be distended but not obstructed (Table 6.7). The classic findings of hydronephrosis, hydroureter, and megacystis have also been identified in a number of other pathologic states, such as reflux, prune belly syndrome, and the megacystic–microcolon–intestinal hypoperistalsis syndrome (MMIHS). In the megacystis microcolon syndrome, an abnormality in muscle structure and function is seen exclusively in female fetuses. It is frequently a lethal anomaly. Other abnormalities associated with urinary tract pathology are those associated with a persistent clora, syndrome that involves the both the gastrointestinal and the lower genitourinary tracts. Many variants of cloacal anomalies have been seen. Some Müllerian anomalies, especially unicornuate uterus, may be associated with renal agenesis or complex urinary tract anomalies.

Ureterocoeles can be seen on antenatal sonography.[60] Both unilateral and bilateral disease have been noted with obstruction of the upper urinary tract. Most cases have not been associated with anhydramnios and/or lethal outcomes. Partial obstruction, often of a duplex system, has been identified. The sonographic appearance is of a thin-walled sonolucent mass that fills the bladder and may be divided into two or more compartments. Garmel et al.[61] reported on two fetuses out of five in which previously recognized ureterocoeles dis-

TABLE 6.6. *Causes of an enlarged fetal urinary bladder*

- Posterior urethral valves
- Urethral stricture
- Urethral agenesis
- Prune belly syndrome
- Persistent cloaca
- Megacystis–microcolon–intestinal hypoperistalsis syndrome
- Maternal drugs: muscle relaxants

TABLE 6.8. *Ultrasonographic findings in fetuses with renal duplex anomalies*

- Length of the kidney (including the upper pole)
- "Cyst" surrounded by a rim of parenchyma (upper pole)
- Kidney with two noncommunicating renal pelves
- Dilated ureter, usually draining the upper pole
- Echogenic cystic structure in bladder

Modified from Abuhamad AZ, Horton CE, Horton SH, Evans AT, Renal duplication anomalies in the fetus: clues for prenatal diagnosis. Ultrasound Obstet Gynecol 1996;7:174–177.

appeared. All five fetures had recognizable ureterocoeles and both hydronephrosis and hydroureter. In the two with disappearing ureterocoeles, postnatal evaluation revealed persistent hydronephrosis in either an upper or lower pole segment of a duplex kidney. In one case repetitive evaluations in the first 4 months of life were required to confirm the ureterocoele. Both infants ultimately required surgery for either excision of the ureterocoele or for an upper pole heminephrectomy.

Abuhamad et al.[62] reported similar findings of hydroureter and ureterocoele in seven fetuses who had a duplex kidney. They also observed that the affected kidney was longer in the sagittal plane than the 95th percentile for gestational age. The authors established five criteria for assessing the fetal duplex system (Table 6.8). Postnatal confirmation of the ureterocoele was established in all seven babies.

Extrinsic compression of the urinary tract, as in type 3 sacrococcygeal teratomas (those that invade the pelvis and lower fetal abdomen) or hydrocolpos, may cause obstruction of one or more components of the lower urinary tract. In addition, some tumors may occur in the renal fossa and can be seen on antenatal ultrasound. Congenital mesoblastic nephroma has been recognized on several occasions and is normally thought to be a benign process. It is often diagnosed as a solid, unilateral renal mass that is not well encapsulated and is often associated with polyhydramnios. Liu et al.[63] reported the combination of hydrops fetalis with mesoblastic nephroma; all three cases ended in fetal or neonatal death. The mechanism of hydrops generation may be obstruction of the portocaval system or, following the development of high-output cardiac failure, secondary to the angiomatous nature of some mesoblastic tumors. Remember that with fetal and neonatal genitourinary tract anomalies, there is an increased probability (9%) that first-degree relatives have occult renal anomalies. Thus all first-degree relatives of the affected infant (proband) should undergo at least some form of noninvasive imaging of the urinary tract.[64]

MEASURING THE GENITOURINARY TRACT

Several researchers have measured the fetal kidneys in both longitudinal and cross-sectional directions.

Grannum et al.[65] were the first to look at the fetal kidney in any detail (Table 6.9). They noted that the ratio of kidney circumference to abdominal circumference remains within the narrow range of 0.27 to 0.30 throughout pregnancy. Hata and Deter[66] provided supplemental data (Table 6.10). The similarity in measurements taken by different investigators allows comparisons to be made between normal and abnormal kidneys[67] (Table 6.11). Most abnormalities are picked up during screening obstetrical ultrasounds. The fetal urinary tract has also been measured[68] (Table 6.12). By 13 weeks of gestation, 92% of kidneys should be visualized on ultrasound.[35]

The clinician must be familiar with the normal anatomy of the fetal genitourinary tract to recognize the abnormal.[4, 8, 69–71] A major problem is the definition of hydronephrosis. The classification of Grignon et al.[72] uses a 10-mm threshold for the grades of calyceal dilation (Table 6.13). When the renal pelvis size exceeds a 10-mm hydronephrosis, a substantial probability for a postnatally recognizable abnormality exists. They developed the system because of the absence of a uniform and specific terminology to describe or quantify fetal hydronephrosis. Grading was always performed when the fetal bladder was empty, because the authors recognized that a full fetal bladder could cause slight dilation of the urinary tract. All neonates known to have fetal hydronephrosis underwent renal ultrasound 3 to 7 days after delivery. Voiding cystourethrography (VCUG) was performed in the 1st month of life in 59 patients (84%). Grignon et al. identified 92 abnormal kidneys in 70 fetuses (out of 34,592 fetal ultrasounds). They noted 28 of 29 fetuses with grade I calyceal dilation were normal after delivery. The remaining grade I kidney progressed to a grade II kidney (UPJ obstruction). Table 6.14 shows the outcome of the 70 fetuses with dilation. Of these, 1 grade IV hyperechoic kidney was found in a fetus with trisomy 13 that was recognized postnatally. Progression of disease was common in the grade II and III kidneys, most of which required surgery (22 of 30). Most authors would agree that development of calyceal scalloping signifies true hydronephrosis (Table 6.14). There is no standard for defining significant renal pelvic dilation.

The frequency of postnatal vesicoureteral reflux raises notion that what constitutes disease to one physician may be interpreted as normal by another; thus some cases of real pathology may be missed. To illustrate this phenomenon, Petrikovsky et al.[73] reviewed 43 fetuses between 18 and 24 weeks of gestation who had pathologic renal pelvic dilation of 6 mm. Because most investigators fail to correlate the effect of fetal bladder filling with the size of the renal pelvis, this group evaluated fetuses before and after bladder emptying. They observed a decrease in renal pelvis dimension from 6.8 ± 1.8 mm before voiding to 4.5 ± 1.6 mm after voiding.

TABLE 6.9. *Size of the kidneys relative to the abdomen at different stages of gestation*

Characteristic	Gestational age, weeks					
	<16 (n = 9)	17–20 (n = 18)	21–25 (n = 7)	26–30 (n = 11)	31–35 (n = 19)	>36 (n = 25)
Fetal Kidney						
Anterior-posterior, mean, cm	0.84	1.16	1.49	1.93	2.20	2.32
Transverse, mean, cm	0.86	1.13	1.64	2.00	2.34	2.63
Circumference, mean, cm	2.79	3.80	5.40	6.58	7.86	8.42
Fetal Abdomen						
Anterior-posterior, mean, cm	2.92	3.73	5.12	6.74	8.50	8.88
Transverse, mean, cm	2.93	3.68	5.12	7.09	8.76	9.68
Circumference, cm						
Mean	9.66	12.37	17.36	22.03	28.11	30.45
SD	1.88	2.28	1.77	1.77	2.31	3.45
KC : AC ratio						
Mean	0.28	0.30	0.30	0.29	0.28	0.27
SD	0.02	0.03	0.02	0.02	0.03	0.04

Modified from Grannum P, Bracken M, Silverman R, et al. Assessment of fetal kidney size in normal gestation by comparison of ratio of kidney circumference to abdominal circumference. Am J Obstet Gynecol 1980;136:249–254.

KC, kidney circumference; AC, abdominal circumference.

TABLE 6.10. *Kidney measurements at different gestational ages*

Gestational age, weeks	AP diameter, cm		Transverse diameter, cm		Length, cm	Circumference, cm	
	Grannum[a]	Bertagnoli[b]	Callan[a]	Grannum[a]	Callan[a]	Bertagnoli[b]	Grannum[a]
12	0.8	—	—	0.9	—	—	2.8
13	0.8	—	—	0.9	—	—	2.8
14	0.8	—	0.9	0.9	1.0	—	2.8
15	0.8	—	0.9	0.9	1.0	—	2.8
16	0.8	—	0.9	0.9	1.0	—	2.8
17	1.2	—	0.9	1.1	1.2	—	3.8
18	1.2	—	0.9	1.1	1.2	—	3.8
19	1.2	—	0.9	1.1	1.2	—	3.8
20	1.2	—	0.9	1.1	1.2	—	3.8
21	1.5	—	1.3	1.6	1.7	—	5.4
22	1.5	1.1	1.3	1.6	1.7	—	5.4
23	1.5	1.2	1.3	1.6	1.7	—	5.4
24	1.5	1.2	1.3	1.6	1.7	2.5	5.4
25	1.5	1.3	1.3	1.6	1.7	2.5	5.4
26	1.9	1.3	1.7	2.0	2.0	2.6	6.6
27	1.9	1.4	1.7	2.0	2.0	2.7	6.6
28	1.9	1.4	1.7	2.0	2.0	2.7	6.6
29	1.9	1.5	1.7	2.0	2.0	2.8	6.6
30	1.9	1.6	1.7	2.0	2.0	2.9	6.6
31	2.2	1.6	2.0	2.3	2.3	3.0	7.9
32	2.2	1.7	2.0	2.3	2.3	3.0	7.9
33	2.2	1.8	2.0	2.3	2.3	3.1	7.9
34	2.2	1.9	2.0	2.3	2.3	3.2	7.9
35	2.2	2.0	2.0	2.3	2.3	3.3	7.9
36	2.3	2.1	2.2	2.6	2.7	3.4	8.4
37	2.3	2.2	2.2	2.6	2.7	3.5	8.4
38	2.3	2.3	2.2	2.6	2.7	3.6	8.4
39	2.3	2.4	2.2	2.6	2.7	3.7	8.4
40	2.3	2.6	2.2	2.6	2.7	3.8	8.4

Modified from Hata T, Deter RL. A review of fetal organ measurements obtained with ultrasound: normal growth. J Clin Ultrasound 1992;20:155–174.

[a]Mean values.
[b]Predicted values.

TABLE 6.11. *Fetal renal size[a]*

Gestational age, weeks	AP diameter, mm		Length, mm	
	Cross section	Longitude	Cross section	Longitude
22	11.3	11.1	24.5	24.4
23	11.7	11.5	25.1	25.0
24	12.1	11.9	25.8	25.7
25	12.6	12.4	26.6	26.4
26	13.1	13.0	27.2	27.2
27	13.7	13.5	28.0	28.0
28	14.3	14.2	28.8	28.8
29	15.0	14.8	29.6	29.6
30	15.6	15.5	30.4	30.4
31	16.4	16.3	31.3	31.3
32	17.2	17.1	32.2	32.2
33	18.0	18.0	33.1	33.1
34	18.9	18.9	34.0	34.1
35	19.9	19.9	35.0	35.1
36	20.9	20.9	36.0	36.1
37	21.9	22.0	37.0	37.1
38	23.1	23.2	38.0	38.2
39	24.3	24.4	39.1	39.3
40	25.5	25.7	40.2	40.4

Modified from Bertagnoli L, Lalatta F, Gallicchio R, et al. Quantitative characterization of the growth of the fetal kidney. J Clin Ultrasound 1983;11:349–356.
[a]Values are ±2 SD ≅2.4.

TABLE 6.13. *Prenatal grading of fetal hydronephrosis after 20 weeks of gestation*

Grade	Calyceal dilation	Size of pelvis, mm
I	Physiologic	<10
II	Normal calyces	10–15
III	Slight dilatation	>15
IV	Moderate dilatation	>15
V	Severe dilatation and atrophic cortex	>15

Modified from Grignon A, Filion R, Filiatrault D, et al. Urinary tract dilation in utero: classification and clinical applications. Radiology 1986;160:645–647.

Approximately 53% of fetuses with a renal pelvis >5 mm when the bladder was full had a normal-appearing renal pelvis after voiding. Petrikovsky suggested that the status of the fetal bladder be considered whenever the renal pelvis is thought to be pathologically dilated. From personal observation, however, it seems that bladder emptying (i.e., contraction) can also increase the size of the renal pelvis. When the renal pelvis enlarges, vesicoureteral reflux must be suspected. It is clear that inconsistencies in the understanding of the natural history and the postnatal prognosis of isolated hydronephrosis require further evaluation. A commitment to postnatal follow-up should be made and the data reported.

Wickstrom et al.[74] followed 82 fetuses (0.72% of 11,340 pregnancies) who had evidence of pyelectasis (defined as an anterioposterior renal pelvic diameter ≥4 mm). In 98 kidneys (60%), the isolated pyelectasis was the first manifestation of pathology that led to multiple uropathies. Specific risk factors associated with the subsequent development of disease were contralateral pyelectasis ($p < .01$), male sex ($p < .01$) and increased kidney length ($p < .001$). Corrective surgery was required in 55% of the fetuses who demonstrated progression of the disease in utero; serial sonography was able to distinguish between progression and nonprogression. Progression was noted in 35 (33%), regression in 26 (25%), and no change in 44 (42%) kidneys. Uropathy was noted in 21 (60%), 6 (23%), and 14 (32%) of the kidneys that showed progression, regression, and no change, respectively. Wickstrom et al. also observed that if the AP diameter was >15 mm between 20 and 25 weeks of gestation the odds of postnatal corrective surgery were 8:1.

During either screening (level I) or referral or targeted (level II) examinations multiple fetal biometric parameters are determined, including the head and abdominal circumferences, femur diaphyseal length, and the transverse diameter of the skull (biparietal diameter; BPD). These measurements are averaged to yield a mean gestational age that may coincide with the time from the mother's last menstrual period (LMP). Gross

TABLE 6.12. *Measurements of the fetal kidney*

Gestational age, weeks	Sample size	AP diameter, mm		Transverse diameter, mm		Length, mm		Circumference, mm		KC : AC	
		Mean	SD	Mean	SD	Mean	SD	Mean	SD	Mean	SD
11	21	3.810	0.535	3.784	0.606	4.234	0.500	10.986	1.208	0.260	0.038
12	40	4.661	0.970	5.044	0.970	5.455	0.850	15.436	1.741	0.284	0.068
13	119	6.179	0.980	6.363	0.934	8.265	1.481	21.877	3.041	0.308	0.067
14	144	7.299	1.121	7.419	0.995	10.312	1.352	27.722	3.143	0.336	0.045
15	93	8.340	0.916	8.461	0.988	11.931	1.260	32.512	3.535	0.340	0.043
16	72	9.594	0.893	9.602	0.851	14.196	1.350	37.420	2.796	0.362	0.049

Modified from Rosati P, Guariglia L. Transvaginal sonographic assessment of the fetal urinary tract in early pregnancy. Ultrasound Obstet Gynecol 1996;7:95–100.
KC, kidney circumference; AC, abdominal circumference.

TABLE 6.14. *Postnatal outcome of fetuses (n = 70) with suspected hydronephrosis on antenatal sonography*

	Antenatal	Postnatal		
Grade[a]	Number of kidneys	Normal	Medical management	Surgical management
I	29	28 (97%)	1 (3%)	0
II	31	15 (48%)	4 (13%)	12 (39%)
III	16	2 (13%)	4 (25%)	10 (62%)
IV	14	0	0	14 (100%)
V	2	0	0	2 (100%)

Modified from Grignon A, Filion R, Filiatrault E, et al. Urinary tract dilation in utero: classification and clinical applications. Radiology 1986;160:645–647.
[a]See Table 6.13.

structure of the brain, chest, abdomen, and limbs is also recorded. Three organizations involved with ultrasound in the United States—American Institute for Ultrasound in Medicine (AIUM),[75,76] American College of Radiology (ACR),[77,78] and American College of Obstetricians and Gynecologists (ACOG)[79]—have specific criteria for sonographic examinations during pregnancy.

AMNIOTIC FLUID ASSESSMENT

During obstetrical ultrasound examinations amniotic fluid is normally seen in reasonable quantities.[80,81] Before the 12th or 13th week of gestation, the amniotic fluid is produced as an osmotic response to active transport of electrolytes across the multiple membranes of the amnion/chorion, umbilical cord, and fetal skin. There is some production of urine late in the first trimester and some turnover by fetal swallowing. By 11 to 12 weeks of gestation, the volume is 50 to 60 mL; and by 16 weeks, it averages 200 mL. At term, the volume is 900 to 1000 mL; however, a wide range of normal volume exists throughout pregnancy.

In early pregnancy, when its presence should be easily ascertainable, the absence of amniotic fluid suggests the presence of a severe fetal renal anomaly or, less common, the presence of unrecognized premature rupture of the membranes (PROM). Two methods of amniotic fluid assessment exist. The first is a subjective method that is operator dependent and based on that individual's prior scanning experience. The volume of fluid is stated in relative terms of absent, low normal, normal, high normal, or markedly increased. The second method attempts to quantitate volume.[82,83] After measuring the vertical depth of fluid in each of the quadrants of the uterus, the physician calculates the amniotic fluid index (AFI) by adding the four values obtained. A commonly used AFI nomogram is given in Table 6.15.[84] This semiquantitative technique has allowed comparative assessments of the same patient to be made by different sonographers. The method of AFI determination is not without its pitfalls. For example, if the physician takes too much time to measure the vertical depths in all quadrants, fetal movement and changes in its position

can displace amniotic fluid, causing an an over or under estimate of the AFI.

Fetal urine formation progressively increases throughout pregnancy; calculations of urine production have been performed (Table 6.16).[85–88] Bladder filling and emptying occurs at 15- to 30-min intervals. The control of amniotic fluid volume depends on the balance between urine production and fetal swallowing (which

TABLE 6.15. *Amniotic fluid index values in normal pregnancy[a]*

Week of gestation	Percentile values				
	2.5th	5th	50th	95th	97.5th
16	73	79	121	185	201
17	77	83	127	194	211
18	80	87	133	202	220
19	83	90	137	207	225
20	86	93	141	212	230
21	88	95	143	214	233
22	89	97	145	216	235
23	90	98	146	218	237
24	90	98	147	219	238
25	89	97	147	221	240
26	89	97	147	223	242
27	85	95	146	226	245
28	86	94	146	228	249
29	84	92	145	231	254
30	82	90	145	234	258
31	79	88	144	238	263
32	77	86	144	242	269
33	74	83	143	245	274
34	72	81	142	248	278
35	70	79	140	249	279
36	68	77	138	249	279
37	66	75	135	244	275
38	65	73	132	239	269
39	64	72	127	226	255
40	63	71	123	214	240
41	63	70	116	194	216
42	63	69	110	175	192

Modified from Moore TR, Cayle JE. The amniotic fluid index in normal human pregnancy. Am J Obstet Gynecol 1990;162:1168–1173.
[a]AFI values are obtained by measuring the vertical depth (in millimeters) of the largest clear amniotic fluid pocket in each uterine quadrant. The values are then added together.

TABLE 6.16. *Third trimester urine output*

Weeks	Urine, mL/h
30	8
32	12
34	16
36	20
38	24
40	27

Modified from Wladimiroff JW, Campbell S. Fetal urine production rates in normal and complicated pregnancy. Lancet 1974;1:151–154.

reduces amniotic fluid volume). Indomethacin, a potent prostaglandin inhibitor that induces intense vasoconstriction within the renal arterial bed, has been used to decrease excessive amniotic fluid volume caused by increased fetal urine production.[88, 89] Other uses of this drug (e.g., as an anti-inflammatory agent for degenerated fibroids or as a tocolytic agent for premature labor) can also induce oligohydramnios.[90, 91] Postnatal renal dysfunction has been observed from both in utero and neonatal indomethacin treatment for inducing closure of the ductus arteriosus.[92] If the fetus has severe anemia from Rh disease, indomethacin should not be used to treat the mother for preterm labor. The combination of severe anemia (hematocrit = 12%) and indomethacin may result in bilateral necrosis of the kidneys and neonatal death.

Angiotensin-converting enzyme (ACE) inhibitors have been reported to cause transient oligohydramnios in utero and anhydramnios and postnatal renal failure, which does not recover after drug therapy is stopped.[93] In these cases, autopsy reveals a lack of proximal renal tubule differentiation. ACE inhibitor use in pregnancy may cause intrauterine growth restriction (IUGR), fetal anoxia, respiratory distress, and hypoplastic calvaria.[94]

THE ABNORMAL FETUS

When the ultrasound examination reveals an abnormality, a detailed evaluation of the entire fetus and uterine contents is required.[95] The size, shape, and number of kidneys; the presence of renal cysts and echogenic tissue; and the presence of amniotic fluid must be determined.[96, 97] A detailed assessment of all other anatomy—including brain, face, and intrathoracic structures (especially the heart and lungs)—is undertaken. There is a good correlation between antenatally diagnosed lesions and those found on autopsy.[98] Discussions of the methods involved in this assessment are available.[4, 99, 100]

Once all organ systems are imaged, the gestational age is calculated from several biometric parameters; internal controls for gestational age rely on measurements of the foot, clavicle, and cerebellum as well as the previously discussed parameters. If the gestational age is less than expected, IUGR may be present. If IUGR or other anomalies are noted, the potential for a chromosomal abnormality, such as trisomy 13, trisomy 18, or fetal triploidy (69 chromosomes), must be considered.[101, 102] Trisomy 13 is often associated with renal cortical cysts; whereas with trisomy 18 and fetal triploidy, cysts are less frequently seen.

Potter's Anhydramnios Sequence

The clinical expression of Potter syndrome or the anhydramnios sequence includes facial anomalies, an excessive amount of skin and subcutaneous tissue, bowing of the legs and inward rotation of the feet, and large spade-like hands.[26] The tip of the nose is classically described as having a "parrot beak" appearance secondary to the turned-down distal tip from pressure applied by the uterine wall and fetal membranes (Fig. 6.17B). The earlobes are drawn forward, so the pinnae appear more upright than usual. The ears are large, flaccid, and pressed close to the sides of the head, and there are suborbital creases.

The major manifestation of the anhydramnios sequence is pulmonary hypoplasia, which results from continued compression of the chest both from within and from without as the limbs and uterine wall apply external pressure to the developing lungs. Internal pressure from the abdominal contents pressing against the diaphragm adds to the force preventing normal lung development. The production and maintenance of lung fluid within the lungs are major components of normal development. When compression prevents these obligatory physiologic processes, pulmonary hypoplasia results. Therefore, one of the most significant issues in fetal evaluation is the assessment of the pulmonary status.

By recognizing potential pulmonary compromise, the obstetrician can arrange for an informed neonatology team to provide for any potential adversity. The prediction of pulmonary hypoplasia is, however, an imprecise art. Nimrod et al.[103] developed the most commonly used method, which requires measuring the abdominal and thoracic circumferences. A thoracic:abdominal (T:A) ratio of ≤80% suggests at least a 90% probability of hypoplastic lungs and neonatal death. Fetuses with a normal T:A value may have oligohydramnios or anhydramnios from long-term premature rupture of the membranes or severe renal insufficiency. Only 10% of such fetuses die secondary to lethal pulmonary hypoplasia. Normal values for thoracic diameters have been reported and may be used to assess fetal chest size.[104] The attempt at predicting the potential outcome in the immediate neonatal period can be helpful when counseling the family about postnatal complications. In some circumstances, infants with severe pulmonary disease may be placed on extracorporeal membrane oxygenation (ECMO), if the disease process is potentially reversible. Long-term survival is then based on the specific disease, and the treatment required to manage the severe renal insufficiency or end-stage renal failure.

The ultrasonographic manifestations of Potter syndrome are the consequences of severe oligohydramnios or anhydramnios; no amniotic fluid is seen. As a result of the increased uterine pressure, the fetal head will be dolichocephalic or flattened in the AP plane. The cephalic index will be <0.72, which is the ratio of the short axis (of the fetal head biparietal diameter or, more properly, the outer parietal diameter) divided by the long axis (the frontal-occipital diameter). The chest will often appear small; there may be an increase in the cardiothoracic ratio often, the heart making up much of the intrathoracic volume. The urinary tract will be abnormal, and its imaging depends completely on the specific disease process. Other malformations (e.g., congenital heart disease with trisomies 13 and 18) or intracranial or extracranial anomalies (e.g., posterior encephalocoele with Meckle–Gruber syndrome) may be present.

Fetal Pyelectasis

Some authors consider isolated mild pyelectasis to be a risk factor for a chromosomal disorder. Multiple criteria exist for what is considered pathologic (Fig. 6.20). Benacerraf et al.[105] defined the abnormal AP diameter as ≥4 mm between 15 and 20 weeks of gestation; ≥5 mm between 20 and 30 weeks, and ≥7 mm between 30 and 40 weeks. Corteville et al.[106] found pyelectasis in up to 25% of fetuses with trisomy 21 compared to 2.8% of normal fetuses. An alternative way to approach the relationship of pyelectasis to chromosomally abnormal fetuses is by looking at the total population with an

TABLE 6.17. *Chromosomal anomalies in 1177 fetuses with mild hydronephrosis*

Population	Number of other abnormalities			
	0	1	2	3+
Patients (n = 1241)	870	223	70	79
Patients with abnormal karyotypes, %	1.1	5.4	22.9	63.3
Patients with trisomy 21 (n = 37)	5	10	10	12
Patients with trisomy 18 (n = 13)	0	0	0	13
Patients with trisomy 13 (n = 18)	0	2	3	13
Patients with other abnormal karyotypes (n = 18)	4	0	3	11
Relative risk	1.6	14.5	44.7	54.3

Modified from Snijders RJM, Sebire NJ, Faria M, et al. Fetal mild hydronephrosis and chromosomal defects: relation to maternal age and gestation. Fetal Diagn Ther 1995;10: 349–355.

abnormal pelvic dimension and ascertaining the incidence of chromosomally abnormal fetuses. Wickstrom et al.[74] found 3 of 82 fetuses with an abnormal renal pelvis to have trisomy 21. They developed an adjusted risk for trisomy 21 based on gestational age and maternal age at recognition of the pyelectasis. Wickstrom et al. noted that the risk increased above the threshold rate (1:250) at 16 to 20 weeks of gestation in women aged 31 to 32 and increased with advancing age.

Snijders et al.[107] reviewed 1177 fetuses who had mild hydronephrosis. Their definition of pyelectasis was an AP diameter of ≥4 mm for fetuses younger than 20 weeks of gestation and ≥5 mm for those between 20 and 26 weeks. No other renal changes could be seen. Isolated hydronephrosis was noted in 805 cases, and karyotypic anomalies were detected in 86 cases (7.3%). In the absence of other anomalies, Snijders et al. found a 1.1% incidence of abnormal chromosomes. Table 6.17 summarizes their data from fetuses with one or more anomalies. The presence of multiple anomalies may suggest a specific genetic syndrome. Occasionally, a final diagnosis can be made only postnatally by biochemical and radiologic investigations or by an autopsy.[69]

Hanna et al.[108] reviewed 3,177 fetuses with sonographic anomalies out of a database of 118,490 karyotypes. Of the 107 cases of renal anomalies, 7 fetuses (6.5%) had karyotypic abnormalities. Of the entire group with abnormal ultrasound studies, 494 (15.5%) had chromosomal abnormalities.

Evaluation of Fetal Chromosomal Anomalies

Three principal methods of prenatal diagnosis exist. The original and most frequently used method is

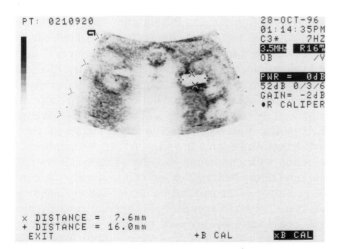

PT: 0210920
28-OCT-96
01:14:35PM
C3* 7HZ
3.5MHz R16
OB /V

PWR = 0dB
52dB 0/3/6
GAIN= -2dB
•R CALIPER

× DISTANCE = 7.6mm
+ DISTANCE = 16.0mm
EXIT +B CAL ×B CAL

FIG. 6.20. Bilateral pyelectasis. The left renal pelvis is just above the upper limits of normal gestational age.

amniocentesis.[109, 110] Under ultrasound sector guidance a 20- or 22-g spinal needle is aseptically inserted into the amniotic sac. Between 20 and 30 mL amniotic fluid is aspirated for karyotype analysis and α-fetoprotein (α-FP) determination. The amniocytes grow sufficiently in 7 to 10 days to provide a karyotype. Amniocentesis is the safest of the invasive techniques; the associated loss rate within 2 weeks of procedure is 0.5%. For traditional amniocentesis performed at 14 to 16 weeks of gestation, the loss rate through the 24th week is 1.8%.

Percutaneous aspiration of fetal urine under ultrasonic guidance is a modification of amniocentesis. The fetal urine contains both renal cells and bladder urothelium, which can be grown to yield reliable cytogenetic analysis.[111] Several authors have reported fetuses with mosaic trisomy 9 in which an isolated dysplastic kidney had the same abnormal karyotype when subsequently studied. Chromosomal data can be obtained from cells aspirated from cystic hygromas and pleural effusions.[112]

The second principal method of prenatal diagnosis is chorionic villus sampling (CVS), which requires that the placenta be located at a site accessible to needle entry either by a single 20-g needle or by an 18-g needle through which a 20-g needle is placed. The 18-g needle serves as an introducer through the uterine wall, which allows free movement of the smaller-bore needle within the placenta. The double-needle technique allows the physician to make multiple passes of the smaller biopsy needle within the placenta without the mother feeling either the pain of the needle's motion against her tissues or the resistance of her tissues to the needle's movement. After villi are aspirated, the separation of the placental tissue from the contaminating maternal decidual tissues can be readily accomplished. The tissue can be grown in standard culture conditions to provide chromosomal data in 7 to 10 days. Some laboratories have the capacity for rapid karyotying by the direct technique.[116] Overnight tissue culture techniques can provide results in 18 to 24 h.

In most major centers, the loss rate from CVS performed at 10 to 13 weeks is 2.5%. The loss rate is calculated from the day of the procedure through the 24th week of gestation. In same circumstances, late in pregnancy and occasionally during labor itself, chorionic tissue can be acquired to give rapid chromosomal information,[117, 118] yielding critical information that can prevent the performance of unnecessary interventions (e.g., C-section, neonatal resuscitation, or other extraordinary intervention). For example, if the neonate was known to have trisomy 18, he or she would not be intubated and ventilated. If such treatment is initiated before the karyotype is analyzed, it may be difficult to discontinue it in some jurisdictions.[119, 120]

The third prenatal diagnostic technique is fetal blood sampling (FBS).[121] Between 0.5 and 1.0 mL blood is aspirated under ultrasonic guidance either from where the cord inserts in the placenta or at the fetal umbilicus.[122, 123] Blood sampling from a free-floating loop of umbilical cord is occasionally required. Several authors[124, 125] have reported on the use of the umbilical portion of the left portal vein (intrahepatic vein), which is present in the center of the fetal liver, for blood sampling and intrauterine transfusion. In most situations, satisfactory samples of blood can be acquired rapidly when no other site is available; however, injury to the liver can occur.[126] If the needle enters the umbilical artery, fetal bradycardia may occur as a result of arterial vasospasm. Direct culture of fetal lymphocytes offers a high-resolution karyotype that is available in 48 to 72 h.

Modern methods of cytogenetics and DNA analysis allow for performance of fluorescent in situ hybridization (FISH). Using multicolored probes for different chromosomes, this advanced method of genetic analysis can provide useful data from fetal blood in 3 to 4 h. The major numerical aberrations (e.g., trisomy 13, 18, and 21 and triploidy) can be rapidly assessed. Other rapid methods of chromosomal analysis, such as polymerase chain reaction (PCR), can be used to amplify small tandem repeats (STR) of chromosome 21 (D21S11).[127] Quantitative analysis of the PCR products demonstrates the advantages of this method as a screen for major chromosomal anomalies; and data are available within 24 h of amniocentesis, CVS, or fetal blood sampling. This method could be used to assay small numbers of cells, such as may be obtained by isolating fetal cells from the maternal circulation.

Percutaneous amnioinfusion can be used to assess the fetus with renal disease and no amniotic fluid (anhydramnios).[128] A needle or catheter is introduced into the amniotic sac, and 400 to 500 mL of a balanced salt solution such as (Ringer's lactate or normal saline) is injected. When the amniotic sac is represented with fluid, it is possible to visualize the fetus, because the tissue–fluid interface allow's examination of the face, limbs, and often the hands and feet. After amnioinfusion, 30 or 35 mL of the freshly instilled fluid can be aspirated for karyotyping. Some investigators[129] have used percutaneous instillation of saline into the fetal peritoneal cavity to evaluate intra-abdominal contents by the creation of ascites. The kidneys especially are enhanced by this procedure and can clearly be seen in their paraspinous location. The major risks with these instillation procedures are rupture of the membranes, infection with cutaneous bacteria (*Staphlococcus* sp.), and fetal injury by direct or indirect trauma to the cord. The creation of an artificial amniotic fluid environment has been used therapeutically to prevent further chest wall compression. This may mitigate additional lung compromise which could lead to pulmonary hypoplasia. Instillation of fluid can be repeated when the amnioinfusion volume decreases.

TABLE 6.18. *Methods of invasive evaluation of the abnormal genitourinary tract*

- Needle aspiration of bladder
- Needle aspiration of dilated renal pelvis
- Bladder catheterization
- Iothalamate clearance testing
- Vesicoinfusion

Renal Evaluation and Therapy

During the 1980s the Fetal Treatment Program at the University of San Francisco initiated multidisciplinary research into the mechanisms of multiple fetal diseases with the potential for in utero correction.[130, 131] The investigations followed the pioneering work of Beck[132] who studied fetal sheep with ureteral obstructions and Tanagho[133–135] who used a silastic tube to occlude fetal sheep ureters and urethras in separate experiments. Both investigators found that the obstructed genitourinary system of the sheep resembled renal dysplasia seen in the human fetus and neonate. The San Francisco group's initial animal experiments and subsequent human evaluation of obstructive urinary tract processes, diaphragmatic hernia,[136–138] congenital cystic adenomatoid malformation,[139] and stem cell transplantation[140, 141] have provided new insights into the evaluation and management of these complex disorders. Crombleholme et al.[142] reported experience with intensive prenatal evaluation by a multispecialty team modeled after the San Francisco program. Their data support the implementation of similar teams for comprehensive evaluation and management of these disease states.

The details of the multiple animal and human experiments have been published.[143] The biochemical data obtained from these studies led to a generalized approximation of kidney function and prognostication of potential postnatal function.[144–153]

Evaluation of the abnormal upper urinary tract has been accomplished by a number of techniques. (Table 6.18) Percutaneous vesicoinfusion has been used to assess the integrity of the bladder.[154] Renal pelvic dilation suggests the presence of reflux but by itself does not lead to a diagnosis of that disease state. Quintero et al.[154] injected saline into the bladder and noted prompt excretion. Slow injection into the bladder with simultaneous observation of the renal pelvis revealed progressive dilation of the renal pelvis. Microbubble admixture confirmed the presence of reflux.

PRENATAL TREATMENT

The current management of the fetus with obstructive uropathy is substantially different from the earliest days of fetal interventional procedures. Bladder shunting

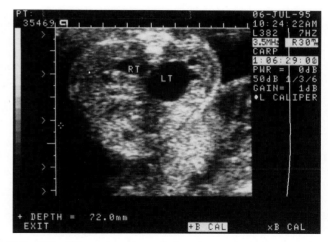

FIG. 6.21. Bilateral pyelectasis in a 23-week-old fetus showing marked dilation of the left renal pelvis with early hydronephrosis.

procedures were performed in fetuses with either poor prognoses secondary to irreversible renal dysplasia or who were otherwise not candidates for intervention[155–160] (Figs. 6.21 and 6.22). Urinary markers now allow repetitive testing of urinary electrolytes,[157] sparing many fetuses from undergoing shunt placement. The initial urine specimen acquired by bladder puncture or vesicocentesis may not reflect the current renal status;[158–160] therefore, follow-up sampling is required to assess the maturing renal function, which is more predictive of long-term function.[161–163]

Fetal urine remains hypotonic throughout gestation, as the ultrafiltrate undergoes reduction in sodium and chloride concentration by selective tubular reabsorption. Urinary sodium decreases with advancing ges-

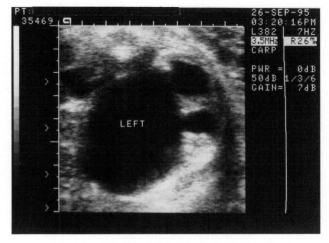

FIG. 6.22. Bilateral pyelectasis in the same fetus shown in Figure 6.21 at 32 weeks of gestation, showing a marked increase in the size of the left renal pelvis with more overt calyceal dilation.

TABLE 6.19. *Prognostic criteria for the fetus with bilateral obstructive uropathy*

Predicted function	Amniotic fluid status at time of initial presentation	Sonographic appearance of kidneys	Fetal urine		
			Sodium, mEq/dL	Chloride, mEq/dL	Osmolarity, mOsm/L
Poor	Moderate to severely decreased	Echogenic to cystic	>100	>90	>210
Good	Normal to moderately decreased	Normal to echogenic	<100	<90	<210

Modified from Glick L, Harrison MR, Golbus MS, et al. Management of the fetus with congenital hydrone-phrosis II: prognostic criteria and selection for treatment. J Pediat Surg 1985;20:367–387.

tational age. The excess free water is not found in the compromised kidney, and an isotonic urine is excreted. When bladder or direct renal sampling is performed, a urinary sodium level of >100 mEq/dL or an osmolality of >210 mOsm/L suggests the presence of renal glomerular damage and impaired tubular function. Glick et al.[148] reported on the reliability of predicting renal function using these criteria (Table 6.19).

Attempts to evaluate in utero renal clearance using iothalamate excretion failed to discriminate between good and bad renal function. The use of serial sampling by Johnson et al.[157] has allowed a more comprehensive evaluation and assessment of the likelihood that in utero therapy will be successful after the third or fourth vesicocentesis (Table 6.20). In another study,[157] the authors noted that a urinary sodium of <100 m Eq/dL, osmolality of <200 mOsm/L, and total protein of <20 mg/dL were associated with good postnatal renal function and absence of renal dysplasia.[164]

Mandebrot et al.[165] determined that a sodium value of >70 mEq/L was the best predictor of poor fetal outcome, whereas a β_2-microglobulin protein of <2.0 mg/L was the most sensitive indicator of normal postnatal renal function. β_2-Microglobulin is a 100-amino-acid protein with an 11,800 dalton molecular weight. It is

filtered entirely by the glomerulus but is completely (99.8%) reabsorbed. Catabolism of the protein occurs in the proximal tubules. Therefore, if a substantive amount of this protein is present in bladder urine, then substantial damage to the nephron has occurred. The concentration of β_2-microglobulin in fetal blood was measured by Cobet et al.[166] who found it had a limited role in the assessment of renal function. Levels of both α_1- and β_2-microglobulin were found to be elevated in 8 of 10 fetuses with severe renal dysplasia; these pregnancies were terminated because of the severity of the disease. The elevated blood levels appear to be secondary to the failure of glomerular filtration to remove the proteins from serum. Reabsorption within the proximal tubules occurs, resulting in low concentrations of the microproteins in the urine. After microprotein uptake by the tubular cells, catabolism occurs within the lysosomes.

Tassis et al.[167] reported that urinary β_2-microglobulin and N-acetyl-β_2-D-glucosaminidase (NAG) have limited roles in the prediction of postnatal renal function for fetuses with isolated hydronephrosis. NAG is a lysosomal hydrolase with a high molecular weight that is not filtered by the glomerulus. When present in urine, it is derived from renal tissue; therefore it is an indicator

TABLE 6.20. *Predictive values of biochemical screening of fetal urine using serial vesicocenteses in obstructive uropathy*

Factor	Sensitivity	Specificity	PPV	NPV	Number[a]
Osmolality	1.00	0.86	0.86	1.00	53
Sodium	1.00	0.82	0.83	1.00	53
Chloride	1.00	0.74	0.78	1.00	53
Calcium	0.95	0.60	0.67	0.94	46
Total globulin	0.92	0.76	0.75	0.93	30
Albumin	0.83	0.80	0.78	0.86	28
Total protein	0.82	0.88	0.86	0.84	46
β_2-Microglobulin	0.68	1.00	1.00	0.81	44
Albumin: total protein ratio	0.75	0.69	0.64	0.79	28
Albumin: total globulin ratio	0.67	0.50	0.50	0.67	28

Data from Johnson M, January 1997.
PPV, positive predictive value; *NPV,* negative predictive value.
[a]Number of cases with documented outcomes used to generate statistical values. Excludes cases in which vesicoamniotic shunts were placed for good prognosis but fetuses experienced shunt complications (displacement, obstructions) associated with loss of function and subsequent adverse renal outcomes.

of renal tubular damage. The presence of both β_2-microglobulin and NAG suggests renal damage to two different mechanisms. In 12 of 33 fetuses, severe isolated hydronephrosis without the presence of an enlarged bladder was seen. Urine sampling on 26 occasions generated values of sodium, calcium, NAG, and β_2-microglobulin that were retrospectively classified as either normal, intermediate, or dysplastic depending on postnatal renal function or histologic studies. The urinary sodium, but not calcium, concentration was directly related to both β_2-microglobulin and NAG. Only sodium and β_2-microglobulin were significantly and similarly higher in both the dysplastic and the intermediately damaged kidneys compared to the normal postnatal controls. In fetuses with isolated hydronephrosis, only the most severe forms of renal failure were suggested by elevated levels of sodium, calcium, β_2-microglobulin, and NAG. Because of the decreasing value of these constituents throughout gestational age, a single threshold value of NAG and β_2-microglobulin for discriminating between fetuses with renal damage and those with normal function is unlikely to be accurate.

Tassis et al.[168] reported serum β_2-microglobulin levels in 53 control fetuses with a mean of 3.4 mg/L. No correlation with gestational age was seen. The 95% confidence intervals were 2.0 to 4.9. Elevated levels were seen in the 14 fetuses with genitourinary anomalies and in the 5 fetuses with a unilateral disorder. In the 4 fetuses with normal postnatal renal function however, the β_2-microglobulin levels were normal. The authors concluded that impaired renal function is predicted by the elevated concentrations of β_2-microglobulin. The raised levels in the unilaterally damaged kidney suggest that the compensatory function of the normal kidney is not complete. Larger series will be required to assess the validity of serum sampling in the antenatal evaluation of renal function, because there is a close correlation between urinary sodium and β_2-microglobulin levels. Urinary sampling is intrinsically safer and less complex than is fetal blood sampling.

Bussieres et al.[169] assessed the fetal urinary content of insulin-like growth factor 1 (ILGF-1) and its associated binding protein 3 in patients with bilateral obstructive uropathies. Markedly increased levels of the protein (18,159 pg/mL) was seen in the 11 fetuses (group 1) with sonographic evidence of severe oligohydramnios or renal dysplasia. A total of 10 patients (group 2) had postdelivery creatinine levels of >0.6 mg/dL and a mean protein level of 1,574 pg/mL. The 16 infants (group 3) with serum creatinine levels of <0.6 mg/dL had a mean protein level of 35 pg/mL. The authors suggested that binding protein 3 may have a significant predictive value for evaluating tubular dysfunction after fetal renal injury. They confirmed Glick et al.'s work, because group 1 fetuses had urinary sodium levels of >100 mmol/L (mean = 123 mmol/L) and β_2-microglobulin levels of

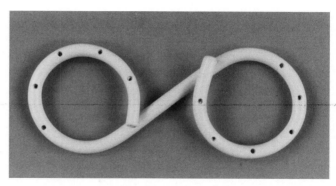

FIG. 6.23. The double-pigtail Harrison catheter showing multiple drainage ports.

>12 mg/L (mean = 19.5 mg/L). No overlap in the concentrations of sodium and β_2-microglobulin was noted between group 2 (means = 59 mEq/L and 5.7 mg/L), respectively and group 3 (means = 46 mEq/L and 0.4 mg/L, respectively). Bussieres et al. speculated that the increase in urinary ILGF-1 and its binding protein may be the consequence of increased filtration and/or decreased reabsorption in the proximal tubule, indicating tubular dysfunction.

Holzgreve et al.[170, 171] analyzed standard fetal urinary electrolytes via polyacrylamide gel electrophoresis (PAGE) using sodium dodecyl sulfate (SDS) as a detergent. Molecules between 10×10^3 and 20×10^3 daltons can be separated and stained with amidoblack using this technique. An increase in urinary micromolecular proteins (<60,000 molecular weight) indicates impairment of tubular reabsorption; in normal pregnancies only small quantities are seen. Holzgreve et al.[172] used SDS-PAGE to examine a series of 21 fetuses with severe dysplasia. For 4 of these fetuses, the authors noted that Glick et al.'s criteria were incorrect in predicting the ultimate outcome.

Occasionally, a large hydronephrotic kidney or perinephric urinoma may obstruct the fetal gastrointestinal tract, causing polyhydramnios, uterine distention, and preterm labor. Therapeutic decompression of the urinoma or hydronephrotic kidney can effectively resolve this fetal–maternal problem.[57] Several questions need to be asked and answered when considering treatment for a specific fetal problem.[173]

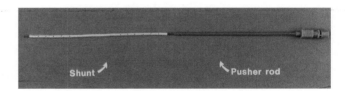

FIG. 6.24. The Harrison catheter placed on a delivery needle. Note the pusher rod above the catheter.

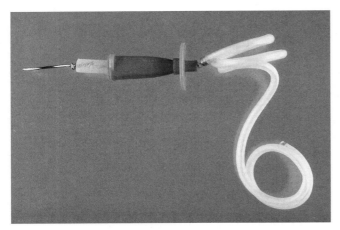

FIG. 6.25. The double-pigtail Rodeck catheter on its supporting guide wire.

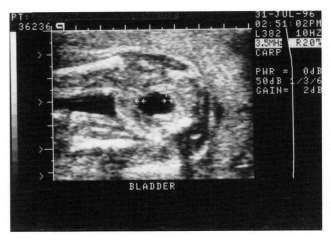

FIG. 6.27. Axial view of a normal fetal bladder.

• What is the natural history or outcome of the condition?

• If treatment does not occur until after birth at term, will further damage occur to the fetus?

• Would preterm delivery of this fetus maximize outcome when term delivery presents the potential for great damage?

• Is a procedure technically possible for the condition?

• Will the proposed procedure change the natural history of the lesion?

• What maternal and fetal risks will occur if the procedure is carried out?

• Just because the procedure can be done, should it be done in this patient?

Evolution of Bladder Shunting

In the past, interventional procedures for fetal urinary tract disorder used the Harrison double-pigtail catheter to divert the lower urinary tract and kidney via in utero nephrostomy and to drain other fluid-filled spaces.[174, 175] The major difficulty in placing the Harrison catheter was its over-the-needle positioning (Figs. 6.23 and 6.24).

Because of a design flaw, the catheter could not be withdrawn for another attempt at placement. A through-the-needle catheter improved placement; however, because it did not have double-pigtail coils, it was easily dislodged from its intravesical location. This catheter was replaced by a double-pigtail catheter that was positioned transluminally in a large-bore needle.

Currently, the Rodeck catheter is preferred for shunting procedures.[176] This catheter has a pigtail memory and is passed through a trocar needle using a pusher rod (Figs. 6.25 and 6.26). The catheter may be placed into the peritoneal cavity to drain ascitic fluid and into the pleural space to drain pleural effusions.[177–179] Tomlinson et al.[180] have used bladder shunting in one patient to correct hemodynamic abnormalities that would have likely lead to an in utero death. The large bladder (72 × 76 × 52 mm) filled the entire peritoneal cavity, displacing the diaphragm superiorly. Increased vascular resistance was noted in the umbilical arteries, which were compressed against the anterior abdominal wall.

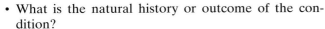

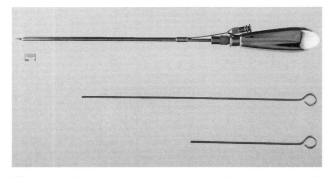

FIG. 6.26. The closed delivery system of the Rodeck needle along with short and long pusher rods.

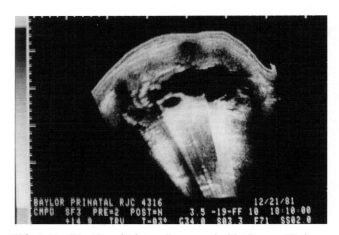

FIG. 6.28. Bladder of a fetus diagnosed with trisomy 13 showing marked distention with anhydramnios.

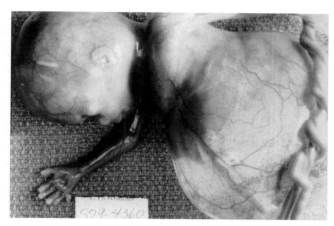

FIG. 6.29. Transillumination of a 19-week-old-fetus showing substantial vesicomegaly generated from urethral atresia. The extra digit was a family trait.

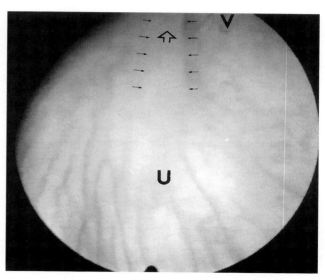

FIG. 6.30. In utero urethroscopy showing the ventral urethra (*U*), plicae urethrali (*small arrows*), and verumontanum (*open arrow*). Once these anatomical landmarks are identified, the obstructing posterior urethral valves (*V*) can be demonstrated dorsal and lateral to the verumontanum. Printed with permission from M. Johnson and R. Quintero, Wayne State University School of Medicine.

Cardiac hemodynamics improved immediately after shunting. Urinary tract obstruction has also been relieved by an in utero nephrostomy tube[181] (Figs. 6.27–6.29). Table 6.21 shows that complications of vesicoamniotic shunting are quite real and frequent. Data from a group at Wayne State University reveal the significant risks in placing a shunt.[182] Of 68 fetuses evaluation resulted in a decision to shunt 31. For 29 fetuses, shunts were placed in one insertion, and 2 fetuses required two insertions. Of the 31 successful shunts, 15 had mechanical complications, including 11 that migrated: 8 entered into the intra-amniotic compartment, and 3 moved into the peritoneal cavity. Urinary ascites occurred in 8 fetuses, and bowel herniation was seen in 3. A total of 5 fetal deaths occurred after shunting: 2 fetus were lost to intrauterine fetal death (one at 1.5 and the other at 6.0 weeks), 1 was lost to chorioamnionitis, and 2 deaths were caused by PROM (one at 3 and the other at 4 weeks after shunt placement). Continuing evaluation of both the procedure and the shunt design is required to improve outcomes.

One recent issue involves changes in fetal response to invasive procedures. Before and after invasive fetal procedures—including shunting, intrahepatic vein sampling and transfusions, and ovarian cyst puncture—Teixeira et al.[183] noted a significant change in the middle cerebral artery pulsatility index (PI). Compared to the controls, who underwent invasive uterine procedures with cord sampling at the placental umbilical cord insertion, there was a fall in the PI. These data are consistent with a reduction in fetal vascular resistance in response to painful fetal procedures, and confirm earlier work that revealed an increase in fetal stress hormone output during fetal needling procedures.[184]

The lack of an effective and optimal shunt prompted investigators to revive earlier fetoscopic approaches to urinary tract obstruction. The original instruments were of small caliber (2.2 to 3.0 mm) and visualization was poor. Reece et al.[185, 186] pioneered the use of both fetoscopy and embryofetoscopy to evaluate and treat the fetus in the first and second trimesters. Modern fiberoptic instruments allow excellent visualization of the fetus, and transluminal laser fibers have made possible new intrauterine and intravesical procedures.[187] Quintero et al.[188, 189] investigated the use of needlescopes for visualization of intra-amniotic fetal anatomy and for human fetal laparoscopy. This technology has also been applied to the fetus for cystoscopy and endoscopic fulguration of the posterior urethral valves (Fig. 6.30). Infusion and aspiration of a small amount of sterile saline through the endoscope's sideport assists in documenting the tympanic character of the obstructing valves before resection is attempted. Failure to clearly identify these

TABLE 6.21. *Complications of vesicoamniotic shunts*

Condition	Number	Shunted, % (*n* = 31)	Unshunted, % (*n* = 37)
Preterm labor	24	71	50
Premature rupture of membranes	10	32	6
Chorioamnionitis	2	6	13
Fetal death	2	6	25

Reprinted with permission from Freeman AL, Johnson MP, Hassan S, et al. Complications of vesicoamniotic shunts. Paper presented at the 16th meeting of the International Fetal Medicine and Surgery Society, Girdwood, AK, June 1997.

landmarks may indicate the presence of a different obstructing lesion, such as urethral atresia, for which resection should not be attempted. Endoscopic guidance for muscle biopsies[190] and laser surgery for twin–twin transfusion syndromes[191] have improved fetal diagnosis and therapy. Few needlescopic procedures have been performed; as a result of its investigational nature, its value for fetal surgery and therapy is not yet known. The fetal therapy group at the University of California, San Francisco is now exploring the use of multiple laparoscopic ports in fetal sheep as an improvement over open procedures (M. Harrison, personal communication, 1998). The next several years will see an increase in knowledge of these techniques through animal investigations and human fetal procedures. The most critical issue will continue to be proper selection of patients who may benefit from an invasive procedure and exclusion of patients who do not require such procedures.

ETHICAL ASPECTS OF PRENATAL DIAGNOSIS

The ethical implications of fetal surgery continues to be the most important area of concern for all investigators regardless of the specific area being considered. The absence of controlled randomized studies presents a dilemma, as different groups of investigators devise surgical approaches to specific fetal problems. The age-old question of technology—If a procedure can be done, should it be done?—is still the most important question a physician can ask after the initial evaluation is complete. All risks must be considered carefully in discussions with the family.

The ethical considerations of the fetus as a patient have been explored by Chervenak and McCullough.[192, 193] The major areas of ethical studies involve theology and religion and the practice of medicine. Religious ethics can exclude many individuals and families in complex medical situations, because not everyone has a religious perspective to draw on. Physicians must recognize the reality that medicine is a secular profession whereas the society they serve is morally pluralistic.[194, 195] This subject is crucial in prenatal diagnosis and fetal therapy, and thoughtful discussions that are applicable to all branches of clinical medicine have been published.[119, 120, 165, 166, 196–198]

OUTCOMES OF ANTENATAL DIAGNOSIS

Multiple antenatal series have generated follow-up outcomes, and one major unifying theme is evident. Many second-trimester fetuses recognized as having significant renal pelvis dilation (using variable definitions) are noted in postnatal evaluations to have vesicoureteral reflux (VUR). Bargy[199] reviewed 116 cases diagnosed with an AP diameter of 7 to 10 mm before 26 weeks of gestation and 10 to 15 mm after 26 weeks. No other malformations were present in these fetuses. At follow-up, infants with no evidence of disease at birth (spontaneous regression), had a 1.8% incidence of VUR compared with the general French population frequency of 0.4%. A total of 53 infants maintained the pyelectasis throughout pregnancy. Of this group, 21 resolved spontaneously, 28 underwent surgical correction, and 5 are in continuing medical follow-up with progression of disease. Feather et al.[200] suggested that primary VUR is inherited in an autosomal dominant manner; thus it is one of the most common inherited disorders. Between 1 and 2% of asymptomatic children will be found to have VUR on screening.

Bierkens et al.[201] reviewed 18 fetuses suspected of having early urethral obstruction syndrome (EUOS). After serial follow-up, 11 were terminated. Pathologic findings of pulmonary hypoplasia and severe renal disease were found in 9 of the 11. Of the remaining 7 fetuses, 2 were delivered preterm and 5 at term. All 7 neonates died secondary to hypoplastic lungs. Given the overall outcome, including a failed attempt at vesicoamniotic shunting, the authors concluded that EOUS is lethal.

Podevin et al.[202] reviewed the efficiency of antenatal diagnosis for predicting postnatal management of urinary malformations. Of 142 fetuses, 7 were diagnosed as having a chromosomal anomaly. Multiple other anomalies were seen in these fetuses. A total of 107 survived to term, and the others died in utero. Of 103 pyelectasis cases, 21.4% were abnormal postnatally. Pyelectasis was diagnosed if the AP diameter was >4 mm in the second trimester and >8 mm at 32 weeks of gestation. If only hydronephrotic kidneys (Grignon's classification) are considered, a positive predictive value of 66% was achieved. Table 6.22 lists the prenatal diagnosis and the number of postnatal confirmations. Podevin et al. also found a substantial number of infants with VUR after obtaining cystourethrograms at 1 month of age. The authors concluded that postnatal evaluation was critical for detecting, following, and managing this anomaly.

Langer et al.[6] reviewed 2170 consecutive ultrasound scans for upper urinary tract dilation and detected 95 anomalies (4.4%); 60% of the sample were male. They defined the mean pelvic dilation as >5 mm before 28 weeks of gestation and >10 mm after 28 weeks. A total of 89 of the 95 fetuses were evaluated postnatally; 13 had an obstructed gentiourinary tract, and 29 with persistent postnatal findings had no evidence of obstruction. Bilateral pelvic dilation was noted in 54.7% of the 95 fetuses detected via ultrasound. The authors noted that if renal pelvic dilation was <10 mm before 28 weeks of gestation, neonate was almost always normal. If renal pelvic dilation was >10 mm in the third trimester, postnatal evaluation was indicated.

TABLE 6.22. *Prenatal renal anomalies*

Anomaly	Ultrasound diagnosis	Final diagnosis
Upper Urinary Tract		
Hydronephrosis	58	31
Renal dysplasia	52	56
Duplex kidney	12	9
Polycystic kidney	6	6
Renal agenesis	4	8
Ureterocele	4	5
Vesicoureteric reflux	0	21
Transitional pyelectasis[a]	80	0
Lower Urinary Tract		
Urethral disorders	17	19
Absent bladder	2	0

Modified from Podevin G, Mandelbrot L, Vuillard E, et al. Outcome of urological abnormalities prenatally diagnosed by ultrasound. Fetal Diagn Ther 1996;11:181–190.
[a]Considered normal.

Kubota et al.[96] reviewed 55 cases of antenatally diagnosed uropathies and found an 81% correlation between the diagnoses made predelivery and postdelivery. Upper tract dilation (33 of 55) and renal dysplasia (15 of 55) made up 87% of all cases. Gunn et al.[203] reviewed 3856 antenatal ultrasound scans done after 28 weeks of gestation. Genitourinary tract anomalies were noted in 313 fetuses; significant defects were seen in 55 infants. Upper urinary tract dilation was evident in 7.7% (298 of 3856) and was transient in 72% (216) cases. Surgical correction was required in 16 of 23 fetuses with recognized obstruction. Overall, significant renal anomalies were identified in 14.3 of 1000 births, which permitted early treatment of the asymptomatic newborn and reduced later renal parenchymal damage. Given the value of the third-trimester scan, the authors suggested that all women undergo sonographic examination so that kidney damage can be prevented.

One of the most important issues is determining the affect of antenatal diagnosis on subsequent outcome. Wiener et al.[204] reviewed the records from two university hospitals and one private hospital from 1970 to 1992. Of 555 pyeloplasties, 240 (43%) were performed on children younger than 12 years of age. A statistically significant increase in the number of the procedures performed in the 1st year of life was seen after 1981. The frequency of procedures in children between 1 and 6 years of age did not change, and the number of pyeloplasties performed in children aged 7 to 12 substantially decreased. The authors concluded that modern imaging techniques have not caused the overdiagnosis of UPJ obstruction but have increased earlier recognition, which has likely resulted in less long-term damage from silently progressive obstructive disease. Van Savage and Mesrobian[205] found that antenatal recognition allowed for corrective surgery and improved the ultimate out-

come of the kidney in renal duplication anomalies. In contrast only 2 of 16 (12.5%) children who underwent surgery at a mean age of 5 years had a renal-sparing procedure.

A Paris group published the results of a study extending from 1986 to 1992.[206, 207] From that population of 167 patients, complete follow-up was available in 157. A total of 63 fetuses were lost to termination of pregnancy, 2 fetuses died in utero with multiple malformations, and 21 died as neonates. Of the remaining infants, 2 died within the first 6 months of life. At 1 year of age 69 children were still alive; 67 of which had isolated obstruction without other malformations. Complete follow-up consisted of a clinical examination in pediatric nephrology, radiographic and ultrasonographic evaluation of the urinary tract, and serial biochemical evaluation and bacteriologic analysis. Postnatal renal function was abnormal in 26 children. Of the 41 normal infants, 12 had posterior urethral valves; 18, bilateral UPJ obstruction; 3, prune belly syndrome; 6 bilateral megaureter; and 2, isolated megacystis. A total of 32 children (78%) underwent corrective surgery. Table 6.23 lists the reference values for urinary compounds in fetuses with bilateral obstructive uropathy who were free of clinical symptoms in infancy and whose serum creatinine was <50 μmol/L at 1 to 2 years of age. Because it is both unethical and impossible to assess the urine of truly normal fetuses, these data represent fetuses who not only survived but also had normal renal parenchyma on prenatal ultrasound (93%) and normal amniotic fluid volume (90%). Therefore, these numbers reflect an appropriate approximation to normal renal development.

The current resolution capabilities of obstetrical ultrasound have the potential to allow physicians to assess

TABLE 6.23. *Reference values for analytes in fetal urine (n = 41)*

Variable	Mean ± SD	95% Confidence interval
Gestational age[a]	32 ± 4	
Protein, g/L	0.04 ± 0.07	0.00–0.22
β_2-Microglobulin, mg/L	0.96 ± 1.2	0.00–3.3
Urea, mmol/L	8.7 ± 2.9	4.4–15
Creatinine, μmol/L	216 ± 68	105–363
Ammonia, μmol/L	695 ± 410	225–1900
Sodium, mmol/L	50 ± 9	31–64
Chloride, mmol/L	50 ± 7	36–66
Glucose, mmol/L	0.15 ± 0.19	0.00–0.74
Calcium, mmol/L	0.65 ± 0.36	0.10–1.52
Phosphate, mmol/L	0.15 ± 0.25	0.00–0.88

Reprinted with permission from Muller F, Dommergues M, Bussieres L, et al. Development of human renal function: reference intervals for 10 biochemical markers in fetal urine. Clin Chem 1996;42:1855–1860.
[a]Weeks of amenorrhea.

anomalies of the genitourinary tract and to begin intervention procedures. The major problem in the United States is the absence of routine scanning at a level of sophistication that allows for a great recognition of antenatal disorders that can be evaluated and managed before delivery and of disorders that require sequential follow-up with or without surgical intervention. Further studies will help clarify and refine the diagnostic and prognostic capabilities.

REFERENCES

1. Fine RN. Diagnosis and treatment of fetal urinary tract abnormalities. J Pediatr 1992;121:333–341.
2. Hadlock FP, Deter RL, Carpenter RJ, et al. Sonography of fetal urinary tract anomalies. Am J Roentgenol 1981;137:251–257.
3. Rizzo N. Prenatal diagnosis of genitourinary tract malformations. Fetal Ther 1986;1:108–111.
4. Romero R, Pilu G, Jeanty P, et al. Prenatal diagnosis of congenital anomalies. East Norwalk, CT: Appleton & Lange, 1989.
5. Helin I, Persson PH. Prenatal diagnosis of urinary tract abnormalities by ultrasound. Pediatrics 1986;78:879–883.
6. Langer B, Simeoni U, Montoya Y, et al. Antenatal diagnosis of upper tract dilation by ultrasonography. Fetal Diagn Ther 1996;11:191–198.
7. Mandell JJ, Blyth BR, Peters CA, et al. Structural genitourinary defects detected in utero. Radiology 1991;178:193–196.
8. Filly RA. Sonographic anatomy of the normal fetus. In: Harrison MR, Golbus MS, Filly RA, eds., The unborn patient: prenatal diagnosis and treatment. 2nd ed. Philadelphia: Saunders, 1990;92–130.
9. Scott JE, Renwick M. Urological anomalies in the Northern Region Fetal Abnormality Survey. Arch Dis Child. 1993;68:22–26.
10. Moretti M, Magnani C, Calzolari E, Roncarati E. Genitourinary tract anomalies: neonatal medical problems. Fetal Ther 1986;1:114–115.
11. Corteville JE, Gray DL, Crane JP. Congenital hydronephrosis: correlation of fetal ultrasonographic findings with infant outcome. Am J Obstet Gynecol 1991;165:384–388.
12. Arger PH, Coleman BG, Mintz MC. Routine fetal genitourinary tract screening. Radiology 1985;156:485–489.
13. Livera LN, Brookfield DSK, Egginton JA, Hawnaur JM. Antenatal ultrasonography to detect fetal renal abnormalities: a prospective screening programme. Br Med J 1985;298:1421–1423.
14. Chitty LS. Ultrasound screening for fetal anomalies. Prenatal Diagn 1995;15:1241–1257.
15. O'Rahilly R, Muller F. Human embryology and teratology. 2nd ed. New York: Wiley-Liss, 1996.
16. Moore KL. Essentials of human embryology. Philadelphia: Decker, 1988.
17. Potter EL, Osathanondh V. Normal and abnormal development of the kidney. In: Mostofi FK, Smith DE, eds. The kidney monographs in pathology. Baltimore: Williams & Wilkins, 1966:1–16.
18. Osathanondh V, Potter EL. Pathogenesis of polycystic kidneys: historical survey, Arch Pathol 1964;77:459–466.
19. Osathanondh V, Potter EL. Pathogenesis of polycystic kidneys: type 1 due to hyperplasia of interstitial portions of collecting tubules. Arch Pathol 1964;77:466–473.
20. Osathanondh V, Potter EL. Pathogenesis of polycystic kidneys: type 2 due to inhibition of ampullary activity. Arch Pathol 1964;77:474–484.
21. Osathanondh V, Potter EL. Pathogenesis of polycystic kidneys: type 3 due to multiple abnormalities of development. Arch Pathol 1964;77:485–501.
22. Osathanondh V, Potter EL. Pathogenesis of polycystic kidneys: type 4 due to urethral obstruction: survey of results of microdissection. Arch Pathol 1964;77:502–509.
23. Osathanondh V, Potter EL. Pathogenesis of polycystic kidneys: survey of results of microdissection. Arch Pathol 1964;77:510–513.
24. Glassberg KI, Stephens FD, Lebowitz RL, et al. Renal dysgenesis and cystic disease of the kidney: a report of the Committee on Terminology, Nomenclature and Classification, Section of Urology, American Academy of Pediatrics. J Urol 1987;138:1085–1092.
25. Risdon RA. Development, developmental defects, and cystic diseases of the kidney. In: Heptinstall RH, ed., Pathology of the kidney. 4th ed., Boston; Little, Brown, 1992;1:93–168.
26. Bernstein J, Risdon RA, Gilbert-Barness E. Renal system. In: Gilbert-Barness E, ed. Potter's pathology of the fetus and infant. New York: Mosby, 1997;869.
27. Rapola J. The kidneys and urinary tract. In: Wigglesworth JS, Singer DB, eds., Textbook of fetal and perinatal pathology. Boston: Blackwell Scientific, 1991.
28. Wisser J, Hebisch G, Froster U, et al. Prenatal sonographic diagnosis of recessive polycystic kidney disease (ARPKD) during the early second trimester. Prenatal Diagn 1995;15:868–871.
29. Walker D, Fennell R, Garin E, Richard G. Spectrum of multicystic renal dysplasia: diagnosis and management. Urology 1978;6:433–436.
30. Peral B, San Millan JL, Ong ACM, et al. Screening the 3′ region of the polycystic kidney disease 1 (PKD1) gene reveals six novel mutations. Am J Hum Genet 1996;58:86–96.
31. Peral B, Gamble V, Strong C, et al. Identification of mutations in the duplicated region of the polycystic kidney disease 1 gene (PKD1) by a novel approach. Am J Hum Genet 1997;60:1399–1410.
32. Ravine D, Gibson RN, Walker RG, et al. Evaluation of ultrasonographic diagnostic criteria for autosomal dominant polycystic kidney disease 1. Lancet 1994;343:824–827.
33. Jain M, LeQuesne GW, Bourne AJ, Henning P. High-resolution ultrasonography in the differential diagnosis of cystic diseases of the kidney in infancy and childhood: preliminary experience. J Ultrasound Med 1997;16:235–240.
34. Pressler LB, Burbige KA, Connor JP. Molecular advances in pediatric urology. Urol 1995;46:888–898.
35. Avni EF, Dacher JN, Stallenberg B, et al. Renal duplications: the impact of prenatal ultrasound on diagnosis and management. Eur Urol 1991;20:43–48.
36. Winters WD, Lebowitz RL. Importance of prenatal detection of hydronephrosis of the upper pole. Am J Roentgenol 1990;155:125–129.
37. Rosati P, Guariglia L. Transvaginal sonographic assessment of the fetal urinary tract in early pregnancy. Ultrasound Obstet Gynecol 1996;7:95–100.
38. Meizner I, Yitzhak M, Levi A, et al. Fetal pelvic kidney: a challenge in prenatal diagnosis? Ultrasound Obstet Gynecol 1995;5:391–393.
39. Mackenzie FM, Kingston GO, Oppenheimer L. The early diagnosis of bilateral renal agenesis using transvaginal sonography and color Doppler ultrasonography, J Ultrasound Med 1994;13:49–51.
40. Zalen-Sprock MM, Van Vugt JMG, Van Den Harten JJ. Early second trimester diagnosis of sirenomelia. Prenatal Diagn 1995;15:171–177.
41. DeVore GR. The value of color Doppler sonography in the diagnosis of renal agenesis. J Ultrasound Med 1995;14:443–449.
42. Mandell J, Paltiel HJ, Peters CA, Benacerraf BR. Prenatal findings associated with a unilateral nonfunctioning or absent kidney. J Urol 1994;152:176–178.
43. Peters CA, Gaertner RC, Carr MC, Mandell J. Fetal compensatory renal growth due to unilateral ureteral obstruction. J Urol 1993;150:597–600.
44. Mandell J, Peters CA, Estroff JA, et al. Human fetal compensatory renal growth. J Urol 1993;150:790–792.
45. Koff SA, Peller PA. Diagnostic criteria for assessing obstruction in the newborn with unilateral hydronephrosis using the renal growth-renal function chart. J Urol 1995;154:662–666.
46. Mesrobian HGJ, Rushton HG, Bulas D. Unilateral renal agenesis may result from in utero regression of multicystic renal dysplasia. J Urol 1993;50:793–796.

47. Ashley DJB, Mostofi FK. Renal agenesis and dysgenesis. J Urol 1960;83:211–230.
48. Deter RL, Hadlock FP, Gonzales ET, et al. Prenatal detection of primary megaureter using dynamic image ultrasonography. Obstet Gynecol 1980;56:759–762.
49. Rosenak D, Meizner I. Prenatal sonographic detection of single and double umbilical artery in the same fetus. J Ultrasound Med 1994;13:992–994.
50. Brumfield CC, Guinn D, Davis R, et al. The significance of non-visualization of the fetal bladder during an ultrasound examination to evaluate second trimester oligohydramnios. Ultrasound Obstet Gynecol 1996;8:186–191.
51. Sebire NJ, Von Kaisenberg C, Rubio C, et al. Fetal megacystis at 10–14 weeks of gestation. Ultrasound Obstet Gynecol 1996;8:387–390.
52. Adzick NS, Harrison MR, Flake AW, DeLorimier AA. Urinary extravasation in the fetus with obstructive uropathy. J Pediatr Surg 1985;20:608–615.
53. Ghidini A, Strobelt N, Lynch L, Berkowitz RL. Fetal urinoma: a case report and review of its clinical significance. J Ultrasound Med 1994;13:989–991.
54. Hadlock FP, Deter RL, Garcia-Prats J, et al. Fetal ascites not associated with Rh incompatibility: recognition and management with sonography. AJR Am J Roentgenol 1980;134:1225–1230.
55. Hatjis CG. In utero diagnosis of spontaneous fetal urinary bladder rupture. J Clin Ultrasound 1993;21:645–647.
56. Fernbach SK, Feinstein KA, Zaontz MR. Urinoma formation in posterior urethral valves: relationship to later renal function. Pediatr Radio 1990;20:543–545.
57. Seeds JW, Cefalo RC, Herbert WNP, Bowes WA. Hydramnios and maternal renal failure: relief with fetal therapy. Obstet Gynecol 1984;64(Suppl):26S–29S.
58. Sepulveda W, Berry SM, Romero R, et al. Prenatal diagnosis of congenital megalourethra. J Ultrasound Med 1993;12:757–760.
59. Smith DP, Felker RE, Noe HN, et al. Prenatal diagnosis of genital anomalies. Urology 1996;47:114–117.
60. Athey PA, Carpenter RJ, Hadlock FP, Hedrick TD, Ultrasonic demonstration of ectopic ureterocoele. Pediatrics 1983;71:568–571.
61. Garmel SH, Crombleholme TM, Cendron M, et al. The vanishing fetal ureterocoele: a cause for concern? Prenatal Diagn 1996;16:354–356.
62. Abuhamad AZ, Horton CE Jr, Horton SH, Evans AT. Renal duplication anomalies in the fetus: clues for prenatal diagnosis. Ultrasound Obstet Gynecol 1996;7:174–177.
63. Liu YC, Mai YL, Chang CC, et al. The presence of hydrops fetalis in a fetus with congeital mesoblastic nephroma. Prenatal Diagn 1996;16:363–365.
64. Roodhooft AM, Birnholz JC, Holmes LB, Familial nature of congenital absence and severe dysgenesis of both kidneys. N Engl J Med 1984;310:1341–1345.
65. Grannum P, Bracken M, Silverman R, Hobbins JC. Assessment of kidney size in normal gestation by comparison of ratio of kidney circumference to abdominal circumference. Am J Obstet Gynecol 1980;136:249–254.
66. Hata T, Deter RL. A review of fetal organ measurements with ultrasound: normal growth. J Clin Ultrasound 1992;20:155–174.
67. Bertagnoli L, Lalatta F, Gallicchio R, et al. Quantitative characterization of the growth of the fetal kidney. J Clin Ultrasound 1983;11:349–356.
68. Bronshtein M, Kushnir O, Ben-Rafael Z, et al. Transvaginal sonographic measurement of fetal kidneys in the first trimester of pregnancy. J Clin Ultrasound 1990;18:299–301.
69. Winter RM, Knowles SAS, Bieber FR, Baraitser M. The kidneys and urinary tract. In: The malformed fetus and stillbirth: a diagnostic approach. New York: Wiley, 1988.
70. Seeds JW, Azizkhan RG. Urinary tract malformations. In: Congenital malformations: antenatal diagnosis, Perinatal Management, and Counseling. Rockville, MD: Aspen, 1990: 319–367.
71. Mahony BS. Ultrasound evaluation of the fetal genitourinary system. In: Callen PW, ed., Ultrasonography in obstetrics and gynecology. 3rd ed. Philadelphia: Saunders, 1994: 389–419.
72. Grignon A, Filion R, Filiatrault D, et al. Urinary tract dilation in utero: classification and clinical applications. Radiology 1986;160:645–647.
73. Petrikovsky BM, Cuomo MI, Schneider EP, et al. Isolated fetal hydronephrosis: beware the effect of bladder filling. Prenatal Diagn 1995;15:827–829.
74. Wickstrom E, Maizels M, Sabbagha RE, et al. Isolated fetal pyelectasis: assessment of risk for postnatal uropathy and Down syndrome. Ultrasound Obstet Gynecol 1996;8:236–240.
75. American Institute of Ultrasound in Medicine. Guidelines for performance of the antepartum obstetrical ultrasound examination, 1991. J Ultrasound Med 1991;10:576–578.
76. American Institute of Ultrasound in Medicine. Guidelines for performance of the ultrasound examination of the female pelvis. J Ultrasound Med 1996;15:800–802.
77. American College of Radiology. Antepartum obstetrical ultrasound examination guidelines. Sept 1986.
78. Nelson NL, Filly RA, Goldstein RB, Callen PW. The AIUM/ACR antepartum obstetrical sonographic guidelines: expectations for detection of anomalies. J Ultrasound Med 1993; 4:189–196.
79. American College of Obstetricians and Gynecologists. Ultrasonography in pregnancy. [Technical Bulletin No. 187]. Washington, DC: ACOG, Dec 1993.
80. Doubilet PM, Benson CB. Ultrasound evaluation of amniotic fluid. In: Callen PW, ed. Ultrasonography in obstetrics and gynecology. 3rd ed. Philadelphia: Saunders, 1994;475–486.
81. Callen PW, Filly RA. Amniotic fluid evaluation. In: Harrison MR, Golbus MS, Filly RA, eds., The unborn patient: prenatal diagnosis and treatment. 2nd ed. Philadelphia: Saunders, 1990;139–150.
82. Phelan JP, Ahn MO, Smith CV, et al. Amniotic index measurements during pregnancy. J Reprod Med 1987;32:601–604.
83. Phelan JP, Smith CV, Broussard P, Small M. Amniotic fluid volume assessment using the four quadrant technique in the pregnancy between 36 and 42 weeks gestation. J Reprod Med 1987;32:540–542.
84. Moore TR, Cayle JE. The amniotic fluid index in normal human pregnancy. Am J Obstet Gynecol 1990;162:1168–1173.
85. Wladimiroff JW, Campbell S. Fetal urine production rates in normal and complicated pregnancy. Lancet 1974;1:151–154.
86. Campbell S, Wladimiroff JW, Dewhurst CJ. The antenatal measurement of fetal urine production. Br J Obstet Gynaecol 1973;80:680–686.
87. Kirshon B. Fetal urine output in polyhydramnios. Obstet Gynecol 1989;73:240–242.
88. Kirshon B, Moise KJ Jr, Wasserstrum N, et al. Influence of short term indomethacin therapy on fetal urine output. Obstet Gynecol 1988;72:51–53.
89. Kirshon B, Mari G, Moise KJ. Indomethacin therapy in the treatment of symptomatic polyhydramnios. Obstet Gynecol 1990;75:202–205.
90. Marpeau L, Bouillie J, Barrat J, Milliez J. Obstetrical advantages and perinatal risks of indomethacin: a report of 818 cases. Fetal Diagn Ther 1994;9:110–115.
91. Moise KJ, Huhta JC, Sharif BS. Indomethacin in the treatment of premature labor. N Engl J Med 319:327–331.
92. Simeoni U, Messer J, Weisburd P, et al. Neonatal renal dysfunction and intrauterine exposure to prostaglandin synthesis inhibitors. Eur J Pediatr 1989;148:371–373.
93. Barr M Jr, Cohen MM Jr. ACE inhibitor fetopathy and hypocalvaria: the kidney–skull connection, Teratology 1991; 44:485–495.
94. Cunniff C, Jones KL, Phillipson J, et al. Oligohydramnios sequence and renal tubular malformation associated with maternal enalapril use. Am J Obstet Gynecol 1990;162:187–189.
95. Grannum PA. The genitourinary tract. In: Nyberg DA, Mahony BS, Pretorius DH, eds., Diagnostic ultrasound of fetal anomalies: text and atlas. Baltimore, 1990;433–483.
96. Kubota M, Suita S, Shono T, et al. Clinical characteristics and natural history of antenatally diagnosed fetal uropathy: an analysis of 55 cases. Fetal Diagn Ther 1996;11:275–285.
97. Johnson CE, Elder JS, Judge NE, et al. The accuracy of antenatal ultrasonography in identifying renal abnormalities. Am J Dis Child 1992;146:1181–1184.
98. Chescheir NC, Reitnauer PJ. A comparative study of prenatal

diagnosis and perinatal autopsy. J Ultrasound Med 1994; 13:443–450.

99. Hill LM. The sonographic detection of trisomies 13, 18, and 21. Clin Obstet Gynecol 1996;39:831–850.

100. Crane JP. Ultrasound evaluation of fetal chromosome disorders. In: Callen PW, ed., Ultrasonography in obstetrics and gynecology. 3rd ed. Philadelphia: Saunders, 1994;35–51.

101. Nicolaides KH, Cheng HH, Abbas AC, Campbell S. Ultrasonographically detectable markers of fetal chromosomal abnormalities. Lancet 1992;340:704–707.

102. Nicolaides KH, Cheng HH, Abbas A, et al. Fetal renal defects: associated malformations and chromosome defects. Fetal Diagn Ther 1992;7:1–11.

103. Nimrod C, Davies D, Stanislaw I, et al. Ultrasound prediction of pulmonary hypoplasia. Obstet Gynecol 1986;68:495–498.

104. Chitkara U, Rosenberg J, Chervenak FA, et al. Prenatal sonographic assessment of the fetal thorax: normal values. Am J Obstet Gynecol 1987;156:1069–1074.

105. Benacerraf BR, Mandell J, Estroff JA, et al. Fetal pyelectasis: a possible association with Down syndrome. Obstet Gynecol 1990;76:58–60.

106. Corteville JE, Dicke JM, Crane JP. Fetal pyelectasis and Down syndrome: is amniocentesis warranted? Obstet Gynecol 1992;79:770–772.

107. Snijders RJM, Sebire NJ, Faria M, et al. Fetal mild hydronephrosis and chromosomal defects: relation to maternal age and gestation. Fetal Diagn Ther 1995;10:349–355.

108. Hanna JS, Neu RL, Lockwood DH. Prenatal cytogenetic results from cases referred for 44 different types of abnormal ultrasound findings. Prenatal Diagn 1996;16:109–115.

109. Lemke RR, Cyr DR, Mack LA. Midtrimester genetic amniocentesis with simultaneous ultrasound guidance. J Clin Ultrasound 1985;13:371–374.

110. NICHD Amniocentesis Registry. Midtrimester amniocentesis for prenatal diagnosis: safety and accuracy. JAMA 1976;236: 1471–1476.

111. Anderson RL, Golbus MS. Bladder aspiration. In: Chervenak FA, Isaacson GC, Campbell S, eds., Ultrasound in obstetrics and gynecology. Boston: Little, Brown, 1993;1273–1275.

112. Costa D, Borrell A, Margarit E, et al. Rapid fetal karyotype from cystic hygroma and pleural effusions. Prenatal Diagn 1995;15:141–148.

113. Smidt-Jensen S, Hahnemann N. Transabdominal fine needle biopsy from chorionic villi in first trimester. Prenat Diagn 1984;4:163–170.

114. Smidt-Jensen S, Permin M, Philip J. Randomized comparison of amniocentesis and transabdominal and transcervical chorion villus sampling. Lancet 1992;340:1237–1244.

115. MRC Working Party on the Evaluation of Chorion Villus Sampling. Medical Research Council European trial of chorion villus sampling. Lancet 1991;337:1491–1499.

116. Simoni G, Brambati B, Danesino C. Efficient direct chromosome analysis and enzyme determinations from chorionic villi sampling in the first trimester of pregnancy. Hum Genet 1983;63:349–357.

117. Holzgreve W, Miny P, Gerlach B, et al. Benefits of placental biopsies for rapid karyotyping in the second and third trimesters (late chorionic villus sampling) in high-risk pregnancies. Am J Obstet Gynecol 1990;162:1188–1192.

118. Smidt-Jensen S, Lundsteen C, Lind A-M, et al. Transabdominal chorionic villus sampling in the second and third trimesters of pregnancy: chromosome quality, reporting time, and feto-maternal bleeding. Prenatal Diagn 1993;13:957–970.

119. Fletcher JC, Jonson AR. Ethical considerations in fetal treatment. In: Harrison MR, Golbus MS, Filly RA, eds., The unborn patient: prenatal diagnosis and treatment. 2nd ed. Philadelphia: Saunders, 1990:14–18.

120. Robertson JA. Legal considerations of fetal treatment. In: Harrison MR, Golbus MS, Filly RA, eds., The unborn patient: prenatal diagnosis and treatment. 2nd ed. Philadelphia: Saunders, 1990;19–25.

121. Daffos F, Capella-Pavlovsky M, Forestier F. Fetal blood sampling during pregnancy with use of a needle guided by ultrasound: a study of 606 consecutive cases. Am J Obstet Gynecol 1985;153:655–660.

122. Donner C, Rypens F, Paquet V, et al. Cordocentesis for rapid karyotype: 421 consecutive cases. Fetal Diagn Ther 1995; 10:192–199.

123. Nicolaides KH, Rodeck CH, Gosden CM. Rapid karyotyping in non-lethal malformations. Lancet 1986;1:283–286.

124. Nicolaides K, Nicolini V, Fisk N, et al. Fetal blood sampling from the umbilical vein for rapid karyotyping in the second and third trimesters. Br J Radiol 1991;64:505–509.

125. Nicolini U, Nicolaidis P, Fisk NM, et al. Fetal blood sampling from the intrahepatic vein: analysis of safety and clinical experience with 214 procedures. Obstet Gynecol 1990;76:47–53.

126. Sturgiss SN, Wright C, Davison JM, Robson SC. Fetal hepatic necrosis following blood sampling from the intrahepatic vein. Prenatal Diagn 16:866–869.

127. Pertl B, Yau SC, Sherlock J, et al. Rapid molecular method for prenatal detection of Down's syndrome. Lancet 1994;343:1197–1198.

128. Gembruch U, Hansmann M. Artificial instillation of amniotic fluid as a new technique for the diagnostic evaluation of cases of oligohydramnios. Prenat Diagn 1988;8:33–46.

129. Nicolini U, Santolaya J, Hubinont C, et al. Visualization of fetal intraabdominal organs in second trimester severe oligohydramnios by intraperitoneal infusion. Prenat Diagn 1989;9:191–194.

130. Harrison MR, Golbus MS, Filly RA, eds. The unborn patient: prenatal diagnosis and treatment. 2nd ed. Philadelphia: Saunders, 1990.

131. Harrison MR, Adzick NS, Flake AW. Prenatal management of the fetus with a correctable defect. In: Callen PW, ed. Ultrasonography in obstetrics and gynecology. 3rd ed. Philadelphia: Saunders, 1994;536–547.

132. Beck AD. The effect of intrauterine urinary obstruction upon the development of the fetal kidney. J Urol 1971;105:784–789.

133. Tanagho EA. Surgically induced partial urinary obstruction in the fetal lamb. I. Technique. Invest Urol 1972;10:19–24.

134. Tanagho EA. Surgically induced partial urinary obstruction in the fetal lamb. II. Urethral obstruction. Invest Urol 1972; 10:25–34.

135. Tanagho EA. Surgically induced partial urinary obstruction in the fetal lamb. III. Ureteral obstruction. Invest Urol 1972; 10:35–43.

136. Harrison MR, Ross NA, DeLorimier AA. Correction of congenital diaphragmatic hernia in utero. III. Development of a successful surgical technique using abdominoplasty to avoid compromise of umbilical blood flow. J Pediatr Surg 1983;18:331–338.

137. Harrison MR, Adzick NS, Longaker MT, et al. Successful repair in utero of a fetal diaphragmatic hernia after removal of herniated visceral from left thorax. N Engl J Med 1990;322:1582–1584.

138. Adzick NS, Harrison MR, Glick PL, et al. Diaphragmatic hernia in the fetus: prenatal diagnosis and outcome in 94 cases. J Pediatr Surg 1985;20:357–361.

139. Harrison MR, Adzick NS, Jennings RW, et al. Antenatal intervention for congenital cystic adenomatoid malformation. Lancet 1990;336:965–967.

140. Harrison MR, Crombleholme TM, Slotnick NR, et al. In utero transplantation of fetal liver hematopoietic stem cells in monkeys. Lancet 1989;2:1425–1427.

141. Crombleholme TM, Bianchi DW. In utero hematopoietic stem cell transplantation and gene therapy. Semin Perinatol 18:376–385.

142. Crombleholme TM, D'Alton M, Cendron M, et al. Prenatal diagnosis and the pediatric surgeon: the impact of prenatal consultation on perinatal management. J Pediatric Surg 1996; 31:156–163.

143. Harrison MR, Filly RA. The fetus with obstructive uropathy: pathophysiology, natural history, selection, and treatment. In: Harrison MR, Golbus MS, Filly RA, eds., The Unborn patient: prenatal diagnosis and treatment. 2nd ed. Philadelphia: Saunders, 1990;328–393.

144. Harrison MR, Ross NA, Noall R, deLorimier AA. Correction of congenital hydronephrosis in utero. I. The model: fetal urethral obstruction produces hydronephrosis and pulmonary hypoplasia in fetal lambs. J Pediatr Surg 1983;18:247–256.

145. Harrison MR, Nakayama DK, Noall R, deLorimier AA. Correction of congenital hydronephrosis in utero. II. Decompression

reverses the effects of obstruction on the fetal lung and urinary tract. J Pediatr Surg 1982;17:965–974.

146. Harrison MR, Filly RA, Parer JT, et al. Management of the fetus with urinary tract malformation. JAMA 1981;246:635–639.

147. Adzick NS, Harrison MR. The unborn surgical patient. Curr Prob Obstet Gynecol Fertility 1995;179–215.

148. Glick PL, Harrison MR, Golbus MS, et al. Management of the fetus with congenital hydronephrosis: II. Prognostic criteria and selection for treatment. J Pediatr Surg 1985;20:376–387.

149. Glick PL, Harrison MR, Noall RA, Villa RL. Correction of congenital hydronephrosis in utero. III. Early mid-trimester urethral obstruction produces renal dysplasia. J Pediatr Surg 1983;18:681–687.

150. Glick PL, Harrison MR, Adzick NS, et al. Correction of congenital hydronephrosis in utero. IV. In utero decompression prevents renal dysplasia. J Pediatr Surg 1984;19:649–657.

151. Crombleholme TM, Harrison MR, Golbus MS, et al. Fetal intervention in obstructive uropathy: prognostic indicators and efficacy of intervention. Am J Obstet Gynecol 1990;162:1239–1244.

152. Crombleholme TM. Invasive fetal therapy: current status and future directions. Semin Perinatol 1994;18:385–397.

153. Crombleholme TM, Harrison MR, Langer JC. Early experience with open fetal surgery for congenital hydronephrosis J Pediatr Surg 1988;23:1114–1121.

154. Quintero RA, Johnson MP, Arias F. In utero sonographic diagnosis of vesicoureteral reflux by percutaneous vesicoinfusion. Ultrasound Obstet Gynecol 1995;6:386–389.

155. Manning FA, Harrison MR, Rodeck C. Catheter shunts for fetal hydronephrosis and hydrocephalus: report of the international fetal surgery registry. N Engl J Med 1986;315:336–340.

156. Golbus MS, Filly RA, Callen PW, et al. Fetal urinary tract obstruction: management and selection for treatment. Semin Perinatol 1985;9:91–97.

157. Johnson MP, Bukowski TP, Reitleman C, et al. In utero surgical treatment of fetal obstructive uropathy: a new comprehensive approach to identify appropriate candidates for vesicoamniotic shunt therapy. Am J Obstet Gynecol 1994;170:1770–1779.

158. Nicolaides KH, Cheng HH, Snijders RJM, Moniz CF. Fetal urine chemistry in the assessment of obstructive uropathy. Am J Obstet Gynecol 1992;166:932–937.

159. Nicolini U, Fisk NM, Rodeck C. Fetal urine biochemistry: an index of renal maturation and dysfunction. Br J Obstet Gynecol 1992;99:46–50.

160. Wilkins IA, Chitkara U, Lynch L, et al. The non-predictive value of fetal urinary electrolytes: preliminary report of outcomes and correlations with pathologic diagnosis. Am J Obstet Gynecol 1987;157:694–698.

161. Evans MI, Sacks AJ, Johnson MP, Robichaux AG. Sequential invasive assessment of fetal renal function and the intrauterine treatment of obstructive uropathies. Obstet Gynecol 1991;77:545–550.

162. Johnson MP, Corsi P, Bradfield W, et al. Sequential urinalysis improves evaluation of fetal renal function in obstructive uropathy. Am J Obstet Gynecol 1995;173:59–65.

163. Muller F, Dommerques M, Mandelbrot L, et al. Fetal urinary biochemistry predicts postnatal renal function in children with bilateral obstructive uropathies. Obstet Gynecol 1993;82:813–820.

164. Qureshi F, Jacques SM, Seifman B, et al. In utero fetal urine analysis and renal histology correlate with the outcome in fetal obstructive uropathies. Fetal Diagn Ther 1996;11:306–312.

165. Mandelbrot L, Dumez Y, Muller F, Dommerques M. Prenatal prediction of renal function in fetal obstructive uropathies. J Perinat Med 1991;19(Suppl 1):283–287.

166. Cobet G, Gummelt T, Bollmann R, et al. Assessment of serum levels of α-1-microglobulin, β-2-microglobulin, and retinol binding protein in the fetal blood. A method for prenatal evaluation of renal function. Prenat Diagn 1996;16:299–305.

167. Tassis BM, Trespidi L, Tirelli AS, et al. In fetuses with isolated hydronephrosis, urinary β_2-microglobulin and N-acetyl-β-D-glucosaminidase (NAG) have a limited role in the prediction of postnatal renal function. Prenat Diagn 1996;16:1087–1093.

168. Tassis BMG, Trespidi L, Tirelli AS, et al. Serum β_2-microglobu-

lin in fetuses with urinary tract anomalies. Am J Obstet Gynecol 1997;176:54–57.

169. Bussieres L, Laborde K, Souberbielle JC, et al. Fetal urinary insulin-like growth factor 1 and binding protein 3 in bilateral obstructive uropathies. Prenatal Diagn 1995;15:1047–1055.

170. Holzgreve W, Lison A, Bulla M. SDS-PAGE as an additional test to determine fetal kidney function prior to intrauterine diversion of urinary tract obstruction. Fetal Ther 1989;4:93–96.

171. Holgreve W. Verbesserte kriterien zur pranatalen Beurteilung der nierenfunktion bei fetalen harnwegsobstrultionen. Dtsch Ges Gynakol Geburtshilfe 1990;4:30–32.

172. Holzgreve W, Lison A, Bulla M, Evans M. Protein analysis to determine fetal kidney function. Am J Obstet Gynecol 1991;164:336.

173. Kogan B. The fetus with obstructive uropathy: alternative approaches. In: Harrison MR, Golbus MS, Filly RA, eds., The unborn patient: prenatal diagnosis and treatment. 2nd ed., Philadelphia: Saunders, 1990;399–402.

174. Evans MI, Drugan A, Manning FA, et al. Therapeutic intrauterine corrections of fetal anomalies. In: Gleicher N, ed., Principles and practice of medical therapy in pregnancy. 2nd ed. Norwalk, CT: Appleton & Lange, 1992.

175. Blanch G, Walkinshaw SA, Hawdon JM. Internalization of pleuroamniotic shunt causing neonatal demise. Fetal Diagn Ther 1996;11:32–36.

176. Nicolini U, Rodeck CH, Fisk NM. Shunt treatment for fetal obstructive uropathy. Lancet 1987;2:1338–1339.

177. Seeds JW, Bowes WA. Results of treatment of severe fetal hydrothorax with bilateral pleuroamniotic catheters. Obstet Gynecol 1986;68:577–579.

178. Rodeck CH, Fisk NM, Fraser DI, Nicolini U. Long term in utero drainage of fetal hydrothorax. N Engl J Med 1988;319:1135.

179. Blott M, Nicolaides KH, Greennough A. Pleuroamniotic shunting for decompression of fetal pleural effusions. Obstet Gynecol 1988;71:798–800.

180. Tomlinson MW, Johnson MP, Gonclaves L, et al. Correction of hemodynamic abnormalities by vesicoamniotic shunting in familial congenital megacystis. Fetal Diagn Ther 1996;11:46–49.

181. Pinckert TL, Kiernan SC. In utero nephrostomy catheter placement. Fetal Diagn Ther 1994;9:348–352.

182. Freeman AL, Johnson MP, Hassan S, et al. Complications of vesicoamniotic shunts. Paper presented at the 16th meeting of the International Fetal Medicine and Surgery Society, Girdwood, AK, June 1997.

183. Teixeira J, Fogliani R, Giannakoulopoulos X, et al. Fetal haemodynamic stress response to invasive procedures. Lancet 1996;347:624.

184. Giannakoulopoulos X, Sepulveda W, Koutis P, Fetal plasma cortisol and β-endorphin response to intrauterine needling. Lancet 1994;344:77–81.

185. Reece EA, Hobbins JC. Embryoscopy: an evolving technology for early prenatal diagnosis. In: Chapman M, Grudzinkas G, Chard T, eds., The embryo: normal and abnormal development and growth. New York: Springer-Verlag, 1991:123–140.

186. Reece EA, Homko C, Goldstein I, Wiznitzer A. Toward fetal therapy using needle embryofetoscopy. Ultrasound Obstet Gynecol 1995;5:281–285.

187. Quintero RA, Reich H, Puder KS, et al. Brief report: umbilical cord ligation of an acardiac twin by fetoscopy at 19 weeks of gestation. N Engl J Med 1994;330:469–471.

188. Quintero RA, Hume R, Johnson MP. Percutaneous fetal cystoscopy, and endoscopic fulguration of posterior urethral valves. Am J Obstet Gynecol 1995;172:206–209.

189. Quintero RA, Romero R, Johnson MP, et al. In utero percutaneous cystoscopy in the management of fetal lower obstructive uropathy. Lancet. 1995;346:537–540.

190. Evan MI, Quintero RA, King M, et al. Endoscopically assisted, ultrasound guided fetal muscle biopsy. Fetal Diagn Ther 10:167–172.

191. Ville Y, Hyett J, Hecker K, Nicolaides K. Preliminary experience with endoscopic laser surgery for severe twin–twin transfusion syndrome. N Engl J Med 1995;332:224–227.

192. Chervenak FA, McCullough LB. Ethical issues in obstetric ultrasound. In: Chervenak FA, Isaacson GC, Campbell S, eds., Ultra-

sound in obstetrics and gynecology. Boston: Little, Brown, 1993:277–283.

193. Chervenak FA, McCullough LB, What is obstetric ethics. In: Chervenak FA, McCullough LB, eds., Ethical dilemmas in obstetrics. Clin Obstet Gyncecol 1992;35:709–719.

194. Englehardt HT Jr. The foundations of bioethics. 2nd ed. New York: Oxford University Press, 1996.

195. Brody B. Life and death decision making. New York: Oxford University Press, 1988.

196. Marteau TM. Towards informed decisions about prenatal testing: a review. Prenatal Diagn 1995;15:1215–1226.

197. Goldsmith JP, Ginsberg HG, McGettigan MC. Ethical decisions in the delivery room. Clin Perinatol 1996;23:529–550.

198. Murray TH. Moral obligations to the not-yet-born: the fetus as patient. Clin Perinatol 1987;14:329–343.

199. Bargy F. Le devenir des petites dilatations des voies urinaires depistees avant la naissance. In: ed., Diagnostic and prise en charge des affections foetales Paris: Prenatal Editions Diffusions Vigot, 1996;195–199.

200. Feather S, Woolf AS, Gordon I, et al. Vesicoureteric reflux: all in the genes? Lancet 1996;348:725–728.

201. Bierkens AF, Feitz WFJ, Nijhuis JG, et al. Early urethral obstruction sequence: a lethal entity? Fetal Diagn Ther 1996;11:137–145.

202. Podevin G, Mandelbrot L, Vuillard E, et al. Outcome of urological abnormalities prenatally diagnosed by ultrasound. Fetal Diagn Ther 1996;11:181–190.

203. Gunn TR, Mora JD, Pease P. Antenatal diagnosis of urinary tract abnormalities by ultrasonography after 28 weeks gestation: incidence and outcome. Am J Obstet Gynecol 1995;172:479–486.

204. Wiener JS, Emmert GK, Mesrobian HG, et al. Hydronephrosis: antenatal and postnatal diagnosis: are modern imaging techniques over diagnosing ureteropelvic junction obstruction? J Urol 1995;154:659–661.

205. Van Savage JG, Mesrobian HGJ. The impact of prenatal sonography on the morbidity and outcome of patients with renal duplication anomalies. J Urol 1995;153:768–770.

206. Muller, F, Dommergues M, Bussieres L, et al. Development of human renal function: reference intervals for 10 biochemical markers in fetal urine. Clin Chem 1996;42:1855–1860.

207. Daikha-Dahmane F, Dommergues M, Muller F, et al. Development of human fetal kidney in obstructive uropathy: correlations with ultrasonography and urine biochemistry. Kidney 1997; 52:21–32.

CHAPTER 7

Imaging the Urinary Tract in Children

Sandra K. Fernbach

The urinary tract can be imaged with many modalities: radiography, nuclear medicine, ultrasound (US), CT, and MRI. Each type of examination offers unique and complementary ways of answering specific questions about the anatomy and function of the kidneys and bladder. This chapter briefly reviews each of the more commonly used studies and presents a rational mode of imaging children with common urologic problems, including neonatal hydronephrosis (HN), hydroureteronephrosis (HUN), urinary tract infection (UTI), renal mass, and neurogenic bladder.

The choice of modality for evaluating renal anomalies or diseases is both personal and institutional. That is, the information necessary to plan treatment can be provided by a number of studies. Which are used depends on the physician's training and comfort with each modality and the strengths of the imaging department.

IMAGING TECHNIQUES

Excretory Urography

The number of excretory urograms (EUs) performed, even in pediatric centers, has diminished in proportion to the development and use of other imaging techniques. EU, however, can provide much anatomic and functional information with little ionizing radiation. Optimal performance requires familiarity with congenital anomalies and acquired abnormalities of the genitourinary tract and the methods and procedures to treat them, review of earlier studies, appropriate clinical information, and experience in doing EU in children.

The pediatric EU requires fewer films than it does in adults; the number is kept low by monitoring the examination and directing the film sequence to answer specific questions, those that will affect treatment. For example, oblique films and renal tomograms may show focal renal scarring but are of little value for the child who has undergone successful ureteral reimplantation and is infection free. In contrast, delayed films (or CT) may be needed to detect a poorly functioning, or ectopi-

cally inserting ureter when evaluating a female child who suffers from dribbling (Fig. 7.1).

Most EU can be accomplished with four or less films. A reasonable protocol would be a scout film; a film of the kidneys shortly after contrast material injection to see the parenchyma; and a full abdominal radiograph about 10 min later to demonstrate the kidneys, ureters, and bladder.[1-3] Occasionally, e.g., after ureteral reimplantation or for children with recurrent UTI, the EU may consist of only one film after contrast material injection, provided that the film completely demonstrates normal anatomy or no change from an earlier EU, if available (Fig. 7.2).[4]

When a recent abdominal radiograph is available, the scout film need not be performed. Although some authors question the value of a scout film, it may provide pertinent information that will be lost once the contrast material is within the urinary tract (calculi, status of the spine) or may indicate that the study should be rescheduled (barium in the gastrointestinal tract from an earlier examination) (Fig. 7.3).

Most pediatric institutions use low osmolality contrast material, despite its high cost, because there is less discomfort during injection, less nausea and vomiting, and a decreased incidence of minor contrast reactions, especially hives and wheezing.[5-7]

The technique for performing EU in children is different from that in adults. Little if any bowel preparation is needed. Compression devices (to externally impede ureteral drainage and enhance opacification of the ureters) are rarely used. A bladder catheter may be necessary in a child with known or possible vesicoureteral reflux (VUR) or in a patient who is unable to empty the bladder to improve drainage of the upper urinary tract.

Cystography

Both the direct nuclear cystogram (NCG) and the radiographic voiding cystourethrogram (VCUG) require that the bladder be catheterized. The details of

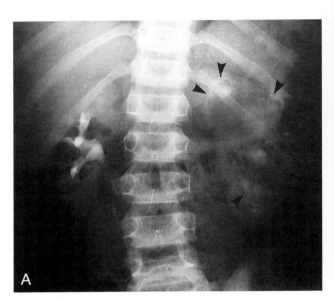

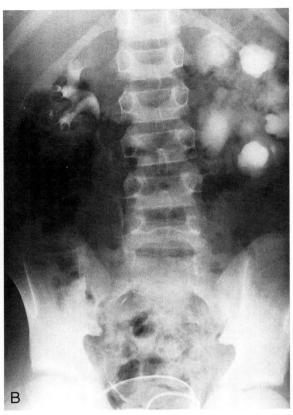

FIG. 7.1. A, The early EU film, centered on the kidneys, showing a normal right kidney. On the left, the dilated pelvicaliceal system has failed to fill with contrast, compressing the parenchyma at its periphery and producing circles of contrast, termed caliceal crescents (*arrows*). **B,** On the delayed EU film of the same patient, the left pelvicaliceal system is opacified and dilated. The left ureter is not visualized, suggesting obstruction at the ureteropelvic junction.

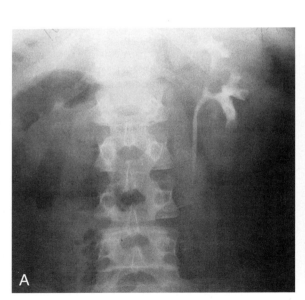

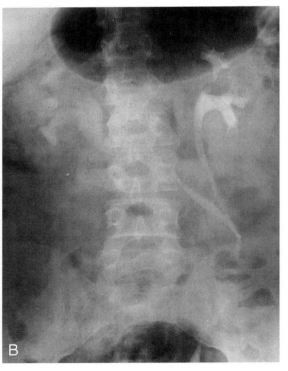

FIG. 7.2. A, An EU study performed about 10 weeks after excision of a paraureteral diverticulum and reimplantation of the right ureter showing a normal left kidney and no function of the right kidney, which previously was normal. **B,** After the patient underwent a right-to-left transureterouretostomy, the EU demonstrates that the right kidney can concentrate contrast, which filled a moderately dilated pelvicaliceal system and normal ureter.

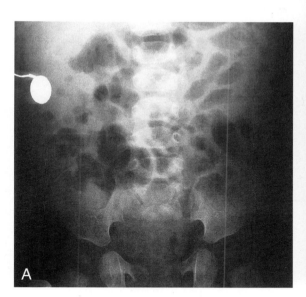

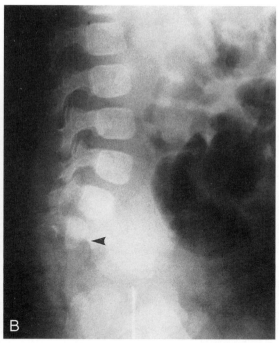

FIG. 7.3. Scout film for a voiding cystourethrogram (VCUG) in 6-month-old girl with renal failure and HUN of unknown cause showing that the sacrum is malsegmented and missing its distal segments. **B,** The lateral view of the spine showing the stubby sacrum, which is missing multiple segments (*arrow*).

each technique are available in the literature.[8–10] Many institutions use an 8-Fr feeding tube for VCUG so that the bladder neck will not become occluded by the balloon of a retention catheter and the child can spontaneously void. A retention catheter is often used for NCG, because visualization of the urethra is not part of the study.

During NCG, an isotope—usually technetium 99m (^{99m}Tc) pertechnetate or ^{99m}Tc chelated to sulfur col-loid—is introduced into the bladder. Using the same catheter, saline is dripped into the bladder; the kidneys and bladder are continuously monitored by a gamma camera beneath the supine child until voiding occurs or another predetermined end point is reached (Fig. 7.4). During VCUG, iodinated contrast material is instilled into the bladder, and a relatively predetermined series of images is performed under fluoroscopic guidance (Fig. 7.5).[10] For a female child with VUR, for example,

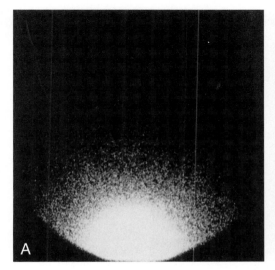

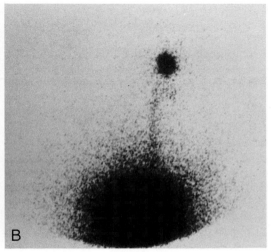

FIG. 7.4. A, A normal NCG showing the isotope filled-bladder surrounded by a corona of emitted radiation and no isotope in the ureters. **B,** An abnormal NCG showing isotope in the right ureter and pelvicaliceal system.

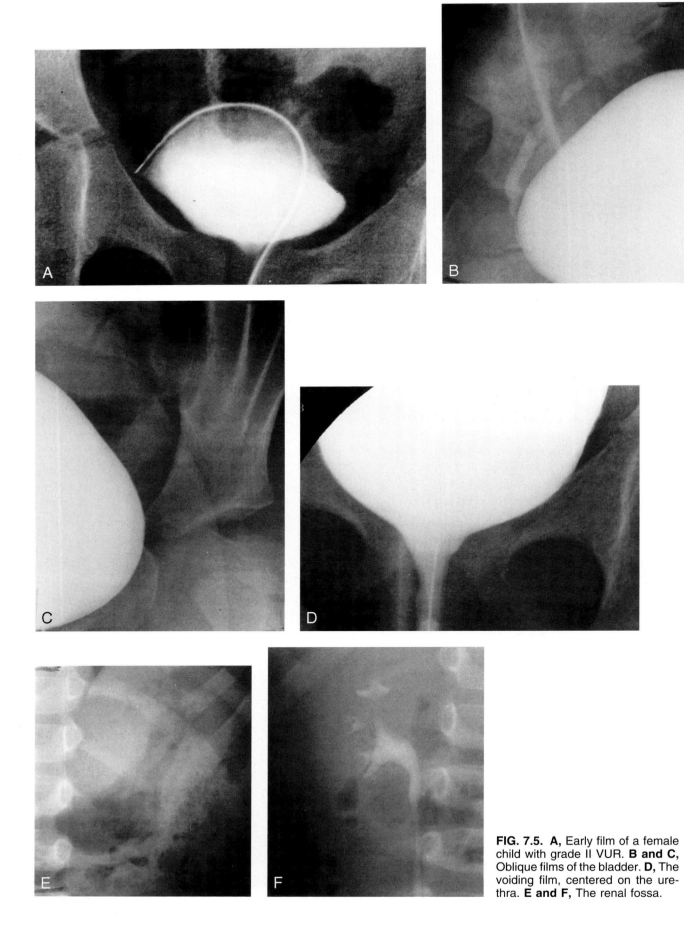

FIG. 7.5. A, Early film of a female child with grade II VUR. **B and C,** Oblique films of the bladder. **D,** The voiding film, centered on the urethra. **E and F,** The renal fossa.

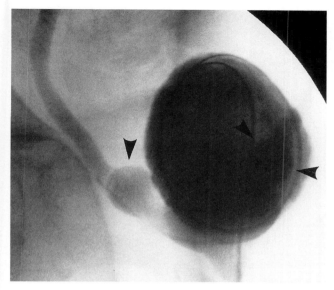

FIG. 7.6. VCUG of a 3-year-old child showing bilateral bladder diverticula (*arrows*) into which the ureters insert and bilateral grade 4 reflux (not shown). Both were missed on earlier NCG studies.

the series would include an early film to exclude ureterocele or mucosal abnormality and oblique films of the bladder to demonstrate the ureterovesical junction (and spare the contralateral ovary from direct radiation exposure). The oblique films can also determine if a diverticulum is undermining the ureterovesical junction. Next a voiding film is taken; it is centered on the urethra, sparing the ovaries from direct radiation. Finally, each renal fossa is filmed, and fluoroscopy of the bladder is performed to assess the completeness of voiding.

The NCG characterizes VUR as mild, moderate, or severe and determines the volume at which VUR occurs. Although some anatomic detail is lost, attention to secondary signs may allow diagnosis of congenital anomalies, such as ureterocele or VUR into a lower pole of a duplex system. If the child does not void (i.e., the bladder is drained via the catheter), VUR may be missed; approximately 20% of VUR occurs only during voiding. Familiarity with the technique used in one's institution is important, because a child with multiple UTIs but a negative NCG may benefit from a radiographic VCUG (Fig. 7.6).

Vesicoureteral reflux detected with VCUG is graded according to the classification system of the International Reflux Study (IRS) (Fig. 7.7).[11] This system distinguishes grades based on the extent of reflux, the dilation of the ureter, and the fullness of the pelvicaliceal system. It allows explicit communication among radiologists and urologists and has prognostic value regarding the possibility of spontaneous resolution of the reflux in both single and duplex systems.[12] Intrarenal VUR does not change the grade of the VUR, is more often seen in the very young, and is a visual indication of one pathway by which infection can enter the renal parenchyma. The IRS grading system should not be used when coexistent obstruction of the renal pelvis or ureter has produced dilatation of the collecting system (Fig. 7.6). Vesicoureteral reflux may delineate the upper tracts and differentiate between complete and incomplete duplication of the ureters when this is unclear after US or EU (Fig. 7.8).

A nuclear cystogram may be favored over radiographic VCUG in children with a low suspicion of anatomic abnormality, e.g., girls with a recurrent UTI but limited symptoms and for screening siblings of known refluxers (especially those with scarring).[13,14] Children whose prior VCUG demonstrated reflux alone and those who have undergone ureteral reimplantation may also be followed with NCG. The possibility of urethral lesions in boys (polyps, valves, diverticula) mandates that they undergo VCUG (Fig. 7.9). Attention to fluoroscopic technique and the use of digital and pulsed fluoroscopy may sufficiently decrease the gonadal dose so that the radiation dose of VCUG is now 10 times less than that for conventional voiding cystourethrography.[8–10,15,16]

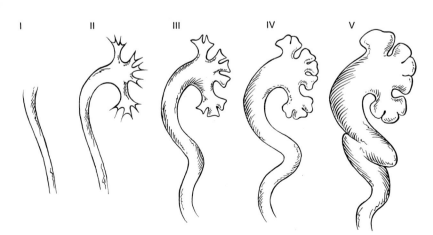

I II III IV V

FIG. 7.7. International Reflux Study grading system for VUR.

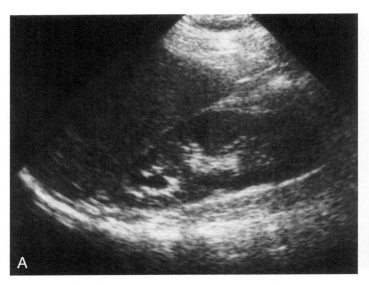
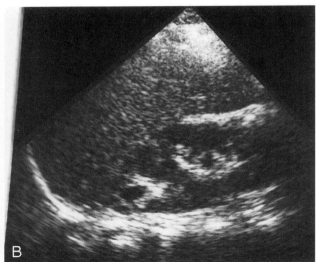
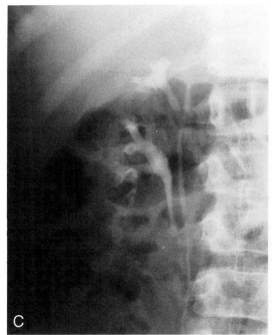
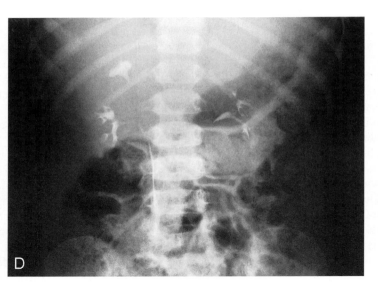

FIG. 7.8. Sagittal view US studies of a complete **(A)** and incomplete **(B)** ureteral duplication demonstrating that the central renal echo complex is separated by parenchyma. EU studies showing both right kidneys of a complete **(C)** and incomplete **(D)** duplication. **E,** VUR into the upper pole confirming the complete ureteral duplication seen in parts A and C. **F,** Reflux into both segments of the kidney indicating the incomplete duplication seen in parts B and D.

Renal Scintigraphy

The varied physiology of the agents to which ^{99m}Tc can be attached allows radionuclide renal scanning to provide diverse information about the kidneys. ^{99m}Tc avoids the high gonadal exposure incurred when iodine 131 (^{131}I) labeled iodohippurate is trapped in obstructed segments of the upper urinary tract. Using ^{99m}Tc has several other advantages: It is inexpensive, is more

readily available than ^{123}I (another iodine isotope with a lower radiation dose) and produces high-quality images. ^{123}I is a cyclotron produced isotope of iodine that emits less radiation than does ^{131}I.

The radiopharmaceutical ^{99m}Tc-labeled diethylenetriamine penta-acetic acid (DTPA) is excreted by glomerular function and can be used to evaluate renal function and renal blood flow.[17, 18] DTPA, administered with a diuretic (e.g., furosemide), is also used to determine the postnatal function and relative degree of obstruction of

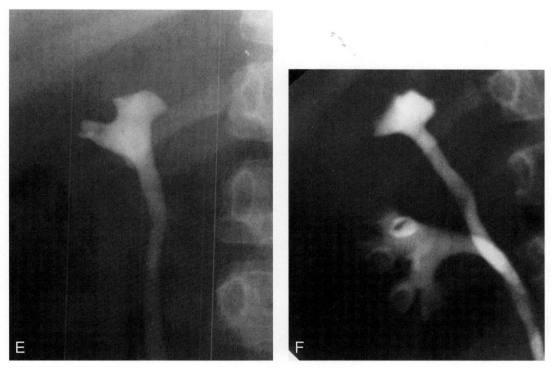

FIG. 7.8. *Continued.*

kidneys in children with prenatally diagnosed HN.[18-24] The data obtained from diuretic-enhanced DTPA renal scans, however, are variable, depending on the age and degree of hydration of the child, and do not always parallel the results of the more invasive Whitaker test.[20]

^{99m}Tc-labeled mercaptoacetyl triglycine (MAG-3), a pharmacological analogue of orthoiodohippurate and para-aminohippurate, produces images of excellent quality, even when renal function is compromised, and can be used to evaluate tubular function and measure renal plasma flow (Fig. 7.10).[25, 26] The criteria developed for diagnosing obstruction with DTPA can be applied to MAG-3.

Obstructive abnormalities can be imaged and quantified at any age; however, attention to technique is important, especially in the neonate, when glomerular filtration rate is relatively low and concentrating ability is poor. One protocol of diuretic renography stresses the value of hydrating the child before and during the study, keeping the bladder empty via a catheter, and giving the diuretic at a specific time.[26] With these rigid criteria, diuretic renography, usually conducted with ^{99m}Tc-MAG-3, can be an excellent, reproducible technique for evaluating the kidneys' function and degree of obstruction (Fig. 7.11).[27] Unilateral disease is especially easy to evaluate because the contralateral normal kidney can serve as a control.

Two radiopharmaceuticals are commonly used to image the cortex in children with suspected acute pyelo-nephritis or questionable parenchymal scarring: ^{99m}Tc-dimercaptosuccinic acid (DMSA) and ^{99m}Tc-glucohepto-nate (Fig. 7.12).[28-33] Imaging with ^{99m}Tc-DMSA also permits measurement of relative renal function. To enhance image quality, children with known or suspected VUR may need a bladder catheter placed before isotope injection. Interobserver variability in the interpretation may affect the usefulness of the DMSA scan.[32]

Renovascular hypertension is an uncommon problem in childhood. Administration of an angiotensin-converting enzyme (ACE) inhibitor, usually captopril, before renal scintigraphy with ^{99m}Tc-DTPA or ^{99m}Tc-MAG-3, is a valuable way to detect a narrowed renal artery.[33] Other techniques, such as Doppler US and digital subtraction angiography, have also been successful for evaluating renovascular hypertension.[34, 35]

^{99m}Tc-pertechnetate is used to evaluate the child with an acutely painful scrotum. Pinhole blood pool scans soon after the intravenous injection of the isotope document perfusion of the testis; later scans are used to differentiate inflammatory processes from acute torsion or missed testicular torsion (Fig. 7.13).[36, 37] Correlation with the clinical history is vital because testicular hematoma, abscess, and tumor can each have a similar appearance to torsion on imaging.

Ultrasound

In many clinical settings, ultrasound is preferred over EU for the initial evaluation of children with UTIs; for

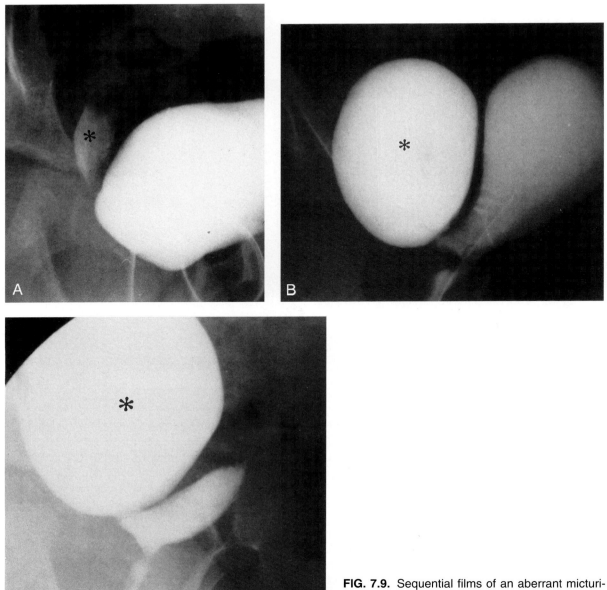

FIG. 7.9. Sequential films of an aberrant micturition into a bladder diverticulum showing enlargement of the diverticulum (*asterisks*) during voiding.

screening the kidneys of children with specific skeletal, cardiac, or gastrointestinal anomalies; for evaluating children with prenatally diagnosed HN, abdominal mass, proteinuria, or hematuria; and for directing renal biopsy, cyst or abscess drainage, or percutaneous catheter placement. US demonstrates urinary tract dilation well and can be used to evaluate the urinary tract after pyeloplasty and ureteroneocystostomy (Fig. 7.14).[38]

US-detected dilatation is usually described subjectively as mild, moderate, or severe. This limits accurate communication of meaningful patient data and accurate interpretation of published surgical reports. The Society for Fetal Urology (SFU) developed a classification sys-

tem to describe the degree of pelvicaliceal and ureter dilation; this system is increasingly being employed by other investigators (Fig. 7.15).[20, 21, 39, 40] At grade 0, the fat about the renal pelvis defines the pelvis; no fluid is within it. Successively higher grades have greater distention of the pelvicaliceal system and, ultimately, thinning of the parenchyma.

Doppler US is used to observe and measure renal blood flow in children with hypertension, renal transplant, and possible infarction or renal vein thrombosis. The resistive index is a calculated measure of pulsatile blood flow and has been used to evaluate abnormal renal vasculature, obstructed kidneys, transplanted kidneys, and kidneys affected by systemic diseases.[41] Doppler US

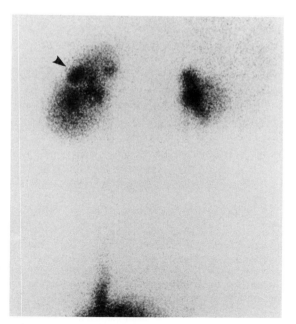

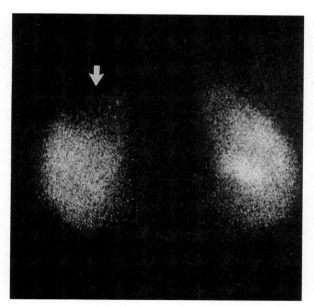

FIG. 7.10. Posterior ⁹⁹ᵐTc-MAG-3 scan showing scarring from VUR. The right kidney has less functioning parenchyma than does the left. Note the subtle parenchymal scarring, resulting in a caliceal system that projects along the periphery of the left kidney (*arrow*).

FIG. 7.12. ⁹⁹ᵐTc-glucoheptonate of a child with pyelonephritis and scarring demonstrating a focal defect (*arrow*) in the infected left upper pole.

may be difficult to perform in a child who is uncooperative or breathing rapidly.

In general, US is insensitive to changes of acute pyelonephritis.[28, 29] Color Doppler and power Doppler enhance detection of blood flow and make it possible

to see the decreased blood flow associated with acute pyelonephritis, the pathophysiology that is responsible for the cortical defects identified with renal scintigraphy.[42] These techniques are not yet in widespread clinical use.

It is important to image the bladder whenever there is an indication to perform a renal ultrasound.[43] An abnormality detected within the bladder may clarify the

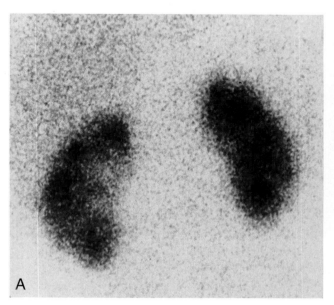

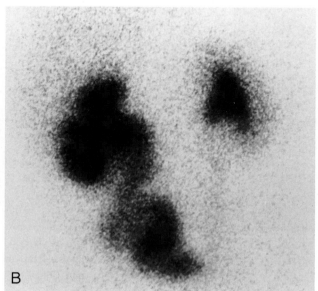

FIG. 7.11. Early ⁹⁹ᵐTc-MAG-3 study of a male neonatal who was prenatally diagnosed with HUN, was postnatally diagnosed with primary megaureter, and has a normal VCUG. The right kidney is normal, and the left has a central photopenic region. **B,** Late image of the same patient demonstrating dilatation of the entire upper tract.

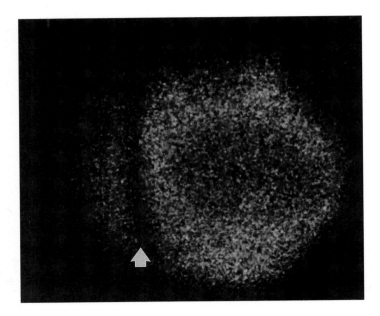

FIG. 7.13. Testicular scan of an 11-year-old showing increased isotope in the periphery of the scrotal sac and a central cold area. The vertical marker (*arrow*) is placed on the median raphe and indicates the degree of enlargement of the left testis and scrotal sac.

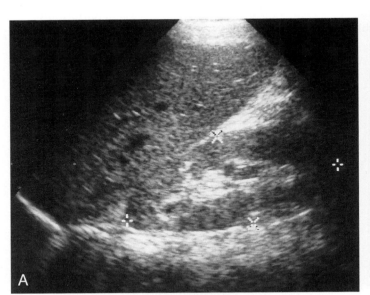

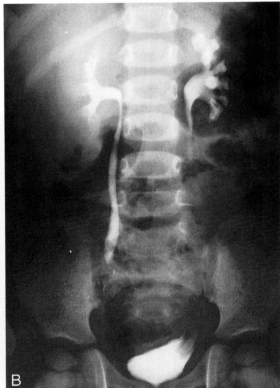

FIG. 7.14. A, Sagittal view US of a normal left kidney. **B,** EU showing normal kidneys and ureters. Note the dilatation of the right ureter to the level of the iliac vessels, a normal variant, and the reimplantation site on the left side of the bladder.

Normal calyces

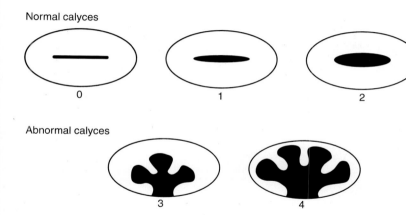

Abnormal calyces

FIG. 7.15. The grading system of the Society for Fetal Urology for hydronephrosis. Reprinted with permission from Fernbach SK, Maizels M, Conway JJ. Ultrasound grading of hydronephrosis: introduction to the system used by the Society for Fetal Urology. Pediatr Radiol 1993;23:478–480.

renal process, e.g., when a ureterocele is seen beneath a dilated kidney and ureter (Fig. 7.16). If the bladder is incompletely filled, intravesical structures may be missed, the bladder wall will be poorly characterized, and retrovesical structures (including the distal ureter) will be hard to image. Thus the child should drink ample volumes of fluids or receive an intravenous fluid bolus before the renal ultrasound and is asked to refrain from voiding.

An overly filled bladder can impede urine passage from the ureter and create or enhance HN or HUN. When HN or HUN is detected and the bladder is full, the bladder must be emptied (by voiding or catheterization) and the kidneys rescanned to determine if the condition persists or resolves.

Ultrasound has been used to study congenital lesions of the genitourinary tract and acquired processes other than infection, such as tumor. US of the acutely painful scrotum has been successful, although imperfectly so, at

differentiating torsion, which demonstrates diminished blood flow, from inflammatory processes, which usually increase vascularity.[44] Testicular torsion is most common in infant and preteen boys.

Computed Tomography

Helical and spiral CT technology have decreased scanning times so that patient motion and breathing are less likely to degrade image quality than in the past. The presence of small, poorly functioning, or ectopic kidneys can be sought with CT. Calcifications within the kidneys or adjacent tumors are better seen with CT than with plain films or MRI. Cysts and fat within the kidneys and renal masses are well shown.

Intravenous contrast material, usually of low osmolality and given as a bolus, provides excellent corticomedullary definition. Abnormal enhancement of the parenchyma occurs with acute pyelonephritis and may

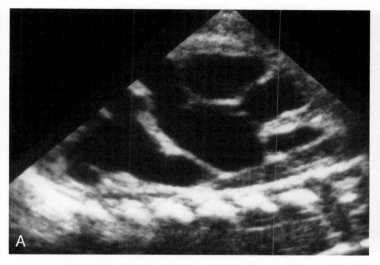

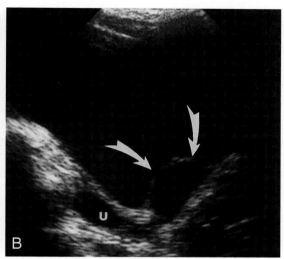

FIG. 7.16. A, Sagittal view US of a female fetus with ureteral duplication and ectopic ureterocele. Note the hydronephrotic upper and lower poles. **B,** Transverse view of the bladder of the same patient demonstrating the thin-walled ureterocele (*arrows*) emanating from the upper pole ureter (U). The lower pole orifice cannot be seen.

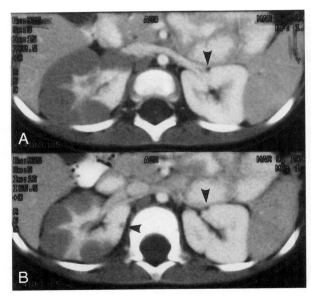

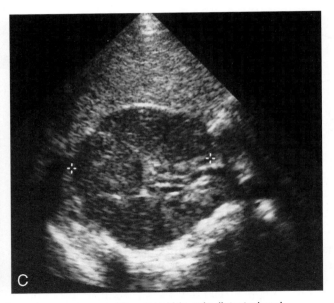

FIG. 7.17. A and B, CT studies showing the normal renal parenchyma of the right kidney is distorted and displaced centrally. Smaller nonenhancing foci of nephroblastomatosis are present bilaterally (*arrows*). **C,** Transverse renal US study at the level of the hilum (as in part B) showing an enlarged kidney. Note the abnormal tissue has the same echogenicity as the kidney.

make CT as sensitive and as specific for infection as cortical scintigraphy.[42, 45]

CT has replaced EU in the evaluation of all but medically unstable patients with abdominal trauma because it images the renal pedicle, the kidney, and the perirenal tissues at the same time as it does other abdominal organs. A scout CT film, performed after the abdominal CT scan, shows the kidneys and bladder like an EU.

Mass lesions (cysts, renal parenchymal tumors, and infiltrative tumors) may deform the caliceal pattern, obstruct the renal pelvis, or fail to enhance (Fig. 7.17). The status (displaced, encased, or occluded) of the major and minor vessels is well delineated (Fig. 7.18). Intra-abdominal metastatic disease can be assessed at the same time as the primary tumor.

Magnetic Resonance Imaging

MRI generally takes longer than any of the other modalities. To ensure patient cooperation and lack of motion, the child usually needs to be sedated, which adds time, cost, and risk to the examination. For these reasons, MRI is not performed as frequently as is CT for children with a suspected tumor.

MRI superbly delineates the retroperitoneal and vascular structures.[46–48] US, especially with Doppler (or color Doppler) to evaluate the blood vessels, may provide sufficient information to plan treatment, especially because many masses are not malignancies. The ability of MRI to see primary tumor and possible intracaval extension without intravenous contrast material is of value when evaluating a child with suspected Wilms

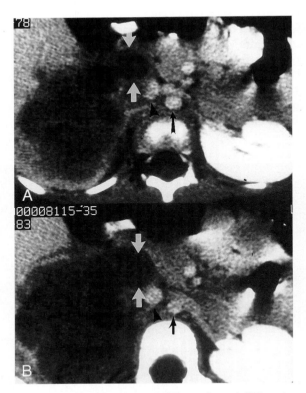

FIG. 7.18. Contrast-enhanced CT studies of Wilms tumor with clot in the inferior vena cava showing the intrarenal mass fails to enhance and distorts the adjacent parenchyma. Contrast fills the aorta (*black arrow*), smaller vessels, and superior mesenteric vein (*arrowhead*). The lumen of the inferior vena cava (*white arrows*) contains a clot and fails to opacify.

tumor who had an equivocal US study. Bone marrow involvement may be sought or incidentally detected when imaging a child with neuroblastoma. The ability to produce direct images, rather than reconstructions, in the sagittal and coronal planes has increased acceptance of the technique by clinicians uncomfortable with cross-sectional imaging.

CLINICAL SETTINGS FOR IMAGING

Neonatal Hydronephrosis

Widespread use of prenatal US has created a new patient population for both pediatric urologist and radiologist: the asymptomatic neonate with HN or HUN. The definition of prenatal HN should be precise to protect the parents from unnecessary concern and the child from unnecessary tests. Clinicians using age-related measurements of the renal pelvis (≥5 mm at 18 to 20 weeks of gestation, ≥8 mm at 34 weeks of gestation) found that renal pelvis dilatation was not a good indicator of postnatal pathology, especially for the presence of VUR.[49] A more commonly used definition of prenatal HN considers a renal pelvis >1 cm in the AP plane on US performed after the 20 weeks of gestation to be abnormal. Less dilatation resolves either prenatally or postnatally and has been infrequently associated with renal pathology.[23]

Approximately 80% of HN/HUN patients are boys, a marked contrast to the female predominance of UTIs later in childhood.[19, 20, 22, 50–55] Prenatal resolution of HN and HUN occurs in about 30% of fetuses.[19, 20] Three entities are commonly responsible for true prenatal HN and HUN: ureteropelvic junction obstruction; VUR; and nonobstructive, nonspecific HN.[50–56] As many as 30% of patients are found to have primary VUR only or primary VUR in association with ureteropelvic junction obstruction or ureterovesical junction obstruction.[19, 51–54] Infants with primary (aperistaltic) megaureter are often detected before symptoms develop (Fig. 7.19).[22, 57] Tables 7.1 and 7.2 list the causes of HN and HUN, respectively, in the neonate.

Sometimes it is difficult to differentiate prenatal HN from multicystic dysplastic kidney, normal hypoechoic medullary pyramids, and duplication with obstructed upper pole.[55, 56] Cystic renal masses may look like other cystic masses of the abdomen and pelvis. Multicystic dysplastic kidney can be recognized prenatally (although confirmation of the diagnosis may require postpartum imaging) and accounts for 2 to 10% of renal anomalies detected in utero.[19, 24, 53, 55] Postnatally, ^{93m}Tc-DMSA scanning is used to help differentiate HN from MCKD, although a few multicystic dysplastic kidneys retain a small degree of function (Fig. 7.20).[58]

Regardless of the presumed diagnosis, postnatal studies are necessary to confirm that an abnormality is pres-

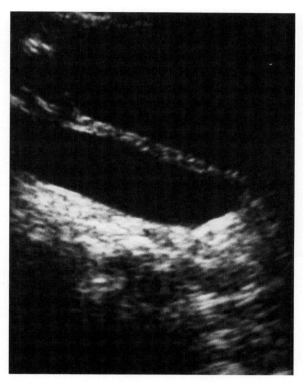

FIG. 7.19. Longitudinal view US of primary megaureter taken behind the bladder demonstrating a ureter with markedly enlarged caliber.

TABLE 7.1. *Causes of hydronephrosis in the neonate*

- Common
  Ureteropelvic junction obstruction
  Ureteral duplication
      Upper pole obstructed
      Lower pole VUR
  VUR
- Uncommon
  Retrocaval ureter
  Ureteral valves
- Spurious
  Lucent medullary pyramids
  Multicystic dysplastic kidney

TABLE 7.2. *Causes of hydroureteronephrosis in the neonate*

- Common
  Ectopic insertion of the upper pole ureter
  Ectopic or orthotopic ureterocele
  Posterior urethral valves
  Primary megaureter
  Vesicoureteral reflux
- Uncommon
  Infection
  Neurogenic bladder
  Prune belly syndrome
  Urethral obstruction other than posterior urethral valves

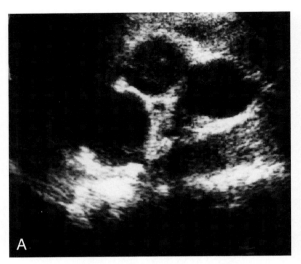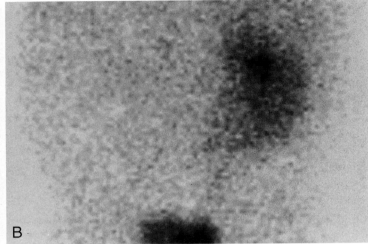

FIG. 7.20. **A,** Sagittal view renal US of a multicystic dysplastic kidney showing multiple fluid-filled structures throughout the renal pelvis. Both multicystic dysplastic kidney (hydronephrotic variant) and hydronephrosis have this appearance. **B,** ^{99m}Tc-MAG-3 scan indicating that the kidney has no function and is thus multicystic dysplastic.

ent, to characterize it more fully, and to diagnose concurrent or associated genitourinary problems. The purpose of all studies is to guide therapy so that loss of renal function owing to obstruction or UTI is prevented. Thus neonates with HN or HUN are given antibiotic prophylaxis until the studies have been completed and a diagnosis (with specific treatment) has been rendered. Despite this precaution, some neonates with prenatally detected anomalies do develop a UTI.[59]

The more problematic patients are those with hydronephrosis but good renal function that persists past the neonatal period. Later testing may reveal that some of these children ultimately will lose function and require surgical intervention.[60, 61] Children with obstruction detected when studies are performed after a UTI has developed or as part of family screening undergo the same evaluation for HN as those diagnosed prenatally. One approach to imaging children with a prenatal diagnosis of HN or HUN is shown in Figure 7.21.

Postnatal evaluation begins with a urinary tract US; this should not be performed immediately after birth, because HN or HUN may be less obvious and hence missed in the immediate postnatal period owing to physiologic oliguria. One report notes that some children with HN or HUN might be missed even when studied 1 week after birth and recommends delaying the screening US until the child is 6 weeks old.[50] Because the yield from the early US is quite high and because early detection of a significant group of neonates enables timely, specific treatment, I usually do US shortly after the 1st week of life.

The grading system developed by the SFU has become increasingly used by clinicians studying children

with prenatal HN or HUN (Fig. 7.15).[20, 39] Standardized testing and criteria have allowed urologists to pool data and show that, in hundreds of cases, similar management is being recommended for this group of children.[62] One study found that the SFU system with US was more useful for evaluating neonates with HN than other tests, including ^{99m}Tc-DTPA renography, Whitaker test, antegrade pyelography, and EU.[20]

A VCUG should always be performed in children with true prenatal HN or HUN, even if the postnatal US is normal, because significant VUR can cause intermittent hydronephrosis. One variation in technique for the VCUG that is gaining popularity is the cyclic VCUG.[63] For this study, the bladder is filled several times to monitor several voiding episodes. A routine

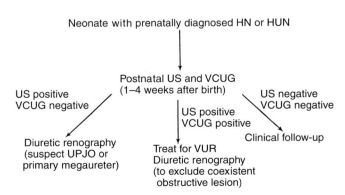

FIG. 7.21. Evaluating the neonate with hydronephrosis or hydroureteronephrosis. UPJO, ureteropelvic junction obstruction.

VCUG, with standard views, is performed during the first cycle of bladder filling and voiding.[10] At the completion of subsequent voids, the renal fossae are imaged. This increases the likelihood of detecting VUR, which may be intermittent—thus missed in only one cycle of bladder filling—and yet still may have the potential to produce renal infection and scars. Cyclic NCG has also been advocated in neonates.[64]

Renal scintigraphy with ^{99m}Tc-DTPA or ^{99m}Tc-MAG-3 can evaluate the degree of obstruction, if any, and assess relative function of the kidneys.[18, 25–27, 62] The neonate has a diminished ability to concentrate urine and a relatively lower glomerular filtration rate but valid data can be obtained in this period when the testing is performed under optimal conditions. Whenever possible, nuclear renography should be delayed until the child is at least 1 month old.[26] Some obstructed kidneys show supranormal renal function; this finding occurs more often on the right and may be artifactual, the result of failure to properly subtract the background activity of the liver.[65]

Urinary Tract Infection

Imaging of the child with UTI is expensive and invasive. It should be performed without hesitation when indicated but avoided when not.[66] The diagnosis of UTI, to be correct, must be based on a properly obtained and handled specimen. A diagnosis based on a bagged urine collection or clean-catch urine left standing at room temperature is suspect, and additional cultures should be performed before imaging.

The very young child with UTI may not have symptoms referable to the urinary tract and instead may present with fever and lethargy. Neonates and children with normal prenatal US may present with UTI owing to anatomic lesions. Even in older children, the symptoms and laboratory findings may make differentiation between upper urinary tract infection (pyelonephritis) and lower urinary tract infection (cystitis, urethritis) difficult. This distinction is of major concern, because cystitis, even if recurrent, has few sequelae; whereas pyelonephritis, with or without VUR, can produce renal scarring.

Imaging is directed to answering specific questions: *(a)* Is there an anatomic problem? If so, where? *(b)* Is there a functional problem? If so, where? *(c)* Has the infection produced problems (e.g., renal scarring, acute pyelonephritis, bladder thickening, pseudotumor)? *(d)* How will the findings affect management? Anatomic problems include ureteropelvic junction obstruction, megacalices, caliceal diverticulum, abnormal development of the ureterovesical junction resulting in VUR, primary megaureter, bladder diverticulum, and obstructive lesions of the urethra. Functional problems include inability to empty the bladder completely, infrequent voiding, and bladder–sphincter dyssynergia. The common denominator of the anatomic and functional lesions is that urinary stasis, a precursor of infection, is present to some degree.

US is frequently the first imaging study performed during or after a UTI. In addition to assessing renal lengths (compared to normal controls), US can detect kidney stones (result of or nidus of UTI) and dilatation that may be caused by obstruction or reflux. UTI can be associated with debris in the renal pelvis (pus, fungus ball, precipitated salts) and thickening of the walls of the renal pelvis (Fig. 7.22). Gray scale US is poor at detecting changes of acute pyelonephritis, such as focal or diffuse edema, loss of definition of the corticomedul-

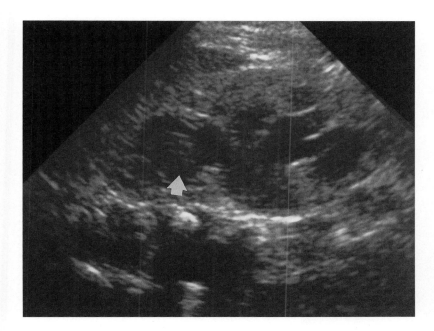

FIG. 7.22. Sagittal view renal US of candidiasis (fungus balls) of the kidney showing echogenic debris within the pelvicaliceal system. Note the debris within the caliceal system of the upper pole (*arrow*).

lary junction, and increased or decreased echogenicity of the parenchyma.[28, 29] Initial edema from the UTI may be difficult to appreciate if the renal length falls within the range of normal; and late scarring may be best diagnosed if a baseline ultrasound is done when edema has resolved, at least several days after treatment was initiated.[67] Renal scars are poorly shown on US images, and measurements of renal length may not be good indicators of global scarring.[68, 69] The bladder must be carefully assessed because it may have an anatomic abnormality predisposing it to infection or may have secondary changes of infection.

Color and power Doppler have been used during acute UTIs to detect regions of hypoperfusion that parallel the isotope-poor areas seen on cortical scintigraphy.[41] Changes in the appearance of pyelonephritic kidneys have also been seen on both CT and MRI studies, but these techniques are not commonly used to diagnose pyelonephritis.[41, 44]

Normal-appearing anatomy on US does not obviate the need for cystography, because significant VUR can be present without urinary tract dilatation or detectable renal scarring.[68] Scarring may also be the result of prior reflux (which was outgrown or surgically treated) or, rarely, from hematogenous pyelonephritis.

Nuclear scintigraphy and EU have different and often complementary roles. Acute pyelonephritis and secondary scars are well demonstrated with cortical-specific isotopes (Fig. 7.12), such as technetium 99m–labeled glucoheptonate and DMSA.[29–33, 69] EU is rarely abnormal acutely and rarely shows small scars, unless tomography is performed or the scarring is severe (Fig. 7.23). EU can, however, provide treatment-important information, especially with complex anomalies, and remains a useful modality.[1, 2, 70]

If the clinician believes that intravenous antibiotics are necessary for treating all children with pyelonephritis, not just infants or those in whom vomiting precludes oral medications, scintigraphy with cortical agents is the best modality available for documenting parenchymal infection.[71] Although it has been shown that the majority of cortical defects (acute pyelonephritis and scarring) are detected in children without VUR, infants, who have unspecific symptoms and a tendency to scar, are more likely to have VUR than are older children. In addition, the majority of children with VUR have abnormal DMSA scans, children with UTI and VUR are more likely to have cortical defects and renal scarring than those without VUR, the association of cortical defects with VUR is strongest in the children younger than 2 years old, and intervention in children with VUR can reduce parenchymal scarring.[71–76] These facts make cystography a rational part of the workup for children with UTIs.

Traditionally, children were imaged only after the UTI had subsided and antibiotic treatment had been in place for several weeks. The reasoning for this was twofold: a concern that children would reflux infected urine, increasing the risk of severe sepsis, and the belief that the current UTI could be the cause of, rather than be the result of, the VUR. Recognition that VUR was occurring regardless of imaging and documentation of the fact that UTI does not cause VUR have led clinicians to rethink this approach. More recently, children have been studied subacutely when confirmation of appropriate antibiotic administration is available.

The advantages of studying children, especially inpatients, during the early stages of a UTI include (a) the study is likely to be performed and does not rely on parental compliance, (b) proper treatment is started

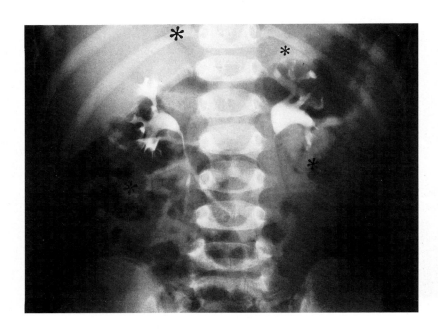

FIG. 7.23. EU showing left renal scarring from prior pyelonephritis and a normal right pelvicaliceal system and ureter. Note that on the left the calices are mildly clubbed and close to the parenchymal edge, indicating scarring. The left kidney is much smaller than the right (*stars*).

early, (c) parental education about VUR can be given and reinforced, and (d) there is no delay in obtaining a urological consult if needed.

The incidence of VUR depends on the age, sex, and race of the population studied. Because VUR may resolve with age, it is expected that younger children are more likely to reflux than are older children. Black children are less likely to have VUR than are white children.

Children with VUR who undergo ureteral reimplantation will need postoperative evaluation. US may detect new HN postoperatively, and NCG may exclude residual VUR. A US study done in the early postoperative period may show ureteral dilation secondary to residual edema at the site of reimplantation. If the dilation is no greater than the maximal dilation of the ureter seen on the preoperative cystogram, there is generally no immediate concern; repeat US is obtained several weeks later. Diuretic renography might also be obtained to assess whether drainage seems satisfactory. Because the overall success of ureteral reimplantation is high, not all surgeons routinely perform postoperative cystography, reserving the test for patients with clinical problems.

Renal Tumors

The age of the child at presentation is important in the differential diagnosis of renal tumors. Some masses are common in the neonate; others typically arise later (Table 7.3). Because almost any tumor may present at any age, meticulous imaging is an important aid for diagnosis and treatment planning.

Specific clinical features may aid in the preoperative diagnosis. A young child who presents with a renal mass after treatment of a posterior fossa brain tumor is likely to have a rhabdoid tumor of the kidney; the renal tumor may precede the neural tumor or occur without it.[77, 78] Children with certain syndromes or anomalies (horseshoe kidney), especially those with isolated hemihypertrophy, sporadic aniridia, or Beckwith–Wiedemann syndrome have an increased incidence of Wilms tumor (Table 7.4).[79, 80] They should undergo renal US every 3 months during the periods of greatest risk. Screening can be discontinued when the risk of developing a Wilms tumor lessens, defined as the 8th birthday for children with hemihypertrophy and/or Beckwith–Wiedemann syndrome and the 5th birthday for those with sporadic aniridia.[81] It is interesting that some physicians suggest that screening has not changed the size or stage of tumors at presentation in this population.[82]

Imaging is performed to help classify and stage the tumor preoperatively and, more important, to help plan any surgery. All abdominal masses are evaluated using a number of criteria:

• Tumor or other cause of renal enlargement
• Renal or extrarenal tumor

TABLE 7.3. *Pediatric renal masses by age*

• Neonates and Infants (birth to 1 year)
  Hydronephrosis[a]
  Multicystic dysplastic kidney[b]
  Congenital mesoblastic nephroma[b]
  Renal vein thrombosis[b]
  Multilocular cystic nephroma[b]
  Autosomal recessive polycystic kidney disease[c]
  Nephroblastomatosis[c]
  Retroperitoneal (nonrenal) teratoma[a]
• Toddlers (1–5 years)
  Hydronephrosis or hydroureteronephrosis[a]
  Wilms tumor[a]
  Neuroblastoma[a]
  Rhabdoid tumor of the kidney[a]
  Autosomal recessive polycystic kidney disease[c]
  Cystic disease of tuberous sclerosis[c]
  Infiltrative processes (leukemia, lymphoma, storage diseases)[c]
  Nephroblastomatosis[c]
• Children (6–11 years)
  Wilms tumor[a]
  Clear cell sarcoma of the kidney[a]
  Infiltrative processes (leukemia, lymphoma, storage diseases)[c]
  Cystic disease of tuberous sclerosis[c]
  Autosomal recessive/dominant polycystic kidney disease (late/early presentation)[c]
• Preteens and Teenagers (12–19 years)
  Wilms tumor[a]
  Renal cell carcinoma[b]
  Medullary carcinoma[b]
  Neuroblastoma (intrarenal)[b]
  Infiltrative processes (leukemia, lymphoma)[c]
  Autosomal dominant polycystic kidney disease[c]

[a]Unilateral or bilateral.
[b]Usually unilateral.
[c]Usually bilateral.

TABLE 7.4. *Syndromes associated with Wilms tumor*

Syndrome	Characteristics
Beckwith–Wiedemann	Macrosomia at birth, macroglossia hemihypertrophy, nesidioblastosis; tumors: Wilms, adrenal, gonadoblastoma
Drash (Denys–Drash)	Autosomal dominant nephritis, pseudohermaphroditism; tumors: 50% of patients develop Wilms
Perlman	Autosomal recessive macrosomia at birth, nesidioblastosis, renal dysplasia including nephroblastomatosis, mental retardation
Wilms tumor, aniridia, genitourinary abnormalities, and mental retardation (WAGR)	

Data from Knudson AG. Introduction to the genetics of primary renal tumors in children. Med Pediatr Oncol 1993;21:193 and Herman TE, McAlister WH. Perlman syndrome: report of a case with additional radiographic findings. Pediatr Radiol 1995;25:S70.

- Unilateral or bilateral
- Focal or diffuse
- Solid, cystic, mixed
- Presence of calcification
- Extrarenal involvement
  Direct extension
  Intravascular extension
  Lymphadenopathy
  Vascular encasement or displacement

In addition, it is important to exclude any congenital anomaly of the contralateral kidney because absence of or severe damage to the kidney might compel a parenchymal-sparing procedure on the side with tumor.

Many tumors can be adequately characterized using one technique alone; US, CT, and MRI usually delineate the tumor and adjacent structures so well that no additional imaging is necessary.[47] The choice of modality depends on the strengths of those performing the study. Additional imaging may be needed to verify the findings of the first, especially when the tumor has an atypical appearance.

The inferior vena cava must be imaged because Wilms tumor grows into it in about 5% of pediatric cases. Neuroblastoma can invade the vena cava also, but does so less frequently (Fig. 7.18).[83, 84] Large right-sided masses may compress the inferior vena cava, making it difficult to see on standard US. When this occurs, color Doppler imaging or imaging with CT or MRI may be useful.

Wilms Tumor

Wilms tumor (WT) accounts for about 5% of all pediatric malignancies. It is typically unilateral, large, and intrarenal.[80] Exophytic and extrarenal Wilms tumor can also occur but are much less frequent.[85] The stage of the tumor is more important than the cell type (Table 7.5), but anaplastic variants have a poor prognosis over-

TABLE 7.5. *Staging of Wilms tumor[a]*

Stage	Description
I	Tumor limited to kidney; complete surgical excision
II	Tumor extends beyond kidney into lymph nodes, inferior vena cava clot; complete surgical excision
III	Residual tumor in abdomen after surgery or spillage at surgery; not resectable
IV	Hematogenous metastases to lung, liver, bone, brain
V	Bilateral renal involvement at diagnosis

[a]Modified from the National Wilms Tumor Study III. Breslow N, Sharples K, Beckwith J, et al. Prognostic factors in the non metastatic, favorable histology Wilms' tumor. Results of the Third National Wilms' Tumor Study. Cancer 1991;68:2345–2353.

all.[86] Currently, the 5-year cure rate for stage I and II tumors is >80%.

Despite the advances in imaging, the average size (10 cm in diameter) at presentation has not changed significantly in the last few decades because referral for imaging usually depends on clinical detection of the mass (Fig. 7.18). Similarly, urine screening for neuroblastoma, routine in parts of Canada and Japan, has increased the number of tumors detected in the young but has not changed the number of higher-stage tumors found in older children.[87]

About 5% of children with Wilms tumor have bilateral disease; 65% of these have bilateral disease at presentation. Failure of normal primitive renal tissue to involute—nephroblastomatosis—is associated with an increased incidence of WT and is present in up to 100% of children with bilateral tumor. Nephroblastomatosis is well seen on contrast-enhanced CT (Fig. 7.17) and MRI.[46, 88, 89] Nephroblastomatosis is generally followed with US, because repeated CT may, through radiation, increase the incidence of malignant change and MRI is too expensive to be performed repeatedly for screening.

All parameters of tumor involvement are well shown by MRI, but this is not as widely performed as CT for imaging renal tumors, perhaps because CT is more readily available, even at institutions that have MRI scanners; motion artifacts are rare with spiral or helical CT scanners; and MRI requires deep and prolonged sedation, with its attendant costs and risks.

Recommendations for follow-up imaging of children with WT remain controversial. For example, some clinicians believe that chest radiographs are sufficient to detect metastatic lung disease, but others prefer the more sensitive CT scans of the chest.[90, 91] Most children receive, at a minimum, the imaging required by the chemotherapy protocol in which they are enrolled.

Recommendations for surgery are also controversial. Because 7% of children with bilateral WT had the contralateral tumor missed at imaging, some physicians recommend that visual inspection of the contralateral kidney remain a standard surgical procedure; however, in one study only 14 bilateral tumors were missed in a population of >2000 children with Wilms tumor.[91] Some surgeons believe that the ability to detect tumors of the contralateral kidney via palpation is about the same as with imaging and argue against exposing and palpating the contralateral kidney.[92, 93]

Neuroblastoma

Neuroblastoma arises in the retroperitoneum in 50% of children; in 50% of these, the tumor is of adrenal origin. An adrenal mass (cystic or solid) detected on late prenatal US is likely to be an adrenal hemorrhage but may be a neuroblastoma (frequently cystic in this population) or other adrenal tumors.[94] Cystic neuro-

TABLE 7.6. *Evans staging of neuroblastoma*

Stage	Description
I	Tumor limited to tissue/organ of origin; complete surgical excision
II	Tumor extends beyond tissue/organ of origin; unilateral involvement
III	Tumor extends across midline
IV	Disseminated disease; bony and soft tissue metastases
IV-S	Stage I or II disease, no bony disease, metastatic disease to soft tissues

From Evans AE. Staging and treatment of neuroblastoma. Cancer 1980;45:1799–1802.

blastoma may decrease in size during the neonatal period, simulating an adrenal hemorrhage; therefore, all newborns with prenatally diagnosed adrenal masses should undergo imaging and measurement of urinary catecholamines.[95]

About 75% of children with neuroblastoma have been diagnosed by the age of 4 years. Neural crest tumors in older children have the more mature histology of ganglioneuroblastoma or ganglioneuroma. Neuroblastoma infiltrates the kidney in about 20% of children and may make the tumor difficult to differentiate from a WT.[96] Age at diagnosis is important for prognosis; children who are younger than 1 year of age at the time of diagnosis have a better rate of survival than those who are diagnosed later. The stage of the tumor (Table 7.6) is another factor determining prognosis as is genetic analysis of the tumor.

Because neuroblastoma can grow into the spinal canal (dumbbell lesion), myelography was once routine in children with bulky paraspinal masses or long tract signs. MRI and CT are now used to demonstrate intraspinal extension. CT is better than MRI at demonstrating calcification, present in about 50% of neuroblastomas (Fig. 7.24).[97, 98] Either CT or MRI can be used to detect encasement of major blood vessels, which is common, or tumor extension into the inferior vena cava, which is rare.[48, 84, 97, 98]

In about 5% of children with neuroblastoma, the tumor arises in the true pelvis. By displacing or encroaching on the bowel and/or bladder, it can produce dysfunction of each, which can mimic neurologic disease produced by tumor within the spinal canal.

Nuclear medicine plays a role in staging neuroblastoma in children. Bone metastases, present in >50% at the time of diagnosis, may be detected with bone scanning agents, usually products labeled with technetium 99m. Bone marrow involvement is equally common, it not imaged routinely, and is usually documented by bone marrow biopsy. The tumor and its metastases may be imaged with metaiodobenzylguanidine (MIBG) labeled with iodine 131 (^{131}I) or ^{123}I.[98, 99] Iodine-labeled MIBG has been used to study the response to treatment when multiple sites of tumor have been detected and to treat the neoplasm by giving the agent in doses that are several orders of magnitude higher than the imaging dose.[99]

Surgical excision of abdominal and retroperitoneal tumors is difficult if there is vascular encasement. Chemotherapy-induced regression or involution of the tumor makes it more amenable to surgery. Occasionally, the adjacent kidney requires removal with residual tumor.

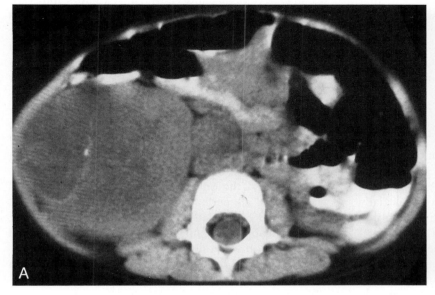
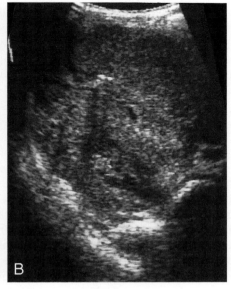

FIG. 7.24. A, CT study showing a neuroblastoma with a well-defined calcification positioned beneath the liver (not shown) adjacent to the psoas muscle. Note the second tumor deposit anterior to the spine. **B,** Transverse view US of the mass showing calcification with posterior acoustic shadowing.

Other Tumors

Congenital Mesoblastic Nephroma

Congenital mesoblastic nephroma (CMN) typically presents as an abdominal mass, usually in a child younger than 3 months of age, and may be associated with hypertension.[101-102] Virtually all tumors are unilateral and focal. CMN has been known to obstruct the stomach before birth, causing polyhydramnios, or after birth, causing feeding problems. Nephrectomy remains the treatment of choice. CMN is generally benign, but cellular variants with a high mitotic rate and/or aneuploidy may recur or rarely metastasize.

Like other intrarenal masses, CMN produces distortion of the pelvicaliceal system on EU, CT, and MRI. The tumor has a rather uniform solid appearance on CT and US. Occasionally, CMN has cystic or calcified components.

Rhabdoid Tumor of the Kidney

Rhabdoid tumor derives its name from its appearance on light microscopy. Patients with this tumor are younger than the usual Wilms tumor patients and do poorly, despite therapy. Posterior fossa CNS tumors are frequently associated with rhabdoid tumors.[77, 78, 86, 90]

Clear Cell Sarcoma of the Kidney

Clear cell sarcoma of the kidney (CCSK) is a rare tumor that occurs in the first decade of life, as a large unilateral mass with cystic spaces.[86, 90, 103] Although CCSK more frequently contains calcifications than does Wilms tumor (25 versus 5%), it accounts for such a small percentage of pediatric renal tumors (about 3%) that any intrarenal tumor with calcification must still be considered to be a WT. CCSK is an aggressive tumor with a poor response to chemotherapy and a tendency to metastasize to bone and brain; follow-up CT and MRI studies of the brain are recommended at 6-month intervals for the first 5 years after diagnosis.[90]

Multilocular Cystic Renal Tumor

Multilocular cystic renal tumor occurs in early childhood and is more common in boys than in girls.[104, 105] There are two types: Cystic nephroma is a benign lesion with septa made up of mature tissues and cystic partially differentiated nephroma is a more aggressive form that has blastemal and embryonal cells within the septa.[104] Nephrectomy, the usual treatment, achieves cure in both. Metastases or associations with anomalies or lesions of other organs have not been reported. At my hospital, one exophytic lesion was treated by excision of tumor (>4000 g) and partial nephrectomy. When the tumor recurred within the kidney several months later, nephrectomy was performed, and the child had no recurrence at the 10-year follow-up.

Renal Cell Carcinoma

Renal cell carcinoma (RCC) is exceedingly rare (about 1% of pediatric renal tumors) and is usually not diagnosed until late in the first or in the second decade of life.[90, 106-108] In contrast to the tumor of similar histology in adults, a high percent of pediatric RCCs (75%) contain calcification. Although hematuria, flank pain, and abdominal mass are common at presentation, few children have all three symptoms. Despite treatment with surgery, radiotherapy, and chemotherapy, RCC has a poorer prognosis than WT; but children with RCC tend to do better than do adults with a similar stage of disease.

Medullary Carcinoma of the Kidney

Medullary carcinoma of the kidney is a rare, recently described tumor that appears after the first decade only in teens with sickle-cell trait. Medullary carcinoma is more common in young adults than in children. It is an infiltrative aggressive lesion; metastases are common at presentation. It has a low cure rate.[109, 110]

Neurogenic Dysfunction of the Bladder

Myelomeningocele

Children with spinal dysraphism (myelomeningocele, lipomeningocele, diastematomyelia, myelocystocele) generally have abnormal innervation of the bladder. The level of the dysraphism does not predict the nature of the bladder dysfunction. Acquired neurogenic bladder may develop in children who have tumors, injury, or degenerative disease of the spinal cord. Once a serious problem has developed, several questions need to be answered to help the clinician protect the kidneys from deterioration and to plan management. (a) Is the bladder capacity normal? Does it hold much less than or more than normal?[111] (b) Is the appearance of the bladder normal or does it have multiple diverticula and cellules? (c) Does the child void spontaneously and to completion? Is there significant postvoid residual? (d) Is there VUR? At low or high bladder volume or during voiding only? (e) Is there HN or HUN?

In the past, the only way to answer these questions was to test all neonates with spinal dysraphism via VCUG and EU, often while the site of spinal closure was still healing.[112] Infants without VUR who could void to completion were allowed to do so; those with a significant postvoid residual or VUR were placed on clean intermittent catheterization (CIC) and prophylactic antibiotics or underwent vesicostomy.[113]

By delaying imaging until a few weeks after surgery, an accurate appraisal of the urinary tract—one not af-

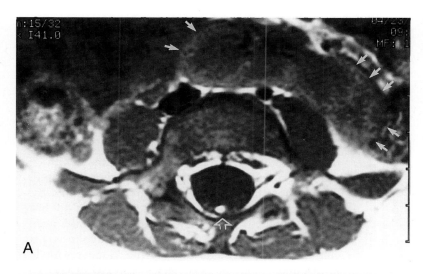

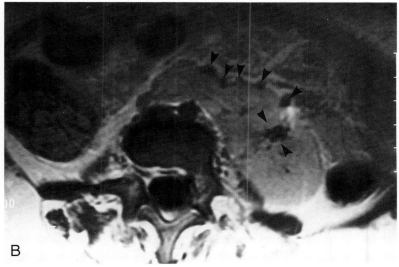

FIG. 7.25. A, Axial view MRI scan showing a thickened fatty filum terminale (*open arrow*) tethering the spinal cord and within the spinal canal. The horseshoe kidney (*arrows*) is anterior to the spine, predominantly to the left. **B,** Axial view MRI scan showing signal voids (*arrows*) along the anterior aspect of the horseshoe kidney and within the parenchyma, which are produced by the multiple renal blood vessels.

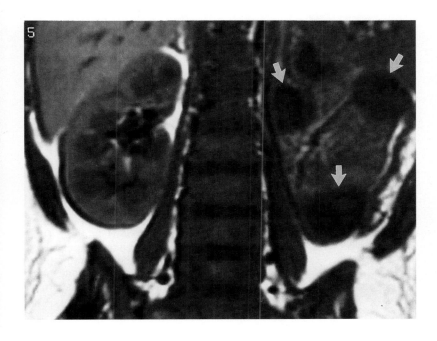

FIG. 7.26. Coronal view MRI scan showing the mesentery simulating dysplastic renal parenchyma and the bowel loops (*arrows*) simulating cysts. On the right, the corticomedullary differentiation is well demonstrated.

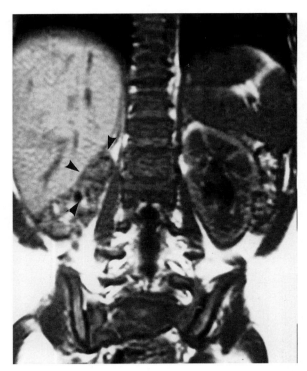

FIG. 7.27. Coronal view MRI scan showing small right kidney (*arrows*) caused by multiple UTIs. The left kidney is normal in size and appearance.

fected by recent surgery on the spinal cord—can be obtained. By using NCG and US, the treatment-necessary information can be obtained with much less gonadal irradiation.[112]

Urodynamic evaluation of the bladder is valuable for planning treatment. High-pressure bladders, defined as those with leakage or voiding at pressures >40 cm H_2O, are more apt to be associated with VUR and deterioration of the upper tracts than are low-pressure bladders.[114–116] Upper urinary tract evaluation must be done periodically (once a year) in all children with neurogenic dysfunction of the bladder and more often (every 4 to 6 months) in those with high-pressure bladders, on CIC, or with VUR.

Ultrasound has, in most instances, replaced EU for interval studies. When measuring the kidneys with US, the clinician must use a normal comparative group developed for this population; children with spinal dysraphism, even without VUR or UTI, tend to have smaller kidneys than do other children of similar age.[117]

If the child's habitus (size, scoliosis, or kyphosis) precludes adequate visualization of the kidneys with US ultrasound, it may be necessary to use EU or CT. The status of the kidneys can often be gleaned by reviewing recent MRI or CT studies of the spinal cord or canal, done to exclude retethering of the cord, hydromyelia, or syringomyelia (Figs. 7.25–7.27).[118] Children with dysraphism beginning in the thoracic region frequently have thoracolumbar kyphosis, atrophy of the psoas muscles, and inferior and medial displacement of the kidneys, known as pseudohorseshoe kidney (Fig. 7.28).[119] A similar change in the renal axis and medial displacement of the kidneys have been noted in some children with caudal regression.

The appearance of the bladder on VCUG, may provide information about the neurologic status of the bladder. An inferior position (sagging) of the bladder neck suggests lower motor neuron denervation of the external urethral (urinary) sphincter and flow, implying that the bladder is associated with low outlet resistance and

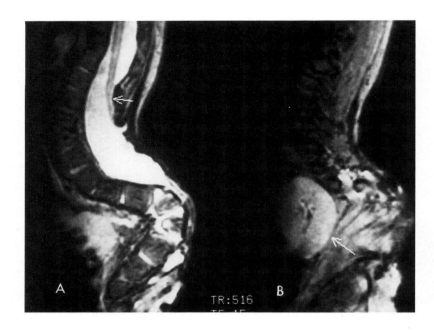

FIG. 7.28. A, Sagittal view MRI scan showing an enlarged thecal sac (*bright white area*). The spinal cord (*arrow*) is tethered along its posterior aspect. **B,** Sagittal view MRI scan showing that the kidney (*arrow*) is displaced inferiorly and has filled the recess produced by the sharply kyphotic lumbar spine.

is unlikely to be associated with deterioration of the upper urinary tract.[120] On the other hand, abnormal upper motor neuron function can cause an imbalance between sphincter and detrusor contraction (bladder–sphincter dyssynergia). This phenomenon is associated with high bladder pressure, VUR, inability to empty the bladder to completion, and reflux of contrast into the prostate and seminal vesicles (Fig. 7.29). The bladder may have an abnormal shape and be studded with cellules and diverticula. The narrowing of the urethra produced by bladder–sphincter dyssynergia is similar in appearance on VCUG to that of urethral fibrosis; electromyography and urodynamics can help differentiate between dyssynergia and fibrosis. All of these abnormalities are best confirmed by properly done videourodynamics, which allows direct correlation of the findings with measurements of pressure and muscle activity.[121]

The child with any spinal cord lesion needs similar evaluation of the urinary tract because of the potential of neurogenic bladder dysfunction. In addition, children acutely immobilized after spinal injury may develop renal calculi and hematuria because of abrupt changes in their calcium metabolism. These stones are frequently tiny and are seen better with US or CT than with plain films; they may enter and obstruct the ureter (Fig. 7.30). Children with myelodysplasia develop stones in hydro-

nephrotic segments, in bladder diverticula; and on staples, sutures, and even pubic hairs introduced during CIC. I have seen pediatric cases of xanthogranulomatous pyelonephritis (and parenchymal calculi) only in myelomeningocele patients.

Because up to 40% of children with spinal dysraphism have some type of latex allergy and to prevent patients from developing this problem through repeated exposure, latex-free products should be used when studying and examining this population.[122–124] The allergic response may be manifest by hives, respiratory distress, and even profound circulatory collapse. In addition to the obvious supplies that must be replaced, such as catheters and gloves, it may be prudent to screen and change tourniquets and even toys. Similar allergies have been reported in children who have undergone multiple operations for congenital genitourinary anomalies or who have had an indwelling urinary catheter.

Some children with a normal spine and spinal cord and a normal neurologic examination of the lower extremities have abnormal bladder function.[124–126] The nonneurogenic neurogenic bladder (Hinman bladder) is one that functions abnormally in the absence of a detectable neurologic lesion.[126] The abnormally high bladder pressures are associated with VUR and, in some patients, a trabeculated bladder like that of myelodyplastic chil-

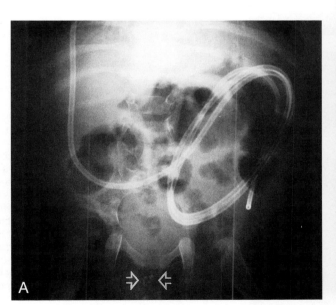
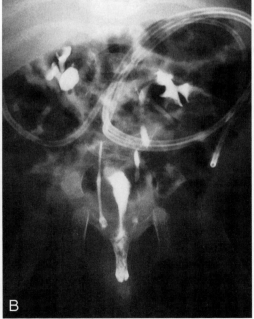

FIG. 7.29. A, Scout film of a 7-month-old with meningomyelocele. The spinal deformity is not well visualized but is indicated by the dislocated hips and shunt tubing. The light exposure enhances visualization of the multiple calculi in the prostatic urethra (*arrows*). **B,** EU of the same patient demonstrating the abnormal axis of both kidneys, the nondilated ureters, and the small-capacity bladder (which has emptied into the prostatic urethra).

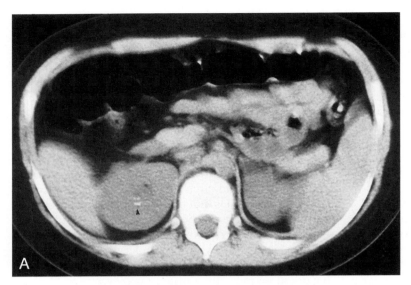

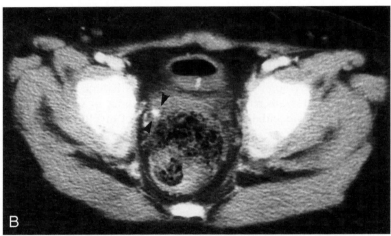

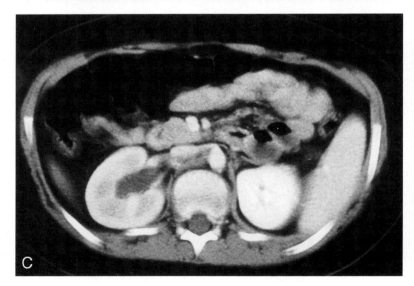

FIG. 7.30. Renal calculi—CT **A,** Noncontrast axial view CT scan through the kidneys of 9-year-old boy with a severe femur fracture showing multiple tiny calculi (*arrow*) in the right kidney. Several were also noted in the left (not shown). **B,** Noncontrast CT scan through the bladder showing another tiny calculus (*arrows*) that is obstructing the distal right ureter. **C,** Contrast CT scan through the kidneys demonstrating classic signs of acute obstruction on the right, including delayed opacification of the parenchyma, enlargement of the kidney, and mild dilatation of the pelvicaliceal system.

dren. The diagnosis is based on clinical dysfunction of the bladder and bowel, urodynamic or videourodynamic function, and imaging of the spinal cord.

REFERENCES

1. Smellie JM, Ridgen SPA, Prescod NP. Urinary tract infection: a comparison of four methods of investigation. Arch Dis Child 1995;72:247–250.
2. Smellie JM. The intravenous urogram in the detection and evaluation of renal damage following urinary tract infection. Pediatr Nephrol 1995;9:213–219.
3. Shanon A, Feldman W, McDonald P, et al. Evaluation of renal scars by technetium-labeled dimercaptosuccinic acid scan, intravenous urography, and ultrasonography: a comparative study. J Pediatr 1992;120:399–403.
4. Leonidas JC, Schwartz R, Schwartz AM, et al. The one-film urogram in urinary tract infection in children. AJR Am J Roentgenol 1983;141:61–64.
5. Cohen MD, Smith JA. Intravenous use of ionic and nonionic contrast agents in children. Radiology 1994;191:793–794.
6. Nybonde T, Wahlgren H, Brekke O, et al. Image quality and safety in pediatric urography using an ionic and non-ionic iodinated contrast agent. Pediatr Radiol 1994;24:107–110.
7. Lebowitz RL. Questions and answers. AJR Am J Roentgenol 1994;163:990.
8. Willi U, Treves S. Radionuclide voiding cystogram. Urol Radiol 1983;5:161–173.
9. Conway JJ, King LR, Belman AB, Thorsen T Jr. Detection of vesicoureteral reflux with radionuclide cystography. AJR Am J Roentgenol 1972;115:720–727.
10. Leibovic SJ, Lebowitz RL. Reducing patient dose in voiding cystourethrography. Urol Radiol 1980;2:103–106.
11. International Reflux Study Committee. Medical versus surgical treatment of primary vesicoureteral reflux: a prospective international reflux study in children. J Urol 1981;125:227–283.
12. Ben-Ami T, Gayer G, Hertz M, et al. The natural history of reflux in the lower pole of duplicated collecting systems: a controlled study. Pediatr Radiol 1989;19:308–310.
13. Strife JL, Bisset GS III, Kirks DR, et al. Nuclear cystography and renal sonography: findings in girls with urinary tract infection. AJR Am J Roentgenol 1989;153:115–119.
14. Noe HN. The current status of screening for vesicoureteral reflux. Pediatr Nephrol 1995;9:638–641.
15. Buonomo C, Treves ST, Jones B, et al. Silent renal damage in symptom-free siblings of children with vesicoureteral reflux: assessment with technetium Tc 99m dimercaptosuccinic acid scintigraphy. J Pediatr 1993;122:721–723.
16. Cleveland RH, Constantinou C, Blickman JG, et al. Voiding cystourethrography in children: value of digital fluoroscopy in reducing radiation dose. AJR Am J Roentgenol 1992;152:137–142.
17. Kleinman PK, Diamond DA, Karellas A, et al. Tailored low-dose fluoroscopic voiding cystourethrography for the reevaluation of vesicoureteral reflux in girls. AJR Am J Roentgenol 1994;162:1151–1154.
18. Sarkar SD. Diuretic renography: concepts and controversies. Urol Radiol 1992;14:79–84.
19. Blachar A, Blachar Y, Livne PM, et al. Clinical outcome and follow-up of prenatal hydronephrosis. Pediatr Nephrol 1994;8:30–35.
20. Kletscher B, de Badiola F, Gonzalez R. Outcome of hydronephrosis diagnosed antenatally. J Pediatr Surg 1991;26:455–459.
21. Koff SA, Campbell K. Nonoperative management of unilateral neonatal hydronephrosis. J Urol 1992;148:525–531.
22. Cozzi F, Madonna L, Maggi E, et al. Management of primary megaureter in infancy. J Pediatr Surg 1993;28:1031–1033.
23. Grignon A, Filion R, Filiatrault D, et al. Urinary tract dilatation in utero: classification and clinical applications. Radiology 1986;160:645–647.
24. Owen RJ, Lamont AC, Brookes J. Early management and post-natal investigation of prenatally diagnosed hydronephrosis. Clin Radiol 1995;51:173–176.
25. Pickworth FE, Vivian GC, Franklin K, Brown EF. 99TcM-mercapto acetyl triglycine in paediatric renal tract disease. Br J Radiol 1992;65:21–29.
26. Society for Fetal Urology and Pediatric Nuclear Medicine Council. The "well tempered" diuretic renogram: a standard method to examine the asymptomatic neonate with hydronephrosis or hydroureteronephrosis. J Nucl Med 1992;33:2047–2051.
27. Chung S, Majd M, Rushton HG, Belman AB. Diuretic renography in the evaluation of neonatal hydronephrosis: is it reliable? J Urol 1993;150:765–768.
28. Bjorgvinsson E, Majd M, Eggli KD. Diagnosis of acute pyelonephritis in children: comparison of sonography and 99mTc-DMSA scintigraphy. AJR Am J Roentgenol 1991;157:539–541.
29. Traisman ES, Conway JJ, Traisman HS, et al. The localization of urinary tract infection with 99mTc glucoheptonate scintigraphy. Pediatr Radiol 1986;16:403–406.
30. Rushton HG, Majd M. Dimercaptosuccinic acid renal scintigraphy for the evaluation of pyelonephritis and scarring: a review of experimental and clinical studies. J Urol 1992;148:1726–1732.
31. Conway JJ, Cohn RA. Evolving role of nuclear medicine for the diagnosis and management of urinary tract infection. J Pediatr 1994;124:87–90.
32. Patel K, Charron M, Hoberman A, et al. Intra- and interobserver variability in interpretation of DMSA scans using a set of standardized criteria. Pediatr Radiol 1993;23:506–509.
33. Taylor A, Nally JV. Clinical applications of renal scintigraphy. AJR Am J Roentgenol 1995;164:31–41.
34. Garel L, Dubois J, Robitaille P, et al. Renovascular hypertension in children: curability predicted with negative intrarenal Doppler US results. Radiology 1995;195:401–405.
35. Tonkin IL, Stapleton FB, Roy S III. Digital subtraction angiography in the evaluation of renal vascular hypertension in children. Pediatrics 1988;81:150–158.
36. Melloul M, Paz A, Lask D, et al. The value of radionuclide scrotal imaging in the diagnosis of acute testicular torsion. Br J Urol 1995;76:628–631.
37. Middleton WD, Siegel BA, Melson GL, et al. Acute scrotal disorders: prospective comparison of Doppler US and testicular scintigraphy. Radiology 1990;177:177–181.
38. Paduano L, Carini C, Alessandrini H. Validity of ultrasonography for postoperative monitoring in pediatric urology. J Urol 1996;155:1053–1056.
39. Maizels M, Riesman ME, Flom LS, et al. Grading nephroureteral dilatation detected in the first year of life: correlation with obstruction. J Urol 1992;148:609–614.
40. Fernbach SK, Maizels M, Conway JJ. Ultrasound grading of hydronephrosis: introduction to the system used by the Society for Fetal Urology. Pediatr Radiol 1993;23:478–480.
41. Palmer JM, DiSandro M. Diuretic enhanced duplex Doppler sonography in 33 children presenting with hydronephrosis: a study of test sensitivity, specificity, and precision. J Urol 1995;154:1885–1888.
42. Dacher JN, Pfister C, Monroc M, et al. Power Doppler sonographic pattern of acute pyelonephritis in children: comparison with CT. AJR Am J Roentgenol 1996;166:1451–1455.
43. Fernbach SK, Feinstein KA. Abnormalities of the bladder in children: imaging findings. AJR Am J Roentgenol 1994;162:1143–1150.
44. Yazbeck S, Patriquin HB. Accuracy of Doppler sonography in the evaluation of acute conditions of the scrotum in children. J Pediatr Surg 1994;29:1270.
45. Talner LB, Davidson AJ, Lebowitz RL, et al. Acute pyelonephritis: can we agree on terminology? Radiology 1994;192:297–305.
46. Gylys-Morin V, Hoffer FA, Kozakewich H, Shamberger RC. Wilms tumor and nephroblastomatosis: imaging characteristics at Gadolinium-enhanced MR imaging. Radiology 1993;188:517–521.
47. Shady KL, Siegel MJ, Brown JJ. Preoperative evaluation of intraabdominal tumors in children: gradient-recalled echo vs spin-echo MR imaging. AJR Am J Roentgenol 1993;161:843–847.
48. Dietrich RB, Kangarloo H, Lenarsky C, Feig SA. Neuro-

blastoma: the role of MR imaging. AJR Am J Roentgenol 1987;148:937–942.

49. Walsh G, Dubbins PA. Antenatal renal pelvis dilatation: a predictor of vesicoureteral reflux? AJR Am J Roentgenol 1996;167:897–900.

50. Clautice-Engle T, Anderson NG, Allan RB, Abbot GD. Diagnosis of obstructive hydronephrosis in infants: comparison sonograms performed 6 days and 6 weeks after birth. AJR Am J Roentgenol 1995;164:963–967.

51. Zerin JM, Ritchey ML, Chang ACH. Incidental vesicoureteral reflux in neonates with antenatally detected hydronephrosis and other renal abnormalities. Radiology 1993;187:157–160.

52. Zerin JM. Hydronephrosis on the neonate and young infant: current concepts. Semin Ultrasound CT MR 1994;15:306–316.

53. Coret A, Morag B, Katz M, et al. The impact of fetal screening on indications for cystourethrography in infants. Pediatr Radiol 1994;24:516–518.

54. Paltiel HJ, Lebowitz RL. Neonatal hydronephrosis due to primary vesicoureteral reflux: trends in diagnosis and treatment. Radiology 1989;170:787–789.

55. Bernstein GY, Mandell J, Lebowitz RL, et al. Ureteropelvic junction obstruction in the neonate. J Urol 1988;140:1216–1221.

56. Mandell J, Blyth BR, Peters CA, et al. Structural genitourinary defects detected in utero. Radiology 1991;178:193–196.

57. Meyer JS, Lebowitz RL. Primary megaureter in infants and children: a review. Urol Radiol 1992;14:296–305.

58. Kirks DR, Kaufman RA. Function within mesoblastic nephroma: imaging-pathologic correlation. Pediatr Radiol 1989;19:136–139.

59. Daucher JN, Mandell J, Lebowitz RL. Urinary tract infection in infants in spite of prenatal diagnosis of hydronephrosis. Pediatr Radiol 1992;22:401–404.

60. Peters CA. Urinary tract obstruction in children. J Urol 1995;154:1874–1883.

61. Rickwood AMK, Harney JV, Jones MO, and Oak S. "Congenital" hydronephrosis: limitations of diagnosis by fetal ultrasonography. Br J Urol 1995;75:529–530.

62. Maizels M, Mitchell B, Kass E, et al. Outcome of nonspecific hydronephrosis on the infant: a report from the registry of the Society for Fetal Urology. J Urol 1994;152:2324–2327.

63. Paltiel HJ, Rupich RC, Kiruluta G. Enhanced detection of vesicoureteral reflux in infants and children with use of cyclic voiding cystourethrography. Radiology 1992;184:753–755.

64. Fettich JJ, Kenda RB. Cyclic direct radionuclide voiding cystography: increasing reliability in detecting vesicoureteral reflux in children. Pediatr Radiol 1992;22:337–338.

65. Gluckman GR, Baskin LS, Bogaert GA, et al. Contradictory renal function measured with mercaptoacetyltriglycine diuretic renography in unilateral hydronephrosis. J Urol 1995;154:1486–1489.

66. Lebowitz RL. The detection and characterization of vesicoureteral reflux in the child. J Urol 1992;148:1640–1642.

67. Pickworth FE, Carlin JB, Ditchfield MR, et al. Sonographic measurement of renal enlargement in children with acute pyelonephritis and time needed for resolution: implications for renal growth assessment. AJR Am J Roentgenol 1995;165:405–408.

68. Stokland E, Hellstrom M, Hansson S, et al. Reliability of ultrasonography in identification of reflux nephropathy in children. Br Med J 1994;309:235–239.

69. Kass EJ, Fink-Bennett D, Cacciarelli AA, et al. The sensitivity of renal scintigraphy and sonography in detecting nonobstructive acute pyelonephritis. J Urol 1992;148:606–608.

70. Hansen A, Wagner AA, Lavard LD, Nielsen JT. Diagnostic imaging in children with urinary tract infection: the role of intravenous urography. Acta Pediatr 1995;84:84–89.

71. Seigle R, Nash M. Is there a role for renal scintigraphy in the routine evaluation of a child with a urinary infection? Pediatr Radiol 1995;25:S52–S53.

72. Ditchfield MR, deCampo JF, Nolan TM, et al. Risk factors in the development of early renal cortical defects in children with urinary tract infection. AJR Am J Roentgenol 1994;162:1393–1397.

73. Hellstrom M, Jacobsson B, Marild S, Jodal U. Voiding cystourethrography as a predictor of reflux nephropathy in children

with urinary-tract infection. AJR Am J Roentgenol 1989;152:801–804.

74. Connor JP. DMSA scanning: a pediatric urologist's point of view. Pediatr Radiol 1995;25:S50–S51.

75. Slovis TL. Is there a single most appropriate imaging workup of a child with an acute febrile urinary tract infection? Pediatr Radiol 1995;25:S46–S49.

76. Blickman JG, Taylor GA, Lebowitz RL. Voiding cystourethrography: the initial radiologic study in children with urinary tract infection. Radiology 1985;156:659–662.

77. Chung CJ, Lorenzo R, Rayder S, et al. Rhabdoid tumors of the kidney in children: CT findings. AJR Am J Roentgenol 1995;164:697–700.

78. Agrons GA, Kingman KD, Wagner BJ, Sotelo-Avila C. Rhabdoid tumor of the kidney in children: a comparative study of 21 cases. AJR Am J Roentgenol 1991;156:1029–1032.

79. Green DM, Breslow NE, Beckwith JB, Norkool P. Screening of children with hemihypertrophy, aniridia, and Beckwith-Wiedemann syndrome in patients with Wilms tumor: a report from the National Wilms Tumor Study. Med Pediatr Oncol 1993;21:188–192.

80. Babyn P, Owens C, Gyepes M, D'Angio GJ. Imaging patients with Wilms tumor. Hematol Oncol Clin North Am 1995;9:1217–1252.

81. Beckwith JB. Certain conditions have increased incidence of Wilms' tumor. AJR Am J Roentgenol 1995;164:1294–1295.

82. Craft AW, Parker L, Stiller C, Cole M. Screening for Wilms' tumour in patients with aniridia, Beckwith syndrome, or hemihypertrophy. Med Pediatr Oncol 1995;24:231–234.

83. Federici S, Galli G, Ceccarelli PR, et al. Wilms' tumor involving the inferior vena cava: preoperative evaluation and management. Med Pediatr Oncol 1994;22:39–44.

84. Day DL, Johnson R, Cohen MD. Abdominal neuroblastoma with inferior vena caval tumor thrombus: report of three cases (one with right atrial extension). Pediatr Radiol 1991;21:205–207.

85. Andrews PE, Kelalis PP, Haase GM. Extrarenal Wilms' tumor: results of the National Wilms' Tumor Study. J Pediatr Surg 1992;27:1181–1184.

86. White KS, Grossman H. Wilms' and associated renal tumors of childhood. Pediatr Radiol 1991;21:81–88.

87. Nishi M, Miyaki H, Takeda T, et al. Cases of neuroblastoma missed by the mass screening programs. Pediatr Res 1989;26:603–607.

88. Fernbach SK, Feinstein KA, Donaldson JS, Baum ES. Nephroblastomatosis: comparison of CT with US and urography. Radiology 1988;166:153–156.

89. White KS, Kirks DR, Bove KE. Imaging of nephroblastomatosis: an overview. Radiology 1992;182:1–5.

90. D'Angio GJ, Rosenberg H, Sharples K, et al. Position paper: imaging methods for primary renal tumors of childhood: cost versus benefits. Med Pediatr Oncol 1993;21:205–212.

91. Cohen MD. Current controversy: is computed tomography scan of the chest needed in patients with Wilms' tumor? Am J Pediatr Hematol Oncol 1994;16:191–193.

92. Ritchey ML, Green DM, Breslow NB, et al. Accuracy of current imaging modalities in the diagnosis of synchronous Wilms' tumor. Cancer 1995;75:600–604.

93. Kessler O, Franco I, Jayabose S, et al. Is contralateral exploration of the kidney necessary in patients with Wilms tumor? J Urol 1996;156:693–695.

94. Koo AS, Koyle MA, Hurwitz RS, et al. The necessity of contralateral surgical exploration in Wilms tumor with modern noninvasive imaging: a reassessment. J Urol 1990;144:416–417.

95. Ferraro EM, Fakhry J, Aruny JE, Bracero LA. Prenatal adrenal neuroblastoma. Case report with review of the literature. J Ultrasound Med 1988;7:275–278.

96. Croitoru DP, Sinsky AB, Laberge JM. Cystic neuroblastoma. J Pediatr Surg 1992;27:1320–1321.

97. David R, Eftekhari F, Lamki N, et al. The many faces of neuroblastoma. Radiographics 1989;9:859–882.

98. Berdon WE, Ruzal-Shapiro C, Abramson SJ, Garvin J. The diagnosis of abdominal neuroblastoma: relative roles of ultrasonography, CT, and MRI. Urol Radiol 1992;14:252–262.

99. Paltiel HJ, Gelfand MJ, Elgazzar AH, et al. Neural crest tumors: I-123 MIBG imaging in children. Radiology 1994;190:117–121.
100. Parisi MT, Matthay KK, Huberty JP, Hattner RS. Neuroblastoma: dose-related sensitivity of MIBG scanning in detection. Radiology 1992;184:463–467.
101. Bolande RP, Brough AJ, Izant RJ. Congenital mesoblastic nephroma of infancy. Pediatrics 1967;40:272–276.
102. Hartman DS, Lesar MSL, Madewell JE, et al. Mesoblastic nephroma: radiologic-pathologic correlation of 20 cases. AJR Am J Roentgenol 1981;136:69–74.
103. Glass RB, Davidson AJ, Fernbach SK. Clear cell sarcoma of the kidney: CT, sonographic and pathologic correlation. Radiology 1991;180:715–717.
104. Agrons GA, Wagner BJ, Davidson AJ, Suarez ES. Multilocular cystic renal tumor in children: radiologic-pathologic correlation. RadioGraphics 1995;15:653–669.
105. Madewell JE, Goldman SM, Davis CJ Jr, et al. Multilocular cystic nephroma: correlation in 58 patients. Radiology 1983;146:309–321.
106. Aronson DC, Medary I, Finlay JL, et al. Renal cell carcinoma in childhood and adolescence: a retrospective survey for prognostic factors in 22 cases. J Pediatr Surg 1996;131:183–186.
107. Kabala JE, Shield J, Duncan A. Renal cell carcinoma in childhood. Pediatr Radiol 1992;22:203–205.
108. Freedman AL, Vates TS, Stewart T, et al. Renal cell carcinoma in children: the Detroit experience. J Urol 1996;105:1708–1710.
109. Davidson AJ, Choyke PL, Hartman DS, Davis CJ Jr. Renal medullary carcinoma associated with sickle cell trait: radiologic findings. Radiology 1995;195:83–85.
110. Davis CJ Jr, Mostofi FK, Sesterhenn IA. Renal medullary carcinoma. The seventh sickle cell nephropathy. Am J Surg Pathol 1995;19:1–11.
111. Berger RM, Maizels M, Moran GC, et al. Bladder capacity (ounces) equals age (years) plus 2 predicts normal bladder capacity and aids in diagnosis of abnormal voiding patterns. J Urol 1983;129:347–349.
112. Fernbach SK, Conway JJ. The evolving uroradiologic evaluation of the lower urinary tract in neonates with myelomeningocele. Urol Radiol 1987;9:141–145.
113. Joseph DB, Bauer SB, Colodny AH, et al. Clean intermittent catheterization of infants with neurogenic bladder. Pediatrics 1989;84:78–82.
114. Flood HD, Ritchey ML, Bloom DA, et al. Outcome of reflux in children with myelodysplasia managed by bladder pressure monitoring. J Urol 1994;152:1574–1577.
115. Hernandez RD, Hurwitz RS, Foote JE, et al. Nonsurgical management of threatened upper urinary tracts and incontinence in children with myelomeningocele. J Urol 1994;152:1582–1585.
116. Zawin JK, Lebowitz RL. Neurogenic dysfunction of the bladder in infants and children: recent advances in the role of radiology. Radiology 1992;182:297–304.
117. Gross GW, Thornburg AJ, Belinger MF. Normal renal growth in children with myelodysplasia. AJR Am J Roentgenol 1986;146:615–617.
118. Williamson MR, Glasier CM, Chadduck WM, et al. MRI in the evaluation of spina bifida patients in the remote period after meningomyelocele repair. Pediatr Radiol 1989;19:442–443.
119. Zerin JM, Lebowitz RL, Bauer SB. Descent of the bladder neck: a urographic finding in denervation of the urethral sphincter in children with myelodysplasia. Radiology 1990;174:833–836.
120. Fernbach SK, Davis TM. The abnormal renal axis in children with spina bifida and gibbus deformity—the pseudohorseshoe kidney. J Urol 1986;136:1258–1260.
121. Saxton HM. Urodynamics: the appropriate modality for the investigation of frequency, urgency, incontinence, and voiding difficulties. Radiology 1990;175:307–316.
122. Zerin JM, McLaughlin K, Kerchner S. Latex allergy in patients with myelomeningocele presenting for imaging studies of the urinary tract. Pediatr Radiol 1996;26:450–454.
123. Ellsworth PI, Merguerian PA, Klein RB, Rozycki AA. Evaluation and risk factors of latex allergy in spina bifida patients: is it preventable? J Urol 1993;150:691–693.
124. Banta JV, Bonanni C, Prebluda J. Latex anaphylaxis during spinal surgery in children with myelomeningocele. Develop Med Child Neurol 1993;35:543–548.
124. Koff SA. Relationship between dysfunctional voiding and reflux. J Urol 1992;148:1703–1705.
125. Fernandez ET, Reinberg Y, Vernier, et al. Neurogenic bladder dysfunction in children: a review of pathophysiology and current management. J Pediatr 1994;124:1–7.
126. Hinman F. Nonneurogenic neurogenic bladder (the Hinman bladder)—15 years later. J Urol 1986;136:768–777.

CHAPTER 8

Prenatal and Perinatal Nephrology: Compensatory Renal Growth

Robert L. Chevalier

RENAL FUNCTION IN THE FETUS

Renal function in the fetus depends on the progression of renal embryogenesis and maturation. Urine production by the metanephros begins between the 10th and 12th week of gestation. Although the contribution of fetal urine to the amniotic fluid volume is minimal during the first half of gestation, there is a progressive increase in the second half of gestation; flow rates average 50 mL by the 40th week of gestation (Fig. 8.1).[1] Although the kidneys do not contribute significantly to maintenance of fetal homeostasis, the renal contribution to amniotic fluid volume in the third trimester is important for normal pulmonary development. Thus fetal oliguria or anuria leads to Potter syndrome, including facial abnormalities, limb deformities, and pulmonary hypoplasia.[2]

Formation of the metanephros begins during the 5th week of gestation; and nephrogenesis is completed by 34 to 36 weeks of gestation. The period of most rapid nephrogenesis occurs in midgestation, which is the earliest that kidneys can be detected reliably by ultrasonography. Renal vascular resistance is markedly elevated in the fetus compared to the postnatal period; and the ratio of renal blood flow : cardiac output at 20 weeks of gestation is 0.02, whereas the ratio in the postnatal period is 10-fold higher.[3] The low renal blood flow during fetal life is related to the decreased cross-sectional area of the glomerular vasculature and the increased arteriolar tone.[4,5] The high renal vascular resistance in fetal and early neonatal life is in part the result of increased sympathetic tone and increased activity of the renin–angiotensin system.

Studies in experimental animals indicate that glomerular blood flow and glomerular filtration rate (GFR) are proportionately greater in juxtamedullary nephrons than in superficial cortical nephrons, after the centrifugal maturation of the metanephric kidney.[6] Glomerular filtration rate in the preterm infant is <10 mL/min/ 1.73 m^2 until after 34 weeks of gestation (when nephrogenesis is complete) (Fig. 8.2).[7]

Although the fetus cannot produce a concentrated urine, fetal urine sodium content is normally <100 mEq/ L; chloride, <90 mEq/L; and osmolality <200 mOsm/ L.[8] These values may be useful in determining the severity of renal impairment from congenital obstructive uropathy, wherein higher values are consistent with poor renal outcome.[9,10] More recently, inappropriately high levels of certain amino acids in fetal urine have been related to renal dysplasia and poor fetal outcome.[11]

In summary, the fetus produces a large volume of hypotonic urine that has a relatively high sodium content. These high rates of diuresis and natriuresis contribute significantly to amniotic fluid volume in the third trimester, an important factor in pulmonary maturation. As discussed below, however, preterm infants may develop hyponatremia from persistent diuresis and natriuresis without adequate sodium replacement. Because urine output is directly related to glomerular maturation, impairment of renal maturation can interfere with intrauterine renal function, resulting in postnatal renal dysfunction. Recent studies have shown that both angiotensin II and prostaglandins, well known as vasoactive compounds, are also important growth factors in the developing kidney.[12,13] There is increasing evidence that administration of angiotensin-converting enzyme (ACE) inhibitors or nonsteroidal anti-inflammatory drugs (NSAIDs) interferes with human fetal renal development.[14,15]

POSTNATAL RENAL DEVELOPMENT

After birth, the homeostatic priorities for the infant change dramatically. In the fetus, solute excretion and fluid balance are regulated by the placenta; after birth

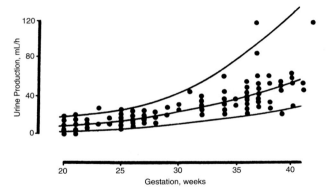

FIG. 8.1. Hourly fetal urine production rate measured by maternal real-time ultrasonography, including individual measurements (*solid circles*), mean, and 95% confidence intervals. Reprinted with permission from Rabinowitz R, Peters MT, Vyas S, et al. Measurement of fetal urine production in normal pregnancy by real-time ultrasonography. Am J Obstet Gynecol 1989;161:1264–1266.

these functions are shifted to the infant's kidneys. Although high rates of urine flow and sodium excretion are necessary for fetal development (particularly pulmonary maturation), for the first several days of the life, the neonate undergoes a physiologic diuresis and natriuresis in which the extracellular fluid space of the fetus is reduced to that compatible with extrauterine life. The proportional magnitude of the diuresis and natriuresis is inversely related to gestational age. Thus the perinatal weight loss of very low birth weight infants can be as high as 15% of body weight, compared to 5% in term infants.[16] After this re-equilibration of extracellular fluid volume, the infant must drastically alter its homeostatic

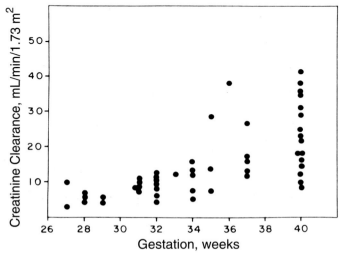

FIG. 8.2. Creatinine clearance for infants born at 27 to 40 weeks of gestation, measured at 24 to 40 h of life. $r = 0.643$; $p < .001$. Reprinted with permission from Siegel SR, Oh W. Renal function as a marker of human fetal maturation. Acta Paediatr Scand 1976;65:481–485.

strategy to avidly conserve sodium, which is necessary for normal somatic growth. Thus term infants are in a significant positive sodium balance, and most of the sodium is deposited in the growing skeleton.

Glomerular Filtration Rate

Immediately after birth, renal blood flow increases as much as 10-fold.[17] There is a redistribution of blood flow toward the outer cortex of the kidney,[18] and vasodilatation is related in part to increased renal prostaglandin production.[19] In term infants, the GFR doubles during the 1st week of life.[20] Because nephrogenesis is not complete before 34 weeks of gestation, GFR rises slowly in very low birth weight infants. After 34 weeks of gestation, however, there is a more rapid rise in GFR. This is the result of a reduction in renal vascular resistance,[19] increase in renal perfusion pressure, increase in glomerular permeability, and increase in glomerular filtration surface area.[21] The increase in surface area for filtration has been shown to be the single most important variable accounting for the postnatal increase in GFR in experimental animals.[6]

The most readily available measure of GFR, serum creatinine concentration, reflects maternal levels immediately after birth. The serum creatinine concentration normally decreases by 50% during the 1st week of life in term babies; and GFR gradually increases, reaching adult levels by 2 years of age (>90 mL/min/1.73 m²).[22] Although very low birth weight infants have a slow start, GFR does reach that of age-matched term infants by 9 months of age.[23]

Measurement of GFR in the neonate is complicated by the difficulty in obtaining accurately timed urine collections and the inherent inaccuracy of plasma creatinine concentration measurement. Because precision of creatinine concentration determinations may vary by 0.3 mg/dL, calculation of GFR in the neonate may be overestimated or underestimated by as much as 100%, even if urine collection is complete. In addition, the normal range of GFR increases markedly during the first 2 months of life (Fig. 8.3). In general, the plasma creatinine concentration should be <1 mg/dL in term infants by the end of the 1st week of life, but owing to low GFR, plasma creatinine concentration may not fall below 1.5 mg/dL during the 1st month of life in very low birth weight infants.[24] The most helpful approach to monitoring GFR in neonates is to check serial plasma creatinine concentrations. Thus a progressive increase in plasma creatinine concentration indicates an abnormal GFR, regardless of gestational age.

A convenient method for tracking GFR in infancy is to estimate the corrected creatinine clearance (Ccr) by using a formula based on the patient's body length.[25] The formula predicts the creatinine clearance in milliliters per minute per 1.73 m²:

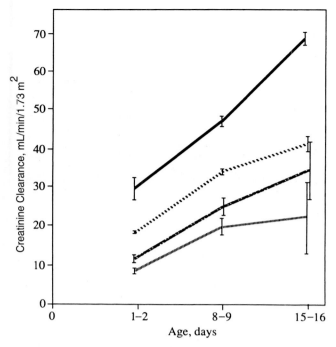

FIG. 8.3. Creatinine clearance for preterm and term infants, measured at 1 to 16 days of life. *Vertical hatched line,* 1000 to 1500 g; *slanted hatched line,* 1501 to 2000 g; *broken line,* 2001 to 2500 g; *solid line,* term. Reprinted with permission from Bueva A, Guignard JP. Renal function in preterm neonates. Pediatr Res 1994;36:572–577.

$$Ccr = K \times L/Pcr$$

where K is a constant (0.33 for preterm infants and 0.45 for term infants), L is body length in centimeters, and Pcr is the plasma creatinine concentration in milligrams per deciliter. The values for creatinine clearance determined by this formula should be compared with the expected age-related normal values (Fig. 8.3).

If a more accurate determination of GFR is desired, technetium 99 diethylenetriamine penta-acetic acid (^{99}Tc-DTPA) can be injected intravenously, and plasma concentration of the isotope can be measured with concurrent scintigraphy to determine the isotope accumulation by each kidney. The limitations of this technique are that venous access is required and the infant must lie still during the scan for accurate counts to be obtained. It should be noted that calculation of GFR by ^{99}Tc-DTPA clearance should be corrected for adult surface area by multiplying the measured value by 1.73 and dividing by the patient's calculated surface area (in square meters).

Sodium Homeostasis

There is a significant difference between renal sodium handling of preterm infants and of term infants. This is related to the maturity of the kidneys and the fact that the kidneys of preterm infants are better adapted to

fetal than to extrauterine life. Thus preterm infants <35 weeks of gestational age are prone to develop sodium wasting and hyponatremia and need sodium supplementation of 3 to 5 mEq/kg/day.[26, 27] In contrast, term infants have enhanced distal tubular sodium reabsorption secondary to high circulating renin, angiotensin, and aldosterone levels and a diminished renal response to atrial natriuretic peptide. In addition, neonates have an attenuated natriuresis after acute sodium loading and may become edematous if given excessive daily sodium supplements.[28]

Note that infants with congenital abnormalities of renal development, including hydronephrosis and renal dysplasia, may have impaired tubular sodium reabsorption and may actually be salt wasters. It is critical to recognize this and to provide adequate sodium supplements, as somatic growth may otherwise be impaired. More important, there is some preliminary evidence that sodium deficiency in the early postnatal period may affect central nervous system development; the consequences for neural development may not be appreciated until the child is older.[29]

In the oliguric neonate (urine flow <1 mL/kg/h), tubular sodium reabsorption should be avid. The fractional sodium excretion (*FE*Na) provides a measure of

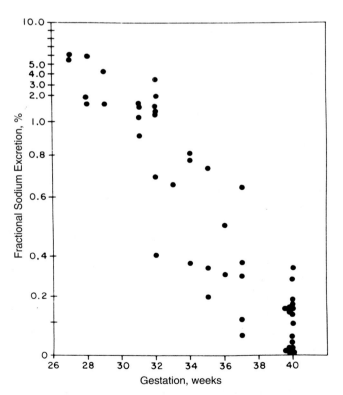

FIG. 8.4. Fractional sodium excretion for infants born at 27 to 40 weeks of gestation, measured at 24 to 40 h of life. $r = 0.755$; $p < .001$. Reprinted with permission from Siegel SR, Oh W. Renal function as a marker of human fetal maturation. Acta Paediatr Scand 1976;65:481–485.

the fraction of filtered sodium that is excreted in the final urine.

This can be calculated from a random urine sample for sodium concentration (U_{Na}) and creatinine concentration (U_{Cr}) and a concurrent plasma sample for sodium concentration (P_{Na}) creatinine concentration (P_{Cr}).

$$FE_{Na} = 100\%(U_{Na} \times P_{Cr})/(P_{Na} \times U_{Cr})$$

As shown in Fig. 8.4, fractional sodium excretion decreases progressively with increasing postconceptional age. Except for very low birth weight infants with a gestational age of <30 weeks, urine fractional sodium excretion in the oliguric infant should be <2.5 (assuming that no diuretics have been given within several hours of the measurement) (Fig. 8.5).[30]

Renal Concentrating Capacity

Compared to the adult, the neonate produces a dilute urine (<50 mOsm/L); maximal concentrating capacity

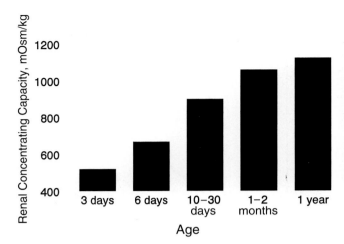

FIG. 8.6. Increasing renal concentrating capacity in the term neonate. Data from Polacek E. The osmotic concentration ability in healthy infants and children. Arch Dis Child 1965;40:291–305. Reprinted with permission from Chevalier RL. Developmental renal physiology of the low birth weight pre-term newborn. J Urol 1996;156;714–719.

is limited to 600 to 700 mOsm/L but reaches adult levels within the first month of life (Fig. 8.6).[16]

In very low birth weight infants, the maximal concentrating capacity may not exceed 500 mOsm/L. There are a number of factors contributing to this limited concentrating capacity: relatively shorter loops of Henle, decreased availability of solute (urea) to generate the medullary gradient, and a reduced responsiveness of the collecting ducts to vasopressin.[31, 32]

Acid–Base Balance

The tubular threshold for bicarbonate reabsorption is lower in the neonate than in the adult. In fact, plasma total carbon dioxide concentrations as low as 15 mEq/L are normal in the neonate (Fig. 8.7).[33] For this reason, the diagnosis of renal tubular acidosis may be difficult in the newborn. Moreover, excretion of an acid load is also limited in the neonate, although it becomes similar to that of the adult within 4 to 6 weeks after birth.[34]

Maturation of Other Tubular Functions

Tubular glucose transport is suppressed at birth and increases rapidly in the first postnatal weeks. The fractional excretion of glucose is quite high in preterm infants who are younger than 34 weeks of gestation.[35] The most frequent cause of glucosuria in the neonate, however, is excessive administration of dextrose in intravenous fluids.

Calcium and phosphorus metabolism also change rapidly in the postnatal period. Parathyroid hormone is suppressed at birth, causing a reduction in serum calcium and a secondary increase in parathyroid hormone

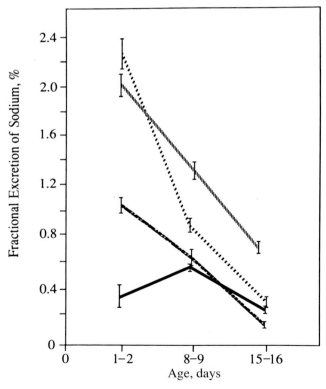

FIG. 8.5. Fractional sodium excretion for preterm and term infants, measured at 1 to 16 days of life. *Vertical hatched line,* 1000 to 1500 g; *slanted hatched line,* 1501 to 2000 g; *broken line,* 2001 to 2500 g; *solid line,* term. Reprinted with permission from Bueva A, Guignard JP. Renal function in preterm neonates. Pediatr Res 1994;36:572–577.

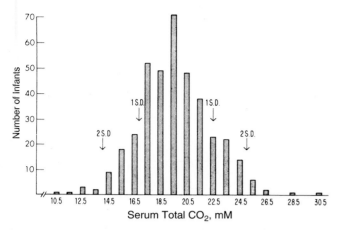

FIG. 8.7. Serum total carbon dioxide in low birth weight infants during the 1st month of life. Mean $\cong$ 20 mM; normal range (± 2 SD) = 14.5 to 24.5 mM. Reprinted with permission from Schwartz GJ, Haycock GB, Chir B, et al. Late metabolic acidosis: a reassessment of the definition. J Pediatr 1979;95:102–107.

release. Serum phosphorus concentration is higher in the neonate than in the older infant and child; and tubular phosphate reabsorption is also elevated in the preterm infant:[35] a serum phosphorus concentration <4 mg/dL is abnormal and should be investigated. To determine whether renal phosphate conservation is defective, the tubular reabsorption of phosphorus (TRP) can be calculated as follows:

$$TRP = 100\%[1 - (U_{PO_4} \times P_{Cr})/(P_{PO_4} \times U_{Cr})]$$

where creatinine and phosphate in the urine (U_{Cr}, U_{PO_4}) and plasma (P_{Cr}, P_{PO_4}) can be measured in a random urine sample. After the 1st week of life, the TRP should exceed 95% in term infants and 75% in preterm infants.[36] Values less than these levels indicate a renal proximal tubular defect or hyperparathyroidism.

As in the case of glucose, proximal tubular amino acid reabsorption is also lower in the neonate than in the older child or adult. Generalized amino aciduria is, therefore, normal in the neonate; when evaluating the neonate for suspected renal tubular defects, it is important to compare urinary amino acid results to those of age-matched normal infants.[37, 38]

Calcium Excretion

Calcium excretion in the neonate differs from that in the older infant and child. The urinary calcium : creatinine ratio in the older child is normally <0.2;[39] the ratio in the term infant can be as high as 0.4, and in the preterm infant it may reach 0.8.[36] Neonatal hypercalciuria is most frequently the result of administration of calciuric drugs, such as furosemide or glucocorticoids used in the management of bronchopulmonary dysplasia. Severe hypercalciuria in these infants has been asso-

ciated with the development of nephrocalcinosis and nephrolithiasis,[40] which may result in renal dysfunction beyond the neonatal period.[33] If diuretics are required for the management of bronchopulmonary dysplasia, chlorothiazide may be substituted for furosemide, thereby reducing urinary calcium excretion.

PRENATAL AND PERINATAL REGULATION OF RENAL FUNCTION

Renin–Angiotensin System

The renin–angiotensin system (RAS) has long been known to play a central role in the regulation of blood pressure and sodium homeostasis. Angiotensin II is also now recognized as an important growth factor for the kidney and cardiovascular system. The RAS is markedly activated in the fetus and early postnatal period. Although renin is normally localized to the juxtaglomerular region in the adult, it is present along the entire renal vasculature in the fetus;[41, 42] and plasma renin activity increases in the perinatal period.[43, 44] The mechanism for increased plasma renin activity at birth may include a rise in prostaglandin synthesis[45] or contraction of the extracellular fluid volume consequent to physiologic postnatal natriuresis.[46]

In addition to these changes in renin production, the adrenal response to angiotensin changes during fetal and early postnatal life. Although furosemide infusion does not increase plasma renin activity or plasma aldosterone concentration in the fetus, it does increase both in the neonate (Fig. 8.8).[43] In response to hemorrhage, there is a greater increase in plasma renin activity, plasma angiotensin II concentration, and plasma aldosterone concentration in late gestation than in early gestation.[47] Natriuresis following acute volume

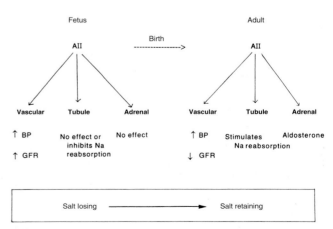

FIG. 8.8. Developmental changes in the response to angiotensin II (All). BP, blood pressure. Reprinted with permission from Lumbers ER. Functions of the renin-angiotensin system during development. Clin Exp Pharmacol Physiol 1995; 22:499–505.

expansion is normally blunted in the neonate compared to the adult, but inhibition of angiotensin II receptors in the neonate markedly enhances the natriuretic response to volume expansion, suggesting a significant role for angiotensin II in neonatal sodium conservation.[48] As shown in Figure 8.8, the response of the fetal RAS is geared to maintaining a natriuretic state and thereby to maintaining the urinary contribution to the amniotic fluid.[49] In contrast, in the neonate and adult, sodium conservation is stimulated by activation of the RAS (Fig. 8.8).

GFR in the fetus and neonate critically depends on vasoconstriction of the efferent arteriole maintained by angiotensin II. Therefore, exposure of the fetus or neonate to ACE inhibitors can result in a marked drop in GFR that can lead to acute renal failure (Fig. 8.9).[50] Extreme caution must, therefore, be exercised when using ACE inhibitors (e.g., captopril or enalapril) in the neonatal period. The initial dose of captopril in the neonate is <10% that in the older infant or child.[51] Because a reduction in functioning renal mass will further accentuate the dependence of GFR on efferent arteriolar tone, neonates with reduced renal mass are at a relatively greater risk for functional impairment secondary to ACE inhibition.

Atrial Natriuretic Peptide

Atrial natriuretic peptide (ANP) is secreted by cardiac myocytes and has direct renal effects, including increasing GFR, natriuresis, diuresis, and vascular permeability.[52] Although the precise role of ANP in the

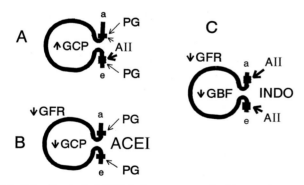

FIG. 8.9. Control of GFR in the neonate. **A,** Glomerular capillary pressure (*GCP*) is maintained by greater angiotensin (*AII*) vasoconstriction at the efferent (*e*) than the afferent (*a*) arteriole, but the effects are attenuated by concurrent vasodilation mediated by prostaglandins (*PG*). **B,** ACE inhibitors (*ACEI*) (e.g., captopril) allow unopposed vasodilation by PGs, thereby reducing GCP and GFR. **C,** Indomethacin (*INDO*) reduces PG synthesis, allowing unopposed AII-mediated vasoconstriction and resulting in reduced glomerular blood flow (*GBF*). Reprinted with permission from Chevalier RL. Developmental renal physiology of the low birth weight pre-term newborn. J Urol 1996;156:714–719.

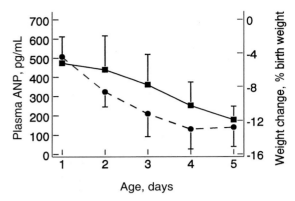

FIG. 8.10. Plasma ANP concentration and fractional change in body weight for nine preterm infants in the first 5 days of life. There was a significant correlation between body weight and plasma ANP concentration (*r* = 0.64; *p* < .02). Data from Bierd TM, Kattwinkel, Chevalier RL, et al. The interrelationship of atrial natriuretic peptide, atrial volume, and renal function in premature infants. J Pediatr 1990;116:753–759.

regulation of sodium homeostasis has not been elucidated, plasma ANP concentration is higher in the fetal circulation than in the maternal circulation.[53, 54] Acute volume expansion in the fetus has been shown to raise plasma ANP concentration.[55] Fetal atrial tachycardia or fetal hypoxia also increases plasma ANP levels.[56, 57] Circulating ANP may adjust blood volume in these pathologic states by increasing vascular permeability.

There is an immediate decrease in atrial ANP content at birth and a subsequent increase in the early postnatal period.[58] Plasma ANP concentration, on the other hand, is elevated at birth and decreases with maturation (Fig. 8.10).[59, 60] Studies in preterm infants suggest that ANP may play a role in the physiologic postnatal natriuresis and diuresis (Fig. 8.10).[61] After the transient natriuretic phase, however, the neonate is in a state of positive sodium balance necessary for rapid growth. It is not surprising, therefore, that the renal response to infused ANP is lower in the fetus and neonate than in the adult.[62–65] Experimental studies have shown that sodium loading during the neonatal period increases the renal natriuretic response to ANP.[66] These findings suggest that the altered neonatal response to ANP and angiotensin II represents a homeostatic adaptation for maintaining sodium conservation and is not a functional limitation of the immature kidney.

Vasopressin

Vasopressin—or antidiuretic hormone (ADH)—is a vasoconstrictor as well as a mediator of water transport in the collecting duct. The collecting duct in the fetus is less responsive to circulating vasopressin than that in the adult, possibly because of a lower density of receptors, which increase in the neonatal period.[67, 68] In addition to the reduced vasopressin receptor density, increased renal prostanoid synthesis in the perinatal period antagonizes the effects of vasopressin on the collecting duct.[69] In the postnatal period, after which the collecting ducts become fully responsive to vasopressin, inappropriate ADH production can occur as a result of birth asphyxia, intracranial hemorrhage, or respiratory distress syndrome, leading to hyponatremia.[70–72]

Prostaglandins

Circulating concentrations of prostaglandins are elevated in the fetus and neonate.[73] Vasodilatory prostaglandins appear to play a significant role in renal hemodynamics in early development, and maternal administration of NSAIDs (e.g., indomethacin) can result in severe intrauterine renal insufficiency that can persist after birth.[13, 74] Moreover, prolonged administration of NSAIDs during pregnancy can interfere with renal development.[13]

Administration of indomethacin to newborns with patent ductus arteriosus commonly reduces GFR, resulting in oliguria (Fig. 8.9).[73] This vasoconstrictor effect of NSAIDs can be magnified further in infants who have renal impairment or a single functioning kidney. For this reason, parents of infants with these conditions should be cautioned to avoid NSAIDs for the routine treatment of fever and pain.

Nitric Oxide

Nitric oxide has been recently recognized as an important vasodilatory compound in the kidney, in addition to regulating tubuloglomerular feedback and natriuresis.[75] In third-trimester sheep fetuses, endogenous nitric oxide production contributes to the maintenance of renal blood flow.[76] In neonatal pigs, endogenous nitric oxide synthesis contributes to renal vasodilation, possibly in response to increased local angiotensin II production.[77]

RESPONSE OF THE FETUS AND NEONATE TO DECREASED RENAL MASS

A reduction in functioning renal mass in the fetus and neonate is almost always secondary to a congenital renal malformation or perinatal vascular accident. In an early study of infants with unilateral multicystic dysplastic kidneys, it was concluded that compensatory renal growth does not begin until after birth.[78] That study was based on the estimation of functional renal mass by intravenous pyelography, which is unreliable in the neonate. More recent studies of fetuses with unilateral renal agenesis or multicystic kidney reveal that a single functioning kidney is significantly larger than the kidneys

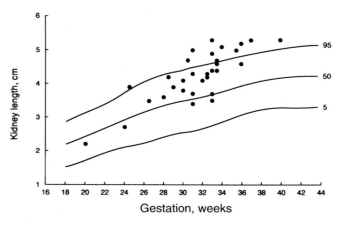

FIG. 8.11. Length of the normal kidney in 21 fetuses with unilateral multicystic dysplastic kidney or unilateral renal agenesis (*solid circles*) compared to the 5th, 50th, and 95th percentiles for fetuses with two normal kidneys. The single functioning kidney was significantly longer than the kidneys of normal fetuses ($p = .001$). Reprinted with permission from Glazebrook KN, McGrath FP, Steele BT. Prenatal compensatory renal growth: documentation with US. Radiology 1993: 189:733–735.

of control fetuses (Fig. 8.11).[79, 80] These reports show conclusively that compensatory renal growth can begin prenatally, when excretory function is provided by the placenta. It is, therefore, likely that signals, such as growth factors (or reduction in growth inhibitors), mediate adaptive growth by the developing kidney.

Experimental studies demonstrate that compensatory renal growth in the neonate is significantly greater than that in the adult.[81–83] In contrast to a hypertrophic response in the adult, renal hyperplasia is also stimulated by contralateral nephrectomy in early development.[84, 85] Although most of the compensatory renal growth is a result of an increase in tubular mass,[86, 87] glomerular hypertrophy also occurs in the neonate.[88] Although older studies suggested that compensatory renal growth after unilateral nephrectomy in neonatal rats involves formation of new nephrons,[89] this theory has now been disproven.[90, 91]

Functional adaptation by the remaining nephrons after renal mass is reduced in early development is also greater than that resulting from nephron loss in the adult. In dogs undergoing 75% reduction in renal mass at birth, GFR was not different from that of sham-operated litter mates at 6 weeks of age.[92] In contrast, dogs undergoing renal ablation at a later age had GFRs less than half that of sham-operated litter mates.[92] Uninephrectomy in neonatal rodents results in acceleration of the normal sequence of functional nephron maturation, so that the compensatory increase in the single nephron GFR is greater in the less-mature superficial nephrons than in the more-mature juxtamedullary nephrons.[93, 94] Thus function follows compensatory renal growth in early postnatal development. For this reason, serial sonographic measurements of renal length may provide early information regarding compensatory growth and even of the functional status of the contralateral kidney. An accelerated rate of renal growth occurs when the contralateral renal function contributes <15% of the total.[95]

PROGRESSION OF RENAL INSUFFICIENCY IN EARLY DEVELOPMENT

Since the 1980s, a number of investigators have related glomerular hyperfiltration and glomerular hypertrophy to the progression of renal insufficiency.[96, 97] Because compensatory renal growth and function are proportionately greater in the neonate than in the adult, the risk for hyperfiltration and glomerulosclerosis may be even greater when nephron loss occurs in early development. There is evidence that reduced renal mass results in greater proteinuria and glomerulosclerosis in early development than in adulthood.[94, 98, 99] Although not proven conclusively, intrauterine growth retardation appears to be associated with a reduced number of nephrons and with an increased incidence of hypertension in later in life.[100] Moreover, unilateral renal agenesis may be associated with glomerulosclerosis and progressive renal insufficiency.[101–103] In another study, more than 25% of children with unilateral nephrectomy had decreased GFR and proteinuria as adults.[104]

An experiment in nature has been provided by oligomeganephronia, a rare form of renal hypoplasia in which the number of nephrons is <50% of normal in each kidney. In this condition, glomeruli become markedly hypertrophic and sclerotic, progressing to renal failure in childhood.[101, 105] A central issue remains: What is the critical number of nephrons below which glomerulosclerosis and progressive reduction in GFR are inevitable? Long-term studies of large numbers of patients will be required to answer this. Regardless of the answer, an improved understanding of the factors regulating normal and adaptive renal growth is necessary to develop new strategies for maintaining functioning renal mass in the fetus and newborn.

REFERENCES

1. Rabinowitz R, Peters MT, Vyas S, et al. Measurement of fetal urine production in normal pregnancy by real-time ultrasonography. Am J Obstet Gynecol 1989;161:1264–1266.
2. Potter EL. Normal and abnormal development of the kidney. Chicago: Year Book, 1972.
3. Rudolph AM, Heymann MA. Circulatory changes during growth in the fetal lamb. Circ Res 1970;26:289–299.
4. Ichikawa I, Maddox DA, Brenner BM. Maturational development of glomerular ultrafiltration in the rat. Am J Physiol 1979;236:F465–F471.
5. Robillard JE, Nakamura KT, Wilkin MK, et al. Ontogeny of renal hemodynamic response to renal nerve stimulation in sheep. Am J Physiol 1987;252:F605–F612.
6. Spitzer A, Brandis M. Functional and morphologic maturation of the superficial nephrons: relationship to total kidney function. J Clin Invest 1974;53:279–287.
7. Siegel SR, Oh W. Renal function as a marker of human fetal maturation. Acta Paediatr Scand 1976;65:481–485.
8. Crombleholme TM, Harrison MR, Golbus MS, et al. Fetal intervention in obstructive uropathy: prognostic indicators and efficacy of intervention. Am J Obstet Gynecol 1990;162:1239–1244.
9. Evans MI, Sacks AJ, Johnson MP, et al. Sequential invasive assessment of fetal renal function and the intrauterine treatment of fetal obstructive uropathies. Obstet Gynecol 1991;77:545–550.
10. Johnson MP, Bukowski TP, Reitleman CI, et al. In utero surgical treatment of fetal obstructive uropathy: a new comprehensive approach to identify appropriate candidates for vesicoamniotic shunt therapy. Am J Obstet Gynecol. 1994;170:1770–1779.
11. Eugene M, Muller F, Dommergues M. Evaluation of postnatal renal function in fetuses with bilateral obstructive uropathies by proton nuclear magnetic resonance spectroscopy. Am J Obstet Gynecol 1994;170:595–602.
12. Friberg P, Sundelin B, Bohman SO, et al. Renin-angiotensin system in neonatal rats: induction of a renal abnormality in response to ACE inhibition or angiotensin II antagonism. Kidney Int 1994;45:485–492.
13. Kaplan BS, Restaino I, Raval DS, et al. Renal failure in the neonate associated with in utero exposure to non-steroidal anti-inflammatory agents. Pediatr Nephrol 1994;8:700–704.
14. Shotan A, Widerhorn J, Hurst A, Elkayam U. Risks of angiotensin-converting enzyme inhibition during pregnancy: experimental and clinical evidence, potential mechanisms, and recommendations for use. Am J Med 1994;96:451–456.
15. Van der Heijden BJ, Carlus C, Narcy F. Persistent anuria, neonatal death, and renal microcystic lesions after prenatal exposure to indomethacin. Am J Obstet Gynecol 1994;171:617–623.
16. Hansen JD, Smith CA. Effects of withholding fluid in the immediate postnatal period. Pediatrics 1953;12:99–113.
17. Aperia A, Herin P. Development of glomerular perfusion rate and nephron filtration rate in rats 17–60 days old. Am J Physiol 1975;228:1319–1325.
18. Aperia A, Broberger O, Herin P. Renal hemodynamics in the perinatal period: a study in lambs. Acta Physiol Scand 1977;99:261–269.
19. Gruskin AB, Edelmann CM Jr, Yuan S. Maturational changes in renal flow in piglets. Pediatr Res 1970;4:7–13.
20. Guignard JP, Torrado A, DaCunha O, Gautier E. Glomerular filtration rate in the first three weeks of life. J Pediatr 1975;87:268–272.
21. John E, Goldsmith DI, Spitzer A. Quantitative changes in the canine glomerular vasculature during development: physiologic implications. Kidney Int 1981;20:223–239.
22. Rubin MI, Bruck E, Rapaport M. Maturation of renal function in childhood: clearance studies. J Clin Invest 1949;28:1144–1155.
23. Vanpee M, Blennow M, Linne T. Renal function in very low birth weight infants: normal maturity reached during early childhood. J Pediatr 1992;121:784–788.
24. Trompeter RA, Al-Dahhan J, Haycock GB, et al. Normal values for plasma creatinine concentration related to maturity in normal term and preterm infants. Int J Pediatr Nephrol 1983;4:145–148.
25. Schwartz GJ, Brion LP, Spitzer A. The use of plasma creatinine concentration for estimating glomerular filtration rate in infants, children, and adolescents. Pediatr Clin North Am 1987;34:571–590.
26. Engelke SC, Shah RL, Vasan U, Raye JR. Sodium balance in very low-birth-weight infants. J Pediatr 1978;93:837–841.
27. Roy RN, Chance GW, Radde IC, et al. Late hyponatremia in very low birthweight infants (< 1.3 kilograms). Pediatr Res 1976;10:526–531.
28. Kim MS, Mandell J. Renal function in the fetus and neonate. In: King LR Jr, ed., Urologic surgery in neonates and young infants. Philadelphia: Saunders, 1988:41–58.
29. Haycock GB. Sodium homeostasis during early development: pathophysiology and clinical significance [Abstract]. Pediatr Nephrol 1996;10:C101.
30. Mathew OP, Jones AS, James E, et al. Neonatal renal failure: usefulness of diagnostic indices. Pediatrics 1980;65:57–60.

31. Stanier MW. Development of intra-renal solute gradients in foetal and postnatal life. Pfluegers Arch 1972;336:263–270.

32. Schlondorff D, Weber H, Trizna W, Fine LG. Vasopressin responsiveness of renal adenylate cyclase in rewborn rats and rabbits. Am J Physiol 1978;234:F16–F21.

33. Svenningsen NW. Renal acid-base titration studies in infants with and without metabolic acidosis in the postnatal period. Pediatr Res 1974;8:659–672.

34. Kerpel-Fronius E, Heim T, Sulyok E. The development of the renal acidifying processes and their relation to acidosis in low-birth-weight infants. Biol Neonate 1970;15:156–168.

35. Arant BS Jr. Developmental patterns of renal functional maturation compared in the human neonate. J Pediatr 1978;92:705–712.

36. Karlen J, Aperia A, Zetterstrom R. Renal excretion of calcium and phosphate in preterm and term infants. J Pediatr 1985; 106:814–819.

37. Brodehl J. Renal hyperaminoaciduria. In: Edelmann CM Jr, ed., Pediatric kidney disease. Boston: Little, Brown, 1978:1047–1079.

38. Rossi R, Danzebrink S, Linnenburger K, et al. Assessment of tubular reabsorption of sodium, glucose, phosphate and amino acids based on spot urine samples. Acta Paediatr 1994;83:1282–1286.

39. Moore ES, Coe FL, McMann BJ, Favus MJ. Idiopathic hypercalciuria in children: prevalence and metabolic characteristics. J Pediatr 1978;92:906–910.

40. Jacinto JS, Modanlou HD, Crade M. Renal calcification incidence in very low birth weight infants. Pediatrics 1988;81:31–35.

41. Gomez RA, Chevalier RL, Sturgill BC, Maturation of the intrarenal renin distribution in Wistar-Kyoto rats. J Hypertens 1986;4(suppl 5):S31–S33.

42. Gomez RA, Lynch KR, Sturgill BC, et al. Distribution of renin mRNA and its protein in the developing kidney. Am J Physiol 1989;257:F850–F858.

43. Siegel SR, Fisher DA. Ontogeny of the renin-angiotensin-aldosterone system in the fetal and newborn lamb. Pediatr Res 1980;14:99–102.

44. Fiselier T, Monnens L, van Munster P, et al. The renin angiotensin aldosterone system in infancy and childhood in basal conditions and after stimulation. Eur J Pediatr 1984;143:18–24.

45. Joppich R, Hauser I. Urinary prostacyclin and thromboxane A2 metabolites in preterm and full-term infants in relation to plasma renin activity and blood pressure. Biol Neonate 1982;42:179–184.

46. Aperia A, Broberger O, Herin P, Zetterstrom R. Sodium excretion in relation to sodium intake and aldosterone excretion in newborn pre-term and full-term infants. Acta Paediatr Scand 1977;68:813–817.

47. Robillard JE, Gomez RA, Meernik JG, et al. Role of angiotensin II on the adrenal and vascular responses to hemorrhage during development in the fetal lambs. Circ Res 1982;50:645–650.

48. Chevalier RL, Thornhill BA, Belmonte DC, Baertschi AJ. Endogenous angiotensin II inhibits natriuresis following acute volume expansion in the neonatal rat. Am J Physiol 1996;270:R393–R397.

49. Lumbers ER. Functions of the renin-angiotensin system during development. Clin Exp Pharmacol Physiol 1995;22:499–505.

50. Martin RA, Jones KL, Mendoza A, et al. Effect of ACE inhibition on the fetal kidney: decreased renal blood flow. Teratology 1992;46:317–321.

51. O'Dea RF, Mirkin BL, Alward CT, Sinaiko AR. Treatment of neonatal hypertension with captopril. J Pediatr 1988;113:403–406.

52. Goetz KL. Physiology and pathophysiology of atrial peptides. Am J Physiol 1988;254:E1–E15.

53. Castro LC, Law RW, Ross MG, et al. Atrial natriuretic peptide in the sheep. J Dev Physiol 1988;10:235–246.

54. Yamaji T, Hirai N, Ishibashi M. Atrial natriuretic peptide in umbilical cord blood: evidence for a circulation hormone in human fetus. J Clin Endocrinol Metab 1988;63:1414–1417.

55. Robillard JE, Weiner C. Atrial natriuretic factor in the human fetus: effect of volume expansion. J Pediatr 1988;113:552–556.

56. Nimrod C, Keane P, Harder J, Atrial natriuretic peptide production in association with nonimmune fetal hydrops. Am J Obstet Gynecol 1988;159:625–628.

57. Cheung CY, Brace RA. Fetal hypoxia elevates plasma atrial natriuretic factor concentration. Am J Obstet Gynecol 1988; 159:1263–1268.

58. Dolan LM, Young CA, Khoury JC, Dobrozsi DJ. Atrial ntriuretic factor during the perinatal period: equal depletion in both atria. Pediatr Res 1989;25:339–341.

59. Weil J, Bidlingmaier F, Dohlemann C, et al. Comparision of plasma atrial natriuretic peptide levels in healthy children from birth to adolescence and in children with cardiac diseases. Pediatr Res 1986;20:1328–1331.

60. Kikuchi K, Shiomi M, Horie K, et al. Plasma atrial natriuretic polypeptide concentration in healthy children from birth to adolescence. Acta Paediatr Scand 1988;77:380–384.

61. Bierd TM, Kattwinkel J, Chevalier RL. The interrelationship of atrial natriuretic peptide, atrial volume, and renal function in premature infants. J Pediatr 1990;116:753–759.

62. Hargrave BY, Iwamoto HS, Rudolph AM. Renal and cardiovascular effects of atrial natriuretic peptide in fetal sheep. Pediatr Res 1989;26:1–5

63. Brace RA, Bayer LA, Cheung CY. Fetal cardiovascular, endocrine, and fluid responses to atrial natriuretic factor infusion. Am J Physiol 1989;257:R580–R587.

64. Braunlich H, Solomon S. Renal effects of atrial natriuretic factor in the rats of different ages. Physiol Bohemoslov 1987;36:119–124.

65. Chevalier RL, Gomez RA. Renal effects of atrial natriuretic peptide infusion in young and adult rats. Pediatr Res 1988;24:333–337.

66. Muchant DG, Thornhill BA, Belmonte DC, Chronic sodium loading augments the natriuretic response to acute volume expansion in the preweaned rat. Am J Physiol 1995;269:R15–R22.

67. Robillard JE, Weitzman RE. Developmental aspects of the fetal response to exogenous arginine vasopressin. Am J Physiol 1980;238:F407–F414.

68. Rajerison RM, Butten D, Jard S. Ontogenic development of kidney and liver vasopressin receptors. In: Spitzer A, ed., The kidney during development: morphology and function. New York: Masson, 1982:249–256.

69. Melendez E, Reyes JL, Escalante BA, Melendez MA. Development of the receptors to prostaglandin E2 in the rat kidney and neonatal renal functions. Dev Pharmacol Ther 1990;14:125–134.

70. Kaplan SL, Feigin RD. Inappropriate secretion of antidiuretic hormone complicating neonatal hypoxic ischemic encephalopathy. J Pediatr 1978;92:431–433.

71. Moylan F, Herin J, Ktishnamoorthy K. Inappropriate antidiuretic hormone secretion in premature infants with cerebral injury. Am J Dis Child 1978;132:399–402.

72. Stern P, LaRochette F Jr, and Little, G. Role of vasopressin in water imbalance in the sick newborn. Kidney Int 1979;16:956–959.

73. Reyes JL, Melendez E. Effects of eicosanoids on the water and sodium balance of the neonate. Pediatr Nephrol 1990;4:630–634.

74. Buderus S, Thomas B, Fahnenstich H, Kowalewski S. Renal failure in two preterm infants: toxic effect of prenatal maternal indomethacin treatment? Br J Obstet. Gynaecol 1993;100:97–98.

75. Bachmann S, Mundel P. Nitric oxide in the kidney: synthesis, localization, and function. Am J Kidney Dis 1994;24:112–129.

76. Bogaert GA Kogan, BA, Mevorach RA. Effects of endothelium-derived nitric oxide on renal hemodynamics and function in the sheep fetus. Pediatr Res 1993;34:755–761.

77. Solhaug MJ, Wallace MR, Granger JP. Endothelium-derived nitric oxide modulates renal hemodynamics in the developing piglet. Pediatr Res 1993;34:750–754.

78. Laufer I, Griscom NT. Compensatory renal hypertrophy: absence in utero and development in early life. AJR Am J Roentgenol 1971;113:464–467.

79. Glazebrook KN, McGrath FP, Steele BT. Prenatal compensatory renal growth: documentation with US. Radiology 1993;189:733–735.

80. Mandell J, Peters CA, Estroff JA, Human fetal compensatory renal growth. J Urol 1993;150:790–792.

81. Dicker SE, Shirley DG. Compensatory renal growth after unilateral nephrectomy in the newborn rat. J Physiol 1973;228:193–202.

82. Hayslett JP. Functional adaptation to reduction in renal mass. Physiol Rev 1979;59:137–164.

83. Shirley DG. Developmental and compensatory renal growth in the guinea pig. Biol Neonate 1976;30:169–180.

84. Karp R, Brasel JA, Winick M. Compensatory kidney growth after uninephrectomy in adult and infant rats. Am J Dis Child 1971;121:186–188.

85. Phillips TL, Leong GF. Kidney cell proliferation after unilateral nephrectomy as related to age. Cancer Res 1967;27:286–292.

86. Hayslett JP, Kashgarian M, Epstein FH. Functional correlates of compensatory renal hypertrophy. J Clin Invest 1968;47:774–799.

87. Horster M, Kemler BJ, Valtin H. Intracortical distribution of number and volume of glomeruli during postnatal maturation in the dog. J Clin Invest 1971;50:796–800.

88. Olivetti G, Anversa P, Melissari M, Loud AV. Morphometry of the renal corpuscle during postnatal growth and compensatory hypertrophy. Kidney Int 1980;17:438–454.

89. Bonvalet JP, Champion M, Wanstok F, Berjal G. Compensatory renal hypertrophy in young rats: increase in the number of nephrons. Kidney Int 1972;1:391–396.

90. Kaufman JM, Hardy R, Hayslett JP. Age-dependent characteristics of compensatory renal growth. Kidney Int 1975;8:21–26.

91. Larsson L, Aperia A, Wilton P. Effect of normal development on compensatory renal growth. Kidney Int 1980;18:29–35.

92. Aschinberg LC, Koskimies O, Bernstein J, et al. The influence of age on the response to renal parenchymal loss. Yale J Biol Med 1978;51:341–345.

93. Chevalier RL. Functional adaptation to reduced renal mass in early development. Am J Physiol, 1982;242:F190–F196.

94. Ikoma M, Yoshioka, T, Ichikawa I, Fogo A. Mechanism of the unique susceptibility of deep cortical glomeruli of maturing kidneys to severe focal glomerular sclerosis. Pediatr Res 1990;28:270–276.

95. O'Sullivan DC, Dewan PA, Guiney EJ. Compensatory hypertrophy effectively assesses the degree of impaired renal function in unilateral renal disease. Br J Urol 1992;69:346–350.

96. Brenner BM, Meyer TW, Hostetter TH. Dietary protein intake and the progressive nature of kidney disease: the role of hemodynamically mediated glomerular injury in the pathogenesis of progressive glomerular sclerosis in aging, renal ablation, and intrinsic renal disease. N Engl J Med 1982;307:652–659.

97. Fogo A, Ichikawa I. Evidence for the central role of glomerular growth promoters in the development of sclerosis. Semin Nephrol 1989;9:329–342.

98. Celsi G, Bohman S, Aperia A. Development of focal glomerulosclerosis after unilateral nephrectomy in infant rats. Pediatr Nephrol 1987;1:290–296.

99. Okuda S, Motomura K, Sanai T, Influence of age on deterioration of the remnant kidney in uninephrectomized rats. Clin Sci 1987;72:571–576.

100. Brenner BM, Chertow GM. Congenital oligonephropathy and the etiology of adult hypertension and progressive renal injury. Am J Kidney Dis 1994;23:171–175.

101. Bhathena DB, Julian BA, McMorrow RG, Baehler RW. Focal sclerosis of hypertrophied glomeruli in solitary functioning kidneys of humans. Am J Kid Dis 1985;5:226–232.

102. Kiprov DD, Colvin RB, McCluskey RT. Focal and segmental glomerulosclerosis and proteinuria associated with unilateral renal agenesis. Lab Invest 1982;46:275–281.

103. Wikstad I, Celsi G, Larsson L, et al. Kidney function in adults born with unilateral renal agenesis or nephrectomized in childhood. Pediatr Nephrol 1988;2:177–182.

104. Argueso LR, Ritchey ML, Boyle ET Jr, et al. Prognosis of children with solitary kidney after unilateral nephrectomy. J Urol 1992;148:747–751.

105. Elema JD. Is one kidney sufficient? Kidney Int 1976;9:308.

CHAPTER 9

Molecular Basis of Pediatric Urologic Disease

Leslie Kushner and Mark A. Rich

Today's physicians have witnessed dramatic changes in the way they practice medicine and treat patients. These clinical changes coincide with advances in molecular biology that have changed our perception of living systems and our approach to the ancient art of healing. Historically, medical practitioners diagnosed patients by characterizing clinical presentations and associated symptoms of an ailment. The search for appropriate treatment was primarily empirical and focused on palliation or prevention of symptoms. The surge of knowledge in molecular medicine requires that the modern physician have a fundamental understanding of cellular processes and of the molecular basis of disease. This chapter provides an overview of the concepts of molecular biology as they apply to urologic disease in children.

BASIC CONCEPTS

To understand the application of molecular biology to pediatric urologic disease, it is necessary to understand some of the basic concepts of cellular function and regulation. The fundamental processes of all cells are regulated at several levels, including cell division, transcription, translation, and intercellular communication.

Cell division is fundamental to all developmental processes of the human organism. It is an essential component of normal growth as well as cancerous growth. During cell division, DNA is replicated in such a way that each daughter cell contains a full complement of the genome after cell division. The genome is a complete set of genes that incorporates all the DNA sequences. That DNA is the genetic material was demonstrated by key experiments performed by Avery, Macleod and McCarty in 1944.[1] It was not until 1953, however, that Watson and Crick[2,3] proposed the double-helical structure of complementary DNA polynucleotide strands. The double-helix of DNA is made up of two DNA strands, each forming a right-handed helix about the same axis. The two strands, running in opposite directions, are held together by hydrogen bonds between specific base pairs. That is, an adenine in one chain pairs with a thymine in the other and a guanine in one chain pairs with a cytosine in the other, resulting in complementary strands. This strict rule of complementary nucleotide base pairing ensures the accuracy of copying genetic information during replication, which results in daughter cells with the same set of genes after cell division.

A gene is the smallest functional sequence of DNA containing the information necessary for the cellular biosynthesis of a specific protein. The DNA sequence of the gene functions as a template for the transcription of a complementary strand of RNA. RNA that encodes a protein is called messenger RNA (mRNA). Thus mRNA leaves the nucleus, enters the cytoplasm of a cell, and is translated into a specific protein with a specific function (Fig. 9.1). In a diploid cell, a gene consists of two alleles. That is, a cell has two DNA sequences that can potentially encode the same functional protein.

The human genome is estimated to contain 50,000 to 100,000 genes on 23 pairs of chromosomes, one of which includes the sex-determining chromosomes X and Y. These genes are responsible for all the functional aspects of the organism's life, including reproduction, embryogenesis, development, growth, health, homeostatis, aging, disease, and death. Currently, the function of only a small portion of these genes is understood.

All of the processes mentioned—cell division, replication, transcription, translation, and the specific function of each protein—are regulated in complex ways by protein–protein and protein–nucleic acid interactions. DNA contains sequences that provide important regulatory information. These include sequences that bind specific proteins that together determine when and whether a gene will be transcribed, which DNA strand will be transcribed, and where transcription will begin and end. In addition, sequences of DNA that determine single mRNAs are not continuous. The regions that code for amino acids (exons) are interrupted by regions that are spliced out of the transcribed RNA before trans-

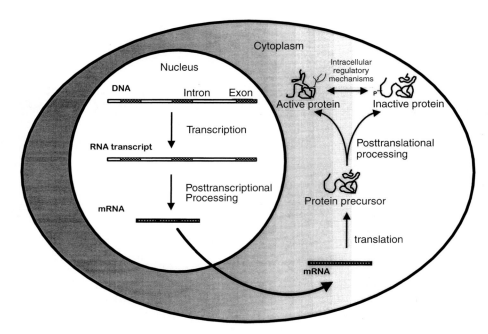

FIG. 9.1. The flow of information in all cells is from DNA to RNA to protein.

lation (Fig. 9.2). This allows alternate sequences of RNAs to be included in the resultant mRNA by replacing one exon with another during posttranscriptional processing, as if these alternate exons were cassettes of information. In this way, transcripts are spliced to change the sequence and length of the mRNA. The process of translation of mRNA to protein is also regulated. In addition, the translated protein can be modified by interaction with other proteins in such a way as to affect its function.

Regulation of these processes, from DNA replication and transcription to protein function, accounts for cell variability in function and morphology. The specific reg-

ulatory mechanisms not only differ among cell types but also vary during different stages of development. Activation and timing of the regulation of gene expression are critical in normal cell differentiation and development, although an interruption or mistake in the regulation of gene expression or in the sequence expressed may result in disease.

STEROID RECEPTORS

Steroid or glucocorticoid receptors modulate cell metabolism, growth, and development by regulating tran-

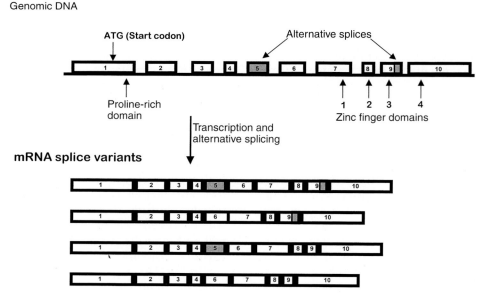

FIG. 9.2. The arrangement of the exons and introns of the Wilms' tumor gene. Alternative RNA splicing can produce four different proteins.

scription of specific genes. They make up a superfamily of nuclear receptors with highly conserved DNA sequences and structural homology.[4] The prototypical steroid receptor contains a hormone-binding domain, a DNA-binding domain, and a transcription-activating domain (Fig. 9.3). Each of these nuclear receptors has high affinity and specificity for a distinct hormone, such as androgen, estrogen, progestin, a mineralocorticoid, a glucocorticoid, or retinoic acid. The hormone-receptor complex binds to a specific DNA sequence in the target genes that regulates transcription.[5]

The demonstration that steroid receptors bind to specific sequences of DNA depended on both purification of steroid-receptor proteins and the development of the molecular biological technique called footprinting.[6] If a sequence of DNA is radioactively labeled, its size can be determined by its electrophoretic movement in gel (gel electrophoresis). In DNA footprinting, a sequence of DNA is labeled at one end of a single strand, and the DNA is digested with DNase. The fragments are identified by electrophoresis in a polyacrylamide gel. If the labeled DNA is allowed to bind protein before digestion with DNase, the protein will protect its DNA-binding sequence from digestion (Fig. 9.4). The protected sequence can then be identified.

A mutation in a steroid hormone receptor gene results in hormonal resistance, characterized by partial or complete absence of the hormone effects, despite normal or increased hormone production.[7] Examples central to sexual development and fertility are the molecular defects identified in patients with androgen receptor resistance.[8–10] Normal male phenotypic development requires transcriptional regulation by the testosterone- and dihydrotestosterone-receptor complexes.[11–13] The

action and potency of the two principal androgens— testosterone and dihydrotestosterone (DHT)—are not equivalent, even though their effects are mediated by the same receptor (Fig. 9.5). Testosterone, a lipophilic molecule, is thought to passively traverse the lipid bilayer of the cell membrane. Once in the cytoplasm, testosterone either binds the androgen receptor or is converted by the enzyme 5-α-reductase to DHT. Dihydrotestosterone binds the same androgen receptor with greater affinity and transforms the hormone-receptor complex into a configuration that binds DNA more efficiently. In concert, both androgen-receptor complexes drive male phenotypic development.[14]

Clinically, androgen-resistance syndromes are phenotypic disorders of sexual development characterized by a 46,XY karyotype, bilateral testes, normal testosterone secretion, and regression of mullerian structures. At the molecular level, androgen resistance is the result of a defective 5-α-reductase or a defective androgen receptor.[15, 16] Mutations in the androgen receptor can result in a nonfunctional receptor that fails to bind androgen efficiently and/or fails to bind DNA and regulate gene transcription.[17] Disorders of the androgen receptor produce a clinical spectrum of phenotypic abnormalities that range from a normal physical appearance (although patients are often infertile) to a phenotypic female with complete testicular feminization. The clinical spectrum of androgen-resistance syndromes depends on the magnitude of the amount of normal binding of the androgen–androgen receptor complex to its specific regulatory sequence on DNA. Such binding may range from nonexistent to decreased but qualitatively normal binding.[18] Patients with absence of binding, which may be the result of: 1) a deletion of the entire androgen receptor gene[19] or 2) absence of transcription; and/or transla-

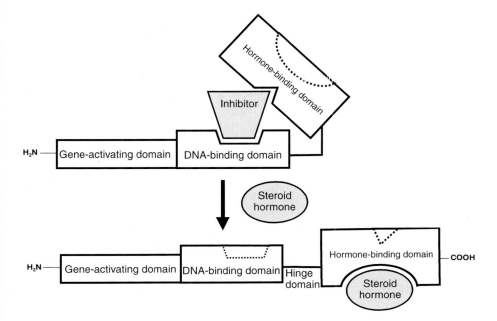

FIG. 9.3. A prototypical steroid hormone receptor.

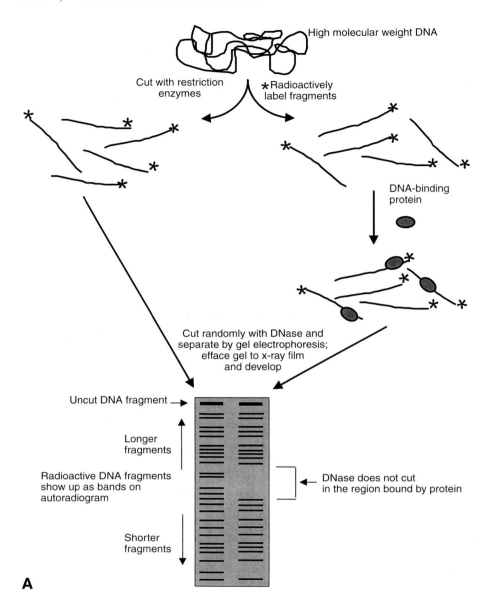

FIG. 9.4. DNA footprinting. **A,** The method by which DNA footprinting is employed to identify the sequence bound by a specific protein. **B,** Photograph of autoradiogram of footprint showing bonding of WT1 zinc fingers domain to the GF-II P3 promoter. **C,** Corresponding sequences protected from DNase digestion by WT1 are indicated by thick lines. Consensus bonding elements for WT1, in the human sequence, are underlined. [**(B)** and **(C)** were courtesy of Drummond IA, Madden SL, Rohwer-Nutter P, Bell GI, Sukhatme VP, Rauscher III FJ, Science 1992;257:674. Used with permission.]

tion of a receptor that binds hormone[20] appear clinically as complete testicular feminization. Mutations in the coding region of the androgen receptor gene, which result in loss of the highly conserved DNA or hormone-binding domains, have also been identified.[21] The androgenreceptor gene has been mapped to the X chromosome (bands Xq11–12);[22] therefore, males have only one copy of the gene. Thus androgen-receptor resistance (androgen-insensitivity syndrome) is a sex-linked recessive disorder.

GROWTH FACTORS

Cell proliferation is orchestrated by a complex sequence of events that begin in the environment surrounding the cell, affect the cell surface, and result in signals to the apparatus controlling replication in the nucleus. Trophic factors, including hormones, cytokines, and growth factors, bind specific cell surface receptors that signal the normal cell to proliferate. These factors may be synthesized and secreted from cells in distant organs and circulated (endocrine), they may be synthesized and secreted from different cell types within the same organ or tissue (paracrine), or they may be synthesized and secreted from the same cell responding to the signal (autocrine).[23]

Interactions between growth factors and their receptors trigger intracellular signal pathways (signal transduction) that culminate in activation or repression of gene expression. Growth factor receptors have an extracellular ligand-binding domain and an intracellular domain responsible for signal transduction. The intracellular domain of most growth factor receptors contains a tyrosine or serine or threonine kinase, the function of

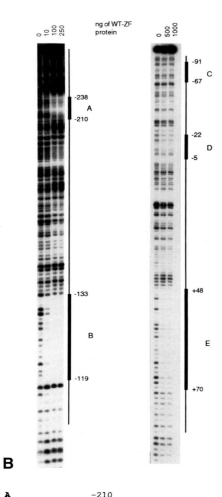

ng of WT-ZF protein

B

```
          -238        A                    -210
HUMAN  CCCACCCAGCCTCGCCCCCGCGCACCCCCCAGCCCCTGCGACCGCCGCCCCCCCCCCCCGGGGCCCCAGGGCCCC.AGCCC
MOUSE  CACAGCCCCCCCCCATCTTTGCCACCAGGCACTCCACTCCCCCCCCCCCACCCCAACCCCCGTGCCCAGGGCCCCCGACCC
RAT    ............................CCATTCCCCCCTCCCCCAACGGCAACCCCCGTGCCCAGGGCCCCGGACCC

       -162                      -133 B        -119
HUMAN  GCACCCCCCGCCCCGCTCTTGGCTCGGGTTGCGGGGGCGGGCCGGGGGCGGGGCGAGGGCTCCGCGGGCGCCCATTGGCG
MOUSE  GCATTCCC.GCGTGGCTC.......GAGTTGCGGGGGCGGGCCCGGGGCGGGGCGAGGGC.CTGCGGACGCCCATTGGCG
RAT    GCATTCCCCCCGTGGCTC.......GAGTTGCGGGGGCGGTCCCGGGGCGGGGCAAGGGCCCTGCGGACGCCCATTGGCG

       -82
HUMAN  CGGGCGCGAGGCCAGCGG...CCCCGCGCGGCCCTGGGCCGCGGCTGGCGCGACTATAAGAGCCGGGCGTGGGCGCCCGC
MOUSE  CGGGCGTAAGGCCAGCGGGGCCCGAGCGGGCGCCGAGCCGCGCGGGGTGGCGCGGCTATAAGAACCGGGCGTTGGCGCCCGG
RAT    CGGGCGTAAGGCCAGCGGGGCCCGAGCGGGCGCCGAGCCGCGCGGGGTGGCGCGGCTATAAGAACCGGGCGTTGGCGCCCGG

           +1 Transcription Start                        +48        E        +70
HUMAN  AGTTCGCCTGCTCTCCGGCGGAGCTGCGTGAGGCCCGGCCGGCCCCGGCCCCCCCCTTCCGGCCGCCCCCGCCTCCTGGC
MOUSE  AGTTCGCCTGCTCTCCGGCGGAGCTGCGTGAGGCCAGGCCGGCCCCCG.GCCCCCCTTCCGGCCGCCCCCGCCTCCTGGC
RAT    AGTTCGCCTGCTCTCCGGCGGAGCTGCGTGAGGCCAGGCCGGCCCCCGGCCCCCCCCTTCCGGCCGCCCCCGCCTCCTGGC
```

C

FIG. 9.4. *Continued.*

which is crucial for a cellular response to growth factor binding.[24]

A number of growth factors have been implicated in the process of nephrogenesis. These include the insulin-like growth factors (IGFs),[25–27] transforming growth factor α (TGF-α),[28] transforming growth factor β (TGF-β),[29] epidermal growth factor (EGF),[30] platelet-derived growth factor (PDGF),[31] neurotrophins,[32–35] hepatocyte growth factor (HGF),[36, 37] and basic fibroblast growth factor (bFGF).[38] A connection between growth factors and cancer has emerged with the identification of certain proto-oncogenes as growth factor receptors. For exam-

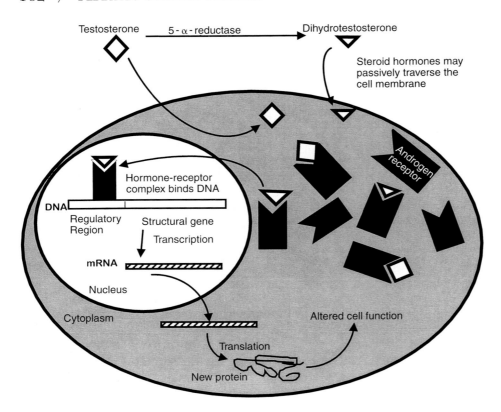

FIG. 9.5. Androgen receptor binding.

ple the c-*met* proto-oncogene was identified as the receptor for HGF[39] and the c-*ret* proto-oncogene was identified as the receptor for glial-derived neurotrophic factor (GDNF).[34]

The importance of genes encoding growth factors, as well as other gene products, in development can be gauged by experiments in which the specific gene is deleted. This method of targeted gene replacement results in a transgenic animal in which the gene of interest is altered, added, or deleted.[40] In brief, a recombinant DNA containing the sequence to be inserted is microinjected into a fertilized egg (usually of a mouse) (Fig. 9.6). The recombinant DNA integrates into the organism's chromosomal DNA. The injected eggs are implanted in a foster mother and allowed to develop. The resulting transgenic animal, if it carries the transgene in its germ cells, can be bred to produce transgenic progeny. A transgene can be constructed so that it results in an organism with a functional deletion of a specific gene. Such transgenic animals are called "knock outs" because the gene has essentially been knocked out of the animal. This molecular tool has been used to evaluate the importance of certain growth factors in renal development.

The IGFs are synthesized primarily in liver and circulate in plasma associated with IGF-binding proteins. The IGFs, however, are also synthesized and secreted from renal cells, suggesting that these factors function in both endocrine and paracrine fashion.[41, 42] During renal development, IGF-II is expressed in undifferentiated

mesenchyme and IGF-I is expressed during the outbranching of ureteric buds.[43] The IGF-I receptor—which binds insulin, IGF-I, and IGF-II—is differentially expressed with greater levels of expression on ureteric bud epithelium.[44] Transgenic mice deficient in expression of IGF-II,[45] IGF-I, and/or IGF-IR[46] have normally developing kidneys, suggesting functional redundancy for the IGF–IGF receptor system in renal development.

EGF and TGF-α are both ligands of the EGF receptors, encoded by the c-*erb* and c-*erb* B2 proto-oncogenes.[47] Both are renal mitogens that induce tubulogenesis of renal cells or metanephrogenic mesenchyme in culture.[48–50] The addition of anti-TGF-α to metanephros in organ culture results in inhibition of ureteric bud branching.[28]

The developing metanephric mesenchyme and the epithelial-mesenchymal surface of the developing kidney express TGF-β_1.[29] In culture, TGF-β inhibits growth and differentiation of the metanephric blastema, whereas anti-TGF-β stimulates tubulogenesis.[29] Similarly, TGF-β blocks HGF-induced tubulogenesis of cultured Makin-Darby canine kidney (MDCK) cells.[51]

Expression of PDGF occurs in differentiated epithelial cells and glomerular mesangium, whereas its receptor is expressed in mesenchyme, endothelium, interstitium, and mesangium during nephrogenesis.[31] Transgenic mice deficient in either the PDGF-B chain or the PDGF-β receptor are lacking glomerular mesangial cells.[52]

The observation that metanephric differentiation is

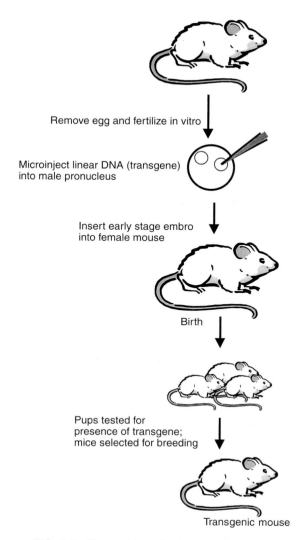

FIG. 9.6. The making of a transgenic mouse.

Remove egg and fertilize in vitro

Microinject linear DNA (transgene) into male pronucleus

Insert early stage embro into female mouse

Birth

Pups tested for presence of transgene; mice selected for breeding

Transgenic mouse

induced by neuronal tissue prompted investigation into the role of neurotrophic factors and their receptors in nephrogenesis.[53, 54] The *trk* family of proto-oncogenes has been demonstrated to be receptors for the neurotrophins.[55–57] Differentiating cortical mesenchyme expresses *trkB*, whereas the low-affinity *trk*[75] is expressed in undifferentiated mesenchyme and developing podocytes.[58] Antisense *trk*[75], which blocks the expression of *trk*[75], inhibits branching of the ureteric bud.[32] Renal development, however, is not affected in transgenic mice lacking *trk*[75] expression,[59] suggesting functional redundancy of its role in nephrogenesis. On the other hand, transgenic mice lacking expression of GDNF have renal agenesis,[35] demonstrating a requirement for GDNF for renal development. GDNF is highly expressed in metanephric mesenchyme, whereas its receptor, encoded by the c-*ret* proto-oncogene, is highly expressed in the Wolffian duct and on ureteric bud epithelium. Interaction between GDNF and its receptor is thought to medi-

ate the induction of ureteric bud branching.[60] Transgenic mice lacking expression of the protein product of c-*ret* exhibit renal and ureteral hypoplasia.[61]

HGF is mitogenic and morphogenic for renal epithelial cells *in vitro*.[62, 63] HGF has been shown to stimulate differentiation of metanephric mesenchymal cells, which also express this growth factor.[64, 65] The receptor for HGF (the product of the c-*met* gene) is highly expressed in metanephric epithelium and in the ureteric bud.[37] The role of HGF in nephrogenesis is demonstrated by experiments in which anti-HGF antibodies are shown to block condensation of metanephric mesenchyme and inhibit ureteric bud branching.[36, 37] Renal development, however, is not affected in transgenic mice lacking expression of HGF.[66]

Basic fibroblast growth factor is known to play a role in embryogenesis, angiogenesis, and wound healing. It has been shown to stimulate secretion of HGF from human mesenchymal cells in tissue culture.[67] In addition, bFGF stimulates the expression of the Wilms' tumor gene (*WT1*), which is required for nephrogenesis, and c-*met* in embryonic metanephrogenic mesenchyme.[38] bFGF is required for induction of tubule formation in cultured renal mesenchyme.[38]

ONCOGENES AND PROTO-ONCOGENES

The concept of an oncogene originated with the discovery that certain RNA viruses (retroviruses) contain genes that encode proteins that cause transformation of normal cells into cancer cells (transformation).[68] These transforming-retroviral oncogenes are highly homologous to genes present in normal cells.[69] The homologous genes present in normal cells were termed proto-oncogenes because they required changes in their sequence (mutation) or levels of expression to initiate transformation.[70, 71] Proto-oncogenes are highly expressed during carcinogenesis, often in a mutated or aberrantly regulated form. Most of these genes are expressed in noncancerous tissue and are necessary for normal cellular function. A number of proto-oncogene protein products have been identified as specific growth factor receptors and thus have a direct role in normal cellular proliferation and differentiation. These include the proto-oncogenes c-*erb*, c-*erb* B2, c-*met*, c-*ret*, and c-*trk*, discussed above. A number of other proto-oncogenes function in intracellular signal transduction and transcriptional regulation during the cell cycle and thus have a role in normal cellular division and differentiation.

The *myc* family of proto-oncogenes have a demonstrated role in nephrogenesis.[72] Cortical metanephric mesenchyme expresses c-*myc*, N-*myc* expression is confined to the developing outer renal cortex, and L-*myc* is expressed in branching ureteric bud.

Overexpression of the N-*myc* protein owing to amplification of the N-*myc* proto-oncogene is the most common abnormality identified as an unfavorable prognostic marker for neuroblastoma.[73, 74] Neuroblastoma constitutes 8 to 10% of all childhood malignancies and has an incidence of 1 in 10,000 births. The tumor is generally found in young children, and clinical presentation is before age 2 in 60% of cases. Adrenal neuroblastoma is a neoplasm that arises from alteration of normal neural crest stem cell and neuroblast differentiation. The clinical behavior of this tumor varies from benign spontaneous maturation to aggressive, relentless malignant progression. Although a number of cytogenetic abnormalities have been detected in neuroblastomas,[75–78] the most prevalent corresponds to the amplified N-*myc* gene integrated into chromosomal DNA.[79] The chromosomal location of the inserted amplified DNA may contain up to 1,000 copies of the N-*myc* gene.

The proto-oncogene *trkA*, which encodes the receptor for nerve growth factor (NGF), may also be overexpressed in neuroblastoma.[55, 80] Expression of the *trkA* gene is inversely correlated with expression of N-*myc* in neuroblastoma.[81] Hence, it is not surprising that neuroblastoma with high levels of *trkA* expression, and without amplification of N-*myc* predicts a favorable outcome.[82]

N-*myc* mRNA expression is also increased in Wilms' tumors;[83] however, the gene is not amplified in Wilms' tumors. This suggests that the increased expression of N-*myc* in this tumor is due to some improperly controlled transcriptional regulatory event.

Amplification of a sequence of DNA is easily detected using the molecular biological Southern analysis technique (Fig. 9.7).[84] In this technique, DNA is cut with a specific restriction endonuclease, which is an enzyme that cuts DNA at a specific internal sequence.[85] The DNA fragments obtained are separated by gel electophoresis and transferred to a special filter. The DNA on the filter is hybridized to a labeled probe that contains a sequence of DNA or RNA complementary to the sequence of interest. A similar technique in which RNA is electrophoretically separated and detected by hybridization with a labeled probe is called a Northern analysis.[86] These two techniques have been used to distinguish between Wilms' tumor and neuroblastoma in pediatric renal tumor.[87] Northern analysis can demonstrate increased expression of the N-*myc* gene in both Wilms' tumors and neuroblastoma. Southern analysis, however, can distinguish between increased expression owing to increased transcription of a single copy of N-*myc* (as in Wilms' tumor) or increased expression owing to N-*myc* gene amplification (as in neuroblastoma) (Fig. 9.8).

TUMOR-SUPPRESSOR GENES

The observation that certain tumors are much more common in some families than in others suggested a role for inherited tumor formation. The two-hit theory of oncogenesis,[88] hypothesizes that certain heritable dis-

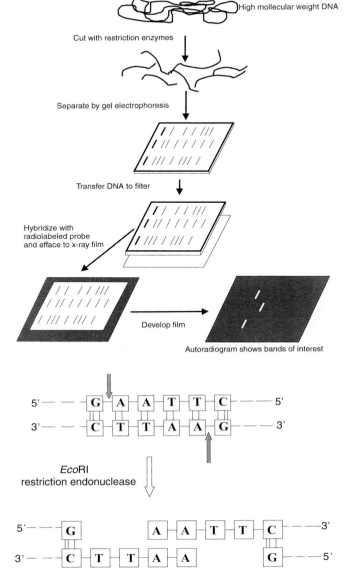

FIG. 9.7. Southern analysis. **A,** The method of Southern analysis. **B,** Mechanism of action of restriction endonuclease EcoRI.

eases resulting in tumor are caused by two mutational events, at least one of which is inherited as a germ-line mutation. That is, the first hit was an inherited mutation in a single allele of a gene that would then be present in all cells of the developing individual, making the individual heterozygous for the defect. Tumor developed only after a second independent mutational event in the other allele that resulted in loss of heterozygosity (Fig. 9.9).

Wilms' tumor, the most common renal tumor of childhood, is associated with the presence of a specific chromosome deletion on the short arm of chromosome 11 (band 11p13). In many patients, this deletion has been observed at the cytogenetic level.[89] Although most cases

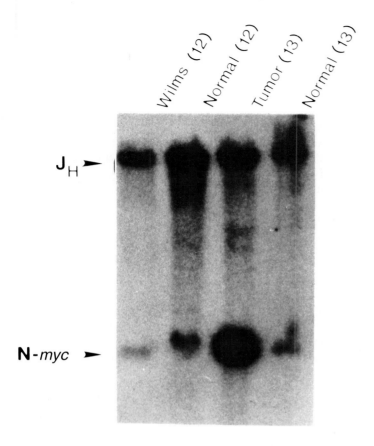

JH ▶

N-*myc* ▶

FIG. 9.8. Southern analysis to detect *N-myc* gene amplification apparent in neuroblastoma (lane C) but not Wilms' tumor (lane A). [Courtesy of Nisen PD, Rich MA, Gloster E, Valderrama E, Sarr O, Shende A, Lanzkowsty P, Alt FW, Cancer 1988;61:1821.]

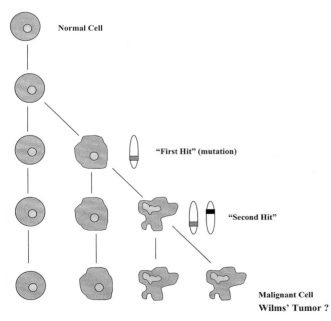

Normal Cell

"First Hit" (mutation)

"Second Hit"

Malignant Cell
Wilms' Tumor ?

FIG. 9.9. Two-hit transformation of a normal cell.

are unilateral and occur sporadically, the earlier age of onset of bilateral and familial Wilms' tumor[90] and Wilms' tumors associated with syndromes such as Wilms' tumor, aniridia, gentiourinary malformations, mental retardation (WAGR); (Beckwith–Wiedemann syndrome (macroglossia, organomegaly, hemihypertrophy, omphalocele); and Denys–Drash syndrome (intersex disorder, mixed gonadal dysgenesis nephropathy, Wilms' tumor) suggest the role of a specific inherited mutation as the first hit. The observed linkage of aniridia (localized to a deletion of a specific region of chromosome 11) with Wilms' tumor helped narrow down the specific location of the inherited defect responsible for a predisposition for Wilms' tumor, because patients with both aniridia and Wilms' tumor had a large deletion at band 11p13.[91]

The Wilms' tumor-suppressor gene (*WT1*) has been mapped to band 11p13.[92] This gene is deleted in patients with WAGR complex and carries a mutation in many patients with Wilms' tumor and Denys–Drash syndrome.[93–99] Although the development of Wilms' tumor apparently requires two mutant alleles for the *WT1* gene, patients with Denys–Drash syndrome are heterozygous for *WT1* mutations.[100] This suggests that the abnormal protein produced by the mutant allele interferes with the function of the normal protein produced by unaffected allele, a phenomenon called dominant negative mutation. Recent evidence suggests that putative self-association regions of the WT1 protein are required to observe dominant negative activity, indicating that the expressed mutant protein encoded by the mutant allele associates with the expressed wild-type WT1 protein to inhibit its activity.[101]

At the molecular level, the WT1 gene encodes a DNA-binding protein that regulates gene transcription. The WT1 protein is a transcriptional modulator of genes containing a specific consensus sequence to which the protein binds. This consensus sequence is identical to the sequence recognized by the transcription activator EGR1, an early growth response gene.[102] In addition, there is evidence that this protein has the capacity to dimerize.[103] The gene encoding the protein is composed of 10 exons (Fig. 9.2). There are two alternative splice sites that give rise to four different protein products.[104]

Transcriptional inhibition of distinct target genes by WT1 has been demonstrated. The transcription of the IGF-II, IGFR-I, PDGF-A, and PAX2 genes are repressed by WT1 binding to the promoter region of those genes.[105–108] These genes are all overexpressed in Wilms' tumor. Thus a lack of developmentally appropriate and tissue-specific transcriptional repression has been implicated as a potential mechanism of Wilms' tumorigenesis.

The paired-box gene PAX2 is a transcription factor expressed in the condensing metanephric tubules and ureteric bud epithelium.[109] Transgenic mice lacking expression of PAX2 or overexpressing PAX2 exhibit renal abnormalities.[110, 111] In addition, antisense to PAX2, which blocks expression of this gene, inhibits metanephric mesenchyme to epithelial conversion in vitro.[112] The PAX2 protein has been shown to bind to the promoter region of the WT1 gene, resulting in transcriptional activation.[113, 114]

WT1 represses the transcription of bcl-2, which codes for a protein that suppresses apoptotic cell death, a process necessary for normal renal devlopment.[115, 116] It is likely that this function of WT1 is responsible for its inhibition of p53-mediated apoptosis.[117] In addition, there is evidence for direct interaction between the p53 and WT1 proteins, resulting in altered function of each protein.[117, 118]

During normal devlopment, WT1 gene expression is tissue specific; the highest levels are identified in developing kidney and genitalia.[119] Specifically, it is expressed in condensed renal mesenchyme and podocytes.[120] Transgenic mice lacking expression of WT1 have a failure of kidney development,[121] demonstrating the requirement of WT1 expression for nephrogenesis. It is likely that during kidney development WT1 gene product acts as a transcription factor in concert with other specific renal regulatory genes normally involved in kidney cell proliferation and blastemal differentiation.

Loss of heterozygosity for a region at band 11p15, but not band 11p13, has been shown for a number of Wilms' tumors.[122, 123] Mutation at this locus is especially prevalent in Wilms' tumor associated with Beckwith–Wiedmann syndrome (BWS).[124, 125] In this syndrome, loss of heterozygosity of the band 11p15 locus is often the result of paternal imprinting.[126] That is, only the paternal allele (which in this case is defective) is expressed. In the case of BWS, patients actually lose the maternal allele and the paternal allele is duplicated, a process called acquired paternal isodisomy. Although the identity of the specific defective gene at band 11p15 is unknown, there are two likely candidates. The IGF-II gene maps to the band 11p15 locus and is paternally imprinted.[127, 128] IGF-II is a known fetal growth factor required for nephrogenesis,[27] and it is overexpressed in Wilms' tumor.[129, 130] The H19 gene also maps to the 11p15 region, and its expression level vary similarly to IGF-II,[131, 132] suggesting coregulation of the expression of these two genes. H19 is highly expressed in developing kidney.[133] Reduced expression of H19 owing to epigenetic inactivation in Wilms' tumor is thought to result in overexpression of IGF-II.[134, 135]

A number of sporadic cases of Wilms' tumors have loss of heterozygosity for a locus on chromosomal region 16q.[136] An additional putative familial Wilms' tumor gene locus has been identified on chromosomal region 17q in a single large kindred.[137] The detection of loss of heterozygosity at these loci and the fact that analysis of several kindred with familial Wilms' tumor show no defects in loci on chromosome 11 suggest that other genes may be involved in Wilms' tumorigenesis.[138–141] This is not surprising considering the complex cascade of regulation of expression of multiple gene products likely to be necessary for nephrogenesis.

CONCLUSION

The mechanism of interaction among growth factors such as bFGF, HGF, and IGF, receptors such as the androgen receptor and the c-met, trk gene products, transcription factors such as WT1 and bcl-2, and enzymes regulating renal and testicular development, growth, and function is only now being elucidated. The advances in molecular biology as applied to pediatric renal disease may be expected to have a major effect on understanding the diseases of interest to the pediatric urologist. These advances have already resulted in more powerful diagnostic tools and will, most certainly, yield new clinical approaches to treatment and prevention of pediatric urologic diseases.

ACKNOWLEDGMENTS

Dr. Kushner is supported by NIH DK49450 and a grant from the Muriel and Howard Weingrow family foundation.

REFERENCES

1. Avery OT, MacLeod CM, McCarty M. Studies on the chemical 1. Avery nature of the substance inducing transformation of pneumonococcus types. J Exp Med 1944;79:137–158.
2. Watson JD, Crick FHC. Molecular structure of nucleic acids: a structure for deoxyribose nucleic acid. Nature 1953;171:737–738.
3. Watson JD, Crick FHC. Genetical implications of the structure of deoxyribonucleic acid. Nature 1953;171:738–740.
4. Evans RM. The steroid and thyroid hormone receptor superfamily. Science 1988;240:889–895.
5. Yamamoto, KR. Steroid receptor regulated transcription of specific genes and gene networks. Ann Rev Genet 1985;19:209–252.
6. Galas D, Schmitz A. DNase footprinting: a simple method for the detection of protein-DNA binding specificity. Nucleic Acid Res 1978;5:3157–3170.
7. Lazar MA. Steroid and thyroid hormone receptors. Endocrinol Metab Clin North Am 1991;20:681–685.
8. Brown TR, Lubahn DB, Wilson EM, et al. Functional characterization of naturally occurring mutant androgen receptors from subjects with complete androgen insensitivity. Mol Endocrinol 1990;4:1759–1772.
9. McPhaul MJ, Marcelli M. Molecular defects in the androgen receptor causing androgen resistance. J Invest Dermatol 1992; 98(Suppl 6):97S–99S.
10. Kasumi H, Komori S, Yamasaki N, et al. Single nucleotide substitution of the androgen receptor gene in a case with receptor-positive androgen insensitivity syndrome (complete form). Acta Endocrinol 1993;128:355–360.
11. Grino PB, Griffin JE, Wilson JD. Testosterone at high concentrations interacts with human androgen receptor similarly to dihydrotestosterone. Endocrinology 1990;126:1165–1172.
12. Deslypere JP, Young M, Wilson JD, McPhaul MJ. Testosterone and 5 α-dihydrotestosterone interact differently with the androgen receptor to enhance transcription of the MMTV-Cat reporter gene, Mol Cell Endocrinol 1992;88:15–22.
13. Zhou ZX, Lane MV, Kemppainen JA, et al. Specificity of ligand-dependent androgen receptor stabilization: receptor domain interactions influence ligand dissociation and receptor stability. Mol Endocrinol 1995;9:208–218.
14. Wiener JS, Teague JL, Rothe DR, et al. Molecular biology and function of the androgen receptor in genital development. J Urol 1997;157:1377–1386.
15. Peterson RE, Imperato-McGinley J, Gautier T, Sturla E. Male pseudohermaphroditism in 5α-reductase deficiency. Am J Med 1977;62:170–199.
16. Griffin JE, Wilson JD. The androgen resistance syndromes: 5-alpha-reductase deficiency, testicular feminization, and related disorders. In: Scriver CR, Beaudet AL, Sly WS, Vales D, eds., The metabolic basis of inherited disease. New York: McGraw-Hill, 1989:1919–1944.
17. Quigley CA, De Bellis A, Marschke KB, et al. Androgen receptor defects: historical, clinical, and molecular perspectives. Endocrine Rev 1995;16:271–321.
18. Griffin JE, Durrant JL. Qualitative receptor defects in families with androgen resistance: failure of stabilization of the fibroblast cytosol androgen receptor. J Clin Endocrinol Metab 1982;55:465–474.
19. Quigley CA, Friedman KJ, Johnson A. Complete deletion of the androgen receptor gene: definition of the null phenotype of the androgen insensitivity syndrome and determination of carrier status. J Clin Endocrinol Metab 1992;74:923–927.
20. Nakao R, Haji M, Yanase T. A single amino acid substitution (met786-Val) in the steroid-binding domain of human androgen receptor leads to complete androgen insensitivity syndrome. J Clin Endocrinol Metab 1992;74:1152–1157.
21. Marcelli M, Zoppi S, Grinok PB, et al. A mutation in the DNA-binding domain of the androgen receptor gene causes complete testicular feminization in a patient with receptor-positive androgen resistance. J Clin Invest 1991;87:1123–1126.
22. Brown CJ, Goss SJ, Lubahn DB, et al. Androgen receptor locus on the human X chromosome: regional localization to Xq11–12 and description of a DNA polymorphism. Am J Hum Genet 1989;44:264–269.
23. Mendley SR, Toback FG. Autocrine and paracrine regulation of kidney epithelial cell growth. Ann Rev Physiol 1988;51:33–50.
24. Schlessinger J, Ullrich A. Growth factor signaling by receptor tyrosine kinases. Neuron 1992;9:383–391.
25. Liu ZZ, Wada J, Alvares K, et al. Distribution and relevance of insulin-like growth factor-I receptor in metanephric development. Kidney Int 1993;44:1242–1250.
26. Wada J, Liu ZZ, Alvares K, et al. Cloning of cDNA for the α subunit of mouse insulin like growth factor-I receptor and the role of the receptor in metanephric development. Proc Natl Acad Sci U S A 1993;90:10360–10364.
27. Rogers SA, Ryan G, Hammerman MR. Insulin-like growth factors I and II are produced in the metanephros and are required for growth and development in vitro. J Cell Biol 1991;113:1447–1453.
28. Rogers SA, Ryan G, Hammerman MR. Metanephric TGF-α is required for renal organogenesis in vitro. Am J Physiol 1992; 262:F533–F539.
29. Rogers SA, Ryan G, Purchio AF, Hammerman MR. Metranephric transforming growth factor-β_1 regulates nephrogenesis in vitro. Am J Physiol 1993;264:F996–F1002.
30. Weller A, Sorokin L, Illgen EM, Ekblom P. Development and growth of mouse embryonic kidney in organ culture and modulation of development by soluble growth factor. Dev Biol 1991; 144:248–261.
31. Daniel TO, Kumjian DA. Platelet-derived growth factor in renal development and disease. Semin Nephrol 1993;13:87–95.
32. Sariola H, Saarma M, Sainio K, et al. Dependence of kidney morphogenesis on the expression of nerve growth factor receptor. Science 1991;254:571–573.
33. Durbeej M, Soderstrom S, Ebendal T, et al. Differential expression of neurotrophin receptors during renal development. Development 1993;119:977–989.
34. Trupp M, Arenas E, Fainzilber M, et al. Functional receptor for GDNF encoded by the c-ret proto-oncogene. Nature 1996;381:785–789.
35. Sanchez MP, Silos-Santiago I, Frisen J, et al. Renal agenesis and absence of enteric neurons in mice lacking GDNF. Nature 1996; 382:70–75.
36. Santos OF, Barros EJ, Yang XM, et al. Involvement of hepatocyte growth factor in kidney development. Dev Biol 1994;163:525–529.
37. Woolf AS, Kolatsi-Joannou M, Hardman P, et al. Role of hepatocyte growth factor/scatter factor and the met receptor in the early development of the metanephros. J Cell Biol 1995;128:171–184.
38. Perantoni A, Dove LF, Karavanova I. Basic fibroblast growth factor can mediate the early inductive events in renal development. Proc Natl Acad Sci U S A 1995;92:4696–4700.
39. Bottaro DP, Rubin JS, Faletto DL, et al. Identification of the hepatocyte growth factor receptor as the c-met proto-oncogene product. Science 1991;251:802–804.
40. Palmiter RD, Brinster RL. Germ line transformation of mice. Ann Rev Genet 1986;20:465–499.
41. Bortz JD, Rotwein P, DeVol D, et al. Focal expression of insulin-like growth factor I in rat kidney collecting duct. J Cell Biol 1988;107:811–819.
42. Aron DC, Rosenzweig JL, Abboud HE. Synthesis and binding of insulin-like growth factor I by human glomerular mesangial cells. J Clin Endocrinol 1989;68:585–591.
43. Rotwein P, Pollock KM, Watson M, Milbrandt JD. Insulin-like growth factor gene expression during rat embryonic development. Endocrinology 1987;121:2141–2144.
44. Smith EP, Sadler TW, D'Ercole AJ. Somatomedins/insulin-like growth factors, their receptors and binding proteins are present during mouse embryogenesis. Development 1987;101:73–82.
45. Dechiara TM, Efstratiadis A, Robertson EF. A growth-deficient phenotype in heterozygous mice carrying an insulin-like growth factor II gene disrupted by targeting. Nature 1990;345:78–80.
46. Liu JP, Baker J, Perkins AS, et al. Mice carrying null mutations of the genes encoding insulin-like growth factor I (IGF-1) and type 1 IGF receptor (IGF1R). Cell 1993;75:59–72.
47. Downward J, Yarden Y, Mayes E, et al. Close similarity of epidermal growth factor receptor and verb-B oncogene protein sequences. Nature 1984;307:521–527.

48. Avner ED. Polypeptide growth factors and the kidney: a developmental perspective. Pediatr Nephrol 1990;4:345–353.
49. Taub M., Wang Y, Szczesny TM, Kleinman HK. Epidermal growth factor or transforming growth factor α is required for kidney tubulogenesis in matrigel cultures in serum-free medium. Proc Natl Acad Sci U S A 1990;87:4002–4006.
50. Perantoni AO, Dove LF, William CL. Induction of tubules in rat metanephrogenic mesenchyme in the absence of an inductive tissue. Differentiation 1991;48:25–32.
51. Santos OFP, Nigam SK. HGF-induced tubulogenesis and branching of epithelial cells is modulated by extracellular matrix and TGF-β. Dev Biol 1993;160:293–302.
52. Soriano P. Abnormal kidney development and hematological disorders in PDGF-β-receptor mutant mice. Genes Dev 1994;8:1888–1896.
53. Grobstein C. Trans-filter induction of tubules in mouse metanephric mesenchyme. Exp Cell Res 1956;10:424–440.
54. Sariola H, Ekblom P, Henke-Fahle S. Embryonic neurons as in vitro inducers of nephrogenic mesenchyme. Dev Biol 1989;132:271–281.
55. Kaplan DR, Hempstead BL, Martin-Zanca D, et al. The trk protogene product: a signal transducing receptor for nerve growth factor. Science 1991;252:544–556.
56. Klein R, Nanduri V, Jing SA, et al. The trkB tyrosine protein kinase is a receptor for brain-derived neurotrophic factor and neurotrophin-3. Cell 1991;66:395–403.
57. Lamballe F, Klein R, Barbacid M. trkC, a new member of the trk family of tyrosine protein kinases, is a receptor for neurotrophin-3. Cell 1991;66:967–979.
58. Durbeej M, Soderstrom S, Ebendal T, et al. Differential expression of neurotrophin receptors during renal development. Development 1993;119:977–989.
59. Lee K-F, Lik E. Huber J, et al. Targeted mutation of the gene encoding the low affinity NGF receptor p75 leads to deficits in the peripheral sensory nervous system. Cell 1992;69:737–749.
60. Robertson K, Mason I. The GDNF-RET signalling partnership. Trends Genet 1997;13:1–3.
61. Schuchardt A, D'Agati V, Larsson-Blomberg L, et al. Defects in the kidney and enteric nervous system of mice lacking the tyrosine kinase receptor ret. Nature 1994;367:380–383.
62. Ishibashi K, Saski S, Sakamoto H, et al. Hepatocyte growth factyor is a paracrine factor for renal epithelial cells: stimulation of DNA synthesis and NA,K-ATPase activity. Biochem Biophys Res Commun 1992;182:960–965.
63. Montesano R, Matsumoto K, Nakamura T, Orci L. Identification of a fibroblast-derived epithelial morphogen as hepatocyte growth factor. Cell 1991;67:901–908.
64. Karp SL, Ortiz-Arduan A, Li S, Neilson EG. Epithelial differentiation of metanephric mesenchymal cells after stimulation with hepatocyte growth factor or embryonic spinal cord. Proc Natl Acad Sci U S A 1994;91:5286–5290.
65. Sonnenberg E, Meyer D, Weidner KM, Birchmeier C. Scatter factor/hepatocye growth factor and its receptor, the c-met tyrosine kinase, can mediate a signal exchange between mesenchyme and epithelia during mouse development. J Cell Biol 1993;123:223–235.
66. Schmidt C, Bladt F, Goedecke S, et al. Scatter factor/hepatocyte growth factor is essential for liver development. Nature 1995;373:699–702.
67. Roletto F, Galvani AP, Cristiani C, et al. Basic fibroblast growth factor stimulates hepatocyte growth factor/scatter factor secretion by human mesenchymal cells. Cell Physiol 1996;166:105–111.
68. Bishop JM. Cellular oncogenes and retroviruses. Ann Rev Biochem 1983;52:301–354.
69. Stehelin D, Varmus HE, Bishop JM, Vogt PK. DNA related to the transforming gene(s) of avian sarcoma viruses is present in normal avian DNA. Nature 1976;260:170–173.
70. Takeya T, Hanafusa H. Structure and sequence of cellular gene homologous to the RSV src gene and the mechanism for generating the transforming virus. Cell 1983;32:881–890.
71. Blair DG, Oskarsson M, Wood TG, et al. Activation of the transforming potential of a normal cell sequence: a model for oncogenesis. Science 1981;212:941–943.
72. Mugrauer G, Ekblom P. Contrasting expression patterns of three members of myc family of proto-oncogenes in the developing and adult mouse kidney. J Cell Biol 1991;112:13–25.
73. Nisen PD, Waber P, Rich MA, et al. N-myc oncogene RNA expression in neuroblastoma. J Natl Cancer Inst 1988;80:1633–1637.
74. Seeger R, Brodeur G, Sather A, et al. Association of multiple copies of the N-myc oncogene with rapid progression of neuroblastoma. N Engl J Med 1985;313:1111–1116.
75. Fong CT, Dracopoli NC, White PS, et al. Loss of heterozygosity for the short arm of chromosome 1 in human neuroblastomas: correlation with N-myc amplification. Proc Natl Acad Sci U S A 1989;86:3753–3757.
76. Caron H, VanSluis P, DeKrader J, et al. Allelic loss of chromosome 1p as a predictor of unfavorable outcome in patients with neuroblastoma. New Engl J Med 1996;334:225–230.
77. Suzuki T, Yokota J, Mugishima H, et al. Frequent loss of heterozygosity on chromosome 14q in neuroblastoma. Cancer Res 1989;49:1095–1098.
78. Plantaz D, Mohapatra G, Matthay KK, et al. Gain of the chromosome 17 is the most frequent abnormality detected in neuroblastoma by comparative genomic hybridization. Am J Pathol 1997;150:81–89.
79. Schwab M, Alitalok K, Klemphauer K, et al. Amplified DNA with limited homology to myc cellular oncogene is shared by human neuroblastoma tumor. Nature 1983;305:245–248.
80. Brodeur GM. TRK-A expression in neuroblastomas: a new prognostic marker with biological and clinical significance. J Natl Cancer Inst 1993;85:344–345.
81. Christiansen H, Christiansen NM, Wagner F, et al. Neuroblastoma: inverse relationship between expression of N-myc and NGF-r. Oncogene 1990;5:437–440.
82. Nakagawara A, Arima-Nakagawara M, Scavarda N, et al. Association between high levels of expression of the trk gene and favorable outcome in human neuroblastoma. New Engl J Med 1993;328:847–854.
83. Nisen PD, Zimmerman K, Cotter S, et al. Enhanced expression of the N-myc gene in Wilms' tumors. Cancer Res 1986;46:6217–6222.
84. Southern EM. Detection of specific sequences among DNA fragments separated by gel electorphoresis. J Mol Biol 1975;98:503–517.
85. Nathans D, Smith HO. Restriction endonucleases in the analysis and restructuring of DNA molecules. Annu Rev Biochem 1975;44:273–293.
86. Alwine JC, Kemps DJ, Stark GR. Method for detection of specific RNAs in agarose gels by transfer to diazobenzyloxymethyl-paper and hybridization with DNA probes. Proc Nat Acad Sci U S A 1977;74:5350–5354.
87. Nisen PD, Rich MA, Gloster E, et al. N-myc oncogene expression in histopathologically unrelated bilateral pediatric renal tumors. Cancer 1988;9:1821–1826.
88. Knudson AG. Mutation and cancer: statistical study of retinoblastoma. Proc Natl Acad Sci U S A 1971;68:820–824.
89. Riccardi VM, Sujansky E, Smith AC. Chromosomal imbalance in the aniridia-Wilms' Tumor association: 11p interstitial deletions. Peadiatrics 1978;61:604–610.
90. Knudson AG, Strong LC. Mutation and cancer: a model for Wilms' tumor of the kidney. J Natl Cancer Inst 1972;48:313–324.
91. Francke V, Holmes LB, Atkins L, Riccardi VM. Aniridia-Wilms' tumor association: evidence for specific deletion of 11p13. Cytogenet Cell Genet 1979;24:185–192.
92. Call KM, Glaser T, Ito Y, et al. Isolation and characterisation of a zinc finger polypeptide gene at the human chromosome 11 Wilms' tumor locus. Cell 1990;60:509–520.
93. Haber DA, Buckler AJ, Glaser T, et al. An internal deletion within an 11p13 zinc finger gene contributes to the development of Wilms' tumor. Cell 1990;61:1257–1269.
94. Cowell JK, Wadey RB, Haber DA, et al. Structural rearrangements of the WT1 gene in Wilms' tumor cells. Oncogene 1991;5:595–599.
95. Tadokoro K, Fujii H, Ohshima A, et al. Intragenic homozygous deletion of the WT1 gene in Wilms' tumor. Oncogene 1992;7:1215–1221.
96. Coppes MJ, Liefers GJ, Paul P, et al. Homozygous somatic WT1

point mutations in sporadic unilateral Wilms' tumor. Proc Natl Acad Sci U S A 1993;90:1416–1419.

97. Pelletier J, Breuning W, Kashtan CE. Germline mutations in the Wilms' tumor suppressor gene are associated with abnormal urogenital development in Denys Drash Syndrome. Cell 1991;67:437–447.

98. Breuning W, Bardeesy N, Silverman BL, et al. Germline intronic and exonic mutations in the Wilms' tumor gene (WT1) affecting urogenital development. Nature Genet 1992;1:144–148.

99. Baird PN, Santos A, Groves N, et al. Constitutional mutations in the WT1 gene in patients with Denys Drash syndrome. Hum Mol Genet 1992;1:301–305.

100. Little MH, Williamson KA, Manners M, et al. Evidence that WT1 mutations in Denys-Drash syndrome patients may act in a dominant negative fashion. Hum Mol Genet 1993;2:259–264.

101. Holmes G, Boterashvili S, English M, et al Two N-terminal self-association domains are required for the dominant negative transcriptional activity of WT1 Denys-Drash mutant proteins. Biochem Biophys Res Commun 1997;233:723–728.

102. Madden SL, Cook DM, Morris JF, et al. Transcriptional repression mediated by the WT1 Wilms' tumor gene product. Science 1991;253:1550–1553.

103. Reddy JC, Morris JC, Wang J, et al. WT1 mediated transcriptional activiation is inhibited by dominant negative mutant proteins. J Biol Chem 1995;270:10878–10884.

104. Haber DA, Sohn RL, Buckler AJ, et al. Alternative splicing and genomic structure of Wilms' tumor gene WT1. Proc Natl Acad Sci U S A 1991;86:9618–9622.

105. Drummond IA, Madden SL, Rohwer-Nutter P, et al. Repression of the insulin-like growth factor-II gene by Wilms' tumor suppressor WT1. Science 1992;257:674–678.

106. Werner H, Re GG, Drummond IA, et al. Increased expression of the insulin like growth factor 1 receptor gene, IGF1R, in Wilms' tumor is correlated with modulation of IGF1R promoter activity by the WT1 Wilms' tumor gene product. Proc Natl Acad Sci U S A 1993;90:5828–5832.

107. Wang, Madden SL, Deuel TF, Rauscher FJ III. The Wilms' tumor gene product, WT1 represses transcription of the platelet derived growth factor A-chain gene. J Biol Chem 1992;267: 21999–22002.

108. Ryan G, Steele-Perkins V, Morris JF. Repression of Pax-2 by WT-1 during normal kidney development. Development 1995;121:867–875.

109. Gruss P, Walther C. Pax in development. Cell 1992;69:719–722.

110. Keller SA, Jones JM, Boyle A, et al. Kidney and retinal defects (Krd), a transgene-induced mutation with a deletion of mouse chromosome 19 that includes the Pax2 locus. Genomic 1994;23:309–320.

111. Dressler G, Wilkinson FE, Rothenpieler U, et al. Deregulation of Pax-2 expression in transgenic mice generates severe kidney abnormilities. Nature 1993;326:65–67.

112. Rothenpieler UW, Dressler GR. Pax-2 is required for mesenchyme-to-epithelium conversion during kidney development. Development 1993;119:711–720.

113. Mcconnell MJ, Cunliffe HE, Chua LJ, et al. Differential regulation of the human Wilms'-tumor suppressor gene (WT1) promoter by two isoforms of PAX2. Oncogene 1997;14:2689–2700.

114. Dehbi M, Ghahremani M, Lechner M, et al. The paired-box transcription factor, PAX2, positively modulates expression of the Wilms' tumor suppressor gene (WT1). Oncogene 1996;13: 447–453.

115. Hewitt SM, Hamada S, McDonnell TJ, et al. Regulation of the proto-oncogenes bcl-2 and c-myc by the Wilms' tumor suppressor gene WT1. Cancer Res 1995;55:5386–5389.

116. Koseki C, Herzlinger D, Al-Awqati Q. Apoptosis in metanephric development. J Cell Biol 1992;119:1327–1333.

117. Maheswaran S, Englert C, Benett P, et al. The WT-1 gene product stabilizes p53 and inhibits p53-mediated apoptosis. Genes Dev 1995;9:2143–2156.

118. Maheswaran S, Park S, Bernard A, et al. Physical and functional interaction between WT1 and p53 proteins. Proc Natl Acad Sci U S A 1993;90:5100–5104.

119. Pritchard-Jones K, Fleming S, Davidson D, et al. The candidate Wilms' tumor gene is involved in genitourinary development. Nature 1990;346:194–197.

120. Pelletier J, Schalling M, Buckler AJ, et al. Expression of the Wilms' tumor gene, WT1 in the murine urogenital system. Genes Dev 1991;5:1345–1356.

121. Kreidberg JA, Sariola H, Loring JM, et al. WT-1 is required for early kidney development. Cell 1993;74:679–691.

122. Mannens M, Slater RM, Heyting C, et al. Molecular nature of genetic changes resulting in loss of heterozygosity of chromosome 11 in Wilms' tumor. Hum Genet 1988;81:41–48.

123. Reeve AE, Sik SA, Raizis AM, Fernberg EP. Loss of allelic heterozygosity at a second locus on chromosome 11 in sporadic Wilms' tumour cells. Mol Cell Biol 1989;9:1799–1803.

124. Koufos A, Grundy P, Morgan K, et al. Familial Wiedemann-Beckwith syndrome and a second Wilms' tumor locus both map to 11p15.5. Am J Hum Genet 1989;44:711–719.

125. Ping AJ, Reeve AE, Law DJ, et al. Genetic linkage of Beckwith-Wiedemann Syndrome to 11p15. Am J Hum Genet 1989;44: 720–723.

126. Henry I, Bonaitie-Pellie C, Chehemsse V, et al. Uniparental paternal disomy in a genetic cancer predisposing syndrome. Nature 1991;351:665–667.

127. Ohlsson R, Nystrom A, Pfeiffer-Ohlsson S, et al. IGF2 is parentally imprinted during human embryogenesis and in the Beckwith-Wiedemann syndrome. Nature Genet 1993;4:94–97.

128. Giannoukakis N, Deal C, Paquette J, et al. Parental genomic imprinting of the human IGF2 gene. Nature Genet 1993;44:98–101.

129. Reeve AE, Eccles MR, Wilkins RJ, et al. Expression of insulin-like growth factor II transcripts in Wilms' tumor. Nature 1985; 317:258–260.

130. Scott J, Cowell JK, Robertson ME, et al. Insulin like growth factor II gene expression in Wilms' tumour and embryonic tissues. Nature 1985;317:260–262.

131. Goshen R, Rachmilewitz J, Schneider T, et al. The expression of the H19 and IGF2 genes during human embryogenesis and placental development. Mol Reprod Dev 1993;34:374–379.

132. Ohlsson R, Hedborg F, Holmgren L, et al. Overlapping patterns of IGF2 and H19 expression during human development: biallelic IFG2 expression correlates with a lack of H19 expression. Development 1994;120:361–368.

133. Lustig O, Ariel I, Ilan J, et al. Expression of the imprinted gene H19 in the human fetus. Mol Reprod Dev 1994;38:239–246.

134. Moulton T, Crenshaw T, Hao Y, et al. Epigenetic lesions at the H19 locus in Wilms' tumour patients. Nature Genet 1994;7: 440–447.

135. Steenman MJC, Rainer S, Dobry CJ, et al. Loss of imprinting of IGF2 is linked to reduced expression and abnormal methylation of H19 in Wilms' tumour. Nature Genet 1994;7:433–439.

136. Maw MA, Grundy P, Millow LJ, et al. A third Wilms' tumor locus on chromosome 16q. Cancer Res 1992;52:3094–3098.

137. Rahman N, Arbour L, Tonin P, et al. Evidence for familial Wilms' tumor gene (FWT1) on chromosome 17q12-q21. Nature Genet 1996;13:461–463.

138. Grundy P, Koufos A, Morgan K, et al. Familial predisposition to Wilms' tumor does not map to the short arm of chromosome 11. Nature 1988;336:374–376.

139. Huff V, Compton DA, Chao LY, et al. Lack of linkage of familial Wilms' tumour to chromosome band 11p13. Nature 1988;336: 377–378.

140. Schwartz CE, Haber DA, Stanton VP, et al. Familial predisposition to Wilms' tuomur does not segregate with the WT1 gene. Genomics 1991;10:927–930.

141. Huff V, Amos CI, Douglass EC, et al. Evidence for genetic heterogeneity in familial Wilms' tumor. Cancer Res 1997;57: 1859–1862.

CHAPTER 10

Clinical Genetics and Heritable Disorders in Urology

Bruce R. Korf

Application of the tools of molecular genetics is rapidly changing the practice of medicine. No area of medical science will remain untouched, because genetics factors influence the development and function of all systems of the body. Although a specialty area of medical genetics has evolved to deal with clinical genetic issues, basic knowledge of genetic mechanisms and the tools of genetics is necessary for every practitioner. Physicians will increasingly be in the position to recognize disorders that have a genetic basis and to interpret genetic laboratory tests.

Genetics already has a well-established role in urology. The urinary system is subject to genetically determined congenital malformations, inborn errors of metabolism, disorders of function, and tumors. This chapter provides an introduction and approach to genetic disorders in urology, and reviews the major modes of genetic transmission; the important tools available for clinical genetics, including laboratory studies; and the principal inherited urologic disorders.

MODES OF GENETIC TRANSMISSION

The human genome consists of an estimated 80,000 genes, distributed on 23 pairs of chromosomes. Males have an X and a Y chromosome, whereas females have two X chromosomes. An individual inherits one copy of each nonsex (autosomal) chromosome from each parent and, therefore, one copy of each autosomal gene from each parent. Men transmit a Y to their sons and an X to their daughters.

Genes function by directing the production of specific proteins (Fig. 10.1). The genetic material, DNA, consists of a sequence of four bases: adenine (A), guanine (G), cytosine (C), and thymine (T). The base sequence of a particular gene is copied in the nucleus as messenger RNA (mRNA), which is then translated in the cytoplasm into a protein. The order of amino acids assembled into the protein is determined by the base sequence; each amino acid is encoded by a triplet of bases.

The basis for genetic variation, including genetic disease, is the occurrence of differences in DNA sequences between individual copies of a particular gene. An individual may have two identical copies (alleles) of a gene at a specific DNA locus (be the homozygous state) or may have copies that differ in their base sequences (the heterozygous state). Some of the differences in base sequences do not greatly affected the function of the gene and may be polymorphisms, variations in base sequences that are relatively common in the population. Other times, the changes may alter gene expression, thereby producing a visible (phenotypic) change the organism. Between the two copies of a gene in an individual, the effects of one may prevail over the other: The copy that is expressed is said to be dominant; the other is recessive.

The two major modes of single-gene transmission are dominant and recessive; and patterns of transmission differ, depending on whether the gene is autosomal or located on a sex chromosome (the X or Y). A dominant trait is expressed in the heterozygous state. An affected individual has one copy of the mutant gene and transmits the gene, on average, to 50% of his or her offspring (Fig. 10.2). For an autosomal trait, males and females may be affected equally and may transmit the trait to sons or daughters. In some individuals, the mutant dominant allele may not be expressed, which is referred to as nonpenetrance. Also, the degree of phenotypic expression may vary from person to person in the population. Penetrance is sometimes age dependent, in which case the likelihood of phenotypic expression increases with age. This is seen, for example, in adult polycystic kidney disease.

In contrast, a recessive trait is expressed only in the homozygous state (Fig. 10.3). This requires that both parents at least be carriers of the trait, i.e., are heterozy-

171

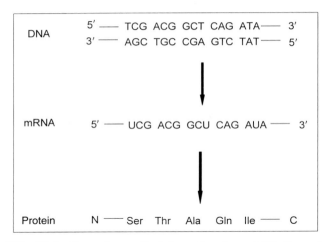

FIG. 10.1. Flow of genetic information from DNA through RNA to protein. Modified from Korf BR. Human genetics: a problem-based approach. Blackwell Science, 1996.

gous for the mutant gene. Carriers will not manifest the trait themselves, but when both partners are carriers there is 25% risk that each offspring will be homozygous for the disorder. For rare autosomal recessive traits, the likelihood that both partners will carry the same mutant

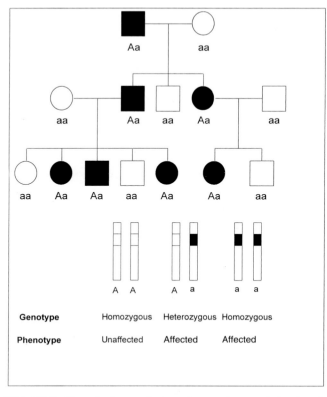

FIG. 10.2. Genetic transmission of an autosomal dominant gene. □, male; ○, female; *solid symbol,* affected; *A,* dominant allele; *a,* recessive allele. Modified from Korf BR. Human genetics: a problem-based approach. Blackwell Science, 1996.

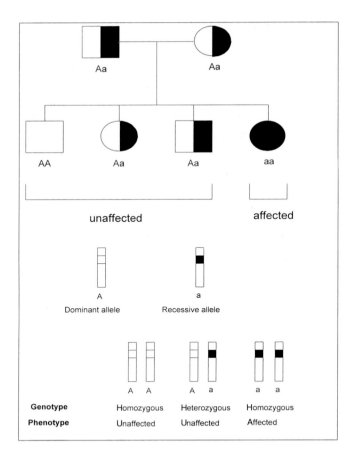

FIG. 10.3. Genetic transmission of an autosomal recessive gene. *Half-solid symbol,* unaffected carrier.

allele is increased if they have a common ancestor, i.e., they are consanguineous. On the other hand, not all consanguineous couples have children with recessive disorders, and not all recessive disorders occur among offspring of consanguineous couples. A child with a recessive disorder owing to consanguinity will have two identical mutant copies of the gene, derived from the common ancestor. Molecular genetic studies have shown, however, that most genetic disorders result from a variety of types of changes in the same gene, each disrupting function, albeit in a different way. Often, therefore, a person with a recessive disorder will have two different mutant alleles, one inherited from each parent. This is referred to as compound heterozygosity (Fig. 10.4).

The principles of dominant and recessive transmission also apply to sex-linked genes, but the patterns of transmission are distinctive (Fig. 10.5). An X-linked recessive trait is most likely to be expressed in a male, who has only one X chromosome (hemizygous). On average, a carrier female passes the gene to half her offspring; of these, the sons express the trait and the daughters become carriers. There is no male-to-male transmission because a father passes only a Y chromosome to his

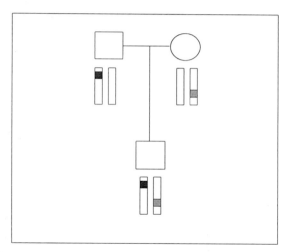

FIG. 10.4. For an individual to have compound heterozygosity, the parents must be heterozygous for a different mutation at the same DNA locus. Although the offspring has a mutation of both alleles, the two mutations are different.

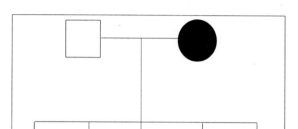

FIG. 10.6. Genetic transmission of an X-linked lethal dominant gene. Modified from Korf BR. Human genetics: a problem-based approach. Blackwell Science, 1996.

sons. Only rarely will females be homozygous, assuming that the trait itself is rare.

In contrast, an X-linked dominant trait will be expressed in both heterozygous females and hemizygous males. There is no male-to-male transmission, but the male will pass the trait to all of his daughters. Some X-linked dominant traits are lethal in the hemizygous state (Fig. 10.6). Only females are affected; males who inherit such a mutant gene are miscarried early in fetal development.

There is another source of genetic information in the cell that may also be responsible for genetic disease. This is the mitochondria, each of which contains multiple copies of a 16.5 thousand base pair circular DNA

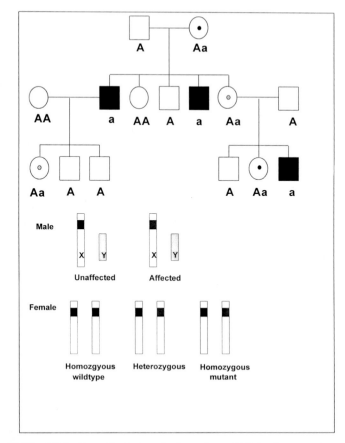

FIG. 10.5. Genetic transmission of an X-linked recessive gene. Modified from Korf BR. Human genetics: a problem-based approach. Blackwell Science, 1996.

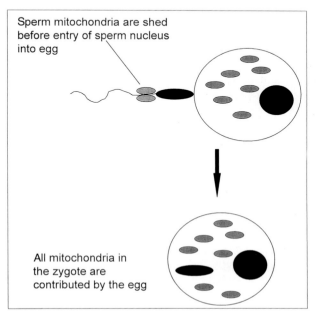

FIG. 10.7. All mitochondria in the zygote are contributed by the oocyte. Thus all mitochondrial traits are maternally inherited. Modified from Korf BR. Human genetics: a problem-based approach. Blackwell Science, 1996.

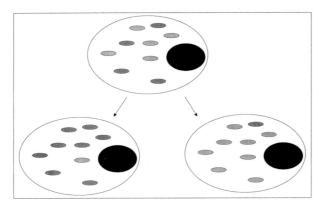

FIG. 10.8. Mutant mitochondria (*dark ovals*) and wild-type mitochondria (*light ovals*) segregate randomly and may co-exist within the same cell. Modified from Korf BR. Human genetics: a problem-based approach. Blackwell Science, 1996.

molecule. This DNA encodes 13 subunits of mitochondrial proteins involved in energy metabolism along with transfer RNA (tRNA) and ribosomal RNA (rRNA) needed for protein synthesis.[1] Genes in the cell nucleus, however, encode most mitochondrial proteins.

The entire complement of mitochondrial DNA is passed via the egg cell; the sperm sheds its mitochondria on fertilization. Thus mitochondrial traits display a pattern of maternal transmission: The mother passes her mitochondria to all her offspring, but the father does not pass on any (Fig. 10.7). Because each cell contains multiple mitochondria, each with multiple copies of mitochondrial DNA, an individual with a mitochondrial mutation generally has a mixture of mutant and normal mitochondria in each cell (heteroplasmy) (Fig. 10.8). Because mitochondria segregate passively on cell division, the proportion of mutant to normal mitochondria in a daughter cell is random. Cells with a high proportion of mutant mitochondria fail to metabolize energy. The list of disorders caused by mitochondria mutations is growing (Table 10.1). Generally these disorders are characterized by the failure of structures that depend heavily on oxidative phosphorylation, especially the brain and muscle.

Most of the genetic traits described so far are relatively rare, although collectively they contribute significantly to human pathology. Genetic factors also influence more common traits, such as hypertension and cancer, but do so in a subtler manner. Most common traits are the result of a complex interaction between multiple genes and environmental factors (multifactional inheritance). Such traits tend to cluster in families but usually do not display simple patterns of transmission. Multifactorial traits must also be considered in sporadic congenital malformations. Counseling in such instances is usually empirical. Indentification of the genes involved in multifactorial inheritance is a major challenge and is part of the ongoing effort to characterize the human genome. This area promises to have the largest affect on the population, as the genetic basis of common disorders comes to light.

APPROACH TO MEDICAL GENETIC PROBLEMS

Family History

The most important tool in genetic diagnosis is readily available to every clinician: the family history. Even if more complex genetic issues are referred to specially trained individuals, such referral occurs only if the clinician is aware of a family history of similar problems or of the potential for genetic transmission. Questions about the family history should be part of every medical history, and a pedigree should be constructed. These measures can lead to identification of the pattern of transmisson, although the expression of traits may vary among members of a family. Furthermore, family members may not reveal important information unless they are directly questioned. Often it is necessary to obtain

TABLE 10.1. *Disorders associated with mitochondrial dysfunction*

Disorder	Features	Type of mutation
Kearns–Sayre syndrome	Ophthalmoplegia, heart block, high cerebrospinal fluid protein	Deletion of mitochondrial DNA
Mitochondrial myopathy, encephalopathy, lactic acidosis, and stroke-like episodes		Mitochondrial point mutations in tRNA
Myoclonus epilepsy associated with ragged-red fibers	Encephalopathy	Mitochondrial point mutations in tRNA
Leber hereditary optic neuropathy	Sudden loss of central vision	Various mitochondrial point mutations
Leigh disease	Encephalopathy, brainstem dysfunction	Various mitochondrial or nuclear gene mutations
Myopathy–hypertrophic cardiomyopathy	Muscle weakness	Various mitochondrial point mutations
Infantile encephalopathy	Lethal	Mitochondrial point mutations

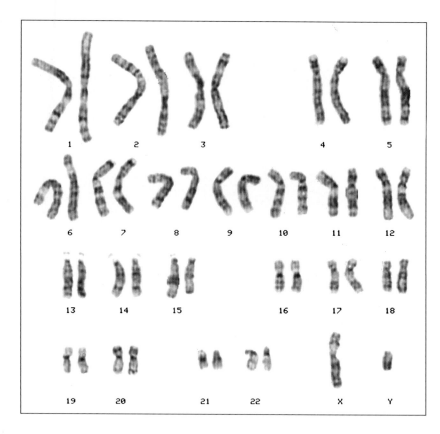

FIG. 10.9. The normal male karyotype. Reprinted with permission from B-L Wu, Brigham and Women's Hospital, Children's Hospital, and Massachusetts General Hospital Cytogenetics Laboratory.

medical records to better document the medical history of a relative.

Cytogenetics

The ability to examine the structure of chromosomes is the oldest laboratory test available for genetic analysis. Usually, chromosomes are examined in dividing cells obtained from peripheral blood lymphocytes, although cultured fibroblasts or fetal cells may also be used. It is standard to stain chromosomes, which elicits banding patterns that enable each chromosome to be identified and arranged as a Karyotype (Fig. 10.9). In this way, major abnormalities of chromosome number or structure can be identified.

Numerical anomalies are the most obvious problems and were the first to be characterized. The most common liveborn autosomal mumerical anomalies are the trisomies (Table 10.2): 21 (Down syndrome), 13 (Patau syndrome), and 18 (Edwards syndrome). Sex chromosome aneuploidies include monosomy X (Turner syndrome), XXY (Klinefelter syndrome), XXX, and XYY. Other chromosome changes include deletions, duplications, inversions, and translocations. The latter involve exchanges of genetic material between two or more chromosomes. If no material is lost or gained, the translocation is said to be balanced and may be phenotypically silent. A balanced carrier, however, faces a risk

of transmission of unbalanced chromosomes to an offspring.

Chromosomal analysis in indicated in any child with two or more unrelated congenital anomalies or who has a clinical recognized chromosomal syndrome. It should also be offered to couples who have experience two or more first-trimester miscarriages to look for a balanced translocation or inversion (Table 10.3).

Classical chromosome analysis reveals both numerical anomalies and relatively large structural re-

TABLE 10.2. *Chromosomal abnormalities compatible with live birth*

Syndrome	Chromosome abnormality	Urologic features
Wolf–Hirschhorn	Deletion of 4p	Hypospadias, renal anomalies
Cri du chat	Deletion of 5p	Renal anomalies
Trisomy 8	Mosaic trisomy 8	Cryptorchidism
Trisomy 9p	Trisomy 9p	Rare
Patau	Trisomy 13	Polycystic kidneys
Edwards	Trisomy 18	Ectopic kidney, hydronephrosis
Down	Trisomy 21	Rare
Klinefelter	47, XXY	Testicular atrophy
Turner	45,X	Ovarian dysgenesis
Triple X	47,XXX	None
XYY	47,XYY	None

TABLE 10.3. *Indications for chromosomal analysis*

• Recognized chromosomal syndrome
• Two or more apparently unrelated congenital anomalies
• Unexplained mental retardation
• Family history of chromosome rearrangement
• Two or more unexplained miscarriages

arrangements, but recently techniques have been developed to reveal more subtle changes. The principal approach is fluorescence in situ hybridization (FISH), which employs samples of cloned DNA labeled with a fluorescent tag (Fig. 10.10). Single-stranded cloned DNA is hybridized with chromosomal DNA on a microscope slide. The probe DNA binds to its homologous sequence on the chromosome and can be visualized under a fluorescence microscope. This technique is used to help identify rearranged chromosomes and has been instrumental in the identification of small deletions (Fig. 10.11). Recently, submicroscopic deletions have been associated with several syndromes (Table 10.4).[2] These disorders are easily detected by FISH but are usually missed via routine chromosomal analysis.

Molecular Genetics

The ability to isolate individual genes to study their structure has revolutionized the approach to human genetics. It is expected that the entire human genome will have been mapped and genes identified during the first decade of the twentieth century, having an enormous effect on medical practice. The identification of a gene responsible for a genetic disorder leads to improved means of diagnosis and provides insights into the pathogenesis, which may result in new means of therapy.

Molecular diagnostic tests may be performed either by direct detection of a gene mutation or by genetic

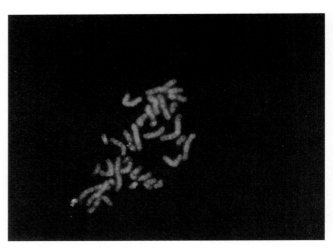

FIG. 10.11. FISH was used to identify a deletion of chromosome 22 involved in velocardiofacial (VCF) syndrome. The normal chromosome 22 lights up with two separate probes, one in the VCF region and one in the control region. A chromosome with a deletion should light up with only the control probe. Reprinted with permission from S Weremowicz, Brigham and Women's Hospital, Children's Hospital, and Massachusetts General Hospital Cytogenetics Laboratory.

linkage analysis.[3,4] Before a mutation can be directly discovered, the gene must be cloned and the pathogenic mutation must be detectable. A linkage study involves tracking the mutation through a family using a genetic marker that is near the gene of interest. The study can be done before the gene is cloned; but unlike direct mutation analysis, it requires a family study.

The technique used for direct mutation analysis depends on the specific gene. In some cases only one or very few mutations account for all affected individuals. This is the case, for example, with sickle-cell anemia, which lends itself to relatively straightforward testing. In other cases, for example, custic fibrosis, a variety of mutations can occur, and multiple tests must be performed to detect pathogenic changes. Finally, in some instances, a wide diversity of mutations may occur in different affected individuals, making routine diagnostic testing difficult. More efficient mutation screening strategies for these cases must be developed.

Genetic linkage strategies are based on the use of polymorphic marker genes that are located near the gene of interest. Such polymorphisms consist of phenotypically silent sequence variants that are common in the population. The basic approach is illustrated in Fig. 10.12. In the figure, the father in generation II is affected with dominant disorder. He inherited the mutant gene from his mother along with the A allele of the marker gene. His partner is homozygous for the B marker allele. His children who inherit A also inherit the disorder, and those who inherit B are unaffected. The exceptions are children whose DNA underwent genetic recombination, allowing them to inherit A with the nonmutant

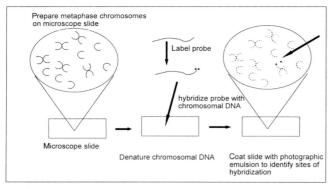

FIG. 10.10. For the FISH technique, DNA from chromosomes in metaphase is fixed on a glass slide, denatured into single strands, and reacted with fluorescently labeled single-stranded probe DNA. Modified from Korf BR. Human genetics: a problem-based approach. Blackwell Science, 1996.

TABLE 10.4. *Syndromes associated with microdeletions*

Syndrome	Features	Chromosome region
Williams	Characteristic facies, supravalvar aortic stenosis, developmental impairment	7q11.23
Langer–Giedion	Exostoes, abnormal facies, developmental delay	8q24.1
Wilms tumor, aniridia, genitourinary abnormalities, and mental retardation (WAGR)		11p13
Retinoblastoma and mental retardation		13q14
Prader–Willi	Hypotonia, developmental delay, obesity	15q12
Angelman	Seizures, abnormal movements, mental retardation	15q12
α-Thalassemia and mental retardation		16p13.3
Rubinstein–Taybi	Microcephaly, characteristic facies, mental retardation	16p13.3
Smith–Magenis	Mental retardation, characteristic facies	17p11.2
Miller–Dieker	Lissencephaly, characteristic facies	17p13.3
Hereditary susceptibility to pressure palsies	Peripheral neuropathy	17p12
Alagille	Intrahepatic biliary atresia, peripheral pulmonic stenosis, characteristic facies	20p11.23
DiGeorge and velocardiofacial	Palatal anomalies, contruncal cardiac anomalies, thymic hypoplasia, parathyroid hypoplasia	22q11.2
Steroid sulfatase deficiency and Kallman	Ichthyosis, anosmia	Xp22.3

gene or vice versa. Although this may lead to a diagnostic error, the probability of recombination can be measured in a genetic linkage study. This provides an estimate of the accuracy of a linkage-based diagnosis. The occurrence of genetic recombination can also be detected if markers that flank the gene of interest are used.

Molecular diagnostic techniques can help confirm a suspected genetic diagnosis or provide prenatal or presymptomatic diagnosis. Diagnosis must be accompanied by genetic counseling that explains the disorder, its natural history and risks, and the available options. Presymptomatic tests must be offered with sensitivity to the risks, including psychological damage, stigmatization, and discrimination.

Molecular studies have revealed a remarkable diversity of types of mutations and some unexpected biologic phenomena. Researchers have identified a growing number of genes that include stretches of trinucleotides repeated up to fifty times; the exact number of repeats is polymorphic (Fig. 10.13). Gross expansion of the repeat number results in clinically important phenotypes, such as fragile X syndrome and Huntington disease.[5]

Sometimes the maternal and paternal contribution of a gene are not equally expressed. Such genes are termed imprinted. Deletion of a gene derived from the parent

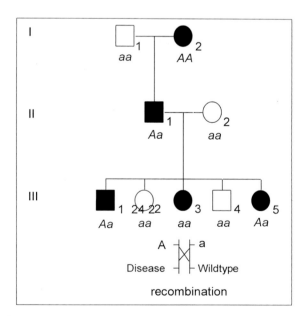

FIG. 10.12. A genetic linkage study can help diagnose a dominant disorder. A marker gene with two alleles (A and a) is closely linked to the disease gene. See text for details. Modified from Korf BR. Human genetics: a problem-based approach. Blackwell Science, 1996.

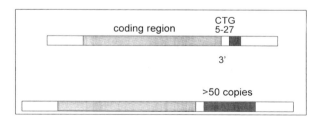

FIG. 10.13. Note the stretch of 5 to 17 copies of the CGT triplet in the 3' untranslated region of the gene (*top*). Expansion of this region, sometimes to hundreds of repeats, underlies myotonic dystrophy (*bottom*). Modified from Korf BR. Human genetics: a problem-based approach. Blackwell Science, 1996.

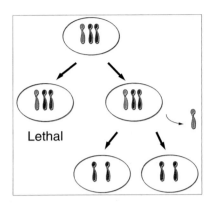

FIG. 10.14. Generation of uniparental disomy by loss of a chromosome from a trisomic embryo. The trisomic cell line dies off, but the disomic cell line has both copies of the chromosome (derived from a single parent). Modified from Korf BR. Human genetics: a problem-based approach. Blackwell Science, 1996.

whose copy is expressed will produce an abnormal phenotype. For example, Prader–Willi syndrome Angelman syndrome are both associated with deletions of part of chromosome 15 (Table 10.4). Deletions responsible for Prader–Willi syndrome are of paternal origin, whereas those responsible for Angelman syndrome are of maternal origin. In some instances, instead of a deletion, two copies of chromosome 15 may be inherited from the same parent if (uniparental disomy) (Fig. 10.14). If the two copies are maternal from the mother, the individual has Prader–Willi; if they are from the father, the individual has Angelman syndrome. Several other imprinted regions have been identified (Table 10.5), although uniparental disomy for nonimprinted regions may have no clinical effect.[7]

Prenatal Diagnosis

A number of approaches have been developed for detecting congenital anomalies and genetic disorders prenatally. Ultrasound can be used to identify some congenital malformations, including those of the kidneys, ureters, bladder, and genitalia. High-resolution studies can be done in the second and third trimesters

TABLE 10.5. *Chromosome regions associated with genomic imprinting*

Chromosome band	Clinical effects
15q12	Prader–Willi or Angelman syndrome
11p	Beckwith–Wiedemann syndrome
7q	Short stature (Russell–Silver syndrome)
14	Short stature, developmental delay

and may prompt genetic diagnosis, planning for the birth of a child with complex needs, and even fetal therapy.

Prenatal genetic testing requires access to fetal tissue, which is usually obtained between 10 and 12 weeks of gestation by chorionic villus biopsy or between 16 and 18 weeks by amniocentesis (Table 10.6). In some centers, early amniocentesis is done at 11 or 12 weeks. Chorionic villus biopsy offers an earlier diagnosis than amniocentesis but is associated with a slightly higher risk of complications (1 versus 0.5%). Fetal tissue obtained by either approach can be used for chromosomal analysis, biochemical testing, and molecular diagnosis.

Indications for prenatal testing include a family history of a genetic disorder or advanced maternal age (defined as ≥35 years) (Table 10.7). The latter is owing to a maternal age-related risk of chromosomal trisomy. Increasingly, screening tests are being offered that, if positive, prompt chorionic vilus sampling or amniocentesis. Such tests include ultrasound and maternal serum screening for α-fetoprotein, human chorionic gonadotrophin, and unconjugated estriol. High α-fetoprotein levels may indicate an open neural tube defect or other congenital anomaly. These tests can also detect trisomy 21 and 18. Couples should be informed about the availability of screening tests for autosomal recessive disorders that may be prevalent in their ethnic population—such as Tay–Sachs disease and hemoglobin disorders (e.g., sickle-cell and thalassemia)—and for other relatively common disorders—such as cystic fibrosis (Table 10.8).

Genetic Counseling

Parents of a fetus identified with a genetic disorder should be offered counseling. Genetic counseling explains the natural history of the genetic disorder; describes its mode of genetic transmission; outlines options, including treatment and termination of pregnancy; helps with the adjustment to the decisions that are made. Medical professionals with special training in clinical genetics include physicians who are certified by the American Board of Medical Genetics and genetic counselors who are certified by the American Board of Genetic Counseling. Expertise in genetic disorders should be available at all major medical centers, although recognition of the need for referral always rests with the physician who is caring for the patient.

GENETIC DISORDERS AFFECTING THE GENITOURINARY SYSTEM

This section provides an overview of the major classes of genetic diseases that are of urologic interest.

Congenital Anomalies

Congenital anomalies of the urogenital system are common components of multiple congenital anomaly

TABLE 10.6. *Approaches to sampling fetal tissue for genetic diagnosis*

Procedure	Approach	Timing, weeks of gestation	Benefits	Risk of miscarriage
Chorionic villus biopsy	Transcervical or transabdominal biopsy of the placenta	10–12	Early diagnosis	1%
Amniocentesis	Transabdominal sampling of amniotic fluid	16–18	Safe; large experience	0.5%
Peripheral umbilical blood sampling	Sampling of the fetal umbilical vein	After 18	Rapid cytogenetic diagnosis later in pregnancy	1–2%

syndromes, including chromosomal, single-gene, and multifactorial disorders. Dysplastic or absent kidneys can occur as an autosomal dominant[8] or recessive trait, sporadically as a multifactorial trait, or as part of associations—such as vetebral defects, imperforateanus, tracheosophageal fistula, and radial and renal dysplasia (VATER) and Müllerian duct, unilateral renal agenesis, and anomalies of the cervicothoracic somites (MURCS). Ureteral anomalies and obstructive uropathy may also be involved. Ectopic kidney or horseshoe kidney often occurs with other congenital anomalies and is sometimes genetically determined. A child born with renal agenesis or dysplasia should be carefully examined for signs of other congenital anomalies; if the renal anomaly appears to be sporadic, both parents should be examined by ultrasound to explore the possibility of an autosomal dominant trait. Vesicoureteral reflux may be inherited as an autosomal dominant trait or may be multifactorial. There is evidence for linkage of a locus for vesicoureteral reflux to the HLA region on chromosome 6 in some families[9] and to the *pax2* gene in others.[10]

Hypoplasia of the bladder occurs along with renal disorders that result in decreased urine output. Bladder agenesis is a component of sirenomelia. Bladder diverticula may be seen in individuals with connective tissue disorders, such as cutis laxa and Ehler–Danlos syndrome. Distension of the bladder may be caused by posterior urethral valves, which can be a component of multiple congenital anomaly syndromes or occur sporadically as a multifactorial trait. Congenital anomalies of the external genitalia can reflect a combination of genetic and/or hormonal origins. Hypospadias are usually multifactorial traits but may be part of an X-linked recessive androgen insensitivity syndrome.

Polycystic kidney may be inherited as either an autosomal dominant or a recessive trait. A gene on chromosome 16 (*pkd1*) accounts for > 90% of the autosomal-dominant inheritance,[11] and a gene (*pkd2*) on chromosome 4 accounts for most of the balance (although rare families may have a trait that does not map to either site).[12] The *pkd1* gene has been cloned;[13] it codes for a protein referred to as polycystin.

Disorders of Function

Functional disorders include renal tubular defects and glomerulonephropathies. The former encompass a group of entities characterized by defective renal tubular absorption of either glucose, specific amino acids (cystine, neutral amino acids, imioamino acids, glycine, dicarboxylic amino acids), phosphate, or bicarbonate. The mitochondrial disorders lead to generalized failure of tubular reabsorption and hence renal Fanconi syndrome.[13] Inherited glomerulopathies include Alport syndrome and congenital nephrosis. Alport syndrome is genetically heterogeneous, with both X-linked and autosomal forms. The gene *col4A1* codes for a collagen subunit and has been implicated in the X-linked form.[14] Congenital nephrosis is a rare autosomal recessive trait most common in Finland.

TABLE 10.7. *Common indications for prenatal genetic diagnosis*

- Advanced maternal age (≥35 years at delivery)
- Previous history of child with chromosomal abnormality
- Known carrier of balanced chromosome rearrangement
- Known carrier of single-gene genetic disorder
- Evidence of fetal anomaly by ultrasound
- Abnormal maternal biochemical screen results

TABLE 10.8. *Disorders for which carrier screening is commonly offered*

Disorder	Screening method	Target populations
Tay–Sachs disease	Enzyme analysis	Ashkenazi Jews, French Canadians
Canavan disease	DNA	Ashkenazi Jews
Cystic fibrosis	DNA	All (especially whites)
Sickle-cell anemia	Hematological	Blacks
Thalassemia	Hematological	Mediterraneans, Africans, Asians
Gaucher	DNA	Ashkenazi Jews

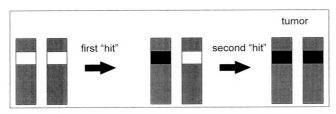

FIG. 10.15. Mutation of both copies of the *WT1* tumor-suppressor gene leads to Wilms tumor. This occurs through successive hits, in which first one copy is mutated and then the other is. Modified from Korf BR. Human genetics: a problem-based approach. Blackwell Science, 1996.

Tumors

Wilms tumor is an embryonal tumor of the kidney and represents one of the paradigms of the tumor-suppressor mechanism of oncogenesis. The responsible gene, designated *WT1*,[15] has been mapped to band 11p initially on the basis of rare individuals with Wilms tumor, aniridia, genitourinary anomalies, and mental retardation (WAGR) who had cytogenetically visible deletions of band 11p. Loss of the wild-type allele was demonstrated in Wilms tumors, establishing that the gene functions as a tumor suppressor, in which loss of both copies of the mutant gene underlies oncogenesis (Fig. 10.15). A heterozygous mutation for *WT1* underlies (Denys–Drash syndrome, which includes diffuse mesangial sclerosis of the kidney, Wilms tumor, and male pseudohermaphroditism.[16] Wilms tumor has also been seen as a manifestation of syndromes of congenital overgrowth, including Beckwith–Wiedemann syndrome and hemihypertrophy. Children with these disorders should be screened for Wilms tumor and hepatoblastoma by regular ultrasound study and measurement of serum α-fetoprotein levels. Renal cell carcinoma can occur either sporadically or as a component of inherited disorders such as von Hippel–Lindau syndrome and tuberous sclerosis.

SUMMARY

Genetic disorders of the genitourinary system are important and common causes of genitourinary dysfunc-

tion. Molecular genetic studies have disclosed the pathogenesis of many single-gene disorders and will likely reveal the basis for multifactorial disorders as well. It will be increasingly important for the urologist to recognize the genetic contribution to these disorders and to obtain appropriate genetic tests and refer families for genetic counseling.

REFERENCES

1. Johns DR. Seminars in medicine of the Beth Israel Hospital, Boston—mitochondrial DNA and disease. N Engl J Med 1995;333:638–644.
2. Schmickel RD. Contiguous gene syndromes: a component of recognizable syndromes. J Pediatr 1986;109:231–241.
3. Korf B. Molecular diagnosis (first of two parts). N Engl J Med 1995;332:1218–1220.
4. Korf B. Molecular diagnosis (second of two parts). N Engl J Med 1995;332:1499–1502.
5. Warren ST. The expanding world of triplet repeats. Science 1996;271:1374–1375.
6. Hall JG. Genomic imprinting: Review and relevance to human disease. Am J Hum Genet 1990;46:857–873.
7. Ledbetter DH, Engel E. Uniparental disomy in humans: development of an imprinting map and its implications for prenatal diagnosis. Hum Mol Genet 1995;4:1757–1764.
8. McPherson E, Carey J, Kramer A, et al. Dominantly inherited renal adysplasia. Am J Med Genet 1987;26:863–872.
9. Izquirdo L, Porteous M, Paramo PG, Connor JM. Evidence for genetic heterogeneity in hereditary hydronephrosis caused by pelvioureteric junction obstruction, with one locus assigned to chromosome 6p. Hum Genet 1992;89:557–560.
10. Sanyanusin P, Schimmenti LA, McNoe LA, et al. Mutation of the PAX2 gene in a family with optic nerve colobomas, renal anomalies and vesicoureteral reflux. Nature Genet 1995;9:358–363.
11. Reeders ST, Breuning MH, Davies KE, et al. A highly polymorphic DNA marker linked to adult polycystic kidney disease on chromosome 16. Nature 1985;317:542–544.
12. Peters DJM, Spruit L, Saris JJ, et al. Chromosome 4 localization of a second gene for autosomal dominant polycystic kidney disease. Nature Genet 1993;5:359–362.
13. Internat Polycystic Kidney Dis Consort Polycystic kidney disease: The complete structure of the PKD1 gene and its protein. Cell 1995;81:289–298.
14. Barker DF, Hostikka SL, Zhou J, et al. Identification of mutations in the COL4A5 collagen gene in Alport syndrome. Science 1990;248:1224–1227.
15. Pritchard-Jones K, Fleming S, Davidson D, et al. The candidate Wilms' tumour gene is involved in genitourinary development. Nature 1990;346:194–197.
16. Pelletier J, Bruening W, Kashtan CE, et al. Germline mutations in the Wilms' tumor suppressor gene are associated with abnormal urogenital development in the Denys-Drash syndrome. Cell 1991;67:437–447.

CHAPTER 11

Ureteropelvic Junction Obstruction

George F. Steinhardt

It seems ironical that a condition whose causation remains unclear should be so well documented in terms of investigation, diagnosis, and surgery and that its treatment should be so successful.

—P. H. O'Reilly

Although the level of the upper ureter and renal pelvis is the most common site for a congenital genitourinary obstruction, meaningful surgical intervention was not routinely possible before the development of reliable imaging techniques. Nevertheless, early surgeons did encounter hydronephrotic kidneys during renal explorations. Trendelenburg, who worked in the late 1800s, is given credit for the first reconstruction of an obstructed kidney (the patient died from a colonic perforation), because most of the early ureteropelvic junction (UPJ) obstructions were treated with simple nephrectomy.[1] By 1890, adequate experience had been gained to provide enough material for discussion of the pathologic anatomy, successful reconstructive techniques, and assessment of surgical success.[2] Most early repairs relied on simple Heineke–Mikilutz type maneuvers (popularized by Fenger[3]) that caused a longitudinal incision through the narrow segment to be closed in a horizontal fashion. Early illustrations show sutures pulling the renal pelvis together without any attempt to close the pelvis to the ureter in a mucosal–mucosal fashion (Fig. 11.1).

Nephropexy was the most common renal operation in the early part of the twentieth century, because ptotic kidneys were thought to cause many constitutional symptoms besides pain. The lack of imaging techniques no doubt resulted in many early surgeons finding obstructed and hydronephrotic kidneys at the time of exploration in patients presenting with flank pain. Regardless, it is likely that suppuration and pyonephrosis were the most common surgical findings associated with UPJ obstructions, because early surgeons had as their only tools urinalysis (from both voided and ureteral catheter specimens) and the physical examination to guide them.

After Roentgen's 1894 discovery of x-rays and Voelcker and von Lictenberg's development of radiopaque silver colloid contrast in 1906, routine demonstration of normal and pathologic urologic anatomy with retrograde pyelography became possible and then commonplace. The development of retrograde pyelography in the first two decades of the twentieth century and then intravenous pyelography (developed by Swick) in 1929 allowed urologic surgeons to more accurately delineate the pathologic anatomy before surgery.[4] With this information and improved surgical techniques, the knowledge of obstruction progressed from anecdotal experience to a systematic appraisal of surgical indications, techniques, and outcomes. Ormond[5] noted that, although successful repair of obstructed kidneys was more common than poor outcome, failure occasionally meant death or almost certain lifelong disability.

In 1891 Kuster successfully repaired a UPJ obstruction by ligating the renal pelvis below the obstruction and transposing the upper ureter to the renal pelvis with a side-to-side anastomosis. Nevertheless, most early surgeons were reluctant to completely separate the ureter from the pelvis, and most early repairs used maneuvers that left at least part of the narrowed ureter intact. In 1936, Foley[6] described the results of 20 pyeloplasties (with only 2 deaths) using a Y repair. In 1946, Anderson and Hynes[7] published their experience with an operation that required complete transection of the upper ureter, subsequent spatulation of the ureter, and trimming of the redundant pelvis. Although their operation was initially done to treat ureteral obstructions deriving from a retrocaval ureter, the principle of transection and reanastomosis has worked well for UPJ obstruction. This step foward defined the highly successful technique most commonly used today to repair this lesion.

Although the second half of the twentieth century has seen no treatment technique as effective as the Anderson–Hynes pyeloplasty, there has been an explosion of information relating directly to the pathogenesis and diagnosis of UPJ obstruction. Newer endoscopic treatments are not yet as effective as open techniques (at least in children) but promise to make the treatment of this interesting lesion a topic of continuing interest and excitement.

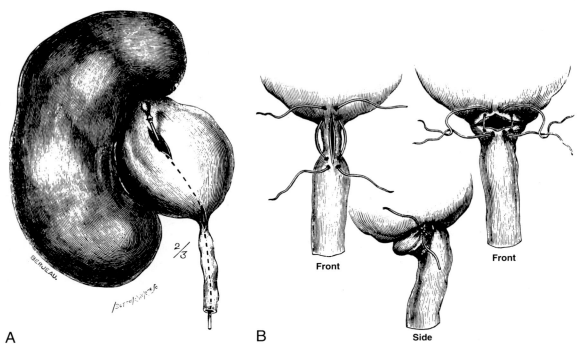

FIG. 11.1. Early depiction of a pyeloplasty using a Heineke–Mikilutz repair without mucosal–mucosal approximation. **A,** The probe is placed through the UPJ to facilitate the incision. **B,** Approximating sutures of fine silk are used to draw the edges together. Reprinted with permission from Morris H. On the origin and progress of renal surgery. Philadelphia: Blakiston's, 1989.

EMBRYOLOGY

The ureter branches off the Wolffian duct quite early in embryonic development, inducing the development of the metanephric blastema. Classic embryologists attributed the narrowing to extrinsic compression by adjacent vascular structures.[8] A detailed study of human embryos between 5 and 23 mm (vertex–coccyx length) with a gestational age of 28 to 41 days demonstrated a normal process in the ureter of luminal obstruction and subsequent recanalization. By 6 weeks of gestation, this process is generally complete.[9] Using ultrastructural techniques, later workers confirmed the obstruction of the developing ureter after a period of patency and the subsequent recanalization before the metanephric production of urine.[10]

The recanalization process is discontinuous and multicentric. Circumferential muscularization of the ureter occurs with continued remodeling of smooth muscle fibers from a predominantly circular pattern in the newborn to the adult pattern. In the adult, the closely packed muscle bundles are oriented obliquely, and there are many fiber crossings (oblique mesh).[11] Kidneys with UPJ obstruction demonstrate disarrayed fibers and an absolute decrease in smooth muscle fibers at the apparent location of the obstruction. Fibrosis, although seen, is not invariably present. Using a rabbit model, Cheng et al.[12] demonstrated that experimentally induced UPJ obstruction in the neonate resulted in increases in lamina muscularis thickness and in the collagen:smooth muscle ratio. They found that reversal of the experimental partial obstruction normalized the ratio.

Issues of cellular differentiation are central in the biologic sciences, and investigators worldwide are increasingly able to probe the mysteries of development with molecular biologic tools. Growth factors are protein kinases present in fetal tissue that stimulate various cellular processes that ultimately control development. No unified-picture of renal or ureteral development has emerged from this research; but as each growth factor is studied in turn, researchers obtain more glimpses of the possible pathways by which normal ureteral and renal growth are controlled. Wang et al.[13] investigated the pathophysiology of UPJ obstruction with both immunohistochemistry and reverse transcription–polymerase chain reaction techniques. They found that specific antibodies to the markers of normal neuronal development PGP 9.5 (a general neuronal marker), S100 (a nerve supporting cell marker), synaptophysin (a synapse vesical marker), and nerve growth factor receptor were all decreased within the muscle bundles in ureteropelvic junctions removed at surgery for symptomatic obstruction. The authors concluded that defective innervation with diminished synaptive vesical expression may be a major factor in the development of obstruction in the involved kidneys.

Dressler et al.[14] showed that one of the earliest genes activated in the kidney mesenchyme upon induction by the ureteric bud is transcription factor *Pax-2*. The *Pax* genes encode important developmental regulatory proteins that are expressed coincidentally with early epithelial differentiation and proliferation. Other researchers have shown various roles for oncogenes, such as *c-ret* and *kdn-1* and *wt1* in the development of normal kidney. It seems likely that the pathologically narrowed upper ureter commonly found at the time of pyeloplasty will be shown to be the result of a perturbation in the prenatal cascade of growth factors, transcription factors, and other gene products necessary for normal development. Indeed, when assessed for transforming growth factor β (TGF-β), upper ureters from pyeloplasty specimens are found to have increased activity and the upregulation of this growth factor. This may account for the hypertrophic smooth muscle growth deposition typically seen in the obstructed renal pelvis.[15] Stimulation of one growth factor is not likely to be the ultimate explanation for kidney obstruction; nevertheless, it is this type of inquiry that will explain the occurrence of UPJ obstruction within the next few years.

ANATOMY

Probably, no surgical lesion is more straightforward than the obstruction found at the junction of the upper ureter and the renal pelvis. The lesion is uncomplicated, with few extraneous details. Renal pelvic dilation is almost the sine quo non of UPJ obstruction. The occurrence of a crossing lower pole vessel at the level of the obstruction engendered discussion about the cause of the lesion among early surgeons and anatomists. Their reports considered whether the obstruction was the result of compression of the vessel, which compromised normal luminal diameter, leading to permanent ureteral narrowing as a secondary phenomena. Approximately one-third of the cases, even in early reports, were found to have this lower pole vessel in relation to the obstruction.[16] Stephens[17] suggested that these vessels were neither accessary nor aberrant. The obstruction in such kidneys may derive from an arrest of the rotation of the kidney as it ascends to the flank. If the lower pole artery forms before the normal rotation and gains entry into the hilus anteriorly, the pelvis may become vulnerable to compression by the lower pole artery. Radiographically, the ureter is located below the UPJ but above the crossing vessel and can retain contrast on a urogram, and giving a double-bubble appearance.

The presence of a vessel in the area of the UPJ has assumed more importance with the advent of endourologic intervention for urinary obstruction. A recent detailed study[18] has shown that the anterior surface of the renal pelvis is associated with a lower pole vessel in 65% of cases whereas the posterior surface is in contact with a vessel in 6% of the kidneys examined. This information is relevant for those wishing to incise the UPJ endoscopically, because the only safe incision is lateral.

With or without a crossing vessel, the involved kidney will demonstrate varying degrees of hydnephrosis, and the renal pelvis will be dilated to the level of narrowing or kinking. Below the narrow segment, which usually is at least probe patent (Fig. 11.2), the ureter usually assumes a more normal caliber. There are many structural variations on this general theme that often have surgical relevance. In many cases, the dilated renal pelvis demonstrates a box configuration, and the ureter inserts high in the renal pelvis. The dilated renal pelvis usually appears medially and is contiguous with the hydronephrotic renal space within the kidney. It is believed that this extra expansion of the renal pelvis serves as a compliant system that modulates any pressure changes caused by the narrowed outflow tract, thereby preserving function in the kidney.[19] In some cases, there is little extra renal pelvis imaged and all the dilation above the narrowed segment occurs intrarenally at the expense of the renal parenchyma. It is common in these cases, and surgically significant, to note the kidney is often posteriorly or anteriorly malrotated (Figs. 11.3 and 11.4).

Although fusion abnormalities of the kidney are embryologically related to rotational problems, note that horseshoe, fused, and ectopic kidneys can all be associated with obstruction at the level of the ureter and the renal pelvis. In such kidneys, the ureter may

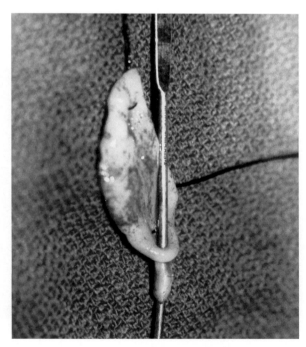

FIG. 11.2. A segment removed from the area of the UPJ showing the typical probe patency found at the time of pyeloplasty in most patients.

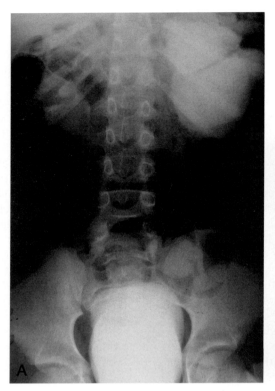

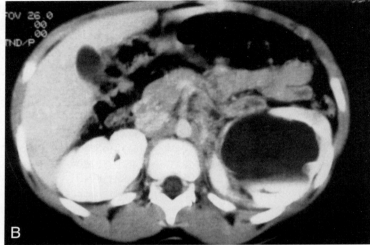

FIG. 11.3. A, Excretory urogram of a 10-year-old girl showing a hydronephrotic left kidney. **B,** CT scan of the same patient showing little extrarenal dilation. The hydronephrosis is all intrarenal and the renal pelvis seems to be oriented anteriorly.

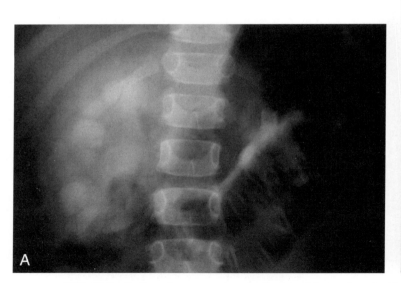

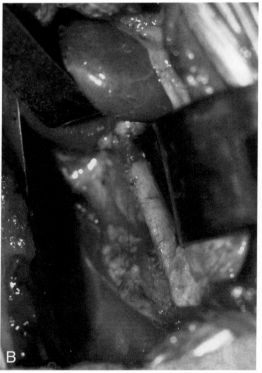

FIG. 11.4. A, Excretory urogram of a 5-year-old showing significant hydronephrosis of the right kidney. No renal pelvis can be seen extending medially beyond the renal sinus. **B,** Interoperative view of the same patient demonstrating the posterior rotation of the kidney; little extrarenal pelvis is present at the point of the ureteral insertion. The ribbon retractor is pulling the lower pole of the kidney anteriorly.

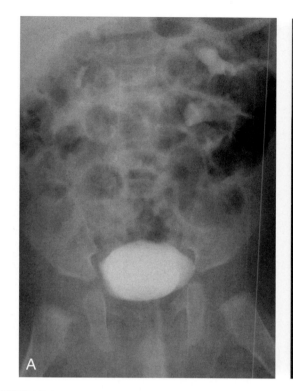

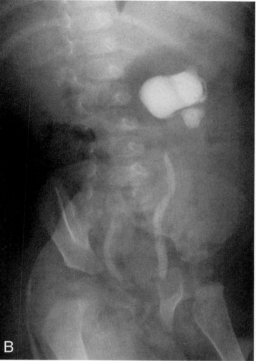

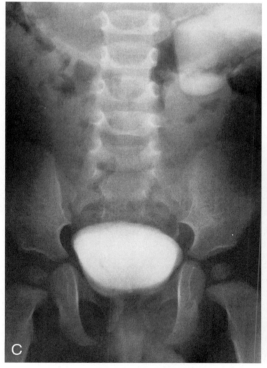

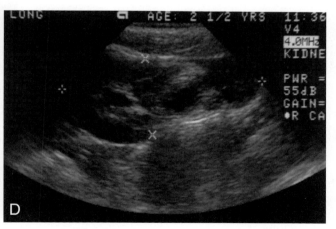

FIG. 11.5. A, Excretory urogram of an infant boy who had fetal uropathy, in the form of bilateral mild hydronephrosis, showing a left-sided duplication with little dilation of the lower pole moiety. **B,** An interval voiding cystourethrogram (VCUG) demonstrating bilateral reflux and lower pole hydronephrosis. **C,** Excretory urogram, taken when the patient was 2 years old, showing a dramatic decompensation of the lower pole. **D,** Ultrasound, performed after a lower pole pyeloplasty, showing improvement in the lower pole hydronephrosis.

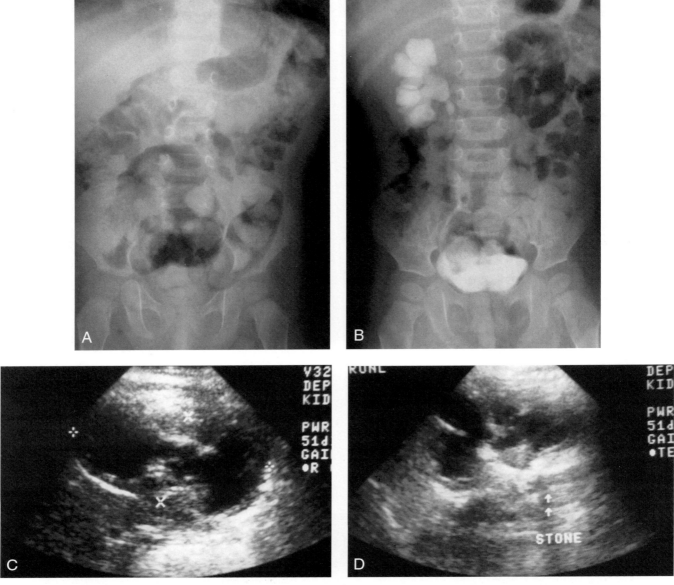

FIG. 11.6. A, X-ray of the kidneys, ureter, and bladder (KUB) of a 3-year-old girl with a urinary tract infection showing a stone located at the UPJ in the right kidney. **B,** A urogram of the same patient suggesting significant hydronephrosis secondary to a UPJ obstruction; the contrast obscured the stone. **C,** Ultrasound longitudinal view showing a typical hydronephrotic kidney. **D,** Ultrasound medial view clearly showing the stone as the cause of the hydronephrosis.

also have a high insertion in the renal pelvis, and the concept of providing dependent drainage of the reconstructed unit is sometimes difficult. Nephrectomy is a common outcome.[20]

Although the embryologic and molecular mechanisms of UPJ obstruction are still being elucidated, it is apparent that the obstructing process is frequently bilateral. In a review[21] of fetally diagnosed uropathies, 10 of 28 babies born with UPJ obstructions had bilateral involvement. Bilateral UPJ obstruction is common; however, <5% of patients require bilateral repair. The

bilateral nature of the process also explains the occurrence of a UPJ obstruction in one kidney and multicystic dysplasia in the other. Multicystic dysplasia derives from a complete obstruction of the upper ureter, resulting in nonfunction and cystic degeneration of that kidney;[22] and kidneys so affected simply have UPJs with total occlusion of the upper ureter rather than just narrowing.

Approximately 15% of kidneys with UPJ obstructions are subserved by ureters that demonstrate vesicoureteral reflux;[23] and often this finding complicates clinical management, particularly if urine infection is present.

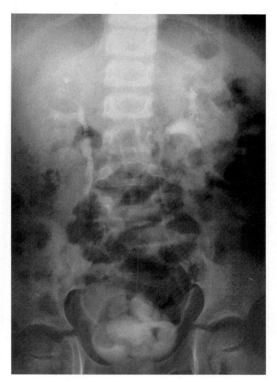

FIG. 11.7. Oestling folds, seen as convolutions of the upper right ureter, do not contribute to any significant urinary obstruction.

In such cases, the correct management plan consists of correcting the most severe of the anomalies first, and addressing the less significant problem later. Some surgeons have performed ureteroneocystostomy and upper urinary tract surgery on the same unit at one sitting.[24] Given the anatomic realities of the blood supply of the ureter, however, few authors would recommend this dramatic approach unless dictated by extreme clinical circumstances.

It is possible for a pediatric patient to have an obstruction at both the ureteropelvic and the ureterovesical junctions. The recommendation is to repair the UPJ obstruction first, because distal ureteral surgery is necessary in only a few children.[25] Duplication anomalies can lead to obstruction at the UPJ in either the upper or the lower poles. The upper pole obstruction is a decidedly uncommon event,[26] and the lower pole obstruction is occasionally seen. In duplicated kidneys with lower pole obstruction, the coexistence of lower pole reflux complicates the picture and may contribute to the progression of the hydronephrosis seen in the lower pole (Fig. 11.5).

In children, most obstructions at the level of the UPJ are congenital and intrinsic, and the concern about urothelial neoplasm is rarely warranted. Occasionally, however, a kidney that seems to have a typical UPJ obstruction will, on close scrutiny, have a benign fibroepithelial polyp in the area of the UPJ, which can lead to some

confusion.[27] Urinary stones can look like a UPJ obstruction (Fig. 11.6). Oestling folds are residua of fetal renal development. Although they may resemble UPJ obstruction, there is usually no significant renal pelvic dilation or hydronephrosis; and in most cases, this radiographic curiosity warrants little concern[28] (Fig. 11.7). Finally, there can sometimes be such massive dilation of the renal pelvis and kidney that the entire flank and abdomen are filled with the dilated renal unit (Fig. 11.8). Such giant hydronephrosis is not invariably associated with poor renal function; even though the renal concentrating ability is usually impaired, creatinine clearance can be satisfactory.[29]

PATHOPHYSIOLOGY

Although surgeons have historically devoted energy and attention to the repair of hydronephrotic kidneys, it is interesting and possibly relevant to consider the pathophysiology of obstructive uropathy. UPJ obstruction isolates the obstructive lesion to the level of the kidney and provides a good model for investigating the long-term physiologic effects of urinary obstruction. Classically, investigation of urinary obstruction followed the experimental creation of complete ureteral obstruction to assess the effect on the physiologic variables of renal function. Reviews of obstructive nephropathy emphasized the upward transmission of ureteral pressure in an obstructed kidney and the subsequent effects on tubular pressure, tubular function, renal blood flow (RBF), and glomerular filtration rate (GFR).[30–32] Collating data obtained from years of experimentation with various physiologic models in different laboratories, Gillenwater[33] concluded that urinary obstruction results in the impairment of all renal functions except urinary dilution.

If the function of the kidney is impaired by urinary obstruction, it is clear that the impairment does not derive directly from the transmission of the pressure up into the nephron. Even in the earliest studies, it was shown that the elevation of ureteral pressure above a certain point had no further effect on intratubular pressure.[34] With complete ureteral ligation, there is a rise in renal pelvic pressure, which is only transitory; and over a period of hours, the renal pelvic pressure falls in concert with RBF.[35] Regarding the effects of pressure in clinical circumstances, the intrapelvic pressure in patients with UPJ obstruction is most often in the normal range or perhaps even low when assessed at the time of surgery.[36] The expansion of the renal pelvis that follows urinary obstruction is protective in that the capacious collecting system allows dampening out of the pressure effects in the kidney. By assessing the relationship between intrapelvic pressure and urinary flow, Koff[37] demonstrated that not all UPJ obstructions are equivalent, because the restriction to flow can

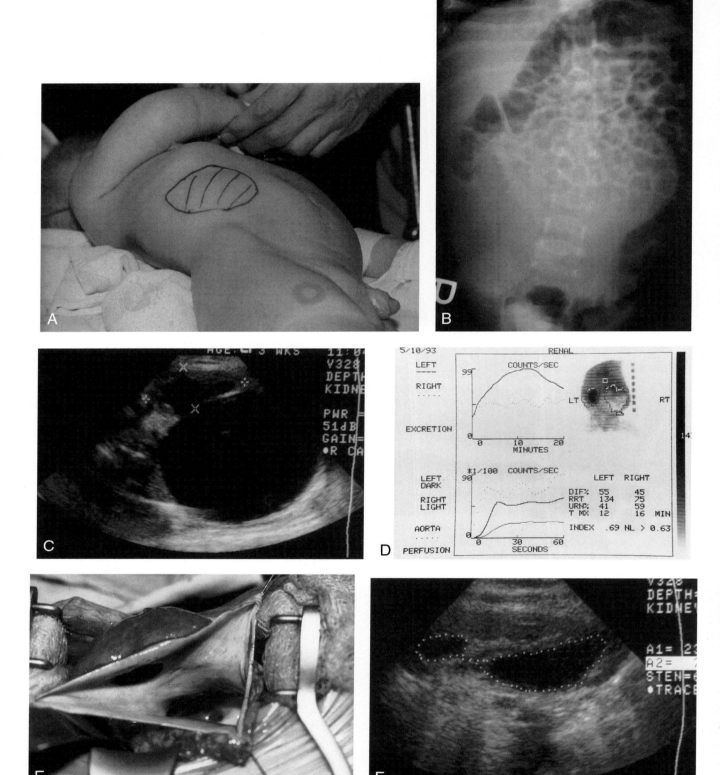

FIG. 11.8. A, The right-sided abdominal mass of a male neonate outlined at the time of surgery. **B,** KUB demonstrating significant displacement of abdominal contents by the dilated renal pelvis. **C,** Ultrasound longitudinal view showing the massive extrarenal expansion of the renal pelvis with adequate renal parenchymal thickness. **D,** Myelin-associated glycoprotein 3 (MAG-3) scan suggesting that 45% of the total renal function is derived from the right kidney. **E,** Interoperative view. **F,** Postoperative ultrasound demonstrating resolution of the massive hydronephrosis.

be either pressure dependent or flow dependent. In flow-dependent obstruction, the flow through the UPJ increases linearly with increases in intrapelvic pressure. This type of obstruction is most commonly seen in cases that demonstrate intrinsic narrowing of the UPJ. Volume-dependent obstructions are found more often with extrinsic obstructions, such as kinks, angulations, crossing bands, and lower pole vessels. In volume-dependent obstruction, the filling of the renal pelvis can become self-obstructing, limiting flow out of the pelvis at a rate greater than that predicted by the modest increase in intrapelvic pressure.[37]

Regardless of the nuances relating renal pelvic compliance and renal function, it is clear that urinary obstruction is not a benign process. Renal damage does occur; and at least from an experimental viewpoint, the decrease in renal function attendant to obstruction seems physiologically dictated by increases in the renal elaboration of vasoconstrictors, such as angiotensin II (AII), thromboxane A_2 (TXA_2) and antidiuretic hormone (ADH).[38] The changes in renal perfusion after obstruction are not equally distributed between cortical and medullary nephrons,[39] and a great deal of experimentation has been performed to try to discern the regulatory mechanisms involved in this redistribution of blood flow and the subsequent changes in glomerular dynamics. Studies show that release of complete ureteral obstruction of 24 h of duration results in a near-normal GFR when studied 60 days after the release. The total number of filtering nephrons, however, is decreased in the postobstructed kidney, indicating a significant increase in the single nephron GFR (SNGFR) of the remaining nephron units.[40] The mechanisms behind these changes in glomerular dynamics are most certainly initially owing to the local production of eicosanoids—mainly prostacyclin and PGE_2—and their total effect on afferent and efferent glomerular arteriolar vascular resistence.[41] It is obvious that these changes, in turn, determine the net effect on renal clearance or GFR.

Tubular functions are also changed by obstruction, but the effects of obstruction on distal tubular and collecting duct physiology may not be as quantitatively significant as the effect on deep nephron function.[42] Insight into the mechanisms of renal impairment can be gained by experimentally inducing complete ureteral obstruction via ligation; however, complete obstruction is seen only rarely clinically. Using perhaps the largest series of congenital UPJ obstructions, Johnson et al.[43] showed that the lumen of the ureter was at least probe patent in all but 4 of 219 cases. This obstruction must, of necessity, be considered partial. Experiments of partial rather than complete obstruction thus have more relevance regarding the pathophysiology of UPJ obstruction in children.

Models of partial ureteral obstruction have been de-

veloped and used in many species.[44-46] Such studies suggest that the total GFR of the obstructed kidney is somewhat decreased, although not as much as the decrease in the overall number of functioning nephrons. This implies an adaptive increase in the SNGFR of the remaining nephrons, presumably owing to changes in the local elaboration of vasoactive peptides and cytokines.[47, 48] Anatomically, chronic partial ureteral obstruction seems to produce the greatest obstructive change (i.e., hydronephrosis) in the 1st or 2nd week; after that, there seems to be no further enlargement in the size of the kidney and there is good preservation of most parameters of renal function.[49-51]

Morsing and Persson[52] showed that partial obstruction in rats resulted in no measurable impairment of renal function or change in tubular glomerular feedback (TGF) under conditions of normovolemia. Using extracellular volume expansion, they demonstrated a major suppression in urinary output from the hydronephrotic kidney; in normal kidneys, volume expansion results in a resetting of the TGF so that fluid and electrolyte reabsorption in the ascending limb of Henle are decreased. This allows for the net excretion of the volume and electrolyte surplus deriving from the fluid expansion. The authors postulated a resetting of the TGF system so that the expected increase in water and electrolyte excretion does not occur with obstruction. The obstructed kidney is thus protected from increases in pelvic pressure that would occur if the TGF system were unimpaired. In these experiments thromboxane blockade resulted in higher urine flow rates in the obstructed kidneys, with subsequent increases in the renal pelvic pressure. The paradoxical resetting of the TGF mechanism when partial obstruction occurs derives from a redirection of prostaglandin synthesis from vasodilatory PG to vasoconstrictive TX, perhaps mediated by bradykinin. This and other[53] experimental models suggest that the factors that cause hydronephrosis also cause the elaboration of many vasoactive peptides in the kidney, which ultimately modulate glomerular dynamics and tubular function. Obviously, changes in glomerular dynamics ultimately affect function. What is becoming increasingly clear from molecular biological techniques is that, in addition to effects on renal and glomerular circulation, the increase in these vasoactive substances has important ramifications for the microstructure and cellular milieu of the kidney as well.

Significant urinary obstruction invariably results in tubular dilation, glomerulosclerosis, inflammation, and fibrosis. Although not absolute, there is a good correlation between the severity of these histologic changes and the function remaining in the affected kidneys.[54] Sclerotic glomeruli and fibrosis are reliably localized to areas of the kidney that demonstrate the most inflammatory infiltrate.[55] The infiltrate consists mostly of mononuclear cells in both cortex and medulla. The cells are predominantly macrophages, although a small number of T cells are present.[56] The arrival of the infiltrating cells closely corresponds with the decrease in RBF and GFR after obstruction. Obstructed kidneys also demonstrate increases in cyclo-oxygenase activity and increased thromboxane synthetase.[57, 58] It is clear that that monocytic infiltration has a role in changing the eicosanoid elaboration in the kidney, which in turn acts locally to decrease the GFR.

The activation of the renin–angiotensin system (RAS), however, is also a major determinant of decreases in renal function associated with partial obstruction. Neonatal partial ureteral obstruction in guinea pigs produces histologic changes of obstruction and decreases in renal function. Administration of the angiotensin-converting enzyme (ACE) inhibitor enalapril not only maintained RBF in partially obstructed kidneys at 3 weeks postobstruction but also prevented the histologic changes of glomerulosclerosis in this model.[59] The effects of obstruction are not all ischemic. Obstruction does activate the RAS, and because of its intense vasoconstrictor action, the resulting increase in AII leads to decreases in GFR. It is becoming increasingly clear, however, that AII profoundly affects the expression of growth factors in the developing kidney that ultimately are responsible for the changes in the histology.

TGF-β refers to a family of multifunctional peptides that promote extracellular matrix (ECM) deposition. In addition, TGF-β inhibits ECM degradation by stopping production of proteinase inhibitors and decreasing expression of degradative enzymes, such as collagenase. Obstruction upregulates the renal expression of genes that encode for components of the RAS.[60] AII is not only a renal vasoconstrictor but also a chemoattractant for monocytes and macrophages.[61] Upregulation of TGF-β is apparent in these infiltrating cells, and the degree of upregulation correlates directly with fibrosis and collagen deposition in obstructed kidneys.[62] The fibrosis and microscopic deterioration of the kidney can be prevented by administration of ACE inhibitors.[63] Experiments suggest that AII has a central role in the development of tubulointerstial fibrosis in obstructed kidneys, because inhibition ameliorates the severity of the leukocytic infiltration, the impairment of RBF, and the severity of fibrosis in obstructed kidneys. Other growth factors may be relevant, too. A series of experiments with fetal opossum showed that administration of insulin-like growth factor 1 (IGF-1) decreased the fibrosis in obstructed fetal kidneys.[64] Apoptosis, or programmed cell death, also has been documented in experimental urinary obstruction; and the process seemed partly controlled by epidermal growth factor (EGF).[65]

It is unlikely that a single growth factor or cytokine is ultimately responsible for all the structural and functional changes found in obstructed kidneys. Nevertheless, the preservation of renal structure and the prevention of interstitial fibrosis in urinary obstruction are worthy goals. The continued study of the cascade of molecular events that occur after urinary obstruction may lead to a nonsurgical means of treating urinary obstruction.

NATURAL HISTORY

All reports describing the clinical findings of patients with UPJ obstruction note that the condition is more common in boys than in girls and more common on the left side than on the right.[66, 67] Historically, the most common presenting symptom in patients with UPJ obstruction was pain, which was reported by approximately 50% of patients. Urinary tract infection (UTI) was generally the second most common presenting complaint, followed by hematuria. The majority of patients were children, and only 25% of those diagnosed with UPJ obstruction were <1 year old. Of those infants, almost half had an abdominal mass. In only 10 to 15% of patients was the diagnosis of a UPJ obstruction an incidental finding.

Whatever the embryologic cause for the obstruction, the problem can occur bilaterally. Between 15 and 30% of patients demonstrate UPJ obstructions of varying degrees in both kidneys.[68, 69] Although there is no unifying embryologic description, it is regularly observed that vesicoureteral reflux and UPJ obstruction coexist in approximately 10% of patients diagnosed as having a UPJ obstruction.[70]

It has been recommended that when surgery is indicated, the pyeloplasty precede operative intervention on the lower ureter, because there is anecdotal experience that initial reimplantation can be problematic.[71] Clinical judgment is necessary; and if the reflux is more dramatic than the obstruction, it seems reasonable to perform reimplantation initially. Given the common occurrence of both UPJ obstruction and urinary stone disease in adults,[72] it is not surprising that children also can present with both problems. Although the narrowed renal pelvis can be repaired, the stone problem is likely to be recurrent.[73]

Hematuria after minor trauma is a classic presentation of UPJ obstructions, but rupture of an obstructed kidney can also occur after significant blunt trauma resulting in difficult surgical decisions (Fig. 11.9). Exploration is in most cases warranted; but at the time of surgery, the functional potential of the kidney is unknown owing to the urgent presentation. Of all kidneys diagnosed as having a UPJ obstruction, approximately 10% have such poor function that nephrectomy is necessary. In the case of a ruptured hydronephrotic kidney, it is reasonable to try to preserve function; but it is generally believed that repair of a shell of a kidney offers no long-term benefit. The immediate need to close the disrupted parenchyma and reconstruct the obstructed renal pelvis

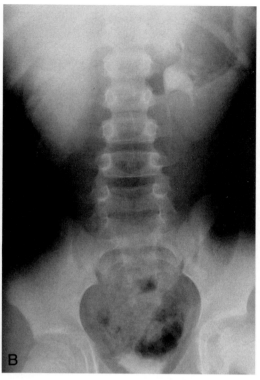

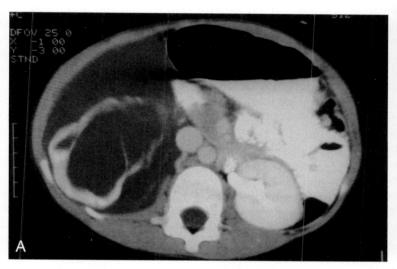

FIG. 11.9. A, CT scan of a patient who presented with blood in his urine after an automobile accident demonstrating marked extravasation of fluid around a hydronephrotic kidney. **B,** Postsurgery, compensatory hypertrophy in the contralateral kidney and poor function in the preserved kidney are noted.

may make conservative surgery seem like a long haul for a short slide. Given the infrequent occurrence of this condition, there are no large series to provide guidance.

Because RAS has a central role in obstructive uropathy, it is surprising that more patients with UPJ obstruction do not present with hypertension.[74] Cure of the hypertension with pyeloplasty is uncertain; but if the kidney warrants surgical intervention, there is a reasonable (20 to 30%) chance that the hypertension could be improved.[75]

The ubiquitous application of sonography for urologic imaging has dramatically changed the evaluation of patients with UPJ obstruction. In 1980, intravenous pyelography (IVP) was the most important study for evaluating possible upper urinary tract obstruction. Although most series at that time mention ultrasound only in passing, the 1980s saw an explosion of the use of this imaging technology, not only for pediatric urologic patients but, more important, for the assessment of fetal development during routine maternal examination.[76] Using ultrasound, clinicians find that 1 in 500 fetuses have a UPJ obstruction.[77] Obstruction is still found in children who present with pain,[78] but today most UPJ obstructions are found incidentally from routine maternal ultrasonography.

In the early 1980s, the sonographic identification of

many infants with obstructions prompted a dramatic increase in the number of neonatal pyeloplasties performed.[79, 80] Initially, newborn pyeloplasty had a reported reoperation rate of 20%;[66] with experience, the results improved. The ease of newborn pyeloplasty stimulated discussion about the necessity of intervention. The old paradigm that surgery cures hydronephrosis is inarguable. The question, however, concerns the natural history of treated (pyeloplasty) versus untreated urinary obstruction in terms of renal function and patient well-being. The question remains unanswered. Lacking this knowledge, many physicians have found it difficult to recommend surgery for asymptomatic infants. The well-documented, observed progression of hydronephrosis from mild to severe in asymptomatic infants is a concern that often prompts the recommendation for surgery.[81, 82] A caveat here is that the newborn does not process much urine, and the degree of dilation increases predictably from the neonatal period to a few weeks of age when the state of hydration normalizes.[83] Patients have been subjected to pyeloplasty because of this so-called deterioration in the kidney, which is actually the result of the infant's changing state of hydration and not intrinsic changes in the basic nature of the anatomic obstruction. Besides this physiologic change, kidneys found to have marked hydronephrosis in the newborn period are a real concern.

Physiologically, the newborn kidney behaves quite differently than does the adult kidney, particularly in the sensitivity of the neonatal kidney to stimulation by the RAS. If renal function could be preserved by relieving the obstruction there is much experimental data suggesting maximal benefit in the youngest of kidneys.[84] Because renal failure caused by obstructive uropathy is a significant clinical problem,[85] it may be reasonable to head off long-term problems with timely pyeloplasty at the time of presentation, even in the asymptomatic infant.[86]

Tapia and Gonzalez[87] suggest that unilateral pyeloplasty not only improves hydronephrosis with relatively few complications, but also significantly increases creatinine clearance (as calculated by the Schwartz formula) and somatic growth. The implication is that unilateral obstruction has negative effects on renal function and on somatic growth. When pairing the operation (pyeloplasty) to the condition (UPJ obstruction), urologists have found a perfect match. With experience, the procedure can be accomplished with few complications, and the inexorable deterioration in renal function can be averted by applying relatively straightforward surgical principles.

The natural history of surgically treated obstruction, however, warrants further discussion. Fortunately, the widespread application of renal sonography for the diagnosis of obstruction coincided with the development of nuclear medicine techniques for assessing this same problem. Clearly, some obstructions that were visualized on the IVP could be repaired, providing improvement in the postoperative urographic function in the kidney.[88] It is not known, however, what this change in visualization means in terms of absolute renal function.

Ultrasound technology has allowed surgeons to diagnose the problem well before any symptoms develop. Quantitative nuclear scintigraphy has provided clinicians with a better method of following-up the results of their interventions. Via nuclear scintigraphy, clinicians can make a quantitative assessment of both the relative function of the kidney and the obstruction to the flow of urine out of the kidney. Intuition suggests a greater likelihood of preserving or increasing the overall function of the involved kidney and enhancing the flow of urine out of the kidney after surgery.[89] Nuclear scintigraphy allows a more objective test of these hypotheses. Although flawed in many respects,[90] the diuretic renal scan still provides the best estimate not only of renal function but also of urine transit time out of the renal pelvis during induced diuresis.

At Children's Memorial Hospital (Chicago, IL), serial nuclear renograms on 75 retrospectively selected patients treated with pyeloplasty demonstrated no change in any of three scintigraphic parameters of renal function that compared preoperative and postoperative measurements.[91] Implied in many papers is an age-dependent sensitivity of the kidney to damage and the thought that the younger the patient, the more likely postoperative improvement in renal function will occur. In this Chicago study, there was no effect of age at initial presentation or manner of presentation in terms of the ultimate renal outcome.

A review of 100 pyeloplasties performed at Children's National Medical Center (Washington, D.C.) disclosed that pyeloplasty improved renal function as measured by isotope renal scan, but this improvement was independent of age at and symptoms at presentation.[92] This suggests that pyeloplasty need not be performed early to avert a loss in renal function over time.

Using not only nuclear medicine scans but also ureteral urine collection as guides to renal function Bratt et al.[93] demonstrated that adult kidneys subjected to pyeloplasty did not demonstrate any improvement in the mean GFR 8 to 10 years after surgery compared to preoperative values for the involved kidney. The authors were able to demonstrate, via ureteral catheterization after desmopressin stimulation, a significant improvement in only the maximum concentrating ability of obstructed kidneys treated surgically. When markedly decreased preoperatively (29% of patients evaluated), the GFR tended to show some improvement postoperatively.

Examining the literature from both an experimental and a clinical perspective, Josephson[94, 95] concluded that the natural history of untreated upper tract obstruction is for the most part not progressive. In all the reports reviewed, the majority of obstructed kidneys had normal RBF and GRF. Of those with decreased function, the magnitude of the decrease was moderate, and the relative contribution of the affected kidney did not vary much with age of presentation. A total of 34% of neonates, 25% of children, and 23% of adults had decreased differential function of the involved kidney at the time of presentation. In a large review of infants with antenatally diagnosed UPJ obstruction, members of the Society of Fetal Urology (SFU) pooled data from >400 patients. Using standardized scanning techniques and sonographic grading, the authors showed that surgery clearly improved the hydronephrosis but not the function of the kidney.[96] This report also suggests that untreated hydronephrotic kidneys do not deteriorate, at least when measured with the well-tempered renogram.

When using nuclear scintigraphy for the assessment of newborns with UPJ obstructions, urologists at Children's Hospital of Philadelphia noted that only 15% of 39 patients required pyeloplasty for deterioration of differential function of the involved kidney when the kidney initially had a differential function >35%.[97] In a retrospective comparison of patients with UPJs in the newborn period and initially good differential function (>35%), the authors found no difference in the ultimate outcome at long-term follow-up between patients who did and did not undergo pyeloplasty. This observation led to the current recommendation for pyeloplasty when the involved kidney contributes <35% of the total renal function on nuclear scan. Neonates with >35% function are followed via serial scintigraphy, and surgery is recommended only when there is a clear deterioration in renal function.[98]

The nuclear scan of neonates diagnosed antenatally with UPJ obstruction shows good preservation of function (usually >35 to 40% of the differential function) in 70 to 90% of patients.[99, 100] Because the natural history of obstruction does not include deterioration for most patients. Those demonstrating good function in the involved kidney are not likely to benefit from surgery (assuming differential renal function on nuclear scan is the most important clinical parameter). Pyeloplasty does improve the amount of hydronephrosis and also probably improves the concentrating ability of the kidney, but some investigators question whether improvement of these parameters is critically important for the patient. It bears stating that surgery does have complications. A recent study of 121 pyeloplasties in adults showed no difference in outcome between age groups. Although the surgery was 98.4% successful, 16.6% of the patients had a recurrence of symptoms on long-term follow-up.[101] Moreover, surgery can have negative consequences. Is the effect on renal function worth the intervention?

For the infants who have impaired renal function on nuclear medicine scans, there is no definitive answer regarding the effect of pyeloplasty on ultimate differential renal function. Nevertheless, the literature suggests that there is no change in the differential function after surgery. Considering the risks of the procedure versus the renal benefits, physicians should be able to make a reasonable case for following all neonates with UPJ obstruction nonoperatively, regardless of the degree of hydronephrosis, the differential renal function on nuclear scan, or the impairment of washout on the diuretic phase of the renogram. Adopting this nonoperative approach for all neonates, Koff and Campbell[102, 103] found that renal units with good initial differential function do not deteriorate on follow-up. For 15 of 16 units with poor initial function, they noted a rapid improvement in the differential function. These data suggest that UPJ obstruction in neonates may be a benign condition that carries a low risk for renal damage. Surgery does not seem to change the function of the kidneys, and many dilated kidneys improve in function with no intervention. No doubt, some of the patients so managed will eventually develop symptoms, such as pain, UTI, and hematuria. As noted, the differential renal function of involved kidneys in patients with symptoms has the same distribution as that in patients who are diagnosed antenatally via maternal sonography.

DIAGNOSIS

The retrograde pyelogram was the first imaging modality that could be used to assess abnormalities of the upper ureter and renal pelvis. The lack of pediatric instrumentation severely limited the procurement of retrograde studies in children, and it was not until the advent of fiberoptic technology that routine pediatric endoscopic assessment was possible. Although instrumentation is now adequate to allow routine imaging of the distal ureter and ureteropelvic junction in all patients, the diagnosis of UPJ obstruction is made with more practical tests. The necessity of a general anesthetic has relegated retrograde pyelography to an adjunctive role, most often used the day of pyeloplasty to confirm the lack of lower ureteral obstruction, which might affect the success of a repair.[104] Such visualization is comforting to the surgeon, but it uses operating room time, theoretically increases the risk of postoperative stricture in males, and adds to the cost. In large series of pyeloplasties in children and adults, the absence of the routine use of retrogrades has had no apparent ill consequences.[105, 106]

The common pattern for patients with UPJ obstruction, is a narrowed ureter at the level of the kidney and not elsewhere. Rarely will a patient have either long segment involvement or functionally significant distal ureteral narrowing. Knowing this common pattern allows the surgeon to comfortably repair the obstruction without visualizing the distal ureter in its entirety.

The excretory urogram is one of the most important tools in evaluating the obstructed kidney. This imaging test provides a rough guide to function of the involved kidney and the normality of the contralateral kidney. Nonfunction on the urogram does not mean that the kidney is beyond salvage.[107] Unfortunately, this has not been always recognized, and in studies of nephrectomy specimens, it is apparent nephrectomy is often performed because of lack of visualization on the IVP.[55] The urogram ideally provides much information about the obstruction that is not attainable by other studies, and this information facilitates operative planning.[108] It is true that infant urograms are compromised somewhat by the relative immaturity of renal function, which impedes adequate visualization of the collecting system. Bowel gas and underlying bony structures also make interpretation of the urogram difficult. Despite drawbacks, the urogram localizes the kidney, renal pelvis, ureter, and exact point of obstruction better than ultrasound and nuclear scanning do. Such localization has great importance in planning the incision. Because many obstructed kidneys are malrotated, the urogram may demonstrate that the obstructed renal pelvis may not present medially. In addition, when parents can see the dramatic dilation revealed by the urogram, they understand the nature of their child's problem.

The urogram does, however, have drawbacks. To obtain high-quality images of the collecting system, the patient should not be well hydrated. Feedings are withheld for 3 to 4 h before the test to ensure adequate visualization of the collecting system; parents are often upset when their child becomes fussy and hungry. The test requires a venipuncture; and in chubby babies, this can be difficult. In an era of consumer awareness, there is a concern about radiation exposure; but most pediatric radiology departments are sensitive to this and try to minimize the number of films taken. Only rarely will a child be subjected to a tomographic study, with its relatively high radiation exposure, that is commonly done in adult patients. As is true in adults, the injection off contrast agents can be nephrotoxic in patients with compromised renal function; and most pediatric radiology departments require a normal serum creatinine level before initiating the study. Anaphylaxis from the contrast injection is always a concern, even though the published rate of serious reactions is quite low (5 per 12,000).[109] Flushing and vomiting are much more common reactions, which parents seem to accept. In today's busy world, the need to get delayed films to achieve adequate visualization of the entire renal pelvis seems a greater inconvenience to parents than do the physical side effects.

The newer nonionic contrast agents seem to be much better in terms of both radiographic visualization and patient tolerance than the older agents.[110] Because these agents are isosmotic with serum, they induce fewer side effects yet preserve the image well. The downside to these newer agents is, of course, higher cost, thus they are not routinely used, despite their obvious superiority.[111]

As noted, ultrasound technology has dramatically changed the way that UPJ obstruction is diagnosed. It goes without saying that the ultrasound demonstrates well the dilation that usually accompanies UPJ obstruction. Ultrasound allows the clinician to measure the thickness of the renal parenchyma and can suggest whether renal disease and dysplasia exist (revealed by an increased echo texture of the parenchyma). Renal sonography requires no injection and has no associated radiation; interpretation is not hampered by bowel gas or bony structures. The technology is increasingly adaptable to the office environment,[112] and it has already revolutionized the diagnosis of UPJ obstruction.

Enough experience with the prenatal assessment of dilated kidneys has been accrued to allow reasonable predictions to be made regarding the ultimate renal outcome of fetal UPJ abnormalities.[113, 114] As a general rule, renal pelvic diameter is easy to measure and provides some prognostic information. Measurements taken at <24 weeks of gestation are difficult to interpret; however, after 24 weeks a renal pelvic diameter >10 mm correlates fairly well with clinically significant postnatal dilation.[115] Studies[116] have documented the correlation between prenatal and postnatal dilation of the renal pelvis and have noted that postnatal dilation correlates poorly with the degree of functional obstruction as determined by IVP and ℞Lasix renography. Because of variability in the renal pelvic anatomy (intrarenal versus extrarenal pelvis), measuring the renal pelvic diameter is not enough to completely assess a kidney. Given the obvious fact that kidneys grow with time, more suitable grading systems seem to be needed. The SFU published a grading system that makes the sonogram more quantitative in the assessment of hydronephrosis.[117] This system, which evaluates the dilation of the calyces in relation to the renal parenchyma, decreases the possibility that the presence of an extrarenal pelvis will unfairly influence the assessment of the kidney. This system has some predictive value, because kidneys with grades 3 and 4 dilations are much more likely to be obstructive on nuclear medicine scans and more likely to be subjected to surgery than are grades 1 and 2.[118] In the study by Maizels et al. pyeloplasty did improve the grade of hydronephrosis although the function on the nuclear scan was not much different postoperatively.

The development of Doppler sonography has added a new dimension to the assessment of kidneys with UPJ obstructions. The presumption is that the vascular resistance in an obstructed kidney will be greater than in dilated but physiologically unaffected kidneys in large part because of the postglomerular vasoconstriction that occurs in significantly obstructed kidneys.[119] With duplex Doppler sonography, intrarenal vasculature can be assessed to determine the resistive index:[120]

$$\text{Resistive index} = (\text{Peak systolic velocity} - \text{End diastolic velocity}) / \text{Peak systolic velocity}$$

Normal kidneys reliably demonstrate resistive indices <0.70, and obstructed kidneys show higher values. There is some indication that stressing the kidney with a furosemide-induced diuresis at the time of assessment can enhance subtle changes in the resistive index of obstructive kidneys, thereby increasing the utility of the assessment.[121] Whatever the future of resistive index determinations, it is clear that ultrasound imaging provides more day-to-day information about kidneys with UPJ obstructions than all other imaging modalities combined. Ultrasound is ideal for following patients with hydronephrosis: It is quick, graphic, reproducible, safe, and user friendly.

Nuclear medicine scanning is also indispensable in the assessment of possibly obstructed kidneys. Technitium 99m (^{99m}Tc) with diethylenetriamine pentaacetic acid (DTPA) is most commonly used in children. Its excretion depends mostly on glomerular filtration, and it lacks significant renal tubular accumulation. Approximately 20% of this tracer is cleared by a single pass through the kidney, giving it a blood clearance half-life ($T_{1/2}$) of about 1.5 h in patients with normal renal function. The cortical image from this nuclide is not exceptional, but both the kidney and the collecting system are visualized well enough to be of value. The newer isotope ^{99m}Tc Mercaptoacetyl triglycine (MAG-3) has been replacing ^{99m}Tc with DTPA as the preferred radionuclide for assessing urinary obstruction. This agent is a better cortical imaging agent than is DTPA and, therefore, provides a better idea of the renal anatomy.[122] The γ-camera can depict sequentially the progress of the nuclide through the kidney, thereby quantitating its arrival, uptake, transit, and elimination.

The ability to determine the differential function of a kidney with a UPJ obstruction is obviously of great benefit.[123] The nuclear scan can provide a quantitative assessment of individual renal function, which is a distinct advantage over the urogram's subjective assessment of differential function. Of equal importance is the quantitative assessment of the washout, or excretion of urine from the involved kidney (Fig. 11.10). The administration of a diuretic during conventional nuclear renography provides a way of measuring the renal pelvis's emptying ability during a time of increased urine flow.[124–126] Most nuclear medicine departments express the renal excretion of urine in terms of the $T_{1/2}$, or the time (after equilibrium has been established in the kidney and following the administration of the diuretic) that it takes for one-half the tracer to empty from the collecting system. This same function can be assessed by the slope of the washout curve generated after diuresis.

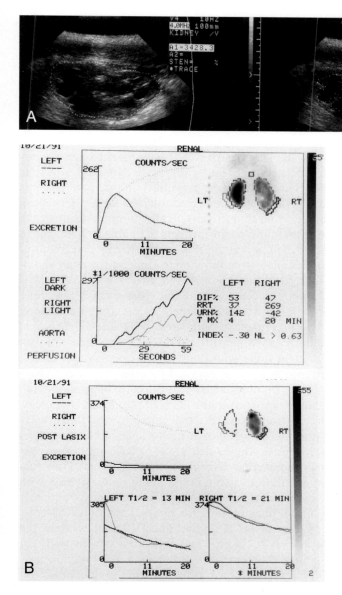

FIG. 11.10. A, Ultrasound study of a 4-year-old girl performed 1 year after she underwent pyeloplasty, which was complicated by persisting drainage that required a nephrostomy tube for 3 months postsurgery. Note the significant dilation within the kidney. On ultrasound, the outside area of the kidney and the isolated hydronephrotic area are compared to derive the cross-sectional area of the kidney that is renal tissue, not urine. In Figure 11.10, approximately 63% of the cross-sectional area is renal parenchyma. This measure allows the clinician to make a quantitative follow-up of the hydronephrotic kidney and to calculate renal volumes and derive a differential function based on the ultrasound. B, The diuretic scan showing good preservation of differential function in the kidney (47%) and acceptable washout after ℞Lasix administration ($T_{1/2}$ = 21 min).

There are many pitfalls of renographic studies. Obviously, the patient's state of hydration is important. Poorly functioning kidneys may not respond to the diuretic stimulus in a reliable manner. Capacious collecting systems may accumulate tracer longer than pelves with lesser volumes. In addition, the urine in the pelvis at the start of the test can dilute the isotope, biasing the excretion curve. The timing of diuretic administration is crucial. Optimally, the test should be done when the patient's bladder is empty. Researchers continue to describe the many variables that defy adequate control and tend to lessen the diagnostic utility of the renogram. To minimize variation, a standardized renogram has recently been proposed.[127] The widespread adoption of this standard will not fix the test's inherent problems; however, if hydronephrotic kidneys are assessed in the same way, with the same yardstick, some insight may ultimately be gained regarding the diagnosis of functionally significant urinary obstruction.

The renogram provides contradictory information regarding kidneys with UPJ obstructions. It is a rather common observation that the renal function of a severely hydronephrotic kidney will be significantly greater than the contralateral normal kidney.[128] This paradoxical superfunction seems more apparent when DPTA and MAG-3 are used to demonstrate differential renal function than when dimercaptosuccinic acid (DMSA) is used.[129] There is no good explanation for this observation, and it is clear that nuclear renography—although a cornerstone in the assessment of obstructive uropathy—is still incompletely understood. For all of its drawbacks, diuretic renography is the best available clinical test for establishing the presence of clinically important urinary obstruction and justifying surgical intervention.

Whitaker[130] noted that the primary concern in assessing a hydronephrotic kidney is the demonstration of damaging pressure within the kidney. Percutaneous technology has allowed easy access to dilated kidneys and routine pressure–perfusion studies to be performed. Initially, unequivocal obstruction was thought to be present if a pressure rise >22 cm H_2O could be demonstrated perfusing the kidney at a rate of 10 mL/min. Refinements of the initial test have defined the relative pressure (RP) to be equal to the renal pelvic pressure minus the bladder pressure at a flow rate into the system of 10 mL/min. Long-term follow-up of kidneys tested with Whitaker pressure–perfusion suggests that favorable outcome with nonoperative management is possible if the perfusion pressure is low. Witherow and Whitaker[131] found that kidneys with a RP <15 cm H_2O did not show decreased renal function and increased renal dilation after >5 years of follow-up.

At first glance, this type of assessment seems invaluable in the management of kidneys with UPJ obstructions. Unfortunately, the failures of the pressure–perfusion studies are well documented in the clinical literature.[132] By combining standard Whitaker testing with diuretic renography, Poulsen et al.[133] found that there was no correlation between renal pelvic pressure measurements and isotope washouts from the kidneys that were subjected to pyeloplasty. Their clinical observation has been duplicated in the laboratory with similar conclusions. Pope et al.[134] created partial obstruction in porcine kidneys and studied the animals thoroughly with intrapelvic pressure monitoring, furosemide renography, Doppler sonography, and pressure–perfusion assessment. The intrapelvic pressure correlated well with conventional sonography, but the results of diuretic renography and the Whitaker test were variable and did not accurately define partial ureteral obstruction. Although perfusion testing seems reasonable, needle size, perfusate viscosity, flow rate, and fluid temperature all influence the measurement of RP.[135] Even though percutaneous access is fairly easily established, particularly in hydronephrotic kidneys, the information gained does not seem sufficiently valuable to warrant routine pressure–perfusion testing in most children with UPJ obstruction.

Whitaker testing aside, percutaneous access can provide some important information in patients with high-grade obstruction. It is generally accepted that renal units with <15% differential function on the renogram do not warrant reconstruction and that nephrectomy is indicated. The vagaries of the renogram have already been discussed. If the renogram is obtained at a time when the renal pelvic pressure is great, it is possible that the differential function could be falsely depressed, leading to an unnecessary nephrectomy. Although the use of pressure–perfusion tests to establish the diagnosis of obstruction may be flawed, the timely placement of a percutaneous nephrostomy tube can provide radiographic demonstration of the anatomic details of the UPJ and, by letting the kidney drain for a few days, allow the direct measurement of creatinine clearance, or absolute function, of the involved kidney.[136] This gold standard assessment of renal function obstruction can be of great value when planning the operative procedure for renal units with marginal function.

CT has revolutionized genitourinary imaging in adult patients, especially in the fields of trauma and oncology. For children, however, the variability of the urinary anatomy is of paramount importance; and sonography and contrast studies will always prove superior in assessing congenital deformities in this area. UPJ obstruction in children is commonly found in association with the even minor trauma. Thus CT studies are frequently the initial imaging tests for patients with UPJ obstructions (Fig. 11.11). CT scans like IVP studies, show the dilation of the kidney and collecting system well; but of course, it estimates differential renal function only indirectly by demonstrating the cortical thickness.

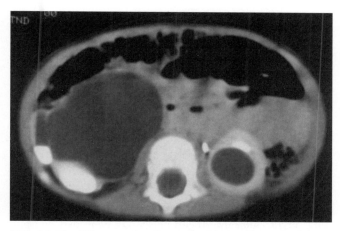

FIG. 11.11. CT scan of a 3-month-old showing a hydronephrotic, but functioning, kidney and a simple renal cyst in the opposite kidney.

New developments in MRI technology have made it possible, at least from a research standpoint, to image kidneys while assessing intracellular metabolic parameters independent of blood flow and tubular function.[137] Cost considerations currently limit the routine use of MRI for evaluating urinary obstruction.

The degree of UPJ obstruction is important for patients, yet none of these tests can tell with certainty which kidneys are obstructed enough to warrant operative intervention. Imaging tests can clearly document kidney dilation, may or may not be associated with a need for surgery. Both the renogram and the pressure–perfusion test can suggest significantly impaired washout of urine from the kidney, but many of this kidneys have no measurable deterioration in any identifiable parameter followed for long periods. Nephrostomy drainage and assessment of creatinine clearance can indicate decreased differential renal function of the involved kidney, which does not necessarily change after surgery. Consequently, decreased function and, therefore, decreased differential function are not necessarily indications for surgery.

Other approaches may discern the presence of damaging UPJ obstruction in kidneys. For example, the clinician may assess the urine for markers of renal stress. Disruption of proximal tubular integrity leads to increased urinary concentrations of β_2-microglobulin (β_2m), which is normally resorbed from the tubular lumen via phagocytosis and lysosomal digestion. An increase in urinary concentrations of β_2m may indicate tubular dysfunction as a result of the obstructive insult: Functionally significant obstruction and recovery from obstruction may be determined by following the urinary concentration of β_2m.[138] The potential for β_2m to be a marker for significant obstruction is quite appealing; however, determination of its levels in obstructed kidneys is not routine, and many diverse insults besides

obstruction, can lead to increased levels of β_2m in the urine. In addition, the immaturity of the nephron and the high fractional excretion of water in neonates contribute to elevated β_2m levels in the absence of any identifiable renal stress.[139] Further observations of the concentration of this protein in urinary obstruction will be necessary before its assessment can have practical application.

N-acetyl-β-D-glucosamindase (NAG) is a tubular lysosomal enzyme present in the urine of children who have various renal diseases. In rats with experimental partial ureteral obstruction, the urinary concentration of NAG increases in the first 2 weeks of obstruction and decreases with the relief of obstruction.[140] In a clinical study, NAG levels in kidneys at the time of pyeloplasty were seven times higher than those in bladder urine from normal control patients. In addition, enzyme levels in the bladder of patients 6 weeks after surgery suggested normalization of NAG excretion.[141]

Although not definitive, studies like these suggest that urinary biochemical markers of renal damage may someday help clinicians diagnose significant urinary obstruction. As noted, biologic modulators of glomerular dynamics and renal histology have been identified. The assessment of urine for growth factors (EGF, platelet-derived growth factor, and TGF β) cytokines, and vasoactive substances may be an important adjunct in evaluating obstructive uropathy in the future.

Clearly, there have been many improvements in the imaging modalities used to assess UPJ obstruction in children. It is also true that many patients are diagnosed prenatally, before they develop symptoms. It is interesting to consider that the widespread use of modern imaging techniques has not lead to an increase in the number of pyeloplasties that are performed. A multi-institutional study investigated the total number of pyeloplasties performed in a well-defined region and found that the total number of operations has remained constant since the late 1970s.[142] The authors found that the number of pyeloplasties conducted in children aged 1 to 6 years increased, whereas the number of children aged 7 to 12 years decreased: Yet the total number performed per year stayed the same.

Comparing the tests often used for establishing the diagnosis of UPJ obstruction in children in 1970 to those currently available could lead to the false impression that the diagnosis of significant urinary obstruction is straightforward. Although dramatic, the explosion of modalities used to image and assess the kidneys of children with UPJ obstruction has done little to indicate which specific renal units would benefit from operative intervention.[143] When looked at critically, the degree of hydronephrosis, impaired isotope washout, or even reduced differential renal function neither defines obstruction nor predicts deterioration.[144]

TREATMENT

There is justifiable interest in defining specific indications for surgery in children with UPJ obstruction. Koff and Campbell[102, 103] argue that aggressive nonoperation is a valid treatment program, particularly for infants, for managing patients with UPJ obstruction. Unavoidably, some UPJ obstructions will need to be repaired no matter what criteria are used to determine operability. Perhaps there was some uncertainty in the first half of the twentieth century about the preferred technique of reconstruction, but it is now clear that the dismembered pyeloplasty is the tried-and-true method to which all other techniques must be compared.

The technique of complete ureteral transection with subsequent reanastomosis to the renal pelvis was first described in the management of a retrocaval ureter, but it was easily adapted for reconstructing the much more common UPJ obstruction.[145] Whether done through lumbotomy,[146] the flank,[147] or an anterior extraperitoneal incision,[148] the essential features of this repair include

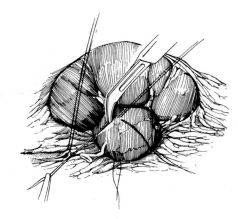

FIG. 11.13. After the dilated pelvis has been exposed and the upper ureter has been transected and spatulated medially, traction sutures are placed on the renal pelvis and the reduction is performed to allow for a dependent anastomosis. Reprinted with permission from Hinman F Jr. Atlas of pediatric urologic surgery. Philadelphia: Saunders, 1994.

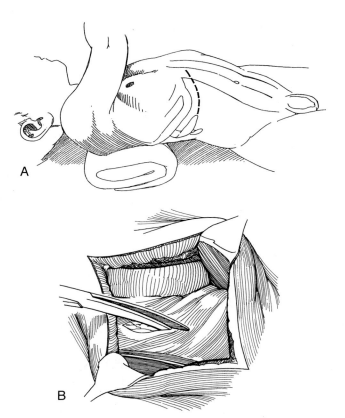

FIG. 11.12. A, Location of the anterior subcostal extraperitoneal incision, the most common incision for pediatric pyeloplasty. **B,** After the muscular layers of the abdominal wall have been incised, the peritoneum is dissected off the transversalis fascia and retracted medially, allowing exposure and incision through the fascia of Gerota. Reprinted with permission from Hinman F Jr. Atlas of pediatric urologic surgery. Philadelphia: Saunders, 1994.

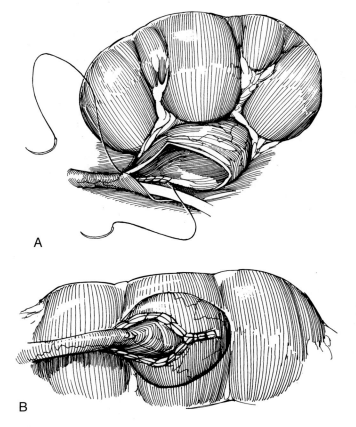

FIG. 11.14. A, A running suture nicely approximates the renal pelvis. A small pediatric feeding tube is passed into the upper ureter to ensure alignment and patency of the anastomosis. **B,** When completed, the ureter is attached to the most dependent portion of the renal pelvis. There should be no kinking of the upper ureter. Reprinted with permission from Hinman F Jr. Atlas of pediatric urologic surgery. Philadelphia: Saunders, 1994.

excision of the narrowed segment of the upper ureter or renal pelvis, lateral spatulation of the upper ureter, and anastomosis to the most dependent portion of the renal pelvis (Figs. 11.12–11.14). The Foley YV-plasty is occasionally useful in the repair of a kidney with a diminutive renal pelvis associated with a high ureteral insertion (Figs. 11.15 and 11.16). The anatomic configuration of a horseshoe kidney is also conducive to the use of this type of nondismembered repair. For most conditions, the Anderson–Hynes (A–H) pyeloplasty has a high success rate with few complications. Virtually all series of pediatric pyeloplasties have used this repair exclusively.[149-152]

There will never be an answer to the question regarding the need for stents and nephrostomy tubes in the postoperative period. It is clear that renal diversion occasionally results in delayed radiographic opening of the anastomosis, thereby prolonging the need for the nephrostomy tube. Although not really a complication, because a good result can still occur, this does nevertheless interfere with the patient's day-to-day routine. Another option is to stent the anastomosis with a double-J catheter, obviating the need for a nephrostomy tube.[153] In children, the need for another procedure to remove the stent diminishes the enthusiasm for this type of drainage. Practitioners who perform pyeloplasties on children tend to leave neither stents nor diversionary tubes.

The overall complication rate with the dismembered repair is quite satisfactory; most series report a success rate of >90 to 95%. Long-term obstruction at the anastomosis can occur; but reoperation for this is low, between 2 and 5% of cases. Bleeding and infection are uncommon following pyeloplasty. In the short term, persistent urinary drainage can occur, which requires internal drainage with a ureteral catheter for correction.[154] There is a belief that prolonged drainage can lead to anastomotic constriction owing to periureteral fibrosis; but if the urinary leakage is controlled as long as necessary with the usual surgical drains, a successful outcome is not compromised.

It is worth repeating that a successful outcome does not always mean an improvement in the differential renal function as measured by renography. In most cases, the A–H procedure improves the degree of hydronephrosis and washout on the renogram, which is comfort enough for the surgeon. The symptoms of pain, infection, and hematuria, if present before surgery, resolve at the same rate as the degree of hydronephrosis in the involved kidney.

The 1990s saw a revolution in minimally invasive surgical techniques. The anatomic configuration of the typical UPJ obstruction lends itself to these innovative techniques, all designed to increase the luminal diameter of the narrowed ureter or renal pelvis. Percutaneous access to the kidney, which is invariably dilated in

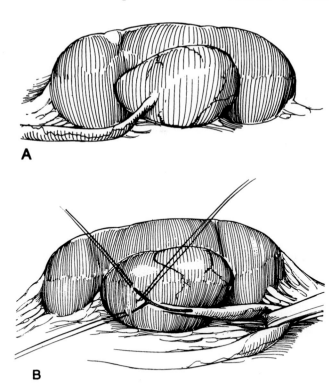

FIG. 11.15. A, The Foley YV-plasty is effective for high insertions of the ureter and when there is little extrarenal pelvis to work with. **B,** For cranial retraction, the Y incision is planned with the help of stay sutures. Reprinted with permission from Hinman F Jr. Atlas of pediatric urologic surgery. Philadelphia: Saunders, 1994.

patients with UPJ obstruction, is straightforward and accomplished without much difficulty. In 1983 Wickham and Kellet[155] established access to a hydronephrotic kidney and performed the first percutaneous pyelolysis. The concept was attractive and the technology available. Soon large series of endopyelotomies in adults were reported with fairly good short- and long-term success.[156]

Although balloon dilation has been tried extensively, incising the narrowed area with a full-thickness cut is more effective.[157, 158] Most reports in adults quote a success rate between 70 and 85% for the endopyelotomy. Encouraged by the adult experience, surgeons applied the principle for the treatment of UPJ obstruction in children.[159] As yet, the success rate for endopyelotomy is not as good as that for open pyeloplasty, but there is hope that further refinements will make the procedure effective. In general, the risks are low; but the newer procedures have refocused attention on the anatomic details relating to the presence of crossing vessels in the area of the UPJ. Laceration of the lower pole vessel, which is in anatomic relationship with the ureter in up to 40% of cases must be avoided.[160] This risk has prompted a rejuvenation of interest in vascular and renal pelvic anatomy and imaging techniques.

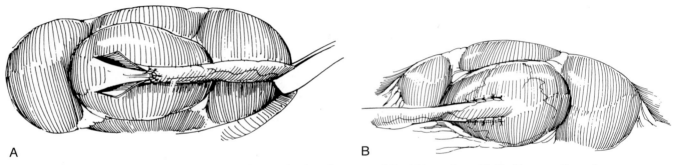

FIG. 11.16. **A,** The apex of the Y is attached to the stem of the Y to make a V. **B,** Closure allows for dependent drainage without dismembering the ureter. Reprinted with permission from Hinman F Jr. Atlas of pediatric urologic surgery. Philadelphia: Saunders, 1994.

Angiograms, endoluminal ultrasound, helical CT scans, and Doppler ultrasound have been used to discern positively and preoperatively the presence of lower pole vessels. None of these assessments has the combination of convenience, accuracy, and low cost; thus the best recommendation is to make sure that all incisions in the ureteral narrowing are directed laterally to minimize the chance for damage to the lower pole vessel.

In a long-term review of adult endopyelotomies, Van Cangh et al.[161] found an average success rate of 73%. When both a crossing vessel and a high-grade hydronephrosis were present, the success rate dropped to 39%; when neither was present, the success rate was 95%. Enough experience has been accrued in the adult population to show that, should an endopyelotomy fail, subsequent open pyeloplasty is slightly more difficult but ultimately no less successful than de novo pyeloplasty.[162]

Although percutaneous access to the kidney is straightforward in hydronephrotic kidneys, the search for minimally invasive techniques has led to the investigation of endoscopic retrograde treatment of UPJ obstructions.[163] Naturally, the technique has been applied to children with appropriate downsizing of the necessary implements.[164,165] At this time, the series are too small and the follow-up too inadequate to determine how the retrograde endopyelotomy compares with the more routine antegrade technique. There is a real concern that the retrograde technique risks significant stricture disease of the lower ureter in adults, a problem that is certainly of more concern with pediatric-sized ureters.

One is limited only by imagination in treating UPJ obstructions with minimally invasive techniques. Laparoscopic dismembered pyeloplasty has been attempted on an anecdotal basis.[166, 167] Four cannula sites are necessary, the operative times are long, and the suture placement is tedious. Nevertheless, many surgeons continue to strive for advancement in the area of minimally invasive procedures, and there is no doubt that improved

techniques will eventually be available. It is worth noting that these methods will not likely have any more effect on differential renal function than does open pyeloplasty. Underscoring this fact Banerjee et al.[168] compared endopyelotomy and pyeloplasty and found that endopyelotomy patients spent less time in the operating room and in the hospital. Urinary drainage occurred with equal frequency in both groups (12% of cases), and the degree of hydronephrosis seemed to improve to the same extent in both groups. No patient in either group, however, demonstrated any significant increase in differential renal function as noted on the ^{99m}Tc-DTPA renal scan.

The roles of endopyelotomy and laparoscopic pyeloplasty are not defined. These techniques may be the preferred methods of management for patients with postoperative obstruction who underwent previous open pyeloplasty.[169] Postoperative obstruction is a difficult problem, and open repair is also difficult. In many cases, the previous trimming of the renal pelvis and the scarring make revision of the anastomosis technically challenging. Faced with these circumstances, surgeons have relocated the ureter to a lower pole calyx via a ureterocalycostomy, as a salvage procedure.[170] For success, the ureter must be anastomosed directly to the calyx, and the overlying renal parenchyma must be trimmed to prevent postoperative obstruction. This technique may require clamping of the renal artery; and in all but the thinnest of kidneys, transfusion may be necessary because of the attendant blood loss. The difficulty of open reoperative surgery in patients with failed pyeloplasty make the minimally invasive aspects of endopyelotomy seem particularly attractive. With postoperative obstruction, the ureter and renal pelvis should already be aligned and remote from any lower pole vessels. The kidney is likely to be dilated, and percutaneous access should not be a problem. The results of endopyelotomy in such circumstances have been good, and most practitioners currently default to the percutaneous techniques for persisting postoperative obstruction.[171]

SUMMARY

Ureteropelvic obstruction is the most common congenital urinary obstruction. It is amenable to surgical repair with a high rate of success and a low rate of complications. In patients with symptoms, the results of surgery are most gratifying. The most difficult aspect of dealing with this lesion is knowing whether intervention is needed. In many cases, the obstruction is not progressive, and many asymptomatic infants and children have done well with observation alone. Clearly, some kidneys do deteriorate and require surgery. There is great interest in identifying the factors related to deterioration and the pathogenesis of renal impairment in obstructive uropathy. These investigations have scientific merit and might provide avenues of nonsurgical treatment. The greatest current need, however, is to find a method for determining which kidneys require operative intervention in asymptomatic patients.

REFERENCES

1. Mathe CP, Pena E. Surgical repair of hydronephrosis. J Urol 1934;36:1.
2. Morris H. On the origin and progress of renal surgery. Philadelphia: Blakiston's, 1898.
3. Fenger C. Demonstration of specimens from operations on the kidney with presentation of patients. Chicago Med Rec 1893;4:64.
4. Witten DM, Myers KGH, Utz DC. Emmett's clinical urography. 4th ed. Philadelphia: Saunders, 1977.
5. Ormond JK. Unsuccessful plastic operations for hydronephrosis. J Urol 1936;36:512.
6. Foley FB. A new plastic operation for stricture at the ureteropelvic junction. J Urol 1936;38:643.
7. Anderson JC, Hynes W. Retrocaval ureter: a case diagnosed preoperatively and treated successfully by a plastic operation. Br J Urol 1949;21:209.
8. Puigvert A. L'hydronephrose chez l'enfant. Facteurs pathogeniques. Acta Urol Belg 1963;31:304.
9. Ruano-Gil D, Coca-Payeras A, Tejedo-Mateu A. Obstruction and normal recanalization of the ureter in the human embryo. Its relation to congenital ureteric obstruction. Eur Urol 1975;1:287.
10. Alcaraz A, Vinaixa F, Tejedo-Mateu A, et al. Obstruction and recanalization of the ureter during embryonic development. J Urol 1991;145:410.
11. Kaneto H, Orikasa S, Chiba T, Takahashi T. Three-D muscular arrangement at the ureteropelvic junction and its changes in congenital hydronephrosis: a stereo-morphometric study. J Urol 1991;146:909.
12. Cheng EY, Maizels M, Chou P, et al. Response of the newborn ureteropelvic junction complex to induced and later reversed partial ureteral obstruction in the rabbit model. J Urol 1993;150:782.
13. Wang Y, Puri P, Hassan J, et al. Abnormal innervation and altered nerve growth factor messenger ribonucleic acid expression in ureteropelvic junction obstruction. J Urol 1995;154:679.
14. Dressler GR, Wilkinson JE, Rothenpieler UW, et al. Deregulation of expression in transgenic mice causes severe kidney abnormalities. Nature 1993;362:65.
15. Maizels M, Sensiber J, Cheng E, et al. Circulating TGF beta distribution and muscle disposition in the human VAT complex in normal fetal renal development in pediatric obstruction. Paper presented at the Annual Meeting of the American Academy of Pediatrics, 1995.
16. Geraghty JT, Frontz WA. A study of primary hydronephrosis. J Urol 1918;2:161.
17. Stephens FD. Ureterovascular hydronephrosis and the aberrant renal vessels. J Urol 1982;128:984.
18. Sampia FJB, Avorito LJA. UPJ stenosis: vascular anatomical background for endopyelotomy. J Urol 1993;150:1787.
19. Koff S. Determinants of progression and equilibrium in hydronephrosis. Urology 1983;21:496.
20. Gleason P, Kelalis P, Husmann D, Kramer S. Hydronephrosis in renal ectopia: incidence, etiology and significance. J Urol 1994;151:1660.
21. Steinhardt GF, Luisiri A, Goodgold H. The long-term outcome of fetally diagnosed uropathies. J Fetal Matern Med 1992;21:277.
22. Glick P, Harrison M, Noah, R. Correction of congenital hydronephrosis in utero III: early midtrimester ureteral obstruction produces renal dysplasia. J Pediatr Surg 1983;18:681.
23. Hollowell J, Altman H, Snyder H, Klackett J. Co-existing UPJ obstruction and vesicoureteral reflux: diagnosis and therapeutic complications. J Urol 1989;142:490.
24. Hensle T, Lattimer J. Urinary tract reconstruction following loop cutaneous ureterostomy. N Y State J Med 1978;78:1392.
25. McGrath MA, Estroff J, Lebowitz RL. The coexistence of obstruction at the ureteropelvic and ureterovesical junctions. AJR Am J Roentgenol 1987;149:403.
26. Ho ESJ, Jerkins GR, Williams M, Noe HN. Ureteropelvic junction obstruction in upper and lower moiety of both complete and incomplete duplex renal systems. Urology 1995;45:503.
27. Greig JD, Asmy AF. An unusual case of pelviureteric junction obstruction. J Pediatr Surg 1992;27:525.
28. Ostling J. The genesis of hydronephrosis: Particularly with regard to the changes at the ureteropelvic junction. Acta Chir Scand 1942;8:72.
29. Green J, Vardy Y, Munichor M, Better OS. Extreme unilateral hydronephrosis with normal glomerular filtration rate: physiological studies in a case of obstructive uropathy. J Urol 1986;136:361.
30. Wilson D. Pathophysiology of obstructive nephropathy. Kidney Int 1980;18:281.
31. Klahr S. Pathophysiology of obstructive nephropathy. Kidney Int 1983;23:414.
32. Klahr S. New insights into the consequences and mechanisms of renal impairment in obstructive nephropathy. Am J Kidney Dis 1991;18:689.
33. Gillenwater J. Hydronephrosis. In: Gillenwater J, Grajhack J, Howard S, Duckett J, eds., Adult and pediatric urology. 3rd ed. St. Louis: Mosby, 1996:1:973–998.
34. Gottschalk C, Mylle J. Micropuncture study of pressures in proximal tubules and peritubular capillaries of the rabbit and their relation to ureteral and renal venous pressures. Am J Physiol 1956;185:430.
35. Vaughn ED, Sorenson E, Gillenwater JY. The renal hemodynamic response to chronic unilateral complete ureteral occlusion. Invest Urol 1970;8:78.
36. Koff SA, Hayden LJ, Cirulli C, Shore R. Pathophysiology of ureteropelvic junction obstruction: experimental and clinical observations. J Urol 1986;136:336.
37. Koff S. The diagnosis of obstruction in experimental hydronephrosis. Invest Urol 1981;19:85.
38. Purkerson ML, Klahr S. Prior inhibition of vasoconstrictors normalizes GFR in postobstructed kidneys. Kidney Int 1989;35:1305.
39. Klahr S, Morrison A, Buerkert J. Effects of urinary tract obstruction on renal function. Contrib Nephrol 1980;23:33.
40. Bander KS, Buerkert J, Martin D, Klahr S. Long term effects of 24-hr unilateral ureteral obstruction on renal function in the rat. Kidney Int 1985;38:614.
41. Yarger W, Schocken D, Harris R. Obstructive nephropathy in the rat. J Clin Invest 1980;65:400.
42. Buerkert J, Head M, Klahr S. Effects of acute bilateral ureteral obstruction on deep nephron and terminal collecting duct function in the young rat. J Clin Invest 1977;59:1055.
43. Johnston JH, Evans JP, Glassberg KI, Shapiro SR. Pelvic hydronephrosis in children: a review of 219 personal cases. J Urol 1977;117:97.
44. Josephson S, Robertson B, Claesson G, Wikstad I. Experimental

obstructive hydronephrosis in newborn rats. I. Surgical technique and long-term morphologic effects. Invest Urol 1980;17:478.

45. Chevalier RL. Chronic partial ureteral obstruction in the neonatal guinea pig. II. Pressure gradients affecting glomerular filtration rate. Pediatr Res 1984;18:1271.

46. Steinhardt G, Salinas-Madrigal L, Farber R, et al. Experimental ureteral obstruction in the fetal opossum. I. Renal functional assessment. J Urol 1990;144:564.

47. Petterson B, Aperia A, Elinder G. Pathophysiological changes in rat kidneys with partial ureteral obstruction since infancy. Kidney Int 1984;26:122.

48. Josephson S, Wolgast M, Ojeteg G. Experimental obstructive hydronephrosis in newborn rats. II. Long term effects on renal blood flow distribution. Scand J Urol Nephrol 1982;16:179.

49. Josephson S, Grossmann G. Partial ureteric obstruction in the pubescent rat. II: Long term effects on renal morphology. Urol Int 1991;47:126.

50. Gonnermann D, Huland H, Schweiker U, Oesterreich FU. Hydronephrotic atrophy after stable mild or severe partial ureteral obstruction: natural history and recovery after relief of obstruction. J Urol 1990;143:199.

51. Josephson S, Lannergren K, Eklof AC. Partial ureteric obstruction in Wearling rats. II: Long term effects on renal function and arterial blood pressure. Urol Int 1992;48:384.

52. Morsing P, Persson EG. Tubuloglomerular feedback in obstructive uropathy. Kidney Int 1991;39:110.

53. Ichikawa I, Brenner B. Local intrarenal vasoconstrictor-vasodilator interactions in mild partial ureteral obstruction. Am J Physiol 1979;236:F131.

54. Elder JS, Stansbrey R, Dahus BB. Renal histological changes secondary to ureteropelvic junction obstruction. J Urol 1995;154:719.

55. Steinhardt GF, Ramon G, Salinas-Madrigal L. Glomerulosclerosis in obstructive uropathy. J Urol 1988;140:1316.

56. Schreiner G, Harris KPG, Purkierson ML, Klahr S. The immunological aspects of acute ureteral obstruction: characterization and kinetics of the immune cell infiltrate in the kidney. Kidney Int 1988;34:487.

57. Morrison AR, Nishikawa K, Needleman P. Unmasking of thromboxane A$_2$ synthesis by ureter obstruction in the rabbit kidney. Nature 1977;269:259.

58. Morrison AR, Nishikawa K, Needleman PO. Thromboxane A$_2$ biosynthesis in the ureter obstructed isolated perfused kidney of the rabbit. J Pharmacol Exp Ther 1978;205:1.

59. Chevalier RL, Sturgill BC, Jones CE, Kaiser DL. Morphologic correlates of renal growth arrest in neonatal partial ureteral obstruction. Pediatr Res 1987;21:338.

60. El Dahr SS, Gee J, Dipp S, et al. Up regulation of the renin-angiotensin system and down regulation of kallikrein in obstructive nephropathy. Am J Physiol 1993;264:F874.

61. Diamond JR, Kees-Folts D, Ding G, et al. Macrophages, monocytes and TGF-β1 in experimental hydronephrosis. Am J Physiol 1994;266:F926.

62. Pimental JL, Sandell CL, Wang S, et al. Role of angiotensin II in the expression and regulation of transforming growth factor-β in obstructive nephropathy. Kidney Int 1995;48:1233.

63. Ishidoya S, Morrissey J, McCracken R, Klahr S. Delayed treatment with enalapril halts tubulointerstitial fibrosis in rats with obstructive nephropathy. Kidney Int 1996;49:1110.

64. Steinhardt GF, Liapis H, Phillips B, et al. Insulin-like growth factor improves renal architecture of fetal kidneys with complete ureteral obstruction. J Urol 1995;154:690.

65. Kennedy WA, Buttyan R, Sawczuk IS. Epidermal growth factor suppresses renal tubular apoptosis following ureteral obstruction. J Am Soc Nephrol 1993;4:738.

66. Synder HM, Lebowitz RL, Colodny AH, et al. Ureteropelvic junction obstruction in children. Urol Clin North Am 1980;7:273.

67. Ahmed S, Sparnon AL, Savage JP, et al. Surgery of pelviureteric obstruction in 101 children over one year of age. Aust NZ J Surg 1986;56:675.

68. Bernstein GT, Mandell J, Lebowitz R, et al. UPJ obstruction in the neonate. J Urol 1988;140:1216.

69. Koyle MA, Ehrlich RM. Management of UPJ obstruction in the neonate. Urology 1988;31:496.

70. Lebowitz RL, Buckman JG. The coexistence of UPJ obstruction and reflux. AJR Am J Roentgenol 1983;140:231.

71. Maizels M, Smith CK, Firlit CF. The management of children with vesicoureteral reflux and ureteropelvic junction obstruction. J Urol 1984;131:722.

72. Husmann DA, Milliner DS, Segura JW. Ureteropelvic junction obstruction with a simultaneous renal calculus: long-term follow-up. J Urol 1995;153:1399.

73. Husmann SA, Milliner DS, Segura JW. Ureteropelvic junction obstruction with concurrent renal pelvic calculi in the pediatric patient: a long-term follow-up. J Urol 1996;156:741.

74. Mizuiri S, Amagasaki Y, Hosaka H, et al. Hypertension in unilateral atrophic kidney secondary to ureteropelvic junction obstruction. Nephron 1992;61:217.

75. Gillenwater JY. Hydronephrosis. In: Gillenwater JJ, Grayhack JT, Howards SS, Duckett JW, eds., Adult and pediatric urology. 1st ed. Chicago: Year Book, 1987;1:691–715.

76. Helin I, Persson PH. Prenatal diagnosis of urinary tract abnormalities by ultrasound. Pediatrics 1986;78:879.

77. Grignon A, Filion R, Filiatrault D, et al. Urinary tract dilatation in utero: classification and clinical applications. Radiology 1986;160:645.

78. Belman AB. Ureteropelvic junction obstruction as a cause for intermittent abdominal pain in children. Pediatrics 1991;88:1066.

79. Murphy JP, Holder TM, Ashcraft KW, et al. Ureteropelvic junction obstruction in the newborn. J Pediatr Surg 1984;19:642.

80. Guys JM, Borella F, Monfort G. Ureteropelvic junction obstructions: prenatal diagnosis and neonatal surgery in 47 cases. J Pediatr Surg 1988;23:156.

81. Noe HN, Magill HL. Progression of mild ureteropelvic junction obstruction in infancy. Urology 1987;30:348.

82. Flashner SC, Mesrobian HG, Flatt JA. Nonobstructive dilation of the upper urinary tract may later convert to obstruction Urology 1993;42:569.

83. Dejter SW Jr, Gibbons MD. The fate of infant kidneys with fetal hydronephrosis but initially normal postnatal sonography. J Urol 1989;142:661.

84. Chevalier RL, El Dahr S. The case for early relief of obstruction in young infants. In: King LR, ed., Urologic surgery in neonates and young infants. Philadelphia: Saunders, 1988;95–118.

85. Warshaw BL, Edelbrock HH, Ettenger RB, et al. Progression to end-stage renal disease in children with obstructive uropathy. J Pediatr 1982;100:183.

86. Perez LM, Friedman RM, King LR. The case for relief of ureteropelvic junction obstruction in neonates and young children at time of diagnosis. Urology 1991;38:195.

87. Tapia J, Gonzalez R. Pyeloplasty improves renal function and somatic growth in children with ureteropelvic function obstruction. J Urol 1995;154:218.

88. Bassiouny IE. Salvage pyeloplasty in non-visualizing hydronephrotic kidney secondary to ureteropelvic junction obstruction. J Urol 1992;148:685.

89. Dowling KJ, Harmon EP, Ortenberg J, et al. Ureteropelvic junction obstruction: the effect of pyeloplasty on renal function. J Urol 1988;140:1227.

90. O'Reilly PH. Diuresis renography 8 years later: an update. J Urol 1986;136:993.

91. MacNeily AE, Maizels M, Kaplan WE, et al. Does early pyeloplasty really avert loss of renal function? A retrospective review. J Urol 1993;150:769.

92. Salem YH, Majd M, Rushton HG, Belman AB. Outcome analysis of pediatric pyeloplasty as a function of patient age, presentation and differential renal function. J Urol 1995;154:1889.

93. Bratt CG, Aurell M, Jonsson O, Nilsson S. Long-term follow-up of maximum concentrating ability and glomerular filtration rate in adult obstructed kidneys after pyeloplasty. J Urol 1988;140:273.

94. Josephson S. Suspected pyelo-ureteral junction obstruction in the fetus: when to do what? I. A clinical update. Eur Urol 1990;18:267.

95. Josephson S. Suspected pyelo-ureteral junction obstruction in the fetus: when to do what? II. Experimental viewpoints. Eur Urol 1991;19:132.

96. Mitchall B, Kasse EN, Maizels MJ. Outcome of non-specific

hydronephrosis in the infant. A report of the Registry of the S.F.U. J Urol 1994;152:2324.

97. Cartwright PC, Duckett JW, Keeting MA, et al. Managing apparent uretopelvic junction obstruction in the newborn. J Urol 1992;148:1224.

98. Blyth B, Snyder HM, Duckett JW. Antenatal diagnosis and subsequent management of hydronephrosis. J Urol 1993;149:693.

99. Freedman ER, Rickwood AM. Prenatally diagnosed pelviureteric junction obstruction: a benign condition? J Pediatr Surg 1994;29:769.

100. Madden NP, Thomas DF, Fordon AC, et al. Antenatally detected pelviureteric junction obstruction. Is non-operation safe? Br J Urol 1991;68:305.

101. Raviv G, Leibovitch I, Shenfeld O, et al. Ureteropelvic junction obstruction: relation of etiology and age at surgical repair to clinical outcome. Urol Int 1994;52:135.

102. Koff SA, Campbell K. Nonoperative management of unilateral neonatal hydronephrosis. J Urol 1992;148:525.

103. Koff SA, Campbell KD. The nonoperative management of unilateral neonatal hydronephrosis: natural history of poorly functioning kidneys. J Urol 1994;152:593.

104. Cockrell SN, Hendren WH. The importance of visualizing the ureter before performing a pyeloplasty. J Urol 1990;144:588.

105. Rushton HG, Salem Y, Belman BA, Majd M. Pediatric pyeloplasty: is routine retrograde pyelography necessary? J Urol 1994;152:604.

106. Connolly J, Gleeson M, Grainger R, et al. Is retrograde ureterography indicated in pelviureteric junction obstruction? Br J Urol 1993;71:148.

107. Taha S, Al-Mohaya S, Abdulkader A, et al. Prognosis of radiologically non-functioning obstructed kidneys. Br J Urol 1988; 62:209.

108. Tamar B, Lebowitz R. Pediatric Uroradiology. In: Retik AB, Cukier J, eds., Pediatric urology. Baltimore: Williams & Wilkins, 1987:12–62.

109. Gooding CA, Berdon LE, Brodeur AE, Rowen M. Adverse reactions to intravenous pyelography in children. AJR Am J Roentgenol 1975;123:802.

110. Katayama H, Yamaguchi K, Kozuka T, et al. Adverse reactions to ionic and nonionic contrast media. Radiology 1990;175:621.

111. Nybonde T, Wahlgren H, Brekke O, et al. Image quality and safety in pediatric urography using an ionic and a non-ionic iodinated contrast agent. Pediatr Radiol 1994;24:107.

112. Maizels M, Zaontz MR, Firlit CF. Role of in-office ultrasonography in screening infarcts and children for urinary obstruction. Urol Clin North Am 1990;17:429.

113. Blachur A, Blachur V, Livne P, et al. Clinical outcome and follow-up of prenatal hydronephrosis. Pediatr Nephrol 1994;8:30.

114. Johnson CE, Elder JS, Judge NE. The accuracy of antenatal ultrasonography in identifying renal abnormalities. Am J Dis Child 1992;146:1181.

115. Anderson N, Clautice-Engle T, Allan R, et al. Detection of obstructive uropathy in the fetus: predictive value of sonographic measurements of renal pelvic diameter at various gestational ages. A J Ar 1995;164:719.

116. Bosman G, Reuss A, Nijman JM, Wladimiroff JW. Prenatal diagnosis, management and outcome of fetal uretero-pelvic junction obstruction. Ultrasound Med Biol 1991;17:117.

117. Fernbach SK, Maizels M, Conway JJ. Ultrasound grading of hydronephrosis: introduction to the system used by the Society for Fetal Urology. Pediatr Radiol 1993;23:478.

118. Maizels M, Mitchell B, Kass E, et al. Outcome of non-specific hydronephrosis in the infarct: a report from the Registry of the Society for Fetal Urology. J Urol 1994;152:2324.

119. Kessler RM, Quevedo H, Lankau CA, et al. Obstructive vs. nonobstructive dilation of the renal collecting system in children: distinction with duplex sonography. AJR Am J Roentgenol 1993;160:353.

120. Chen JH, Pu YS, Liu SP, Chiu TY. Renal hemodynamics in patients with obstructive uropathy evaluated by duplex doppler sonography. J Urol 1993;150:18.

121. Kincaid W, Hollman AS, Azmy AF. Doppler ultrasound in pelviureteric junction obstruction in infants and children. J Pediatr Surg 1994;29:765.

122. Eshima D, Taylor A Jr. Technitium-99m (^{99m}Tc) mercaptoacetyl-triglycine: update on the new ^{99m}Tc renal tubular function agent. Semin Nucl Med 1992;22:61.

123. Belis JA, Belis TE, Lai JC, et al. Radionuclide determination of individual kidney function in the treatment of chronic renal obstruction. J Urol 1982;127:636.

124. O'Reilly PH, Lawson RS, Shields RA, Testa HJ. Idiopathic hydronephrosis—the diuresis renogram: a new non-invasive method of assessing equivocal pelvioureteral junction obstruction. J Urol 1979;121:153.

125. Koff SA, Thrall JH, Keyes JW. Diuretic radionuclide urography: a non-invasive method for evaluating nephroureteral dilatation. J Urol 1979;122:451.

126. Thrall JH, Koff SA, Keyes JW. Diuretic radionuclide renography and scintigraphy in the differential diagnosis of hydroureteronephrosis. Semin Nucl Med 1981;11:89.

127. Conway JJ. Well tempered diuresis renography: its historical development, physiological and technical pitfalls and standardized technique protocol. Semin Nucl Med 1992;22:74.

128. Steckler RE, McLorie GA, Jayanthi VR, et al. Contradictory supranormal differential renal function during nuclear renographic investigation of hydroureteronephrosis. J Urol 1994; 152:600.

129. Groshar A, Issaq E, Nativ O, Livne PM. Increased renal function in kidneys with UPJ obstruction: fact or artifact? Assessment by a vartive single photon emission computerized tomography of dimercapto-succinic acid uptake by the kidneys. J Urol 1996; 155:844–846.

130. Whitaker RH. Methods of assessing obstruction in dilated ureters. Br J Urol 1973;45:15.

131. Witherow R, Whitaker R. The predictive accuracy of antegrade pressure flow studies in equivocal upper tract obstruction. Br J Urol 1981;53;496.

132. Horstman WG, Darcy MD. Intermittent hydronephrosis as a cause of a false-negative pressure-flow study. Cardovasc Intervent Radiol 1991;14:185.

133. Poulsen EU, Frokjaer F, Taagehoj-Jensen F, et al. Diuresis renography and simultaneous renal pelvis pressure in hydronephrosis. J Urol 1987;138:272.

134. Pope JC, Showalter PR, Milam DF, Brock JW. Intrapelvic pressure monitoring in the partially obstructed porcine kidney. Urology 1994;44:565.

135. Toguri AG, Fournier G. Factors influencing the pressure-flow-perfusion system. J Urol 1982;127:1021.

136. Cronan JJ. Contemporary concepts in imaging urinary tract obstruction. Radiol Clin North Am 1991;29:527.

137. Fichtner J, Spielman D, Herfkens R, et al. Ultrafast contrast enhanced magnetic resonance imaging of congenital hydronephrosis in a rat model. J Urol 1994;152:682.

138. Tataranni G, Farineli FR, Zavagtli G, et al. Tubule recovery after obstructive nephropathy relief: the value of enzymuria and microproteinuria. J Urol 1987;138:24.

139. Zanardo V, DaRiol R, Faggian D, et al. Urinary beta-2-microglobulin excretion in prematures with respiratory distress syndrome. Child Nephrol Urol 1990;10:135.

140. Huland H, Gonnermann D, Werner B, Possin U. A new test to predict reversibility of hydronephrotic atrophy after stable partial unilateral ureteral obstruction. J Urol 1988;140:1591.

141. Carr MC, Peters CA, Retik AB, Mandell J. Urinary levels of the renal tubular enzyme N-acetyl-β-D-glucosaminidase in unilateral obstructive uropathy. J Urol 1994;151;442.

142. Wiener JS, Emmert GK, Mesrobian HG, et al. Are modern imaging techniques over diagnosing ureteropelvic junction obstruction. J Urol 1995;154:659.

143. King LR. Hydronephrosis. When is obstruction not obstruction. Urol Clin North Am 1995;22:31.

144. Koff SA. The case for non-operative management of apparent UPJ obstruction. Dial Pediatr Urol 1991;14:5.

145. Anderson JC. Hydronephrosis: a 14 years' survey of results. Proc R Soc Med 1962;55:93.

146. Gonzalez R, Aliabadi H. Posterior lumbotomy in pediatric pyeloplasty. J Urol 1987;137:468.

147. Hendren WH, Radhakrishnan J, Middleton AW. Pediatric pyeloplasty. J Pediatr Surg 1980;15:133.

148. Hinman F. Atlas of pediatric urologic surgery. Philadelphia: Saunders, 1994.
149. Nguyen DH, Aliabadi H, Ercole CJ, Gonzalez R. Nonintubated Anderson–Hynes repair of ureteropelvic junction obstruction in 60 patients. J Urol 1989;142:704.
150. Wolpert JJ, Woodard JR, Parrott TS. Pyeloplasty in the young infant. J Urol 1989;142:573.
151. Sheldon CA, Duckett JW, Snyder HM. Evolution in the management of infant pyeloplasty. J Pediatr Surg 1992;27:501.
152. Deleted.
153. Sibley GNA, Graham MD, Smith ML, Doyle PT. Improving splintage techniques in pyeloplasty. Br J Urol 1987;60:489.
154. Cromie WJ. Complications of pyeloplasty. Urol Clin North Am 1983;10:385.
155. Wickham JEA, Kellet MJ. Percutaneous pyelolysis. Eur Urol 1983;9:122.
156. Motola JA, Badlani GH, Smith AD. Results of 212 consecutive endopyelotomies: an 8-year follow-up. J Urol 1993;149:453.
157. Chandhoke PS, Clayman RV, Stone AM, et al. Endopyelotomy and endoureterotomy with the acucise ureteral cutting balloon device: preliminary experience. J Endourology 1993;7:45.
158. Snow TM, Wells IP, Hammonds JC. Balloon rupture and stenting for pelviureteric junction obstruction: abolition of wasting is a prognostic marker. Clin Radiol 1994;49:708.
159. Figenshau RS, Clayman R, Colburg J, et al. Pediatric endopyelotomy: the Washington University experience. Paper presented at the 90th Annual Meeting of the American Urology Association, Las Vegas, 1995.
160. Streem SB, Geisinger MA. Prevention and management of hemorrhage associated with cautery wire balloon incision of ureteropelvic junction obstruction. J Urol 1995;153:1904.
161. Van Cangh PJ, Wilmart JF, Opsomer RJ, et al. Long-term results and late recurrence after endoureteropyelotomy: a critical analysis of prognostic factors. J Urol 1994;151:934.
162. Motola JA, Fried R, Badlani GH, Smith AD. Failed endopyelotomy: implications for future surgery on the ureteropelvic junction. J Urol 1993;150:821.
163. Meretyk I, Meretyk S, Clayman RV. Endopyelotomy: comparison of ureteroscopic retrograde and antegrade percutaneous techniques. J Urol 1992;148:755.
164. Bolton DM, Bogaert GA, Mevorach RA, et al. Pediatric ureteropelvic junction obstruction treated with retrograde endopyelotomy. Urology 1994;44:609.
165. Tan HL, Roberts JP, Grattan-Smith D. Retrograde balloon dilation of ureteropelvic obstructions in infants and children: early results. Urology 1995;46:89.
166. Peters CA, Schlussel RN, Retik AB. Pediatric laparoscopic dismembered pyeloplasty. J Urol 1995;153:1962.
167. Schuessler WW, Grune MT, Techaunhuey LV, Preminger GM. Laparoscopic dismembered pyeloplasty. J Urol 1993;150:1795.
168. Banerjee GK, Ahlawat R, Dalela D, Kumar RV. Endopyelotomy and pyeloplasty: face to face. Eur Urol 1994;26:281.
169. Kavoussi LR, Meretyk S, Dierks SM, et al. Endopyelotomy for secondary ureteropelvic junction obstruction in children. J Urol 1991;145:345.
170. Ross JH, Streem SB, Novick AC, et al. Ureterocalicostomy for reconstruction of complicated pelviureteric junction obstruction. Br J Urol 1990;65:322.
171. Faerber GJ, Ritchey ML, Bloom DA. Percutaneous endopyelotomy in infants and young children after failed open pyeloplasty. J Urol 1995;154:1495.

CHAPTER 12

Megaureter

Charlotte Massad and Edwin Smith

Early anatomists were aware that the ureter is a muscular tube with a lumen that is fairly consistent in size. In fact, Galen recognized ureteral dilation in association with vesicoureteral reflux as a pathologic change. Modern efforts to understand ureteral dilation initially produced a confusing plethora of terms including megaloureter,[1] ureteral achalasia,[2] aperistaltic distal ureteral segment,[3] refluxing megaureter, obstructed megaureter, and primary obstructive megaureter.[4] Greater specificity was added when Cussen[5] reviewed the normal dimensions of ureters in cadavers aged 30 weeks of gestation to 12 years and determined that normal ureteral diameter in children does not exceed 7 mm. In current practice, however, ureteral dilation is a feature seen on radiographic studies; and exact quantitation of the degree of widening is not necessary. Rather the reflexive question is directed at explaining the cause of the dilation and its effect on renal function.

The term *megaureter* simply means a wide ureter. Most often ureteral widening is caused by either obstruction or reflux. Other disease processes, however (i.e., those associated with excessively high urinary flow rates or high intravesical pressures), can result in ureteral dilation. Clinical evaluation of a megaureter is tailored to identify the underlying cause in each case. Other descriptive terms can then be used to explain the specific type of megaureter. Differences in natural history, histology, and surgical management of specific forms of ureteral enlargement clearly warrant this individualized approach.

PATHOPHYSIOLOGY

The normal ureter is expected to effectively transmit the urinary bolus from the level of the renal pelvis to the urinary bladder at acceptably low pressures. The efficiency with which this task is performed depends on appropriate transmission of the electrical wave between smooth muscle cells to which peristalsis is coupled and satisfactory coaptation of the ureteral wall to propel the urinary bolus. Other factors that affect ureteral transport are urinary volume and bladder pressure; a high intravesical pressure impairs ureteral emptying into the bladder, producing a functional obstruction. Compromise of one or more of these features usually results in ureteral dilation.

For instance, the primary obstructive megaureter contains a distal ureteral segment that fails to propagate the peristaltic wave. The static urine both distends the upper urinary tract and reduces luminal coaptation. Functional ureteral obstruction often occurs with the high vesical pressures of neurogenic and posterior urethral valve bladders. When bladder pressures exceed contractile ureteral pressures under these conditions, a gradient is produced that reduces ureteral emptying. Reflux alters ureteral efficiency by both ureteral distension and by augmentation of the volume of urine that must be moved back to the bladder.

High urinary flow rates, as seen with diabetes insipidis, may overwhelm the maximum transport of the ureter by peristalsis. Initially, the ureter responds to increased urinary volume by increasing the frequency of peristalsis. Next, the volume of individual boluses increases. And, finally, there is a coalescence of the urinary boluses that ultimately produces columnar flow without luminal coaptation.

CLASSIFICATION

To enhance the accuracy and uniformity in nomenclature a classification scheme for widened ureter was proposed in 1976 by the Section of Urology of the American Academy of Pediatrics, the Society for Pediatric Urologic Surgeons, and the Society for Pediatric Urology.[6] This scheme has been generally accepted and facilitates discussion of specific disease entities. Megaureters are logically divided into three primary categories: refluxing megaureters; obstructed megaureters; and nonrefluxing, nonobstructed megaureters. The second tier of classification provides discrimination between primary defects that are ureteral in origin and secondary defects that are extraureteral in origin. This allows the inclusion of other anomalies often associated with ureteral dilation, such as posterior urethral valves and neurogenic bladder. An uncommon, fourth primary variety, the refluxing obstructed megaureter, was described later.

Primary Obstructive Megaureter

The most common cause of the primary obstructive megaureter is an adynamic juxtavesical segment of the ureter that fails to propagate urine flow effectively (Fig. 12.1). This adynamic segment of normal caliber may vary in length from 0.5 to 4.0 cm. Curiously, the lumen of this segment will accept a catheter of appropriate size, and there is no actual anatomical stenosis. Primary obstructive megaureter has a male:female ratio of nearly 4:1; the left side is more often affected. Bilateral involvement is present in about 20% of cases, and association with contralateral renal agenesis has been reported.[7]

Because the aperistaltic ureteral segment with proximal dilation seems analogous to colonic dilation in Hirschsprung disease, a neuropathic cause was initially sought.[8] Unlike the bowel, however, the normal ureter does not contain intramural neural ganglia, and an aberrant ureteral nerve supply has not been demonstrated in association with obstructive megaureter.[9] Instead, histologic studies have shown that the defect is intrinsic to the ureteral wall.

The normal ureteral musculature has been described as braided bundles of muscle fibers arranged in interlacing spirals. Changes in this architecture occur as the ureter approaches the bladder and layers become distinguishable. At this point, an inner longitudinal layer is surrounded by a layer of circularly oriented cells. In older children and adults, an outer layer of longitudinally oriented fibers may also be visible. Examination of the distal aspect of a megaureter may show that this pattern is preserved but that the segment fails to perpetuate a peristatic wave. More often, however, there is a departure from normal histology, and one of three patterns are noted under light microscopy: (a) a predominance of circular smooth muscle; (b) muscle fiber hypoplasia and atrophy, with collagen deposits separating the muscle cells; and (c) mural fibrosis with scant muscle fibers.[10] A consistent finding via electron microscopy is the increased deposition of collagen within the adynamic segment.[11, 12] The result of these changes is the formation of an inelastic collar that impedes the transmission of the urinary bolus. Investigation of the dilated ureter proximal to the adynamic segment has shown an increase in both collagen and elastin.[12, 13] The excess production of these connective tissue elements by ureteral smooth muscle seems to represent a cellular response to obstruction.[14]

Other primary ureteral abnormalities that may produce distal obstruction include ureteral valves, congenital strictures, and ureteral ectopia. A ureteral valve is rare and most often found in the upper ureter, but it may occur distally.[15] Ostling[16] recognized the presence of transverse folds of the upper ureter during fetal development and suggested that their persistence could produce an obstructive lesion. These folds are composed of muscle cells with a urothelial covering and may assume either a cusplike or annular configuration.[17] A persistence of the Chwalle membrane has also been suggested as a cause but does not explain the occurrence of valves away from the transmural tunnel.[18]

Congenital strictures of the distal ureter show true anatomic narrowing and are thereby distinguished from the ureter possessing an adynamic segment. Histologically, the involved segment shows sparse smooth muscle cells and collagen deposition. Faulty muscularization during embryologic development is purported as the cause. Ectopic ureters may be obstructive because of ureteral narrowing or stenosis at the meatus or because of entry amid the muscular fibers of the bladder neck.

Primary Refluxing Megaureter

Primary megaureter associated with reflux occurs when the transmural tunnel of the ureter is deficient and the ureterovesical junction is rendered incompetent. Because refluxing ureters often show a greater degree of dilation by voiding cystourethrography (VCUG) than by ultrasound or intravenous pyelography (IVP), identification of a refluxing megaureter may be a matter of judgment (Fig. 12.2).

According to the Mackie–Stephens[19] theory, the defect occurs because of an excessively caudal origin of the ureteral bud on the mesonephric duct. After union with the vesicoenteric canal, the ureteral orifice migrates to a position that is lateral and lacks detrusor backing. At its cranial end, the ureteral bud may meet a more peripheral zone of the metanephric blastema, and the kidney may show some degree of dysplasia. Antenatally detected hydronephrosis that proves to be vesicoureteral reflux (VUR) is associated with dysmorphic renal development (dysplasia) in as many as one-third of cases. This occurs without an associated urinary tract infection.[20] There is a higher prevalence of refluxing megaureters in males than in females, and bilaterality is common. Although unlikely, spontaneous resolution is possible.

The megaureter–megacystis syndrome represents an extreme form of the primary refluxing megaureter. In this condition massive reflux prevents effective bladder emptying with voiding. There is no evidence of an anatomical or functional bladder outlet obstruction, and the bladder radiographically is smooth walled with a normal bladder neck configuration.[21] The bladder emp-

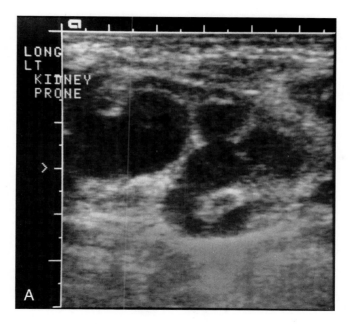

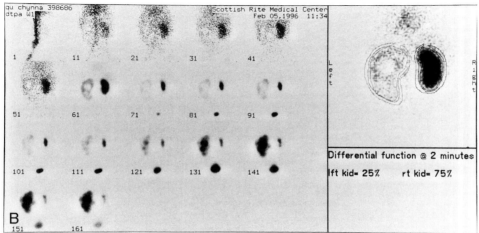

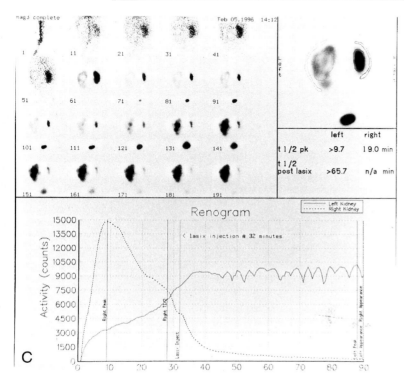

FIG. 12.1. A, Postnatal ultrasound of an obstructed megaureter demonstrating hydroureteronephrosis. **B,** Diethylenetriamine penta-acetic acid ℞Lasix renogram revealing impaired function and drainage. **C,** Time−activity curves from the renogram revealing slow accumulation and no response to ℞Lasix administration. **D,** Retrograde ureterogram demonstrating typical megaureter. **E,** Follow-up renogram after tapered reimplantation demonstrating improved function. **F,** Time−activity curves from the follow-up renogram showing improvement. **G,** Postoperative nuclear cystogram is negative for reflux.

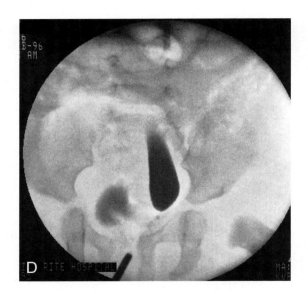

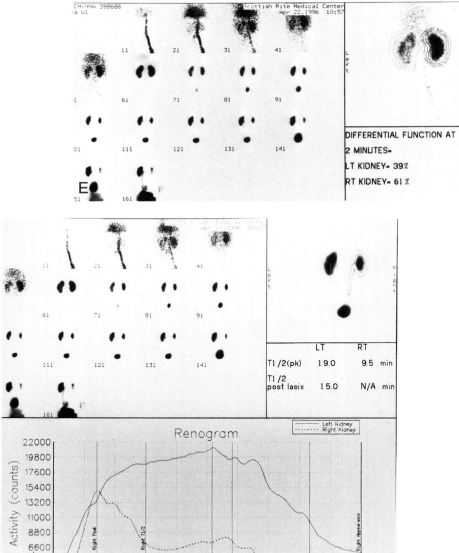

FIG. 12.1. *Continued.*

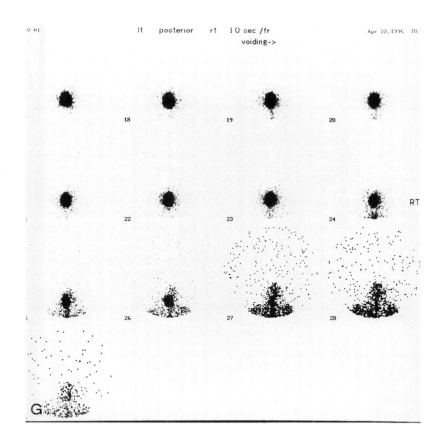

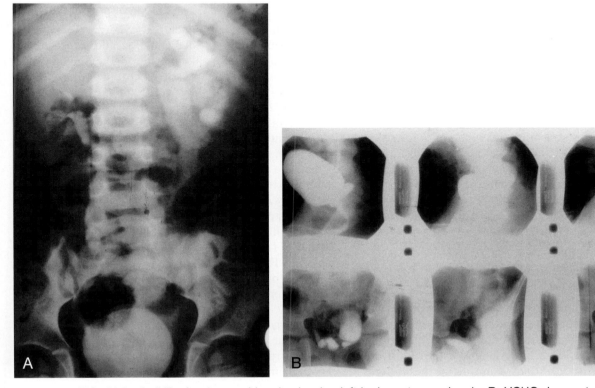

FIG. 12.1. *Continued.*

FIG. 12.2. A, IVP of a 4-year-old male showing left hydroureteronephrosis. **B,** VCUG demonstrating high-grade reflux with periureteral diverticulum.

ties when imaged at the immediate end of voiding, but large urinary residuals develop as a consequence of the back-and-forth passage of urine between the ureters and bladder.

Several investigators have observed that the complication rate for ureteral reimplantation is higher for refluxing megaureters than for obstructive megaureters.[22,23] Although the collagen content of the obstructive megaureter is increased, an even more exaggerated elevation of collagen content has been observed for the refluxing megaureter. Lee et al.[24] observed a twofold increase in the collagen:smooth muscle ratio in refluxing megaureters compared to obstructive megaureters. These ultrastructural derangements offer a reasonable explanation for the high rate of surgical complications seen with reconstruction of a refluxing megaureter.

Primary Nonrefluxing, Nonobstructive Megaureter

Primary nonrefluxing, nonobstructive megaureter may represent a mild variant of the obstructive megaureter with a short, nonstenotic adynamic segment at the most distal aspect of the ureter (Fig. 12.3). This diagnosis is being made with great frequency in this era of prenatal ultrasonography. At birth, an ultrasound will reveal normal renal parenchyma, usually with well-preserved calyces, and ureteral dilation to the level of the bladder. The subsequent VCUG excludes reflux, and the nuclear renogram shows preservation of renal function with a good drainage pattern. Usually, the lower third of the ureter appears the most dilated, and there is little ureteral tortuosity.

Primary Refluxing Obstructive Megaureter

The final category, combining both refluxing and obstructive megaureter, seems an unusual combination. In this condition, the vesicoureteral junction is incompetent and allows reflux through an adynamic distal segment. The VCUG demonstrates faint contrast refluxing into a dilated ureter; and because the ureter empties poorly, delayed images reveal persistent contrast in the collecting system and ureter. An obstructive pattern can be seen on nuclear renogram imaging with a bladder catheter in place.

Secondary Megaureter

Secondary megaureters are acquired as the consequence of forces applied to the ureter and may result in the patterns of obstruction, reflux, or ureteral dilation in the absence of reflux or ureteral obstruction. Obstruction may be produced at any point along the ureteral course by extrinsic processes, such as tumors, retroperitoneal fibrosis, and vascular malformations. Ureteral calculi and, rarely, primary ureteral tumors may also cause obstruction. Finally, obstruction may result as a postsurgical complication, usually as a consequence of ureteral angulation or devascularization of the ureter.

Functional obstruction of the ureter, such as that associated with posterior urethral valves or neuropathic bladder disease, occurs with elevated bladder pressures that impede ureteral emptying. The bilateral hydroureteronephrosis that accompanies posterior urethral valves is expected to show gradual improvement after valve ablation.[25] Despite the considerable hypertrophy of the bladder wall, this alone does not usually impede ureteral emptying. Elevated bladder pressures after valve resection may persist, however, despite complete resolution of the urethral obstruction, a phenomenon described as the valve bladder syndrome.[26] Fibrosis and bladder muscle hypertrophy as a result of bladder outlet obstruction may produce a noncompliant bladder that develops high intravesical pressures at relatively low volumes. These hostile bladder dynamics may be exacerbated when there is a urine-concentrating defect and high urinary flow rates.

Neurogenic dysfunction, most often caused by myelomeningocele, may also produce hostile bladder dynamics that impair ureteral emptying. Parameters that predict upper tract deterioration include detrusor–sphincter dyssynergia, diminished bladder wall compliance, and leak point pressure >40 cm H_2O.[27] Hinman–Allen syndrome (nonneurogenic, neurogenic bladder) may also produce upper tract dilation as a result of functional detrusor–sphincter dyssynergia. Despite the absence of a neurologic defect, these children are unable to relax the external sphincter during voiding and thus have elevated voiding pressures, chronic urinary retention, and reduced bladder wall compliance.[28]

Secondary refluxing megaureter may occur with posterior urethral valves, neurogenic bladder, or Hinman–Allen syndrome. The elevated bladder pressures cause decompensation of the ureterovesical junction. Occasionally, a paraureteral diverticulum is present cephalolateral to the orifice, which may be drawn into the diverticulum with complete loss of the transmural tunnel. With posterior urethral valves, reflux is present in 50% of cases; half are unilateral and half are bilateral. Resolution of reflux may be observed after successful valve ablation. Reflux associated with neurogenic bladder dysfunction may resolve after anticholinergic therapy and intermittent catheterization or after bladder augmentation.

Secondary nonrefluxing, nonobstructed megaureter may occur with persistent ureteral dilation after correction of a refluxing or obstructive megaureter. Although gradual improvement is expected, continued dilation should prompt re-evaluation of ureteral drainage and preservation of renal function.

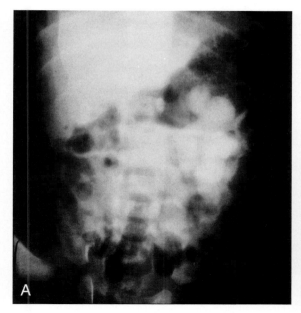

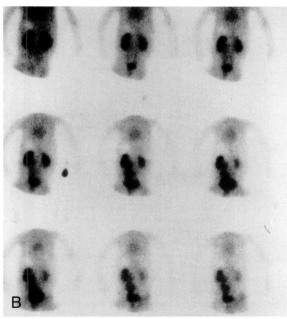

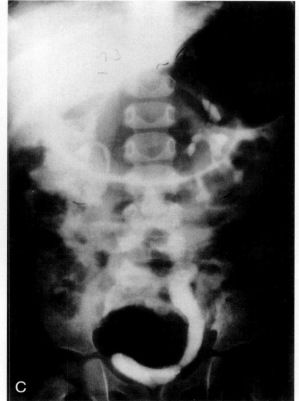

FIG. 12.3. **A,** Early postnatal IVP demonstrating hydroureteronephrosis. The VCUG is negative for reflux. **B,** Diuretic renogram showing good function but statis of urine in the large collecting system and ureter. **C,** IVP taken 1 year later showing spontaneous resolution of hydronephrosis with residual dilation of the distal one-third of the ureter.

Other causes include diabetes insipidus and ureteral atony accompanying gram negative urinary tract infection. The latter is caused by the paralytic effect of bacterial endotoxin on the ureteral smooth muscle.

DIAGNOSIS

A megaureter may be suspected after an abnormal prenatal ultrasound or radiologic evaluation for urinary tract infection, hematuria, abdominal mass, or cyclic abdominal pain. The goal of the evaluation is specific classification of the cause of the enlarged ureter. Ultrasound is an excellent anatomical study that can reveal the degree of dilation of the renal pelvis and calyces, proximal and distal ureteral dilation, atrophy of the renal parenchyma, bladder wall thickness, and presence of intravesical ureteroceles (Fig. 12.4). The timing of neonatal ultrasound performed for the initial evaluation of prenatal hydronephrosis is important, because the transient oliguria that occurs after birth may underestimate even severe degrees of urinary tract dilation. Optimally, the neonatal ultrasound should take place at least 48 hours after birth in a well-hydrated infant.

Intravenous pyelography is also an excellent anatomical study and provides subjective estimation of relative renal function. Unfortunately, young infants often have

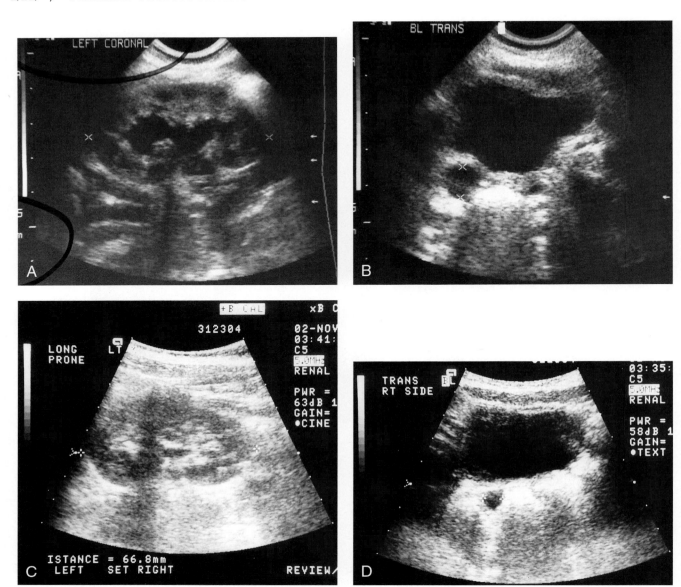

FIG. 12.4. A, Early postnatal ultrasound showing moderate left hydronephrosis. **B,** Transverse imaging at the level of the bladder showing distal ureteral dilation. **C,** Ultrasound study conducted 2 years later showing that the hydronephrosis spontaneously resolved. **D,** Note the distal ureter is still dilated, although less so.

large amounts of intestinal gas, which can obscure detail, especially for poorly functioning renal units. Delayed films are essential for evaluating hydroureteronephrosis, because early films might erroneously suggest a ureteropelvic junction obstruction rather than a ureterovesical junction obstruction. A properly performed VCUG and radiographic images of the spine, pubis, and bladder (early and late filling); voiding images of the bladder, urethra, and renal fossa; and postvoiding images of the bladder are essential for ruling out primary VUR, poste-

FIG. 12.5. A, Early postnatal ultrasound demonstrating severe bilateral hydroureteronephrosis. Note that the VCUG is negative for reflux and posterior urethral valves; the creatinine level is normal. **B,** The 2-min images revealing significant background activity and equal renal function. **C,** Time–activity curves showing slow accumulation and partial response to Lasix administration. **D,** The 2-min images taken 1 year later showing low background activity and equal renal function. **E,** Time–activity curves showing spontaneous improvement in accumulation and drainage of isotope. **F,** Ultrasound study confirming the spontaneous improvement.

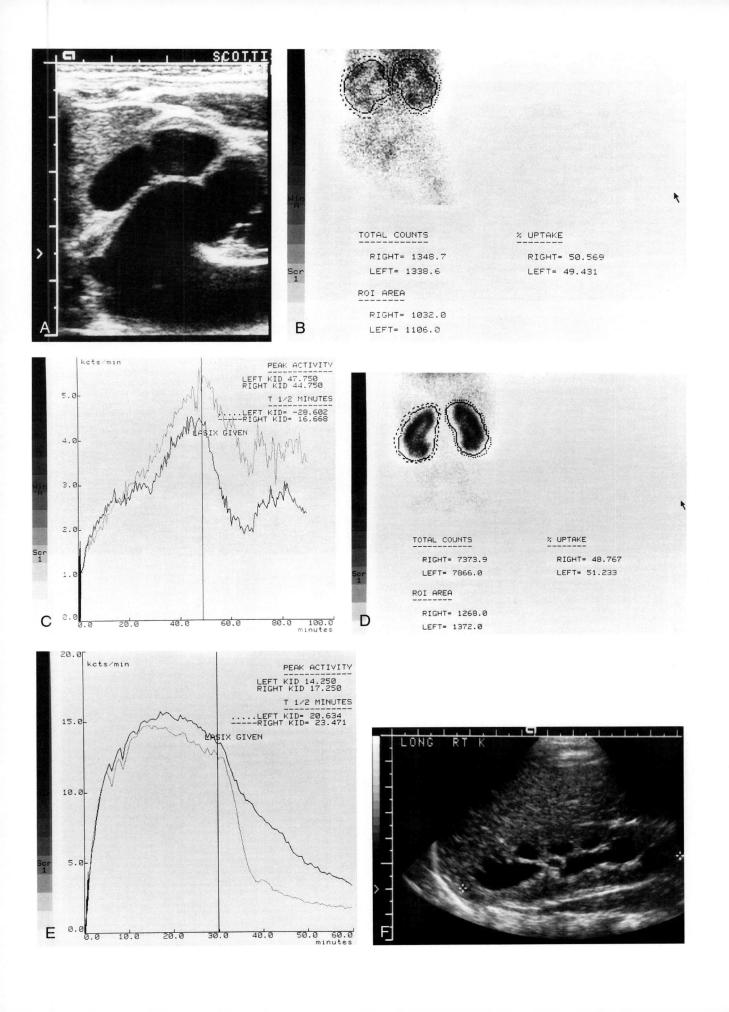

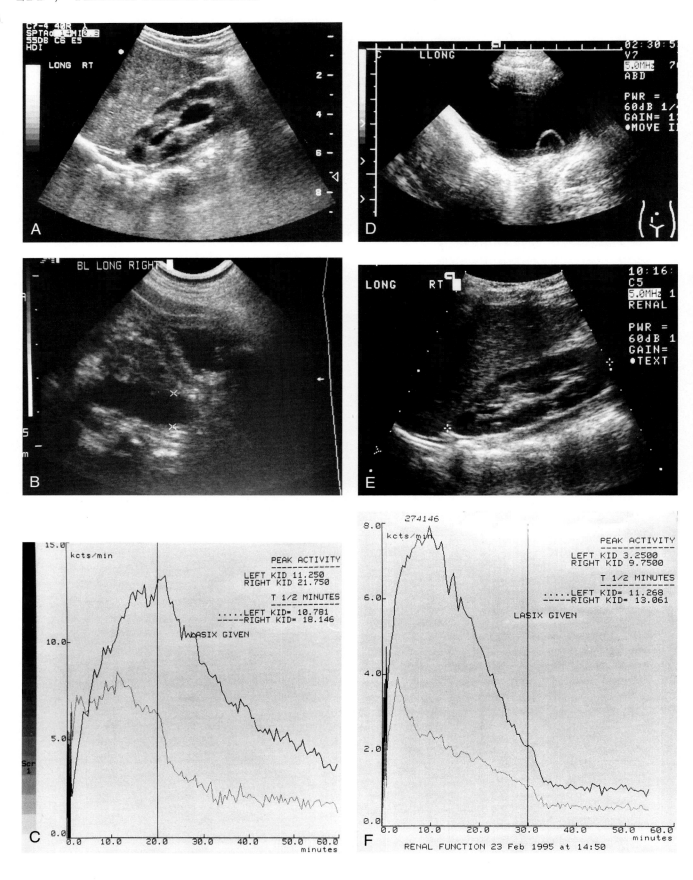

rior urethral valves, bladder diverticulum, neurogenic bladder, ureteroceles, and ectopic refluxing ureters. Generally, the combination of ultrasound and voiding cystourethrogram is adequate to eliminate all possible causes, except primary nonobstructive and primary obstructive megaureters.

Diuretic nuclear renography has replaced contrast excretory renography at many institutions as a valuable aid for objectively establishing differential renal function and for serially monitoring both function and drainage of dilated renal and ureteral units (Fig. 12.5). Diuretic renography involves intravenous injection of a radioisotope after establishing a well-hydrated state with intravenous fluids. After injection, a time–activity curve of the tracer's passage through the kidney and ureter can be generated, and washout patterns are recognized after the administration of an intravenous diuretic. Because the fractional renal uptake of the isotope within the first 3 min after administration is proportional to the glomerular filtration rate (GFR) of each kidney, estimates of differential renal function are obtained. In a nonobstructed system, the differential function should be 50% from each kidney, and the tracer should promptly wash out from the pelvis and ureter. In cases of partial obstruction, there should be retention of tracer proximal to the obstruction. Unfortunately, because diuretic renography is a physiologic study, its accuracy depends on many factors, including renal function (poor function may cause poor washout), capacity and contractility of the renal pelvis and ureter (large systems do not coapt well), state of hydration (dehydration causes prolonged parenchymal transit), and the state of bladder filling (the study should be performed with continuous bladder drainage).

Pressure–perfusion studies (Whitaker tests) can be useful in evaluating equivocal urinary tract obstruction.[29] Generally a nephrostomy tube or needle is placed percutaneously into the renal pelvis, and perfusion of the kidney at high flow rates (10 mL/min) is used to simulate a diuresis and to determine the pressure required to sustain urine flow past the obstruction. A pressure >22 cm H_2O correlates with true obstruction; a pressure <15 cm H_2O suggests no obstruction; and intermediate values are considered indeterminate. Unfortunately, the test does not actually measure or define obstruction. Rather, it records pressures in the renal pelvis during unphysiologically high flow rates. The pressures observed during the study may never occur at normal flow rates, especially if the pelvis and ureter are highly compliant, as is common in children.

Despite an array of anatomical and functional testing, differentiating urinary dilations that are significantly obstructive (requiring surgery) from those that represent mere anatomical variants (with no implications for renal functional deterioration) is no simple task, especially in the newborn. Numerous reports of spontaneous resolution in cases of mild, moderate, and even severe degrees of hydroureteronephrosis have caused clinicians to adopt a conservative approach for the management of neonatal megaureters.[30–34] In the absence of infection, it is rare to see deterioration of renal function during a course of expectant observation with serial ultrasound and diuretic renography. For this reason, most patients receive antibiotic prophylaxis during the period of observation until improvement (either spontaneous or surgical) is realized.[32, 33, 35] Reasonable indications for surgical correction are deterioration of renal function, as measured by renography, and symptoms such as breakthrough pyelonephritis, pain, or calculus formation. As few as 17% of cases in a large series of patients with primary obstructive megaureters required surgical intervention for these indications, whereas 34% of cases experienced spontaneous resolution of difficulties, and 49% of cases reported no symptoms.[33] In this same study, a distal ureteral diameter >10 mm and poor drainage on diethylenetriamine penta-acetic acid (DTPA) renography were highly correlated with the eventual need for surgical correction.

Pitfalls in Diagnosis

Despite the aggregate high sensitivity and specificity of ultrasound, VCUG, IVP, and nuclear renography, sometimes misdiagnosis occurs. An orthotopic ureterocele can be mistaken for primary obstructive or nonobstructive megaureter if the intravesical portion is missed on ultrasound (Fig. 12.6). IVP delineates the cobra head deformity seen with orthotopic ureteroceles. Ectopic ureters can be mistaken for primary obstructive megaureters until cystoscopy reveals the absence of a normal ipsilateral ureteral orifice. Primary obstructive megaureters can occur with ureteral duplication and masquerade as an upper pole ectopic ureter (Fig. 12.7). Ureteropelvic junction obstruction can coexist with obstructive megaureter, and the anatomy of the system may be fully recognized only with retrograde pyelography. Because

FIG. 12.6. Prenatal (A) and postnatal (B) ultrasound studies showing right hydroureteronephrosis and no intravesical defects. C, Diuretic renogram showing good function and mild impairment in drainage. D, Subsequent ultrasound study demonstrating intravesical ureterocele, which was shown to be orthotopic by cystoscopy. The ureterocele was punctured with the Bugbee electrode. Follow-up ultrasound (E) and diuretic renogram (F) showing improvement.

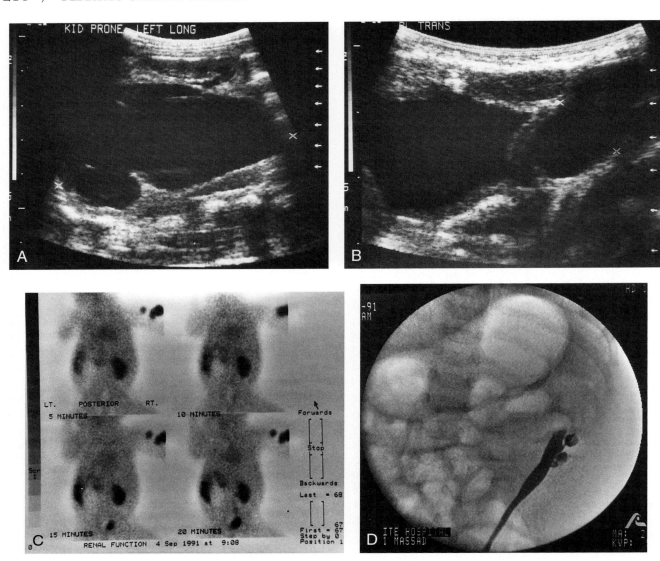

FIG. 12.7. A, Ultrasound study of a newborn male showing a massive hydroureteronephrosis on the left side. **B,** Bladder images showing a large distal ureter but no intravesical abnormality. **C,** Nuclear renogram revealing good function in the lower pole area and impaired function in the upper and more medial area. The VCUG is negative for reflux. **D,** Cystoscopy revealing two normal-appearing left-sided ureteral orifices. Retrograde pyelogram of the most lateral orifice is negative for obstruction. Retrograde ureterogram **(E)** and pyelogram **(F)** for the most medial orifice demonstrating megaureter with a distal adynamic segment. **G and H,** Follow-up ultrasound studies are normal. **I,** Dimercaptosuccinic acid scan showing a rim of function from the previously obstructed segment. **J,** Nuclear cystogram showing no reflux.

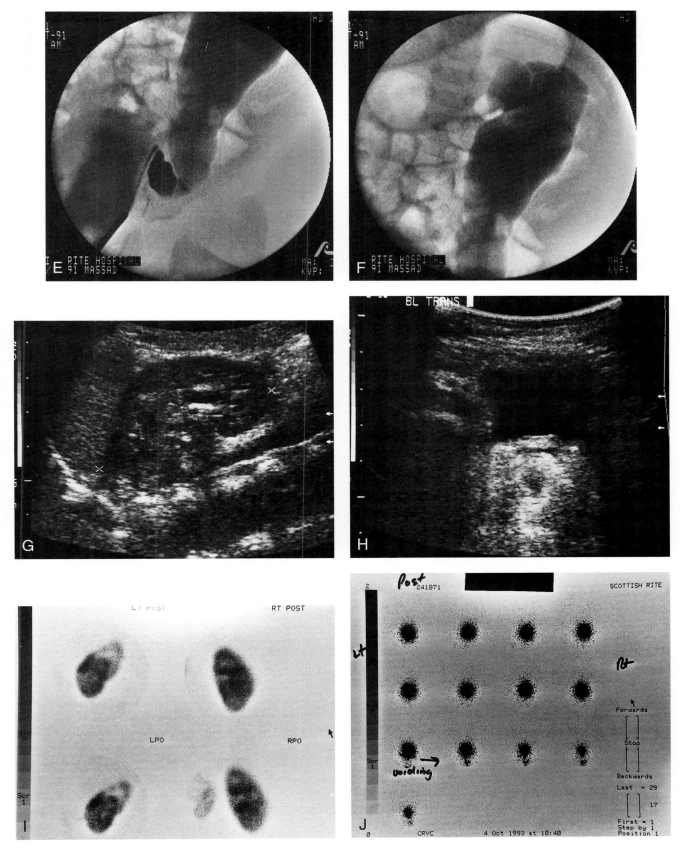

FIG. 12.7. *Continued.*

of these possibilities, the surgical approach to obstructed megaureters should include preliminary cystoscopy and, occasionally, retrograde pyelography to confirm the diagnosis before an incision is made.

SURGICAL MANAGEMENT

If an obstructive megaureter has significant loss of ipsilateral renal function on the initial work-up or subsequently fails nonoperative management (progressive loss of renal function, urinary infection, recurring pain) surgical repair is indicated. The goals of the surgery are removal of the obstructing segment; reduction of the caliber of the portion of the ureter to be reimplanted (while carefully preserving ureteral blood supply); and reimplantation of the tapered segment to prevent reflux, obstruction, and interference with the contralateral ureter.

Approach to the Ureter

Mobilization of the megaureter can be accomplished via an intravesical, an extravesical, or a combination of intravesical and extravesical approaches. For the intravesical approach, the bladder is opened anteriorly through a Pfannenstiel incision. Generally, the ureteral orifice and intramural ureter are normally positioned and easily cannulated with a feeding tube or ureteral stent. A pursestring suture at the orifice facilitates tension and countertension as the ureter is detached from adjacent bladder muscle, and the wide portion of the ureter is continuously mobilized into the bladder through the original muscular hiatus. Fibrous and vascular bands that contribute to ureteral tortuosity can be released serially until enough ureter for the reimplantation has been freed. The temptation to overstraighten the more proximal ureter should be resisted, because this may impair distal ureteral vascularity and does not improve the success of the operation.

The extravesical approach to the megaureter involves a transverse lower abdominal incision, and the bladder is reflected to the contralateral side. The obliterated hypogastric artery is divided, the peritoneum is reflected medially and superiorly, and the ureter is identified underneath. Ureteral mobilization is then carried proximally and distally to the intramural ureter. Completion of the tapering and reimplantation then can be accomplished intravesically or extravesically. Bilateral extravesical mobilization has been associated with transient bladder dysfunction, necessitating continuous or intermittent bladder catheter drainage.

To reduce the complication of postsurgical reflux and possibly increase the efficiency of peristalsis in the lower ureter, some form of caliber reduction is performed. Prevention of reflux requires a 5:1 ratio of tunnel length to ureteral width. Folding techniques, such as Kalicinski

et al.'s and Starr's, reduce the need for prolonged ureteral drainage and perhaps are superior to excisional techniques in regard to preserving ureteral vascularity.[36, 37] The Kalicinski et al. technique of ureteral folding begins with a continuous suture placed at the superior aspect of the tapering; and a 10- to 12-Fr catheter is used to guide the gentle transition to the new meatus (Fig. 12.8). The lateral excluded portion is then wrapped around the remaining ureter with another continuous suture.[38] The Starr technique plicates the ureteral wall, rolling the excess ureter into the lumen[39] (Fig. 12.9).

Excisional reduction of the ureter has the advantage of debulking the muscular ureter[40] (Fig. 12.10); but leaks can occur during the healing process, and it requires 10 to 12 days of stent drainage. Some surgeons confirm ureteral healing with retrograde studies before stent removal. Intravesical fistula formation can be decreased by using tunneling reimplant techniques and by placing the ureteral suture lines against the bladder muscle, not the mucosa. Before excision of a portion of the ureter, the segment is inspected in regard to the preponderance of ureteral vessels. The use of optical magnification is helpful for this part of the procedure. A wedge of ureter is marked out with holding sutures about a 10- to 12-Fr catheter. Overlying adventitia with vessels can be preserved as an overlapping edge. Long, straight scissors are used to trim off the wedge to prevent a ragged edge. Then the ureter is closed in a watertight fashion in two

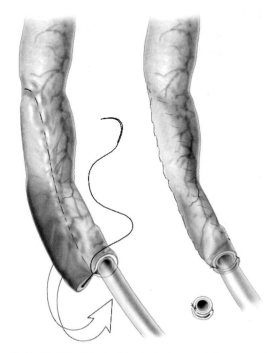

FIG. 12.8. Kalicinski et al.'s technique of lumen reduction of megaureter.

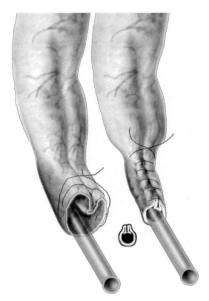

FIG. 12.9. Starr technique for lumen reduction of megaureter.

continuous layers: one a full thickness of the ureter, and the other of overlying adventitia. Leaks can be identified by retrograde injection along with suture line.

Reimplantation techniques are similar to those used for correcting primary vesicoureteral reflux. Depending on bladder size, ureteral caliber, and the unilateral or bilateral nature of the megaureter, one of several tech-

niques can be employed. The Politano–Leadbetter procedure for ureteral reimplantation involves creation of a new vesical hiatus, located superiorly on the posterior bladder wall, by blindly passing the ureter outside the bladder to its new position. The ureter is then tunneled toward the bladder neck under the submucosa. Problems with this procedure include ureteral obstruction with bladder distension (J hooking) and the possibility of peritoneal entry and visceral perforation when blindly creating the new vesical hiatus.

The Lich extravesical approach has been modified for use with megaureter surgery.[41] Bladder distension is adjusted so that intravesical detrusorrhaphy can be made over the mobilized ureter from the ureterovesical junction to the cephalad border of the posterior vesical wall. The bladder mucosa is left intact, and the ureter is then detached and tapered. The ureter is anchored to the caudal aspect of the detrusorrhaphy; and the bladder muscle is reapproximated over the ureter, creating the submucosal tunnel. Stenting the repair is problematic, however, because internal double-J catheters are used, which are removed with a secondary anesthetic 4 to 6 weeks after surgery.

The Glenn–Anderson procedure is an intravesical technique that displaces the vesical hiatus and leaves the submucosal tunnel to extend toward the bladder neck (Fig. 12.11). This can create a long, straight tunnel that superiorly can be cannulated in the future by traditional transurethral techniques.

The Cohen technique of transtrigonal reimplantation of the ureters has become one of the most widely used procedures for megaureter surgery (Fig. 12.12). Additional length of the submucosal tunnel is gained by cross-

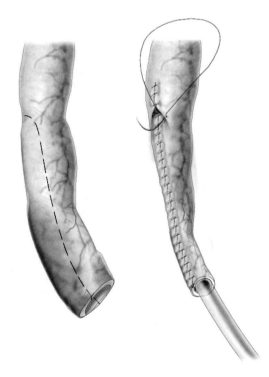

FIG. 12.10. Hendren technique of excisional reduction of megaureter.

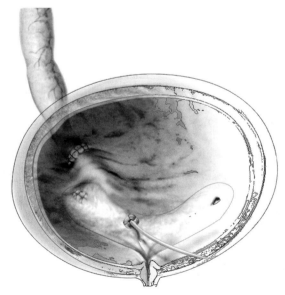

FIG. 12.11. Glenn–Anderson reimplantation of a tapered megaureter with advancement of the neo-orifice toward the bladder neck.

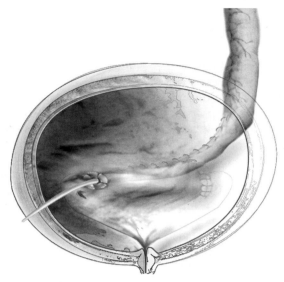

FIG. 12.12. Cohen transtrigonal reimplantation of a tapered megaureter.

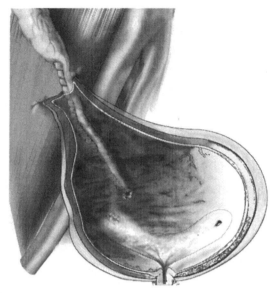

FIG. 12.13. Psoas hitch reimplantation of a tapered megaureter.

ing to the contralateral posterior bladder wall. Care must be taken not to interfere with the opposite ureteral orifice. Ipsilateral ureteral obstruction is rare, probably because of the maintenance of the original vesical hiatus. One drawback to the procedure is that the neomeatus faces laterally on the opposite side of the bladder, possibly confounding future ureteral cannulation per the urethra. Percutaneous access to the bladder is often necessary to aid cystoscopic ureteral access.

Occasionally, function of the kidney supplied by a megaureter will be severely impaired, and nephroureterectomy may be appropriate. In the rare case of renal insufficiency in a small infant, temporary cutaneous ureterostomy can be considered. This may be accomplished at the distal ureter with an end cutaneous ureterostomy or more proximally with a cutaneous pyelostomy or loop cutaneous ureterostomy. Proximal procedures have the advantage of not interfering with the distal ureteral blood supply (which will be important in later reconstruction) but the disadvantage of requiring a second incision for ultimate reconstruction.

Success rates for reimplantation surgery for megaureter are good, although not as high as for nondilating ureters associated with primary reflux. VUR is the most common complication; the incidence is approximately 10% of primary obstructive megaureter repairs. In many cases, postoperative reflux will resolve; sometimes as late as 2 to 3 years after the operation.[35] Observation and use of antibiotic therapy seem reasonable if this is encountered. Persistent obstruction can also complicate megaureter surgery, although it is much less common than reflux, occurring in 2 to 5% of cases. It is thought to be the result of ureteral ischemia and subsequent fibrosis of the tapered segment.

Reoperation for failed megaureter repair is generally approached intravesically and extravesically and can employ stretching the bladder toward a foreshortened ureter by sewing the superolateral aspect of the bladder to the psoas muscle with heavy absorbable suture (Fig. 12.13). If the contralateral ureter is normal (without reflux or obstruction), then a transureteroureterostomy can be performed if the ureteral length has been compromised distally by ischemia.

REFERENCES

1. Caulk JR. Megaloureter: the importance of the ureterovesical valve. J Urol 1923;9:315.
2. Creevy CD. The atonic distal ureteral segment (ureteral achalasia). J Urol 1967;97:457.
3. Swenson O, Fisher JH. The relation of megacolon and megaloureter. N Eng J Med 1955;253:1147.
4. Williams DI, Holme-Moir I. Primary obstructive megaureter. Br J Urol 1970;42:140.
5. Cussen LJ. Dimensions of normal ureter in infancy and childhood. Invest Urol 1967;5:164.
6. Smith ED, Cussen LJ, Glenn J, et al. Report of working party to establish an international nomenclature for the large ureter. In: Bergsma D, Duckett JW Jr, eds., Birth Defects 1977;13:3.
7. Noe HN. The wide ureter. In: Gillenwater JY, Grayhack JT, Howards SS, Duckett JW Jr, eds., Adult and pediatric urology. Chicago: Year Book, 1987;2:1653–1675.
8. Swenson O, MacMahon HE, Jaques WE, et al. A new concept of the etiology of megaureters. New Engl J Med 1952;246:41.
9. Leibowitz S, Bodian M. A study of the vesicle ganglia in children and the relationship to the megaureter megacystis syndrome and Hirshsprung's disease. J Clin Pathol 1963;16:342.
10. McLaughlin AP III, Leadbetter WF, Pfister RC. Reconstructive surgery of primary megaloureter. J Urol 1973;106:86.
11. Notley RG. Electron microscopy of the primary obstructive megaureter. Br J Med 1972;44:29.
12. Hanna MK, Jeffs RD, Sturgess JM, et al. Ureteral structure and ultrastructure. Part II: congenital ureteropelvic junction obstruction and primary obstructive megaureter. J Urol 1976;116:725.

13. Pagano F, Passerini G, Cortivo R, et al. The elastic component of normal and dilated ureters in children: chemical and histochemical characterization. Br J Urol 1976;48:13.

14. Gosling JA, Dixon JS. Functional obstruction of the ureter and renal pelvis. A histological and electron microscopic study. Br J Urol 1978;50:145.

15. Maizels M, Stephens FD. Valves of the ureter as a cause of primary obstruction of the ureter: anatomic, embryologic and clinical aspects. J Urol 1980;123:742.

16. Ostling K. Genesis of hydronephrosis. Acta Chir Scand 1942; 72(Suppl):5.

17. Sant GR, Barbalias GA, Klauber GT. Congenital ureteral valves: an abnormality in ureteral embryogenesis? J Urol 1985;133:427.

18. Chwalle R. The process of formation of cystic dilations of the vesical end of the ureter and of the diverticula of the ureteral ostium. Urol Cutan Rev 1927;31:499.

19. Mackie GC, Stephens FD. Duplex kidneys: a correlation of renal dysplasia with position of the ureteral orifice. J Urol 1975;114:274.

20. Elder JS. Commentary: importance of antenatal diagnosis of vesicoureteral reflux. J Urol 1992;148:1750.

21. Burbige KA, Leibowitz RL, Colodney AH, et al. The megacystis-megaureter syndrome. J Urol 1984;131:1133.

22. Johnston JH, Farlias A. The congenital refluxing megaureter: experiences with surgical reconstruction. Brit J Urol 1975;47:153.

23. Rabinowitz R, Barkin M, Schillinger JF, et al. Primary massive reflux in children. Urol 1979;13:248.

24. Lee BR, Partin AW, Epwstein JI, et al. A quantitative histological analysis of the dilated ureter of childhood. J Urol 1992;148:1482.

25. Glassberg KI, Schneider M, Halter JL, et al. Observations on persistently dilated ureter after posterior urethral valve ablation. Urol 1982;20:20.

26. Bauer SB, Dieppa RA, Labib K, et al. The bladder in boys with posterior urethral valves: a urodynamic assessment. J Urol 1979;121:769.

27. McGuire EJ, Woodside JR, Burden TA, Weiss RM. Prognostic value of urodynamic testing in myelodysplastic patients. J Urol 1977;177:232.

28. Allen TD. The non-neurogenic bladder. J Urol 1977;177:232.

29. Hanna MK, Edwards L. Pressure perfusion studies of the abnormal uretero-vesical junction. Br J Urol 1972;44:331.

30. Mollard P, Foray P, DeGodoy JL, Valignat C. Management of primary obstructive megaureter without reflux in neonates. Eur Urol 1993;24:505.

31. Cozzi F, Madonna L, Maggi E, Piacenti S, et al. Management of primary megaureter in infancy. J Pediatr Surg 1993;28:1031.

32. Baskin LS, Zderic SA, Snyder HM, Duckett JW. Primary dilated megaureter: long-term follow-up. J Urol 1994;152:618.

33. Lui HYA, Dhillon HK, Yeung CK, et al. Clinical outcome and management of prenatally diagnosed primary megaureters. J Urol 1994;152:614.

34. Keating MA, Escala J, Snyder HM, et al. Changing concepts in management of primary obstructive megaureter. J Urol 1989; 142:636.

35. Peters CA, Mandell J, Lebowitz RL, et al. Congenital obstructed megaureters in early infancy: diagnosis and treatment. J Urol 1989;142:641.

36. Bakker HHR, Scholtmeijer RJ, Klopper PJ. Comparison of 2 different tapering techniques in megaureters. J Urol 1988;140: 1237–1239.

37. Ehrlich RM. The ureteral folding technique for megaureter surgery. J Urol 1985;134:668.

38. Kalicinski ZH, Kansy J, Kotarbinska B, Joszt W. Surgery of megaureters—modification of Hendren's operation. J Pediatr Surg 1977;12:183.

39. Starr A. Ureteral plication. A new concept in ureteral tailoring for megaureter. Invest Urol 1979;17:153.

40. Hendren WH. Operative repair of megaureter in children. J Urol 1969;101:491.

41. McLorie GA, Jayanthi VR, Kinahan TJ, et al. A modified extravesical technique for megaureter repair. Br J Urol 1994;74:715.

CHAPTER 13

Posterior Urethral Valves and Other Obstructions of the Urethra

Anthony J. Casale

An obstruction more or less complete, due to the presence of abnormal valves or folds in the posterior urethra has occasionally been described in the literature.
— H. H. Young, R. H. Frontz, and T. C. Baldwin

Although Langenbeck is credited with giving the first recognition of posterior valves in 1802, the description by Young et al.[2] was the premiere scholarly statement of the condition; the classification that they devised is still in use today. Posterior urethral valves are the most common form of congenital urethral obstruction, occurring in 1 in 8,000 to 25,000 live male births.[3,4] There are reported cases of congenital urethral obstruction in the female, but this condition is not embryologically comparable to posterior valves of the male urethra.[5]

The word *valves* is inaccurate, because it implies a structure that has a normal function. It was adopted because these folds or membranes of the posterior urethra act as a passive one-way valve and impair the urine flow primarily in the antegrade direction while allowing easy retrograde flow. These structures are not present in the normal urethra, nor are they a part of normal urethral development.

Young et al. originally described three types of congenital posterior urethral obstruction (Fig. 13.1).

Type I. In the most common type there is a ridge lying on the floor of the urethra, continuous with the verumontanum, which takes an anterior course and divides into two fork-like processes in the region of the bulbomembranous junction. These processes are continued as thin membranous sheets, directed upward and forward which may be attached to the urethra throughout its entire circumference. In the majority of cases of this general type the fusion of the valves anteriorly is not complete, there existing at this point a slight separation of the folds. However, in a few of the cases . . . the anterior fusion

is complete while a cleft exists between the folds posteriorly.[2]

Modern authors believe that most patients have complete fusion of the valves anteriorly, leaving the only channel along the posterior urethra[6] (Fig. 13.2). Nevertheless, Young et al.'s description is remarkable, considering the limitations of endoscopic equipment and the few patients available to them.

Type I valves make up 95% of all posterior urethral obstructions. The membranes may be quite thin and almost transparent or rigid and thick. Pathologically they are made of a fibrous stroma surfaced on each side with transitional epithelium. The degree of obstruction caused by the valves varies considerably, depending on their configuration within the urethra. The embryologic source of these valves is thought to lie in the abnormal insertion of the mesonephric ducts into the fetal cloaca.[7] Evidence of this theory lies in the fact that type I valve patients lack plicae colliculi, mucosal folds found in the normal male urethra that are believed to represent a remnant of the normal pathway of migration of the mesonephric ducts toward the verumontanum.

Young et al.[2] described type II valves, which originate at the verumontanum and pass along the posterior urethral wall toward the bladder neck. They had only one case to study and were no doubt impressed by the similarities of these tissue folds with those distal to the verumontanum in type I. Type II folds are not obstructive but result from hypertrophy of muscle strips of the superficial trigone in response to high-pressure voiding due to obstruction distal to the verumontanum. They are seen in patients with urethral strictures, type I and type III valves, and detrusor–sphincter dyssynergia caused by neurogenic bladder. Although type II valves

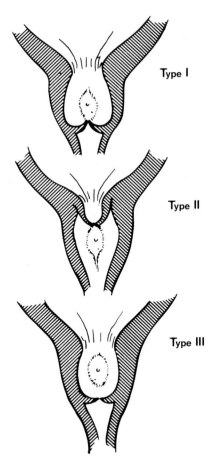

FIG. 13.1. Young et al.'s classification of posterior urethral valves. Reprinted with permission from Kaplan GW and Scherz HC. Infravesical obstruction. In: Kelalis PP, King LR, Belman AB, eds., Clinical pediatric urology. 3rd ed. Philadelphia: Saunders, 1992;2:821–864.

are relatively common, they are probably the result of a pathologic process rather than a cause. Modern urologic theory has established that type II valves do not exist as a pathologic condition.

> There is a third type which has been found at different levels of the posterior urethra and which apparently bears no such relation to the verumontanum as the types just considered. . . . This obstruction was attached to the entire circumference of the urethra, there being a small opening in the center. Incomplete varieties of this type have been described, the most common being a more or less crescentic or semicircular fold crossing the urethra and being attached either to the roof or floor.[1]

A type III posterior urethral valve is actually a membrane lying transversely across the urethra; a small perforation near the center allows some urine to pass, but the valve is a constant partial obstruction (Fig. 13.3). Type III valves differ from type I in that there is resistance to flow in both directions with type III. Both the degree of obstruction and the long-term prognosis appear to be significantly worse in type III. Because

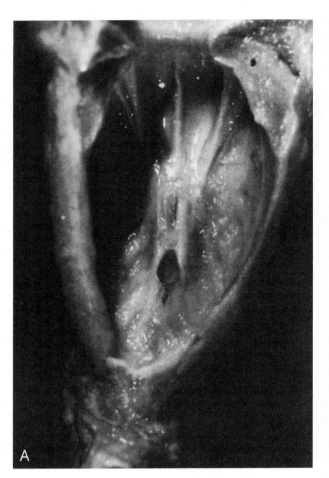

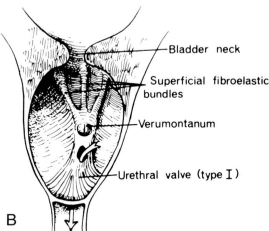

FIG. 13.2. A, An autopsy specimen of type I posterior urethral valves demonstrating the fused valve originating from the verumontanum and the raised folds between the verumontanum and the hypertrophied bladder neck, which Young et al. called type II valves. **B,** The same anatomy, labeled. Reprinted with permission from Gonzales ET. Posterior urethral valves and other urethral anomalies. In: Walsh PC, Retik AB, Stamey TA, Vaughan Jr ED, eds., Campbell urology. 6th ed. Philadelphia: Saunders, 1992:1872–1892.

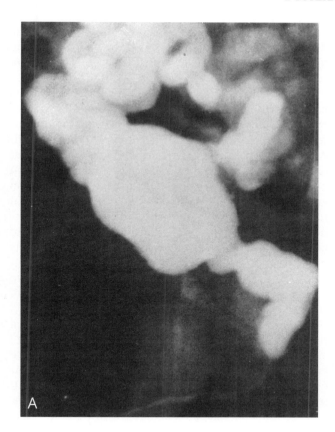

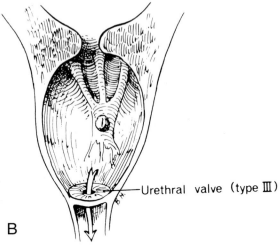

FIG. 13.3. A, A voiding cystourethrogram (VCGU) of a patient with type III posterior urethral valves and severe obstruction. The valve lies transversely across the urethra and is distal to the verumontanum. **B,** The same anatomy, labeled. Reprinted with permission from Gonzales ET. Posterior urethral valves and other urethral anomalies. In: Walsh PC, Retik AB, Stamey TA, Vaughan Jr ED, eds., Campbell urology. 6th ed. Philadelphia: Saunders, 1992:1872–1892.

type III valves have a different appearance and location from type I, the embryologic origins of the conditions are thought to differ. Type II valves are believed to originate from incomplete dissolution of the urogenital portion of the cloacal membrane.[8]

The shape of these membranes may be quite unusual; and if they are thin, they can elongate and extend into the bulbous urethra as a wind-sock valve. Type III valves make up only 5% of the total congenital obstructions of the posterior urethra and are thus rare. In fact, Rosenfeld et al.[9] could find only 17 cases reported in the literature by 1994.

The genetics of posterior urethral valves are poorly understood; but valves have occurred in siblings, twins, and successive generations.[10] The inheritance is probably polygenetic.[11]

PATHOPHYSIOLOGY

Congenital urethral obstruction of the urethra leads to almost global injury to the urinary tract, and the urethra distal to the valves is the only segment spared. The proximal urethra, bladder, ureters, and kidneys are affected in varying degrees, depending closely on the severity of the urethral obstruction. The prostatic urethra develops by the eighth week of life from the urogenital sinus, and the valves must develop during or after this period.[12] Although the exact embryologic cause of valves is still speculative, it appears that obstruction usually develops early in the second trimester after normal differentiation of the urinary tract, which is then forced to mature in the face of high interluminal pressure.

The nature of injury to the lower urinary tract seems solely caused by high-pressure voiding and storage of urine. Histologic studies of the bladder of fetuses with valves have demonstrated hypertrophy and hyperplasia of the detrusor muscle and increased connective tissue. The ratio of muscle to connective tissue, however, is the same as in normal bladders. Analysis of these connective tissue changes have yielded some conflicting results. Ewalt et al.[13] showed that type I collagen decreased and type III collagen increased in bladder muscle placed under strain. This contrasts with a study by Kim et al.[14] who examined valve bladders and found more type I than type III collagen. Because type I collagen is stiffer than type III, it seems that an increased ratio of type I collagen would decrease compliance and limit bladder capacity. Although the exact pathohistology is still debated, it is clear that valve patients have some of the most dysfunctional and abnormal-appearing bladders encountered in neonates. Most of the gross histologic changes in bladder structure resolve with relief of the obstruction, but bladder dysfunction persists into adulthood in many patients.

High intraluminal pressure is the cause of the damage to the proximal urethra and bladder neck. The prostatic urethra dilates in the face of high voiding pressures, and sometimes its capacity can approach that of the bladder. The verumontanum is distorted and the ejaculatory ducts may be dilated, permitting reflux of urine into the vas deferens. The bladder neck is rigid and hypertrophied. The high, thickened bladder neck was once thought to be a source of the obstruction, but it is now recognized that these bladder neck changes are secondary and will resolve once the urethral valves are destroyed and the obstruction is relieved.

The cause of injury to the upper urinary tract is more controversial. There is no question that high intraluminal pressures play a significant role in this process and are involved in the development of vesicoureteral reflux, ureterectasis, hydronephrosis, and renal damage found in most patients. These changes often resolve when the valve obstruction is relieved and the pressures are lowered. There are variations in the structure and competency of the ureterovesical junction, which play a major role in protecting the upper tract from the high pressures generated in the bladder. The pressure can lead to dilation of the upper tracts and to renal injury. The more functional the ureterovesical junction, the more protection is provided to the ureter and kidney on that side.

The nature of injury to the kidney in posterior urethral valves is complex. Renal damage in congenital obstruction appears to have two components. Some damage, described as obstructive uropathy, is caused by increased pressure and is potentially reversible. Other damage, renal dysplasia, may be a result of increased pressures early in fetal life or may be owing to abnormal embryologic development. Renal dysplasia is not reversible.

Renal dysplasia is a histologic diagnosis based on findings that include disorganization of the renal parenchyma and the presence of embryonic tubules, cartilage, cysts, and mesenchymal connective tissue. Some degree of dysplasia is found in almost all patients with posterior urethral valves. The type of dysplasia that occurs in valves is microcystic and occurs primarily in the peripheral cortical zone.[7]

Some authors believe that renal dysplasia is the result of high pressures affecting the maturation of the primitive metanephric blastema. There is some experimental evidence to support this view in animal models. Beck[15] and Glick et al.[16] showed that dysplastic changes occurred in the kidneys of lambs subjected to experimental fetal urinary obstruction. Maizels and Simpson[17] demonstrated dysplasia in chick embryonic kidneys after fetal ureteral obstruction. The consensus from these studies is that obstruction early in development can lead to dysplasic changes within the fetal kidney.

Henneberry and Stephens,[18] on the other hand, contend that dysplasia is a primary embryologic malformation that is the result of an abnormal position of the primitive ureteral bud along the mesonephric duct. They studied the position of the ureteral orifice in both valve and nonvalve patients with vesicoureteral reflux and found a strong relationship between dysplastic kidneys and an abnormal position of the ureteral orifice. The authors concluded that this relationship determines the degree of dysplasia within the kidney and defines the ultimate potential of the kidney for normal function, regardless of management.

In addition to dysplasia, virtually all valve patients have some degree of obstructive uropathy. This form of renal injury is expressed in both glomerular and tubular dysfunction and is potentially treatable. Glomerular filtration is decreased in valve patients just as in any other obstruction of the urinary tract. Increased intraluminal pressures eventually cause decreased renal perfusion and filtration. Early on, these changes are somewhat reversible; and immediate relief of the urethral obstruction is the first step after confirming the diagnosis of urethral valves. The prevention of progressive effects of obstruction is the basis for early diagnosis and treatment. Some degree of fibrosis and scarring within the parenchyma usually persists, but unlike dysplasia, obstructive uropathy is potentially reversible.

The injury from urethral valves also involves the renal tubules. Tubular damage results in failure to concentrate and acidify the urine normally in up to 59% of valve patients.[19] Parkhouse and Woodhouse[20] found tubular impairment may exist without decreased glomerular filtration rates. Concentrating defects are a form of nephrogenic diabetes insipidus and result in pathologically high urine output, independent of the patient's state of hydration. Sodium loss is high, and patients are prone to electrolyte imbalances. Infants with concentrating defects are fragile, because they easily become dehydrated if they cannot maintain enough oral intake to compensate for their obligatory urine output. Simple illnesses, such as gastroenteritis, are a problem because the kidneys are unable to conserve water and salt appropriately.[21] Pathologically high urine output also puts a strain on the ureters and bladder and often contributes to persistent hydronephrosis and exacerbates bladder dysfunction.

Most valve patients have hydronephrosis, which may be the result of obstruction or reflux. High pressures within the bladder may be transmitted to the ureters and kidneys either indirectly, by distorting the ureterovesical junction and impairing drainage at that level, or directly, through hydrostatic pressure. Another possible cause is an abnormal ureteral bud, which results in a dysplastic kidney and an ectatic collecting system.

Hydronephrosis may also be associated with vesicoureteral reflux. As with nonrefluxing hydronephrosis, the structure and function of the ureterovesical junction play important roles. Reflux is usually secondary to the bladder outlet obstruction due to valves and subsequent high bladder pressures. In some cases paraureteral diverticuli develop and contribute to reflux by further distorting the ureterovesical junction. Reflux may also be the result of an abnormal ureteral bud, leading to an ectopic ureteral orifice. Henneberry and Stephens[18] studied a series of fetuses and newborn infants with valves and found a significant incidence of ectopic ureteral orifices, which would explain reflux even in the absence of valves.

There are several variants in the pathologic process that are actually protective of renal function and decrease morbidity and mortality. All involve a form of pop-off valve or pressure-release mechanism. Urinary ascites, large bladder diverticuli, and massive unilateral reflex allow urine to escape the vice of the obstructed bladder, decreasing pressure on at least one renal unit and thus preserving function in that kidney.[22] Hoover and Duckett[23] identified the relationship of valves, unilateral reflex, and renal dysplasia as the VURD syndrome and outlined its potential protective effects on the contralateral kidney.

CLINICAL PRESENTATION

Posterior urethral valve patients present with a wide variety of symptoms that range from conditions incompatible with life to minor voiding dysfunction.[24] The presentation is age dependent.

Antenatal diagnosis by maternal ultrasound screening has become the most common method of identifying valve patients. Signs of fetal distress and intrauterine growth failure may accompany the common anatomic findings of a dilated bladder, hydroureteronephrosis, and oligohydraminos. Ultrasound screening is not foolproof, and a significant number of valve patients are missed when the maternal screening is done early in pregnancy.

Neonates present with a variety of clinical problems. The most profound and life-threatening is pulmonary distress, which accounts for almost all of the patient mortality in valve patients today.[25] Oligohydramnios secondary to decreased fetal urine production early in pregnancy leads to pulmonary hypoplasia, which may be untreatable even with heroic measures such as extracorporal oxygenation.[26] The exact pathophysiology is unclear but includes physical restriction of fetal breathing movements, leading to a small chest cavity and reduced chest wall musculoskeletal motion.[27] Other contributing factors are decreased branching of the bronchial tree and fewer alveoli, owing to restricted pressures and flow of amniotic fluid in the peripheral lung buds during development or possibly a failure to provide enough of an amniotic fluid substance necessary to promote alveolar development. Infants may be stillborn, progress to full respiratory failure within 48 h despite maximal ventilatory efforts, or may have transient pulmonary insufficiency that resolves with time and support.

Neonates may also present with signs of intrauterine growth retardation, failure to thrive, lethargy, and poor feeding; all signs of severe systemic illness. Urinary tract infection and urinary sepsis may lead to fever and vomiting. On physical examination, the infant may be pale and floppy with a palpable mass or masses in the abdomen, representing a distended bladder or hydronephrotic kidneys. There may be other signs of oligohydramnios, such as Potter's facies, limb deformities, and pressure contractures over the knees and elbows. The abdomen may be distended by urinary ascites, a complication of valves that makes up 40% of ascites in the newborn.[28] The high intraluminal pressure leads to extravasation of fetal urine, usually across a renal fornix. The retroperitoneal urine can then enter the peritoneal cavity directly or by transudation across the peritoneum (Fig. 13.4). Most patients strain to void with an intermittent stream; but this is not a reliable sign, and some infants with valves have been reported to have a normal void stream.[29] As a rule, the most severely affected patients present in the neonatal period, presumedly due

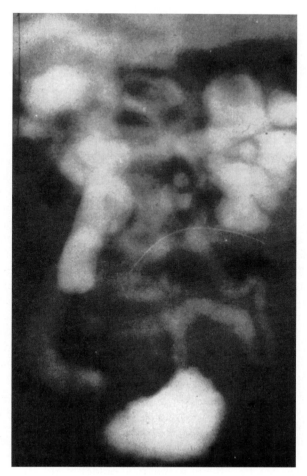

FIG. 13.4. A voiding cystourethrogram (VCUG) of a neonate with neonatal ascites owing to posterior urethral valves. Note the extravasation of contrast from the right kidney. Reprinted with permission from Casale AJ. Early ureteral surgery for posterior urethral valves. Urol Clin North Am 1990;17:364.

to advanced renal insufficiency and often urinary tract infection.[30]

Older infants and children either present with urinary tract infection or voiding disorders, such as urinary frequency, a dribbling stream, and incontinence. Occasionally, a child will present with the systemic signs of renal insufficiency: failure to thrive, vomiting, and hypertension. The majority of older patients complain primarily of incontinence and sometimes have a history of urinary tract infection; these patients often have good renal function.

INITIAL DIAGNOSTIC EVALUATION

Antenatal evaluation via maternal ultrasound has become commonplace in the United States. Approximately 80% of women undergo at least one screening ultrasound during pregnancy. The technology has improved greatly since the first reported ultrasound diagnosis of a fetal urologic anomaly in 1970, and the fetal urinary tract imaging is approaching the quality of that obtainable in infants.[31] Posterior urethral valves is the third most common antenatal genitourinary diagnosis made, after ureteropelvic junction obstruction and megaureter; it accounts for about 10% of all cases of fetal uropathy diagnosed in utero.[32] In the 1990s up to two-thirds of infants with posterior urethral valves were identified by antenatal ultrasound.[33]

Ultrasound is not foolproof either in sensitivity or in specificity. In one review, of 42 patients diagnosed with valves whose mothers had at least one ultrasound during pregnancy, only 45% were detected by antenatal ultrasound.[34] The remaining patients presented within the first 6 months of life with significant complications associated with urethral valves. The timing of the ultrasound examination seems critical, because 92% of the 36 patients scanned before 24 weeks of gestation were not identified as having obstructive uropathy. Hutton et al.[35] reviewed 31 patients whose valves were diagnosed prenatally and found that 55% were diagnosed by 24 weeks of gestation. The remaining 45% had a normal ultrasound at a median age of 18 weeks of gestation but were diagnosed with hydronephrosis later, at a median age of 30 weeks. Likewise, Jee et al.[36] found that 11 valve patients who presented as neonates had a normal ultrasound late in pregnancy. These studies suggest that screening for fetal uropathy should be done after 24 weeks of gestation and that, in some cases, hydronephrosis develops later in fetal life.

Although ultrasound is reasonably sensitive in detecting fetal hydronephrosis, the specific urologic diagnosis may be difficult to make. Shoulder et al.[37] studied 18 fetuses who were diagnosed with bilateral hydronephrosis and found that the correct diagnosis was made in 66% of cases. The differential diagnosis of valves includes prune belly syndrome, bilateral ureteropelvic junction obstruction, bilateral severe vesicoureteral reflux, bilateral ureterovesical junction obstruction, congenital urethral atresia, and anterior urethral valves. The classic abdominal ultrasound findings in patients with posterior urethral valves are bilateral hydroureteronephrosis associated with a distended bladder, a thickened bladder wall, and dilated posterior urethral and bladder neck[38] (Fig. 13.5).

Studying male fetuses with bladder distension and bilateral hydroureteronephrosis, Kaefer et al.[39] found that renal echogenicity predicted an obstructive processes and helped in the diagnosis of valves. They noted that of fetuses with bilateral hydroureteronephrosis and distended bladders, 87.5% of valve patients had increased renal echogenicity at a mean age of 26 weeks of gestation, whereas none of the patients with nonobstructive conditions (e.g., megacystis–megaureter association) displayed increased echogenicity. The same predictive value was true of oligohydraminos. Even in the absence of these diagnostic criteria, any male fetus with bilateral hydroureteronephrosis and decreased amniotic fluid volume have valves at the top of the list of diagnostic possibilities.

In the neonate and older child, the diagnostic evaluation is simple. The infant should undergo a renal and bladder ultrasound as soon as possible, which must be followed with a voiding cystourethrogram (VCUG). Once the diagnosis is suspected in a sick infant, a catheter should be placed to drain the bladder, even before radiographic examination. If the patient does not have bladder outlet obstruction, the catheter may be removed after a negative VCUG.

Ultrasound imaging of the posterior urethra from the perineal approach has been used in an attempt to diagnose valves via a noninvasive manner. Good et al.[40]

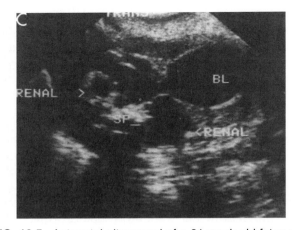

FIG. 13.5. Antenatal ultrasound of a 21-week-old fetus with posterior urethral valves. Note the bilateral hydroureteronephrosis and distended bladder. Reprinted with permission from Cendron M, Elder JS, Duckett JW. Perinatal urology. In: Gillenwater JY, Grayhack JT, Howards SS, Duckett JW, eds. Adult and Pediatric Urology. 3rd ed. St. Louis: Mosby, 1996;3:2075–2169.

compared the perineal ultrasound images obtained in infants with valves with those of normal children. They measured bladder wall thickness and the posterior urethral diameter before and during voiding. All three measurements were significantly greater in the valve patients; and in more than half of valve patients, the actual valve leaflets were visible on ultrasound. Although not applicable for many patients, perineal ultrasound may have a role in screening older children suspected of having valves.

Bladder wall thickness is clearly increased in patients with posterior urethral valves, but ultrasound measurements of the bladder wall are somewhat subjective and depend on the volume of urine in the bladder at the time. Kaefer et al.[41] helped clarify this measurement by studying the bladder thickness index, the ratio of the bladder wall thickness to the inner diameter of the bladder. They found the index to be reliable in predicting the presence of bladder outlet obstruction.

The VCUG remains the gold standard in the diagnosis of any type of urethral obstruction and should be obtained as soon as the patient's clinical condition allows the study to be done. Many neonates with valves are too ill at birth for a trip to the radiology department and require intensive support and resuscitation. As long as the bladder is adequately drained with a catheter, the infant can wait for the diagnosis to be established with a VCUG.

The VCUG of valve patients is different from that of normal controls in the posterior urethra, the bladder, and often the upper tracts. The importance of obtaining views of the urethra during voiding cannot be overemphasized. The appearance of the bladder and upper tracts may be identical in patients with neurogenic bladder and valves. The visualization of the posterior urethra is the critical diagnostic point. If the patient does not void with filling, then the Credé maneuver should be attempted.

The type I valve is usually visible as a linear flap across the urethra, extending obliquely from the level of the verumontanum posteriorly to a point more distal on the anterior urethral wall. The flow of contrast is limited to a posterior channel, which is usually quite narrow (Fig. 13.6). Type III valves are more perpendicular to the urethra and cause obstruction distal to the verumontanum. Both types are best visualized on the lateral projection; and both can cause similar changes in the proximal urethra and bladder, although Rosenfeld et al.[9] have reported that in type III valves the posterior urethra may be minimally dilated and beaklike.

The posterior urethra is dilated, often massively, and may be larger than the bladder itself, particularly on images taken late in voiding. The Christa urethralis and the verumontanum may be prominent, and there may be reflux of contrast into the ejaculatory ducts or seminal

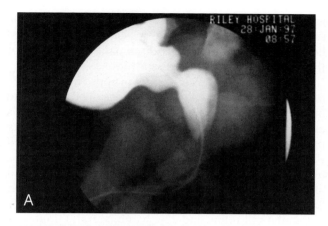

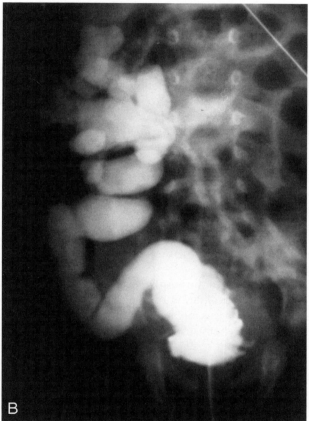

FIG. 13.6. **A,** Urethral view VCUG of a neonate with type I posterior urethral valves. Demonstrating a dilated posterior urethra and hypertrophied bladder neck. The contrast ends abruptly at the valves, and there is a catheter in the distal normal urethra. **B,** Abdominal view of the same patient shows a small trabeculated bladder with severe vesicoureteral reflux on the right.

vesicles. Frequently, a posterior diverticulum of the urethra or bladder neck exists. The bladder neck is thick and prominent, and the channel into the bladder is anteriorly displaced.

The bladder is thick walled and trabeculated. Often there are multiple saccules or diverticuli on the lateral aspects. The actual bladder volume may be surprisingly small compared to the mass, which may be palpated before catheterization. This discrepancy is a result of the thickened mass of detrussor muscle.

Vesicoureteral reflux is present in approximately 50% of valve patients at the time of diagnosis. Today, because most valve patients are diagnosed in utero and VCUGs are obtained soon after birth, the incidence of reflux may increase. In a large series, Churchill et al.[25] found the incidence of reflux to be 40%; the incidence was higher in neonates (52%) than in patients diagnosed after 1 year of age (31%). Hoover and Duckett[23] studied 82 patients with valves and found 48% with reflux: 24% had unilateral reflux and 22% had bilateral. Of interest was the preponderance of left-sided reflux in the unilateral cases (80%). Many patients with unilateral reflux have associated dysplasia and VURD syndrome, which occur in 15 to 20% of valve patients.

Radionuleide renal scans have become an invaluable tool for assessing renal function and planning management. Myelin-associated glycoprotein 3 (MAG-3) is the favored isotope, because of its ability to provide functional data along with visual images of the parenchyma and collecting system. Because of the relative immaturity of neonatal renal function, scans in the newborn may not be optimal, but they provide data about renal perfusion and function. In patients with reflux care must be taken to keep the bladder as empty as possible to avoid artifactual function from refluxed isotope. Gravity drainage of the catheter may not keep the bladder empty in the face of a diuresis induced by the isotope or diuretic, and it may be necessary to aspirate the bladder catheter manually during the scan.

Laboratory evaluation of newly diagnosed valve patients should focus on renal function and electrolyte status. Serum chemistries in the newborn do not clearly reflect the infant's renal function during the first 48 h after birth. The mother's kidneys, in effect, dialyze the fetus via the placenta; and only after this effect has been removed, can the infant's renal function be assessed. Elevations in serum creatinine and blood urea nitrogen (BUN) are usual, and associated metabolic acidosis is reflected in a decrease in serum bicarbonate levels. Hyperkalemia may present an acute threat to the infant's survival and is often the first priority in treatment. The urinalysis usually demonstrates some tubular injury in the patient's inability to concentrate the urine. The most critical finding in the urinalysis is evidence of infection in the presence of nitrites and leukocytes. Once the catheter is placed, the urine should be sent for culture and the patient started on broad-spectrum antibiotics. The choice of antibiotics should take into account the potential compromised renal function, and nephrotoxic antibiotics must be used with extreme caution or avoided completely.

INITIAL MANAGEMENT

Once the diagnosis of posterior urethral valves is suspected, the first treatment is to relieve the obstruction. In newborns or patients with urinary tract infection, a catheter should be placed immediately and followed as appropriate by the radiographic evaluation. For older children who are not acutely ill, a renal ultrasound and VCUG can be performed first to confirm the diagnosis before any treatment is undertaken. Neonates can be catheterized with a small feeding tube (3.5 or 5 Fr). Foley catheters have been used successfully but have also been associated with poor upper tract drainage owing either to volume displacement of the balloon or to irritation of the bladder by the balloon.[42] It is important to confirm that the catheter has been placed within the bladder. It must irrigate easily; if there is any doubt about its location, a one-shot cystogram should be done to identify its position. In severe valve cases with pulmonary hypoplasia, catheter drainage is the only reasonable urologic treatment until the pulmonary status has improved. A bedside ultrasound can confirm the presence of renal pathology and hydronephrosis, but VCUG may need to be delayed.

Neonatology has contributed greatly to the decreased mortality in valve patients in the 1980s and 1990s. The initial management of the severe pulmonary, metabolic, infectious, and nutritional problems in these patients requires a dedicated team of pediatric medical specialists including a pediatric urologist. Infants with severe posterior urethral valves may require maximal ventilatory support, extracorporal membrane oxygenation, dialysis, and parenteral nutrition for prolonged periods.[43] Even with the most aggressive management and latest technology, some patients succumb to their pulmonary hypoplasia.[44] The stage of initial resuscitation carries the highest mortality risk for modern valve patients, and there are few deaths subsequently until the complications of end-stage renal disease, dialysis, and transplantation eventually become issues.

After the patient is stabilized and the diagnostic workup completed, the pediatric urologist must decide how to provide permanent relief of the obstruction. Historically, valves were destroyed with open procedures or suprapubic catheters were left in place for prolonged periods.[1, 45] These treatment methods often damaged the urethra or bladder and had a high mortality, because of urinary infection or progressive renal failure. They have been replaced with either initial endoscopic ablation of the valve or a temporary proximal diversion of the urine, followed months later with endoscopic ablation and reconstruction.

Methods of primary valve ablation include disruption with the Whitaker hook, a 6-Fr instrument with what looks like a crochet hook on the end.[46, 47] The instrument is passed into the urethra and may be used blindly or under fluoroscopic control to hook and disrupt the valves. For urologists who prefer to have direct vision of the procedure, a pediatric cystoscope may be passed and a bugbee electrode used to incise the valves (Fig. 13.7). Alternatively, an infant resectoscope may be used with a hook or flattened loop to incise the valves. Experienced surgeons can use a Nd-YAG laser to cut the valves.[48] If the patient's urethra is too small to easily admit the instrument, a perineal urethrostomy may be used to access the valves for ablation or the cystoscope may be passed in the antegrade manner through a suprapubic site.[49]

The exact point of incision of the valves is a matter of opinion; some pediatric urologists believe the valves may be incised once at the 12 o'clock position, whereas others contend two incisions at 4 and 8 o'clock positions are better. The point of the surgery is to disrupt the ability of the valves to obstruct the flow of urine from the bladder, and it has been my experience that some patients can be adequately treated with two incisions, but others require the 12 o'clock incision as well. It is not necessary to resect the valves; and in fact, most experts note that resection with a loop electrode can

lead to urethral damage and stricture formation. If the procedure has been particularly difficult or there is bleeding, the catheter may be left in place for 24 h; but this is not usually necessary.

In the past, the complication of urethral stricture following primary valve ablation was common, particularly in infants. Today, modern instruments allow safe access in all but the smallest urethras. For very small infants and for cases in which primary ablation is not the best option, a cutaneous vesicostomy may initially be performed; then valve ablation can be performed months later.

Proponents of vesicostomy as initial treatment of valves have shown it to be a safe and efficient method with long-term results that are equal to those of primary ablation[50] (Fig. 13.8). Vesicostomy is a good option in some valve patients with severe reflux. Krahn and Johnson[51] reviewed 50 infants who underwent vesicostomy for a variety of diagnoses, including urethral valves. More than 90% of these patients showed improvement or stabilization of the upper urinary tract. Vesicostomy is not without complications, however; and Noe and Jerkins[52] found a 40% complication rate in 35 patients including 3 who required surgery. The most common

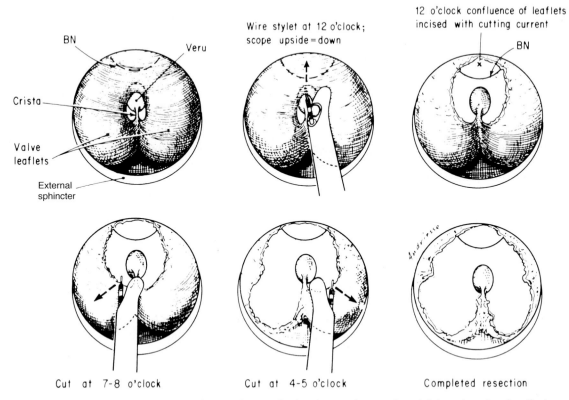

FIG. 13.7. Endoscopic ablation of posterior urethral valves using a wire stylet and ureteral catheter. The same method of incising valves may be used with an infant resectoscope and a wire electrode. *BN,* bladder neck. Reprinted with permission from Hendren WH. Urethral valves. In: Ashcraft KW, Holder TM, eds., Pediatric surgery. 2nd ed. Philadelphia: Saunders, 1993:668.

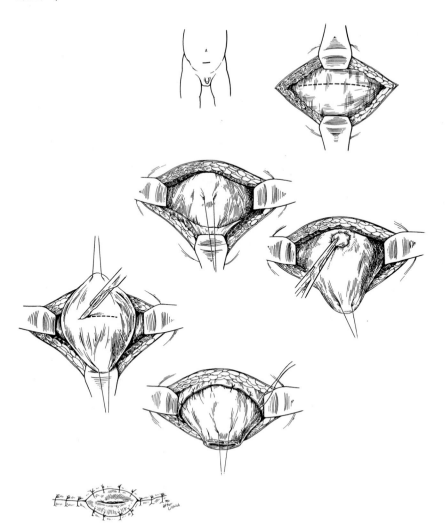

FIG. 13.8. Cutaneous vesicostomy. It is important to open the bladder near the dome and to suture it to the fascia and the skin to help prevent prolapse. Reprinted with permission from Retik AB, Colodny AH, Bauer SB. Pediatric urology. In: Paulson DF, ed., Genitourinary surgery. New York: Churchill Livingstone, 1984;2:867.

problem encountered in valve patients with vesicostomies was severe urinary infection. Despite earlier fears that the bladder would contract permanently when decompressed, this study and others have shown that patients treated with a temporizing vesicostomy did not lose bladder capacity.

A final option in initial management of valve patients is diversion above the level of the bladder, with either a cutaneous ureterostomy or a pyelostomy. There has been much debate over which initial treatment of valves will yield the best long term renal function and upper tract drainage. High-loop ureterostomy, introduced in the 1950s, efficiently drains the upper tracts while helping control infection.[53] Sometimes ureterostomy left patients with difficult reconstructive problems; but considering the technology of the times, it was a major step forward. As new endoscopes were developed, primary valve ablation became safer and easier. In 1966, Johnson[54] showed that infants treated endoscopically experienced improvement of their upper tracts and renal function. Once endoscopic ablation was established as a

reasonable alternative to upper tract diversion, proponents of each approach debated the question vigorously over the following decades.

Krueger et al.[55] presented data showing that infants treated primarily with ureterostomy had better somatic growth and ultimate renal function than did patients treated only by endoscopic valve ablation. Reinberg et al.[56] and Hendren[57] demonstrated that the results of primary ablation and vesicostomy are similar to those of ureterostomy; however, ureterostomy patients have the added problems of a flank stoma and must face several reconstruction surgeries. Some surgeons believe strongly in the benefits of an externally drained upper urinary tract, but no one has yet established that upper tract diversion is superior to primary ablation of valves or a vesicostomy. Currently, both approaches yield similar results in the long term, but patients who undergo upper tract diversion must undergo more surgical procedures.

Most pediatric urologists proceed with an initial transurethral valve ablation and follow the improvement of hydronephrosis and renal function (Fig. 13.9). In patients who respond with dropping creatinine levels and decreasing hydronephrosis, nothing else is done at this time. There are a few patients who fail to improve despite successful valve ablation. Their upper tracts continue to drain poorly through the ureterovesical junction, and renal function does not improve. If the bladder drains adequately and upper tract function does not improve after a reasonable amount of time, then an upper tract diversion may help maximize renal function improvement. The kidneys have the best opportunity to improve in the first few months of life, and there is evidence that they may actually continue to produce new cells during this time.[58, 59] Thus it is logical to relieve obstruction as soon as possible to allow optimal renal development. Although upper tract diversion may initially improve renal function, it appears to have no significant effect on long-term outcome.

The timing of upper tract intervention is a matter of judgment; but if there is no clear improvement of severely impaired renal function 10 days after valve ablation, then upper tract diversion may be considered. Improvement is usually measured by following serum creatinine and the severity of the hydronephrosis. Patients who have a serum creatinine level ≤2.0 generally can be watched, even in the face of hydronephrosis. Patients who have a creatinine level >2.0 after valve ablation can be followed for 7 to 10 days; if hydronephrosis persists, then upper tract diversion is an option. Upper tract diversion may also be useful in the rare patient with recurrent urinary infection who fails medical management. I prefer a low loop ureterostomy with upper tract diversion. This allows adequate upper tract drainage and makes reconstruction less complicated. The proximal end of the ureter can be reimplanted into the bladder, and the distal end can be removed or used as a continent stoma, if necessary. Before upper tract diversion is considered, all questions about the ability of the bladder to empty efficiently must be answered. Only in cases of persistent renal insufficiency and hydronephrosis, when the bladder empties well, should ureterostomy be considered. If the bladder is contributing to the upper tract problems, then a vesicostomy may be a better alternative.

The timing for urinary tract reconstruction in patients who have undergone vesicostomy or upper tract diversion depends on the child's renal and bladder function. The success of transplantation and the complication rate are more favorable in children older than 6 years. If end-stage renal disease is inevitable once the urinary

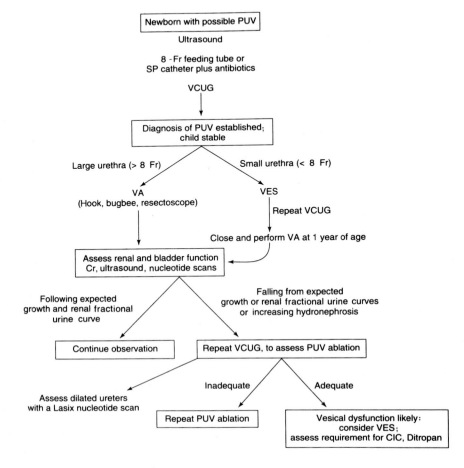

FIG. 13.9. Current initial treatment plan in an infant with posterior urethral valves (*PUR*). The role of upper tract diversion has diminished but may still be helpful in select patients. *U/S,* ultrasound; *SP,* suprapubic; *VA,* valve ablation; *VES,* vesicostomy; *Cr,* creatinine; *Fx,* fraction; *CIC,* clean intermittent catheterization. Reprinted with permission from Smith GHH, Duckett JW. Urethral lesions in infants and children. In: Gillenwater JY, Grayhack JT, Howards SS, Duckett JW, eds. Adult and pediatric urology. 3rd ed. St. Louis: Mosby, 1996;3:2422.

tract is internalized, it is best to wait until transplantation can be conducted.[60] Let the child use diapers or a stomal bag instead of pushing marginal kidneys into failure before dialysis and transplantation are practical. These management decisions are best made by a medical team that includes pediatricians, pediatric nephrologists, pediatric urologists, and transplant surgeons along with the family.

MANAGEMENT OF VESICOURETERAL REFLUX IN VALVE PATIENTS

Between 50 and 70% of patients with posterior ureteral valves have vesicoureteral reflux at the time of diagnosis.[61] Scott[62] examined a series of 46 patients with valves and found reflux in 72% of patients and 53% of ureters. Reflux was bilateral in 32% of patients. Reflux in valve patients is often secondary to increased intravesical pressure. The initial treatment of this reflux is to relieve the voiding obstruction from the valves, thereby lowering bladder pressure. It is also necessary to prevent infection by prescribing maintenance antibiotics. Between 20 and 32% of refluxing ureters resolve after valve ablation; resolution may occur up to 3 years later.[61, 62]

If the reflux persists or if infections occur even when the patient is on antibiotics, the physician must study the bladder to evaluate intravesical pressures and the ability of the bladder to empty adequately. If bladder function is abnormal, then anticholinergic therapy, a vesicostomy, or repeat valve ablation may be necessary before consideration is given to repair of the vesicoureteral reflux. Surgery to repair reflux in the valve patient is limited to patients who have breakthrough infections and fail medical therapy and those with reflux so severe that it interferes with bladder emptying.[3] Persistent low-grade reflux in the absence of infection need not be repaired, if the bladder function is adequate. Ureteral reimplantation conducted before the bladder has had an opportunity to rehabilitate carries a high complication rate (15 to 30%).[61, 63]

The special association of unilateral reflux into a nonfunctional kidney with dysplasia and posterior urethral valves, or VURD syndrome, was described by Hoover and Duckett[23] in 1982 (Fig. 13.10). They found this association in 13% of valve patients reviewed. The refluxing nonfunctioning kidney was on the left in 92%. Patients with the VURD association have a better prognosis than valve patients with bilateral reflux. The nonrefluxing kidney is spared the high pressures generated within the bladder by the severe reflux on the dysplastic side. This reflux acts as a pop-off valve to lower intraluminal pressures and protect the nonrefluxing kidney.

The long-term protective effects of VURD have been brought into question recently by Cuckow et al.,[64] who followed patients for up to 10 years. They found the glomerular filtration rate (GFR) to be significantly de-

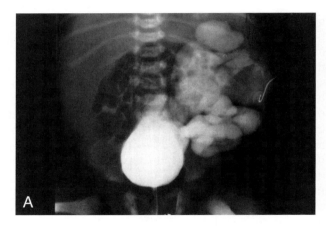

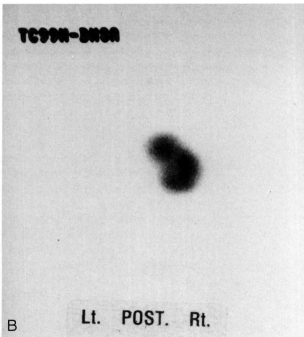

FIG. 13.10. **A,** VCUG in a patient with posterior urethral valves and the VURD syndrome. Severe unilateral reflux is associated with renal dysplasia on the refluxing side. **B,** Nuclear scan demonstrating nonfunction of the refluxing renal unit and reasonable function of the contralateral kidney.

creased in valve patients 5 to 8 years of age and the serum creatinine level to be normal in only 30% of patients aged 8 to 10 years. Although the renal prognosis of children with the VURD syndrome is better than that for patients with valves and bilateral reflux, these patients are still at significant risk for renal dysfunction throughout their life and should be followed accordingly.

In the past, the refluxing nonfunctional renal unit was removed when the patient was 2 to 3 years old. Today, the refluxing unit is often retained until adequate bladder function is established, because of the potential to use this segment for a ureteral augmentation of the bladder if necessary.[65] The ureter is the best material available for augmentation cystoplasty, because the bladder will be completely lined with urothelium and the surgery may be extraperitoneal.[66] Kim et al.[67] examined a series of valve patients in whom poorly functioning kidneys were left in place and reflux was repaired, if necessary. The authors note that in the absence of hypertension and pyelonephritis, the poorly functioning kidneys may be left alone. When surgery is needed to correct reflux in a poorly functioning contralateral kidney, reimplantation of both ureters is a reasonable option instead of nephrectomy.

PERSISTENT HYDRONEPHROSIS IN THE VALVE PATIENT

At diagnosis, almost all patients with posterior urethral valves have significant hydroureteronephrosis. Scott[62] found hydronephrosis, including reflux, in 96.5% of patients, which was bilateral in 78%. In some patients, the hydronephrosis will resolve soon after the valves are ablated and the bladder pressures are reduced. Nonrefluxing upper tract dilation subsided after valve ablation in 49% of patients. In many patients, however, the upper tracts remain dilated, despite successful valve ablation and adequate bladder emptying.

Hulbert and Duckett[68] found that 25% of valve patients aged 5 to 15 years have hydronephrosis without evidence of obstruction on diuretic renography. The question of whether there is simultaneous obstruction at the ureterovesical junction and at the posterior urethra is still difficult to answer.

Whitaker[69] studied the upper urinary tracts of 170 patients with posterior urethral valves and found that 70 (41%) remained grossly dilated and without reflux after treatment. Retrograde pyelograms and percutaneous antegrade pyelograms did not answer the question of obstruction in all cases. He developed the antegrade infusion test, which involves perfusing saline into the renal pelvis via a nephrostomy tube (usually placed percutaneously) at 10 mL/min. The difference between the renal pelvic pressure and the bladder pressure is then determined. Whitaker found that few patients had increased intrarenal pressures, even when infused, and concluded significant obstruction at the ureterovesical junction was rare.

Tietjen et al.[70] presented data on 25 valve patients who underwent the antegrade infusion test on their distal ureters months after proximal ureteral diversion and before reconstruction. The authors noted obstruction at the ureterovesical junction in only two ureters, demonstrating that 92% of the ureterovesical junctions in their series were satisfactorily functional; the median perfusion pressure was 3 cm H_2O.

These studies support the theory that eventually the ureterovesical junction will drain adequately in almost all patients, although the junction may be functionally obstructed before the valves are treated and for some time after treatment. The improvement in upper tract drainage depends on the bladder's recovery from high pressures owing to outlet obstruction.

Apart from the ureterovesical junction, bladder dysfunction may have a profound effect on the persistence of hydronephrosis, as Mitchell[71] described for valve bladder syndrome. Some children with posterior urethral valves have persistent bladder dysfunction despite successful relief of the obstruction. These patients have thick-walled, poorly compliant bladders that maintain high resting pressures. They have decreased sensation and are comfortable at bladder pressures sufficient to cause persistent hydronephrosis.

Glassberg et al.[72] categorized the hydronephrotic upper tracts of valve patients into three types: those that drain efficiently independent of bladder volume, those that drain efficiently with the bladder empty but are obstructed when the bladder is full, and those that are obstructed independent of bladder volume. Smith and Duckett[29] reviewed 100 cases of valves and applied these criteria. They found only 4 cases with obstructed ureters independent of bladder volume, and all these patients had previous ureteral reimplants.

Although the antegrade infusion test remains the gold standard for diagnosing obstruction, it is invasive and usually requires an anesthetic. The diethylenetriamine penta-acetic acid (DTPA) or MAG-3 nuclear scan with diuretic is a less invasive test, which provides considerable insight into the obstruction. A standardized scan, known as the "well-tempered" renogram, was developed to allow comparison of data among centers.[73] The scan provides split function of the two kidneys, and the progression of the isotope through the kidneys and upper tracts can be measured and represented as in terms of half-life. Scans can be done with serum sampling, and total GFR can be calculated. Scans should be done in a well-hydrated patient and with a catheter in the bladder.

Hydronephrosis in the absence of infection and with adequate low-pressure drainage poses little risk to the patient or the kidney. This type of hydronephrosis tends to decrease with time and can be safely watched for years. Prophylactic antibiotic coverage may be a wise choice in some cases.

BLADDER FUNCTION

Detrusor injury from posterior urethral valves varies with the degree of bladder outlet obstruction. Initially, the bladder is thick and trabeculated and often has saccules or diverticuli. The bladder contracts reflexively with great force, and sometimes the presence of a catheter will cause a tetanic bladder contraction that prevents urine flow from the upper tracts. This contraction can be relieved by removing the catheter after valve ablation or vesicostomy, and occasionally anticholinergics will help. Although the posterior urethra shows signs of normalization after a few days, the bladder may appear abnormal and function poorly for months. Urodynamics are often difficult to interpret in infants, particularly in the presence of reflux. The clinician is usually left to focus on the upper tracts and renal function while waiting for bladder function to improve.

Incontinence is a problem for most young children with a history of valves. Smith et al.[74] reviewed 100 patients and found that 81% had delay in achieving urinary control, defined as both day and night dryness by age 5. Parkhouse et al.[75] found that only 55% of 87 patients with valves were dry by age 5. Churchill et al.[25] presented an extensive series in which 53% of patients were continent by age 12. The prognosis for continence improves in adolescence, and all of Parkhouse et al.'s patients were completely dry by age 16, and all but one of Smith et al.'s patients were continent by age 20. In the past, incontinence was often thought to be the result of sphincter injury from valve ablation, but today this injury is rare. Incontinence is usually caused by a combination of poor bladder compliance, detrusor instability, and polyuria. Most patients have an inability to concentrate their urine owing to tubular damage. Renal tubular damage leads to increased free water loss and urine volumes two to four times normal, which may overwhelm the bladder's limited ability to compensate.

Peters et al.[76] identified three abnormal urodynamic patterns in valve patients: myogenic failure, detrusor hyperreflexia, and poor compliance associated with small capacity. Myogenic failure results in poor bladder contractility and increased postvoid residual urine. Children with myogenic failure void by doing the Valsalva maneuver, and double-voiding may aid emptying. Some of this group will eventually need intermittent catheterization. As part of the evaluation, it is necessary to rule out valve remnants and strictures that may interfere with emptying. Patients with detrusor hyperreflexia have good emptying but suffer from urgency and incontinence owing to uninhibited bladder contractions. They respond well to anticholinergic therapy. Patients with small, poorly compliant bladders may respond somewhat to anticholinergics but many eventually need augmentation cystoplasty.

Holmdahl et al.[77] presented urodynamic data gathered from a group of valve patients who were followed through adolescence and young adulthood. They found that the three described patterns of bladder dysfunction overlapped in the majority of patients. In most patients, a predominant pattern could be identified, but the pattern changed with age. The authors concluded that the patterns are simply stages in the development of the bladder and identified the trend for age-related patterns of bladder dysfunction in valve patients. In infants and young patients, poor compliance dominates; whereas in older children, instability with uninhibited detrusor contractions develops. In postpuberty valve patients, the instability resolves and myogenic failure with large bladder volumes and poor sustained voiding contraction predominates. The incidence of incontinence follows this pattern, and many young children are bothered by day and night wetting; almost all patients became continent after puberty. In most patients, the valve bladder is one in transition: from poorly compliant and hyperreflexic as an infant to unstable as a child to poorly contractile as an adult.

Holmdahl et al.[78] used natural-filling cystometry in boys and found that valve patients had bladder instability during the day and stable bladders at night. Night studies revealed increased bladder capacity and decreased voiding pressures. In childhood, problems of compliance, detrussor instability, incontinence, and reflux can benefit from anticholinergic therapy. Urodynamics should be used to guide this therapy and to avoid myogenic failure, which occurs later in life.[79]

There is a recent debate concerning the effect of initial treatment on long-term bladder function. Lome et al.[80] and Tanagho,[81] for example, presented data suggesting that upper tract diversion can lead to bladders with decreased capacity. Close et al.[82] demonstrated that primary valve ablation results in improved bladder compliance and normalization of bladder appearance on VCUG compared to patients treated with upper tract diversion. Likewise, fewer patients needed bladder augmentation, and the early continence rate was higher in the group treated with valve ablation. When the groups were compared for eventual renal function, diversion offered no significant improvement. If renal function is equally protected by primary valve ablation and upper tract diversion, then it is reasonable to choose the initial treatment that gives the best chance for bladder rehabilitation. Primary ablation and even vesicostomy allow the bladder to fill and empty in a cyclic manner. Some authors now believe that this cycling in early life is important for developing optimal bladder function. Mitchell and Close[12] described a "window for healing" of the bladder, which occurs in the first few months of life and is not available later. To round out the debate, Kim et al.[33] presented urodynamic data on 32 valve patients treated with either valve ablation, vesicostomy, or upper diversion. Although the size of the treatment groups was not large, the authors could find no deleterious effects to the bladder from upper tract diversion. The effect of initial treatment of posterior urethral valves on eventual bladder function is still under investigation, and more data are needed to resolve the question.

GLOMERULAR INJURY AND RENAL INSUFFICIENCY

The foremost goal in managing the urethral valve patient is to maintain and maximize renal function. In children, sufficient renal function is necessary not only to clear water and metabolic waste but also to provide an adequate metabolic environment to allow the child to grow. The kidneys must be able to grow along with the child to keep up with increased metabolic demands.

In normal babies, the GFR increases rapidly after birth from 25 mL/min/1.73 m^2 at birth to 50 mL/min/1.73 m^2 at day 12, to 105 mL/min/1.73 m^2 at age 1 year. The GFR continues to increase slowly until age 2.[84] Early changes in the GFR are thought to be caused by increased blood pressure and decreased renal vascular resistance, which lead to increased hydrostatic pressure in the glomerular bed. Also contributing to this change is increasing permeability of the basement membrane of the glomeruli owing to increasing surface area and a changing permeability constant.[85] The GFR increases more rapidly in the neonatal period than at any time during life, which is why relief of obstruction soon after birth is so beneficial to the kidney.[86] After 1 year of life, renal function improves in proportion to increasing body surface area.

Renal insufficiency in valve patients is caused by several factors, including varying degrees of permanent damage owing to dysplasia. Dysplasia not only affects function early in life but may limit the potential of the kidney to grow appropriately along with somatic growth. The kidneys may also suffer progressive damage as a result of obstruction and infection.[87, 88] These factors are important if the diagnosis is delayed. Bladder dysfunction with high-pressure reflux acts as a form of obstruction, often leading to infection and renal damage. The effect of hyperfiltration as a form of progressive injury has been recognized in animal models and may apply to humans as well.[89] As somatic growth outstrips renal growth and function, patients experience proteinuria, hypertension, and glomerularosclerosis. Poorly controlled hypertension also accelerates renal deterioration.

End-stage renal disease (ESRD) is defined as the degree of renal dysfunction that requires dialysis or transplantation or that leads to death owing to renal failure. ESRD occurs in 25 to 51% of valve patients, and the onset falls into two age groups.[60, 90, 91] One-third of patients will need dialysis in the first few months of life, and the other two-thirds will reach ESRD in their late teen years.[90]

The effect of initial treatment on eventual renal function has long been debated. Krueger et al.[55] evaluated patients who presented as neonates and were treated either with upper tract diversion or primary valve ablation. The two groups had similar renal function, but the group treated with diversion seemed to have better somatic growth.

Reinberg et al.[56] later reported a group of 40 valve patients of which 19 underwent upper tract diversion and 21 had either fulguration or primary valve ablation. Of the group who underwent diversion, ESRD developed in 63%, compared to the primary ablation and vesicostomy group in which ESRD developed in 33%. Body growth was below the 25th percentile in 79% of the diversion group and 48% of the ablation group. In Reinberg et al.'s study, growth depended only on renal function and was not predicted by treatment.

Tietjen et al.[70] reported 26 valve patients treated with proximal urinary diversion. They found that 85% had dysplasia on renal biposy. After upper tract diversion, the median nadir creatinine level at 1 year was 1.0; at 9 years later, 58% of these patients had significant renal dysfunction, and 42% reached ESRD.

These studies support the position that initial treatments—upper tract diversion, primary valve ablation, vesicostomy—are equally effective in preserving renal function and providing the metabolic conditions to allow renal and somatic growth. The degree of renal dysplasia is probably the most important factor in determining the ultimate renal function; and unfortunately, dysplasia is not presently treatable.

ANTENATAL DIAGNOSIS AND TREATMENT OF URETHRAL VALVES

Urologic anomalies are present in 1 in 500 fetal ultrasound examinations.[92] Most patients with posterior urethral valves are now diagnosed by antenatal ultrasound. The ability to diagnose and possibly treat urinary obstruction in utero has developed with the technology of ultrasound imaging. The antenatal diagnosis of posterior urethral valves is based on a male fetus with bilateral hydroureteronephrosis; a dilated, thick-walled bladder; and a dilated posterior urethra. Oligohydraminos is variable. Ultrasound screening depends on the skill of the operator and also on the age of the fetus. The accuracy of ultrasound in detecting valves is proportional to the fetal age, and valves may be missed in scans done <24 weeks of gestation. Even when hydronephrosis and a distended bladder are detected, the diagnostic accuracy is marginal. The differential diagnosis includes prune belly syndrome and severe vesicoureteral reflux.

Hydronephrosis may occur without severe renal damage, and the relationship between oligohydraminos and pulmonary hypoplasia is variable. There are prognostic factors that can be measured during fetal life, including increased echogenicity of the renal parenchyma; decreased amount of amniotic fluid; and decreased fetal urinary sodium, chloride, and osmolarity. Hutton et al.[93] studied the prognostic value of the appearance of the urinary tract during pregnancy. They found that the presence of marked hydronephrosis during the second trimester predicted chronic renal failure or death in 89% with a median follow-up of 5.7 years. Other findings that correlated with poor outcome were echogenic kidneys, cystic parenchymal changes, and the late development of oligohydraminos.

If the diagnosis of valves is probable then the decision must be made regarding possible intrauterine intervention. In the early 1980s, physicians were excited about the possibility of relieving urinary tract obstruction before brith. The most common form of intervention has been the coiled stent, placed to drain the fetal bladder urine directly into the amniotic cavity. Technical problems with placing shunts and maintaining their position, along with the uncertainty of the diagnosis made the benefit of these procedures uncertain, and complications occurred in 44% of 73 patients reviewed in the International Fetal Surgery Registry[94] (Fig. 13.11). Risks to

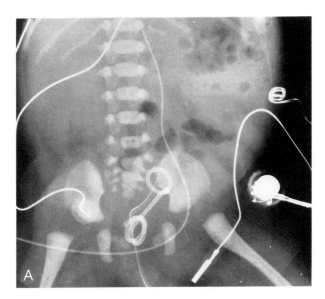

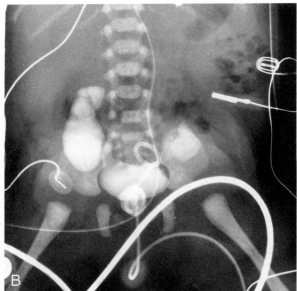

FIG. 13.11. Abdominal x-ray **(A)** and cystogram **(B)** of a newborn with posterior urethral valves who had undergone fetal bladder shunting. The shunt migrated so that one end was within the bladder and the other end was in the anterior pelvis. It did not exit the skin or drain the bladder.

the fetus included inducing premature labor and the introduction of infection and a foreign body into the amniotic environment. Maternal risks must also be weighed and involve bleeding and damage to the uterus, which may endanger future pregnancies.

Despite the efforts of several dedicated researchers, fetal intervention has remained a rare event and has been relegated to a few specialized centers. The widespread application of this new technology has never occurred, primarily owing to the lack of objective evidence that intrauterine intervention improves either renal or pulmonary function. Dysplasia is the most profound form of renal damage, and most data indicate that it occurs too early in development for successful treatment to make a difference in the ultimate outcome of renal development. The decision to intervene in a case of antenatal hydronephrosis is difficult in the most experienced hands.

Ongoing work in intrauterine intervention continues. Freedman et al.[95] studied 13 patients diagnosed prenatally with posterior urethral valves: 7 patients had good fetal urine parameters, and 6 were shunted in utero. Of these, 5 survived, and 4 had good renal function. Of the remaining 6 patients with poor urine parameters, 3 were shunted; 2 of these fetuses died, and all survivors are in renal failure. Although fetal urine parameters and ultrasound features help predict outcome, their effect on management is still controversial, because they may measure previously determined renal dysfunction. The question remains whether fetal shunting actually alters outcome. Physicians continue to search for a pathologic process that can be treated with intrauterine intervention; but it seems that once the diagnosis has been made, the potential for therapeutic intervention has passed (if it ever existed).

PROGNOSTIC INDICATORS

Renal dysplasia is an untreatable condition, and the degree of dysplasia within a kidney accurately determines its potential growth and function. Dysplasia, strictly speaking, is a histologic diagnosis; but renal ultrasound helps predict its presence. Increased parenchymal echogenicity and the presence of cysts are the earliest signs of dysplasia. Sanders et al.[96] reported that patients with urethral obstruction had small echogenic kidneys that contained some small cysts in some cases and no detectable cysts in others. This contrasts with the appearance of dysplasia in obstructions of the ureteropelvic junction that produced a large kidney with multiple large cysts. In assessing the echogenicity of the renal parenchyma, physicians can use the liver and spleen as controls, because the density of these organs on ultrasound is similar to kidney. Ultrasound can also be used to measure the thickness of the renal parenchyma, which helps predict the eventual renal potential.

Hulbert et al.[97] correlated loss of the ability to visualize the corticomedullary junction on ultrasound early in life with poor long-term renal function (Fig. 13.12).

The measurable degree of renal insufficiency at the time of diagnosis and during the 1st year of life have helped predict outcome of renal function. Warshaw et al.[63] reported that a nadir serum creatinine level ≤0.8 mg/dL during the 1st year of life correlated with good long-term renal function. Conner and Burbige[98] found the same relationship with a nadir creatinine level of 1.0 mg/dL in the 1st year. Denes et al.[99] reviewed 32 valve patients diagnosed as infants who were treated with either valve ablation or vesicostomy. The authors noted the creatinine levels at diagnosis, after 4 days of catheter drainage, and at the nadir during the 1st year of life. After a mean follow-up of 10 years, Denes et al. found that two patient groups emerged: one group had a GFR of <70 mL/min/1.73 m² and the other had a

GFR >70. Group 1 had an initial creatinine level of 3.6 mg/dL and a postcatheter drainage level of 2.4. This contrasts with group 2, who had creatinine levels of 1.3 mg/dL at diagnosis and 0.6 after catheter drainage. These early creatinine levels correlated well with 1st-year nadir levels of 1.7 in group 1 and 0.4 in group 2. These studies support the concept that early measurements of renal function predict the degree of irreversible renal damage and eventual renal function.

Age at the time of diagnosis has long been identified as a predictor of the severity of the condition and ultimate outcome. In the past, infants who presented at <1 year of age were more likely to have a poor long-term outcome than those patients who presented later in childhood. Since the initiation of widespread fetal ultrasound screening, most patients are now identified in utero. Early detection and improved neonatal care have lowered the mortality of newborns with valves from almost 50% to between 3 and 10%.[25, 84, 100]

The long-term outcome in terms of renal function, however, has not been improved. The incidence of renal failure in patients detected prenatally has been reported at 64%[101] and 19%.[35] Hutton et al.[35] studied whether the gestational age at diagnosis had an effect on renal failure and survival. They reviewed 32 patients diagnosed with valves prenatally and found that of those patients diagnosed before 24 weeks of gestational age, 53% had a poor outcome, including death, ESRD, and chronic renal failure. Only 7% of patients detected after 24 weeks of age had a poor outcome and renal failure. In all of the later cases, there had been a previously normal ultrasound performed at a median gestational age of 18 weeks. The authors concluded that the diagnosis of valves at a gestational age of <24 weeks carries a significantly worse prognosis a diagnosis later in pregnancy. This probably relates to the timing of the obstructive process in relationship to developing renal and pulmonary function.

The presence of reflux in valve patients carries a poor prognosis. Johnson[102] presented a series of valve patients in which the mortality was 57% with bilateral reflux, 17% with unilateral reflux, and 9% with no reflux. Parkhouse et al.[75] followed 88 patients for 11 to 22 years and found that 58% of valve patients with bilateral reflux eventually had poor renal function compared to 21% of other valve patients. Churchill[102B] stated that all patients with valves and significant bilateral reflux must be considered to have severe disease.

In the future, predicting outcomes in individual valve patients may lie at the genetic level. Brock et al.[103] analyzed the genotypes of the renin–angiotensin system in patients with progressive renal disease. Patients who have evidence of renal scarring and decreased renal function have a significantly increased incidence of a deletion mutation in the gene coding for angiotensin-converting enzyme. Because the genetic information is

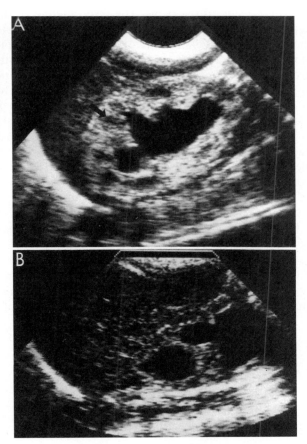

FIG. 13.12. A, Renal ultrasound of an infant with posterior urethral valves demonstrating a preserved corticomedullary junction. **B,** Renal ultrasound of an infant with posterior urethral valves who does not have a visible corticomedullary junction. Loss of this feature carries a poor prognosis for long-term renal function. Reprinted with permission from Cendron M, Elder JS, Duckett JW. Perinatal urology. In: Gillenwater JY, Grayhack JT, Howards SS, Duckett JW, eds. Adult and pediatric urology. 3rd ed. St. Louis: Mosby, 1996;3:2131.

present at birth, this finding may allow physicians to predict outcome at the time of diagnosis. The potential for treatment, either through gene therapy or enzyme replacement therapy, is equally dramatic.

TRANSPLANTATION AND POSTERIOR URETHRAL VALVES

Up to 50% of patients with posterior urethral valves will reach ESRD in their lifetime, and most of these individuals will need dialysis or transplantation during childhood. Renal transplantation is the preferred method of treating children with ESRD to allow for optimal growth and quality of life. Because the bladder function is markedly abnormal in the majority of severe valve patients and the transplant kidney depends on the recipient's bladder, there has been some concern about the effect of bladder function on transplant success.

Reinberg et al.[104] presented data that demonstrated a significant decrease in both transplant graft survival and graft function in patients who had posterior urethral valves compared to a group with ESRD caused by reflux nephropathy. The principal cause of kidney loss was chronic rejection, and the relationship between rejection and bladder function was not apparent. Churchill et al.[105] also supported the concept that patients with posterior urethral valves have decreased transplant graft survival and proposed that this was owing to decreased bladder compliance and increased storage pressures. The actual cause of graft loss was not provided, and the series covered many patients treated before the common use of such vital modern concepts such as augmentation cystoplasty and intermittent catheterization.

More encouraging reports have been presented by Bryant et al.[106] and by Solomon et al.[107] Both studies found no decrease in transplant graft survival in patients with posterior urethral valves at follow-up of 8 to 10 years. Both groups did find a statistically significant increase in serum creatinine levels in valve patients compared to controls. This was a late phenomenon and occurred after 3 years in Bryant et al.'s study and 6 years in Solomon et al.'s.

Ross et al.[108] presented another series of transplanted valve patients and found no difference in graft survival or function at the 5-year follow-up. The authors found urologic complications in 19% of patients, including urethral strictures, stones, and urinary retention. Five patients had irritative voiding symptoms, and four of these had pretransplant bladder capacities of ≤50 mL. Four of the five lost the graft to chronic rejection in the absence of other complaints. Although it is clear that renal transplantation can be performed successfully in patients with a history of posterior urethral valves with comparable graft survival, these patients present risks that are not present for other transplant patients. The transplanted valve patient deserves closer follow-up of

bladder function, and the relationship between bladder function and rejection remains to be defined.

ANTERIOR URETHRAL VALVES

There are rare cases of congenital obstruction of the anterior urethra. Obstruction may be caused by a form of urethral diverticulum or a discrete valve leaflet. It has not been established whether they are two separate entities or variations of the same anomaly. The first case of anterior urethral valves in the English literature was presented by Watts[109] in 1906; there have been few reported cases since.[110, 111]

Obstructing valves can occur throughout the anterior urethra in nearly equal distribution. Diverticuli of the anterior urethra are clearly the most common of this rare group of disorders. There is a defect of the corpus spongiosum, leaving a thin-walled urethra. The urethra dilates during voiding and balloons ventrally, causing a saccular mass that is palpable and sometimes visible on the ventral side of the penis. The distal margin of the defect forms a flap that is flexible enough to fold into the lumen during voiding and obstruct the flow of urine at the junction of the diverticulum and the normal distal urethral (Fig. 13.13). The proximal urethra, bladder, and upper urinary tract are involved to varying degrees. The effect of anterior urethral valves may be as severe as those found in the posterior urethra.

The embryology of anterior urethral valves has not been delineated. They seem to derive from an incomplete fusion of the urethral plate and incomplete formation of the corporus spongiosum. They are embryologically distinct from the much more common valves of the posterior urethra.

Patients with this disorder often suffer from a weak urinary stream, urinary infection, or incontinence. Today, one-third of anterior urethral valve patients present with voiding symptoms, one-third with antenatal hydronephrosis, and one-third with a visible urethral diverticulum[112] (Fig. 13.14). The diverticulum appears as a soft,

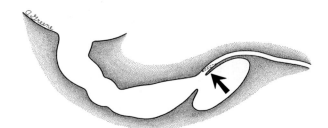

FIG. 13.13. Anterior urethral diverticulum. Note how the distal lip of the diverticulum acts as an obstructing urethral valve (*arrow*). Reprinted with permission from Retik AB, Colodny AH, Bauer SB. Pediatric urology. In: Paulson DF, ed., Genitourinary surgery. New York: Churchill Livingston, 1984;2:837.

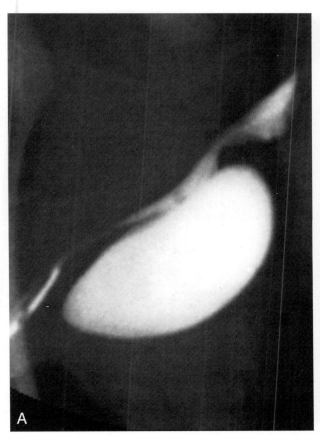
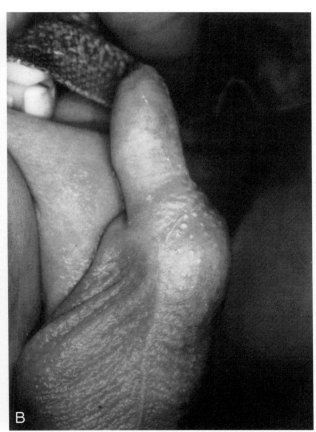

FIG. 13.14.

elongated, midline mass on the ventrum of the penis, which will increase in size during and after voiding. Palpation of the mass may result in drainage of urine from the meatus owing to manipulation of the diverticulum and valve.

Diagnosis of anterior urethral valves depends on VCUG or cystoscopy. It is often difficult to pass a catheter through the diverticulum, because it will tend to miss the small proximal urethra and coil within the diverticulum. Often an injection of contrast into the diverticulum helps the physician visualize the proximal urethra and guide the catheter. A coude-tip catheter can be useful in these patients. The dorsal wall of the urethra is usually flat and straight; and if the catheter can be directed along the dorsal urethral plate, it will pass into the bladder.

Treatment of anterior urethral valves parallels those of the posterior urethra. Obstruction must be relieved with a catheter, and the patient should be treated for infection and metabolic problems as necessary. Catheter drainage must be continued until the patient is stable enough for surgery. In patients with severe renal compromise or poor upper tract function and in very small infants, a temporary vesicostomy or upper tract diversion may be appropriate.[113]

In less severe cases, primary ablation or open excision of the valve is best. When the diverticulum is small and the proximal urethra appears functional, a transurethral incision of the valve leaflet can be performed using a pediatric resectoscope and a hook or wire to incise the valve at its midpoint. These valves are frequently assymmetric and consist of one flap or leaflet.[114] In cases for which transurethral ablation is performed, it is important to avoid the thin wall of the diverticulum, which, if injured, can lead to formation of a urethrocutaneous fistula.

If the diverticulum is so large that it will drain poorly even if the distal obstruction is relieved, then an open excision of the valve and tapering of the diverticulum is a good option.[115] This will leave the patient with a more normal-size urethra and will facilitate normal voiding. This is more complex surgery with a higher complication rate, including stricture, fistula, and urinary extravasation.

There are even more rare anterior urethral valves

that are not associated with urethral diverticula. They can occur as an anterior urethral membrane or a valve of the fossa navicularis.[116] These cases can be successfully treated transurethrally.

The long-time outcome of patients with anterior urethral valves is superior to that of posterior urethral obstruction. The severity of hydronephrosis in anterior valves is much less, and they are associated with chronic renal failure in <5% of cases compared to posterior valves, which carry a >30% incidence of ESRD.[117]

URETHRAL POLYPS

There are rare cases of intermittent obstruction of the urethra by fiberoepithelial polyps of the urethra or bladder. These have been reported exclusively in males and are benign.[118] They are usually seen in young children who have signs of intermittent dysuria and a weak stream. Some cases have been discovered from urinary infection or hematuria. About half of reported cases have associated hydronephrosis or reflux. Polyps usually originate in the posterior urethra, often near the verumontanum, but have been described in the anterior urethra as well.[119] The origin of fibroepithelial polyps is unclear; and although their association with the verumontanum suggests an embryologic origin possibly related to failed mullerian regression, the fact that they usually present in children between ages 7 and 9 years indicates that some may be acquired lesions.[117]

Diagnosis of urethral polyps requires persistence and suspicion. If the polyp occurs at the bladder neck, it may intermittently act as a ball valve from the bladder into the urethra and the VCUG may sometimes be negative (Fig. 13.15). A child with persistent severe intermittent voiding complaints may need a repeat VCUG and cystoscopy to make the diagnosis. Because these polyps often have a long stalk, they may move a consid-

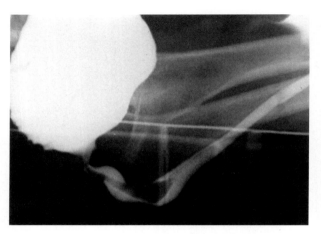

FIG. 13.16.

erable distance within the urethra, creating a filling defect that can be pushed proximally with the catheter to flow more distally during voiding (Fig. 13.16).

Treatment of urethral polyps is usually transurethral resection. An open resection may be appropriate in polyps of the anterior urethra. If the polyp is to be excised transurethrally, I prefer to use a pediatric resectoscope and a right-angle wire. This wire can be used to hook the base of the stalk; a quick burst of cutting current will amputate the polyp. Just as in posterior urethral valves, a loop electrode is likely to make contact with the urethral wall and could lead to stricture formation. Polyps have not been reported to recur once excised.[117]

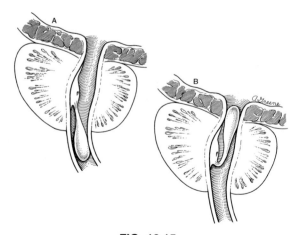

FIG. 13.15.

REFERENCES

1. Deleted.
2. Young HH, Frontz RH, Baldwin TC. Congenital obstruction of the posterior urethra. J Urol 1919;3:289.
3. Casale AJ. Early ureteral surgery for posterior urethral valves. Urol Clin North Am 1990;17:361.
4. Atwell JD. Posterior urethral valves in the British Isles: a multicenter BAPS review. J Pediatr Surg 1983;18:70.
5. Nesbit RM, McDonald HP Jr, Busby S. Obstructing valves in the female urethra. J Urol 1964;91:79.
6. Dewan PA, Zappala PG, Ransley PG, et al. Endoscopic reappraisal of the morphology of congenital obstruction of the posterior urethra. Br J Urol 1992;70:439.
7. Gonzales ET Jr. Posterior urethral valves and other urethral anomalies. In: Gillenwater JY, Grayhack JT, Howards SS, Duckett JW Jr, eds., Adult and pediatric urology. 3rd ed. St Louis: Mosby, 1996:1872–1892.
8. Field PL, Stephens FD. Congenital urethral membranes causing urethral obstruction. J Urol 1974;111:250.
9. Rosenfeld B, Greenfield SP, Springate JE, et al. Type III posterior urethral valves: presentation and management. J Pediatr Surg 1994;29:81.
10. Hanlon-Lundberg KM, Verp MS, Loy G. Posterior urethral valves in successive generations. Am J Perinatol 1994;11:37.
11. Livne PM, Delaune J, Gonzales ET Jr. Genetic etiology of posterior urethral valves. J Urol 1983;130:781.
12. Mitchell ME, Close CE. Early primary valve ablation for posterior urethral valves. Semin Pediatr Surg 1996;5:66.

13. Ewalt DH, Howard PS, Blyth B, et al. Is lamina propria matrix responsible for normal bladder compliance? J Urol 1992;148:544.

14. Kim KM, Kogan BA, Massad CA, et al. Collagen and elastin in the obstructed fetal bladder. J Urol 1991;146:528.

15. Beck AD. The effect of intra-uterine urinary obstruction upon the development of the fetal kidney. J Urol 197;105:784.

16. Glick PL, Harrison MR, Noall RA, et al. Correction of congenital hydronephrosis in utero. II. Early mid-trimester ureteral obstruction produces renal dysplasia. J Pediatr Surg 1983;18:20.

17. Maizels M, Simpson SB. Primitive ducts of renal dysplasia induced by culturing ureteral buds denuded of condensed renal mesenchyme. Science 1983;219:509.

18. Henneberry MO, Stephens FD. Renal hypoplasia and dysplasia in infants with posterior urethral valves. J Urol 1980;123:912.

19. Dinneen MD, Duffy PG, Barratt TM, et al. Persistent polyuria after posterior urethral valves. Br J Urol 1995;75:236.

20. Parkhouse HF, Woodhouse CRJ. Long-term status of patients with posterior urethral valves. Urol Clin North Am 1990;17:373.

21. Gonzales ET Jr. Posterior urethral valves and bladder neck obstruction. Urol Clin North Am 1978;3:57.

22. Rittenberg MH, Hulbert WC, Snyder HM III, et al. Protective factors in posterior urethral valves. J Urol 1988;140:993.

23. Hoover DL, Duckett JW Jr. Posterior urethral valves, unilateral reflux, and renal dysplasia: a syndrome. J Urol 1982;128:994.

24. Hendren WH. Posterior urethral valves in boys. A broad clinical spectrum. J Urol 1971;106:298.

25. Churchill BM, McLorie GA, Khoury AE, et al. Emergency treatment and long-term follow-up of posterior urethral valves. Urol Clin North Am 1990;17:343.

26. Detjer S, Gibbons D. The newborn valve. In: Gonzales ET, Roth DR, eds., Common problems in pediatric urology. Houston: Mosby, 1990:76.

27. Landers S, Hanson TN. Pulmonary problems associated with congenital renal malformations. In: Gonzales ET, Roth DR, eds., Common problems in pediatric urology. Houston: Mosby 1990:85.

28. Adzick NS, Harrison MR, Flake AW, et al. Urinary extravasation in the fetus with obstructive uropathy. J Pediatr Surg 1985;20:608.

29. Smith GHH, Duckett JW Jr. Urethral lesions in infants and children. In: Gillenwater JY, Grayhack JT, Howards SS, Duckett JQ Jr, eds., Adult and pediatric urology. 3rd ed. St Louis: Mosby, 1996;3:2411–2443.

30. Dinneen MD, Duffy PG. Posterior urethral valves. Br J Urol 1996;78:275.

31. Garrett WJ, Grunwald G, Robinson DE. Prenatal diagnosis of fetal polycystic kidney by ultrasound. J Obstet Gynecol 1970; 10:7.

32. Thomas DFM, Gorddon AC. Management of prenatally diagnosed uropathies. Arch Dis Child 1989;64:58.

33. Greenfield SP. Posterior urethral valves—new concepts. Editorial. J Urol 1997;157:996.

34. Dinneen MD, Dhillon HK, Ward HC, et al. Antenatal diagnosis of posterior urethral valves. Br J Urol 1993;72:364.

35. Hutton KAR, Thomas DFM, Arthur RJ, et al. Prenatally detected posterior urethral valves: is gestational age at detection a predictor of outcome? J Urol 1994;152:698.

36. Jee LD, Rickwood AMK, Turnock RR. Posterior urethral valves. Does prenatal diagnosis influence prognosis? Br J Urol 1993;72:830.

37. Sholder AJ, Maizels M, Depp R, et al. Caution in antenatal intervention. J Urol 1988;139:1026.

38. Cremin BJ. A review of the ultrasonic appearances of posterior urethral valve and ureteroceles. Pediatr Radiol 1986;16:357.

39. Kaefer M, Peters CA, Retik AB. Increased renal echogenicity: a sonographic sign in differentiating between obstructive and nonobstructive etiologies of in utero bladder distension. J Urol 1997;158:1026.

40. Good CD, Vinnicombe SJ, Minty IL, et al. Posterior urethral valves in male infants and newborns: detection with US of the urethra before and during voiding. Radiology 1996;198:387.

41. Kaefer M, Barnewolt C, Retik AB, et al. The sonographic diagnosis of infravesical obstruction in children: evaluation of bladder wall thickness indexed to bladder filling. J Urol 1997;157:989.

42. Jordan GH, Hoover DL. Inadequate decompression of the upper tracts using a Foley catheter in the valve bladder. J Urol 1985;134:137.

43. Gibbons MD, Horan JJ, Dejeter SW, et al. Extracorporal membrane oxygenation: an adjunct in the management of the neonate with severe respiratory distress and congenital urinary tract anomalies. J Urol 1993;150:434.

44. Nakayama DK, Harrison MR, de Lorimier AA. Prognosis of posterior urethral valves presenting at birth. J Pediatr Surg 1986;21:43.

45. Gonzales ET Jr. Alternatives in the management of posterior urethral valves. Urol Clin North Am 1990;17:335.

46. Whitaker RH, Sherwood T. An improved hook for destroying posterior urethral valves. J Urol 1986;135:531.

47. Chandna JB, Dickson BA, Gough D. The Whitaker hook in the treatment of posterior urethral valves. Br J Urol 1996;78:783.

48. Ehrlich RM, Shanberg A. Neodymium-YAG laser ablation of posterior urethral valves. Dial Pediatr Urol 1988;11:29.

49. Zaontz MR, Firlit CF. Percutaneous antegrade ablation of posterior urethral valves in premature or underweight term neonates: an alternative to primary vesicostomy. J Urol 1985;134:139.

50. Walker RD, Padron M. The management of posterior urethral valves by initial vesicostomy and delayed valve ablation. J Urol 1990;144:1212.

51. Krahn CG, Johnson HW. Cutaneous vesicostomy in the young child: indications and results. Urology 1993;41:558.

52. Noe HN, Jerkins GR. Cutaneous vesicostomy experience in infants and children. J Urol 1985;134:301.

53. Johnston JH. Temporary cutaneous ureterostomy in the management of advanced congenital urinary obstruction. Arch Dis Child 1963;38:161.

54. Johnston JH. Posterior urethral valves; an operative technique using an electric auriscope. J Pediatr Surg 1966;1:583.

55. Krueger RP, Hardy BE, Churchill BM. Growth in boys with posterior urethral valves. Urol Clin North Am 1980;7:265.

56. Reinberg Y, de Castano I, Gonzalez R. Influence of initial therapy on progression of renal failure and body growth in children with posterior urethral valves. J Urol 1992;148:532.

57. Hendren WH. Complications of ureterostomy. J Urol 1978; 120:269.

58. Mayor G, Genton R, Torrado A, et al. Renal function in obstructive nephropathy: long-term effects of reconstructive surgery. Pediatrics 1975;58:740.

59. Hayslett JP. Effect of age on compensatory renal growth. Kidney Int 1983;23:599.

60. Sheldon CA, Churchill BM, McLorie GA, et al. Evaluation of factors contributing to mortality in pediatric renal transplant recipients. J Pediatr Surg 1992;27:629.

61. Hulbert WC, Duckett JW Jr. Posterior urethral valve obstruction [AUA Update Series]. American Urology Association, 1992; II: Lesson 26.

62. Scott JES. Management of congenital posterior urethral valves. Br J Urol 1985;57:71.

63. Warshaw BL, Hymes LC, Trulock TS, et al. Prognostic features in infants with obstructive uropathy due to posterior urethral valves. J Urol 1985;133:240.

64. Cuckow PM, Dinneen MD, Risdon RA, et al. Long-term renal function in the posterior urethral valves, unilateral reflux and renal dysplasia syndrome. J Urol 1997;158:1004.

65. Bellinger MF. Ureterocystoplasty: a unique method for vesical augmentation in children. J Urol 1993;149:811.

66. Landau EH, Jayanthi VR, Khoury AE, et al. Bladder augmentation: ureterocystoplasty versus ileocystoplasty. J Urol 1994; 152:716.

67. Kim YH, Horowitz M, Comes AJ, et al. The management of unilateral poorly functioning kidneys in patients with posterior urethral valves. J Urol 1997;158:1001.

68. Hulbert WC, Duckett JW. Current views on posterior urethral valves. Pediatr Ann 1988;17:31.

69. Whitaker RH. The ureter in posterior urethral valves. Br J Urol 1973;45:395.

70. Tietjen DN, Gloor JM, Husmann DA. Proximal urinary diversion in the management of posterior urethral valves: is it necessary? J Urol 1997;158:1008.

71. Mitchell ME. Persistent ureteral dilation following valve resection. Dial Pediatr Urol 1982;5:8.
72. Glassberg KI, Schneider M, Haller JO, et al. Observations on persistently dilated ureter after posterior urethral valve ablation. Urology 1982;20:20.
73. Society for Fetal Urology and Pediatric Nuclear Medicine Council. The "well tempered" diuretic renogram: a standard method to examine the asymptomatic neonate with hydronephrosis or hydroureteronephrosis. J Nuc Med 1992;33:2047.
74. Smith GHH, Canning DA, Schulman SL, et al. The long-term outcome of posterior urethral valves treated with primary valve ablation and observation. J Urol 1996;155:1730.
75. Parkhouse HF, Barratt TM, Dillon MJ, et al. Long-term outcome of boys with posterior urethral valves. Brit J Urol 1988;62:59.
76. Peters CA, Bolkier M, Bauer SB, et al. The urodynamic consequences of posterior urethral valves. J Urol 1990;144:122.
77. Holmdahl G, Sillen U, Hanson E, et al. Bladder dysfunction in boys with poster urethral valves before and after puberty. J Urol 1996;155:694.
78. Holmdahl G, Sillen U, Bertilsson M, et al. Natural filling cystometry in small boys with posterior urethral valves: unstable valve bladders become stable during sleep. J Urol 1997;158:1017.
79. Kim YH, Horowitz M, Combs AJ, et al. Management of posterior urethral valves on the basis of urodynamic findings. J Urol 1997;158:101.
80. Lome LG, Howat JM, Williams DI. The temporarily defunctionalized bladder in children. J Urol 1972;108:469.
81. Tanagho E. Congenitally obstructed bladders: fate after prolonged defunctionalization. J Urol 1974;111:102.
82. Close CE, Carr MC, Burns MW, et al. Lower urinary tract changes after early valve ablation in neonates and infants: is early diversion warranted? J Urol 1997;157:984.
83. Kim YH, Horowitz M, Combs A. Comparative urodynamic findings after primary valve ablation, vesicostomy, or proximal diversion. J Urol 1996;156:673.
84. Aperta A, Broberger O, Thodenius K. Development of renal control of salt and fluid homeostasis during the first year of life. Acta Paediatr 1975;64:393.
85. Yared A, Ichikawa I. Renal blood flow and glomerular filtration rate. In: Holliday MA, Barratt TM, Vernier RL, eds., Pediatric nephrology. 2nd ed. Baltimore: Williams & Wilkins, 1987:52.
86. King LR, Coughlin PW, Bloch EC, et al. The case for immediate pyeloplasty in the neonate with ureteropelvic junction obstruction. J Urol 1984;132:725.
87. McGuire EJ, Woodside JR, Borden TA, et al. Prognostic value of urodynamic testing in myelodysplastic patients. J Urol 1981;126:205.
88. Schaeffer AJ. Infections of the urinary tract. In: Walsh PC, Retik AB, Stamey YA, et al., eds., Campbell's urology. Philadelphia: Saunders, 1992:760.
89. Brenner BM, Meyer TW, Hostetter TH. Dietary protein intake and the progressive nature of kidney disease: the role of hemodynamically mediated glomerular injury in the pathogenesis of progressive glomerular sclerosis in aging, renal ablation, and intrinsic renal disease. N Engl J Med 1982;307:652.
90. Smith GHH, Duckett JW Jr, Canning DA. Posterior urethral valves, a cohort with a 20-year follow-up. J Urol 1994;151:275.
91. Smith GHH, Canning DA, Schulman SL, et al. The long term outcome of posterior urethral valves treated with primary valve ablation and observation. J Urol 1996;155:1730.
92. Colodny AH. Antenatal diagnosis and management of urinary abnormalities. Pediatr Clin North Am 1987;34:1365.
93. Hutton KAR, Thomas DFM, Davies BW. Prenatally detected posterior urethral valves: qualitative assessment of second trimester scans and prediction of outcome. J Urol 1997;158:1002.
94. Elder JS, Duckett JW, Snyder HM. Intervention for fetal obstructive uropathy: has it been effective? Lancet 1987;2:1007.
95. Freedman AL, Bukowski TP, Smith CA. Fetal therapy for obstructive uropathy: specific outcomes diagnosis. J Urol 1996;156:720.
96. Sanders RC, Nussbaum AR, Solez K. Renal dysplasia: sonographic findings. Radiology 1988;167:623.
97. Hulbert WC, Rosenberg HK, Cartwright PC, et al. The predictive value of ultrasonography in evaluation of infants with posterior urethral valves. J Urol 1992;148:122.
98. Connor JP, Burbige KA. Long-term urinary continence and renal function in neonates with posterior urethral valves. J Urol 144:1209.
99. Denes ED, Barthold JS, Gonzalez R. Early prognostic value of serum creatinine levels in children with posterior urethral valves. J Urol 1997;157:1441.
100. Williams DI. Congenital valves in the posterior urethra. Br Med J 1954;1:623.
101. Reinberg Y, De Castano I, Gonzalez. Prognosis for patients with prenatally diagnosed posterior urethral valves. J Urol 1992;148:125.
102. Johnson JH. Vesicoureteric reflux with urethral valves. Br J Urol 1979;51:100.
102B. Churchill BM, Khoury AE, McLorie GA. Posterior urethral valves. Acta Urol Belg 1989;57:435.
103. Brock JW, Adams M, Hunley T, et al. Genotyping of the renin angiotensin system: identifying potential risk factors linked to progressive renal failure in childhood urologic disease. Paper presented at the meetings of the American Association of Pediatrics, Urology Section, New Orleans, 1997.
104. Reinberg Y, Gonzalez R, Fryd D, et al. The outcome of renal transplantation in children with posterior urethral valves. J Urol 1988;140:1491.
105. Churchill BM, Sheldon CA, McLorie GA, et al. Factors influencing patient and graft survival in 300 cadaveric pediatric renal transplants. J Urol 1988;140:1129.
106. Bryant JE, Joseph DB, Kohaut EC, et al. Renal transplantation in children with posterior urethral valves. J Urol 1991;146:1585.
107. Solomon L, Fontaine E, Gagnawoux M, et al. Posterior urethral valves: long-term renal function consequences after transplantation. J Urol 1997;157(3):992.
108. Ross JH, Kay R, Novick AC, et al. Long-term results of renal transplantation into the valve bladder. J Urol 1994;151:1500.
109. Watts SH. Johns Hopkins Hosp Rep 1906;13:49.
110. Williams DI, Retik AB. Congenital valves and diverticula of the anterior urethra. Brit J Urol 1969;41:228.
111. Firlit RS, Firlit CF, King LR. Obstructing anterior urethral valves in children. J Urol 1978;119:819.
112. Van Savage JG, Khoury AE, McLorie GA, et al. An algorithm for the management of anterior urethral valves. J Urol 1997;158:1030.
113. Rushton HG, Parrott TS, Woodware JR, et al. The role of vesicostomy in the management of anterior urethral valves in neonates and infants. J Urol 1987;138:107.
114. DeCastro R, Battaglino F, Casolari E, et al. Valves of the anterior urethra without diverticulum: description of three cases. Pediatr Med Chir 1987;9:211.
115. Tank ES. Anterior urethral valves resulting from congenital diverticula. Urology 1987;30:467.
116. Scherz HC, Kaplan GW, Packer, MG. Anterior urethral valves in the fossa navicularis in children. J Urol 1987;138:1211.
117. Kaplan GW, Scherz HC. Infravesical obstruction. In: Kelalis PP, King LR, Belman AB, eds., Clinical pediatric urology. 3rd ed. Philadelphia: Saunders, 1992:821–864.
118. Kearney LP, Lebowitz RL, Retik AB. Obstructive polyps of the posterior urethra in boys: embryology and management. J Urol 1979;122:802.
119. Foster RS, Weigel JW, Mantz RA. Anterior urethral polyps. J Urol 1980;124:125.

CHAPTER 14

Effects of Obstruction on the Detrusor

Congenital and Acquired

Michael A. Keating

Despite the apparent simplicity of its function, the urinary bladder is a true hydrodynamic marvel. Although not as dramatic in its action as the heart or as debilitating with dysfunction as the brain, the expectations of the bladder and its sphincters are extremely high. The acts of retaining large volumes of urine at low pressures (so-called compliance), maintaining continence, and then expelling those contents to completion are extraordinary in their complexity. When abnormal, debilitating incontinence or recalcitrant secondary hydronephrosis serve as unfortunate reminders of the importance of normal bladder function. It is little wonder that these same characteristics will probably never be replicated by enteric replacements, cultured tissue, or artificial prostheses.

Outlet obstruction presents a formidable threat to the unique abilities of the bladder. Table 14.1 lists and classifies a variety of causes of obstruction. Drawing firm conclusions about their sequelae can be challenging for two reasons. First, by nature, each obstruction is variable in severity. Timing of the onset of obstruction is also key. The implications regarding detrusor damage of posterior urethral valves for the developing fetal bladder differ from those of increased sphincter resistance to the transitional bladder during toilet training of a toddler or gradual prostatic enlargement of a mature male. As a consequence, obstruction—like most urologic diseases—results in a spectrum of histopathologic, urodynamic, and medical manifestations. Second, the effects of obstruction on the detrusor are described in the literature as a collage of clinical and experimental studies. The latter include elegant physiologic, pharmacologic, and molecular analyses that offer a challenge in interpretation to investigators and, at times, seem marginally germane to some practicing clinicians.

This chapter summarizes the evolving understanding of the interplay between obstruction and the bladder. It will become apparent that the end organ's contemporary response far surpasses yesterday's simplistic notion of sequential hypertrophy or hyperplasia, connective tissue deposition, noncompliance, and eventual detrusor decompensation (Table 14.2). The discussion is, by necessity, compartmentalized. Actually, outlet obstruction appears to elicit a multifactorial response from the detrusor, each of which contributes in some interrelated way to variable degrees of bladder dysfunction. Understanding the biomechanics of and contributors to normal bladder function is instrumental to discussing the consequences of obstruction on its various components.

NORMAL BIOMECHANICS

Compliance measures the difference in intravesical pressure, which is affected by changes in bladder volume. When the normal bladder is filled at physiologic rates, pressures <10 cm H_2O are sustained until capacity. Intrinsic properties of bladder muscle and its supporting matrix appear to be largely responsible, because acute denervation does not appreciably alter this response initially.[1] The same two components, muscle and matrix, are responsible for the forces, tonus, and elasticity that ultimately dictate detrusor compliance.

Tonus defines the state of tension that results from the perpetual activity of any muscle's contractile elements. This continuous stress is influenced by the ultrastructural composition of detrusor smooth muscle and the interactive roles of its contractile proteins (myosin, actin, and tropomyosin). Cytoskeletal elements such as elastin also contribute. The autonomic nervous system undoubtedly exerts some modification of tonus, but the organ has intrinsic tone in the absence of neuronal influence. Denervated rabbit bladders, for example,

TABLE 14.1. *Causes of bladder outlet obstruction*

- Congenital
  Posterior urethral valves
  Anterior urethral valves
  Megalourethra
  Urethral atresia
  Ureterocele
  Sphincter dyssynergia
- Acquired
  Urethral stricture
  Sphincter or bladder dysfunction
  Sphincter dyssynergia (trauma)
  Bladder stone
  Benign prostatic hypertrophy

demonstrate increased compliance when bathed in calcium channel blockers, a response contingent on intrinsic contractile mechanisms and/or intracellular electrical activity.[2] A number of tissue factors may also play a role, including opioids, prostaglandins, and vasoactive intestinal polypeptide. Any alteration in receptor density, sensitivity, and factor manufacture or uptake could conceivably disrupt the delicate biomechanical balance required of tonus and normal bladder function.

Elasticity largely reflects the makeup of the bladder's passive elements. The main contributors are collagen and elastin, although mucopolysaccharide ground substance and noncontractile components of smooth muscle also play roles. The detrusor is not an ideal spring whose force increases linearly with elongation. Instead, as with many biomaterials, a nonlinear relationship between action and response exists. Force rises slowly with the initial stretch but more rapidly once a certain degree of lengthening has occurred. The rapidity of deformation also affects the organ's response and accounts for its viscoelasticity. Fast stretch typically generates greater force, which will gradually relax if the muscle length is kept constant. Similar characteristics allow the detrusor to regain force after rapid shortening and initial loss of tension.[3]

Role of Collagen

Collagen is the major structural protein in the body, and alterations in its extracellular deposition are repeatedly cited in studies of bladder outlet obstruction and the noncompliant bladder.[4] This ubiquitous substance provides tensile strength for smooth muscle and the scaffold for its contraction; a role similar to that of intramuscular tendons for skeletal muscle.[5] The orientation of collagen may be far more important to an organ's compliance than its elasticity, or lack thereof; and matrix deposition appears to affect function and responsiveness. For example, apparently random fiber arrangements of collagen in rabbit aorta become uniformly aligned with increases in intraluminal pressure. It seems plausible that the bladder's collagen reacts similarly and accounts for the increases in intravesical pressure seen when functional capacity is exceeded.[6]

Collagen is a fibrillar protein characterized by a taut helix composed of three entwined polypeptides, or α chains. More than 20 genetically determined α chains have been identified that, in different combinations, result in the 15 collagen subtypes. Chains are assembled intracellularly and are secreted as large procollagen molecules. These precursors are then cleaved by hydroxylation and glycosylation and readied for fiber formation through covalent intermolecular cross-linking. Progressive insolubility leads to increased stability and tensile strength.[7]

Subtypes of collagen I and III have received a great deal of attention owing to their roles in normal and abnormal bladder function (Table 14.3). These two major interstitial collagens typically appear together, but tissue-specific predispositions exist. Function follows form and fiber distribution. For example, type I collagen forms thick fibers; provides strong tensile strength; and is ideal for denser, less compliant connective tissues (e.g., tendon, skin, and bone), where it predominates. In contrast, type III collagen is made of thinner fibers and is more abundant in resilient tissues that must distend (e.g., uterus, smooth muscle and arterial media of intestine).[8]

The ontogeny of collagen and its developmentally regulated integration into bladder structure has been studied in normal fetuses. Form may also follow function, and collagen fibers apparently distribute in response to the need required of the developing organ.

TABLE 14.2. *Factors contributing to the bladder's response to obstruction*

- Matrix
  Accumulation and disorganized deposition alter the passive bladder characteristics seen with normal filling and stretch
  Acts as barrier to the transfer of nutrients or transmitters between the neurovascular bundle and the muscle
  Impairs discrete conduction pathways existing in the detrusor, altering the intercellular interactions essential for contraction and relaxation
- Muscle
  Hypertrophy, perhaps in concert with hyperplasia, alters the contractile abilities and leads to hypertonicity
  Continual injury and repair, with matrix as its expression, alters normal dynamics
- Neuroeffector
  End organ injury leads to lower-motor lesion-type insults, with progressive atrophy and fibrosis
  Alterations in the abilities of the transmitters and/or receptors, caused by relative changes in muscular configuration and matrix deposition
  Changes in the electronic characteristics of the leiomyocytes and their adjacent nerves (resting potentials, passive transmission)

TABLE 14.3. *Major components of bladder extracellular matrix*

- Collagen
  Major structural protein of the body
  Provides tensile strength and scaffold for muscle
  Type I
    Thick fibers, extreme strength, minimal compliance
  Type III
    Thin fibers, some compliance
  Type IV
    Localized to basement membrane
- Elastin
  High elasticity
  Allows stretching and recoil
  Little strength
- Fibronectin
  Ubiquitous glycoprotein
  Mediates cell adhesion and differentiation and fibrin and heparin binding

Interestingly, the ratio of type I (thick) to type III (thin) collagen decreases with age; the change is thought to be related to muscular development and is consistent with the response required with increases in capacity.[9] In keeping with this trend, fetal compliance has been shown to increase during gestation until term, then decrease with aging.[10] Bovine bladder shows similar patterns of predictable regulation. Collagen type I expression is significantly downregulated postnatally, whereas collagen type III reaches a nadir in the early postnatal period but increases in the adult.[11]

The exact role of smooth muscle cells in abnormal collagen deposition in the bladder remains to be fully defined, but parallels with other systems are easily drawn. Protein production by smooth muscle appears to be the rule. For example, the decreased compliance of the vasculature found with pulmonary hypertension is associated with a change in smooth muscle phenotypes, causing alterations in collagen and elastin expression. Models of striated muscle respond similarly if their innervation is changed.[12]

Collagen is not the inert substance it seems to be when the gristled wall of a thickened neuropathic bladder is incised. Instead, like most proteins in the body, the substance undergoes cyclic deposition and uptake under the action of enzymes; here, collagenases. Preliminary studies suggest that the expression and activation of collagenases (type IV matrix metalloproteinases 2 and 9) are developmentally regulated and may play a role after partial outlet obstruction.[13] Subtle differences in collagen types, either as the result of alterations in production or breakdown, may explain functional variations among normal and diseased tissues.

Role of Elastin

Elastin, the other major component of extracellular matrix, is thought to be largely responsible for the rate of change in form (i.e., elasticity) of connective tissue.[14] Filaments of this polypeptide form fibers that become extensively cross-linked after being excreted into the extracellular space. Existing as random coils within an organ's walls, these fibers provide high elasticity that allows rubber band–like stretching and recoil. Little tensile strength results. Given its behavior, elastin should allow an organ additional compliance. It has been shown that the number of elastin fibers increases with age, perhaps a reflection of the need for additional compliance to accommodate capacity.[9] This increase, however, may not be as beneficial as first supposed. As elastic fibers age, they begin to fray and exhibit an increased affinity for polar amino acids and calcium salts, both possible indicators of fibrosis.[15] Elastin weaves an extensive network within the lamina propria of the detrusor that, in theory, may contribute to the refolding of collagen fascicles during bladder contractions.[16] The interaction between detrusor smooth muscle and extracellular proteins, such as elastin and collagen, which are three-dimensionally organized throughout the bladder,[17] undoubtedly plays an important role in normal and abnormal bladder dynamics.

The Bladder Wall

Each of the four distinctive layers of the bladder wall—urothelium, lamina propria, submucosa, and detrusor muscle—probably contributes in some way to the organ's compliance. In addition, the serosa may play a much larger role than supposed in cases of bladder dysfunction in which thickening and fibrosis are noted.[18] The serosa also partakes in the structural remodeling and differentiation process that occurs after partial outlet obstruction. Mesenchymal cells that reside in this layer have been implicated as progenitors of myofibroblasts.[19] These are then transformed into smooth muscle cells that group into bundles, depending on the density of regional innervation.[20] Clinically, the release of neuropathic detrusor that is seen after incising this investing layer can sometimes be impressive. It is plausible that serosa compromises distension and decreases compliance.

The contribution of urothelium to compliance in vivo remains to be defined. In vitro characteristics are revealing. Cultured urothelial cells manufacture collagen types I and III as well as fibronectin, a component of the matrix that promotes cellular adhesion and the binding of other elements of the extracellular matrix. When strain is applied to cultures, type I collagen increases.[21] In addition, it is becoming increasingly clear that the urothelial layer is instrumental to normal bladder development. In the fetal rat, primordial bladder mesenchyme will not differentiate into mature smooth muscle in the absence of urothelium. Adult urothelium is able to exert similar inductive effects on smooth muscle.[22]

The effect the increased pressures of obstruction on complex epithelial–mesenchymal interactions in embryonic and fetal tissue is unknown. Peptide growth factors have been implicated as the signal mediators. It may be significant that alterations of oncogenes (c-*myc*, c-*los*, H-*ras*, K-*ras*) and fibroblast-growth and -transforming factors have been noted after acute bladder outlet obstruction.[23] These and other types of growth factors are also differentially regulated during bladder development and have been shown to play a role in the repair of urothelial injury and, perhaps, the bladder's response to obstruction.[24]

Finally, the absorptive characteristics of urothelium in the face of obstruction deserve mention. Transitional epithelium is not the impermeable layer once thought. Instead, active ion transport and permeability to a variety of medications (including antineoplastics and anticholinergics) are now recognized.[25, 26] Whether the increased pressures of outlet obstruction are able to weaken or disrupt cellular adhesion and urothelial tight junctions, cause changes in the bladder mucosa's sulfated polysaccharide protective barrier, or alter one or more of its active transport systems have not been studied.[27] If hypertonic urine broached this crucial barrier, it takes little imagination to envision the damage that would occur to the underlying musculature, especially in the fetus. It has been shown that the subepithelial vasculature increases in diameter after obstruction, perhaps an injury response to tissue hypoxia.[28]

The contribution of the bladder's intermediate layers—the lamina propria and submucosa—to normal bladder dynamics is probably also underestimated. The lamina propria demonstrates a fairly uniform lacework pattern under electron microscopy, and its matrix is replete with fibroblasts and collagen subtypes I and III.[29] In the normal bladder, antibody localization to these matrix components is much more intense in the lamina propria and adjacent submucosa than in the underlying muscle. In contrast, intense localization shifts to the adjacent detrusor in neuropathic bladders.[16] A variable response to insult by the different layers of the bladder appears to be the rule. Aging also makes a difference. The submucosa is composed primarily of connective tissue containing the nervous and vascular supply to the muscle. Collagen is organized into distinct bundles that are interwoven to form larger fascicles. This architecture changes with aging and is unrecognizable after severe obstruction; these findings may have implications for compliance and detrusor function.

Bladder Muscle

The muscle of the bladder, with exception of the trigone, is arranged in large, coarse bundles composed of smaller bundles that are widely separated, freely cross planes, and appear to have no hierarchical organization.

Bundles are supported by connective tissue containing collagen and elastin, as well as other matrix. The syncytial arrangement that results is ideal for coordinated evacuation and maintaining low pressure, despite lumenal distension. The seemingly random alignment probably also plays a role in the excitatory propagation of bladder contractions.

Detrusor Excitation

Smooth muscle excitation occurs over both neurogenic and myogenic pathways, although the bladder may not be typical in this regard. Nerves that exist in the adventitia as neuronal bundles initiate neurogenic excitation. These branch within the muscularis to terminals containing synaptic vesicles that store a variety of neurotransmitters. Specific distribution and integration remain the focus of ongoing research. Myogenic pathways are even less well defined. Electron microscopy shows intermediate junctions between individual cells and zones of close (sarcolemma) apposition. The gap junctions usually associated with cells that electrically couple have not been demonstrated in the human bladder, although they are found in the bladder muscle of other species.[30] Some investigators believe that cell-to-cell excitatory coupling may not exist. The default alternative, a 1:1 ratio of nerve endings and muscle fiber, however, has never been shown; and a looser pattern of intramural innervation is probably required to allow for structural deformation. Regardless of their cause(s), normal bladder contractions depend on complex interactions that could be easily disrupted by abnormal matrix deposition, alterations in end organ muscular responsiveness, or microneuronal or macroneuronal injury.

Ultrastructurally, excitation causes a rise in intracellular calcium that depends on both the entrance of the ion through receptor-operated channels and its stimulated release from the sarcoplasmic reticulum. Calcium initiates the cyclic phosphorylation and ratcheting actions of myogenic contractile proteins, including myosin, actin, and tropomyosin. Muscle contractility can change if the isoforms of these proteins are altered in heart and skeletal muscle.[12] The bladder is probably similarly affected, although the biochemical and functional significance of its different isoforms is unknown. In skeletal muscle, isoform makeup correlates with active and passive force generation and shortening velocity. Significant shifts in myosin isoforms are seen in developing rabbit bladder at a time when smooth muscle cells in the detrusor wall are increasing in size and proliferating.[31] In addition, the myosin heavy chains of rabbit bladder undergo changes in translation and transcription under the influence of obstruction. These return to normal upon removal of transient obstruction.[32] Like any phasic muscle, the bladder develops some active myogenic response to unopposed stretch. Subtle alterations in the detrusor's electrophysiologic properties and network and faulty regulation or response of its contractile elements conceivably result from obstruction.[33]

At the gross neuronal level, coordinated voiding depends on viscerosomatic integration among autonomic (sympathetic and parasympathetic) pathways to the bladder and urethra and somatic pathways supplying the external urinary sphincter.[34] Damage to this innervation occurs in varying degrees with myelomeningocele, the most common congenital cause of neuropathic bladder in children. The bladder and its sphincters are both usually affected by upper or lower motor neuron lesions in various combinations. The bladders of some myelodysplastic children, however, are obviously secondarily damaged by functional obstruction from classic dyssynergia and/or abnormal electromyographic responsiveness of the external urinary sphincter.[35] Parallels can be drawn with the neuropathic bladder caused by upper spinal cord injuries, an acquired lesion. The sequelae of primary denervation injuries exceeds the scope of this discussion, although the bladder is different from skeletal muscle in this regard. Motor horn cells exert a trophic influence on the latter. Classic lower motor neuron lesions result in paralysis, atrophy, and eventual fibrosis. A similar end organ effect with lumbosacral decentralization has been theorized for the urinary bladder, despite its smooth muscle composition and autonomic innervation. For example, hypocompliance and areflexia are common findings in children with spina bifida and damage of the conus medularis and/or spinal roots.[36] In addition, morphometric analysis of stillborn fetuses suggest that insult to the bladder from myelodysplasia occurs early in development, before the effects of recurrent infection or detrusor–sphincter dyssynergy (implicated in the neuropathic bladders of older myelodysplastic children) occur.[37] It is interesting that outlet obstruction may injure this innervation in retrograde fashion with a similar end result.

DEVELOPMENTAL CONSIDERATIONS

Outlet obstruction has different implications for the bladder at various stages in its development. The resiliency and response of the primitive myoblasts of the fetal bladder are different from those of mature myocytes in the adult bladder. Matrix deposition in the immature organ and its excitatory system response also appear to differ.[38] The spectrum of acuity and severity of obstruction obviously plays a role. It becomes difficult to draw parallels among the gradual compromise of the outlet provided by benign prostatic hypertrophy in adults; nearly occlusive urethral valves in the fetus; and for that matter, the obstructed bladders of animals, from which the bulk of pertinent research originates. Most experimental models acutely obstruct the bladder outlet. Constricting bands of uniform diameter may not

provide the standard for uniform partial obstruction desired; a fact borne out by the variable results reported in many contemporary studies. In addition, species-specific differences exist that must be taken into account. Despite these drawbacks, preliminary work in this area is revealing, and theoretical insight of the human condition warrants discussion.

Smooth muscle first appears in the human bladder at 7 weeks of gestation, developing from mesenchymal cells at the apical dome of the bladder.[39] Dispersion begins; and by 12 weeks of gestation, the cells of the fundus are arranged in discreet bundles. Near normal organization is seen by week 17. An increase in smooth muscle bulk begins at week 21 and continues through gestation and postnatally until adult proportions are reached. Myoblasts have been studied in skeletal and cardiac muscle. They too have a mesenchymal origin and undergo fusion and similar maturation. The maturation of muscle in these organs requires normal innervation, thyroid hormone, and probably other growth hormones. The bladder is probably no different at the macroscopic level as well as at the microscopic level, at which developmental regulation of contractile proteins is evident and obstruction causes alterations in its isoform synthesis (Fig. 14.1).

The autonomic nervous system plays an important and nearly symbiotic role in normal bladder development. Studies of sensory and adrenergic neuronal maturation in a variety of organ systems suggest that visceral innervation is incomplete at birth. Once axons reach an organ, synapses are formed that allow access of growth

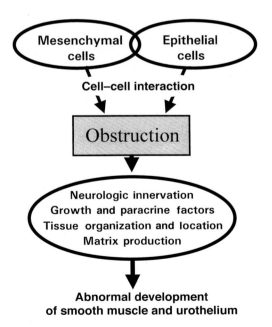

FIG. 14.1. Bladder outlet obstruction may affect several factors crucial to bladder development, including tenuous cell–cell interactions and contractile protein differentiation.

factors produced by the target tissues, where receptor systems are formed before innervation. Nerves not reaching the recipient organ and its nutrient(s) involute. Nerve growth factor (NGF) appears to be instrumental to the mechanism so crucial to neuronal survival and maturation. NGF is undetectable in fetal rat bladders and is not stored in peripheral nerves. At birth, an elevation in the neurotropin occurs in synch with closure of the urachus and increases in bladder distension. Adrenergic innervation increases with NGF levels, which appear to change in relation to axonal uptake and mRNA transcription by the neurons. At 4 weeks of life, catecholamine-labeled fibers and norepinephrine appear.[40] Notably, newborn guinea pigs die with urinary retention if they are immune to neurotropin. Hypertensive rats, whose vascular smooth muscle produce excessive amounts of the substance, develop increased noradrenergic innervation and urinary frequency.

Functional studies of the developing bladder demonstrate a significant change in contractility during this same period of development.[41] It is interesting that this also correlates to a significant shift in smooth muscle myosin isoenzymes, which determine contractility responses in other types of muscle. Adrenergic innervation to the bladder may play a role in this regulation.[42] Other studies have suggested that neurotransmitters, such as acetylcholine, not only accomplish initiation of a contraction but also function as growth factors in bladder muscle cell cultures.[43] Correlates with lower motor denervation injuries to striated muscle are obvious. Outlet obstruction that causes alterations in recipient smooth muscle phenotype, its innervation, and its reception to neurotropins and other growth factors may not normalize if a critical period of neuromuscular plasticity has passed.

Finally, the onset of urine production and response to cyclic stretching and emptying play roles in normal bladder dynamics. Bovine bladders are much less compliant in the first timester than later in gestation.[44] Perhaps it is not surprising that the greatest rise in capacity occurs when fetal urinary output is dramatically increasing. Clinically, females with bilateral ectopic ureters typically have rudimentary, small-capacity bladders. The irreparable bladder plate sometimes found with classic exstrophy is also suggestive. In animals, urinary diversion results in the downregulation of muscarinic receptors and decreased bladder compliance.[45] The amount of urethral resistance required for normal bladder dynamics obviously straddles a fine line between underdistension and overdistension.

THE POSTOBSTRUCTIVE BLADDER

Histoanatomy and Dynamics

Traditionally, the origin of the poorly compliant bladder was summarized by the myogenic theory, by which outlet obstruction induces smooth muscle hypertrophy or hyperplasia followed by connective tissue replacement, ultimately resulting in abnormal contractility, decreased compliance, and detrusor decompensation. Although probably true in part, this notion is now modified by a neuroexcitatory explanation by which primary alterations in reflex pathways or the destruction of intramural innervation contribute to the decreases in compliance or detrusor instability often associated with outlet obstruction. Presently, elements of both will continue to form the basis of theories of the end organ effects of bladder obstruction. Clinical and experimental studies of obstruction have demonstrated transformations in the muscular, matrix, and neuroeffector components of the affected detrusor. Although discussed individually, these changes occur concurrently and are as intimately involved in the response to outlet obstruction as they are in normal bladder dynamics.

Muscle

Smooth muscle hypertrophy typifies the bladder's reaction to partial outlet obstruction. The extent of increase in visceral muscle mass is a function of the degree of obstruction, the timing of its onset, and its duration. Acutely, animal bladders exhibit a marked increase in mass when partially obstructed. Although some of this represents perioperative inflammation, significant increases persist in the face of more extended (6-month) obstructions.[2] Histochemical analysis shows that most of this increase is not collagen, although collagen deposition occurs. Increased intracellular RNA and endoplasmic reticulum (both measures of protein synthesis) are found and indicate that the majority of the increase is smooth muscle hypertrophy.[46] Increases in nuclear size, the nuclear : cytoplasmic ratio, and cellular length have also been cited as additional signs of hypertrophy.[47, 48] A variety of growth factors, including fibroblast growth factor, epidermal growth factor (EGF), and transforming growth factor β (TGF-β), have been shown to play a role in this response.[49]

Hyperplasia of the bladder smooth muscle probably also occurs, though mitosis has not been documented but only inferred from changes in cellular and nuclear counts.[18] Quantitative studies of leiomyocytes in rabbit bladders have reportedly shown hyperplasia and hypertrophy.[50] In rats, time-induced thymidine labeling, a marker for DNA synthesis, immediately increases in the urothelium and connective tissue after partial obstruction. Smooth muscle labeling is less intense and is delayed.[51] Regardless of the animal chosen, hypertrophy and hyperplasia are closely regulated during normal development, and an age-related response to obstruction has also been noted. Young guinea pig bladders show increased DNA and an apparent hyperplastic response. In contrast, hypertrophy predominates with advanced age.[33] In addition, fetal sheep bladders obstructed early in gestation (at 60 days; term = 140 days) demonstrate both processes by morphometric analysis. Partial obstructions produced later in gestation produce similar increases in mass, but the lack of DNA changes suggests hyperplasia alone.[52]

Hyperplasia and hypertrophy may not provide a panacea to obstruction. Although an individual hypertrophied bladder cell could theoretically generate stronger contractions than a normal bladder, two consistent features of myohypertrophy may compromise contractions of the whole bladder. Hypertrophic cells exhibit distorted morphology, including abnormal interlocking of their tapered ends, that could limit their ability to shorten; and there is exaggerated spacing between individual cells caused by collagen that could impede transmission of the contraction through mechanical coupling.[53] A change in the function of smooth muscle cells, from contraction to involvement with collagen synthesis, has also been postulated.[54]

The permanence of the muscular changes that occur appears related to the duration of obstruction, although it cannot yet be determined when a bladder becomes irreparably damaged. On the microscopic level, the degree of hypertrophy is found to be proportional to the length of obstruction in rabbits.[47] It is interesting that the number of enlarged cells and the nuclear morphology returned to normal a few months after release of partial obstructions lasting 20 and 40 days. More prolonged or severe obstruction imprinted deleterious irreversible changes, although great plasticity is present. In another study of rat bladder ultrastructure, a 10-fold increase in muscular volume occurred with obstruction. After relief of the obstruction, 80% of the hypertrophic muscle mass was lost, although there was no degeneration of cells or nerve endings. Muscle cell size did not return to normal, and some fine ultrastructural features remained altered.[55]

Cellular physiology and metabolism are also affected. Partial outlet obstruction has been shown to decrease blood flow and high-energy phosphates in the tissue of rabbit bladders after 2 weeks of obstruction.[56] After 90 days of partial obstruction, rat bladders were found to adapt metabolically to a similar insult with significant changes in the isoform patterns of lactate dehydrogenase.[57] Reversible patterns were found in bladders transiently obstructed for only 10 days. This response was presumably a reflection of compromised oxygen supply from prolonged voiding times and increased detrusor pressure. Decreased oxidative metabolism also appears to be responsible for the significant changes in the mitochondrial genetic systems and enzymatic activity that have been noted after obstruction.[58–60]

Muscular degeneration and regeneration, rare findings in normal bladders, are consistent features of partially obstructed bladders and may account for some of the nuclear alterations that occur with this condition. With filling alone, the canine bladder experiences a significant decrease in blood flow and oxygen tension with or without outlet obstruction. These become markedly decreased when bladder contractions are directed against a closed bladder neck.[61] An element of ischemia must play a role in the metabolic changes discussed above and may be important in the pathophysiology of the injury incurred by the neuropathic bladder. It is enticing to view partial obstruction as a chronic injury state for the detrusor. The healing response that occurs and allows for early compensation can scar the organ permanently and ultimately impair its performance with its cumulative effect.[62, 63] The development of trabeculations, where increases in connective tissue and smooth muscle are collected, is an ominous sign that permanent functional damage has occurred.[64] Factors that allow some bladders to safely compensate for obstruction and others to deteriorate to full-blown myogenic failure form the basis for future research.

Finally, alterations of bladder muscle at the molecular level have also been described. The detrusor hypertrophy of obstruction is associated with the downregulation of myosin heavy chain expression and changes in myofilament gene expression.[65] In addition, the composition of the various isoforms of actin is altered in the hypertrophic response to obstruction.[66] The smooth muscle dedifferentiation and altered matrix expression that occur contribute to decreased smooth muscle contractility primarily and/or by its disruption of muscular excitability.[67]

Recent studies have looked at the role growth factors and co-factors play in the detrusor muscular response and collagen deposition.[68] Studies of angiotensin II (AII), an octapeptide that helps regulate sodium balance, blood volume, and vascular tone through the renin–angiotensin loop, offer insight. Angiotensin II causes the upregulation of several secondary growth factors (e.g., platelet-derived growth factor, TGF-β), which have well-recognized effects on cell function and proliferation. A number of in vitro studies have shown that the protein also induces contraction and tone in the bladders of dogs, rats, rabbits, and humans.[69, 70] Administration to cultured stromal cells produces an increase in cell number and thymidine labeling.[71] When catopril—which blocks the conversion of AI to AII by inhibiting their converting enzyme—was given to rabbits, considerably less postobstructive changes are seen compared to controls who did not receive the medication. Changes include reductions in serosal hyperplasia and collagen, which suggests some involvement in smooth muscle growth regulation and collagen production.[72] Muscle hypertrophy is not similarly affected, however; and species-specific variability exists.[73, 74] Angiotensin II is probably only one of many factors that help regulate the bladder's response to obstruction (Fig. 14.2).

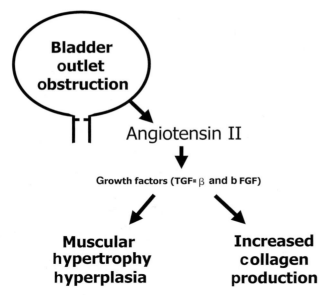

FIG. 14.2. Hypothetical sequence of how outlet obstruction causes AII production. The interplay of growth factors leads to increased matrix production and muscle response. *bFGF,* bovine fibroblast growth factor.

Matrix

Alterations that occur in the interstitium of the bladder's wall may overshadow the long-term functional significance of the initial hyperplastic or hypertrophic response of its leiomyocytes.[9, 75, 76] Matrix deposition likely represents the response of smooth muscle to increased work and/or overdistension. Intercellular disruption and subsequent healing occur in a repetitive fashion with detrimental results. At first thought to originate from fibroblasts, connective tissue manufacture by smooth muscle has now been shown in other organs. Bladder is probably no different. Cellular behavior and matrix production are influenced by mechanical forces (e.g., stretch, sheer) in addition to traditional environmental factors (e.g., temperature, pH). Biaxial deformation was initially found to increase fibronectin production from cultures of pulmonary artery endothelium.[77] Using the same device, physicians noted that urothelial cell cultures subjected to stress produced increased amounts of collagen as well as fibronectin.[21]

Several less sophisticated studies support the concept that alterations in connective tissue deposition decrease bladder compliance. The concentration of collagen may not change significantly because of increases in the thickness of the adjacent musculature,[15] but absolute increases do occur. Matrix type and orientation, however, may have more important implications for compliance than the absolute amount of matrix. In a study of obstructed fetal bladders, a relative decrease in collagen was noted, and a marked increase in the ratio of type I : type III isoforms accompanied the change. Increased

collections of elastin with abnormal thickness and tortuosity were also found.[9]

Matrix orientation and distribution determine tissue compliance and dynamics in other tissues, and there is no reason to believe the bladder is an exception. Skin flexibility, for example, stems from its collagen's combination of random coiling and wicker-work intermeshing, whereas tendons exhibit a singular axis of collagen orientation that provides tensile strength. In contrast, disrupted histoanatomy and disoriented connective tissue infiltration are common light microscopic findings in the walls of hypertrophied bladders affected by obstruction. Electron microscopy shows widened intracellular spaces and apparent loss of muscle cell junctions. Progressively exaggerated deposits of elastin and collagen are found within interstitial spaces.[48] These types of abnormalities in arrangement undoubtedly affect some aspect of the tonus and elasticity characteristics of the detrusor, the functional and electrical continuity of its musculature, or both (Fig. 14.3).

Molecular studies have shown that collagen production is, in part, transcriptionally regulated; and parallel rises in mRNA are seen in urodynamically proven noncompliant bladders.[78] Expression of the genes of both type I and type III collagen are upregulated with obstruction. It is interesting that these alterations have been described as starting in the superficial layers of the bladder wall. Deeper penetration is noted as the pathologic process progresses.[79] Altered proteolytic balance may also play a role. Surgically obstructed fetal bovine bladders demonstrated less interstitial collagenase activity than did normal controls and higher levels of inhibitors of proteins responsible for collagen degradation.[80]

Neuroeffectors

The effects of obstruction are not caused solely by alterations in noncellular matrix in many patients; a fact underscored by the improvements in bladder capacity and compliance seen with pharmacologic manipulation. Secondary neuromuscular damage occurs in ways that are only now being defined.

A reduction in nerve density is found in the obstructed bladders of humans and other animals and may account for the impaired contractile response seen in functional studies.[81, 82] Most investigators believe this is a relative reduction and is a consequence of increased bladder wall thickness. Although nerve loss occurs acutely, it is transient and reversible. Neuroreceptors have also been studied in experimental models, but species variability exists. A fourfold decrease in muscarinic cholinergic receptors was noted in rabbit bladders after 1 week of partial obstruction. Concomitant morphologic changes were not quantitiated, but receptor density returned to normal once the obstruction was removed.[83] In contrast,

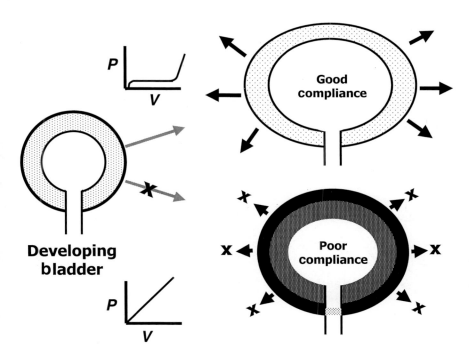

FIG. 14.3. Bladder tonus and elasticity are both affected by outlet obstruction. Reorganization of connective tissue impairs compliance, causing the bladder to tighten as it is stretched. Extracellular matrix accumulation could also affect nerve conduction or detrusor muscle interaction.

an increase in cholinergic density occurred in partially obstructed rat bladders, although the number of receptors per smooth muscle cell did not change appreciably.[84] Adrenergic receptors are also affected by obstruction.

From early muscle strip studies in dogs, it has been suggested that chronic bladder outlet obstruction either downregulates β (relaxation) receptors or upregulates α (contraction) receptors.[85] These types of findings are similar to the autonomic imbalances that are seen with decentralization injuries. Regardless of receptor density changes, recent studies have implicated an intrinsic partial denervation and postjunctional receptor supersensitivity as causes of the detrusor instability that commonly accompanies obstruction.[86] Such instability has been noted in more than half of men with prostatic hyperplasia and obstructive symptoms. It may also underscore the instability that accompanies the functional outlet obstruction found with bladder dysfunction.

Mild obstructions can result in increased contractile force, whereas severe obstruction can lead to marked contractile dysfunction. These phenomena are being studied at the cellular level and seem to be partly related to altered calcium translocation and intracellular release. When variably obstructed rat detrusor is stimulated, it releases intracellular free calcium in amounts that parallel its contractile response.[87] Obstruction can also create a blunted response in the movement of calcium into the myocyte and its release from intracellular storage sites.[88] The role of the sarcoplastic reticulum (SR) seems particularly important in this regard. A progressive reduction in activity of the SR calcium pump has been shown in the detrusor of rabbits that digressed from a compensated to decompensated state.[89] This sce-

nario would hinder the active sequestration of the ion, a finding consistent with tissue hypoxia and decreased intracellular ATP. In the partially obstructed bladder, defects in calcium regulation may well trigger a positive-feedback process that generates cyclical alterations of the ion, causing instability.[90] Alterations in contractile proteins may also contribute to detrusor hypercontractility.[91]

Urologists will hear more about neural plasticity in the future as studies of bladder obstruction shift their focus from the end organ response to that of the bladder's central and peripheral neural pathways. Electrophysiologic and retrograde tracing data suggest that an enhancement of the spinal micturition reflex occurs with obstruction. This finding conceivably accounts for the instability that often accompanies obstruction.[92] The mechanism of neural change may depend on an injury signal from the bladder; and neurotrophic factors, such as nerve growth factor, are implicated in such recruitment.[93]

EXPERIMENTAL OBSERVATIONS AND CLINICAL CORRELATES

Acute partial obstructions of the bladder cause vesical overdistension and ischemia in experimental models. A period of acute decompensation is followed by recovery and structural remodeling in some bladders. Other bladders become permanently decompensated. Muscular and neuronal degeneration are common in all cases. After 3 to 7 days of obstruction, rabbit bladders show loss of cholinergic and adrenergic nerves and disruption of neuroeffector junctions, in addition to increases in

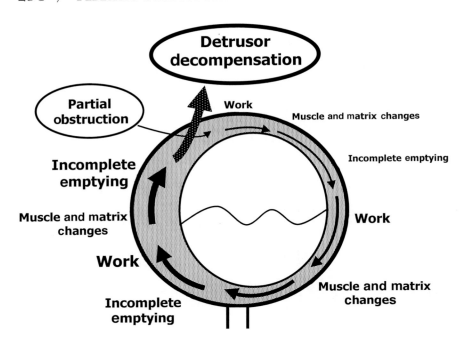

FIG. 14.4. Partial obstruction begins a cycle of progressive injury and functional impairment, which may lead to myogenic failure.

bladder mass. Localization differences in DNA synthesis suggest a reorganization of the relationships among smooth muscle, connective tissue, and neuroeffectors. In favorable cases, axonal regeneration and junctional re-establishment gradually occur, giving testament to the organ's neuromyogenic regenerative abilities.[94] Removal of the obstruction results in apoptosis of the previously responsive urothelial and connective tissue elements, growth factor increases, and restoration of function.[95] Similar findings are seen in dogs, although axonal lysis and organelle loss are uncommon except in extended, severe obstructions.[96] Anatomic restoration results in preservation of nerve conduction, but the bladder's functional status is permanently altered in all but the mildest cases.[75]

Why some bladders are able to compensate and others cannot is unclear. Indelible dysfunction must result from one or more of the alterations discussed earlier. The acuity of congenital and functional outlet obstructions is difficult to gauge. Although most obstructions seem to occur gradually, their temporal effects may be somewhat acute, especially if affecting the initiation and coordination of key sequences in bladder development. What is apparent from animal studies is that the longer an outlet obstruction remains, the greater the likelihood that irreversible changes to the detrusor muscle, extracellular matrix, and neuroeffectors will occur. Fixed obstructions, such as urethral valves, are usually more ominous in their sequelae than are transient obstructions, such as the external sphincter found with bladder dysfunction. The most severe cases of transient problems (Hinman syndrome), however, are associated with neuropathic bladders as severe as any seen with valves and

similar urodynamic cases in their lesser grades of dysfunction.

Impaired contractility and decreased compliance are the functional abnormalities found almost uniformly in muscle strip studies, whole bladder mounts, and in vivo evaluations of obstructed bladders.[18, 82, 97] Poor compliance and impaired contractility are related to the duration of obstruction. Both increase in proportion to the degree of hypertrophy and deposition of inert tissues.[98] Severely hypertrophied bladders are less able to generate high intravesical pressures than are normal bladders and those with only mild hypertrophy. Animal models provide functional correlates of the progression of uropathy sometimes seen in clinical practice. Partially obstructed rabbit bladders generate similar maximal pressures as control bladders; however, they are not able to sustain those pressures to the same degree.[94] As a result, obstructed bladders empty incompletely; and resting pressures become progressively elevated, requiring more work on the part of the detrusor. In the worst-case scenario, decreased functional capacity and progressively larger postvoiding residual volumes lead to total bladder decompensation from myogenic failure (Fig. 14.4).

The variable urodynamic situation found with posterior urethral valves offers an interesting clinical correlate to the detrusor's variable response to outlet obstruction. In one study, three bladder patterns were identified in a group of 41 patients. Hyperreflexia, small capacity with poor compliance, and myogenic failure with overflow incontinence occurred in nearly equal amounts.[99] Some clinicians believe that these are variations of the same basic pattern, which change with time;[100]

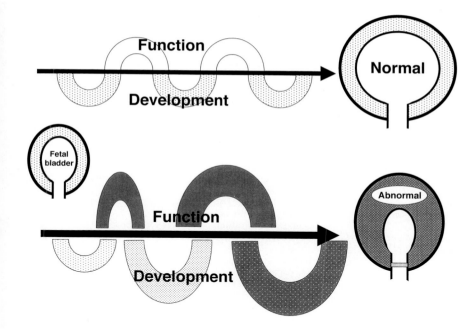

FIG. 14.5. Function and development are intimately and dynamically related. A change in one influences a change in the other, often with irreversible effects.

essentially, these patterns represent transformational stages in the natural history of obstruction.

A partial explanation for the spectrum may lie with the type of work required of the developing bladder. Valve bladders accompanied by natural pop-offs (e.g., massive reflux) do volume work. Myogenic failure is common, undoubtedly exacerbated by incomplete emptying. In contrast, bladders without pop-offs are required to do isometric work during development. Small capacities and poor compliance are typical.[101] Cyclic stretching, filling, and emptying play a key role in normal bladder development. Although intrinsic damage has already occurred, early valve ablation helps restore favorable components of work, giving the bladder its best hope for recovery.[102]

SUMMARY

The implications of outlet obstruction to the bladder can be dissected into individual responses but must be regarded as a sum of the whole. Obstruction alters the muscle, matrix, and neuroeffectors of the detrusor. These affect function and are, in turn, affected by function in an intimately involved dance. And so the cycle continues, in some cases evolving into a vortex of bladder dysfunction (Fig. 14.5). Static interpretations of microanatomy, biochemical analyses, and cytometrograms offer but one frame in a dynamic, ever-changing process.

REFERENCES

1. Langely LL, Whiteside JA. Mechanisms of accommodation and tone of urinary bladder. J Neurophysiol 1951;14:147–155.
2. Levin RM, Goldman M, Wein AJ. Effect of isoproterenol and EGTA on the volume-pressure relationship of the in-vitro whole bladder preparation. Neurourol Urodynam 1984;3:133–137.
3. Guyton AC. Smooth muscle. In: Guyton AC, ed., Textbook of medical physiology. Philadelphia: Saunders, 1986:136–149.
4. Macarak EJ, Ewalt D, Baskin L, et al. The collagens and their urologic implications. Adv Exp Biol 1995;385:173–177.
5. Gabella G. Arrangement of smooth muscle cells and intramuscular septa in the tenia coli. Cell Tissue Res 1977;184:195–212.
6. Kondo A, Susset JG. Viscoelastic properties of bladder. Invest Urol 1974;11:459–465.
7. Miller EJ, Gay S. The collagens: an overview and update. In: Cunningham LJ, ed., Methods in enzymology. Orlando, FL: Academic Press, 1987;144:3–42.
8. Burgeson RE. New collagens, new concepts. Ann Rev Cell Bio 1988;4:551–577.
9. Kim KM, Kogan BA, Massad CA, et al. Collagen and elastin in the normal fetal bladder. J Urol 1991;146:524–527.
10. Koo HP, Macarak EJ, Zderic SA, et al. The ontogeny of bladder function in the fetal calf. J Urol 1995;154:283–287.
11. Koo HP, Howard PS, Chang SL, et al. Developmental expression of interstitial collagen genes in fetal bladder. J Urol 1997; 158:954–961.
12. McConnell JD. Detrusor smooth muscle development in the bladder's response to outlet obstruction. Dial Pediatr Urol 1989;12(12):9–12.
13. Sutherland RS, Baskin LS, Elfman F, et al. The role of type IV collagenases in rat bladder development and obstruction. Pediatr Res 1997;41:430–434.
14. Sandberg LB, Soskel NT, Leslie JG. Elastin structure, biosynthesis and relation to diseased states. N Engl J Med 1981; 304:566–579.
15. Cortivo R, Pagano F, Passerini G, et al. Elastin and collagen in the normal and obstructed urinary bladder. Br J Urol 1981;53:134–137.
16. Ewalt DH, Howard PS, Blythe B, et al. Is lamina propria matrix responsible for normal bladder compliance? J Urol 1992; 148:544–549.
17. Murakumo M, Ushiki T, Abe K, et al. Three-dimensional arrangement of collagen and elastin fibers in the human urinary bladder: a scanning electron microscopic study. J Urol 1995; 154:251–256.
18. Ghoniem GM, Regnier CH, Biancani P, et al. Effect of vesical outlet obstruction on detrusor contractility and passive properties in rabbits. J Urol 1986;135:1284–1289.

19. Buoro S, Ferrarese P, Chiavegato A, et al. Myofibroblast-derived smooth muscle cells during remodeling of rabbit urinary bladder wall induced by partial outflow obstruction. Lab Invest 1993;69:589–602.
20. Pampinella F, Roelofs M, Castellucci E, et al. Time-dependent remodeling of the bladder wall in growing rabbits after partial outlet obstruction. J Urol 1997;157:677–682.
21. Baskin L, Howard PS, Macarak E. Effect of physical forces on bladder smooth muscle and urothelium. J Urol 1993;150:637–641.
22. Baskin LS, Hayward SW, Young P, et al. Role of mesenchymal-epithelial interactions in normal bladder development. J Urol 1996;156:1820–1827.
23. Chen MW, Krasnapolsky L, Levin RM, et al. An early molecular response induced by acute overdistension of the rabbit urinary bladder. Mol Cell Biochem 1994;132:39–44.
24. Baskin LS, Sutherland R, Thomson AA, et al. Growth factors in bladder wound healing. J Urol 1997;157:2388–2395.
25. Lewis SA. The mammalian urinary bladder: it's more than accommodating. News Physiol Sci 1986;1:61–68.
26. Brendler CB, Radebaugh LC, Mohler JL. Topical oxybutinin chloride for relaxation of dysfunctional bladders. J Urol 1989;141:1350–1352.
27. Wilson CB, Leopard J, Cheresh DA, et al. Extracellular matrix and integrin composition of the normal bladder wall. World J Urol 1996;14(Suppl 1):30–37.
28. Boels PJ, Arner A, Malmquist U, et al. Structure and mechanics of growing arterial microvessels from hypertrophied urinary bladder in rat. Pflugers Arch Eur J Physiol 1994;426:506–515.
29. Levy BJ, Wight TN. Structural changes in the aging submucosa: new morphologic criteria for the evaluation of the unstable human bladder. J Urol 1990;144:1044–1055.
30. Dixon J, Gosling J. Structure and innervation of human bladder. In: Torrens M, Morrison JFB, eds., The physiology of the lower urinary tract. Berlin: Springer-Verlag, 1987:3–22.
31. McConnell JD, Robertson JB, Abernathy BB, et al. Myosin heavy chain heterogeneity in the developing rabbit bladder. J Urol 1988;139:258–264.
32. Wang ZE, Gopalakurup SK, Levin RM, et al. Expression of smooth muscle myosin in urinary smooth muscle during hypertrophy and regression. Lab Invest 1995;73:244–251.
33. Mostwin JL. The obstruction of electrical properties in urinary bladder smooth muscle. Dial Pediatr Urol 1993;16(3):7–8.
34. Steers WD. Physiology and pharmacology of the bladder and urethra. In: Walsh PC, Retik AB, Vaughn ED Jr, Wein AJ, eds., Campbell's urology. Philadelphia: Saunders, 1998:870–915.
35. Bauer SB, Hallet M, Khoshobin S, et al. The predictive value of urodynamic evaluation in the newborn with myelodysplasia. JAMA 1984;252:650–652.
36. McGuire EJ, Woodside JR, Borden TA, et al. Prognostic value of urodynamic testing in myelodysplastic patients. J Urol 1981;126:205–209.
37. Shapiro E, Becich MJ, Perlman E, et al. Bladder wall abnormalities in myelodysplastic bladders: a computer assisted morphometric analysis. J Urol 1991;145:1024–1029.
38. Rohrmann D, Monson FC, Damaser MS, et al. Partial bladder outlet obstruction in the fetal rabbit. J Urol 1997;158:1071–1074.
39. Matsuno T, Todunaka S, Koyanagi T. Muscular development in the urinary tract. J Urol 1984;132:148–152.
40. Steers WD. Role of NGF in bladder innervation during development. Dial Pediatr Urol 1996;19(11):9–12.
41. Levin RM, Malkowitz SB, Jacobwitz D, et al. The ontogeny of the autonomic innervation and contractile response of the urinary tract. J Pharmacol Exp Ther 1981;219:250–257.
42. Boone TB, Ewalt DH, McConnell JD, et al. Effects of sympathetic denervation and thyroid hormone on myosin heavy chain isoforms in the neonatal rabbit bladder. J Urol 1989;141:324–329.
43. Gong C, Kennedy WA, Devaud CM, et al. The effect of cholinergic stimulation on cultured smooth muscle. J Urol 1997;157:676–681.
44. Coplen D, Macarek EJ, Levin RM, et al. Developmental changes in the fetal bovine bladder physiology. J Urol 1994;151:1391–1395.
45. Chun AL, Ruzich JV, Wein AJ, et al. Functional and pharmacological effects of ureteral diversion. J Urol 1989;141:403–407.
46. Malkowicz SB, Wein AJ, Elbadawi A, et al. Acute biochemical and functional alterations in the partially obstructed rabbit urinary bladder. J Urol 1986;136:1324–1329.
47. Brent L, Stephens FD. A quantitative study of smooth muscle cells in reflux, obstructed and triad bladders. Invest Urol 1975;12:503–508.
48. Gilpin SA, Gosling JA, Barnard RJ. Morphological and morphometric studies of the human obstructed trabeculated urinary bladder. Br J Urol 1985;57:525–529.
49. Buttyan R, Chen MW, Levin RM. Animal models of bladder outlet obstruction and molecular insights into the basis for the development of bladder dysfunction. Eur Urol 1997;32(Suppl 1):32–39.
50. Brent L, Stephens FD. The response of smooth muscle cells in the rabbit urinary bladder to outflow obstruction. Invest Urol 1975;12:494–502.
51. Saito M, Hypolite JA, Wein AJ, et al. Effect of partial outflow obstruction on rat detrusor contractility and intracellular free calcium concentration. Neurourol Urodyn 1994;13:297–305.
52. Peters CA, Vasavada S, Dator D, et al. The effect of obstruction on the developing bladder. J Urol 1992;148:491–496.
53. Elbadawi A, Meyer S, Malkowicz SB, et al. Effects of short-term partial bladder outlet obstruction on the rabbit detrusor: an ultrastructural study. Neurourol Urodyn 1989;8:89–96.
54. Gosling JA. Modification of bladder structure in response to outflow obstruction and aging. Eur Urol 1997;32(Suppl 1):9–14.
55. Gabella G, Uvelius B. Reversal of muscle hypertrophy in the rat bladder after removal of urethral obstruction. Cell Tissue Res 1994;277:333–339.
56. Lin AT, Chen MT, Yang CH, Chang LS. Blood flow of the urinary bladder: effects of outlet obstruction and correlation with bioenergetic metabolism. Neurourol Urodyn 1995;14:285–292.
57. Polysanska M, Arner A, Malmquist U, et al. Lactate dehydrogenase activity and isoform distribution in the rat urinary bladder: effects of outlet obstruction and its removal. J Urol 1993;150:543–545.
58. Zhao Y, Levin RM, Levin SS, et al. Partial outlet obstruction of the rabbit bladder results in changes in the mitochondrial genetic system. Mol Cell Biochem 1994;141:49–55.
59. Hsu TH, Levin RM, Wein AJ, et al. Alterations of mitochondrial oxidative metabolism in rabbit urinary bladder after partial outlet obstruction. Mol Cel Biochem 1994;141:21–26.
60. Hypolite JA, Longhurst PA, Haugaard N, et al. Effect of partial outlet obstruction on 14C-adenine incorporation in the rabbit urinary bladder. Neurourol Urodyn 1997;16:201–208.
61. Azadzoi KM, Pontari M, Vlachiotis J, et al. Canine bladder blood flow and oxygenation: changes induced by filling, contraction and outlet obstruction. J Urol 1996;155:1459–1465.
62. Mayo ME, Lloyd-Davies RW, Shuttleworth KED, et al. The damaged human detrusor: functional and electron microscopic changes in disease. Br J Urol 1973;45:1116–1125.
63. Keating MA, Levin RM. Experimental observations. Dial Pediatr Urol 1989;12(12):4–6.
64. Gosling JA, Dixon JS. Structure of trabeculated detrusor smooth muscle in cases of prostatic hypertrophy. Urol Int 1980;35:351–355.
65. Cher ML, Abernathy BB, McConnell JD, et al. Smooth-muscle myosin heavy-chain isoform expression in bladder-outlet obstruction. World J Urol 1996;14:295–300.
66. Kim YS, Wang Z, Levin RM, et al. Alterations in the expression of the beta-cytoplasmic and the gamma-smooth muscle actins in hypertrophied urinary bladder smooth muscle. Mol Cell Biochem 1994;131:115–1124.
67. Lin VK, McConnell JD. Molecular aspects of bladder outlet obstruction ADV Exp Med Biol 1995;385:65–74.
68. Chen MW, Levin RM, Buttyan R. Peptide growth factors in normal and hypertrophied bladder. World J Urol 1995;13:344–388.
69. Tanabe N, Ueno A, Tsujimoto G. Angiotensin II receptors in the rat urinary bladder smooth muscle: type I subtype receptors mediate contractile response. J Urol 1993;150:1056–1059.
70. Andersson KE, Hedlund H, Stahl M. Contractions induced by angiotensin I, angiotensin II, and bradykinin in isolated muscle from the human detrusor. Acta Physiol Scand 1992;145:253–259.

71. Cheng EY, Grammatopoulos T, Lee C, et al. Angiotensin II and bFGF induce neonatal bladder stromal cell mitogenesis. J Urol 1996;15:593–597.

72. Cheng EY, Lee C, Decker RS, et al. Captopril (an inhibitor of angiotensin converting enzyme) inhibits obstructive changes in the neonatal rabbit bladder. Urology 1997;50:465–471.

73. Persson K, Pandita RK, Waldeck K, et al. Angiotensin II and bladder obstruction in the rat: influence on hypertrophic growth and contractility. Am J Physiol 1996;271:R1186–1192.

74. Cheng EY. Bladder development and function. Dial Pediatr Urol 1997;20(9):4–5.

75. Mayo ME, Hinman F. Structure and function of the rabbit bladder altered by chronic obstruction or cystitis. Invest Urol 1976;14:6–9.

76. Uvelius B, Mattiasson A. Collagen content in the rat urinary bladder subjected to infravesical outflow obstruction. J Urol 1984;132:587–590.

77. Gorfien SF, Winston FK, Thibault LE, et al. Effects of biaxial deformation on pulmonary artery endothelial cells. J Cell Physiol 1989;139:492–500.

78. Kaplan EP, Richier JC, Howard PS, et al. Type III collagen messenger RNA is modulated in non-compliant human bladder tissue. J Urol 1997;157:2366–2369.

79. Tekgul S, Yoshino K, Bagli D, et al. Collagen types I and III localization by in situ hybridization and immunohistochemistry in the partially obstructed young rabbit bladder. J Urol 1996;156:582–586.

80. Peters CA, Freeman MR, Fernandez CA, et al. Dysregulated proteolytic balance as the basis of excess extracellular matrix in fibrotic disease. Am J Physiol 1997;272:R1960–1965.

81. Gosling JA, Gilpin SA, Dixon JS, et al. Decrease in autonomic innervation of human detrusor muscle in outflow obstruction. J Urol 1986;136:501–504.

82. Speakman MJ, Brading AF, Gilpin RJ, et al. Bladder outflow obstruction: a cause of denervation supersensitivity. J Urol 1987;138:1461–1466.

83. Levin RM, Memberg W, Ruggieri MR, et al. Functional effects of in vitro obstruction on the rabbit urinary bladder. J Urol 1986;135:847–851.

84. Nilvebrandt L, Ekstrom J, Malmbert L. Muscarinic receptor density in the rat urinary bladder after denervation hypertrophy and urinary diversion. Acta Pharmacol Toxicol 1986;59:306–314.

85. Rohner TJ, Hannigan JD, Sanford EJ. Altered in vivo adrenergic responses of dog detrusor muscle after chronic bladder outlet obstruction. Urology 1978;11:357–361.

86. Sibley GN. Developments in our understanding of detrusor instability. Br J Urol 1997;80(Suppl 1):54–61.

87. Saito M, Longhurst PA, Murphy M, et al. 3H-thymidine uptake by the rat urinary bladder after partial outflow obstruction. Neurourol Urodyn 1994;13:63–69.

88. Yoon JY, Zderic SA, Duckett JW, et al. Effect of partial outlet obstruction in the biphasic response to field stimulation at different concentrations of calcium. Pharmacology 1994;49:167–172.

89. Zderic SA, Rohrmann D, Gong C, et al. The decompensated bladder. II: evidence for loss of sarcoplasmic reticulum function after bladder outlet obstruction in the rabbit. J Urol 1996;156:587–592.

90. Fry CH, Wu C. The cellular basis of bladder instability. Br J Urol 1998;81:1–8.

91. Shell JT, Tansey MG, Word RA, et al. Myosinlight chain kinase phosphorylation: regulation of the Ca2t sensitivity of contractile elements. Adv Exp Med Biol 1991;304:129–138.

92. Steers WD, DeGroat WC. Effect of bladder outlet obstruction on micturition reflex pathways in the rat. J Urol 1988;140:864–871.

93. Steers WD, Tuttle JB, Creedon DJ. Neurotrophic influence of the bladder following outlet obstruction: implications for the unstable bladder. Neurourol Urodyn 1989;8:395–403.

94. Levin RM, High J, Wein AJ. The effect of short-term obstruction on urinary bladder function in the rabbit. J Urol 1984;132:789–791.

95. Levin RM, Wein AJ, Buttyan R, et al. Update on bladder smooth-muscle physiology. World J Urol 1994;12:226–231.

96. Sehn JT. The ultrastructural effect of distension on the neuromuscular apparatus of the urinary bladder. Invest Urol 1979;16:369–375.

97. Williams JH, Turner WH, Sainsbury GM, et al. Experimental model of bladder outflow tract obstruction in the guinea pig. Br J Urol 1993;71:543–554.

98. Kato K, Monson FC, Longhurst PA, et al. The functional effects of long-term outlet obstruction on the rabbit urinary bladder. J Urol 1990;143:600–606.

99. Peters CA, Bolkier M, Bauer SB, et al. The urodynamic consequences of posterior urethral valves. J Urol 1990;144:122–126.

100. Holmdahl G, Sillen U, Hanson E, et al. Bladder dysfunction in boys with posterior urethral valves before and after puberty. J Urol 1996;155:694–698.

101. Kaefer M, Keating MA, Adams MC, et al. Posterior urethral valves, pressure pop-offs and bladder function. J Urol 1995;154:708–711.

102. Close CE, Carr MC, Burns MW, et al. Lower urinary tract changes after early valve ablation in neonates and infants: is early diversion warranted? J Urol 1997;157:984–988.

CHAPTER 15

Diagnostic Maneuvers to Differentiate Obstructive from Nonobstructive Ureteral Dilation

Linda M. Dairiki Shortliffe

Evaluating the dilated urinary tract associated with so-called hydronephrosis or hydroureteronephrosis is often thought tantamount to evaluating for urinary tract obstruction. This is not the case. Urinary tract dilation is a normal physiologic response to physiologic phenomena and, as such, may be caused by increased urinary tract pressures and obstruction but also may be related to hormonal, pharmacologic, and flow issues. When urinary tract dilation is associated with increased urinary tract pressures, however, urinary tract dilation may herald obstruction and impending loss of renal function. It is for this reason that determining the cause(s) of urinary tract dilation is important.

With the widepsread use of fetal and neonatal ultrasonography, increasing numbers of asymptomatic children are being diagnosed with urinary tract dilation. Only if the causes of urinary tract dilation are differentiated and diagnosed can patients be managed and treated appropriately. Specifically, urinary tract dilation must be found as obstructive or nonobstructive. Although tests and algorithms for determining obstruction exist, there are no gold standards. Moreover, physiologic studies suggest that obstruction is a relative phenomenon (low urinary flow may not be associated with high intraluminal pressure, whereas high urinary flow may be) and occurs in a range from partial to complete. It is thus important to identify or develop tests for optimizing the diagnosis of obstruction and defining when and how often obstruction occurs.

DEFINING OBSTRUCTION

There is no single test that makes the diagnosis of urinary tract obstruction. Although radiologic obstruction has been observed in association with a dilated collecting system on excretory urography, renal ultrasonography, and nuclear renogram, no standard parameters are used to define obstruction. Urodynamic parameters for obstruction with elevated renal pelvic pressures under defined flow criteria, as outlined in the Whitaker test, have also been questioned as being nonphysiologic. In the past, urinary tract dilation, delayed renal pelvic drainage, and increased renal pelvic pressure have been used to define obstruction. There have been instances in which a radiographic picture has been corrected surgically whether or not it demonstrated physiologic obstruction.

A physiologic definition of obstruction is the finding of substantially higher pressure above the restriction than below it; there is, therefore, a considerable differential pressure. For instance, in the case of a ureteral (or ureteropelvic junction or ureterovesical junction) obstruction, the renal pelvic pressure should be higher than the bladder pressure when obstruction exists. Unless there is complete obstruction, the conditions under which this pressure differential occurs will also be determined by the rate of urinary flow and extent of bladder fullness. Exactly when these conditions of restricted flow lead to renal deterioration must be determined.

In 1987 Koff[1] gave a practical definition of urinary tract obstruction: "Any restriction to urinary outflow that left untreated will cause progressive renal deterioration." This defines clinically significant obstruction, even though the actual parameters that define the restriction are left unspecified. This lack of specification emphasizes that a wide range—from nonobstruction to total obstruction—may exist, but conditions (such as urinary flow rate or bladder fullness) associated with urinary tract dilation that cause a clinically significant restriction in one situation may be clinically insignificant in another.

It becomes important, therefore, to consider three questions when examining a dilated urinary tract: (a) Is the urinary tract abnormal? (b) What is the cause of the dilation? (c) Will the dilation damage the kidney?

FACTORS AFFECTING URINARY TRACT DILATION

Multiple factors affect urinary tract dilation. Although it has long been recognized that obstruction and vesicoureteral reflux are causes of urinary tract dilation, other factors, such as changes in smooth muscle compliance (as influenced by age, hormonal response, or drugs) infection, urinary flow rate, and/or bladder fullness may be as important as obstruction in causing urinary tract dilation.

Bladder Fullness

Clinical studies in humans suggest that bladder fullness can alter the anatomy and function of the upper urinary tract[2,3] (Fig. 15.1). Whitaker[4] emphasized that bladder pressure may affect upper tract urinary flow and for that reason states that the bladder should be kept empty during the Whitaker test. It has also been suggested that bladder drainage after pyeloplasty may protect the ureteropelvic anastomosis from increased pressure and extravasation.[5]

When excretory urograms of full and empty bladders are compared, caliceal, renal, pelvic, and ureteral dila-

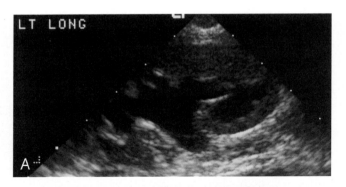

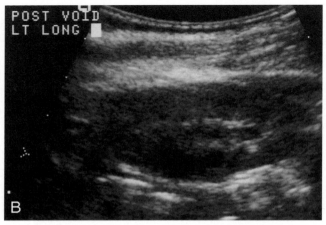

FIG. 15.1. A, Renal ultrasound study of a 3-month-old girl showing a left pelvocaliectasis. There is a full bladder; VCUG showed no vesicoureteral reflux. **B,** After voiding, the same kidney has minimal pelvocaliectasis.

tion are associated with a full bladder.[3] Renal pelvic pressure has been found to rise as the bladder approaches fullness and when voiding occurs.[6] During the diuretic renogram, moreover, as full bladder may cause the study to be falsely interpreted as showing obstruction.[7,8]

Urinary Flow Rate

Animal studies confirm that renal pelvic pressures increase with high urinary flow rates.[6,9,10] It is also known that urinary tract dilation is associated with conditions in which chronically elevated urinary flow rates occur, such as diabetes insipidus and lithium treatment. The extent to which renal immaturity and poor renal concentrating ability related to renal insufficiency and urinary tract infection contribute to high flow rates is often difficult to evaluate.

Infection

It has been observed radiologically that during acute pyelonephritis the renal pelvis and ureter may undergo so-called nonobstructive dilation.[11-14] In some studies, ureteral dilation has been associated with acute urinary tract infection.[15,16] The exact cause for this dilation is unknown, but animal studies have shown that renal pelvic and bladder pressures are abnormally elevated during acute urinary tract infection, particularly with higher urinary flows.[17] During these infections, the renal pelvic pressure was commonly higher than the bladder pressure, suggesting that nonobstructive pyelonephritis is nonexistent.

Whether the cause of urinary tract dilation during infection is from a bacterial toxin effect of the smooth muscle or some other urodynamic effect of inflammation on the smooth muscle is unclear.[16,18] Infections caused by highly adhering bacteria (generally the more uropathogenic organisms) are more commonly associated with ureteral dilation than less pathogenic organism or those associated with asymptomatic bacteruria.[16] The overall effect may be to create a functional obstruction to urinary flow and changes in deposition of type I and type IIA collagen, making the bladder stiffer than normal. Furthermore, these factors may increase the severity of previous dilation when such a system becomes infected (Fig. 15.2).

Hormonal

Dilation of the renal pelvis and ureter occurs during pregnancy in almost all normal women and has been described as the "physiologic hydronephrosis and hydroureter of pregnancy."[19] Usually this dilation starts during the second trimester and has been attributed to hormonal, physiologic, and obstructive changes.[19-22]

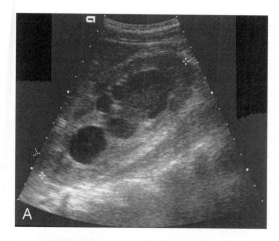

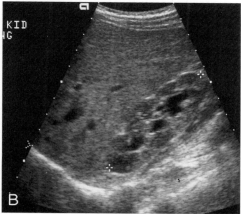

FIG. 15.2. A, Ultrasound study performed during acute pyelonephritis showing hydroureteronephrosis. **B,** A few months after the infection was treated, the same kidney has decreased dilation. The bladder was moderately full in both studies.

Other studies have found that this increased dilation may be caused by increased bladder capacity and increased urinary tract compliance, which may be related to hormonal changes in estrogen and progesterone.[23] The contribution of this hormonal factor to the fetus and neonate is unknown.

Age

With the common use of antenatal ultrasonography, hydronephrosis has been found as frequently as 1 in 500 births.[24] Although this dilation is easily detected ultrasonographically, often the dilation resolves spontaneously by birth. In patients with persistent dilation, however, differentiating between dilation that causes significant urinary tract obstruction and dilation that causes no physiologic or pathologic sequelae may be difficult, because the smooth muscle in the infant urinary tract may differ from that in the adult or older child.

In infants in whom antenatal hydronephrosis is de-

tected but resolves by or shortly after birth, there is clearly a transitional hydronephrosis. The causes of this physiologic or transitional hydronephrosis in the newborn are unclear; but physiologic factors such as incomplete bladder emptying and increased bladder compliance at term may contribute to its development.[25–27]

Obstruction

As already emphasized, urinary tract obstruction is but one cause of urinary tract dilation, albeit possibly the most significant. Urinary tract obstruction at any level—urethra, bladder outlet, ureterovesical junction, ureteropelvic junction—is usually associated with urinary tract dilation proximal to the site of obstruction. This is caused by elevation of the intraluminal pressure above the point of obstruction, which acts as a restriction to urinary flow and can cause distention of the system in response to increased pressure.[28]

The amount of dilation is usually related to the degree of obstruction and the compliance of the system. Thus an extrarenal pelvis associated with a ureteropelvic junction obstruction may show greater pelvic dilation for the same level of restriction than will an intrarenal pelvis. The degree of calyceal dilation and renal damage may be greater in the latter, however, because of the lack of pelvic compliance and the resulting higher intraluminal pressures.

Vesicoureteral Reflux

Vesicoureteral reflux is often accompanied by urinary collecting system dilation that depends on the volume of reflux, and reflux is in part graded by the degree of collecting system dilation. This dilation is caused by ureteral turbulence associated with both retrograde and antegrade peristalsis of urine.[28] In low to moderate degrees of reflux, however, the dilation is unrelated to increased pressures, because pelvic pressures are the same in both refluxing and nonrefluxing systems.

EVALUATION

The evaluation of hydronephrosis most commonly occurs after fetal hydronephrosis is detected on antenatal ultrasound. In other situations, hydronephrosis may be discovered after evaluation of a childhood urinary tract infection, localized flank pain, or a palpable flank mass.

However the diagnosis is made, obstructive and nonobstructive dilations need to be differentiated. To distinguish between the two, it is necessary first to understand the factors that contribute to nonobstructive urinary tract dilation and, second, to selectively eliminate those factors to improve the chances of making the correct diagnosis. For instance, if a urinary infection caused the initial evaluation, it is important to recognize that the infection itself may have caused the urinary tract dilation. If the dilation persists months after the infection has resolved, it may then be correctly evaluated and interpreted. Some tools for evaluating urinary tract dilation are discussed, with an emphasis on precautions to be taken and pitfalls to be avoided while performing the test.

History

The clinical history is important because the conditions under which hydronephrosis is detected may affect the interpretation of its significance. The child's history may start before gestation, if the pregnancy was achieved through in vitro or hormonal manipulation techniques; and gestational and neonatal drug exposures are usually pertinent. For instance, muscle relaxants given for neonatal intubation may cause urinary tract relaxation. In addition, a family history for other genitourinary or genetic disorders should be sought.

Any fetal imaging, usually ultrasound, should be examined for signs of urinary tract and/or bladder abnormalities. Obviously, posterior urethral valves may cause hydronephrosis; but other data relating to external genitalia, amniocentesis, and karyotyping are important as well. Associated abnormalities, such as spina bifida or cardiac abnormalities, may also help assess the hydronephrosis and its cause. Once antenatal hydronephrosis is detected, serial antenatal ultrasounds are usually obtained to follow the progression of the dilation and to detect if bladder filling and emptying occur normally.

When interpreting radiologic imaging of the neonate, the physician should note that the reason for the imaging may influence the interpretation and significance of the dilation. If images were initially obtained to evaluate infection, the dilation will appear worse the closer the studies were performed to the time of the infection. Conditions with poor bladder emptying, such as neurogenic bladders, or high urinary flow rates, such as diabetes insipidus, may suggest specific causes of the dilation but also influence the interpretation of the degree of dilation.

Radiologic Imaging

Infants and children with significant urinary tract dilation need further evaluation. Because the specific studies differ, depending on the resources and professionals available in the hospital or institution, urologists should understand how their institution performs the studies and should inform the radiologist of the patient's clinical problems and potential abnormalities. Thus meaningful studies can be obtained and interpreted correctly.

Renal and Bladder Sonography

Renal ultrasonography is usually the first study to demonstrate urinary tract dilation, although the condition may be found serendipidously on other studies performed to examine other problems. Today, high-resolution Doppler ultrasonography is probably the most frequently used initial modality for assessing the urinary tract. Because ultrasonography is independent of renal function, it is useful for detecting even severe hydronephrosis in which little or no renal function is present. For this reason it can be used successfully to define the renal anatomy of infants in whom renal-concentrating ability and function may be suboptimal for contrast studies.

Imaging the bladder is an essential portion of urinary tract ultrasonography. As noted, urinary tract dilation may be affected by the status of the bladder. Only by imaging the bladder, can the most distal and intravesical portions of the ureter be seen. By seeing ureteral dilation against the full bladder, the physician can outline the level of dilation. Ureteroceles and occasionally posterior urethral valves may be diagnosed or suggested from ultrasonographic findings.

For infants and children, ultrasonographic details are important for detecting the dilation and detailing the extent of the problem. When evaluating antenatally detected dilation, the clinician must consider that the degree of dilation is affected by the infant's state of hydration and renal function. As a result, studies performed within the first few days of life may show little dilation, because breast-fed neonates may be relatively dehydrated and have immature renal function. As emphasized, the urinary tract may show increased dilation when the bladder is full, so pediatric urinary tract ultrasonography should include the bladder. For comparison, serial ultrasonography must be performed with the bladder similarly filled and empty.

In the 1990s, Doppler sonography was investigated as a means of evaluating renal hydronephrosis. Doppler sonography has the capability of obtaining physiologic information about renal vascular resistance. Because a pattern of renovascular changes are known to occur with urinary tract obstruction, it has been suggested that measuring intrarenal renovascular resistance may give additional insight into renal obstruction.

$$\text{Resistive index} = \frac{\text{Peak systolic velocity} - \text{End diastolic velocity}}{\text{Peak systolic velocity}}$$

Collecting system obstruction is usually associated with three distinct phases: an initial and transient rise in renal blood flow, with vasodilatation lasting for a few hours; followed by decreased renal blood flow and elevated collecting system pressures in response to the renal vascular resistance; and after 5 to 6 h, a continued rise in renal vascular resistance and decreased or normal urinary collecting system pressures. Because most obstructive pediatric hydronephroses are chronic, these kidneys should have increased renovascular resistance and increased Doppler-derived resistive indices. Clinical studies have shown that elevated resistive indices correlate with obstruction.[30, 32]

Clinical studies support a correlation between elevated resistive indices and partial obstruction and note a correlation between improvement (or decrease) in the resistive index and relief of obstruction after surgical correction. On the other hand, resistive indices that define obstruction have been inconsistent.[31–33] Some investigators have suggested that comparing the resistive index of a hydronephrotic kidney with the contralateral nonhydronephrotic one may be more reliable than are absolute resistive indices.[32]

Other investigators have suggested that the resistance index is age dependent and of limited value when there is medical renal disease and marked parenchymal loss.[30] As a result, resistive indices are not universally used, even though they may confirm other findings.

Voiding Cystourethrogram

Because the most frequent anatomic abnormality causing some degree of urinary tract dilation is vesicoureteral reflux (VUR), the first study performed after hydronephrosis is detected is usually the voiding cystourethrogram (VCUG). This procedure is meant to be a physiologic study demonstrating voiding, thus the techniques used to perform the study are important. The bladder is filled under gravity pressure of about 1 m H_2O through a feeding tube (not a balloon-retained urethral catheter), which is usually placed transurethrally until voiding is observed.[35, 36] Voiding must occur for the study to be meaningful. The VCUG is the most important study for detecting VUR, but it will also show filling defects and bladder and urethral abnormalities that may relate to urinary tract dilation.

Diuretic Radionuclide Renography

Although there have been problems with interpreting and performing the diuretic renogram, it is probably the most frequently used test for distinguishing obstructive from nonobstructive hydronephrosis. The test measures and quantifies at least two factors that allow assessment of urinary tract obstruction: relative differential renal function and renal (and collecting system) uptake with subsequent workout of the dilated segment. Diuretic renography is based on monitoring the renal uptake and urinary clearance of a intravenously injected radioisotope, followed by intravenous injection of a diuretic agent. Because there has been controversy relating to the reliability of the test, recommendations have

been made to standardize the study parameters and decrease factors that may lead to test variability. These points have been emphasized by several investigators.[35–37]

The diuretic renogram suggests obstruction if there is delayed renal uptake of the radionuclide and delayed excretion. Multiple factors may affect the renogram curve as a quantitative measure of radioisotope washout from the dilated collecting system, including degree of obstruction, urinary flow rate, hydrational status, dose and choice of diuretic agent, bladder fullness, urinary tract compliance, renal maturity or dysfunction, technical factors related to renography (patient positioning, radiopharmaceutical, patient movement, timing of diuretic injection, definition of region of interest) and—probably most important—interpretation of the data.[36] Performing this test is often delayed until after the 1st month of life, when some renal maturation has been achieved.

Some worthwhile recommendations for standardizing the renography technique and interpretating results were described in the well-tempered renogram studies.[35, 37] In these studies, 2 h before beginning the test, the child is orally hydrated; then an 8-Fr urethral feeding tube is placed to keep the bladder empty. About 15 min before the radionuclide is injected, an intravenous line is inserted and infused with dilute normal saline at 15 mL/kg/h for 30 min, with subsequent infusion at 200 mL/kg/24 h until the test is complete. Technetium 99m-labeled mercaptoacetyl triglycine (^{99m}Tc-MAG-3) is injected (50 μCi/kg), and a renogram time–activity curve is obtained. When the dilated collecting system is at the peak of the renogram curve and full, furosemide is injected intravenously at a dose of 1 mg/kg.

During the study period (from the time of radioisotope injection), time–activity curves are produced for the radionuclide uptake, excretion, and diuretic phases. These are usually graphed as the percent of radioisotope activity in the defined region of interest followed over time. The half-time ($T_{1/2}$) clearance of radionuclide from the renal pelvis during the diuretic phase is measured. When the response to furosemide is delayed or when inadequate isotope gets into the collecting system before the diuretic is injected, the study results may be clarified by giving the furosemide 15 min before the isotope injection.[38]

Even with these standards and precautions, interpretation of the diuretic renogram has been problematic. Although decreased differential renal function usually correlates with some degree of renal functional damage, the renogram time–activity curve may or may not correlate with obstruction. Most excretion curves are interpreted to show no obstruction when the clearance $T_{1/2}$ <10 min, to show significant obstruction when $T_{1/2}$ is >20 min, and as being equivocal for obstruction when $T_{1/2}$ is between 10 and 19 min (Fig. 15.3).

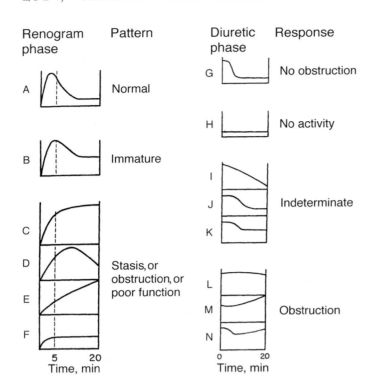

FIG. 15.3. A–F, Characteristic renography time–activity patterns. **G–N,** Characteristic diuretic excretion time–activity patterns. Reprinted with permission from Conway JJ. "Well-tempered" diuresis renography: its historical development, physiological and technical pitfalls and standardized technique protocol. Semin Nucl Med 1992;22:74–84.

Although a decreased differential renal function (10 to 15% lower than the contralateral kidney) associated with an ipsilateral clearance $T_{1/2}$ >20 min suggests obstruction that may benefit from surgical correction, there are no clinical–pathologic studies showing that this kind of time–activity curve indicates ongoing renal damage in individual cases. Furthermore, there are no studies correlating varying degrees of obstruction and renal dysfunction, especially in neonates and young children who may demonstrate renal immaturity. Thus serial renal ultrasonography and diuretic renography performed at prescribed intervals to show progressive hydronephrosis or increasing renal function impairment may be more helpful than single studies in identifying children who may benefit from correction.

Pressure–Perfusion Studies (Whitaker Test)

The Whitaker test was developed to try to distinguish nonobstructive from obstructive urinary tract dilation based on monitoring renal pelvic pressure during established flow rates with an empty bladder.[39] This test allows measurement of a differential pressure across a suspected obstruction. With the patient in the supine position, a rate of infusion of 10 mL/min through a nephrostomy tube is established. A urethral catheter is used to keep the bladder empty, and the intrapelvic pressure and bladder pressures are measured. A differential pressure (renal pelvic–bladder) of 12 to 15 cm H_2O or less is considered normal, and differential pressures >20 to 22 cm H_2O are abnormal and suggest obstruction.

Similar to difficulties with diuretic renography, standards for interpretation and performance in poorly functioning and immature kidneys have not been fully investigated. Specifically, the range of physiologic urinary flow rates in infants and young children has not been well examined and may affect the accuracy of the study.[40] Error may be introduced if the study is terminated before the pelviocaliceal system is completely full, if the bladder is incompletely drained, and if the flow of 10 mL/min is not a physiologic flow for the individual studied (i.e., in certain individuals with poor concentrating ability, a kidney may have urinary flow >10 mL/min).

Although this test has often been cited as the gold standard for diagnosing obstruction, it is not practical for every child because of its invasive nature and associated problems.[41] As a result, pressure–perfusion tests have been used primarily when other tests show confusing or equivocal results. Because each test has its own advantages, disadvantages, and sources of error, any one or the other may be desirable at different times.

Pressure–Flow Studies

Because of the sources of error introduced by urinary tract compliance and the lack of reproducibility of constant perfusion studies, pressure–flow studies of the renal pelvis have been examined. In these studies, the constant pressure used for urinary tract perfusion that is associated with low or no urinary outflow documents obstruction. Some of the problems associated with constant perfusion (Whitaker) studies may be eliminated.[42, 43] Experience with these studies has been limited, however.

MRI and CT

MRI and CT scans may be highly useful for defining the anatomy and renal parenchyma in complex urinary tract abnormalities. Although MRI has been used to determine renal blood flow and demonstrate obstruction experimentally,[44] neither it nor CT has been studied or used for routine evaluation at this time.

RATIONAL APPROACH

After urinary tract dilation has been detected in an infant or child, a rational approach to evaluating the cause of the dilation should be based on the likelihood of findings and the availability and quality of resources. Today, most urinary tract dilation in children is detected by renal and bladder ultrasound. The physician can make an initial determination of the degree and level of dilation from ultrasound studies performed with a full and an empty bladder. If the dilation is antenatally detected, it is important to reconfirm the dilation 3 or more days after birth. Renal and bladder ultrasound studies performed sooner or immediately after birth may underestimate the degree of dilation, because of neonatal dehydration during the first few days of life. If the antenatally detected dilation is severe or bilateral, however, confirmatory and comprehensive renal and bladder ultrasonography should be performed early. For instance, antenatally detected severe bilateral hydroureteronephrosis in an infant boy should be re-evaluated urgently after birth to eliminate a diagnosis of posterior urethral valves.

After renal and bladder ultrasonography, the next step is usually VCUG, because VUR is the most common cause of urinary tract dilation. Furthermore, about 15% of children with ureteropelvic junction obstruction or ureterovesical junction obstruction may also have concomitant VUR. VCUG diagnoses urinary tract dilation associated with reflux and bladder abnormalities, such as ureteroceles.

If the abnormal dilation is unaccounted for by the VCUG and the dilation is significant (more than minor pelviectasis), a carefully performed diuretic renogram to determine differential renal function and the pattern of isotope uptake and excretion may be helpful for evaluating the severity of obstruction. In most instances, this study may be performed when the infant is at least 1 month old, when renal function is more mature to better assess function and excretion patterns without having the difficulties of renal immaturity confusing the evaluation. If relatively minor pelviectasis was seen

on ultrasonography, repeat ultrasonography several months later may help ascertain progression or resolution of the findings.

If the diuretic renogram does not show a significant difference in differential renal function, however, renal and bladder ultrasonography and diuretic renograms performed at prescribed intervals for comparison may help determine whether obstruction is getting worse or better as the child and urinary tract mature. Intervals of re-evaluation are determined by the child's age, severity of the dilation, and the results of the initial studies. For example, more frequent examinations may be necessary for a neonate with moderate to severe dilation and equivocal diuretic renogram findings for obstruction.

Although there are algorithms for deciding between obstructive and nonobstructive dilation of the urinary tract, initial evaluation and re-evaluation should be individualized for the specific child, circumstances, and quality of resources available (Fig. 15.4). Evaluating the urinary tract that is obstructed in all studies and shows moderate to severe hydronephrosis, significantly decreased renal blood flow, and delayed drainage is much easier than evaluating the urinary tract that may be more or less obstructed under different circumstances and gives equivocal findings. In these situations, the physician may not be able to recommend a correction at the time of initial studies. Diagnosis and treatment may need to be made after re-evaluation studies demonstrate that urinary tract dilation is associated with increasing urinary tract dilation and/or loss of renal func-

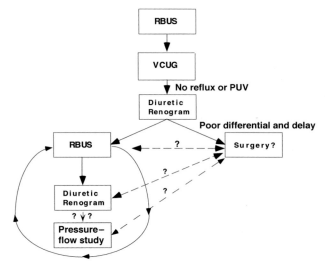

FIG. 15.4. Dilation is usually diagnosed by renal and bladder ultrasonography (*RBUS*); the VCUG is useful for evaluating VUR, posterior urethral valves (*PUV*), and other bladder or urethral abnormalities. If the results of the diuretic renogram are equivocal for urinary tract obstruction, interval surveillance (with periodic re-evaluation) or other studies may be performed before the decision for surgical correction is made.

tion. Because age, urinary flow rate, bladder function, and urinary tract compliance may change in growing children, there is reason to re-evaluate the urinary tract as long as there is urinary tract dilation and the child is growing.

REFERENCES

1. Koff S. Problematic ureteropelvic junction obstruction. J Urol 1987;138:390.
2. Pierce J, Braun E. Ureteral response to elevated intravesical pressures in humans. Surg Forum 1960;11:482.
3. Gill W, Curis G. The influence of bladder fullness on upper urinary tract dimension and renal excretory function. J Urol 1977;117:573.
4. Whitaker R. Clinical assessment of pelvic and ureteral function. Urology 1978;12:146.
5. Wollin M, Duffy P, Diamond D, et al. Priorities in urinary diversion following pyeloplasty. J Urol 1989;142:576.
6. Smyth T, Shortliffe L, Constantinou C. The effect of urinary flow and bladder fullness on renal pelvic pressure in a rat model. J Urol 1991;146:592–596.
7. Gordan I, Mialdea-Fernandez R, Peters A. Pelviureteric junction obstruction. The value of a post-micturition view in 99m Tc DTPA diuretic renography. Br J Urol 1988;61:409–412.
8. Takeda MT, Takahashi H, Hatano A, et al. Correlation of upper and lower urinary tract function in patients with neurogenic bladder: evaluation using simultaneous measurement of cystometry and diuresis renography with full and empty bladder. Neurourol Urodyn 1994;13:243–253.
9. Boyarsky S, Martinez J. Ureteral peristaltic pressures in dogs with changing urine flows. J Urol 1962;87:25.
10. Struthers N. The role of manometry in the investigation of pelvi-ureteral function. Br J Urol 1969;41;129.
11. Kass E, Silver T, Konnak J. The urographic findings in acute pyelonephritis: nonobstructive hydronephrosis. J Urol 1976;116:544.
12. Silver T, Kass E, Thronbury J, et al. The radiological spectrum of acute pyelonephritis in adults and adolescents. Radiology 1976;118:65.
13. Teplick J, Teplick S, Berinson H, et al. Urographic and angiographic changes in acute unilateral pyelonephritis. Clin Radiol 1978;30:59.
14. Lindsell D, Moncrieff M. Comparison of ultrasound examination and intravenous urography after a urinary tract infection. Arch Dis Child 1986;61:81–82.
15. Hellström M, Jodal U, Mårild S, Wettergren B. Ureteral dilatation in children with febrile urinary tract infection or bacteriuria. AJR Am J Roentgenol 1987;148:483–486.
16. Mårild S, Hellström M, Jacobsson B, et al. Influence of bacterial adhesion on ureteral width in children with acute pyelonephritis. J Pediatr 1989;115:265–268.
17. Issa M, Shortliffe L. The effect of bacteriuria on bladder and renal pelvic pressures in the rat. J Urol 1992;148:559–563.
18. Roberts J. Experimental pyelonephritis in the monkey. III. Pathophysiology of ureteral malfunction induced by bacteria. Invest Urol 1975;13:117.
19. Fainstat T. Ureteral dilatation in pregnancy: a review. Obstet Gynecol Surv 1963;18:845.
20. Rasmussen P, Nielsen F. Hydronephrosis during pregnancy: a literature survey. Eur J Obstet Gynecol Reprod Biol 1988;27:249.
21. Roberts J. Hydronephrosis of pregnancy. Urology 1976;8(1):1–4.
22. Sala N, Rubi R. Ureteral function in pregnant women. Am J Obstet Gynecol 1972;112:871.
23. Hsia T-Y, Shortliffe L. Effect of pregnancy of rat urinary tract dynamics. J Urol 1995;154:684–689.
24. Fichtner J, Boineau F, Lewy J, Sibley R, et al. Congenital unilateral hydronephrosis in a rat model: continuous renal pelvic and bladder pressures. J Urol 1994;152:652–657.
25. Mevorach R, Kogan B. Fetal lower urinary tract physiology: in vivo studies. Adv Exp Med Biol 1995;385:85–91.
26. Koo H, Macarak E, Zderic S, Duckett J. The ontogeny of bladder function in the fetal calf. J Urol 1995;154:283–287.
27. Coplen D, Macarak E, Levin R. Developmental changes in normal fetal bovine whole bladder physiology. J Urol 1994;151:1391–1395.
28. Labay P, Boyarsky S. Laboratory models of diseases altering ureteral hydrodynamics. In: Boyarsky S, Gottschalk C, Tanagho E, Zimskind P, eds., Urodynamics, hydrodynamics of the ureter and renal pelvis. New York: Academic Press, 1971:349–351.
29. Angue SK, Prushi RS, Shortliffe LD. The urodynamic relationship between renal pelvic and bladder pressure with varying flow rates in rats with congenital versicaloral reflux. J Urol 1998;160(1):150–156.
30. Platt J. Duplex Doppler evaluation of native kidney dysfunction: obstructive and nonobstructive disease. AJR Am J Roentgenol 1992;158:1035–1042.
31. Cronan J. Contemporary concepts for imaging urinary tract obstruction. Urol Radiol 1992;14:8–12.
32. Brkljacic B, Drinkovic I, Sabljar-Matovinovic M, et al. Intrarenal duplex Doppler sonographic evaluation of native kidney obstruction. J Ultrasound Med 1994;13:197–204.
33. Odorica R, Lindfors K, Palmer J. Diuretic Doppler sonography following successful repair of renal obstruction in children. J Urol 1993;150:774–777.
34. Fung L, Steckler R, Khoury A, et al. Intrarenal resistive index correlates with renal pelvis pressure. J Urol 1994;152:607–611.
35. Society for Fetal Urology and Pediatric Nuclear Medicine Council. The "well tempered" diuretic renogram: a standard method to examine the asymptomatic neonate with hydronephrosis or hydroureteronephrosis. J Nucl Med 1992;33:2047–2051.
36. Majd M. Diuretic renography. In: Ehrlich R, ed., Dialogues in pediatric urology. Pearl River, NY: Miller Associates, 1989;12:6–8.
37. Conway J. "Well-tempered" diuresis renography: its historical development, physiological and technical pitfalls and standardized technique protocol. Semin Nucl Med 1992;22:74–84.
38. English P, Testa H, Lawson R, et al. Modified method of diuresis renography for the assessment of equivocal pelviureteric junction obstruction. Br J Urol 1987;59:10–14.
39. Whitaker R. Methods of assessing obstruction in dilated ureters. Br J Urol 1973;45:15.
40. Fung L, Ae K, McLorie G, et al. Evaluation of pediatric hydronephrosis using individualized pressure flow criteria. J Urol 1995;154:671–676.
41. Kass E, Massoud M, Belman A. Comparison of the diuretic renogram and the pressure perfusion study in children. J Urol 1985;134(1):92–96.
42. Woodbury P, Mitchell M, Scheidler D, et al. Constant pressure perfusion: a method to determine obstruction in the upper urinary tract. J Urol 1989;142:632–635.
43. Itoh K, Nonomura K, Matsuno T, et al. Radionuclide constant pressure perfusion study on measurement of exit urine flow: experimental and preliminary clinical investigations. J Urol 1993;150:420–426.
44. Fichtner J, Spielman D, Herfkens R, et al. Ultrafast contrast enhanced magnetic resonance of congenital hydronephrosis in a rat model. J Urol 1994;152:682–687.

CHAPTER 16

Nonvirilizing Adrenal Disease

J. Lynn Teague and Terry M. Phillis

INTRODUCTION

While congenital adrenal hyperplasia rightly takes prominence in any discussion of pediatric adrenal disease, nonvirilizing adrenal disease (NVAD) in children also presents unique challenges to the pediatric urologist. NVAD encompasses a wide range of both benign and malignant pathologic entities involving medical and surgical processes (Table 16.1). The pediatric urologist involved in treating children with NVAD must therefore be as familiar with the metabolic pathways of adrenal hormone production as he or she is with the anatomy of the gland. Accurate diagnosis can require hormonal evaluation, as well as radiologic and nuclear imaging studies. No other organ the pediatric urologist is called upon to treat presents as formidable a challenge in both medical and surgical treatment.

ADRENAL NEOPLASMS

Neoplasms of the adrenal gland fortunately are rare in children, comprising less than one percent of pediatric tumors. Tumors can arise from both the medullary and cortical portions of the gland and can be benign or malignant. Not all retroperitoneal masses are caused by adrenal neoplasms, and a wide range of differential diagnoses must be considered (Table 16.2).

BENIGN MEDULLARY NEOPLASMS

Ganglioneuroma

The ganglioneuroma is the most mature benign lesion arising from neural crest tissue.[1] Although not malignant, it can become quite large with extensive local spread. By extending through the spinal foramen and compressing the spinal cord, these so-called 'dumbbell' lesions can produce significant neurologic symptoms.[2] Ganglioneuromas can arise de novo from the adrenal medulla, but these lesions may result from the maturation of a malignant neuroblastoma. This maturation occurs both spontaneously and following radiation ther-

apy. Conversely, late degeneration of the lesion into a malignant schwannoma can also occur.[3] Because of their mature nature, ganglioneuromas are rarely metabolically active and generally cause few symptoms.

Ganglioneuroblastoma

Ganglioneuroblastoma is an unusual lesion that is intermediate between ganglioneuroma and neuroblastoma. Both benign ganglioneuroma and apparently malignant neuroblastoma elements are present in this rare tumor.[1] Therapy is based on the predominant histologic pattern. If the lesion appears more mature with predominant ganglioneuroma elements, local excision is generally adequate. If the more ominous neuroblastoma pattern predominates, more aggressive therapy is necessary. See Malignant Medullary Neoplasms for this level of therapy.

Pheochromocytoma

Although pediatric pheochromocytoma (PC) can rarely be malignant,[4] the vast majority of these tumors are benign. Despite their benign nature they can cause significant morbidity, and undiagnosed lesions are associated with a 40% mortality rate.[5] Pediatric PC's represent about 5% of all PC's and usually occur in children eight to nine years of age.[3] These tumors arise from the neural crest cells that migrate to the adrenal medulla and mature into pheochromocytes. Pheochromocytes are metabolically active and produce large amounts of catecholamines that are delivered directly into the bloodstream.[1] Because of this catecholamine excess, these tumors can produce marked hemodynamic symptoms.

Pediatric patients with PC often present with sustained hypertension, in contrast to adults, who often experience paroxysmal elevations of blood pressure.[4] This difference is due to the predominant secretion of norepinephrine in pediatric PC.[2] Systemic symptoms such as nausea, vomiting, and weight loss are also more

TABLE 16.1. *Nonvirilizing adrenal disease*

Medullary neoplasms	Adrenal cysts
Ganglioneuroma	Adrenal hemorrhage
Ganglioneuroblastoma	Ectopy
Pheochromocytoma	Agenesis
Cystic neuroblastoma	Infectious lesions
Neuroblastoma	Endocrine abnormalities
Cortical neoplasms	Cushing syndrome
Adenoma	Conn syndrome
Myelolipoma	Adrenal insufficiency
Cortical carcinoma	
Metastatic lesions	

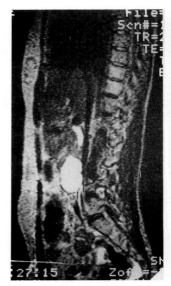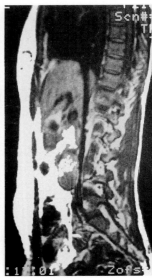

FIG. 16.1. T2-weighted sagittal view on MRI scans showing an extraadrenal pheochromocytoma.

common in children. Children with PC are three times more likely to have bilateral disease and twice as likely to have extraadrenal lesions as adults. The most common extraadrenal site in children is the bladder. Females are affected more commonly in children while the reverse is true for adults.[2]

Once a PC is suspected, radiologic and chemical confirmation of the diagnosis can begin. Since these tumors are of neural crest origin, they can occur anywhere along the sympathetic chain from the neck to the Organ of Zuckerkandel at the aortic bifurcation. The majority, however, occur in the abdomen. Ultrasound of the abdomen and retroperitoneum is a good screening modality, but it can miss small tumors. CT and MRI provide better anatomic detail, but may require sedation or general anesthetic in children. MRI can be particularly helpful in diagnosing a PC, in that these lesions produce a characteristic "light bulb" sign on T2-weighted images (Fig. 16.1). Because of its ability to produce superior anatomic images and more accurately determine the organ of origin for retroperitoneal lesions, MRI is now considered the imaging study of choice for evaluation of adrenal lesions.[5] Nuclear imaging with metaiodobenzyl quanidine (MIBG) can help delineate questionable lesions and has been shown to be highly sensitive and specific in the evaluation of pheochromocytoma.[6]

TABLE 16.2. *Pseudoadrenal masses*

Normal organs
Kidney
Pancreas
Spleen
Lymphadenopathy
Vascular structures
Intraabdominal extralobar pulmonary sequestrations
Extraadrenal retroperitoneal neoplasms
Lymphangioma
Neurofibroma
Lipoma
Lymphoma
Liposarcoma
Fibrosarcoma
Leiomyosarcoma
Malignant fibrous histiocytoma

Biochemical confirmation of pheochromocytoma has traditionally rested on the determination of elevated urinary catecholamine and metanephrine levels. More than 95% of patients with PC will have elevated urinary metanephrines. Lenders et al. recently demonstrated the superiority of plasma metanephrine levels over both plasma catecholamine and urinary metanephrine levels in the diagnosis of patients with PC.[7] In their series of 52 adult and pediatric patients with PC, the sensitivity of plasma normetanephrine and metanephrine in the diagnosis of PC was 100%.

Therapy for PC is based on surgical excision, but this must be preceded by careful volume expansion and alpha and beta blockade.[8] Patients with PC are often severely volume contracted, and at least one week is usually necessary for adequate hydration. Preoperative blood transfusion may be necessary as well. A rapid fall in blood pressure is expected following resection. If this reduction does not occur, the resection may have been incomplete.[9] Follow-up should include monitoring of blood pressure and determination of urinary or plasma metanephrine levels.

Cystic Neuroblastoma

Cystic neuroblastoma is a rare lesion of the adrenal gland with only 31 cases reported.[10, 11] Unlike solid neuroblastoma, it is a benign lesion. The majority of cases have been diagnosed prenatally and the exact origin of these cystic lesions is unclear. It is well known that neuroblastoma in very young children can spontaneously regress, and these lesions may represent degeneration of a solid NB or be the result of hemorrhage within the tumor (Fig. 16.2*A*).

In stark contrast to solid NB, these lesions are generally not metabolically active. Vanillyllmandelic acid and homovanillic acid levels are not elevated in the majority of cases. Diagnosis rests on the radiologic demonstration of an adrenal mass by ultrasound, CT, or MRI followed by complete surgical excision of the lesion.[11] Complete excision is curvature, and no patient who has had complete removal of all gross tumor has had a recurrence.

MALIGNANT MEDULLARY NEOPLASMS

Pheochromocytoma

As noted above, pheochromocytoma is generally a benign lesion with fewer than 2% being malignant.[4] It is very rare in children, with only 8 cases reported. There seems to be little difference between the adult and pediatric varieties. Malignancy may be anticipated if on preoperative radiologic evaluation the lesion is very large with extensive local infiltration.[12] Histologic determination of malignancy is difficult, as there are no microscopic features that are characteristic of malignancy in PC. While mitotic rate, vascular invasion, degree of necrosis, and nuclear pleomorphism have been suggested as histologic indicators of malignancy, none has been proven reliable.[4] Definitive diagnosis of malignancy rests on the demonstration of metastatic disease in soft tissues where neural crest cells are not normally found, such as liver and lung, and in bone.[13] Recurrent PC along the sympathetic chain likely represents synchronous or metachronous disease rather than metastases. Therapy for malignant PC is based initially on complete surgical excision of the tumor. As is the case for benign disease, follow-up should include blood pressure measurements and determination of urinary metanephrines. If either of these is elevated, residual disease must be ruled out. Radiologic evaluation can begin with CT or MRI scan, although either can miss small lesions. MIBG scanning has been shown to have superior sensitivity in locating metastatic disease.[7] Bone scan is helpful for detecting osseous lesions. Adjuvant chemotherapy is usually based on adriamycin or cisplatinum, and has an overall response rate of 50%.[4] While rarely curative, it can provide significant palliation. The use of MIBG combined with I[131] has been successfully used for palliation.[14]

Neuroblastoma

Neuroblastoma (NB) is by far the most common malignancy of adrenal medullary origin and represents 6 to 8% of all pediatric malignancies. It is the most common tumor in infants less than one year old. In addition, it is the most common abdominal neoplasm in children and the second most common solid malignancy overall.

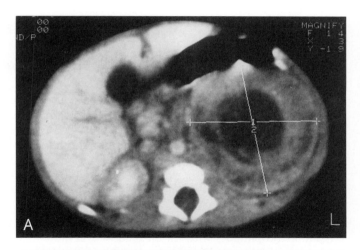

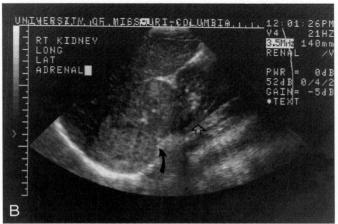

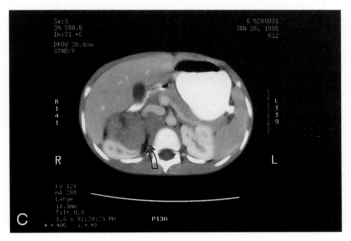

FIG. 16.2. A, CT scan showing a cystic adrenal mass in a neonate. **B,** Sonogram showing the appearance of a neuroblastoma in a 2-year-old girl. *Open arrow,* right kidney; *closed arrow,* neuroblastoma. **C,** CT scan of the patient shown in part B confirming the neuroblastoma above the right kidney (*arrow*).

There is a slight male predominance. NB is an aggressive tumor and is responsible for 15% of all pediatric cancer deaths.[15] Although described in adults, NB is generally a disease of infants and young children. Seventy-five percent of cases occur before 4 years of age and 50% occur before the age of two. It can occur in utero, and prenatal diagnosis based on fetal ultrasound findings and amniotic catecholamine levels has been reported.[16] If the diagnosis is suspected prenatally, the child and mother must be followed closely for signs of preeclampsia (due to transplacental diffusion of catecholamines) or enlargement of the placenta (due to placental metastases).

Children with NB usually present with an abdominal mass, as do patients with the next most common solid tumor in children, Wilms tumor. In contrast to children with Wilms tumor, however, patients with NB generally have more systemic symptoms such as weight loss, fever, malaise, and anorexia. Also unlike Wilms tumor, there is a low incidence of associated anomalies, although skull defects, neurofibromatosis, and Hirschsprung disease are seen more commonly in children with NB. Physical examination shows an irregular upper abdominal mass that often crosses the midline. Hepatomegaly secondary to metastatic disease may be present. The child with NB often appears sickly and irritable, with pallor and generalized wasting. Subcutaneous nodules representing metastatic deposits are present in up to one-third of infants with NB.[2] Laboratory studies may show anemia if bone marrow involvement is extensive. Renal function is generally not compromised and electrolytes are normal.[17]

As is the case with most pediatric abdominal masses, radiologic evaluation begins with ultrasound. A solid suprarenal mass is easily identified sonographically (Fig. 16.2B), but involvement of adjacent organs may be difficult to determine if the mass is large. Intravenous pyelogram classically shows a suprarenal mass with stippled calcification that displaces the ipsilateral kidney caudally. In the past, CT (Fig. 16.2C) was considered the definitive study for evaluation of metastatic disease and was done in all cases. MRI, with its ability to better delineate tissue planes and because of its superior spatial resolution, has now become the imaging modality of choice for staging neuroblastoma[6] (Fig. 16.3). Metastatic spread to the liver is most common in infants, while the bone marrow is a more common site of metastasis in older children. Nuclear medicine imaging with MIBG has been shown to be superior to standard bone scan in the detection of metastatic disease (Fig. 16.4). Neither test is 100% sensitive, however, and all patients with NB must have bone marrow aspiration for complete staging.[17]

The large majority of NB's are metabolically active, secreting significant amounts of catecholamines. This can lead to symptoms comparable to that of pheochro-

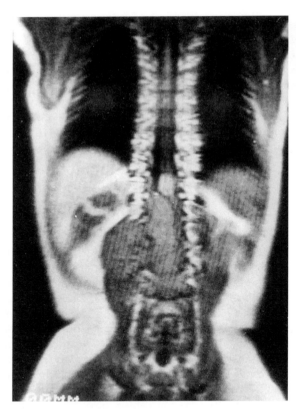

FIG. 16.3. Coronal view MRI scan showing a neuroblastoma with intraspinal extension.

mocytoma, although sustained hypertension is unusual in patients with NB. This may be a result of the metabolism of norepinephrine within the tumor before it is released into the circulation. Over 95% of patients with NB will have an elevation of urinary VMA or HVA, the byproducts of catecholamine breakdown. These markers serve for both diagnosis and follow-up.[18]

As with all neoplasms, accurate staging is critical for prognosis and for guiding therapy. This is hampered in neuroblastoma, however, by competing staging systems. The Evans system, first proposed in 1970, has widespread acceptance. However, it fails to consider surgical resectability of the tumor, which is a major prognostic factor. The Pediatric Oncology Group system and the American Joint Committee on Cancer TMN system have similar shortcomings.[19] In response to this, a new international staging system has been devised (Table 16.3).[20] While accurate staging is critical for prognosis, there are other factors that affect outcome (Table 16.4). The amplification of n-*myc*, a protooncogene derived from chromosome 2, has been shown to have a significant impact on survival. If more than one copy of n-*myc* is present, prognosis is dismal.[21] Ferritin is a serum protein that is produced by NB. Elevated levels correlate with increased tumor activity and poor prognosis. The Shimada index is a histologic grading system that

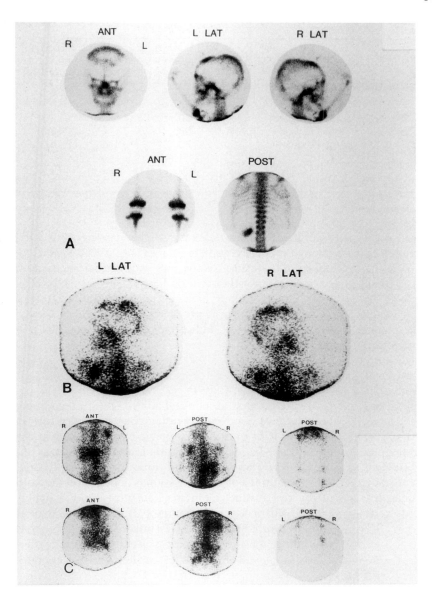

FIG. 16.4. A, Technetium 99m methylene diphosphonate (MDP) scan of a child with stage IV neuroblastoma. **B and C,** Iodine-131 MIBG scan of same child. Both scans demonstrate extensive bony involvement.

TABLE 16.3. *Staging system for neuroblastoma*

International neuroblastoma staging system
I	Localized tumor confined to the area of origin; complete gross excision, $+/-$ microscopic residual disease; identifiable ipsilateral and contralateral lymph nodes negative microscopically
IIA	Unilateral tumor with incomplete gross excision; identifiable ipsilateral lymph nodes negative microscopically
IIB	Unilateral tumor with complete or incomplete gross excision; with positive ipsilateral nonadherent lymph nodes; identifiable contralateral lymph nodes negative microscopically
III	Tumor infiltrating across the midline (vertebral column) with or without regional lymph node involvement; or unilateral tumor with contralateral regional lymph node involvement; or midline tumor with bilateral regional lymph node involvement or extension by infiltration
IV	Dissemination of tumor to distant lymph nodes, bone, bone marrow, liver, or other organs (except as defined in stage IVS)
IVS	Localized primary tumor as in stage I or II with dissemination limited to liver, skin, and/or bone marrow (<10% tumor) in infants younger than one year

TABLE 16.4. *Prognostic factors in neuroblastoma—adapted from Matthay*[16]

Prognostic factor	Favorable	Unfavorable	Survival favorable (percent)	Survival unfavorable (percent)
Age	<2 years	>2 years	77	38
Stage	I, II, IVS	III, IV	90–100	50, 30
Pathology (Shimada)	Favorable	Unfavorable	90	23
Ferritin	<143 ng/ml	>143 ng/ml	83	19
MYCN	1	Amplified (>1)	70	5
Urine VMA/HVA	>1	<1	84	44
DNA index	>1.1	1	100	10
Neuron-specific enolase	<100	>100	79	10

classifies NB as favorable or unfavorable based on a combination of histologic features and patient age.[16]

Therapy for NB is based on a combination of the stage and prognostic factors. Low risk patients (Stage I or II, <1 year old, single copy n-*myc*) have a 95 to 100% survival with complete surgical resection. The addition of chemotherapy and radiation adds little to survival in this fortunate group of patients. Intermediate risk patients (Stage III, IV, IVs, <1 year old, single copy n-*myc*) also have good survival (75 to 90%) with surgical resection followed by chemotherapy and/or radiation therapy. Chemotherapy is most often based on cisplatin, carboplatin, etoposide, ifosfamide, and cyclophosphamide.[22] High-risk patients have poor survival (<30%) regardless of therapy.[16] Megatherapy with autologous bone marrow transplant has been shown to be effective in some high-risk patients.[23] Despite the proven efficacy of complete surgical excision, heroic surgical measures to remove all tumor in these unfortunate patients adds little to overall cure.[24]

BENIGN CORTICAL NEOPLASMS

Adenoma

Adrenal cortical adenomas are rare in children and can be very difficult to differentiate from adrenocortical carcinoma. The average age at presentation is three years for adenomas, in contrast to six years for carcinoma.[25] Adenomas are usually metabolically active. All patients with suspected adenoma should therefore receive a thorough metabolic evaluation. Symptoms related to the tumor will fall into one or more of three categories, depending on the hormone(s) that are being produced in excess. Overproduction of sex steroids results in virilization or feminization. Excess glucocorticoid results in Cushing syndrome, while excess mineralocorticoid will cause hypertension and hypokalemia. Most patients present with a combination of symptoms, with some degree of virilization being most common.[3]

Accurate imaging studies are critical in evaluation of suspected adrenal adenomas, as size (>4 cm) can give some hint as to the possibility of malignancy. Ultra-

sound, CT, and MRI have all been used, with MRI giving the most complete images (Fig. 16.5). While evidence of metastases is the only pathognomonic feature of malignancy, other criteria have been suggested.[26] Mitotic rate (>10 per high-power field) and degree of nuclear pleomorphism are the two most widely accepted histologic features indicative of malignancy with a poor prognosis.

Myelolipoma

Myelolipoma is an unusual adrenal tumor containing both fat and bone marrow elements. It is very rare in children, with only one pediatric case reported in the literature.[27] In adults, diagnosis is usually made at autopsy or on radiologic exam done for another reason. The appearance on imaging studies depends on the ratio of the two distinct elements. On ultrasound, a hyperechoic solid mass is most common. If the lipoma element in the tumor is significant, CT shows distinct fatty areas within the tumor. The tumor is usually confined within a distinct capsule. MRI can often show the distinct fatty

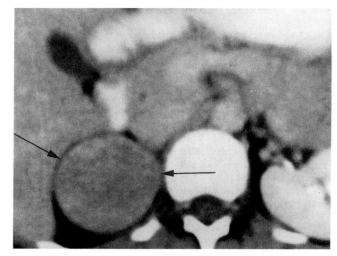

FIG. 16.5. CT scan showing a well-defined adrenal adenoma (*arrows*) just posterior to the vena cava and second portion of the duodenum.

areas within the tumor with greater clarity than CT. Myelolipomas are not metabolically active.[28] This should be confirmed with MIBG scanning and catecholamine studies in any lesion being considered for this diagnosis.

MALIGNANT CORTICAL NEOPLASMS

Adrenocortical carcinoma (ACC) is a very rare tumor in children, with an estimated incidence in the general population of one in 1.7 million.[29] Only 350 cases have been reported in children.[2] As noted above, adrenal carcinoma in children occurs at a slightly older age than adenoma. The left side is more commonly affected, and there is a female-to-male ratio of 4 : 1.[30] These tumors are almost always hormonally active and, as with adenomas, the presenting symptoms are related to the hormone produced.[31] When the symptoms of Cushing syndrome and virilization are both present in a patient with an adrenal tumor, malignancy is to be expected.[32]

Treatment of ACC rests on surgical excision of the mass. Fortunately, ACC in children tends to metastasize later than in adults and may therefore have a better prognosis.[33] Recurrent disease may be successfully excised.[33] Unresectable or metastatic disease is generally refractory to therapy. Mitotane (O, P, DDD) causes necrosis of the adrenal gland and has been used with variable success in patients with disseminated disease.[34,35] Its significant toxicity limits its use, however.

AGENESIS AND ECTOPY OF THE ADRENAL GLANDS

Aberrant adrenal tissue is a common finding[36,37] and has been reported in numerous locations. The most common site is in the retroperitoneum, particularly the area adjacent to the adrenal gland. Because of the intimate anatomic relationship between the developing gonad, kidney, and adrenal, accessory adrenal tissue is commonly found in the kidney, along the route of descent of the gonads, within the gonads themselves, or in hernia sacs. Less common sites include the area near the celiac plexus, attached to the peritoneum, on the uterus, or along the broad ligament. Adrenal rests are believed to be present in 50% of newborn infants and to atrophy within a few weeks.[38] Most of these nodules of adrenal tissue are of little clinical relevance or pathological significance, unless present in an individual with increased levels of ACTH, such as in Cushing or Addison disease. In these instances, the aberrant tissue may undergo hyperplasia and may give rise to a neoplastic process or become functionally active, warranting removal.[38] Adrenal rests are noted in all male patients with congenital adrenal hyperplasia (CAH).[39] It is, therefore, important to recognize this association to avoid unnecessary orchiectomies once an intratesticular mass is identified.[40]

Grossly, the adrenal rests appear as tiny (<4 mm),

yellow, round or oval masses, similar to fat lobules. They are firm and elastic in consistency and are occasionally umbilicated.[41] Some investigators have reported that adrenal rest tissue is found in 3% of pediatric patients undergoing herniorrhaphy, hydrocoelectomy, and orchiopexy.[38,41] The rests are composed of cortex only, usually adult or definitive, without a medulla.[38] Most authors recommend removal of incidentally encountered rests, but special attempts to locate adrenal rest tissue are not indicated. Sonographically, adrenal rests are hypoechoic and minimally disruptive of testicular tissue. They are peripherally located, do not distort the contour of the testicle, and occur surrounded by normal testes in the area of the mediastinum testis.[40] Again, knowledge of these characteristics is valuable when a male patient with a history of CAH presents with an intratesticular or scrotal mass.

Because the liver, kidney, and adrenal glands are enveloped in peritoneum in early gestation, fusion between the adrenal gland and kidney or liver may occur. Analogous to the horseshoe kidney, loss of intervening layers of coelomic epithelium can result in fusion of the limbs of the adrenal gland, creating a "horseshoe" or "circumrenal" adrenal gland.[42]

Bilateral agenesis of the adrenal glands is exceedingly rare and is incompatible with life. Of the small number of reported cases of unilateral adrenal agenesis, almost all are associated with ipsilateral renal agenesis. Early in gestation, the adrenal cortex develops from the mesodermal tissue arising from the coelomic epithelium. The adrenal medulla is derived from the ectoderm in the primitive cells of the sympathetic nervous system. Adrenal development occurs at the thoracic end of the nephrogenic ridge, and the branching ureteral bud occupies the caudal end of the ridge. Failure of the ureteral bud to induce development of the metanephric blastema results in renal agenesis. Failure of the entire nephrogenic ridge to develop, probably by the fourth week of gestation, results in adrenal and renal agenesis. Though the ipsilateral adrenal gland is absent in 8 to 10% of all cases of renal agenesis,[43,44] most cases of renal agenesis will have a normally positioned ipsilateral adrenal gland.

ADRENAL HEMORRHAGE

Neonatal adrenal hemorrhage is a relatively common condition associated with perinatal hypoxia, birth trauma, and coagulation defects. Reported incidence was 1.7 per 1,000 births in 1972, but may be different now that ultrasound is more commonly used in neonatal intensive care units.[45] Recent investigations have concluded that adrenal hemorrhage may occur in as many as 30% of neonatal intensive care admissions.[46] Birth ischemia remains the most common denominator associated with adrenal hemorrhage,[47] but additional possible risk factors include "large for date" babies, infant resuscitative efforts, bradycardia, sepsis, and hypoprothrombinemia. The adrenal gland is prone to hemorrhage in the neonate for several reasons: Three suprarenal arteries feed into a subcapsular plexus consisting of a dense network of arterioles. The venous drainage is limited to a relative few venules in the medullary sinusoids that feed into a single adrenal vein; therefore, a rise in arterial pressure or an increase in venous pressure can result in intraglandular hemorrhage. Stress from illness or from a difficult or traumatic delivery can result in this increased vascular congestion. The right gland is more susceptible to hemorrhage because of its anatomic position beneath the liver and its direct drainage into the inferior vena cava. The left side is protected by the long left renal vein, demonstrated by the fact that less than 10% of cases are bilateral.[48]

The classic triad associated with adrenal hemorrhage consists of a flank mass, anemia, and jaundice within the first week of life. There are sporadic reports of adrenal hemorrhage presenting as acute scrotal swelling from blood dissecting along the subcutaneous and muscular tissues from the retroperitoneum into the scrotum.[49–52] Rarer still are cases of intraperitoneal rupture and vascular collapse. Most infants will have neither symptoms of adrenal insufficiency nor symptoms of massive blood loss. Instead, an abdominal mass is noted on physical examination and may be accompanied by microscopic hematuria. Renal vein thrombosis (RVT) has been associated with adrenal hemorrhage, and it is necessary to image both kidneys, especially in the presence of gross or microscopic hematuria or proteinuria. Though almost an exclusively left-sided phenomenon,[53] RVT can coexist with isolated right-sided adrenal hemorrhage,[54] contralateral adrenal hemorrhage,[55–58] and bilaterally when associated with an inferior vena caval thrombus. Adrenal hemorrhage is usually not accompanied by hypertension. Hypertension may be an indication that there is a coexisting renovascular complication, such as RVT.[54] Recognition of RVT is important because hypertension and renal impairment are noted in long-term follow-up in over half of these patients.[59]

Historically, the intravenous pyelogram (IVP) was used to diagnose adrenal hemorrhage. A kidney displaced caudad with suprarenal shell-like calcifications is thought to be indicative of adrenal hemorrhage. Currently, ultrasound has replaced the IVP as the primary diagnostic imaging study and is fairly precise in the diagnosis of adrenal masses. The typical sonographic finding in adrenal hemorrhage is an echogenic or mixed echogenic/lucent mass that shows progressive echolucency as hemorrhage liquifies after a week[54, 60] (Fig. 16.6). The differential diagnosis includes neuroblastoma, cysts, renal tumors, and ureteral duplication anomalies. Differentiating neuroblastoma from adrenal hemorrhage can be difficult; however, normal urinary catecholamines and serial ultrasound studies that document a change in echogenicity and a decrease in the size of the adrenal mass can safely exclude a neuroblastoma.[52, 60–62] If the mass grows, fails to resolve, or has other characteristics of neuroblastoma in the face of normal urinary

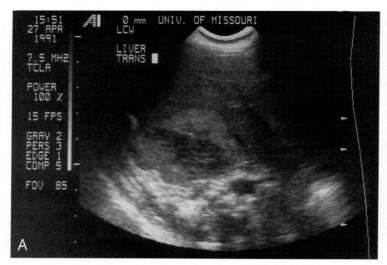

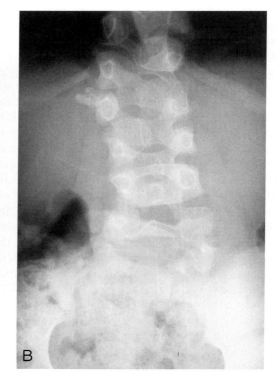

FIG. 16.6. A, Sonogram demonstrating adrenal hemorrhage in a newborn. *Open arrow,* right kidney; *solid arrows,* adrenal hemorrhage. **B,** Follow-up plain film of the abdomen of the same patient showing residual calcification from the adrenal hemorrhage.

catecholamines, consideration for surgical intervention is warranted. It is important to remember that 10% of patients with neuroblastoma have normal homovanellic acid (HVA), and 27.5% have normal vanillylmandelic acid (VMA) levels.[63] CT adds little more than ultrasonography, alone, can provide.[64] Acute or subacute bleeding in an adrenal hemorrhage will be characterized by high attenuation (50 to 90 Hounsfield units) material on CT. The value of MRI has not yet been defined, although there is some thought that it may be a better diagnostic tool in cases of massive hemorrhage associated with a relatively small neuroblastoma.[64]

Rarely, massive adrenal hemorrhage with intraperitoneal rupture is encountered. In these cases of vascular compromise and shock, surgical intervention is necessary. More commonly, the bleeding is slower, shorter, and self-contained, so there is no circulatory insufficiency. In these cases, conservative therapy can be adopted with close monitoring of vital signs as the disorder spontaneously resolves. Adequate hydration is usually all that is necessary, although some infants with bilateral disease will need steroid and blood replacement. Even in severe cases involving both adrenal glands, adrenal function is nearly always restored within 3 months.[65] Sonographic resolution should be documented within one to two months, and adrenal masses that fail to resolve spontaneously should be surgically explored. Suprarenal masses detected in utero can be followed postnatally in a similar fashion to those detected postnatally, assuming that the infant's urinary catecholamines are within normal limits. Fetal adrenal hemorrhage cannot be distinguished from spontaneously resolved neuroblastoma. Though calcifications are more commonly a result of hemorrhage, 50 to 75% of neuroblastomas will also contain calcifications.[60] Stippled calcification or widening of the paravertebral soft tissues is particularly suggestive of neuroblastoma.[66]

ADRENAL CYSTS

Adrenal cysts are rare findings that are usually discovered incidentally during imaging procedures. Most adrenal cysts are unilateral. Calcifications are present in 15% of the cases[67] but do not necessarily imply malignancy. Adrenal cysts can be divided into four groups: parasitic, epithelial, endothelial, and pseudocysts.[68 69] Most reported cases of adrenal cysts in neonates are the result of adrenal hemorrhage, though there is a report of spontaneously resolving, bilateral, nonhemorrhagic cysts.[70] Occasionally, cysts resulting from the spontaneous resolution of perinatal adrenal hemorrhage will persist into adulthood. The encapsulated residua of the hemorrhage represents what are actually pseudocysts, as they lack an epithelial lining. Rarely do adrenal cysts require interventional therapy, though pseudocysts can continue to enlarge and potentially compress adjacent structures,

necessitating surgical removal. Endothelial or lymphangiomatous cysts are the most common variety of adrenal cysts seen in adults,[67] but are rarely encountered in children. Rarely diagnosed in this country, echinococcal disease is the most common cause of parasitic adrenal cysts.

ADRENAL ABSCESS

Most cases of adrenal hemorrhage resolve spontaneously without adverse sequelae. Uncommonly, an adrenal hemorrhage may be complicated by an adrenal abscess. Most investigators believe that the hematoma is seeded by circulating bacteria from maternal infection at the time of delivery.[71] Nosocomial pathogens arising from central venous access appliances may also seed existing perinatal adrenal hemorrhage. Suspicion of an abscess is usually based on the findings of a palpable abdominal mass, jaundice, leukocytosis, fever, microscopic hematuria, and anemia. Prompt diagnosis may prevent the suppurative process from spreading to adjacent organs. Sonographic imaging will typically demonstrate a suprarenal fluid-filled mass with layered debris.[72] Differential diagnosis includes a duplication anomaly, pseudocyst, hematoma, hydronephrosis in an upper pole calyx, cystic or hemorrhagic neuroblastoma, and Wilms tumor.[73]

In the past, treatment of an adrenal abscess was exclusively surgical, by excision of the abscess or incision and drainage. Often, ipsilateral nephrectomy was required. With improved sonographic imaging, guided needle drainage and concomitant intravenous antibiotic therapy may prove to be sufficient.[74]

OTHER INFECTIOUS CONSIDERATIONS

Because of the increased incidence of immunocompromised patients seen in the pediatric population over the last 15 years, a new dimension has been added to disseminated infectious disease. Though there are very few reports of disseminated disease in neonates born with HIV, older children and adolescents with AIDS are at risk for a growing list of disseminated opportunistic infections. Though infrequent, some of these pathogens may infect adrenal tissue. Granulomatous diseases, including tuberculosis, and fungal infections, such as histoplasmosis, blastomycosis, and coccidiomycosis, have all been reported.[75]

ENDOCRINE DISORDERS

Hypercortisolism

Cortisol, the major glucocorticoid in humans, is secreted by both the zona fasciculata and reticularis of the adrenal cortex. Its actions are multiple and varied, and it affects a wide spectrum of cellular function. Glucocorticoids, essential for sustaining life, affect a wide range of metabolic and catabolic processes, including accumulation of glycogen in muscle and liver, amplification of gluconeogenesis, inhibition of bone and collagen formation, suppression of inflammatory and auto-immune activities, augmentation of vascular contractility, and maintenance of glomerular filtration.[67]

Like all steroids, cortisol passively diffuses into cells and binds to high-affinity receptors in the cytosol. This receptor–steroid complex passes into the nucleus where activation results in stimulation of transcription and the synthesis of specific ribonucleic acids and proteins. Ninety percent of circulating cortisol is bound to serum protein, corticosterone-binding globulin (80%), and albumin (10 to 15%). The remainder is free and is the metabolically active form. Adrenocorticotropic hormone (ACTH), produced by the pituitary gland, regulates the release of cortisol from the adrenal cortex. ACTH has a diurnal pattern of release that parallels serum cortisol levels. Loss of this diurnal variation is diagnostic of hypercortisolism and forms the premise upon which the dexamethasone suppression test is founded. Secretion of ACTH is stimulated by stress communicated from the hypothalamus and cerebral cortex. A protein known as corticotropin releasing factor (CRF), that increases circulation of ACTH has also been identified. Other recognized stimulators of ACTH are listed in Table 16.5.

Hypercortisolism can be caused either by pituitary hypersecretion of ACTH (Cushing disease) or from overproduction of glucocorticoids independent of pituitary ACTH (Cushing syndrome). Cushing syndrome can result from adrenal hyperplasia, adenoma, or carcinoma, or from ectopic sources of ACTH. Although 3 of Harvey Cushing's original 15 patients in 1932[76] were children, Cushing disease is quite rare in the pediatric population, and Cushing syndrome is even more uncommon. The Mayo clinic had but 13 children with Cushing syndrome and 46 with Cushing disease in a 40-year period from 1950 to 1990.[77]

It has been stated that adrenal tumors are the predominant cause of Cushing syndrome in children under the age of 7,[78] though the scarcity of the disease does not allow for much generalization regarding predominance.

TABLE 16.5. *Recognized stimulators of ACTH[2]*

Corticotropin releasing factor (CRF)
Oxytocin
Epinephrine
Angiotensin II
Vasoactive intestinal peptide
Serotonin
Atrial naturetic factor
Gamma-aminobutyric acid

It is, however, fairly well-established that, although the cause of ACTH-dependent Cushing syndrome may be an ectopic source in up to 15% of adult cases, it is much less common in children.[79] In the Mayo Clinic series of 13 patients with Cushing syndrome, 5 had adrenocortical carcinomas, 4 had adrenal adenomas, 2 had primary pigmented micronodular hyperplasia, and 2 had ectopic production of ACTH from bronchial carcinoid tumors.[76] There does not appear to be a male or female predominance.

Children with cortisol excess present with many of the signs and symptoms seen in adults, including central obesity, "moon facies" (Fig. 16.7A), striae, hirsuitism (Fig. 16.7B), acne, headaches, and easy bruising. Hypertension, osteopenia, and kidney stones are also frequently encountered. The hallmark of Cushing syndrome in children, however, is growth failure. The majority will report growth arrest with age-adjusted heights well below the average. Puberty is usually not delayed and can be premature. Menstrual irregularities are common.

The 24-hour urine collection for free cortisol determination is considered the single best test for confirming hypercortisolism.[78, 80] Sensitivity and specificity are excellent without the need to draw additional blood or administer medications. If the results are inconclusive, plasma levels of cortisol can be drawn in the morning and evening to look for a break in the normal diurnal pattern. There is considerable overlap, however, between patients with Cushing syndrome and normals, and the sensitivity of the test is thought to be approximately 70%.[76] The 2-day low-dose dexamethasone suppression test has been in use since its development in 1960 by Liddle[81] and has comparable accuracy to the urinary cortisol determination. Dexamethasone, 30 times more potent than cortisol, is given at a dosage of 20 μg/kg/d for 2 days. Normal subjects will have a dramatic decrease in 17-hydroxycorticosteroid, urinary free cortisol and plasma cortisol. Patients are diagnosed with Cushing syndrome if they fail to show a decrease in circulating levels of cortisol or its metabolic products.

Once hypercortisolism is confirmed, differentiation between ACTH-dependent and ACTH-independent disease is determined. The high-dose (2 mg every 6 hours) dexamethasone suppression test is able to differentiate Cushing disease from ectopic ACTH syndrome and ACTH-independent causes of Cushing syndrome.[80, 82] Suppression of 17-hydroxysteroids by 50% from baseline after 2 days of suppression is characteristic of pituitary-dependent disease. Patients with adrenal adenomas or carcinomas and most patients with ectopic sources of ACTH show no suppression. Radioimmunoassays for ACTH have been in use for nearly 20 years, and would appear to be a simpler method than the high-dose dexamethasone suppression test. Limited availability and inability to detect suppressed levels in

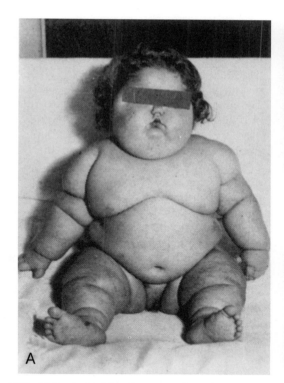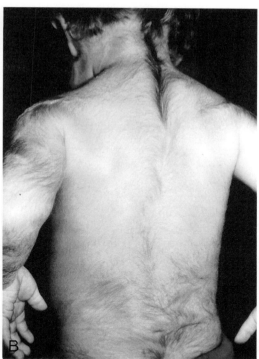

FIG. 16.7. A, Striking features of cortisol excess in a young girl. **B,** Striking hirsuitism in a 3-year-old boy with Cushing's syndrome secondary to a hyperfunctioning adrenocortical carcinoma.

ACTH-independent Cushing syndrome have limited its use in the past, but the advent of two-site immunoassays has improved the sensitivity of the test[76] and the agent is now widely available. Corticotropin releasing hormone (CRH) stimulation tests have been developed with sensitivity and specificity percentages that rival dexamethasone suppression.[82] Reliability in differentiating eutopic from ectopic sources of ACTH and a lack of experience, especially in children, have limited its use.

Differentiation of hyperplasia from adenoma and carcinoma can be difficult, as hyperfunctioning neoplasms can be very small. Patients with hyperplasia can show diffuse thickening and elongation of the limbs of the adrenal or prominent glands bilaterally. A multinodular form of hyperplasia is seen in a small minority of the cases that can be diagnosed by CT alone. Carcinomas can sometimes be suspected on CT findings of necrosis, calcification, and larger size, but none of these is diagnostic.[83] Adenomas have higher lipid content because of their accumulation of cholesterol esters and may be less dense on CT. Most lesions less than 10 Hounsfield units (especially if less than 0) are benign, and those greater than 10 units may be benign or malignant.[84] MRI may be of more benefit when adrenocortical carcinoma is suspected, because of the ability to visualize the inferior vena cava and any tumor thrombus from intravascular extension. When CT is equivocal or hyperplasia is suspected, scintigraphy with 131 I 6-Beta-iodomethyl-19-norcholesterol (NP-59) is recommended. Adenomas are characterized as a unilateral focus of radioactivity.[85] Nodular hyperplasia has a pattern of asymmetric but bilateral adrenocortical NP-59 uptake. Reports of scintigraphy's efficacy in localization of nodular hyperplasia have been excellent.[12, 13] Usually, adrenocortical carcinomas that produce Cushing syndrome do not accumulate sufficient NP-59 for imaging. Instead, they produce a scintigraphic pattern of bilateral nonvisualization, owing to suppression of function of the normal contralateral gland.[85, 86] If these findings are inconclusive, one should proceed with adrenal venous sampling.

The treatment of a hyperfunctioning adrenal adenoma or adrenocortical carcinoma is surgical resection, preferably through an extraperitoneal approach. Careful attention must be paid to the likelihood of suppression of the normal contralateral gland, and immediate adrenal insufficiency is expected upon removal of the affected side. Substitution therapy usually involves the administration of hydrocortisone, in a tapering dose regimen. The contralateral gland may be slow to recover, and substitution therapy may be necessary for up to two years. Sodium supplementation is rarely necessary, since the atrophic adrenal usually produces sufficient aldosterone. Serial urinary cortisol and 17-ketosteroids are monitored in the recovery period. The prognosis for benign disease is excellent; but, despite the tenuous feeling that survival is better in children than in adults,

TABLE 16.6. *Inhibitors of steroidogenesis and their sites of action*

Agent	Site of action
Aminoglutethimide	Blocks conversion of cholesterol to pregnenolone
Metyrapone	Blocks conversion of 11-deoxycortisol to cortisone
Ketoconazole	Blocks the cytochrome P-450 mediated side chain cleavage and hydroxylation in biosynthesis

adrenocortical malignancies are still highly lethal and refractory to adjuvant therapies.[87]

The goal of management in patients with hypercortisolism from adrenal hyperplasia is lowering the daily cortisol to normal levels. Utilization of inhibitors of steroidogenesis is the mainstay of medical therapy. Inhibitors of steroidogenesis and their sites of action are listed in Table 16.6. Patients on aminoglutethimide must be observed for adrenocortical insufficiency, because aldosterone synthesis will also be inhibited. Metyrapone usage usually does not result in salt wasting, because the accumulation of deoxycorticosteroid actively binds to mineralcorticoid receptors.[88] Patients with disease that is refractory to medical management or patients who are unable to tolerate medical therapy may eventually require bilateral adrenalectomy. This results in lifelong adrenal steroid supplementation, including both mineralcorticoid and glucocorticoid replacement, obviously a concern for the pediatric population. In addition, 10 to 20% of patients undergoing bilateral adrenalectomy will subsequently develop pituitary adenomas (Nelson syndrome) because of the lack of hypothalamic/pituitary feedback and high ACTH and related compounds.[89, 90] Long-term follow-up with ACTH levels and sella turcica imaging is recommended in this population.

Hyperaldosteronism

Aldosterone is secreted by the zona glomerulosa of the adrenal cortex and acts upon the ion-exchange mechanism of the distal renal tubule with resultant sodium retention and potassium and hydrogen ion excretion. Control of aldosterone secretion differs from glucocorticoid release in that it is much less sensitive to adrenocorticotropic hormone (ACTH). The primary regulator of aldosterone secretion is the juxtaglomerular apparatus of the kidney. Decreased renal perfusion results in increased secretion of renin, an enzyme that acts upon angiotensinogen to convert it to angiotensin I. A pulmonary tissue enzyme converts angiotensin I to angiotensin II, which is a potent stimulator of the zona glomerulosa and, thus, of aldosterone production. Serum potassium directly affects aldosterone production,

and dopamine has also been recognized as a regulator. Overproduction of aldosterone results in lower blood and tissue levels of potassium, and systemic alkalosis with kaliuresis and large volumes of alkaline urine. Presenting features include headache, weakness of proximal muscle groups, polyuria, tachycardia with or without palpitation, and hypertension. Hyperaldosteronism can be the result of a hyperfunctioning adenoma or carcinoma, or from adrenal hyperplasia.

Hyperaldosteronism (Conn syndrome) is an infrequent finding in the hypertensive adult population, and it is even rarer in children. Most (80%)[91] cases of hyperaldosteronism in adults are secondary to an adrenal adenoma. In contrast, most children have hyperplasia, with a higher incidence of bilaterality.[92, 93] There have only been nine reported cases of aldosteronoma in children, and eight of these were found in girls.[94–102] Though there have been seven reported cases in the adult literature[103] of adrenocortical carcinoma causing hyperaldosteronism, there are no such reported cases in children.[102] A rare familial form of hyperaldosteronism with autosomal dominant transmission has been described with bilateral adrenal hyperplasia.[104]

Though many believe that the true incidence of hypertension in the pediatric population is underestimated, the current incidence is thought to be around 5%.[105] Hypertensive children may present with fatigue, irritability, vomiting, and growth failure. New guidelines comparing body mass indices to blood pressure readings in age-specific percentiles have recently been employed to increase the sensitivity of diagnosing hypertension in children. Nearly 80% of hypertensive children have renovascular or renal parenchymal disease.[106] The possibility of hyperaldosteronism as a cause of hypertension should be entertained when a child presents with hypertension (often severe), polyuria, headaches, and dizziness. Some children will have enuresis or nocturia secondary to the increased urine output. Low serum potassium (often critically low), hypernatremia and alkalosis indicate the need for further diagnostic studies. Hypokalemia can be misdiagnosed as being a result of nephrogenic diabetes insipidus, and the diagnosis should be questioned when the patient is hypertensive, as well as hypokalemic.[102] One should also consider the possibility of hyperaldosteronism in a hypertensive child on diuretic therapy who does not develop hypokalemia or who has difficulty maintaining normal potassium levels while on conventional doses of potassium supplementation.

The best biochemical indicators of aldosteronoma are hypokalemia (<3.0 mEq/L) and anomalous postural decrease in plasma aldosterone concentration.[91] Plasma aldosterone concentration (PAC) before and after saline infusion is also helpful in making the diagnosis. Nonsuppression of plasma aldosterone values to less than 10 ng/dL after infusion of physiologic saline is highly suggestive of hyperaldosteronism. Plasma renin activity (PRA) is suppressed in primary hyperaldosteronism but is elevated in secondary disease. Glucocorticoids in sufficient excess can bind to mineralcorticoid receptors, and other mineralcorticoid syndromes should be excluded with serum cortisol, ACTH, 17-hydroxy-progesterone, dehydroepiandrosterone sulphate, and testosterone.[93]

High-resolution CT with thin cuts (5 mm) have had the highest yield in detecting adrenal masses, but aldosteronomas can be very small and can be missed even when technique is flawless. If CT is inconclusive, scintigraphy with 131 I 6-Beta-iodomethyl-19-norcholestrol (NP-59) is performed. NP-59, like native cholesterol, is transported in the circulation by low-density lipoproteins (LDL). It binds to LDL receptors on adrenocortical cells, which then internalize and esterfy the molecule but do not continue to metabolize it into steroid hormone analogues.[84] This results in imaging confined to the adrenal cortex. NP-59 scintigraphy is used in conjunction with dexamethasone suppression to amplify the functional differences between the secretory capacity of the corticotropin-dependent inner adrenal cortex (including the zona fasciculata and reticularis) and the renin-angiotensin-dependent outer adrenal cortex (zona glomerulosa) and increase the sensitivity of the study. The scintiscan can provide both functional and localization information.[84] Bilateral uptake is diagnostic of hyperplasia, while unilateral uptake is consistent with adenoma. When scintigraphy is inconclusive, venous sampling is indicated. Selective adrenal venous sampling should be able to differentiate a hypersecreting adenoma from hyperplasia in most cases, and arteriography and venography are of little benefit in gaining more diagnostic information. MRI, though offering better tissue characterization, is inferior to CT in spatial resolution[107] and offers no major role in the evaluation of patients with adrenocortical hyperfunction.[108] More work with chemical shift MRI is necessary before we will know if its ability to detect subtle amounts of lipid, characteristic of adenomas, will be of clinical value.

The treatment of choice for aldosteronoma is surgical excision, which should result in cure. Preoperatively, the adenoma should be localized to avoid bilateral exploration, and most are resectable from an extraperitoneal approach.[102] Close monitoring of fluid and electrolyte status and blood pressure are imperative in the immediate postoperative setting. Most patients will see an improvement in the control of their blood pressure within several weeks. Antihypertensives should be withheld accordingly.

For adrenal hyperplasia, medical therapy with spironolactone is preferred. Spironolactone inhibits the action of aldosterone on the distal renal tubule, and thereby corrects the hypokalemia and returns control of blood pressure to the renin-angiotensin system. For cases of bilateral hyperplasia, bilateral adrenalectomy has no place in the management of primary aldosteronism because adrenal insufficiency is significantly more difficult to treat than the hypertension from aldosteronism.

Feminizing Adrenal Tumors

Ninety-five percent of adrenal cortical neoplasms in children, benign and malignant, are hormonally active,[109] and the majority of children present with signs and symptoms of hypercortisolism with or without virilization. Rarely, a functional adrenal neoplasm will secrete androstenedione, which is peripherally converted to estrogen, and a child may present with feminization, as well as Cushingoid features. Though, in general, there is a female predominance in adrenocortical tumors, feminizing tumors affect males twice as often as females.[110] Typical clinical findings at presentation include breast enlargement (the most common finding), galactorrhea, testicular atrophy, accelerated growth, delayed isosexual pubertal development, and advanced bone age.[111] Some male patients may not present until they are referred for decreased libido, erectile dysfunction, oligospermia, or infertility. Menstrual irregularities and vaginal bleeding can occur in girls.

A thorough physical examination of the scrotum and a scrotal ultrasound are mandatory in the male child or adolescent with feminization, to exclude gonadal or extragonadal neoplasms producing chorionic gonadotropin or estrogen. Elevated urinary 17-ketosteroids and serum estradiol, estrogen, and testosterone are necessary to diagnose an adrenal neoplasm. Estradiol is more biologically potent than testosterone, and although testosterone may also be elevated, an elevated estradiol-to-testosterone ratio accounts for feminization. Malignant tumors exhibit elevated urinary 17-ketosteroid more often than benign lesions. A patient suspected of having an adrenal neoplasm can be imaged with either CT or MRI. Evaluation of the abdomen and pelvis is indicated to rule out metastatic disease. There are no reliable predictors of malignancy, though the size of the lesion is the best predictor of the tumor's biologic activity.[109]

Treatment revolves around surgical resection of the tumor. Aggressive resection of a neoplasm thought to be malignant is recommended because of the limited value of adjunctive therapy. Gynecomastia may regress but will persist in more than half of the patients (Fig. 16.8), and early reduction mammoplasty is indicated to preserve psychological well-being. Unfortunately, mortality rates remain high despite aggressive multimodal therapies for pediatric patients with adrenocortical carcinomas.[109] Mitotane has been used effectively in adult patients, but successful experience is lacking in children, and other chemotherapeutic agents have been disappointing.

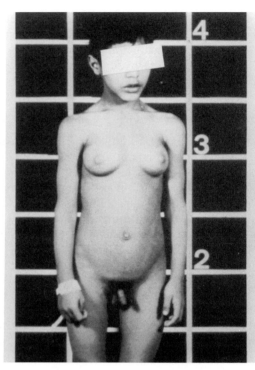

FIG. 16.8. A young boy with gynecomastia secondary to a feminizing adrenal tumor.

ADRENAL INSUFFICIENCY

Adrenal insufficiency (Addison disease) can result from destruction of the adrenal cortex, primary disease, or from disruption of the hypothalamic-pituitary-adrenal axis, secondary disease. Adrenal insufficiency is rare in the pediatric population. In children, adrenal hypoplasia is the most common cause of adrenal insufficiency and is usually encountered in the neonatal period, when the infant is in adrenal crisis. Congenital hypoplasia of the adrenals (CHA) can be an isolated, primary abnormality or can be secondary in association with pituitary hypoplasia, anencephaly,[112, 113] or advanced toxoplasmosis.[114] Most cases of adrenal insufficiency in adults are secondary to autoimmune adrenalitis, which has surpassed tuberculous andrenalitis as the most common cause,[115] and tends to present with more chronic symptoms. Though uncommon, adrenal insufficiency in children can be idiopathic or autoimmune in origin or can result from granulomatous disease, including tuberculosis, sarcoidosis, and fungal infections, such as histoplasmosis, blastomycosis, cryptococcus, and coccidiomycosis. As AIDS has become more prevalent in infants and adolescents, more patients have become susceptible to opportunistic infections and malignancies that may result in adrenal insufficiency. Bilateral adrenal hemorrhage can cause temporary insufficiency but very rarely results in permanent adrenal insufficiency.

The adrenal medulla is not affected and appears normal histologically. In contrast, the entire adrenal cortex is involved in all cases of primary adrenal insufficiency, creating deficiencies in cortisol, aldosterone, and androgens. In secondary disease, aldosterone secretion is minimally disturbed because its production is more dependent on angiotensin II than on corticotropin. There are rare syndromes of isolated glucocorticoid deficiencies in primary adrenal disease. These appear to involve adrenocortical unresponsiveness to ACTH with normal responses to angiotensin II.[116, 117] Cases of CHA have been reported in which the patient initially had only mineralcorticoid deficiency, and the glucocorticoid deficiency became progressively more severe over time. Though this disorder is rare, these children may be misdiagnosed as having acquired adrenal insufficiency.[118] The absence of another autoimmune disorder, present in nearly half of all patients with idiopathic Addison's disease,[119] may raise suspicion of the possibility of CHA.

Children with chronic adrenal insufficiency present much like their adult counterparts, with fatigue, weakness, dizziness, weight loss, anorexia, nausea, vomiting, and diarrhea. Hyperpigmentation of mucosal surfaces is one of the more specific signs of adrenal failure because of the increased circulating levels of corticotropin. Salt craving is also observed in primary disease. Acute insufficiency in newborns with CHA, life-threatening if unrecognized, is characterized by hyponatremia, hyperkalemia, hypoglycemia, and vascular collapse. Before the 1960s, many neonates died with adrenal hypoplasia. Now, many survive because of prompt recognition and appropriate therapy.[118] If an infant with CHA survives beyond two days, the clinical picture may include dehydration, poor feeding, failure to thrive, vomiting, and intractable diarrhea.[120]

There have been over 30 cases of CHA since it was first reported in 1948 by Sikl.[121] To make the diagnosis of CHA, three criteria should be fulfilled: symptoms or biochemical evidence of adrenal insufficiency, lack of substantial urinary secretion of the metabolites of androgens or progesterone to implicate an enzyme block in steroidogenesis, and failure to respond to prolonged administration of corticotropin.[122] The combined weight of the adrenal glands should also be less than one gram or less than 0.1% of the total body weight.[123] The diagnosis of CHA can never really be made with certainty, however, until there is histological confirmation.[118]

Adrenal hypoplasia is suspected when hyponatremia, hyperkalemia, and hypoglycemia are found on serum chemistry studies. Low serum dehydroepiandrosterone (DHEAS) and very low urinary excretion of delta-5 adrenal steroid metabolites demonstrate adrenocortical hypofunction. Poor serum cortisol response after corticotropin stimulation is diagnostic of adrenal failure. The possibility of an enzyme block in adrenal steroidogenesis is excluded if there is an elevation of urinary 17-hydroxyprogesterone or 24-hour ketosteroids. After fluid resuscitation and correction of electrolyte abnormalities, therapy revolves around appropriate replacement of adrenal steroids. Children with secondary adrenal insufficiency will also require growth hormone replacement. Prognosis can vary substantially in infants who survive through the postnatal period because of the association with other congenital abnormalities. Regardless, the prognosis remains poor.

There are two main histological patterns recognized in CHA, a cytomegalic form and a miniature form. If a fetal cortex is found microscopically, it is referred to as the cytomegalic variety. The miniature form is applied when adult adrenal cortex is present but is smaller than normal.[118] The cytomegalic form is predominant in the presence of adequate or elevated levels of circulating ACTH, while the miniature form exists when ACTH is low or absent, as in pituitary hypoplasia or anencephaly.

CHA has been described in infants with other congenital malformations, such as polydactyly, hemihypertrophy, omphalocele, multiple kidneys, and complex cardiac anomalies.[124] CHA has been reported in association with an autosomal-recessive disorder,[125] and in association with X-linked disorders with a deletion in the X chromosome at p21 and p22.[126–128] Other disorders that have a deletion in this area and that have been associated with CHA include Duchenne's muscular dystrophy,[129] glycerol kinase deficiency,[130] ornithine transcarbamylase deficiency,[131] and hypogonadotropic hypogonadism with or without cryptorchidism.[132–133] Clinically, it is important to differentiate between children with glycerol kinase deficiency and CHA from those with CHA alone, because mental retardation can result from hypoglycemia and can be prevented if it is an isolated CHA. At this time, the cause of CHA is unknown. Some factors that have been proposed include maternal steroid ingestion during gestation,[134] low birth weight,[135] prolongation of pregnancy,[136] and maternal preeclampsia.[137]

In families with a suggestive history, maternal urinary estriol levels should be monitored to evaluate the fetus for adrenal insufficiency[120] in hopes of preventing neonatal death. The placenta metabolizes large amounts of 3-Beta-hydroxy-5-ene-C19 steroids (secreted by the normal fetal zone of the adrenal cortex) into estrogen, and low maternal urinary estriol may be a sign of impending fetal adrenal insufficiency. However, this does not exclude placental sulfatase deficiency, a condition that is not harmful to the fetus and, thus, requires no treatment. The best hopes for preventing neonatal death lie in the expectation of and preparation for possible adrenal insufficiency.

Finally, there has been some controversy regarding the possibility of betamethasone nasal drops causing iatrogenic adrenal suppression in children being treated for bronchial asthma or allergic rhinitis. Initial studies that relied on high-dose ACTH tests and failed to show any adrenal effects may not have been sensitive enough to detect subtle impairment in adrenal function. Recent reports of studies using a lower dose of ACTH have raised concerns that inhaled corticosteroids indeed may cause untoward side effects, although the significance remains controversial.[138] The response may vary from child to child, and, at this time, additional corticosteroid administration for children under stressful situations, like surgery, should be withheld unless they have demonstrated more significant adrenal suppression.

REFERENCES

1. Joshi VV, Silverman JF. Pathology of neuroblastic tumors. Semin Diagn Pathol 1994;11(2):107.
2. Snyder H. Adrenal, sympathetic chain, and retroperitoneal tumors. In: Kelalis PP, King LR, Belman AB, eds. Clinical pediatric urology. Philadelphia: W.B. Saunders Co., 1992;2(34):1379–1414.
3. Daneman A. Adrenal neoplasms in children. Semin Roentgenol 1988;23(3):205.
4. Ein SH, Weitzman S, Thorner P, Seagram CG, Filler RM. Pediatric malignant pheochromocytoma. J Pediatr Surg 1994;23(9):1197.
5. Vaughn ED Jr. Pheochromocytoma. In: Seidmon EJ, Hanno PM, eds. Current urologic therapy. Philadelphia: W.B. Saunders Co., 1994;13.
6. Petrus LV, Hall TR, Boechat MI, Westra SJ, Curran JG, Steckel RJ, Kangarloo H. The pediatric patient with suspected adrenal neoplasm: Which radiological test to use? Med Pediatr Oncol 1992;20:53.
7. Gelfand MJ. Meta-iodobenzylguanidine in children. Semin Nucl Med 1993;23(3):231.
8. Lenders JWM, et al. Plasma metanephrines in the diagnosis of pheochromocytoma. Ann Intern Med 1995;123(2):101–109.
9. Turner MC, Lieberman E, De Quattro V. The perioperative management of pheochromocytoma in children. Clin Pediatr 1992;31:583.
10. Revillon Y, et al. Pheochromocytoma in children: 15 cases. J Pediatr Surg 1992;27(7):910.
11. Richards ML, Gundersen AE, Williams MS. Cystic neuroblastoma of infancy. J Pediatr Surg 1995;30(9):1354.
12. Croitoru DP, Sinsky AB, Laberge JM. Cystic neuroblastoma. J Pediatr Surg 1992;27(10):1320.
13. Stringel G, Ein SH, Creighton R. Pheochromocytoma in children—An update. J Pediatr Surg 1980;15:496.
14. James RE, Baker HL Jr, Scanlon PW. The roentgenologic aspects of metastatic pheochromocytoma, AJR 1972;115:783.
15. Manger WM, Gifford RW, Hoffman BB. Pheochromocytoma: A clinical and experimental overview. In: Hickey RC, ed. Current problems in cancer. Chicago: Year Book, 1985;51.
16. Matthay KK. Neuroblastoma: A clinical challenge and biologic puzzle. CA Cancer J Clin 1995;45:179.
17. Jennings RW, LaQuaglia MP, Leong K, Hendren WH, Adzick NS. Fetal neuroblastoma: Prenatal diagnosis and natural history. J Pediatr Surg 1993;28(9):1168.
18. Azizkhan RG, Haase GM. Current biologic and therapeutic implications in the surgery of neuroblastoma. Sem Surg Oncol 1993;9:493.
19. Gorsfeld, JL. Neuroblastoma in infancy and childhood. In: Hays DM, ed. Pediatric surgical oncology. Orlando: Grune and Stratton, 1986;63.
20. Fleming ID. Staging of pediatric cancers: Problems in the development of a national system. Semin Surg Oncol 1992;8:94.
21. Brodeur GM, et al. Revisions of the international criteria for neuroblastoma diagnosis, staging and response to treatment. J Clin Oncol 1993;11:1466.
22. Seeger RC, et al. Association of multiple copies of the n-*myc* oncogene with rapid progression of neuroblastomas. N Engl J Med 1985;313:1111.

23. Cairo MS. The use of ifosfamide, carboplatin and etoposide in children with solid tumors. Semin Oncol 1995;22(3) Suppl 7:23.

24. Ladenstein R, Hartmann O, Pinkerton CR. The role of megatherapy with aurologous bone marrow rescue in solid tumors of childhood. Ann Oncol 1993;4 Suppl 1:45.

25. Kiely EM. Radical surgery for abdominal neuroblastoma. Semin Surg Oncol 1993;9:489.

26. Daneman A, Chan HSL, Martin DJ. Adrenal carcinoma and adenoma in children: A review of 17 patients. Pediatr Radiol 1983;13:11.

27. Evans HL, Vassilopoulou-Sellin R. Adrenal cortical neoplasms—A study of 56 cases. Anat Path 1995;105(1):76.

28. Escuin F, Gomez P, Martinez I, Perez-Fontan M, Selgas R, Sanchez-Sicilia L. Angiomyelolipoma associated with bilateral adrenocortical hyperplasia and hypertension. J Urol 1985;133:655.

29. Hofmockel G, Dammrich J, Manzanilla Garcia H, Frohmuller H. Myelolipoma of the adrenal gland associated with contralateral renal cell carcinoma: case report and review of the literature. J Urol 1995;153:129.

30. Nader S, et al. Adrenal cortical carcinoma. Cancer 1983;52:707.

31. Richie JP, Gittes RF. Carcinoma of the adrenal cortex. Cancer 1980;45:1957.

32. Telander RL, et al. Paediatric endocrine surgery. Surg Clin North Am 1985;65:1560.

33. Al-Salem AH, Abu-Srair HA. Recurrent adrenocortical carcinoma in a 4-year-old girl. Aust N Z J Surg 1993;64:723.

34. Lee PD, Winter RJ, Green OC. Virilizing adrenocortical tumors in childhood. Pediatrics 1985;76:645.

35. Hoffman D, Mattox VR. Treatment of adrenocortical carcinoma with o.P-DDD. Med Clin North Am 1972;56:999.

36. Nelson AA. Accessory adrenal cortical tissue. Arch Pathol 1939;27:955.

37. Schecter DC. Aberrant adrenal tissue. Ann Surg 1968;167:421.

38. Okur H, Kucukaydin M, Kazez A. Ectopic adrenal tissue in the inguinal region in children. Pediatr Pathol Lab Med 1995;15:763.

39. Shanklin DR, Richardson AP, Rothstein G. Testicular hilar nodules in adrenogenital syndrome. Am J Dis Child 1963;106:243.

40. Avila NA, Premkumar A, Shawker TH, et al. Testicular adrenal rest tissue in congenital adrenal hyperplasia: Findings at grayscale and color doppler US. Radiology 1996;198:99.

41. Mares AJ, Shkolnik A, Sacks M, et al. Aberrant (ectopic) adrenocortical tissue along the spermatic cord. J Pediatr Surg 1980;15:289.

42. Burton EM, Strange ME, Edmunds DB. Sonography of the circumrenal and horseshoe adrenal gland in the newborn. Pediatr Radiol 1993;23:362.

43. Gray SW, Skandalakis JE. The embryological basis for the treatment of congenital defects. In: Embryology for surgeons. Philadelphia: W.B. Saunders Co., 1972;553.

44. Ashley DJB, Mostofi FK. Renal agenesis and dysgenesis. J Urol 1962;83:211.

45. Desa DJ, Nicholls S. Haemorrhagic necrosis of the adrenal gland in perinatal infants: A clinicopathological study. J Pathol 1972;106:133.

46. Eklof O, Grotte G, Garulf H. Perinatal hemorrhagic necrosis of the adrenal gland. Pediatr Radiol 1975;4:31.

47. Belman AB, King LR. The pathology and treatment of renal vein thrombosis in the newborn. J Urol 1972;107:852.

48. Hartmann GE, Shochat SS. Abdominal mass lesions in the newborn: Diagnosis and treatment. Clin Perinatol 1989;16(1):123.

49. Yang WT, Ku KW, Metrewell C. Case report: Neonatal adrenal hemorrhage presenting as an acute right scrotal swelling (hematoma)—Value of ultrasound. Clin Radiol 1995;50:127.

50. Putnam MH. Neonatal adrenal hemorrhage presenting as a right scrotal mass. Letter to the Editor. JAMA 1989;261:2958.

51. Giacoia GP, Cravens JD. Neonatal adrenal hemorrhage presenting as scrotal haematoma. J Urol 1990;143:567.

52. Liu KW, Ku KW, Cheung KL, et al. Acute scrotal swelling: A sign of neonatal adrenal hemorrhage. J Paediatr Child Health 1994;30:368.

53. Orazi C, Fariello G, Malena S. Renal vein thrombosis and adrenal haemorrhage in the newborn: Ultrasound evaluation of four cases. J Clin Ultrasound 1993;21:163.

54. Errington ML, Hendry GMA. The rare association of right adrenal haemorrhage and renal vein thrombosis diagnosed with duplex ultrasound. Pediatr Radiol 1995;25:157.

55. Bowen AD, Smazal SF. Ultrasound of coexisting right adrenal hemorrhage in a newborn. J Clin Ultrasound 1981;9:511.

56. Koch KJ, Cory DA. Simultaneous renal vein thrombosis and bilateral adrenal hemorrhage: MR demonstration. J Comput Assist Tomogr 1986;10:681.

57. Lebowitz JM, Belman AB. Simultaneous idiopathic renal hemorrhage and renal vein thrombosis in the newborn. J Urol 1983;129:574.

58. Starinsky R, Manor A, Segal M. Nonfunctioning kidney associated with neonatal adrenal hemorrhage: Report of 2 cases. Pediatr Radiol 1986;16:427.

59. Mocan H, Beattie TJ, Murphy AV. Renal vein thrombosis in infancy: Long-term follow-up. Pediatr Nephrol 1991;5:45.

60. Strouse PJ, Bowerman RA, Schlesinger AE. Antenatal sonographic findings of fetal adrenal hemorrhage. J Clin Ultrasound 1995;23:442.

61. Smith JA, Middleton RG. Neonatal adrenal hemorrhage. J Urol 1979;122:674.

62. Karpe B, Nybonde T. Adrenal hemorrhage versus testicular torsion—A diagnostic dilemma in the neonate. Pediatr Surg Int 1989;4:337.

63. Tuchman M, Ramnaraine MLR, Woods WG, et al. Three years of experience with random urinary homovanillic and vanillylmandelic acid levels in the diagnosis of neuroblastoma. Pediatrics 1987;79:203.

64. Brill PW, Jagannath A, Winchester P, et al. Adrenal hemorrhage and renal vein thrombosis in the newborn: MR imaging. Radiology 1990;170:95.

65. Jojart G, Nagy G, Pasztor J, et al. Bilateral neonatal adrenal hemorrhage associated with hypoadrenalism. Orv Hetil 1981;133:1179.

66. Galatius-Jensen F, Damgaard-Pedersen K. Malignant versus benign paravertebral widening in children. Pediatr Radiol 1981;11:193.

67. Vaughan ED Jr, Blumenfeld JD. The adrenals. In: Walsh PC, Retik AB, Stamey TA, Vaughan ED Jr, eds. Campbell's urology. Philadelphia: W.B. Saunders Co., 1992;2381.

68. Abeshouse GA, Goldstein RB, Abeshouse BS. Adrenal cysts: Review of the literature and report of three cases. J Urol 1959;81:711.

69. Ellis FH, Dawe CJ, Clagett OT. Cysts of the adrenal glands. Ann Surg 1952;136:217.

70. Patti G, Fiocca G, Latini T, et al. Prenatal diagnosis of bilateral adrenal cysts. J Urol 1993;150:1189.

71. Gibbons MD, Duckett JW Jr, Cromie WJ, et al. Abdominal flank mass in the neonate. J Urol 1978;119:671.

72. Carty A, Stanley P. Bilateral adrenal abscesses in a neonate. Pediatr Radiol 1973;1:63.

73. Atkinson GO Jr, Kodroff MB, Gay BB Jr. Adrenal abscess in the neonate. Radiology 1985;155:101.

74. Elder JS, Duckett JW. Perinatal urology. In: Gillenwater JY, Grayhack JT, Howards SS, Duckett JW, eds. Adult and pediatric urology. St. Louis: Mosby Year Book, 1991;1776.

75. Leggiadro RJ, Barrett FF, Hughes WT. Disseminated histoplasmosis of infancy. Pediatr Infect Dis J 1988;7:799.

76. Cushing H. Basophil adenomas of the pituitary body and their clinical manifestations ("pituitary basophilism"). In: Papers relating to the pituitary body, hypothalamus, and parasympathetic nervous system. Springfield: Charles C. Thomas, 1932;113–174.

77. Leinung MC, Zimmerman D. Cushing's disease in children. Endocrinol Metab Clin North Am 1994;23:629.

78. Grua J, Nelson D. ACTH-producing pituitary tumors. Endocrinol Metab Clin North Am 1991;20:319.

79. Leinung MC, Young WF, Whitaker MD, et al. Diagnosis of corticotropin-producing bronchial carcinoid tumors causing Cushing's syndrome. Mayo Clin Proc 1990;65:1314.

80. Carpenter P. Diagnostic evaluation of Cushing's syndrome. Endocrinol Metab Cl North Am 1988;17:445.

81. Liddle GW. Test of pituitary-adrenal suppressibility in the diagnosis of Cushing's syndrome. J Clin Endocrinol Metab 1960;20:1539.

82. Miller J, Crapo L. The biochemical diagnosis of hypercortisolism. Endocrinolog 1994;4:7.
83. Belldegrun A, deKernion JB. What to do about the incidentally found adrenal mass. World J Urol 1989;7:117.
84. Freitas JE. Adrenocortical and medullary imaging. Semin Nuc Med 1995;XXV:235.
85. Gross MD, Shapiro B, Thrall JH, et al. The scintigraphic imaging of endocrine organs. Endocr Rev 1984;5:221.
86. Fig LM, Gross MD, Shapiro B, et al. Adrenal localization in adrenocorticotrophic hormone independent Cushing's syndrome. Ann Intern Med 1988;109:547.
87. Kay R, Schumaker OP, Pank ES. Adrenal cortical carcinoma in children. J Urol 1983;130:1130.
88. Scott HW, Liddle GW, Mulherin JL, et al. Surgical experience with Cushing's disease. Ann Surg 1977;185:587.
89. Cohen KL, Noth RH, Pechinski T. Incidence of pituitary tumors following adrenalectomy. A long-term follow-up study of the patients treated for Cushing's disease. Arch Intern Med 1978; 138:575.
90. Nelson DH. The adrenal cortex: physiological function and disease. Major Probl Intern Med 1980;18:15.
91. Bravo EL. Primary aldosteronism. Urol Clin North Am 1989; 16:481.
92. Grim CE, McBryde AC, Glen JF, et al. Childhood primary aldosteronism with bilateral adrenocortical hyperplasia: Plasma renin activity as an aid to diagnosis. J Pediatr 1967;71:377.
93. Li JT, Shu SG, Chi SC. Aldosterone-secreting adrenal cortical adenoma in an 11-year-old child and collective review of the literature. Eur J Pediatr 1994;153:480.
94. Orndahl G, Hokfelt B, Ljunggren E, et al. Two cases of primary aldosteronism. Comments on differential diagnosis and difficulties in screening. Acta Med Scand 1959;165:445.
95. Crane MG, John E, Holloway JE, et al. Aldosterone secreting adenoma: Report of a case in a juvenile. Ann Intern Med 1961;54:280.
96. Cavell B, Sandegard E, Hokfelt B. Primary aldosteronism due to an adrenal adenoma in a 3-year-old child. Acta Paediatr Scand 1964;53:205.
97. Mora H, Cullen M, Bergada C, et al. Suprarenal adrenal adenoma with virilisation and hyperaldosteronism in a 10-year-old girl. Rev Argent Endocrinol Metab 1965;11:117.
98. Kelch RP, Connors MH, Kaplan SI, et al. A calcified aldosterone secreting producing tumor in a hypertensive, normokalemic, prepubertal girl. J Pediatr 1973;83:432.
99. Kafrouni G, Oakes MD, Lurvey AN, et al. Aldosteronoma in a child with localisation by renal vein aldosterone: Collective review of the literature. J Ped Surg 1975;10:917.
100. Ganguly A, Bergstein J, Grim CE, et al. Childhood primary aldosteronism due to an adrenal adenoma: Preoperative localisation by adrenal vein catheterisation. Pediatrics 1980;65:605.
101. Bryer-Ash M, Wilson DM, Tune BM, et al. Hypertension caused by an aldosterone secreting adenoma: Occurrence in a 7-year-old child. Am J Dis Child 1984;138:673.
102. Agarwala S, Mitra DK, Bhatnager V, et al. Aldosteronoma in childhood: A review of clinical feature and management. J Ped Surg 1994;10:1388.
103. Slee PHTJ, Schaberg A, Brummelen PV. Carcinoma of the adrenal cortex causing primary hyperaldosteronism. Cancer 1983; 51:2341.
104. New MI, Baum CJ, Levine LS. Normograms relating aldosterone excretion to urinary sodium and potassium in the pediatric population: Their application to the study of childhood hypertension. Am J Cardiol 1976;37:658.
105. Loggie JMH, New MI, Robson AM. Hypertension in the pediatric patient: A reappraisal. J Pediatr 1979;94:685.
106. Wigfall DR. Systemic arterial hypertension in children and adolescents. In: Kelalis PP, King LR, Belman AB, eds. Clinical pediatric urology. Philadelphia: W.B. Saunders Co., 1992;1201.
107. Westra SJ, Zaninovic AC, Hall TR, et al. Imaging of the adrenal gland in children. Radiographics 1994;14:1323.
108. Francis IR, Gross MD, Shapiro B. Integrated imaging of adrenal disease. Radiology 1992;184:1.
109. Koyle MA. Feminizing adrenal tumors in children. In: Seidmon EJ, Hanno PM, eds. Current urologic therapy. Philadelphia: W.B. Saunders Co., 1994;8.
110. Neblett WW, Frexes-Steed M, Scott HW. Experience with adrenocortical neoplasms in childhood. Am Surg 1987;53:117.
111. Morales L, Rovira J, Rotterman M, et al. Adrenocortical tumors in childhood: A report of four cases. J Pediatr Surg 1989;24:276.
112. Blizzard RM, Alberts M. Hypopituitarism, hypoadrenalism and hypogonadism in the newborn infant. J Pediatr 1956;48;782.
113. Brewer DD. Congenital absence of the pituitary gland and its consequences. J Pathol Bacteriol 1957;73:59.
114. Le SQ, Kutteh WH. Monosomy 7 syndrome associated with congenital adrenal hypoplasia and male pseudohermaphroditism. Obstet Gynecol 1996;87:854.
115. Oelkers W. Adrenal insufficiency. New Eng J Med 1996;335:1206.
116. Tsigos C, Arai K, Laronico AC, et al. A novel mutation of the adrenocorticotropin receptor (ACTH-R) gene in a family with the syndrome of isolated glucocorticoid deficiency, but no ACTH-R abnormalities in two families with the triple A syndrome. J Clin Endocrinol Metab 1995;80:2186.
117. Moore PSJ, Couch RM, Perry YS, et al. Allgrove syndrome: An autosomal recessive syndrome of ACTH insensitivity, achalasia and alacrima. Clin Endocrinol 1991;34:107.
118. Sills IN, Voorhess ML, MacGillivray MH, et al. Prolonged survival without therapy in congenital adrenal hypoplasia. Am J Dis Child 1983;137:1186.
119. Zelissen PMJ, Bast EJEG, Croughs RJM. Associated autoimmunity in Addison's disease. J Autoimmun 1995;8:121.
120. Batch JA, Montaalto J, Yong ABW, et al. Three cases of congenital adrenal hypoplasia: A cause of salt-wasting and mortality in the neonatal period. J Paediatr Child Health 1991;27:108.
121. Sikl H. Addison's disease due to congenital hypoplasia of the adrenals in an infant aged 3 days. J Patol Bacteriol 1948;60:323.
122. Sperling MA, Wolfsen AR, Fisher DA. Congenital adrenal hypoplasia: An isolated defect of organogenesis. J Pediatr 1973;82:444.
123. Favara BE, Franciosi RA, Miles V. Idiopathic adrenal hypoplasia in children. Am J Clin Pathol 1972;57:287.
124. McMahon H, Wagner R, Weiner D. Acute adrenal insufficiency due to congenital defect. Amer J Dis Child 1957;94:282.
125. Ohlbaum P, Hehunstra PP, Bouchet JL, et al. Insufficience surrenale chroniaue et hyalinose segmentaire et focale famiale: Una nouvelle association. Pediatrie 1986;41:86.
126. Mitchell RG, Rhaney K. Congenital adrenal hypoplasia in siblings. Lancet I 1959;488.
127. Hay ID, Smail PJ, Forsyth CC, et al. Familial cytomegalic adrenocortical hypoplasia. An X-linked syndrome of pubertal failure. Arch Dis Child 1981;56:715.
128. Petersen KE, Bille T, Jacobsen BB, et al. X-linked congenital adrenal hypoplasia: A study of five generations of a Greenlandic family. Acta Paediatr Scand 1982;71:947.
129. Wise JE, Matalon R, Morgan AM, et al. Phenotypic feature of patients with congenital adrenal hypoplasia and glycerol kinase deficiency. Amer J Dis Child 1987;141:744.
130. Guggenheim MA, McCabe ERB, Roig M. Glycerol kinase deficiency with neuromuscular, skeletal and adrenal abnormalities. Am Neurol 1980;7:441.
131. Hammond J, Howard NJ, Brookwell R, et al. Proposed assignment of loci for X-linked adrenal hypoplasia and glycerol kinase genes. Lancet I 1985;54.
132. Prader A, Zachmann M, Ilig R. Luteinising hormone deficiency in hereditary congenital adrenal hypoplasia. J Pediatr 1975; 86:421.
133. Zachmann M, Ilig R, Prader A. Gonadotropin deficiency and cryptorchidism in three prepubertal brothers with congenital adrenal hypoplasia. J Pediatr 1980;97:255.
134. Laverty CRA, Fortune DW, Beischer NA. Congenital idiopathic adrenal hypoplasia. Obstet Gynecol 1973;41:655.
135. Bongiovanni AM, McPadden AJ. Steroids during pregnancy and possible fetal consequences. Fertil Steril 1960;11:181.
136. Szalay CG. Congenital adrenal hypoplasia. J Pediatr 1973;83:169.
137. O'Donohoe NV, Holland PDJ. Familial congenital adrenal hypoplasia. Arch Dis Child 1968;43:717.
138. Broide J, Soferman R, Kivity S. Low-dose adrenocorticotropin test reveals impaired adrenal function in patients taking inhaled corticosteroids. J Clin Endocrinol Metab 1995;80:1243.

CHAPTER 17

Disorders of Renal Position and Parenchymal Development

Richard N. Schlussel

RENAL ECTOPIA

Embryology

Ureteric growth and spinal growth are normally the two factors most responsible for renal ascent. Deranged spinal growth can therefore affect the ultimate position of the kidney. Maizels and Stephens tested this hypothesis by inducing deformities of the caudal trunk in chick embryos.[1] When scoliosis was induced, the chicks had renal ectopia 10 times more often than the chicks without scoliosis. They postulated that the abnormal growth of the spine precluded normal renal ascent and may even have been responsible for renal agenesis and hypoplasia.

Another possible cause of ectopia is an anomalous obstructing blood vessel preventing normal ascent.[2, 3] However there are few descriptions of these vessels seen during surgical exploration of the ectopic kidney. It is possible that such vessels may regress prior to birth as do many other vessels during gestation.

Friedland and DeVries[4] studied a collection of human embryos and, with detailed serial dissections, showed that the developing kidney ascends from the second sacral level to the second lumbar level. This occurs between the fifth and eighth weeks of gestation. These authors attribute ectopia not to interference of the inferior mesenteric artery but to retardation of ureteric growth or inhibition of the growth of the spine. Teratogenic agents that inhibit these growth processes should therefore result in spinal defects and renal ectopia and fusion.

Crossed fused ectopia appears to be a result of the ureteric bud migrating across the midline to interact with the contralateral metanephric blastema. Evidence of this embryologic theory is found in the series of patients with ureteral and renal colic in the setting of crossed renal ectopia.[5] Patients that had ureteral stones in the ureter draining the crossed ectopic kidney developed flank pain on the side of origin of the ureter (i.e.,

the *anephric* side). Consider the case of right to left cross fused renal ectopia. The ectopic ureter maintains its innervation from the right side of the body. A stone in the distal ureter of this crossed ectopic kidney will distend the ureter and stimulate the nerves on the right side of the body and hence the patient will have right flank pain. However, a stone in the crossed ectopic kidney in the same clinical situation will lead to flank pain on the left side. These clinical findings lend support to the theory that crossed fused ectopia is due to ureteral migration and interaction with the contralateral metanephric blastema.

Vascularity

The normally developing kidney obtains its blood supply from varied sources as it ascends. In order, the ascending kidney's blood supply is from the middle sacral artery, the external iliac artery, the common iliac artery and finally the aorta.[6] In renal ectopia, the blood supply to the kidney may arise from a source other than the thoracolumbar aorta such as the iliac artery or sacral artery. The ectopic kidney can even receive vessels from the right and left iliac arteries.[7] Similarly, the ectopic and the crossed ectopic kidney's blood supply is from a local source near its final location. In patients with crossed renal ectopia, there are frequently multiple renal arteries. These varied arteries may arise from the ipsilateral common iliac artery, the contralateral common iliac artery, or the lower lumbar aorta. Arteries arising from the aorta to supply an ectopic kidney can originate from the anterior portion of the aorta or even from the contralateral side of the aorta.[7, 8] Because of the unpredictable nature of the renal blood supply in the ectopic or crossed ectopic kidney, many clinicians advocate a preoperative angiogram in any instance where surgery is being contemplated on the ectopic kidney.

Associated Anomalies

The ectopic kidney may be associated with both urologic and nonurologic anomalies. The ectopic kidney may be subtended by either an ectopic ureter[9-11] or a ureterocele.[12, 13] An ectopic ureter should be suspected when a toilet-trained female child with a normal voiding history complains of continuous dribbling of urine. This ureter is usually draining an upper pole of a duplicated system. However, it may also drain a single system and that kidney commonly is in an ectopic position. Such a kidney is difficult to locate due to its ectopia, small size and usually severely diminished function. It is not surprising that the anomaly of an ectopic ureter is associated with ectopic kidney since ureteral ectopia is thought to be due to an abnormally cephalad takeoff from the mesonephric duct, which may lead to abnormal ureteral migration or altered growth of the ureteral bud with subsequent abnormal renal migration as well. Therefore, Gharagozloo[11] recommends dimercaptosuccinic acid (DMSA) scanning followed by thin cut computerized tomographic (CT) scanning of the area of interest to pinpoint the location of the ectopic kidney.

In renal ectopia, ureteroceles may be found either at the end of the ectopic kidney's ureter or at the end of the orthotopic kidney's ureter. In both scenarios, the ureterocele can cause hydronephrosis of both kidneys as it distorts the trigone and compresses the contralateral ureteral orifice or obstructs the bladder neck.

Malek et al.[3] report a variety of abnormalities in the genitourinary tract associated with an ectopic kidney. In their experience, the contralateral kidney was often affected by either hydronephrosis, malrotation, malfunction or agenesis. Other urinary tract anomalies seen in their series included ipsilateral absence of the trigone (hemitrigone), ectopic ureter, vesicoureteral reflux, urethral stricture and ureteral duplication. The genital anomalies associated with an ectopic kidney include hypospadias and cryptorchidism. Other genital anomalies seen in crossed renal ectopia are absent or atrophic vas deferens, absent seminal vesicles and absence or agenesis of the uterus or vagina.[14] Gleason published a 26% incidence of genitourinary anomalies.[2] Hendren noted that in his series of 9 patients with ectopic kidneys, 4 had posterior urethral valves, 5 had vesicoureteral reflux and 3 had ectopic ureters.[15]

Anomalies of other organ systems are also prevalent. The urologist who cares for a child with an ectopic kidney must keep these anomalies in mind and initiate the appropriate specialist consultation and evaluation. The association of orthopedic anomalies and renal anomalies is well known and include vertebral anomalies (spina bifida, hemivertebra); absence of fingers, sacrococcyx and forearm; rib anomalies; skull asymmetry and a deformed extremity, such as club foot.[3, 14, 16-18]

The child with an ectopic kidney should undergo a cardiac evaluation. The most prevalent of these cardiac anomalies are aortic stenosis and pulmonary stenosis. Atrial septal defects, ventricular septal defects, coarctation of the aorta, tetralogy of Fallot and small left ventricle are also seen.[2, 3, 16]

Gastrointestinal anomalies are also seen more commonly in renal ectopia. Malrotation of the colon and diaphragmatic hernia were found in 10% of these patients along with a variety of single cases of absent cecum, imperforate anus, accessory spleen and anal stricture.[2, 3] Other anomalies include inguinal hernia, otologic abnormalities (preauricular skin tags, low set ears, absent ear) and palatolabial anomalies (harelip, cleft palate).

Location

The most common location of an ectopic kidney is within the true bony pelvis, followed by cross fused, lumbar and rarely thoracic.[2, 3] The kidneys are invariably malrotated in these ectopic positions (Fig. 17.1). This is likely due to the fact that the ascending kidney undergoes ninety degree rotation along its long axis during ascent. In the pelvic position, the renal pelvis is oriented anteriorly. The orthotopic kidney's pelvis is oriented medially. Renal ectopia appears to be more common in males and is found on the left side in 51%, the right side in 37% and bilaterally in 12%.[2] Ten to seventeen percent of patients with an ectopic kidney have a solitary kidney.[2, 3]

Diagnosis

Most cases of renal ectopia remain asymptomatic throughout a person's life. This is supported by the clinical incidence of 1 : 5–10,000 versus the autopsy incidence of 1 : 1,000.[2] The method of presentation of an ectopic kidney in the published literature is likely to

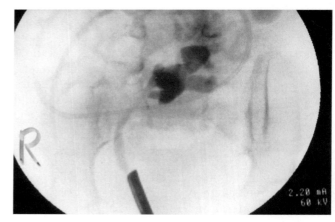

FIG. 17.1. Retrograde pyelography showing an ectopic kidney occupying a pelvic position. Note that the collecting system is malrotated and the calyces are oriented anteriorly.

vary depending on the era of investigation. Prior to the advent of the common use of sonography and computed tomography (CT) scanning, patients with an ectopic kidney presented either with symptoms of pain or fever or the physical finding of a mass. Currently, patients are often diagnosed with an ectopic kidney coincidentally during imaging for other purposes. Nevertheless, the most common presentation remains the symptomatic one with the most common symptoms being abdominal pain, dysuria, fever or a urinary tract infection (UTI). Other presentations include a palpable abdominal mass, evaluation for multiple congenital anomalies, hematuria, incontinence, renal insufficiency or hypertension. The UTIs likely result from urinary obstruction (which may be due to the unrotated collecting system) or vesico-ureteral reflux. Instances of obstruction were found not only at the ureteropelvic junction (UPJ) but at the ureterovesical junction as well. The abdominal pain that is experienced may follow seemingly minor blunt trauma or it can present *de novo* in an acute fashion.[19, 20] Patients may present with a urinary calculus manifested by abdominal or flank pain, hematuria or infection.[9, 21–26]

The first study obtained in the evaluation of a pediatric renal anomaly is a sonogram. The absence of a kidney in its normal fossa raises the possibilities of either renal agenesis or renal ectopia. The examiner should look for a kidney in the predictably ectopic positions mentioned previously, namely pelvic, cross fused, lumbar or thoracic locations. On occasion, the colon that occupies the renal fossa in renal ectopia will be mistaken for a hydronephrotic or dysplastic kidney on sonographic examination. The presence of a flattened adrenal gland in its normal position is a helpful radiologic clue to renal ectopia.[27] This finding correlates with absent renal development in the flank and may be seen with either agenesis or ectopia. Another sonographic finding is the absence of the normal central renal sinus echo complex in the ectopic kidney. In one study this renal sinus echo was absent in two-thirds of the patients and eccentrically located in the other one-third.[28] The sonogram will also demonstrate hydronephrosis, renal stones and fusion if these conditions are present (Fig. 17.2).

An excretory urogram (IVP) may be quite helpful in renal ectopia as it identifies the location and relative function of the kidney while providing an accurate orientation of the collecting system and the course of the ureters. Care must be taken to carefully look for contrast in the collecting system as it may be missed when the ectopic kidney overlies the bones of the pelvis. The IVP is also helpful in assessing the presence of obstruction (Fig. 17.3).

On the scout film, the renal fossa which is vacated by the ectopic kidney will be occupied by the ipsilateral colon.[29–31] This association is so consistent that if an IVP shows nonvisualization of the kidney in the presence of a normally positioned ipsilateral colon, the diagnoses

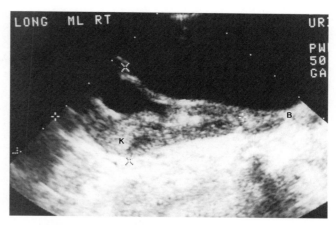

FIG. 17.2. Sonogram showing a pelvic ectopic kidney (*K*) just above the bladder (*B*). Note the moderate pelviectasis.

of ectopia or agenesis can be ruled out. Also, in light of the high incidence of vertebral anomalies, the spine images deserve special attention.

A voiding cystourethrogram (VCUG) or radionuclide cystogram (RNC) should be performed to rule out the possibility of vesicoureteral reflux (Fig. 17.4).

Useful adjuncts in evaluating ectopic kidneys are the nuclear medicine scans employing the agents diethylenetriamine pentaacetic acid (DTPA) or dimercaptosuccinic acid (DMSA). These agents will identify ectopic kidneys which may be missed on other radiologic evaluations due to their small size or their poor function.[11, 32–34] Once the position of the ectopic kidney is established by nuclear scan one can then redirect more focused and detailed imaging with modalities such as ultrasonography or contrast enhanced CT scans to further characterize the kidney. DTPA scan is also helpful in differentiating between the obstructed versus nonobstructed hydronephrotic ectopic kidney.

Management

The management of the ectopic kidney is dictated by the clinical complaints of the patient and whatever threats exist to renal function. One should bear in mind that the majority of patients with renal ectopia will remain asymptomatic throughout their lives. It is also incumbent upon the urologist to remember that other anomalous organ systems often need treatment and that the urologic care needs to be integrated into the patient's overall management. The most pressing anomalies, such as the cardiac and gastrointestinal, often need to be addressed prior to the urologic anomalies.

Armed with the knowledge of the above mentioned renal abnormalities, one can understand how to best direct the patient's evaluation and management. The main goals of treatment are preservation of renal function and minimization of morbidity. As mentioned

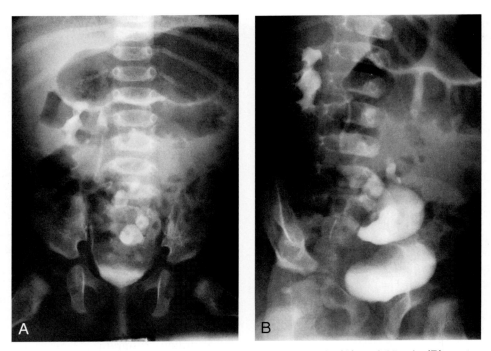

FIG. 17.3. IVP of a child with a left ectopic pelvic kidney at 5 min **(A)** and 25 min **(B)** post-contrast injection. Note the dilated renal pelvis in part B.

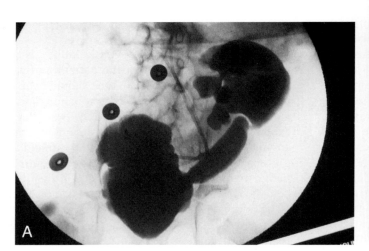

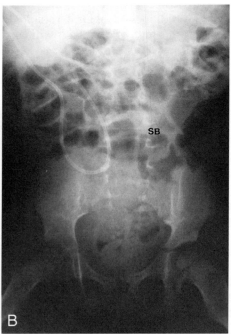

FIG. 17.4. A, VCUG of a child with a left ectopic kidney revealing marked reflux and a secondary ureteropelvic junction obstruction. **B,** Scout film of the same patient showing spina bifida, manifest by widened vertebral interpedicular distances (*SB*).

previously, many ectopic kidneys are associated with ureteral obstruction. Gleason et al. noted that 56% of the ectopic kidneys in their series were hydronephrotic with half due to obstruction.[2] Some of these renal units will have such poor function that nephrectomy is required.[3,15,25] In Gleason's series 14 patients underwent nephrectomy versus 8 patients who had repair of the obstruction. Relief of obstruction at the level of the UPJ can be performed either via standard open pyeloplasty, via endoscopic pyelotomy[35] or, in cases of crossed ectopia, via pyelouretrostomy to the other kidney's ureter. Angiography before surgery is advised to identify any anomalous blood supply in order to prevent vascular injury.

Several anatomical considerations make endoscopic procedures in ectopic kidneys unusually difficult. The crossed ectopic kidney has a long, winding ureter that can make ureteroscopy impractical. Secondly, the risk of vascular injury during percutaneous placement of nephrostomy tubes is increased because of the anomalous location of the renal vessels. Finally, the malrotated ectopic kidney will place a renal pelvis anteriorly making it difficult to access the renal pelvis retroperitoneally.[21]

Several reports in the literature describe urologic neoplasms in patients with ectopic kidneys.[36–38] These usually arise in the kidney but can arise in the ureter as well. It is difficult to know how often tumors occur in ectopic kidneys as these tumors may not be uniformly reported. The ectopic kidney is presumed to be susceptible to tumor formation due to hydronephrosis, infection and stones, which can cause epithelial metaplasia that can lead to neoplasia. The tumors reported in ectopic kidneys include renal adenocarcinoma (including renal mucinous adenocarcinoma), squamous cell carcinoma of the renal pelvis, transitional cell carcinoma and Wilms' tumor. The standard oncologic approaches for these tumors should be performed. Of note is the special situation of a tumor in the cross fused ectopic kidney. One should strive for a plane between the two kidneys that will allow for the least amount of blood loss while also allowing for a complete resection with negative margins and preservation of the remaining kidney. One approach to achieve these goals is the use of bench surgery followed by revascularization of the remnant kidney.[36]

RENAL DYSPLASIA

Embryology

Renal dysplasia is a histologic diagnosis of altered renal development characterized by immature and disordered nephrons. Dysplasia can result from more than one pathologic condition. Many nephrons may fail to form and the microscopic appearance is one of isolated nephrons in a sea of connective tissue. Segments of the

nephrons may be affected and be atrophic or cystic with collars of mesenchyme around the tubules (Fig. 17.5). The aberrant development can only be understood if one has an appreciation of normal renal ontogeny.

Normal kidney formation is dependent on the proper

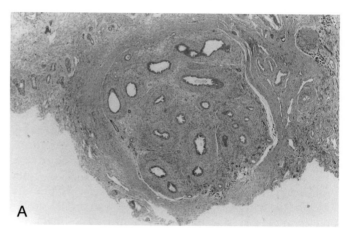

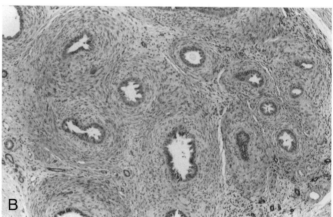

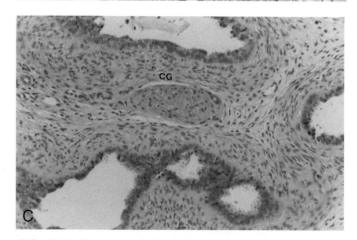

FIG. 17.5. Histologic studies of renal dysplasia as seen on low- **(A)**, medium- **(B)** and high-power **(C)** magnification. Note the typical findings of absent nephrons, increased extracellular matrix, and dilated tubules surrounded by mesenchymal collars. A focus of cartilage (*CG*) is seen on the high-power view.

interaction between the ureteric bud and metanephric blastema. These structures induce one another's development. The free efflux of urine produced by the developing kidney is also necessary for normal growth and development. It is now known that renal development is the end product of a great deal of time-specific gene transcription, translation, and growth factor action. Basement membranes and the extracellular matrix play important roles in renal development. Any alteration in these critical factors will alter the environment necessary for normal renal development.

The ureteric bud originates from the mesonephric duct and meets the undifferentiated metanephric blastema. If this meeting does not occur, the ureteric bud will not be stimulated to divide into the future collecting system and the blastema will not be stimulated to differentiate into the mature kidney. When the ureter meets the primitive renal blastema at a peripheral location, induction occurs, but the renal parenchyma is commonly dysplastic. This has been shown experimentally and it has been observed in the clinical setting. The final position of the ureteral orifice along the trigone or in the bladder neck or urethra is thought to represent the location of the ureteral bud along the mesonephric duct. The more abnormal the position of the ureteral orifice the greater the dysplastic changes are in the kidney.

While the interaction between the ureteral bud and the metanephric blastema is necessary for proper development, it is not sufficient. Extracellular matrix components such as collagen, fibronectin, and laminin are involved in the conversion of the metanephric mesenchyme into epithelium. The extracellular matrix is also involved in stimulating kidney tubule development.[40, 41] While this is an oversimplification of a very complex process, it does explain why inhibitors of extracellular matrix synthesis can cause altered ureteral bud branching.

Several growth factors have been investigated in regards to their role in renal development. These include epidermal growth factor (EGF), transforming growth factor alpha (TGF alpha) and insulin-like growth factors 1 and 2 (IGF-1 and IGF-2) which are expressed during renal development and appear to promote growth and differentiation of the kidney.[40] Nerve growth factor (NGF), hepatic growth factor (HGF), fibroblast growth factor (FGF) and proencephalin A may also play a part in organ formation.[40, 41]

The product of the Wilms' tumor gene (WT-1) works to regulate transcription and its expression is temporally found in the fetal kidney.[42] The WT-1 gene is thought to regulate differentiation of mesenchyme into epithelium as well as control the growth of the renal progenitor cells.

There is some evidence that abnormalities on chromosome 6 may be responsible for multicystic renal dysplasia.[43] Urinary tract obstruction may cause different renal parenchymal abnormalities based on the severity of the obstruction and how soon it occurs in gestation.[39] Presumably, this pathologic process is mediated via alteration of the transcription and translation of the above mentioned genes. Experimental data demonstrate that urinary tract obstruction during gestation may result in dysplasia or hydronephrosis depending on the timing and degree of obstruction.[44] Many feel that multicystic dysplastic kidneys result from total ureteral obstruction-typically at the uretero-pelvic junction. Dysplasia can be associated with obstruction at any level in the urinary tract, including posterior urethral valves,[39] ureteropelvic junction obstruction and the obstructed upper pole moiety due to either an ectopic ureter or a ureterocele.

In summary, the very precise and intricate process of renal development is dependent on a variety of cell-to-cell interactions, interactions with extracellular matrix, growth factors and transcription factors and, likely, additional unknown mediators. Alterations in this special milieu can lead to abnormal renal development and renal dysplasia.

Diagnosis

The diagnosis of renal dysplasia may occur after a radiologic investigation for a UTI, abdominal pain, or an abdominal mass.[45] Imaging of the kidneys is indicated in certain conditions which are known to be associated with renal anomalies (e.g., spina bifida, renal-pancreatic-hepatic dysplasia).[18, 45–49] In evaluating certain obstructive uropathies, such as posterior urethral valves or ectopic ureters, the renal unit may be shown to be dysplastic. Increasingly renal dysplasia is brought to our attention via prenatal sonography.[50–55]

The study that most often alerts us to a possible dysplastic kidney is the sonogram (Fig. 17.6). In the series of Sanders et al., 38 patients with histologically proven

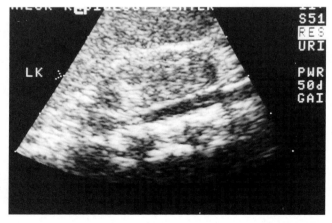

FIG. 17.6. Sonogram of a 1-yr-old showing a left solid dysplastic kidney that measures only 28 mm. The renal parenchyma has increased echogenicity.

dysplasia in 47 kidneys had their sonograms reviewed.[56] Forty of the 47 kidneys had an obstructive etiology for the dysplasia. The obstructions were at the level of the ureteropelvic junction, ureterovesical junction and urethra. When the obstruction was more proximal, the kidneys tended to be larger and associated with larger cysts. Smaller cysts and the absence of cysts were more often seen with distal obstruction. Echogenicity was compared to the renal sinus. Half of the patients had renal parenchyma that was as echogenic as the renal sinus and the other half had parenchyma that was more echogenic than the renal sinus. Only one kidney had normal echogenicity. The echogenicity did not correlate with the level of obstruction. Twelve patients had no parenchyma demonstrable.

Use of the sonogram should help to differentiate a multicystic dysplastic kidney (MCDK) from a UPJ obstruction. In a UPJ obstruction the largest fluid area is medial and this represents the renal pelvis. The smaller radially positioned hypoechoic areas are the dilated calyces. When rotating the transducer to achieve different imaging planes these dilated calyces are seen to communicate with each other via their infundibular connections to the pelvis. The kidney maintains its reniform shape and even in the most severe cases of obstruction, a rim of parenchyma may be seen. In contrast, a multicystic dysplastic kidney has noncommunicating cysts of random size and the largest one is not necessarily medial (Fig. 17.7). There are interfaces between the cysts which do not communicate. The reniform shape is lost and there is usually no discernible renal parenchyma. Whatever solid tissue is seen is usually of increased echogenicity. Renal function of a multicystic dysplastic kidney as measured by DMSA scan is negligible to absent (Fig. 17.8).

In light of the primitive nature of the nephrons in a dysplastic kidney it is not surprising to note that these kidneys have little to no function on studies such as a

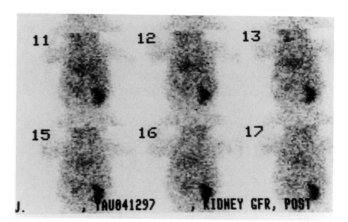

FIG. 17.8. A posterior view DMSA scan of the dysplastic left kidney seen in Figure 17.6 showing no function in the left kidney.

renal scan[56] utilizing either ^{99m}Tc dimercaptosuccinic acid or ^{99m}Tc mercapto-acetyl-tryglicine (MAG-3) or an intravenous pyelogram.[45] The kidneys, however, may have limited function due to some residual normal glomeruli and tubules but this function is severely compromised and is present in fewer than 15% of cases. This function rarely represents more than 5% of total renal function when present.[53] Another modality that may be of use in localizing the dysplastic kidney is magnetic resonance (MR) imaging.[57]

Management

All children with a dysplastic kidney should have a VCUG, as the incidence of reflux in the contralateral kidney is high.[58, 59] Serum chemistries including a blood urea nitrogen (BUN) and creatinine are necessary. A nuclear scan (i.e., DMSA) should be obtained to confirm absence of function in the kidney in question. A functional study such as a DTPA scan or MAG 3 lasix renogram or an IVP is indicated if there is a suspicion of obstruction in the contralateral kidney.

The ultimate question regarding the dysplastic kidney is whether it needs to be removed or not. Clearly if the dysplastic kidney is large enough to cause respiratory or gastrointestinal embarrassment it should be removed expeditiously. This is seen occasionally in the multicystic variety of dysplasia.

In the past, most MCDKs were recognized at birth as a palpable abdominal mass. Imaging studies then could not distinguish between cystic or solid masses efficiently and early surgical removal was recommended. Presently, most MCDKs are found on fetal ultrasound, are small, and are not palpable at birth. This has generated a debate as to what is the proper management of these asymptomatic dysplastic kidneys, but recently there has been a trend towards non-opera-

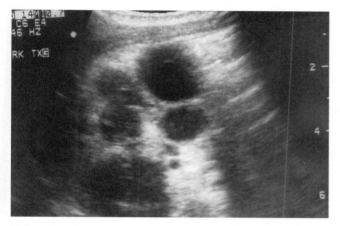

FIG. 17.7. Sonogram of a MCDK showing cysts of varying sizes and minimal highly echogenic parenchyma.

tive treatment since problems attributable to the MCDKs seem to be exceedingly unlikely.

The largest clinical experience with MCDKs is the Multicystic Dysplastic Kidney Registry of the American Academy of Pediatrics Section on Urology.[59] Their 441 patients were registered from nearly 50 hospitals in North America. Nephrectomies were performed in 181 patients and 260 patients were managed conservatively. The natural history of these MCDKs with regards to involution was based solely on sonographic findings. Of the MCDKs followed for 1 to 3 years, 47% decreased in size, 37% remained the same size and 13% disappeared. At 3 to 5 years 23% had disappeared. A greater rate of resolution (albeit in a smaller group of patients) was seen by Orejas et al.; in their series, 75% of the MCDKs involuted.[60] The mean time to involution was 16 months.

In the MCDK registry, no patients required nephrectomy due to infection. The registry has reported no cases of hypertension attributable to the MCDK. There were only 6 cases of tumor formation; 3 were in adults and 3 were in the pediatric age group (ages 10 months, 4 years and 15 years). Based on the low incidence of infections, hypertension and tumors the registry suggests that it is reasonable to manage these patients non-operatively and obtain sonograms every 3 to 6 months in the first year of life, every 6 to 12 months in the next four years and possibly yearly thereafter. Others[51, 60–63] recommend that nephrectomy not be performed in the asymptomatic child with a MCDK.

Further evidence to downplay the neoplastic potential in dysplastic kidneys is Horan's study that analyzed 16 affected individuals.[64] Only 1 kidney had nodular renal blastema and all 16 had a normal diploid DNA pattern.

Nevertheless, there are still proponents for removing the asymptomatic MCDK. Part of their justification is the suspicion that the incidence of hypertension in dysplasia is understated. This may be due to under reporting to the registry and in the literature at large.[65–68] This is based on their own anecdotal evidence of seemingly large numbers of hypertensive patients (each reported 2 to 3 cases of hypertension). Emmert and King state that accurately recorded blood pressures in the small, uncooperative, agitated child is difficult.[65] In addition, parents are often not compliant with follow-up. They postulate that when patients with MCDK do develop hypertension, nephrectomy may not cure the hypertension[62] because the hypertension may have caused chronic contralateral renal arteriolar thickening. Due to the possible underreporting of complications to the registry and the difficulty of obtaining long term follow-up in these patients as well as the possibly irreversible nature of some of these conditions (such as hypertension and tumor formation), there remain advocates for the removal of the asymptomatic kidney.

Long term follow-up data on patients followed pro-spectively are necessary for physicians to make more objective decisions. At the present time, a frank discussion with the families should include the currently available information as well as the gaps in our knowledge. This will allow for consideration of each family's concerns and informed, prudent decision making.

Renal Hypoplasia

Less common than the dysplastic kidney is the small, but otherwise histologically unremarkable renal unit. In some cases, the individualized tubules seem unusually large, so called "oligomeganephronic." Small kidneys without obvious dysplasia are sometimes seen in association with vesicoureteral reflux, especially the more severe variety of reflux that can be recognized prenatally in the male fetus.

No specific therapy is indicated for this condition, but if hypoplasia is present bilaterally, renal insufficiency can result with renal transplantation ultimately being required.

REFERENCES

1. Maizels M, Stephens FD. The induction of urologic malformations. Understanding the relationship of renal ectopia and congenital scoliosis. Invest Urol 1979;17:209–217.
2. Gleason PE, Kelalis PP, Husmann DA, Kramer SA. Hydronephrosis in renal ectopia: incidence, etiology and significance. J Urol 1994;151:1660–1661.
3. Malek RS, Kelalis PP, Burke EC. Ectopic kidney in children and frequency of association with other malformations. Mayo Clin Proc 1971;46:461–467.
4. Friedland GW, de Vries P. Renal ectopia and fusion. Embryologic Basis. Urology 1975;5:698–706.
5. Romans DG, Jewett MA, Robson CJ. Crossed renal ectopia with colic. A clinical clue to embryogenesis. Br J Urol 1976;48:171–174.
6. Daskalakis E, Bouhoutsos J. Crossed renal ectopia without fusion: case report with angiographic study. Br J Surg 1980;67:142.
7. Rubinstein ZJ, Hertz M, Shahin N, Deutsch V. Crossed renal ectopia: angiographic findings in six cases. Am J Roentgenol 1976;126:1035–1038.
8. Ohtsuka A, Kikuta A, Taguchi T, Murakami T. Ectopic kidney in front of the right common iliac artery and its blood vascular supply—a case report. Okajimas Folia Anat Jpn 1993;70:29–34.
9. Sheih CP, Hung CS, Liao YJ, Chen CH, Li YW. Crossed, unfused ectopic kidney with a single ectopic ureter: report of a case. J Formos Med Assoc 1995;94:754–756.
10. Chida N, Orikasa S, Konda R, Takahashi M, Ishidoya S, Ogata Y. Crossed ureteral ectopia with an ectopic blind-ending ureter. Urol Int 1995;55:169–172.
11. Gharagozloo AM, Lebowitz RL. Detection of a poorly functioning malpositioned kidney with single ectopic ureter in girls with urinary dribbling: imaging evaluation in five patients. AJR Am J Roentgenol 1995;164:957–961.
12. Mishra VK, Kapoor R. Crossed fused renal ectopia with crossed single ectopic ureterocele: an unusual presentation. Arch Esp Urol 1995;48:321–323.
13. Farkas A, Earon J, Firstater M. Crossed renal ectopia with crossed single ectopic ureterocele. J Urol 1978;119:836–838.
14. Rivard DJ, Milner WA, Garlick WB. Solitary crossed renal ectopia and its associated congenital anomalies. J Urol 1978;120:241–242.
15. Hendren WH, Donahoe PK, Pfister RC. Crossed renal ectopia in children. Urology 1976;7:135–144.

16. Marshall FF, Freedman MT. Crossed renal ectopia. J Urol 1978;119:188–191.
17. Golomb J, Ehrlich RM. Bilateral ureteral triplication with crossed ectopic fused kidneys associated with the VACTERL syndrome. J Urol 1989;141:1398–1399.
18. Gotoh T, Shinno Y, Koyanagi T. Crossed renal ectopia and asymmetric fused kidney, with special reference to associated vertebral anomalies. Int Urol Nephrol 1987;19:33–40.
19. Fowlis GA, Mee AD, Colbeck R, Twomey B. Acute abdomen—an unusual presentation of crossed renal ectopia. Br J Urol 1994;73:328–329.
20. Connor JM, Brautigan MW. The ectopic kidney in the emergency department. Ann Emerg Med 1987;16:715–717.
21. Chang TD, Dretler SP. Laparoscopic pyelolithotomy in an ectopic kidney. J Urol 1996;156:1753.
22. Culkin DJ, Wheeler JS Jr, Karasis M, Nam SI, Canning JR. Treatment of renal calculus in inferior crossed renal ectopia. Urology 1988;32:424–426.
23. Eichwald M, Wolfe LE. Nephrolithiasis connected with hydronephrosis of a crossed renal ectopia. JAMA 1970;211:117–118.
24. Stubbs AJ, Resnick MI. Struvite staghorn calculi in crossed fused ectopia. J Urol 1977;118:369–371.
25. Dalton DP, Zaontz MR. Giant hydronephrosis in ectopic kidney in a child. Urology 1988;32:323–326.
26. Del Boca C, Colloi D, Ferrari C, Giuberti AC, Guardamagna A, Beretta M. [Transperitoneal nephrectomy of crossed ectopic kidney without fusion associated with stenosis of the pyeloureteral junction and pyelocaliceal staghorn calculi] Nefrectomia transperitoneale di rene ectopico crociato senza fusione con stenosi del giunto pieloureterale e calcolosi a stampo completa secondaria. Minerva Urol Nefrol 1994;46:183–186.
27. Hoffman CK, Filly RA, Callen PW. The "lying down" adrenal sign: a sonographic indicator of renal agenesis or ectopia in fetuses and neonates. J Ultrasound Med 1992;11:533–536.
28. Barnewolt CE, Lebowitz RL. Absence of a renal sinus echo complex in the ectopic kidney of a child: a normal finding. Pediatr Radiol 1996;26:318–323.
29. Curtis JA, Sadhu V, Steiner RM. Malposition of the colon in right renal agenesis, ectopia, and anterior nephrectomy. AJR Am J Roentgenol 1977;129:845–850.
30. Mascatello V, Lebowitz RL. Malposition of the colon in left renal agenesis and ectopia. Radiology 1976;120:371–376.
31. Meyers MA, Whalen JP, Evans JA, Viamonte M. Malposition and displacement of the bowel in renal agenesis and ectopia: new observations. Am J Roentgenol Radium Ther Nucl Med 1973;117:323–333.
32. Applegate K, Connolly L, Treves ST. Tc-99m DMSA imaging of crossed fused ectopia. Clin Nucl Med 1995;20:947–948.
33. Serena A, Duque JJ, Cotero A, Llorens V, Fombellida JC. Radionuclide visualization of a thoracic renal ectopia. Clin Nucl Med 1994;19:1021–1022.
34. Wholey MH, Sostre S, Wong O. Crossed fused ectopic kidneys diagnosed by renal DTPA study. Clin Nucl Med 1994;19:554–556.
35. Bales GT, Jarrard DF, Gerber GS. Ureteroscopic endopyelotomy in an ectopic kidney. Urology 1995;46:104–106.
36. Gerber WL, Culp DA, Brown RC, Chow KC, Platz CE. Renal mass in crossed-fused ectopia. J Urol 1980;123:239–244.
37. Mavromanolakis E, Samonis G, Cranidis A. Mucinous adenocarcinoma arising in the renal pelvis of an ectopic pyelic kidney. Oncology 1995;52:331–333.
38. Urnes T, Muri O Jr. Crossed, non-fused renal ectopia and ipsilateral ureteral carcinoma. A case report. Scand J Urol Nephrol 1979;13:213–215.
39. Gonzalez R, Reinberg Y, Burke B, Wells T, Vernier RL. Early bladder outlet obstruction in fetal lambs induces renal dysplasia and the prune-belly syndrome. J Pediatr Surg 1990;25:342–345.
40. Ekblom P. Rena Development. In: Seldin DW, Giebisch G, eds. The Kidney: Physiology and Pathophysiology, Second Edition. New York: Raven Press, Ltd., 1992:475–501.
41. Burrow CR, Wilson PD. Renal progenitor cells: problems of definition, isolation and characterization [editorial]. Exp Nephrol 1994;2:1–12.
42. Pritchard Jones K, Fleming S, Davidson D, Bickmore W, Porteous D, Gosden C, et al. The candidate Wilms' tumour gene is involved in genitourinary development. Nature 1990;346:194–197.
43. Devriendt K, Fryns JP. Genetic locus on chromosome 6p for multicystic renal dysplasia, pelvi-ureteral junction stenosis, and vesicoureteral reflux [letter; comment]. Am J Med Genet 1995;59:396–398.
44. Peters CA, Carr MC, Lais A, Retik AB, Mandell J. The response of the fetal kidney to obstruction. J Urol 1992;148:503–509.
45. Quinn CM, Kelly DG, Cahalane SF. Renal dysplasia—a clinicopathological review. Br J Urol 1988;61:399–401.
46. Blowey DL, Warady BA, Zwick DL, Ong C. Renal-pancreatic-hepatic dysplasia in siblings. Pediatr Nephrol 1995;9:36–38.
47. Daggilas A, Antoniades K, Palasis S, Aidonis A. Branchio-oto-renal dysplasia associated with tetralogy of Fallot. Head Neck 1992;14:139–142.
48. Hunter AG, Jimenez C, Tawagi FG. Familial renal-hepatic-pancreatic dysplasia and Dandy-Walker cyst: a distinct syndrome? Am J Med Genet 1991;41:201–207.
49. Lurie IW, Kirillova IA, Novikova IV, Burakovski IV. Renal-hepatic-pancreatic dysplasia and its variants. Genet Couns 1991;2:17–20.
50. Gough DC, Postlethwaite RJ, Lewis MA, Bruce J. Multicystic renal dysplasia diagnosed in the antenatal period: a note of caution. Br J Urol 1995;76:244–248.
51. Mesrobian HG, Rushton HG, Bulas D. Unilateral renal agenesis may result from in utero regression of multicystic renal dysplasia. J Urol 1993;150:793–794.
52. Rickwood AM, Anderson PA, Williams MP. Multicystic renal dysplasia detected by prenatal ultrasonography. Natural history and results of conservative management. Br J Urol 1992;69:538–540.
53. Roach PJ, Paltiel HJ, Perez Atayde A, Tello RJ, Davis RT, Treves ST. Renal dysplasia in infants: appearance on 99mTc DMSA scintigraphy. Pediatr Radiol 1995;25:472–475.
54. Robson WL, Leung AK, Thomason MA. Multicystic dysplasia of the kidney. Clin Pediatr Phila 1995;34:32–40.
55. Mandell J, Paltiel HJ, Peters CA, Benacerraf BR. Prenatal findings associated with a unilateral nonfunctioning or absent kidney. J Urol 1994;152:176–178.
56. Sanders RC, Nussbaum AR, Solez K. Renal dysplasia: sonographic findings. Radiology 1988;167:623–626.
57. Li YW, Sheih CP, Chen WJ. MR imaging and sonography of Gartner's duct cyst and single ectopic ureter with ipsilateral renal dysplasia. Pediatr Radiol 1992;22:472–473.
58. Flack CE, Bellinger MF. The multicystic dysplastic kidney and contralateral vesicoureteral reflux: protection of the solitary kidney. J Urol 1993;150:1873–1874.
59. Wacksman J, Phipps L. Report of the Multicystic Kidney Registry: preliminary findings. J Urol 1993;150:1870–1872.
60. Orejas G, Malaga S, Santos F, Rey C, Lopez MV, Merten A. Multicystic dysplastic kidney: absence of complications in patients treated conservatively. Child Nephrol Urol 1992;12:35–39.
61. al Khaldi N, Watson AR, Zuccollo J, Twining P, Rose DH. Outcome of antenatally detected cystic dysplastic kidney disease. Arch Dis Child 1994;70:520–522.
62. Gordon AC, Thomas DF, Arthur RJ, Irving HC. Multicystic dysplastic kidney: is nephrectomy still appropriate? J Urol 1988;140:1231–1234.
63. Menster M, Mahan J, Koff S. Multicystic dysplastic kidney. Pediatr Nephrol 1994;8:113–115.
64. Horan JJ, Lobos MJ, Azumi N, Blair OC, Gibbons MD. Analysis of solid renal dysplasia by flow cytometry: malignant potential? Urology 1993;41:598–601.
65. Emmert GK Jr, King LR. The risk of hypertension is underestimated in the multicystic dysplastic kidney: a personal perspective [see comments]. Urology 1994;44:404–405.
66. Hanna MK. The multicystic dysplastic kidney [letter; comment]. Urology 1995;45:171.
67. Webb NJ, Lewis MA, Bruce J, Gough DC, Ladusans EJ, Thomson AP, et al. Unilateral multicystic dysplastic kidney: the case for nephrectomy. Arch Dis Child 1997;76:31–34.
68. Worck RH, Ibsen H, Andersen CB, Ibsen KK, Rasmussen F. The etiology of hypertension in nonrenovascular unilateral renal disease—two cases of renin induced hypertension in congenital renal dysplasia. Blood Press 1995;4:113–116.

CHAPTER 18

Ureteral Ectopy, Ureteroceles, and Other Anomalies of the Distal Ureter

Douglas A. Husmann

To comprehend the clinical presentations and pathologic findings of distal ureteral abnormalities, it is imperative to understand the embryologic development of this region. This chapter provides a brief review of the embryology of the distal ureter.

EMBRYOLOGIC DEVELOPMENT OF THE TERMINAL URETER

Normal Embryogenesis of the Ureter

At 28 days of gestation the ureteral bud (the anlage of the ureter) arises from the distal mesonephric duct (Fig. 18.1).[1] Following the development of the ureteral bud, the portion of the mesonephric duct distal to its origin is known as the common excretory duct.[1] This latter structure joins the anterior cloaca at the location that will become the bladder neck and separates the anterior cloaca into two segments, the primitive bladder and the urogenital sinus. As the embryo develops the common excretory duct is absorbed into the developing bladder. Because the ureteral bud is in a more distal and medial position than the proximal mesonephric duct, the ureteral bud is the first of these two structures to be absorbed (Fig. 18.1). At the time that the ureteral bud is incorporated into the anterior cloaca a differential (accelerated) growth pattern exists between the primitive bladder and the urogenital sinus. This preferential growth causes the bladder, and subsequently the ureter, to migrate cephalad and laterally, while the mesonephric duct slips to a more caudal and medial position. The opening of the mesonephric duct is eventually absorbed into the posterior urethra. The common excretory duct ultimately develops into the bladder trigone, bladder neck, and proximal posterior urethra. The ureteral bud forms the ureter, renal pelvis, the renal calyceal systems, and the collecting tubules of the kidney. In the male the mesonephric ducts become the ejaculatory ductal

system of the testis. In the female the mesonephric ductal system largely disappears.

The development of the kidney is the result of the interaction between the most cephalad portion of the ureteral bud and the metanephric blastema (a coherent mesodermal cellular mass present in the lower lumbar and upper sacral regions). The interplay between these two structures is critical for the normal development of the kidney.[2]

COMPLETE URETERAL DUPLICATION

Embryologic Development

Complete ureteral duplication occurs when two separate ureteral buds develop from the mesonephric duct.[1] The ureteral bud that is the closest to the anterior cloaca connects to the lower pole of the kidney and is the first absorbed into the developing bladder (Fig. 18.2A). The lower pole ureter moves with the bladder to a more cephalad and lateral position. In contrast, the upper pole ureteral bud stays with the common excretory duct for a longer time interval; this results in its migration to a more medial and caudal position. After bladder development is complete, the lower pole ureter will enter the bladder in a more cranial and lateral position, whereas the upper pole ureter will be more caudal and medial (Fig. 18.2B & C). The ureteral relationship in a completely duplicated system was originally described by Weigert and later modified by Meyer. It is almost invariably present and has been termed the Weigert-Meyer law.[1,3-6]

Incidence and Genetic Transmission

Autopsy findings suggest that complete ureteral duplication occurs in 1 of 500 (0.2%) people.[1,3-6] The right and left collecting systems are affected equally. Whether

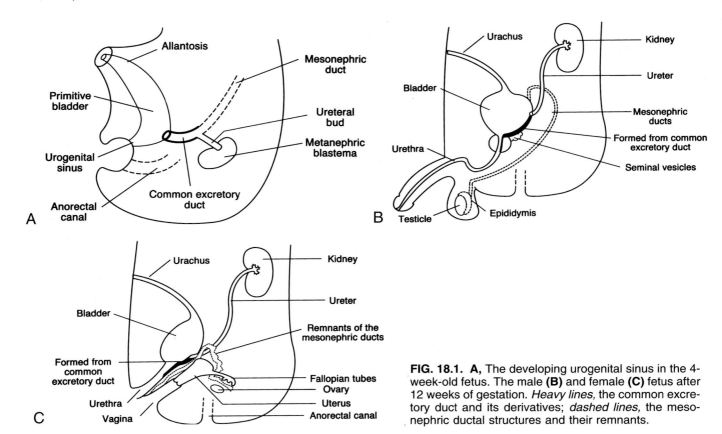

FIG. 18.1. A, The developing urogenital sinus in the 4-week-old fetus. The male **(B)** and female **(C)** fetus after 12 weeks of gestation. *Heavy lines,* the common excretory duct and its derivatives; *dashed lines,* the mesonephric ductal structures and their remnants.

the congenital abnormality is more common in females is open to debate. Clinical studies have suggested that the abnormality is approximately two times more common in females than males.[5] Autopsy findings, however, have been unable to confirm any sexual differences.[4] The discrepancy between the clinical and autopsy data appears to be related to the radiologic workup of symptomatic patients. For example, radiologic evaluations of patients with a history of a urinary tract infection (UTI) reveal that 5% will be found to have a complete ureteral duplication anomaly. Because females are more likely to develop urinary tract infections than males are, duplication anomalies are more likely to be detected in the female population.[4, 5, 7]

When complete ureteral duplication is discovered, the physician should be aware of two associated and pertinent facts. First, if complete ureteral duplication exists on one side there is up to a 40% chance that a complete duplication abnormality will be present on the other side.[8] Significant attention must therefore be given to the contralateral kidney and ureter to rule out the presence of a ureteral anomaly (i.e., ureteral ectopy or ureterocele). Second, ureteral duplication is an inheritable defect transmitted in an autosomally dominant fashion with incomplete penetrance. The risk that a sibling could also be affected by a complete duplication abnormality is approximately 10%.[9–12] Although we do

not recommend familial screening, we think that the physician should ask if the affected child has any siblings. If siblings exist, we inquire whether they have a history of UTIs or urinary incontinence. If the answer to either of these questions is affirmative, we think that screening radiographic studies should be performed.

URETERAL ECTOPY (SINGLE AND DUPLICATED SYSTEMS)

Aberrant Embryologic Development

A ureter is said to be ectopic if its orifice opens distal to the bladder neck, whether it is associated with a single or duplicated system. An ectopic ureteral opening occurs when a ureteral bud arises too high (cephalad) on the mesonephric duct. Because of the delayed incorporation of the ureteral bud into the bladder, the ureteral orifice comes to lie in a more caudal and medial position. The opening of the ureter can be anywhere of the normal position of the mesonephric duct. In the male this "ectopic pathway" extends from the trigone of the bladder to the ejaculatory ducts (Fig. 18.3A).[1, 13, 14] In the female (Fig. 18.3B) the mesonephric ducts involute to form three residual structures, the duct of the epoophron (adjacent to the fallopian tubes), the duct of the paroophoron (adjacent to the body of the uterus), and Gartner's duct (the most distal extent of the mesonephric duct). If the ureter opens ectopically into vestigial remnants of the female mesonephric ductal system, distention of the ductal walls ensue. The distended mesonephric duct will eventually rupture into the adjacent Müllerian ductal system. This results in a communication of the ectopic ureter with the fallopian tubes, uterus, or vagina (Fig. 18.3B).[1, 13–15]

Associated Congenital Abnormalities of Single System Ectopic Ureters

Single system ectopic ureters are frequently found in association with the VACTERL syndrome (vertebral

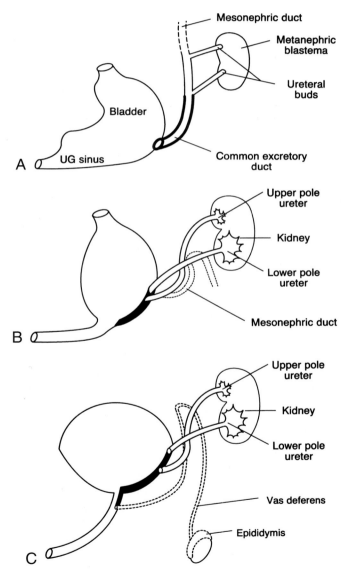

FIG. 18.2. The developing urogenital sinus in a male fetus with a duplication at 4 **(A)**, 7 **(B)**, and 12 **(C)** weeks of gestation. *UG,* urogenital. *Heavy lines,* the common excretory duct and its derivatives; *dashed lines,* the mesonephric ductal structures and their remnants.

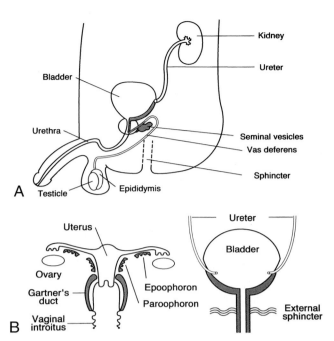

FIG. 18.3. The ectopic pathway (*shaded areas*) in males **(A)** and females **(B)**.

anomalies, anal atresia, cardiac defects, tracheoesophageal fistulas, renal and limb abnormalities). The historical presence of any of the congenital deformities mentioned should raise the physician's index of suspicion for the presence of this anomaly.[16, 17]

Incidence of Single and Duplex System Ectopy

Ectopic ureters are a rare abnormality occurring once in every 4,000 autopsies (0.025% of the population). In general, 80% of ectopic ureters arise from the upper pole of a completely duplicated system, whereas 20% of the ectopic ureters arise from a single system.[5] Ectopic ureters are predominantly diagnosed in the female population, with females having a fourfold to sixfold higher incidence of ureteral ectopia than males. A significant difference between single and duplex system ectopy exists between the sexes. Specifically, in males ureteral ectopy is found in single collecting systems 75% of the time. In contrast, in females, ureteral ectopy is found in completely duplicated systems 85% of the cases.[18–20]

Clinical Presentation (Female)

Over the last decade, half of our female patients diagnosed with an ectopic ureter came to our attention because of a history of fetal hydronephrosis. The remaining 50% had a variety of clinical complaints: constant urinary incontinence (i.e., "the child voids periodically but is still wet all the time"), a palpable abdominal mass, recurrent UTIs, or recurrent vaginitis or vaginal discharge.

Location of Ectopic Ureters (Females)

The most common openings for ectopic ureters in females are the bladder neck or urethra (35%), the vaginal introitus (30%), proximal vagina (25%), the fundus, body or cervix of the uterus (5%), persistent Gartner's duct (4%), or into a urethral diverticulum (1%) (Fig. 18.3B).[22–24, 26] Note: The physician should be acutely aware that all urethral diverticuli found in a prepubertal female should be considered to be associated with an ectopic ureter until proven otherwise.[24]

Clinical Presentation (Males)

Similar to females, fetal ultrasonography has had a significant impact on how and when males with an ectopic ureter present. Males with ureteral ectopy present during the neonatal, prepubertal, or postpubertal time spans. At this time, a third of the males diagnosed with ureteral ectopy come to our attention because of an abnormal finding on fetal ultrasonography. A third present during the prepubertal time span with complaints of recurrent UTIs, intermittent flank pain, gross hematuria, a palpable abdominal mass, or bladder outlet obstruction. The other third present in the postpubertal time period with complaints of UTI, flank or perineal pain, chronic prostatitis, persistent dysuria, pain with ejaculation, or infertility.

Classical teaching regarding an ectopic ureter states that urinary incontinence secondary to ureteral ectopy is never seen in males. This age old dictum is based on the fact that the ectopic ureter enters above the external sphincter in the male (Fig. 18.3A & Fig. 18.4).[20] Exceptions to every rule exist, and rare case reports of urinary incontinence in males secondary to ectopic ureters have been published.[25, 26] Incontinence within these latter patients is caused by the accumulation of the urine within the posterior urethra. Intermittent urinary leakage develops whenever the external sphincter relaxes (Fig. 18.4).

Another classical teaching point regarding ureteral ectopy and the prepubertal male population needs to be addressed. In particular, it has been recommended that prepubertal males with epididymitis undergo complete radiologic evaluation with a voiding cystourethrogram and a renal ultrasound to rule out ureteral ectopy.[5, 18, 27] In the past we vigorously pursued this approach in dozens of patients with little to no significant pathologic findings being discovered. We concur with Siegal and associates that the best way to screen the prepubertal patient with epididymitis is to obtain a urine culture at the time of the symptomatic presentation. If a negative urine culture result is obtained the likelihood

that a significant genitourinary abnormality exists is very small. If, however, a positive urine culture result is obtained, a significant abnormality is present 60% of the time.[28] In essence, a negative urine culture result virtually rules out the presence of a ureteral-Wolffian ductal abnormality and will save the patient and his family the pain and expense of a more complete diagnostic evaluation.

Location of Ectopic Ureters (Males)

The most common locations for ectopic ureter in males are the bladder neck, posterior or prostatic urethra (48%), the seminal vesicles (40%), common ejaculatory duct or prostatic utricle (8%), vas deferens (3%), epididymis (0.5%), and rectum or anal verge (0.5%) (Fig. 18.3A).[18, 21]

Radiologic Findings

Most of our patients with an ectopic ureter have an antenatal ultrasound diagnosis of a renal duplication anomaly, fetal hydronephrosis, or renal agenesis. In these cases confirmation of a congenital renal abnormality is made by obtaining a voiding cystourethrogram and an abdominal ultrasound shortly after birth.

The sonographic diagnosis of a duplex ectopic ureteral system is suggested when upper pole hydronephrosis with ureteral dilation and tortuosity are present. The lower pole system is usually normal. On occasion, however, the lower pole may be dilated because of coexisting lower pole reflux or obstruction. During the sonographic evaluation the sonographer must take care to provide adequate views of the bladder to rule out the presence of a ureterocele as the etiology of the upper urinary tract distortion.

Renal function of the upper pole system can be ascertained by nuclear renography or excretory urography (EXU). Although nuclear scans are frequently useful in these patients, they cannot always separate the upper pole from the lower pole of moiety. Because of this limitation to clearly define the anatomy with renal scans, excretory urography is of sporadic benefit. The classic findings of complete ureteral duplication on EXU are: (a) the inferior and lateral displacement of the functioning lower pole system by the nonfunctional dilated upper pole moiety, the so-called "drooping lily sign," (b) the functional lower pole system has fewer visualized calyces than the normal kidney, and (c) if the upper pole system is functional it will usually consist of two calyceal structures directed 180° opposite of each other, the so-called "hammer head" configuration (Fig. 18.5).

Although we do not routinely use computerized tomography (CT) or magnetic resonance imaging (MRI) to diagnose renal and ureteral ectopy, there are times when these studies are also useful. In particular, we

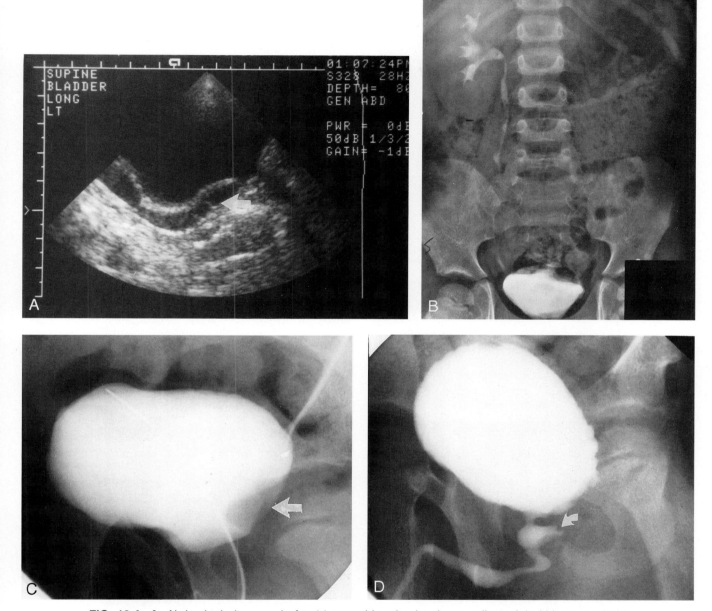

FIG. 18.4. A, Abdominal ultrasound of a 14-year-old male showing a solitary right kidney; a tubular structure is visualized behind the left aspect of the bladder (*arrow*). **B,** Excretory urography confirming a solitary right kidney with compensatory hypertrophy. Voiding cystourethrography revealed a filling defect in the posterior bladder wall (**C,** *arrow*), coexisting with a posterior urethral abnormality (**D,** *arrow*).

have seen several infants with an antenatal diagnosis of unilateral renal agenesis who have had an ectopic kidney with a single system ectopic ureter (Fig. 18.4). If the clinical suspicion of renal ectopy is high and ultrasonography or nuclear renography does not confirm the diagnosis, an MRI or CT study may be of benefit.[29]

When an ectopic ureter is thought to be present, a voiding cystourethrogram is an imperative part of the radiographic evaluation for two reasons. First, in renal duplication associated with upper pole ectopia, approximately 50% of the lower pole ureters will have coexisting vesicoureteral reflux.[20, 30] Second, the presence of reflux into an ectopic ureter alters the surgical approach (see Management of Duplex Systems).

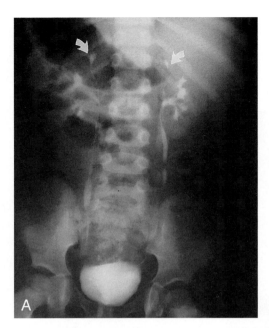

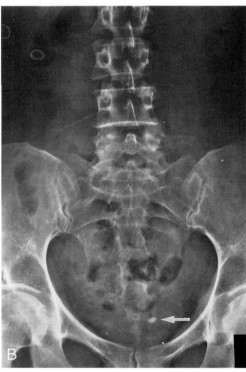

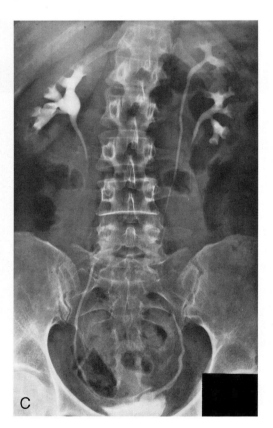

FIG. 18.5. A, Excretory urography of a 12-year-old female showing bilateral duplication anomalies (*arrows*), upper pole hammer head deformities, and lower pole drooping lilies. **B,** Plain film of a 34-year-old female showing a possible radioopaque calculus in the left distal ureter (*arrow*). **C,** Excretory urography showing a complete left duplication with a distal ureteral calculus in an upper pole intravesical ureterocele. Note the obvious hammer head deformity of the functioning upper pole ureter and the lateral and downward displacement of the lower pole system.

Physical Examination and Cystoscopic Findings

A careful physical examination may indicate the ectopic ureteral opening to be located in the anterior lateral portion of the vaginal introitus or parameatal area. If an ectopic opening is not found at the introitus, a cystoscopy is performed. The urethra and bladder neck region are carefully inspected and any suspicious areas probed with a small ureteral (3–4 French) catheter.

If the ectopic opening is found, retrograde injection of a contrast medium is performed to confirm the presence of an ectopic ureter. If the cystoscopic examination does not locate the ectopic opening, vaginoscopy is undertaken. In our experience attempts to locate the ectopic ureter in the proximal vagina are usually unsuccessful. An undue amount of operative time for the vaginoscopic examination should therefore not be expended, especially if prior radiographic evaluations have confirmed the presence of the ectopic ureter.

Pathology (Renal Ectopy)

The classic method of treating an ectopic ureter associated with a renal duplication is by upper pole partial nephrectomy plus or minus distal ureterectomy.[20, 31, 32] The routine use of partial nephrectomy for treatment has been criticized because it does not assess whether the upper pole renal moiety is functioning. This criticism is predominantly based on a pathologic study that revealed normal renal histology in 57% of the upper pole renal moieties that were removed.[33] The finding that more than half of the upper pole systems associated with an ectopic ureter are histologically normal suggests that early surgical repair of the ectopic ureteral system could correct the congenital defect and possibly preserve renal function.[34, 35]

In contrast to the duplex collecting system with upper pole ureteral ectopy, only 10% of the kidneys with a single system ectopic ureter are histologically normal. Pathologic evaluation of kidneys with single system ectopy reveal widespread areas of renal dysplasia in 90% of the affected kidneys.[18, 35]

Management of Duplex Systems

The decision regarding when and how to manage the patient with ureteral ectopy is based on three important facts. What is the age of the child? Is the upper pole moiety functioning? Is vesicoureteral reflux present?

In the infant diagnosed by antenatal ultrasound, we defer definitive surgery until the child is older than 3 months of age. This elective delay allows the infant to recover from the physiologic anemia of the newborn. (Note: A normal newborn will drop hemoglobin for the first 2 months of life, with a physiologic rebound occurring during the third month.[36]) It is our unsubstantiated belief that by delaying surgical repair until after the third month we can decrease the possible need for a blood transfusion. To prevent UTI while awaiting surgery, we administer antibiotic prophylaxis with Amoxicillin or Cepahlexin (12.5 mg/kg/day) until surgery is performed. If for some reason antibiotic suppression is continued beyond the third month we change to sulfamethoxazole/trimethoprim or nitrofurantoin suspension. Using this treatment protocol we have had only rare (<3%) breakthrough UTI among our neonatal patient population.[37] If the neonate (<3 months of age) has an infected obstructed upper pole system, the infant may be temporized by placing a percutaneous nephrostomy tube into the involved kidney; if appropriate antibiotics do not control the sepsis. After the infant's fever (<3 months of age) deferveses, a loop or end cutaneous ureterostomy of the ectopic upper pole system is performed for temporary management. Definitive surgical correction is conducted when the infant is older than 3 months of age. Alternatively, the surgeon may elect to proceed with definitive surgical reconstruction, irrespective of the infant's age.

In a child diagnosed with an ectopic ureter after 3 months of age, we proceed promptly to surgical correction. In general, if the upper pole moiety is nonfunctional and not associated with vesicoureteral reflux a partial nephroureterectomy is performed with removal of the upper pole ureter down to the pelvic brim. The distal ureter is left open to prevent the formation of a loculated abscess from developing. If the nonfunctional upper pole moiety is associated with vesicoureteral reflux, the surgeon must decide between tying off the ureteral stump or performing a distal ureterectomy. The ureteral stump is tied off to prevent the retroperitoneal extravasation of urine with each void. Alternatively, the distal ureter is removed with a second Pfannesteil or Gibson incision to prevent the formation of a urethral diverticulum. Proponents of completely excising a refluxing ureteral stump base their decision on the hypothesis that the refluxing ureteral stump acts as a urethral diverticulum and that will predispose the patient to recurrent UTIs.[20, 38] If a distal ureterectomy is performed care must be taken to prevent injury to the lower pole ureter, the vagina, or the external urethral sphincter mechanism.[20, 31] If the surgeon elects to excise the distal stump, rarely the upper and lower pole ureters cannot be easily separated from each other within the distal common sheath portion. If the common sheath is dense and the distal dissection difficult, a mucosal strip of the ectopic ureter can be left attached to the lower pole ureter. This maneuver helps to prevent an injury to the distal lower pole ureter.[39] Any time a distal ureterectomy is performed, it is mandatory to have a urethral catheter in place at the time of the procedure. The ureter is traced down until it meets the pelvic floor or joins with the urethra. The ureter is not dissected beyond the pelvic floor. If the ureter joins the urethra above the pelvic floor, the ureter is excised and its opening is sutured closed. If the ureter proceeds beyond the pelvic floor, two stay sutures are placed a few millimeters above the pelvic floor, the ureter is transected, and then under direct vision the distal ureter is electrofulgrated. The distal ureter is not fulgrated beyond what we can visualize. The ureter is subsequently sutured closed. In either case the foley catheter is left indwelling for 5 to 7 days to allow for adequate healing.

In patients with a functioning upper pole system, the radiographs are carefully assessed to determine if there is a size disparity between the upper and lower pole ureters. If the two ureters are similar in size, these patients are managed with a upper to lower pole ureteroureterostomy, performed approximately 5 cm outside of the bladder. Cystoscopy, retrograde pyelography and ureteral stent placement into the lower pole ureter are performed before the open procedure. Placement of a ureteral stent into the lower pole ureter significantly helps discern between the two ureters at the time of surgery. If there is a great disparity in size of the two ureters and no lower pole vesicoureteral reflux exists, an upper to lower pole pyelopyelostomy is performed because of technical considerations. In patients with a functioning upper pole system and coexisting lower pole vesicoureteral reflux, a duplicate common sheath urethral reimplantation is carried out. In this latter situation it will frequently be necessary to do a tapering procedure of the upper pole ureter. An alternative is to perform a ureteropyelostomy (upper to lower), total excision of the upper pole ureter, and reimplantation of the lower pole ureter only. This is done through 2 extraperitoneal incisions and, some would argue, avoids the problem of a complex ureteral reimplantation.

Single System Management

Most kidneys (90%) associated with single system ectopic ureter are nonfunctional. If the nonfunctional single system kidney associated with an ectopic ureter is associated with a nonrefluxing ureteral orifice, nephrectomy is the treatment of choice (Fig. 18.4). On occasion preoperative voiding cystourethrography will reveal reflux into the ectopic ureteral orifice, common ejaculatory duct, vas deferens, or epididymis. In these latter situations the ureter should be excised where it enters into the genital tract; this will usually require excision of the ipsilateral common ejaculatory duct and ligation of the involved vas deferens. Failure to ligate the vas and excise the common ejaculatory duct will lead to bouts of recurrent epididymitis.[20] If the kidney has sufficient function to warrant its preservation, ureteral reimplantation of the ectopic ureter into the bladder is recommended.

Bilateral Single System Ectopy: Occurrence, Problems, and Management

Bilateral single system ureteral ectopia is a rare congenital anomaly found more frequently in females than males. This complex anomaly usually coexists with a multitude of other urinary tract abnormalities, such as vesicoureteral reflux, renal dysplasia, urinary incontinence, and rudimentary bladder development.[40–43] In females the degree of urinary continence that is possible after surgical reconstruction is directly related to the proximity of the ectopic ureters to the bladder neck. The closer the ureteral orifices are to the bladder neck the more likely the patient will be continent. In males, the external urinary sphincter will usually allow for some degree of continence after the surgical reconstruction.[40–43] The extent of surgery necessary depends on the degree of urinary continence and how well the bladder has developed. In the simplest cases only bilateral vesicoureteral reimplantation is necessary. Unfortunately, complex reconstruction scenarios are usually the norm. Surgery will generally consist of bilateral ureteral reimplantation, bladder neck reconstruction, and possibly bladder augmentation. In some circumstances the bladder is so rudimentary that primary surgical treatment with urinary diversion is preferred.[42]

URETEROCELES

Aberrant Embryologic Development

A ureterocele is defined as a saccular dilation of the terminal (intravesical) portion of the ureter. Four specific hypotheses exist that attempt to explain how ureteroceles develop.

Chwalle noted that a two-layered membrane completely separated the ureteral bud from the developing urogenital sinus in the early stages of embryo development. Based on this finding he hypothesized that a ureterocele developed from the incomplete or defective breakdown of this membrane (Chwalle's membrane). The saccular dilation found in the terminal ureter was secondary to urine accumulating from a functional kidney located above the site of blockage.[44] Unfortunately, this hypothesis cannot explain all of the variations found with ureteroceles. Specifically, some ureteroceles exist with patulous wide open orifices (no evidence of obstruction) while others are associated with blind-ending ureters with no functioning proximal renal tissue found. In an attempt to explain the variety of ureteroceles seen, three other hypotheses have been promulgated.

Two similar theories are those advanced by Drs. Stephens[45] and Tanagho.[46] Both of these hypotheses state that a proximally displaced ureteral bud is a prerequisite for ureterocele formation. Stephens believes that the displacement of the ureteral bud results in its delayed arrival at the urogenital sinus. Because of this delay the ureter enters the bladder when embryologic expansion of the urogenital sinus is occurring. The distal portion of the ureter is caught up in the cystic expansion of the bladder resulting in saccular deformity of the distal ureter. Tanagho argues that if this hypothesis is accurate all ectopic ureters should invariably be associated with a ureterocele. In an attempt to explain this discrepancy he hypothesized that a proximally located ureteral bud and defective canalization of the ureter must coexist for the embryologic abnormality of a ureterocele to develop.

The final hypothesis regarding ureterocele development arose from the observations of Tokunaka and associates.[47] These investigators evaluated the muscular orientation of the terminal segments of the ureters in individuals with ureteroceles. These studies documented that approximately 90% of their patients had complete absence or severe attenuation of the terminal ureteral musculature. (Note: Ten percent of their patients had completely normal terminal ureteral musculature.) They subsequently hypothesized that a ureterocele was the result of the segmental arrest in the development of the ureteral muscle.

Classification

Although a variety of classification schemes and definitions have been proposed for ureteroceles, we find that only five terms have clinical significance.[45, 48–50]

A *single system ureterocele* arises from a kidney with only one ureter.

A *duplex system ureterocele* refers to a ureterocele arising from the upper pole of a completely duplicated system.

Intravesical ureteroceles are completely located within the bladder. They usually arise from a single collecting system and are more commonly seen in the adult population. The intravesical ureterocele is almost invariably associated with a functioning kidney that has minimal to moderate hydronephrosis (Fig. 18.6*A*).

Ectopic ureteroceles will have some portion of the ureterocele located at the bladder neck or in the urethra. These are ordinarily found in conjunction with a duplex collecting system (Fig. 18.6*B*). Single system ectopic ureteroceles rarely occur. When they occur they are usually found in male infants.

A *cecoureterocele*[45] is a variant of an ectopic ureterocele. In this situation the ureteral orifice lies within the bladder; however, a long, tongue-like projection (cecum) extends submucosally beneath the bladder neck into the urethra. Misdiagnosis and inappropriate treatment of this entity can lead to urinary incontinence or obstruction of the urethra.

Incidence

Autopsy reports reveal that ureteroceles (originating from a single or duplex system) occur in one of every 500 people (0.2%).[51] Most ureteroceles are clinically silent with only 10% of the people with this congenital abnormality developing symptoms.[52, 53]

Clinical Presentation

Over the past two decades there has been a significant change regarding how the child with a ureterocele comes to seek medical attention. In the 1970s the median age of presentation was 4.5 years with most patients having a history of a urinary tract infection. During the 1980s routine use of fetal ultrasonography drastically altered the clinical presentation of this population of patients. Seventy-five percent of the patients diagnosed with a ureterocele come to attention because of an abnormal

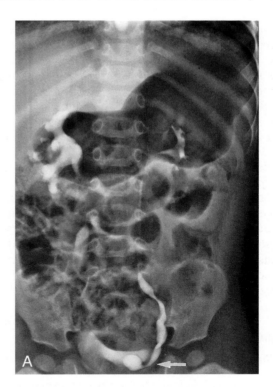

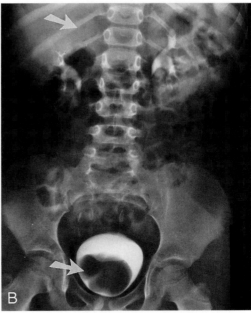

FIG. 18.6. A, A single system intravesical ureterocele. Note that functioning kidney fills the ureterocele with contrast, resulting in a cobra head deformity of the distal ureter (*arrow*). **B,** A right renal duplication associated with a poorly functioning right upper pole system (*upper arrow*). Note the drooping lily appearance of the right lower pole and the large filling defect within the bladder (*lower arrow*) caused by the upper pole ectopic ureterocele.

fetal ultrasound. The median age for the definitive diagnosis of a ureterocele has been reduced to 3 days of life. Less than 25% present after a urinary tract infection.[37]

In addition to antenatal hydronephrosis and urinary tract infection, ureteroceles may become manifest in two other distinctive ways. Occasionally, a neonate will have a palpable abdominal mass as a result of a distended bladder and urinary retention. When this is found the usual cause is a prolapsed ureterocele obstructing the bladder outlet. In female infants a polypoid mass prolapsing out of the urethra should be considered a ureterocele until proven otherwise. In rare circumstances patients with a ureterocele may have urinary incontinence. Incontinence within these patients presumably occurs as a result of the ureterocele inducing a muscular defect in the bladder neck and external sphincter area (in cases of cecosphincteric ureteroceles).[37, 54]

Diagnosis

Radiologic Findings

Prenatal or postnatal ultrasonography will usually depict a renal duplication with pronounced upper pole hydronephrosis. Whether hydronephrosis of the lower pole moiety and the contralateral kidney exists depends on the degree of bladder outlet obstruction caused by the ureterocele and the presence or absence of coexisting vesicoureteral reflux. Careful ultrasonographic evaluation of the bladder will demonstrate a well-defined cystic intravesical mass that can usually be traced back to a dilated ureter.[55, 56]

Voiding cystourethrography (VCUG) is one of the major keys to the diagnosis and treatment of a ureterocele. Experience suggests that a VCUG will demonstrate vesicoureteral reflux into one or more of the renal moieties in approximately 75% of the patients.[37, 57–60] In rare circumstances, reflux has been seen that is usually a result of a patulous ureteral orifice associated with the ureterocele or inadvertent puncture of the ureterocele by the urinary catheter at the time of the VCUG.[37, 61] Occasionally a ureterocele may be misdiagnosed as a paraureteral diverticulum. In these instances the density of the contrast on the voiding cystourethrogram obscures the radiolucent filling defect of the ureterocele. When the bladder is filled with a contrast medium, the ureterocele, because of its poor muscular backing, everts to form what appears to be a "Hutch" or paraureteral diverticulum. The physician is cautioned to consider such a diverticulum as an everted ureterocele until proven otherwise (Fig. 18.7).[57, 58]

Although the accurate diagnosis of a ureterocele may be made with the aforementioned studies, a functional study with an intravenous pyelogram or radionuclide scintography is important in assessing the degree of functioning renal parenchyma associated with the obstructed segment. Whether a functioning renal segment is present appears to be directly related to whether the ureterocele is ectopic or intravesical. Most large series report that only 10 to 25% of the upper poles associated with an ectopic ureterocele are functioning at the time of diagnosis.[56, 62, 66, 67] Irrespective of the type of functional study obtained, the study serves only as a preoperative baseline regarding ultimate renal function. It may not be helpful in predicting the ability of the kidney to recover function after removal of the obstruction.[62, 66, 67]

Management of Single System Intravesical Ureteroceles

Management of the single system intravesical ureterocele depends on two major issues: is the ureterocele truly obstructing and does the involved kidney function. In the presence of a functioning obstructed system the preferred treatment is with low endoscopic incision of the ureterocele (a 2–3 mm incision made on the lower lip of the ureterocele) or transurethral puncture of the ureterocele (1–2 punctures of the lower lip of the ureterocele with a 3 French Bugbee electrode).[68, 69] Either of these treatments will result in successful drainage of the obstructed system, without the development of vesicoureteral reflux, in 90% of the patients. A tapered ureteral reimplantation is reserved for functioning systems that develop high-grade vesicoureteral reflux or have persistent obstruction after these endoscopic procedures. In nonfunctioning kidneys, nephrectomy with aspiration of the ureterocele through the proximal ureter at the time of the surgical procedure is preferred. Surgical extirpation of the ureterocele is unnecessary unless there is coexistent reflux.

Endoscopic Management of the Duplex System Ureterocele (Ectopic Ureterocele)

The appropriate management of an ectopic ureterocele associated with a duplex collecting system has been controversial for several decades. Three major treatment protocols exist: endoscopic management,[66, 68–70] partial nephrectomy and ureterocele aspiration,[37, 60, 71–73] and complete urologic reconstruction (i.e., partial nephroureterectomy, ureterocele excision, or marsupulization with simultaneous ureteral reimplantation).[74–77] Each of these treatment modalities have their advantages and disadvantages. In particular endoscopic incision of ectopic ureteroceles has been reported to have success rates as high as 50% (no persistent obstruction and no reflux).[68] Although endoscopic treatment of an intravesical ureterocele has been highly successful (>90% success, 10 of 11 patients), endoscopic incision for ectopic ureteroceles has been profoundly disappointing. Specifically, we have endoscopically treated

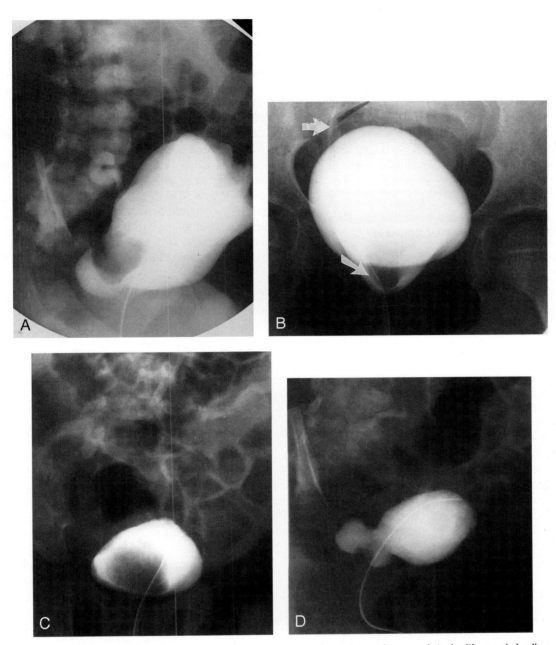

FIG. 18.7. A, Voiding cystourethrogram showing an ectopic ureterocele associated with renal duplication. Note the grade 1 vesicoureteral reflux into the lower pole moiety. **B,** Voiding cystourethrogram showing a left ectopic ureterocele that prolapses into the bladder neck (*lower arrow*), obstructing the bladder during voiding. Note the grade 1 reflux into the contralateral right ureter (*upper arrow*). **C,** Voiding cystourethrogram with the bladder partially filled showing a filling defect due to an ectopic ureterocele. **D,** Voiding cystourethrogram of the same patient shown in part C showing that as the bladder fills with contrast the ureterocele everts. This eversion can be misinterpreted as a "bladder diverticulum."

19 ectopic ureteroceles (17 patients), and had vesicoureteral reflux develop in 12 of 19 (63%) of the upper pole systems. Persistent obstruction of the upper pole was present in 2 of 19 (11%). Only 24% (4 of 17) of our patients had resolution of the obstruction and no development of reflux. Unfortunately, three of the patients whose ureterocele was successfully treated by endo-

scopic therapy required an open procedure because of persistent reflux into the lower pole system or the contralateral kidney. In essence, in only 1 of our 17 patients (6%) was the endoscopic therapy the definitive treatment modality. Similar poor results have been reported by Smith et al. These investigators reported endoscopic management for ectopic ureterocele was the definitive treatment in only 20% (2 of 10) of their patients.[69] Based on these bad results, endoscopic incision of the ectopic ureterocele is recommended in only three circumstances: 1) when an infant has an obstructed and infected upper pole system; 2) in the rare neonate who has progressive renal failure as a result of bladder outlet obstruction caused by an ectopic ureterocele; 3) as part of a planned multistage procedure (i.e., decompression of the ureterocele in the neonate) followed by definitive surgical reconstruction at approximately 18 months of age.

Partial Nephrectomy as Management of the Duplex System Ureterocele (Ectopic Ureterocele)

The simplified or staged urinary reconstruction in the infant with an ectopic ureterocele was popularized by Cendron and Bonhomme in 1968.[71] In this approach the first procedure performed is a partial nephroureterectomy and aspiration of the ureterocele. This simplified approach is based on the concept that decompression of the ureterocele would result in restoration of more normal trigonal anatomy and resolution of any accompanying vesicoureteral reflux or bladder outlet obstruction.[71, 73] The major advantage of this approach is that the difficult dissection of the ureterocele at the bladder neck is avoided in the infant. Theoretically surgical dissection in the older child is easier and reduces the risk of urinary incontinence caused by bladder neck or external urethral sphincter injury. The need for subsequent surgery is chiefly due to the presence of persistent vesicoureteral reflux into the lower poles or the contralateral ureter.[37, 60, 73, 74, 76] Proponents of this approach state that up to 80% of the patients are completely cured by the partial nephrectomy. Although we have been an advocate for this treatment modality, a recent review of our patient data base caused us to have second thoughts regarding routine management of all patients with an ectopic ureterocele by this technique.[37] In our experience, 62% (54 of 87) of the patients managed by this approach required additional surgical procedures. When reviewing our data, we found that the preoperative voiding cystourethrogram enabled the physician to determine who will need additional surgery after the partial nephrectomy (Table 18.1). Specifically, the need for additional surgery is directly proportional to three items: 1) the number of ureteroceles present, 2) the number of renal moieties with vesicoureteral reflux, and 3) the grade of reflux present (Table 18.1). If no vesicoureteral reflux is present on the initial VCUG (grades I and II, i.e., the patient has one or two ureteroceles present and no associated reflux), 87% of the patients will be definitively cured by a partial nephrectomy.[37, 60, 73, 76] Partial nephrectomy will not cure all of the grade I and II patients because 25% of these individuals will develop reflux after surgery. In patients

with the delayed onset of reflux, approximately half will spontaneously resolve their reflux during a 2-year observation period, the remainder will require surgical repair.[37, 60, 73, 76] When preoperative voiding cystourethrograms reveals the presence of low grade reflux, i.e., two of five or fewer, into a single renal moiety (grade IIb), 60% of the patients are definitively treated by partial nephrectomy. If, however, high grade vesicoureteral reflux or reflux into more than one renal moiety is found on the initial VCUG (grade IIb, III, IV), partial nephroureterectomy alone cures only 4% (2 of 45) of our patients (Table 18.1). These findings suggests that partial nephroureterectomy alone is an excellent definitive treatment modality in patients with ureteroceles not associated with reflux or who have only low grade reflux into one renal moiety on the initial VCUG.

Complete Surgical Reconstruction as Management of the Duplex System Ureterocele (Ectopic Ureterocele)

The need for additional surgery after partial nephrectomy has been found to be as high as 60 to 70% by some authors.[37, 74] This has prompted the recommendation that most patients with an ectopic ureterocele would be best treated by complete urologic reconstruction (i.e., partial nephroureterectomy, ureterocele excision, or marsupialization with simultaneous ureteral reimplantation).[74, 75] Unfortunately, reports on the frequency of complications and the success of complete reconstruction are rare. The most complete review is reported by Scherz et al.[74] who noted a success rate of 86% (24 of 28 patients), with four patients needing additional procedures because of persistent vesicoureteral reflux. No median age at the time of the complete reconstruction was given. Opponents of complete reconstruction focus their arguments on the following points. Not all of the patients with an ectopic ureterocele need complete urologic reconstruction. Three possible major complications can occur with a complete repair: devitalization of the lower pole ureter, damage to the continence mechanisms of the bladder, and the development of uretero- or vesico-fistulas.[56, 75, 76, 78] They also argue that treatment of the patient by endoscopic methods or by partial nephrectomy allows the physician to reasses the patient in a stepwise fashion. Reevaluation after decompression of the ureterocele enables the doctor to document that an additional intravesical operation, with its attendant risks, is necessary.

Proponents of complete reconstruction argue that total reconstruction is necessary in most patients. They believe that the simplified approach or treatment with endoscopic methods only delays the inevitable.[37, 69, 74-76] Advocates of complete reconstruction are careful to point out several keys to successful reconstruction. First, all of the ureterocele must be completely excised or marsupialized. Not removing the distal margin of the

TABLE 18.1. *Prognostic classification for ectopic ureteroceles managed by partial nephroureterectomy and aspiration of the ureterocele*

Grade	Preoperative radiologic findings	No. of patients requiring additional surgery or with persistent reflux/ total no. of patients (%)
I	Upper pole ureterocele, no vesicoureteral reflux	8/65 (12)
II	Bilateral upper pole ureteroceles	1/6 (16)
IIa	Upper pole ureterocele, Grade 2 or less vesico- ureteral reflux into 1 renal moiety	6/15 (40)
IIb	Upper pole ureterocele, Grade 3 vesicoureteral re- flux or higher into one renal moiety	5/5 (100)
III	Upper pole ureterocele and any degree of vesico- ureteral reflux into two renal moieties	26/28 (93)
	Bilateral upper pole ureteroceles, and any degree of vesicoureteral reflux into one moiety	3/3 (100)
IV	Upper pole ureterocele and any degree of reflux into three systems	9/9 (100)
	Bilateral ureteroceles any degree of vesicoure- teral reflux into two systems	5/5 (100)

The prognostic classification that allows the physician to determine if a patient should respond to partial nephrectomy alone is based on the number of renal moieties involved with a ureterocele and the presence of vesicoureteral reflux into coexisting renal moieties.[37] (The information expressed in this table is accumulative data from references 37, 60, 73, and 76.)

ureterocele will leave a flap valve or "wind sock" deformity that can obstruct the bladder outlet. Second, if the common sheath is dense and the distal dissection difficult, a mucosal strip of the ectopic ureter can be left attached to the lower pole ureter. This maneuver will eliminate possible devitalization of the ureter.[39] Third, the ureterocele should be treated with complete excision and meticulous reconstruction of the bladder neck or by complete marsupulization of the anterior surface of the ureterocele with tacking of the posterior surface of the ureterocele to the adjacent bladder mucosa. Advocates for reconstruction of the bladder neck hypothesize that to not reconstruct the weakened muscle below the ureterocele could lead to diverticular formation, possible voiding dysfunction, and urinary incontinence.[37,75] Advocates for marsupulization of the ureterocele believe that leaving the posterior wall of the ureterocele intact reduces the risk of iatrogenic injury to the continence mechanisms of the bladder neck.[74,77]

Individualized Treatment for Ectopic Ureteroceles

We recommend that treatment of the patient with an ectopic ureterocele be tailored to the individual. If a functional upper pole moiety is present, an ipsilateral pyelopyelostomy or ureteroureterostomy is performed. Whichever of these procedures is used depends on the size discrepancy between the upper and lower pole ureters and whether the lower pole renal pelvis is intraparenchymal. On occasion, a small functioning upper pole (<15% total renal function) is sacrificed if an attempt

to salvage this portion of the kidney places the lower pole system at undue risk.[62]

In patients with nonfunctioning upper pole systems, treatment is based on the patient's functional renal status, the number of renal moieties involved, and the age of the patient. Specifically, if the child is younger than 18 months of age and the diagnostic evaluation reveals compromised renal function (persistently elevated serum creatinine) or the presence of high-grade vesicoureteral reflux (greater than 2 of 5) into more than one renal moiety (grade IIb, III, or IV) endoscopic incision of the ureterocele and placement of the patient on antibiotic prophylaxis are warranted. Definitive repair is performed at approximately 18 months of age. In the child older than 18 months of age with a prognostic ureterocele grade of IIb, III, or IV complete genitourinary reconstruction is the most definitive and efficacious treatment modality.[37]

In children younger than 3 months of age with a nonfunctioning upper pole system and prognostic ureterocele grade of I, II, or IIa, antibiotic prophylaxis is begun and partial nephroureterectomy is performed at 3 months of age. In the infant or child older than 3 months of age with grade I, II, or IIa partial nephrectomy and aspiration of the ureterocele is undertaken without delay. This approach is preferred because most of these patients (87%) will not need additional surgery after partial nephrectomy. Although endoscopic incision of the ureterocele within this patient population is also a viable alternative, this procedure is not chosen because iatrogenic vesicoureteral reflux will occur in 50 to 60% of the patients.[68] Incision of the ureterocele in this select patient population could result in an additional, and perhaps unnecessary, intravesical procedure.

PSEUDOURETEROCELES

A *pseudoureterocele* is an ectopic ureter that enters into a rudimentary mesonephric ductal structure (Fig. 18.8).[79–82] The potential for misdiagnosing an ectopic ureter as a ureterocele in the fetus or newborn is relatively easy and can lead to improper therapy. On two separate occasions, neonates with ectopic ureters draining into Gartner's Duct misdiagnosed as ectopic ureteroceles have been seen. Treatment of these patients with endoscopic incision of the "ureterocele" within the first week of life, unfortunately, established a vesico-ureteral-vaginal fistula (see Fig. 18.8). The key to preventing this misdiagnosis is an accurate bladder ultrasound that demonstrates the distal extent of the ureterocele or ectopic ureter. If a ureter is seen to extend below the bladder neck, the differential diagnosis should be a cecoureterocele or an ectopic ureter. In these situations, the physician is cautioned not to hasten to incision of the ureterocele until the possibility of an ectopic ureter has been ruled out. To rule out ureteral ectopy historical evidence of chronic urinary incontinence should be ascertained. If the patient's historical information does not definitively answer the question, methylene blue can be injected into the "ureterocele" with cystoscopic or ultrasonic guidance. Careful vaginoscopic evaluation for an ectopic opening of the ureter into the vagina can then be performed.

INVERTED Y URETERS

An inverted Y ureter occurs when two ureteral buds arise from the mesonephric duct but fuse proximally before joining the metablastic nephrema. This results in one single proximal channel with the distal ureter having two lumens (i.e., an inverted y configuration). In most cases the most caudal Y segment inserts ectopically, is atretic, or ends in a ureterocele.[83–88] Patients frequently complain of recurrent infections, pain, or urinary incontinence. The usual surgical treatment is

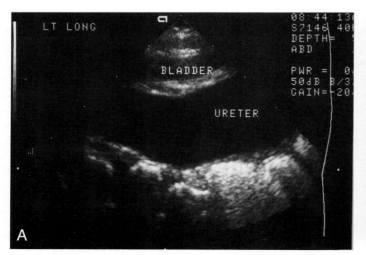

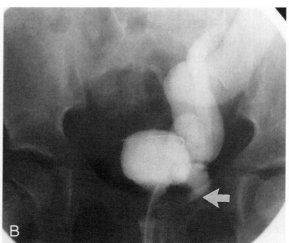

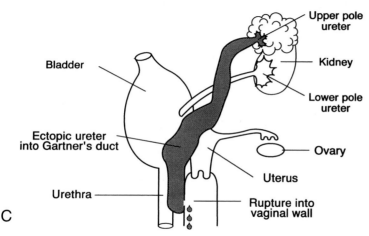

FIG. 18.8. A, Sonogram of a 3-yr-old female showing a dilated distal ureter extending behind the bladder. **B,** Cystogram of the same patient revealing vesicoureteral reflux into both the left lower and the upper pole ureters. Note the extent of the upper pole ureter descending beyond the bladder neck (*arrow*). **C,** The structure of the patient's left ureter.

resection of the most caudal ureteral segment and reimplantation of both ureteral limbs.

URETERAL TRIPLICATION

Ureteral triplication occurs when three separate ureteral buds develop from the mesonephric duct or when two ureteral buds arise from the mesonephric duct with one of the buds having a premature fission.[4] Ureteral triplication has four different classifications:[89, 90]

1. Complete triplication. Three complete ureters arise from the kidney and insert with three separate orifices.
2. Incomplete triplication. Three ureters arise from the kidney. Two of the ureters form a Y configuration and join outside the bladder. Two orifices exist.
3. Trifid ureter. The most common anomaly. Three ureters arise from the kidney, all three unite before entering the bladder. Only one ureteral orifice is present in the bladder.
4. Ureteral triplication caused by an inverse Y duplication. Two ureters arise from the kidney, but as one ureter descends it develops an inverse Y duplication. Three separate ureteral orifices.

Ureteral triplication may be found in association with a ureterocele or ureteral ectopy.[89–91] A ureterocele is usually associated with the middle ureter. Patients usually have a history of urinary infection, incontinence, or pain secondary to obstruction. Surgical treatment is based on surgical reconstruction of the obstructed or ectopic ureteral orifice.

BLIND ENDING URETERS

A blind ending ureter can occur when two ureteral buds arise from the mesonephric blastema with one of the buds not making contact with the metablastic nephrema or alternatively when a solitary ureteral bud premature fissures and one of the ureters does not contact the metablastic blastema. Most blind ending ureteral segments do not cause symptoms and are found incidentally at autopsy. When they cause symptoms patients usually complain of vague abdominal flank pain or recurrent urinary tract infections. Because the lesion is more common in women and is usually located on the right side, several patients with this congenital abnormality have had right-sided flank pain during the second and third trimesters of pregnancy.[92–96]

The diagnosis of a blind ending ureteral segment is often difficult.[94] The ureteral segment does not usually fill on excretory urography and is not commonly identifiable with ultrasonography. On occasion an excretory urogram may reveal ureteroureteral reflux into the blind stump, or the presence of a "ureteral calculus" outside of the collecting system.[92–96] If clinical suspicion for this entity is high, retrograde pyelography is often necessary for diagnosis. Surgical treatment, with excision of the blind ending segment, is pursued only in symptomatic patients.

REFERENCES

1. Snell RS. The urinary system. Boston: Little, Brown and Co., 1975;203–219.
2. Mackie GG, Stephens FD. Duplex kidneys: a correlation of renal dysplasia with position of the ureteral orifice. J Urol 1975;114:274.
3. Gonzales E Jr. Anomalies of the renal pelvis and ureter. In: Kelalis PP, King LR, Belman AB, eds. Clinical Pediatric Urology. Philadelphia: W.B. Saunders Company, 1992;530–579.
4. Bauer SB, Perlmutter AD, Retik AB. Anomalies of the upper urinary tract. In: Walsh PC, Retik AB, Stamey TA, Vaughan ED Jr, eds. Campbell's Urology. Philadelphia: W.B. Saunders, 1992;1402–1424.
5. Snyder HMc III. Anomalies of the ureter, adult and pediatric urology. In: Gillenwater JY, Grayhack JT, Howards SS, Duckett JW, eds. St. Louis: Mosby Year Book, 1991;1831–1862.
6. Nation EF. Duplication of the kidney and ureter. A statistical study of 230 new cases. J Urol 1944;51:456.
7. Hartman GW, Hodson CJ. The duplex kidney and related abnormalities. Clin Radiol 1969;131.
8. Timothy RP, Decter A, Perlmutter AD. Ureteral duplication: clinical findings and therapy in 46 children. J Urol 1971;105:445.
9. Cohen N, Berant M. Duplications of the renal collecting system in the hereditary osteo-onchodysplasia syndrome. J Urol 1976; 89:261.
10. Whitaker J, Danks DM. A study of the inheritance of duplication of the kidneys and ureters. J Urol 1966;95:176.
11. Atwell JD, Cook PL, Howell CJ. Familial incidence of bifid and double ureters. Arch Dis Child 1974;49:390.
12. Babcock JR Jr, Belman AB, Sholnik A. Familial ureteral duplication and ureterocele. Urology 1977;9:345.
13. Stephen FD. Congenital malformations of the rectum, anus, and genitourinary tracts. London: E.S. Livingstone Ltd, 1963.
14. Meyer R. Normal and abnormal development of the urinary tract in the human embryo—a mechanistic consideration. Anat Rec 1946;96:355.
15. Tanagho EA. Embryologic basis for lower ureteral anomalies: a hypothesis. Urology 1976;7:451.
16. Blame CE, Ritchey ML, DiPietro MA, Sumida R, Bloom DA. Single system ectopic ureters and ureteroceles associated with dysplastic kidney. Pediatr Radiol 1992;22:217.
17. Johnson DK, Perlmutter AD. Single system ectopic ureters and ureteroceles with anomalies of the heart, testis and vas deferens. J Urol 1980;123:81.
18. Terai A, Tsuji Y, Terachi T, Yoshida O. Ectopic ureter opening into the seminal vesicle in an infant: a case report and review of the Japanese literature. Inter J Urol 1995;2:128.
19. Schulman CC. The single ectopic ureter. Eur Urol 1976;2:64.
20. Shapiro E. The ectopic ureter, AUA Update Series. Ball TP, ed. Houston: American Urological Association, 1990;242–247.
21. Ellerker AG. The extravesical ectopic ureter. Br J Surg 1958; 45:344.
22. Curranino G. Single vaginal ectopic ureter and Gartner's duct cyst with ipsilateral hypoplasia and dysplasia (or agenesis). J Urol 1982;128:988.
23. Prewitt LH, Lebowitz RL. The single ectopic ureter. Am J Roentgenol 1976;127:941.
24. Vanhoutte JJ. Ureteral ectopia into a Wolffian duct remnant (Gartner's ducts or cysts) presenting as a urethral diverticulum in two girls. Am J Roentgenol 1970;110:540.
25. Williams DI, Royle M. Ectopic ureter in the male child. Br J Urol 1969;41:421.
26. Elaz T, Maline PS. Male duplex urinary incontinence. J Urol 1995;153:470.
27. Mandell J, Bauer SB, Colodny AH, Lebowitz RL, Retik AB. Ureteral ectopy in infants and children. J Urol 1981;126:219.
28. Siegal A, Snyder H, Duckett JW. Epididymitis in infants and

boys: underlying urogenital anomalies and efficacy of imaging modalities. J Urol 1987;138:1100.

29. Gharagozloo AM, Lebowitz RL. Detection of a poorly functioning malpositioned kidney with single ectopic ureter in girls with urinary dribbling: imaging evaluation in five patients. Am J Roentgenol 1995;164:957.

30. Wyly JB, Lebowitz RL. Refluxing urethral ectopic ureters: recognition by the cyclic voiding cystourethrogram. Am J Roentgenol 1984;142:1263.

31. Churchill BM, Abara EO, McLorie GA. Ureteral duplication, ectopy, and ureteroceles. Pediatric Clin North Am 1987;34:1273.

32. Schulman CC. The ureter. In: O'Donnell B, Koff SA, eds. Pediatric Urology. Oxford: Butterwort Heinmann, 1997;397–418.

33. Smith FL, Ritchie EL, Maizels M, et al. Surgery for duplex kidneys with ectopic ureters: ipsilateral ureteroureterostomy versus polar nephrectomy. J Urol 1997;142:532.

34. Monfort G, Guys JM, Coquet M, Roth K, Louis C, Bocciardi A. Surgical management of duplex ureteroceles. J Pediatr Surg 1992;27:634.

35. Patil U, Matthews R. Minimal surgery with renal preservation in anomalous complete duplicated systems: Is it feasible? J Urol 1995;154:727.

36. Glader BE, Schiason G. Anemias. In: Eichenwald HF, Stoder J, eds. Current Therapy in Pediatrics. Toronto: B.C. Decker, 1989;416.

37. Husmann DA, Ewalt DH, Glenski WJ, Bernier PA. Ureterocele associated with ureteral duplication and a nonfunctional upper pole segment: management by partial nephroureterectomy alone. J Urol 1995;154:723.

38. Schlussel RN, Retik AB. Ureteroceles and ectopic ureters. In: Stamey TA, ed. Monographs in Urology. Medical Directions Publishing Company, 1994;27–43.

39. Kroovand RL, Perlmutter AD. A one stage surgical approach to ectopic ureterocele. J Urol 1979;122:367.

40. Williams DI, Lightwood RG. Bilateral single system ureters. Br J Urol 1972;44:267.

41. Noseworthy J, Persky L. Spectrum of bilateral ureteral ectopia. Urology 1982;19:489.

42. Glenn JF. Agenesis of the bladder. JAMA 1997;169:2016.

43. Cox CE, Hutch JA. Bilateral single system ectopic ureter: a report of 2 cases and review of the literature. J Urol 1966;95:493.

44. Chwalle R. The process of formation of cystic dilation of the vesical end of the ureter and of the diverticula at the ureteral ostium. Urol Cutan Rev 1927;31:499.

45. Stephens FD. Cecoureterocele and the embryology and etiology of ureteroceles. Aust NZ J Surg 1971;82:257.

46. Tanagho EA. Ureteroceles: embryogenesis, pathogenesis and management. Urology 1976;7:451.

47. Tokunaka S, Goto T, Koyanagi T, Tsuji I. The morphometric study of ureteroceles: a possible clue to its morphogenesis as evidenced by a locally arrested myogenesis. J Urol 1981;126:726.

48. Uson AC. A classification of ureteroceles in children. J Urol 1961;85:732.

49. Ericsson NO. Ectopic ureteroceles in infants and children. Chir Scand 1954;197(Suppl):1.

50. Glassberg KI, Braren V, Duckett JW, et al. Suggested terminology for duplex systems, ectopic ureters and ureteroceles. J Urol 1984;132:1153.

51. Uson AC, Lattimer JK, Melicow MM. Ureteroceles in infants and children: a report based on 44 cases. Pediatrics 1961;27:971.

52. Malek MS, Kelasis PP, Stickler GB, Burke EC. Observations on ureteral ectopy in children. J Urol 1972;107:308.

53. Malek RS, Kelasis PP, Burke EC. Simple and ectopic ureterocele in infancy and childhool. Surg Gynecol Obstet 1972;134:611.

54. Leadbetter GW Jr. Ectopic ureterocele as a cause of urinary incontinence. J Urol 1970;103:222.

55. Nussbaum AR, Dorst JP, Jeffs RD, Gearhart JP, Sanders RC. Ectopic ureter and ureterocele: their varied sonographic manifestations. Radiology 1986;159:227.

56. Coplen DE, Duckett JW. The modern approach to ureteroceles. J Urol 1995;153:166.

57. Daniels MA, Allen TD. Unsuspected ureterocele and ureteral duplication. J Urol 1994;152:179.

58. Caldamone AA. Editorial comment on: unsuspected ureterocele and ureteral duplication. J Urol 1994;152:181.

59. Share JC, Lebowitz RL. Ectopic ureterocele without ureteral and calyceal dilation (ureterocele disproportion): findings on urography and sonography. AJR 1989;152:567.

60. Caldamone AA, Snyder HMc III, Duckett JW. Ureteroceles in children: follow-up of management with upper tract approach. J Urol 1984;131:1130.

61. Sen S, Beasley SW, Ahmed S, et al. Renal function and vesicoureteral reflux in children with ureteroceles. Pediatr Surg Int 1992;7:192.

62. Levy JB, Vandersteen DR, Morgenstern BZ, Husmann DA. Hypertension following surgical management of renal duplication associated with upper pole ureterocele. J Urol 1997 (pending publication).

63. Rickwood AMK, Reiner I, Jones M, Pournaras C. Current management of duplex system ureteroceles: experience with 41 patients. Br J Urol 1992;70:196.

64. Churchill BM, Sheldon CA, McLorie GA. The ectopic ureterocele: a proposed practical classification based on renal unit jeopardy. J Pediatr Surg 1992;27:497.

65. Schwobel MG. Duplex ureteroceles: Is radical surgery always necessary? Eur J Pediatr Surg 1994;4:207.

66. Tank ES. Experience with endoscopic incision and open unroofing of ureteroceles. J Urol 1986;136:241.

67. Monfort G, Morrisson-Lacombe G, Coquet M. Endoscopic treatment of ureteroceles revisited. J Urol 1985;133:1031.

68. Blyth B, Passerini-Glazel G, Camuffo G, Snyder HMc III, Duckett JW. Endoscopic incision of ureteroceles: intravesical versus ectopic. J Urol 1993;149:556.

69. Smith C, Gosalbez R, Parrott TS, Woodard JR, Broecker B, Massad C. Transurethral puncture of ectopic ureteroceles in neonates and infants. J Urol 1994;152:2110.

70. Rich MA, Keating MA, Snyder HMc III, Duckett JW. Low transurethral incision of single system intravesical ureterocele. J Urol 1990;144:120.

71. Cendron J, Bonhomme C. 31 Cas d'ureter a bouchement ectopique sons-sphincterien chez l'enfant du sexe feminin. J Urol Nephrol 1968;74:1.

72. King LR, Kozlowski JM, Schacht MJ. Ureteroceles in children—a simplified and successful approach to management. JAMA 1983;249:1461.

73. Mandell J, Colodny A, Lebowitz R, Bauer SB, Retik AB. Ureteroceles in infants and children. J Urol 1980;123:921.

74. Scherz HC, Kaplan GW, Packer MG, Brock WA. Ectopic ureteroceles: surgical management with preservation of continence—review of 60 cases. J Urol 1989;142:538.

75. Hendren WH, Mitchell ME. Surgical correction of ureteroceles. J Urol 1989;142:538.

76. Mor Y, Ramon J, Raviv G, Jonas R, Goldwasser B. A 20-year experience with treatment of ectopic ureteroceles. J Urol 1992;147:1592.

77. Johnston JH, Johnson LM. Experiences with ectopic ureteroceles. Br J Urol 1969;41:61.

78. Caldamone AA, Duckett JW. Update on ureteroceles in children. AUA Update. 1984;(Series 3):1.

79. Sumfest JM, Burns MW, Mitchell ME. Pseudoureterocele: potential misdiagnosis of an ectopic ureter as a ureterocele. Br J Urol 1995;75:401.

80. Innes-Williams D, Lillie JG. Functional radiology of ectopic ureterocele. Br J Urol 1972;44:417.

81. Gill B. Ureteric ectopy in children. Br J Urol 1980;52:257.

82. Williams DI. Ectopic ureterocele. Paediatric Urology. London: Butterworths, 1968;210.

83. Schenkman NS, Fernandez EB, Wind G, Irby P. Inverted Y duplication of the ureter associated with a distal limb ectopic to the seminal vesicle. J Urol 1994;152:946.

84. Mosli HA, Schillinger JF, Futter N. Inverted Y duplication of the ureter. J Urol 1986;135:126.

85. Regan TC, Dejter SW. Inverted Y duplication of the ureter with associated ureterocele and bladder outlet obstruction. J Urol 1996;155:642.

86. Beasley SW, Kelly JH. Inverted U duplication of the ureter in

association with ureterocele and bladder diverticulum. J Urol 1986;136:899.

87. Ecke M, Klatte D. Inverted Y ureteral duplication with a uterine ectopy as a cause of ureteric enuresis. Urol Int 1989;44:116.

88. Suzuki S, Tsujimura S, Sugiura H. Inverted Y ureteral duplication with a ureteral stone in atretic segment. J Urol 1977;117:248.

89. Smith I. Triplicated ureter. Br J Surg 1946;34:182.

90. Zoantz MR, Maizels M. Type one ureteral triplication: an extension of the Weigert-Meyer law. J Urol 1985;139:949.

91. Finkel LI, Watts FB Jr, Cobrett DP. Ureteral triplication with a ureterocele. Pediatr Radiol 1983;13:343.

92. Albers DD, Geyer JR, Barnes SD. Clinical significance of blind ending branch of a bifid ureter: report of three cases. J Urol 1971;105:634.

93. Marshall FF, McLoughlin MG. Long blind-ending ureteral duplications. J Urol 1978;120:626.

94. Miller EV, Tremblay RE. Symptomatic blind ending bifid ureters. J Urol 1964;92:109.

95. Rao KG. Blind-ending bifid ureter. Urology 1975;6:81.

96. Sharma SK, Subudhi CL, Kumar S, Bapna BC, Suri S. Ureteric diverticula: ureterodiverticular reflux and yo-yo effect. Br J Urol 1980;52:345.

CHAPTER 19

Anatomic Abnormalities of the Bladder

Phillip F. Nasrallah and Daniel R. McMahon

EMBRYOLOGY

At the fourth fetal week the caudal portion of the hindgut is a dilated chamber called the cloaca. The allantois extends from the upper cloaca into the umbilicus and the mesonephric (Wolffian) duct opens laterally on each side. The ureteric bud is apparent. When cloacal dilatation first appears, a depression of ectoderm (proctodeum) develops at the caudal end of the embryo ventrally. This depression continues to deepen until only a thin membrane remains between the hindgut and the outside of the body.[1] This is the cloacal membrane (Fig. 19.1A).

Between the fifth and sixth fetal week the urorectal septum begins its descent and divides the cloaca into the dorsal rectal segment and the ventral urogenital segment (Fig. 19.1B). This separation is completed before the rupture of the cloacal membrane. At this stage the urogenital sinus is tubular and continuous with the allantois. The ventral portion will form the bladder. The ventral portion also forms the entire urethra in the female and the prostatic and membranous urethra in the male. This urethral portion also receives the metanephric and mesonephric ducts. With rapid growth of the bladder, the terminal portions of these ducts are absorbed so that they come to have separate openings. The mesoderm that surrounds both segments of the early bladder begins to differentiate into smooth muscle and fibroelastic connective tissue. By 12 weeks, the characteristic smooth muscle layers of the urethra and bladder are visible. It is clear embryologically that the detrussor and urethral musculature are of the same origin.[2,3] In both sexes, the bladder develops as an intra-abdominal organ and does not assume a pelvic position until late in childhood.

BLADDER AGENESIS AND HYPOPLASIA

Agenesis of the bladder is an uncommon condition that rarely exists as a solitary anomaly. Campbell reported only seven cases in a study of more than 19,000 autopsies.[4] In all seven cases, other anomalies coexisted. This condition is thought to be secondary to absence of urine filling the developing bladder. In most cases, the ureters enter the urethra, vagina, or rectum. Renal development may vary from total agenesis to bilateral dysplasia. In some instances of bilateral ectopia, the bladder may be present but of such a diminutive volume that it cannot function as a reservoir (Fig. 19.2). The tiny bladder does not distend if the ureters are reimplanted, and the sphincteric mechanism of the bladder neck may be absent. Bladder augmentation is a necessary part of reconstruction.

Absence of the bladder may appear as on prenatal ultrasound. In these cases, significant urinary tract pathology (exstrophy, renal agenesis) results in failure of bladder filling.[5]

URACHUS

The urachus is a fibrous cord that extends from the fibrotic allantoic duct to the dome of the bladder. It is contained within the potential space of Retzius between the transversalis fascia and the peritoneum. During organogenesis, the bladder forms within the abdominal cavity. As development continues, the bladder descends into the pelvis and its apical portion narrows to form the urachus. During the fourth to fifth month of gestation, the epithelial-lined lumen of the urachus normally obliterates. If the lumen does not obliterate completely, a spectrum of urachal abnormalities can occur (Fig. 19.3).

Patent Urachus

A patent urachus produces urinary leakage through the umbilicus. Typically, the diagnosis is made after a neonate is found to have a "wet umbilicus." The differential diagnosis of the wet umbilicus includes omphalitis, patent omphalomesenteric duct (enteroumbilical fistula), granulation of the umbilical stump, infected umbilical vessels, and urachal sinus. The etiology of the

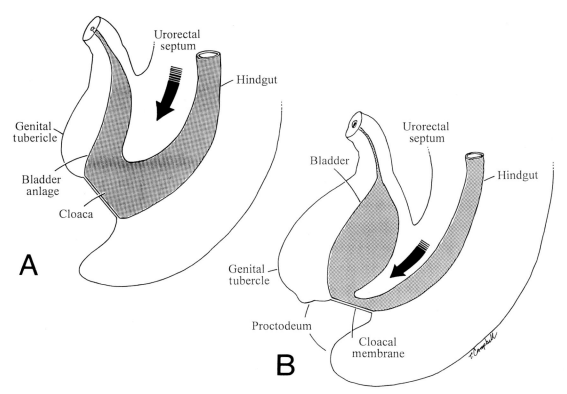

FIG. 19.1. A, The cloaca before the descent of the urorectal septum in the 4th fetal week. **B,** Bladder development depends on the descent of the urorectal septum and on the systematic dissolution of the cloacal membrane.

patent urachus remains unknown. It has been proposed that bladder outlet obstruction produces high intravesical pressure that inhibits the obliteration of the urachal lumen. Patent urachus has been reported in association with prune belly syndrome and posterior urethral valves. However, bladder outlet obstruction is present in only 14% of neonates who have a patent urachus, and most infants with outlet obstruction do not have a patent urachus.[6]

The diagnosis is most effectively made by canalization of the urachal tract and contrast injection under fluoroscopy (Fig. 19.4). A voiding cystourethrogram (VCUG) is a less reliable method of delineating the defect; however, it is useful in ruling out infravesical obstruction.[7] Evaluation of urea nitrogen or the creatinine content of the umbilical fluid is often diagnostic. Ultrasonography may demonstrate the patent channel. Alternatively, the diagnosis can be made by the injection

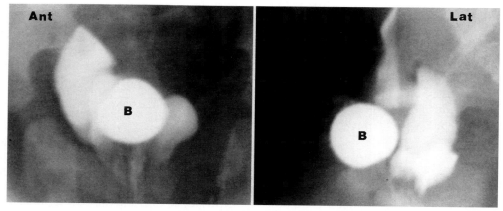

FIG. 19.2. Cystogram of an infant with bilateral ureteral ectopia and bladder hypoplasia. Bladder capacity is approximately 4 mL.

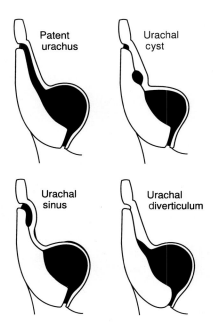

FIG. 19.3. Schematic representation of urachal anomalies. (Modified from Gillenwater J, Grayhack J, Howards S, Duckett J. Adult and Pediatric Urology. St. Louis: Mosby Yearbook, 1996.)

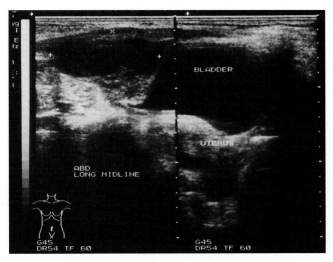

FIG. 19.5. Ultrasound demonstrating patent urachus.

of methylene blue into the sinus tract or the bladder (Fig. 19.5).

Complete excision of the urachus with a cuff of bladder is the accepted treatment. In infants, a small semilunar subumbilical incision provides adequate exposure. In older patients, a transverse midhypogastric incision provides the best access to the dome of the bladder.[8] The umbilicus should be preserved in virtually all patients.

Urachal Sinus

An external urachal sinus is produced when the distal aspect of the urachus retains its lumen while the proximal aspect is fully obliterated. The patient has umbilical inflammation and drainage. Pain and fever may also be present. The differential diagnosis echoes that of the patent urachus. A sinogram should confirm the diagnosis (Fig. 19.6).

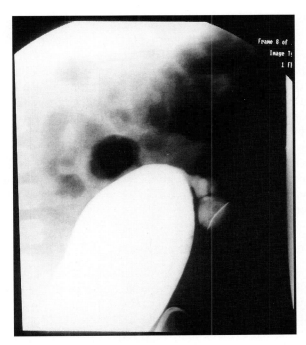

FIG. 19.4. VCUG demonstrating patent urachus.

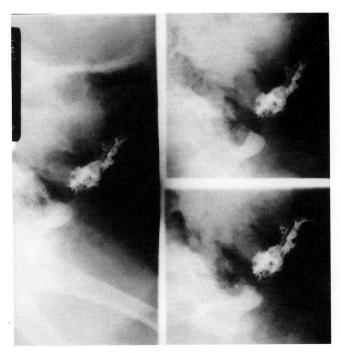

FIG. 19.6. Sinogram of urachal sinus.

Excision of the sinus tract should be deferred until the acute infection and inflammation have abated. Lesions characterized by extensive inflammation are best resected with a midline incision. At times, extension of the inflammatory process may necessitate excision of the adjacent omphalomesenteric duct remnants.[9] Rarely, extensive inflammation necessitates excision of the umbilicus.

Urachal Cyst

If a portion of the urachus maintains its epithelial lining but the proximal and distal limits of the urachal lumen obliterate, a urachal cyst is produced. Desquamation of the epithelium expands the cyst, which may become secondarily infected. *Staphylococcus aureus* is the most common pathogen isolated.[10] The infected cyst can drain into the bladder or to the umbilicus, and an alternating pattern has been observed. Peritonitis secondary to intraperitoneal rupture of the cyst is reported but uncommon.[11]

The diagnosis is best made by ultrasound. Computed tomography (CT) scanning is also effective but carries a higher cost (Fig. 19.7). Small cysts may be treated with primary excision, but larger infected cysts may require initial drainage with subsequent excision.[12] The importance of complete excision is demonstrated by the report of a urachal adenocarcinoma developing in a 15-year-old boy 2 years after he was diagnosed with a urachal abscess that was treated only by local drainage.[13]

Urachal Diverticulum

A urachal diverticulum is produced when only the proximal aspect of the urachus remains patent. Urachal diverticulae are most commonly found as incidental

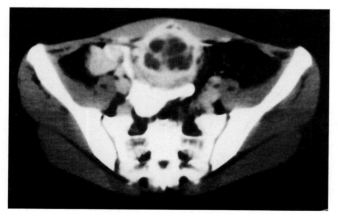

FIG. 19.7. CT scan demonstrating urachal cyst.

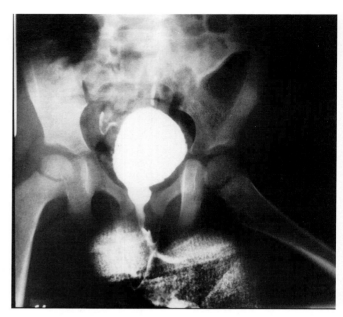

FIG. 19.8. VCUG showing small urachal diverticulum.

findings on a variety of imaging modalities (Fig. 19.8). Large urachal diverticulae are frequently encountered in patients with prune belly syndrome and have been reported in association with severe bladder outlet obstruction. Poor drainage may lead to calculus formation within the diverticulum.[14] Resection is not required if the lesion is small, but excision is indicated if the diverticulum is large and impedes bladder emptying.

BLADDER DIVERTICULUM

Acquired Diverticulum

Acquired bladder diverticula are produced by elevated bladder pressure. The relative weakness of the ureteral hiatus predisposes this area to form diverticula.[15] Acquired diverticula may be found in patients with elevated bladder pressure caused by dysfunctional voiding, neurogenic disease, and bladder outlet obstruction. The term Hutch diverticulum refers specifically to a parahiatal diverticulum that is associated with a neurogenic bladder. The correction of voiding abnormalities with the restoration of low bladder pressure may result in the regression of small parahiatal diverticula.

Congenital Bladder Diverticulum

A congenital bladder diverticulum, like an acquired defect, is the protrusion of bladder mucosa through the muscular wall of the bladder. The differential diagnosis includes secondary diverticula, everted ureterocele, and bladder ears (bladder wings extending into the internal ring in infant males). Primary bladder diverticula are less common than acquired or secondary diverticula but are not rare. Congenital diverticula are more common in boys than girls. A primary diverticulum is usually solitary; if multiple diverticula are present, then the clinician must aggressively rule out obstruction or neurogenic bladder.

The defect is most commonly located cephalad and lateral to the ureteral orifice. The etiology of these defects is unknown; however, the parahiatal location implicates an abnormality in the incorporation of Waldeyer's sheath into the developing bladder.[15] Congenital diverticula have been reported in association with connective tissue disorders, most specifically, Ehlers-Danlos syndrome; however, causality has not been fully confirmed. A conservative approach to diverticula has been advocated for patient with Ehlers-Danlos syndrome.[16] Diverticula have also been associated with fetal alcohol syndrome and Menkes' syndrome.[17, 18]

The diverticulum may incorporate the submucosal ureter and produce vesicoureteral reflux (Fig. 19.9). Large diverticula may produce bladder outlet obstruction with urinary retention[19] or ureteral obstruction.[20] Diverticula that cause infection, reflux, or obstruction should be excised. Excision is facilitated by distending the diverticulum with a gauze pack and a combined intravesical/extravesical approach. Some surgeons advocate routine prophylactic excision of diverticula.

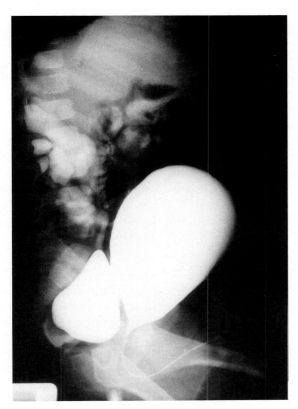

FIG. 19.9. VCUG demonstrating congenital diverticulum with ipsilateral reflux.

Transitional cell carcinoma develops in 2 to 10% of patients with a diverticulum and these tumors have the potential for early extension.[21] Most of the tumors develop after the fifth decade of life.

MEGACYSTIS

Congenital megacystis is a diagnosis of exclusion. The term is accurately applied in the setting of a huge bladder when obstruction, reflux, and other pathology is absent.

Megacystis megaureter syndrome is characterized by a large smooth bladder, dilated ureteral orifices, and dilated refluxing ureters.[22] During micturition, a large volume of urine is transferred to the ureters. This urine is subsequently recycled between the ureters and the bladder. Over time, persistent bladder distention produces an atonic, thin-walled, and dilated bladder.[23] Correction of reflux will often restore normal voiding dynamics. However, ureteral reimplantation in the setting of grossly dilated ureters and a thin detrusor is challenging. A transureteroureterostomy with a unilateral reimplantation should be considered. Initial temporizing vesicostomy may be a reasonable option in select patients.[24]

Megacystis-microcolon-hyperperistalsis syndrome is a functional obstruction of the bladder and intestine. The neuropathology of this condition is poorly understood. The bladder is distended and reflux may be present. The colon is small, the small bowel is dilated, and the entire tract exhibits hypoperistalsis.[25]

BLADDER DUPLICATION

Duplication of the bladder is a rare condition. True duplication consists of two distinct bladder chambers with a ureter entering each chamber. Each bladder is drained by a separate urethra (Fig. 19.10). First described by Nesbit and Bromme in 1933,[26] this condition may be accompanied by diphallia. The duplication may rarely occur in the coronal plane with the extra urethra lying in an epispadiac position (Cheng and Maizels).[27] More commonly, bladder duplication accompanies anomalies of the hindgut. In a review of 20 hindgut duplications by Ravitch and Scott, 12 were associated with bladder duplication.[28]

The embryologic explanation of each anomaly probably lies with the formation and descent of the urorectal septum in the fifth fetal week. This alone cannot account for the constellation of anomalies that usually accompany bladder duplication. Ravitch and others[29] have suggested that bladder duplication represents a form of partial twinning. Campbell proposed a complicated explanation hinging on a septal outgrowth in the sagittal plane that would fuse with the urorectal septum. The timing of this fusion of septa would explain the wide range of hindgut anomalies that are common with blad-

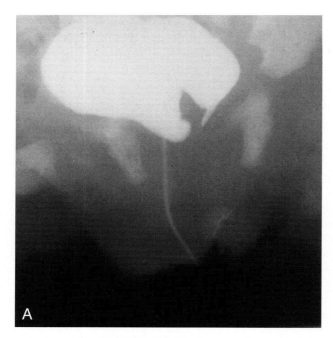

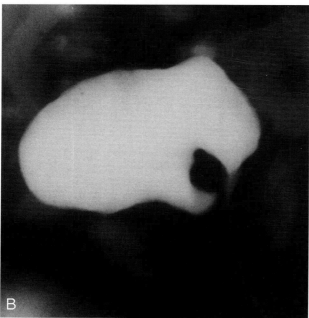

FIG. 19.10. **A and B** Cystograms of a patient with bladder duplication and diphallia. A catheter is visible in each of the urethrae. The duplication is incomplete because the two bladder chambers are communicating.

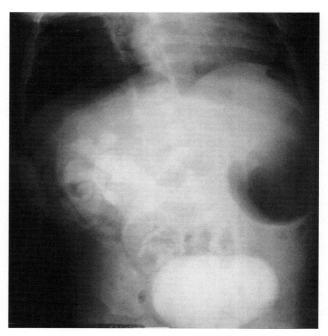

FIG. 19.11. An IVP from the patient in Figure 19.10 showing right hydroureteronephrosis secondary to outlet obstruction of the right hemibladder.

der reduplication. As the embryology suggests, there are several variations in the spectrum of bladder reduplication. A septum may divide the bladder in the sagittal or frontal (transverse) plane. These septa may be complete or partial. A complete sagittal septum may divide the bladder into two halves and cause obstruction to one chamber with resulting hydroureteronephrosis (Fig. 19.11). Incomplete septa are usually nonobstructive in nature. A transverse muscular constriction may divide the bladder into upper and lower chambers similar to an hourglass. The ureter may open into either chamber.

Treatment of bladder duplication is aimed at restoring normal function to the urinary tract. All other anomalies must be managed appropriately and often take priority over the urinary abnormality. A septum causing obstruction must be excised. An accessory bladder in the coronal plane may be excised along with its epispadiac urethra. Caution must be used in dissection of the duplicated urethra lest sphincteric injury occur. Diagnosis in those cases not accompanied by hindgut duplication or by diphallia is usually made during evaluation of an extraurinary meatus, two streams, or of dorsal chordee.

BLADDER POLYPS

Benign polyps in the urinary tract are uncommon. These lesions are most often seen in the renal pelvis or ureter. In children, polyps are most often found in the posterior urethra.[30] When present in the bladder, a polyp may be the cause of hematuria or voiding difficulty.[31] Young described a fibroepithelial polyp in a 35-year-old man with such symptoms.[32] We have seen this lesion in a 4-month-old female infant who had a prolapsing, bleeding urethral mass (Fig. 19.12). Cystography demonstrated the unusual lesion on a long stalk. Endoscopic

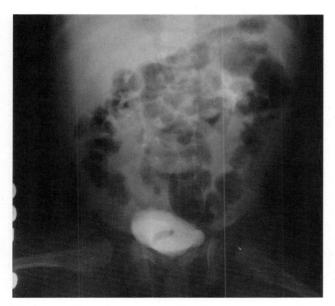

FIG. 19.12. IVP of a 4-month-old girl with hematuria. Negative filling defect in the bladder demonstrates pedunculated polyp.

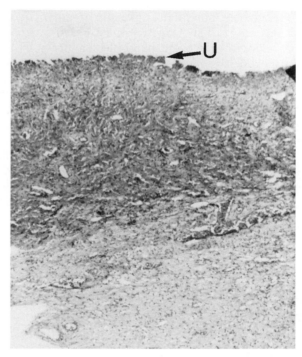

FIG. 19.14. Photomicrograph showing urothelial covering (U) and polyp's fibrous stroma.

removal confirmed the presence of a fibroepithelial polyp (Fig. 19.13).

Bladder polyps have been misdiagnosed as sarcoma botryoides because of their rarity and their presentation with hematuria and prolapse. The polyp is composed of fibrous connective tissue covered by transitional epithelium (Fig. 19.14). This urothelium may be hyperplastic and hemorrhagic. The central portion is hypocellular. Mesenchymal cells with atypical, hyperchromatic nuclei may be found in the lamina propria of the inflamed bladder. Differentiation from sarcoma rests on absence of invasion into the overlying urothelium and lack of mitotic figures and cross striations.

Treatment is simple endoscopic excision. Recurrence has not been reported.

NEPHROGENIC ADENOMA

Nephrogenic adenoma is a rare benign lesion of the bladder that occurs in response to infection or trauma. This condition is more commonly seen in adults, but there have been several reports in pediatric patients. In each an irritative predisposing factor was present. Kay and Lattanzi reported two cases of nephrogenic adenoma after ureteral reimplantation and traumatic vesical fistula.[33] Ureteral reimplantation was seen as the predisposing factor in three other case reports.

Nephrogenic adenoma is seen as multiple papillary projections that closely resembles low grade transitional cell bladder carcinoma. Histologically, this lesion is characterized by structures in the lamina propria resembling nephrogenic tubules. Other components of the nephron are absent. The tubules lack characteristics of urothelium but branching is reminiscent of ureteral bud division seen in embryonic development. The bladder's metaplastic response seen in cystitis cystica, cystitis follicularis, and cystitis glandularis are variations of the metaplastic urothelial changes represented by nephrogenic adenoma.

Clinically, nephrogenic adenoma may present with hematuria or other symptoms of bladder inflammation such as dysuria, urgency, or frequency. Upper tract involvement is rare unless the lesion causes ureteral obstruction or attempts at fulgeration result in severe bladder fibrosis. The lesions can occur anywhere in the bladder and are often multifocal. Nephrogenic adeno-

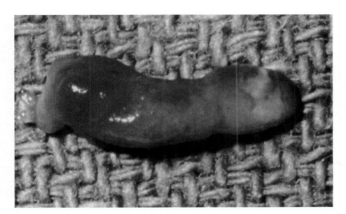

FIG. 19.13. Gross specimen from patient in Figure 19.12.

ma's malignant potential causes the greatest concern with this entity. This fear is justified because nephrogenic adenoma has been found incidentally in cystectomy specimens removed for transitional cell carcinoma. In children, this concern is heightened because of the potential of other irritative and carcinogenic exposure with a life expectancy of 60 or 70 years. However, the progression of nephrogenic adenoma to definite carcinoma has never been documented.

Treatment with endoscopic fulgeration controls this disease for most patients. Periodic cytology and cystoscopy are recommended because this is a proliferative and metaplastic epithelial lesion. Antibiotic prophylaxis is a useful adjunct to therapy.

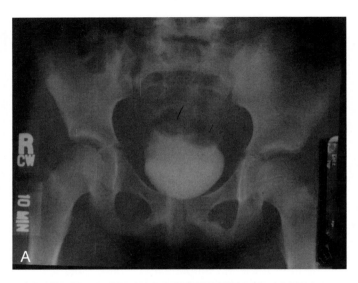

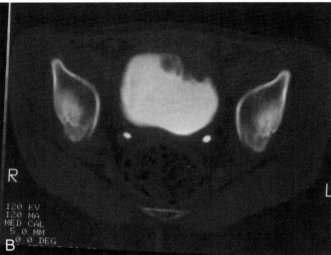

FIG. 19.15. A, Cystogram of an 8-year-old girl with hematuria and large filling defect of the bladder dome. **B,** CT scan of same patient shown in **A** demonstrating a large mass in the dome of the bladder.

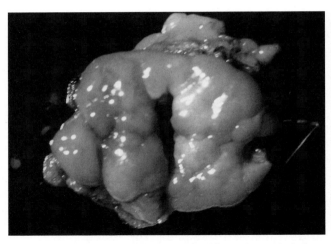

FIG. 19.16. Gross specimen removed from the patient from Figure 19.15. The lesion involved most of the bladder dome and extended through the bladder wall.

INFLAMMATORY PSEUDOTUMOR

Inflammatory pseudotumor (pseudosarcoma) of the bladder was first described in 1985.[34] This is a benign proliferative lesion of the submucosal stroma that can be easily mistaken for a malignant neoplasm, both clinically and histologically. Although more commonly reported in adults, this condition can be seen in children and adolescents. Stark et al. reported two cases in teenage patients.[35] Both had hematuria secondary to a large polypoid and ulcerated mass visualized cystoscopically. Dietrick et al. also reported inflammatory pseudotumor in an 18-year-old man with dysuria, urgency, and hematuria.[36] We have seen an 8-year-old girl with a large lesion at the dome of the bladder that was thought to be a sarcomatous tumor (Fig. 19.15). Endoscopic biopsy was inconclusive. Surgical exploration revealed an inflammatory pseudotumor that was totally excised (Fig. 19.16).

Imaging studies will show a mass of the bladder wall that is often extensive. Extravesical extension and lymphadenopathy are routinely absent. Endoscopy usually reveals a solitary, broad-based, exophytic tumor. Occasionally, these tumors may be large enough to be palpable. There is no sex predilection. Hematuria is the most common mode of presentation. Inflammatory pseudotumor may arise in the presence of chronic irritation (chronic urinary infection or previous surgery), but most occur de novo without predisposing conditions.

Histologically, these cases bear a resemblance to nodular fasciitis, a benign tumor of mesenchymal origin. Microscopically, there are widely separated spindle cells with elongated cytoplasmic processes in a myxoid stroma. There may be a mild inflammatory component (Fig. 19.17). Mitoses are uncommon and these tumors lack the nuclear pleomorphism that characterizes

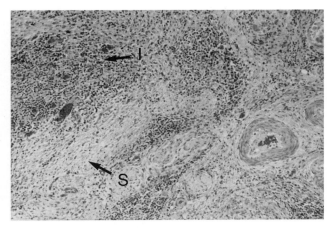

FIG. 19.17. Photomicrograph of the lesion in Figure 19.15. Note the inflammatory infilitrates (I) surrounding the stroma of spindle cells.

mesenchymal tumors. Electron microscopy demonstrates smooth muscle myofibroblastic differentiation with no evidence of skeletal muscle differentiation. For this reason the term "myofibroblastoma" has been suggested as more appropriate, but the term "inflammatory pseudotumor" endures in the literature.

Optimal management rests in local excision because these are benign tumors that have little potential for recurrence. Several cases have been managed with transurethral resection. Segmental resection has been performed in most reported cases. In nodular fasciitis, complete excision is unnecessary for cure. Despite inflammatory pseudotumor's benign nature, the histologic similarity to several malignant lesions make follow-up mandatory. Awareness of this entity and its histologic appearance should prevent radical excision.

REFERENCES

1. Kaplan G, Scherz H. In: Kelalis P, King L, eds. Infravesical Obstruction in Clinical Pediatric Urology. Philadelphia: WB Saunders, 1992;821–823.
2. Stephens F. Congenital Malformations of the Rectum, Anus and Genitourinary Tract. London: E&S Livingstone Ltd., 1963;4–5.
3. Muecke E. Exstrophy, epispadias and other anomalies of the bladder. In: Campbell's Urology, 5th ed. Philadelphia: WB Saunders, 1986;856–858.
4. Sarica K, Kupeli S. Agenesis of the bladder associated with multiple organ anomalies. Int Urol Nephrol 1995;27(6):697–730.
5. Bronshtein M, Bar-Hava I, Blumenfeld Z. Differential diagnosis of the non-visualized fetal urinary bladder by transvaginal sonography in early second trimester. Obstetrics Gynecol 1993; 2:490–493.
6. Herbst WP. Patent urachus. South Med J 1937;30:711.
7. Zacharias A, Mesrobian HO, Balcom A, Cohen R. Ten years experience with urachal anomalies in children. American Academy of Pediatrics Section on Urology, 1996. Abstract 100.
8. Caldamone AA. Excision of urachus. In: Hinman F Jr, ed. Atlas of Pediatric Urologic Surgery. Philadelphia: WB Saunders, 1994.
9. Bauer SB, Retik AB. Urachal and related umbilical disorders. Urol Clin North Am 1978;5:195.
10. Macmillan RW, Schulinger JN, Santulli VT. Piourachus: an unusual surgical problem. J Ped Surg 1973;8:87.
11. Agustein EH, Stabile BE. Peritonitis due to intraperitoneal perforation of infected urachal cyst. Arch Surg 1984;199:1269.
12. Goldman IL, Caldamone AA, Gauderrer M, et al. Infected urachal cysts: a review of 10 cases. J Urol 1988;140:373.
13. Cornil C, Reynolds CT, Kickham CJ. Carcinoma of the urachus. J Urol 1967;98:93.
14. Bandler CG, Milbed AH, Alley JL. Urachal calculus. NY State J Med 1942;42:2203.
15. Stephens FD. The vesicoureteral hiatus and paraureteral diverticula. J Urol 1979;121:786.
16. Stage HH, Tank ES. Primary congenital bladder diverticula in boys. Urology 1992;40(G):536.
17. Havres W, Majewski F, Obling H, et al. Anomalies of the kidneys and genitourinary tract in alcohol embryopathy. J Urol 1980; 124:108.
18. Daly WJ, Rabinovitch HH. Urologic abnormalities with Menkes syndrome. J Urol 1981;126:262.
19. Taylor WN, Alton D, Toguri A, et al. Bladder diverticulum causing posterior urethral obstruction in children. J Urol 1951; 66:692.
20. Lione PM, Gonzales ET. Congenital bladder diverticula causing ureteral obstruction. Urology 1985;25:273.
21. Micic S, Illic V. Incidence of neoplasm in vesical diverticula. J Urol 1983;129:734.
22. Williams DI. Megacystis and megaureter in children. Bull NY Acad Med 1959;35:317.
23. Harrow BR. The myth of the megacystis syndrome. J Urol 1967;98:205.
24. Hsu HS, Duckett JW, Tempelton JM. Experience with urogenital reconstruction of ischiopagus conjoined twins. J Urol 1995; 154:563.
25. Berdon WE, Baker DH, Blanc W. Megacystis microcolon-intestinal hypoperistalsis syndrome: a new cause of intestinal obstruction in the newborn. Report of radiologic findings in five newborn girls. AJR 1976;126:957.
26. Nesbit R, Bromme W. Duplication of the urinary bladder. Am J Roentgenology 1933;30:497.
27. Maizels M, Cheng R. Complete duplication of the bladder and urethra in the coronal plane: case report. J Urol 1996;155:1414–1415.
28. Ravitch M, Scott W. Duplication of the entire colon, bladder and urethra. Surgery 1953;34:843–848.
29. Abrahamson J. Double bladder and related abnormalities. Br J Urol 1961;33:195–241.
30. DeCastro R, Campobasso P, Belloli G, Pavanello P. Solitary polyp of the posterior urethra in children: report on seventeen cases. Eur J Ped Surg 1993;3:92–96.
31. Rubin J, Khanna O, Damjanov I. Adenomatous polyp of the bladder: a rare cause of hematuria in young men. J Urol 1982;126:549–550.
32. Young R. Fibroepithelial polyp of the bladder with atypical stromal cells. Arch Path Lab Med 1986;110:241–242.
33. Kay R, Lattanzi C. Nephrogenic adenoma in children. J Urol 1985;133:99–101.
34. Nochomovitz I, Orenstein J. Inflammatory pseudotumor of the urinary bladder—possible relationship to nodular fasciitis. Two case reports, cytologic observations and structural observations. Am J Surg Path 1985;9:366.
35. Stark G, Feddersen R, Lowe B, Benson C, Black W, Borden T. Inflammatory pseudotumor (pseudosarcoma) of the bladder. J Urol 1989;141:610–612.
36. Dietrick D, Kabalin J, Daniels G, Epstein A, Fielding I. Inflammatory pseudotumor of the bladder. J Urol 1992;148:141–144.

CHAPTER 20

Triad Syndrome and Other Disorders of Abnormal Detrusor Development

David B. Joseph

Triad Syndrome (TS), the clinical association of the thin, flaccid abdominal wall, undescended testes, and distended bladder with hydroureters was originally described by Parker in 1895.[1] In 1901, Osler presented similar findings in a 6-year-old child he described as having the appearance of a "wrinkled prune."[2] Since that time "Prune Belly" has unfortunately become synonymous with this syndrome. This clinical manifestation is also known as the Eagle-Barrett syndrome and the abdominal muscular deficiency syndrome (Fig. 20.1).[3,4]

The classic description of TS occurs in boys with a reported incidence of 1:29 to 40,000 live births.[5] Five percent of children with this syndrome are girls with similar physical findings, but lacking the gonadal abnormality.[6,7] A true association of females with TS has been questioned.

Most cases of TS are sporadic, although familial occurrence has been described.[8,9] TS has been associated with trisomies 13, 18, 21.[10,11,12] With the exception of an increased incidence of TS reported in Nigeria,[8] there does not appear to be an increased association of TS based on race or geographic location.

PATHOGENESIS

There is no single theory of development that incorporates all aspects of TS. The two most commonly recognized theories are based on the occurrence of a primary defect resulting from urethral obstruction as proposed by Stumme,[13] or a primary mesenchymal defect initially suggested by Bardeen.[5]

Urethral Obstruction

The urethral obstruction theory is based on the existence of an obstructing lesion at the junction of the prostatic and membranous urethra in a location similar to that found in association with posterior urethral valves.[5] This temporary obstruction is present long enough to cause compression of the prostatic primordial tissue, allowing for posterior urethral dilation. Subsequently, distention of the bladder results in urinary ascites and degeneration of the abdominal wall muscle. The elevated pressure in the bladder leads to upper urinary tract ectasia and subsequent renal dysplasia. The massive distention of the bladder mechanically prevents the testes from entering the internal ring and descending into the scrotum. Rupture of the obstructing lesion later in development accounts for the lack of an identifiable obstruction in neonates with TS.

Beasley has proposed a transient obstruction in the distal portion of the urethra caused by delay in cannulization of the spongy glanular urethra.[14] This delay would produce a temporary obstruction during weeks 11 to 16 of gestation. The timing of this defect could explain the poor prostatic development that occurs during the 11th week and the persistence of a patent urachus that typically closes at the 15th week. Urinary tract enlargement during the 13th to 15th weeks could also lead to the degenerative changes of the abdominal wall and contribute to the mechanism causing malrotation of the gastrointestinal tract.

The postmortem dissections by Stephens and Gupta of fetal and neonatal specimens affected with TS places the urethral obstruction theory in doubt.[15] They compared the postmortem evaluation of 21 children with TS to 23 children with typical type I and type III posterior urethral valves. The specimens with TS were noted to have abnormal development of the seminal duct vesicles and prostatic glands. Similar abnormalities were not identified in the specimens with posterior urethral valves. They concluded that an obstructive process by itself would not explain many of the changes noted in TS.

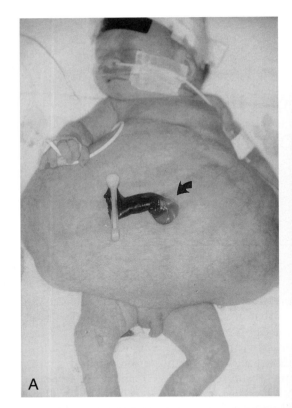

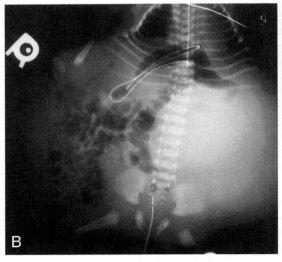

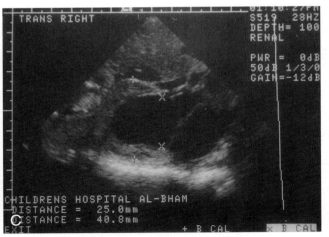

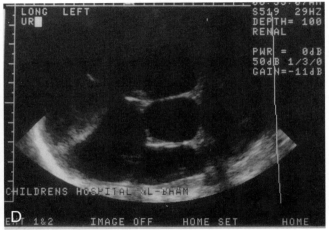

FIG. 20.1. A, Newborn with triad syndrome. Arrow indicates a membrane overlying a patent urachus. **B,** Babygram showing deviation of bowel loops to the right caused by a severely dilated urinary system. Typical rib splaying is also noted. **C,** Transverse image of right kidney showing hydronephrosis and a thin rim of parenchyma. **D,** Longitudinal image of left kidney showing minimal parenchyma, hydronephrosis, and loops of dilated ureter.

Mesodermal Defect

The mesodermal defect theory is based on the premise that abnormal development affects the medial somites and the lateral plate (during the third week of gestation).[5] The mesoderm between these areas contributes to development of the mesonephros, mesonephric (Wolffian) duct, and metanephros. Smooth muscle from the genitourinary and gastrointestinal tract derives from the visceral layer of the lateral plate. Ives proposed that a deficiency in equal distribution of mesoderm results in the development of TS.[9]

Stephens has long been a proponent of the theory that abnormal development of the mesoderm is the cause of TS.[16] This hypothesis is based on postmortem evaluation of children with TS and relates to the finding that the terminal portion of the Wolffian duct is incorporated into the prostatic and membranous urethra.[15] With development there is overexpansion of the Wolffian duct and ureteric bud resulting in the saccular dilation of the prostatic urethra and prostatic hypoplasia. Membranous leaflets in this area result in the appearance of obstructing valves. Dilation of the ureteric bud results in megaureters that meet the metanephric blastema in a peripheral location, ultimately inducing dysplastic renal parenchyma.[17]

The simultaneous failure of myoblasts to migrate from the thoracic somites leads to defects in the abdominal wall.[5] In addition, defective perineal development results in the occurrence of anorectal anomalies and abnormal development of the corpora cavernosa and corpus spongiosum. The mesodermal defect theory does not explain the significant predominance of TS in males, although it has been proposed that there is a greater demand on the mesoderm for differentiation of the Wolffian versus Müllerian system, which subsequently accounts for the male predominance.[4, 9]

SYSTEM FEATURES OF TRIAD SYNDROME

Abdominal Wall

Classic description of TS is based on the wrinkled, lax appearance of the abdominal wall. The muscular deficiency varies from a minor defect with patchy, asymmetric areas of muscular development in the lower abdomen to an extensive deficiency throughout the abdominal wall. When the patient is standing, the asymmetric deficiency is manifested by unusual protuberance and bulging of the abdominal wall. The rectus abdominus is often poorly developed in the lower portion but overall retains a normal blood supply and segmental nerve distribution.[18, 19, 20] The discrepancy in rectus development results in a cephalic displacement of the umbilicus. Microscopic assessment of the abdominal muscles shows areas of normal muscle cells and muscle cells that are enlarged with indistinct borders.[18] Electron microscopy has shown large glycogen aggregates and disorganization of muscle bands.[21]

The abnormal abdominal wall is an obvious cosmetic problem, but in addition, some children have difficulty changing from a supine to sitting position. There may also be an associated delay in ambulation.[22] Deficiency in abdominal wall musculature may also inhibit productive coughing, which can affect an already compromised pulmonary system and result in a higher incidence of upper respiratory infections.

Kidneys

Renal development may be normal, but the kidneys are commonly hypoplastic or dysplastic. Kidneys range in size from small and cystic to grossly hydronephrotic. The degree of hydronephrosis does not necessarily correlate with the degree of hydroureter or megacystis. In addition, there may be good preservation of renal function as might be expected with a mesenchymal defect but not necessarily with an obstructive process.

Renal abnormalities have been broadly categorized into one of three groups.[3–5] The most severely affected

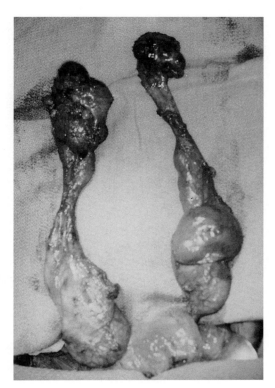

FIG. 20.2. Small dysplastic appearing kidneys with megaureter. Note the tortuous, disproportionate dilation of the distal ureter.

are dysplastic kidneys, characterized by primitive tubules, embryonic mesodermal cysts, and metaplastic cartilage. These kidneys have few nephrons and demonstrate gross parenchymal disorganization. Potter's type II cystic malformations result from an early insult to the nephrogenic blastema, preventing normal development.[23] The second group is characterized by Potter's type IV cystic dysplasia, consisting of subcortical, glomerular, and tubular cysts within fibrous tissue surrounding medullary collecting ducts. This abnormality usually results in smaller kidneys.[4, 5] The third group consists of a combination of Potter's type II and IV cystic dysplasia.[5] The occurrence of renal dysplasia is best explained by the Mackie-Stephens theory of renal development,[17] that is, that dysplasia occurs from abnormal induction of nephrogenic mesenchyme by a defective ureteral bud or vascular ischemia (Fig. 20.2).

Ureters

The ureters are elongated, tortuous, and dilated in appearance. The distal ureter is often asymmetrically involved with significant ectasia. Secondary obstruction may occur because of kinking and folding of the redundant ureter. Primary obstruction has been reported at the ureteropelvic junction and the ureterovesical junction.[19, 20, 24] The ureteral orifices are lateral, often golf

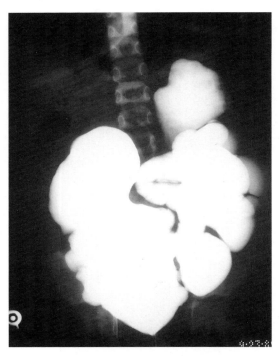

FIG. 20.3. Cystogram showing megacystis with a large urachal cap and grade V vesicoureteral reflux into a tortuous left system.

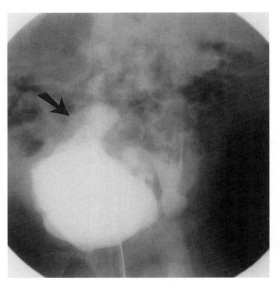

FIG. 20.4. Cystogram showing a large bladder with the appearance of a pseudodiverticulum in the dome (*arrow*), a remnant of the urachus.

hole in appearance, and associated with a diverticulum. Vesicoureteral reflux is the rule, occurring in approximately 75% of children (Fig. 20.3).[25, 26]

Microscopically, there is an increase in fibrous tissue at the expense of normally developed ureteric muscle.[5] Gearhart et al. have shown that children with vesicoureteral reflux have an increased ratio of collagen to smooth muscle fibers in the muscularis layer.[27] This increased fibrous tissue may help explain the poor dynamic characteristics of the ureter that leads to ineffective peristalsis and urinary stagnation.[18, 19, 27] Ehrlich and Brown have reported a degeneration of nonmyelinated Schwann fibers and fewer nerve plexi, which may contribute to decreased ureteral peristalsis.[28] Ureteral abnormalities tend to predominate in the distal portion of the ureter, an observation that should be kept in mind at the time of urinary tract reconstruction.

Bladder

The bladder is often massively enlarged. There is usually the appearance of a pseudodiverticulum in the bladder dome, which is a remnant of the urachus. A patent urachus or urachal cyst is present in 25 to 50% of children (Fig. 20.4).[15, 19, 29]

Stephens and Gupta described two characteristic patterns of the bladder trigone.[15] In one, the trigone was V-shaped with the apex fading into the internal urethral meatus and the ureteral orifices located at the end of a

long cornu. The second pattern was a normal triangular configuration of the trigone with the ureteral orifice situated on the lateral border. The bladder neck was widely patent, and the result was direct continuity of the distended bladder with the posterior prostatic urethra (Fig. 20.5).

Histologically, the bladder wall is thickened, most often from increased collagen deposits. In the presence of true obstruction, muscular hypertrophy may account for some of the detrusor thickening. However, without obstruction there is an increase in the ratio of collagen to muscle fibers.[30] There does not appear to be any

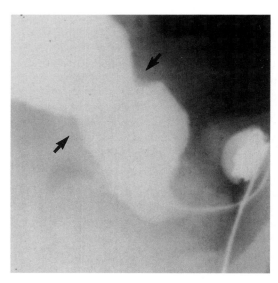

FIG. 20.5. A widely patent bladder neck defined by arrows with direct continuity with the posterior prostatic urethra.

neurologic deficit of the bladder with a normal distribution of ganglion cells noted in the bladder base.[18]

Prostate and Prostatic Urethra

The prostate is hypoplastic, presumably secondary to the failure of epithelial differentiation during development.[15, 31] Histologically, the tubuloalveolar glands are present in sparse populations. As with other components of the urinary system there is an increase in the ratio of fibrous tissue and collagen fibers to smooth muscle. The verumontanum is poorly developed and has been described as flat, totally absent, or replaced by a small, rounded pocket consistent with the utriculus.[15] The utriculus has also been described as a saccule or tubule.[15]

The prostatic urethra is typically characterized as an expanded pouch-like structure caused by extreme dilation of the posterior, caudal, and lateral walls relative to the anterior wall.[5] There is often an abrupt junction between the prostatic and membranous urethra giving the appearance of an obstruction. Stephens and Gupta have described three urethral profile patterns.[15] In the first, the membranous urethra exits anteriorly and is of normal caliber or narrowed with an abnormally high take-off. In the second pattern, the membranous urethra exits distally with an anterior overlying prostatic urethral pouch consistent with a variant of a Young's type I posterior urethral valve. The third group is characterized by a membranous urethra that is dilated and has stenosis or atresia at the level of the perineal membrane in a configuration consistent with Young's type III valve (Fig. 20.6).

Genital Tract

The course of the ductus deferens has been reported to be abnormal from the level of the bladder to the urethra.[15] The seminal ducts may be poorly developed with midline fusion and are straight, sinuous, or ectatic. In a few specimens reviewed by Stephens and Gupta there was a normal convergence of the ductus deferens in a V-fashion from the distal ureter to the hilum of the prostate.[15] The seminal vesicles are often absent and, if present, they appear rudimentary. The vas deferens are narrow and convoluted from the prostate gland to the testes. The attachment of the epididymis to the testis is tenuous and frequently nonexistent.

Anterior Urethra

Anatomic characteristics of the penile urethra cover a spectrum from normal to bulbous dilation to atresia. Measurements of urethral caliber determined from voiding cystourethrograms have shown a distinctly abnormal appearance in boys with TS compared with those

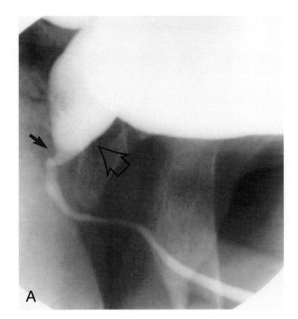

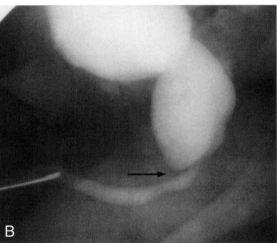

FIG. 20.6. A, Open arrow indicates typical pouch-like posterior urethra with dilation of the caudal wall. Closed arrow shows abrupt junction between prostatic and membranous urethra. **B,** The classic appearance of Young's type I posterior urethral valve (*arrow*).

in normal controls and in boys with posterior urethral valves.[14] Transient obstruction during fetal development has been proposed as a mechanism for some of these changes.[32] A patent urachus is often found when urethral atresia or a true obstruction is present.

Testes

The testes are universally found in an intra-abdominal location in boys with classically described TS. The histologic pattern of TS testes shows absence of spermatogenesis, fewer spermatogonium and Sertoli cells, and Leydig cell hyperplasia.[33, 34] Massad demonstrated atypical germ cells with large nuclei, prominent nucleoli, and alkaline phosphatase staining cystoplasmic membranes suggestive of developmental arrest as the pathogenesis of the undescended testis.[35] Because of the lack of spermatogonia the risk of a germ cell tumor has been considered minimal.[34] However, the histologic similarities with intratubular germ cell neoplasia, noted by Massad et al., reinforce the importance of long-term follow-up to identify possible germ cell neoplasms.[35]

The testes are usually located overlying the ventral aspect of the distal ureter. Gubernacular attachment to the testis occurs proximally at the tail of the epididymis and distally at the pubic tubercle. The gubernaculum itself is histologically normal with a normal neuronal input.[36] To date, there has not been a report of paternity in any man with TS. This could be because of the combined effects of histologic abnormalities of the testes and structural abnormalities of the genital ductal system.

ASSOCIATED ORGAN SYSTEM ANOMALIES

Orthopedic

Associated organ system anomalies occur in 60 to 70% of children with TS.[3–5] This may be explained by abdominal distention that can lead to multiple orthopedic anomalies, especially of the chest wall. On chest radiographs the ribs show a particular splayed appearance, and on physical examination there is protrusion of the upper sternum and depression of the lower sternum (Fig. 20.7). Intrauterine oligohydramnios may lead to lateral dimpling of the elbows and knees. Other skeletal abnormalities include talipes, equinovarus, congenital hip dislocation, calcaneovalgus, polydactylia, syndactylia, and scoliosis.[5, 19] Severe oligohydramnios results in a classic Potter syndrome with low set ears, talipes, bowed limbs, dislocated hips, formed digits, indented thorax, severe pulmonary hypoplasia and arthrogryposis.[5]

Pulmonary

The structural changes of the rib cage, the lax abdominal muscles, and poor development of the diaphragm contribute to a compromised pulmonary toilet resulting in significant upper respiratory infections in many of the children with TS.[37] Initially, the neonatal prognosis depends directly on the degree of pulmonary development. Pneumothorax and pneumomediastinum have been reported in the neonate.[3] Compromised pulmonary development and chronic bronchitis place the child at an increased anesthetic risk.

Cardiac

Patent ductus arteriosus, atrial and ventral septal defects, or tetralogy of Fallot occurs in 10 to 17% of

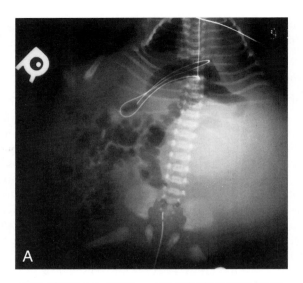

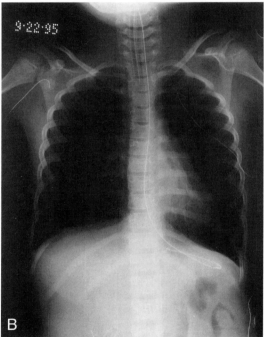

FIG. 20.7. **A,** Typical chest radiograph of newborn showing splayed appearance of lower ribs (chest radiograph of child in Figure 21.1). **B,** Seven-year follow-up on the same child after urinary diversion showing improvement in body habitus and rib flaring.

children.[19, 24] Serious cardiac anomalies may affect early neonatal care and subsequently delay urologic assessment.

Gastrointestinal

Defective fixation of the mid-gut to the posterior abdominal wall and a wide mesentery contribute to malrotation, atresia, volvulus, and stenosis in 30% of children.[19, 24] Gastroschisis, omphalocele, anorectal abnormalities, and splenic torsion also have been reported.[19, 24, 29, 30, 38]

DETRUSOR FUNCTION

Typically, the TS bladder is highly compliant, allowing for an excessive volume of urine stored at low pressure. Decreased detrusor contractility associated with the increased capacity leads to urinary stasis in the lower and upper urinary tract and a predisposition for sepsis. Spontaneous voiding can be achieved but may be at the expense of significant residual urine. Uninfected residual urine rarely leads to upper urinary tract deterioration because of the highly compliant bladder.

Relatively normal voiding pressures and insignificant postvoid residuals have been reported.[38] In a review by Kinahan et al., 44% of boys evaluated were noted to void spontaneously and 56% required intermittent catheterization.[39] With urodynamic assessment the authors described three distinct voiding patterns: normal, with modest postvoid residual; prolonged voiding with low leak point pressure; and an intermittent pattern. In addition, they noted that the ability to void was not affected by previous urinary reconstruction. Initial improvement in voiding after operative bladder reduction was not long lasting. The mean uroflowmetry pattern for children with spontaneous voiding was recorded as voided volume of 285 mL, a peak flow of 20 mL/second, residual volume 60 mL, and a voiding time of 34 seconds.[39] Voiding in these children was often accomplished by increasing intra-abdominal pressure with diaphragmatic contraction or manual suprapubic compression.

The large urachal cap or pseudodiverticulum combined with the capacious bladder capacity has stimulated interest in reductive cystoplasty for the improvement of detrusor function.[40, 41] However, there is little information to support any long-term improvement in the ability to void after reductive cystoplasty.[42] Kinahan showed no improvement in voiding efficiency over an extended period.[39]

SEXUAL FUNCTION

Preservation of the upper urinary tract in children with TS has led to increased survival through puberty and into adulthood. Woodhouse and Snyder surveyed a small group of adult men with TS regarding their sexuality.[43] Those few who responded to the questionnaire were able to achieve normal erections and orgasm. However, most reported retrograde ejaculation. Serum testosterone levels were normal in 66% along with elevated levels of luteinizing hormone and follicle-stimulating hormone. All the men were infertile.

Paternity has not been reported in TS, but it must be kept in mind that most men have had their orchidopexy performed at a later age than currently practiced. With the current philosophy of early orchidopexy it is possible, but not expected, that there will be an impact on spermatogenesis. However, the lack of spermatogonia in biopsied testes and the structural abnormalities of the genital tract will likely hamper the potential for fertility more than the timing of the orchidopexy.

DIAGNOSIS

Fetal sonography has played a major role in early identification of all genitourinary abnormalities. With sophisticated equipment and operator expertise the presence of TS can often be established in utero. A similar constellation of findings can be seen in the fetus with posterior urethral valves or the megacystis megaureter syndrome. Close inspection of the abdominal wall musculature will often hedge the differential diagnosis to that of TS. In utero intervention has been performed in children with TS without practical clinical gain.[44, 45]

In utero diagnosis of TS allows for a planned approach to management, directed by the pediatric urologist. At birth the diagnosis of TS is often obvious because of the pathognomonic physical findings of a loose, lax, wrinkled abdominal wall, flared chest, and undescended testes.

Several classifications of TS have been established based on severity and clinical presentation.[5, 25, 46, 47] For practical purposes, children may be grouped clinically into those with severe, moderate, or mild abnormalities. With severe presentation, survival is often limited by significant respiratory compromise because of pulmonary immaturity or dysplasia and renal dysplasia resulting in a Potter-like syndrome. Children classified with moderate involvement have combined renal and respiratory insufficiencies that mandate close observation and early intervention to minimize their sequela. Monitoring of the urinary system is necessary to prevent progressive renal deterioration secondary to stagnant urinary flow, urinary tract infections, and possible urinary tract obstruction. Urinary reconstruction may play an important role in preventing renal deterioration and recurrent sepsis.[47, 48] Children with mild involvement do not suffer from respiratory or renal compromise. While long-term follow-up is necessary, operative intervention is often limited to orchidopexy and abdominal wall reconstruction.

EVALUATION

A team approach by a pediatric urologist, neonatologist, and nephrologist is required to maximize the chances of a good outcome. On occasion, consultation with a pulmonologist or cardiologist may be required. Initially, the cardiorespiratory status must be established. All neonates should undergo a chest radiograph with particular attention paid to the possibility of a pneumothorax or pneumomediastinum. Cardiac sonography is indicated in selected patients. Aggressive pulmonary treatment may be required to maintain an adequate pulmonary toilet, oxygenation, and prevention of upper respiratory infections.

Urologic evaluation commences with abdominal sonography, assessing the upper and lower urinary tract. Attention should be paid to the degree of hydronephrosis and the volume and echogenicity of the renal parenchyma. Often the distal ureter is significantly more dilated than the proximal ureter; on occasion there is a rather marked transition of ureteral caliber. If the infant is clinically stable and is voiding through the urethra or draining through a patent urachus, further diagnostic testing can be postponed.

Children with renal insufficiency must undergo further testing including a voiding cystourethrogram to determine whether the insufficiency is influenced by true urinary obstruction or stagnant urinary flow. It is most important that any invasive imaging of the lower urinary tract be performed in a sterile environment with the child receiving preprocedural and postprocedural antibiotics. The abnormally dilated urinary system is susceptible to bacteriuria, and it is often difficult to clear once established. For this reason, lower urinary tract instrumentation should be limited and the decision to obtain a voiding cystourethrogram made on an individualized basis. When renal insufficiency and a poor urinary stream are present, urethral obstruction should be considered. Vesicoureteral reflux has been reported in 75% of children with TS.[25, 26]

An initial serum creatinine should be obtained and its trend followed over the first several days of life. A nadir creatine of ≥0.8 mg/dL or a serum creatinine that continues to increase is indicative of renal insufficiency. If the serum creatinine remains stable along with adequate voiding, a tempered management approach can be continued. However, when renal insufficiency is encountered a more aggressive approach may be required. All neonates should have a urine culture obtained at birth and receive oral prophylactic antibiotics.

When functional renal data are required, renal scintigraphy often provides information more objective than conventional intravenous urography. Parenchymal function can be evaluated by Tc-99m dimercaptosuccinic acid (DMSA). Renal clearance and obstruction can be assessed by Tc-99 diethylene triamine pentaacetic acid (DTPA), or Tc-99m mercapto-acetyl-triglycine (Mag 3).

INDICATIONS FOR INTERVENTION

There is no other pediatric urologic condition that requires more individualized patient care than TS. Each child has a unique constellation of problems, each resulting in its own set of considerations. Therefore, no one treatment plan is appropriate for all children. In general, operative management can be divided into three broad categories:[48] reconstruction of the urinary system, abdominal wall reconstruction, and orchidopexy. Controversies surround the benefits of urinary reconstruction as it relates to need, timing, and short- and long-term effect.[42, 49–51] Early aggressive operative intervention in all cases is countered by the fact that renal dysplasia may be inherent, thus preventing any intervention from improving the functional status of the kidneys. In addition, imaging studies depicting significant hydroureteronephrosis do not correlate with obstruction and that entity alone does not mandate reconstruction. Urinary reconstruction is beneficial in the child who has a component of obstructive uropathy and has been shown to have improved renal function with decompression of the urinary system. Reconstruction is also helpful in the child who has progressive hydroureteronephrosis associated with increasing renal compromise and in the child who has urinary tract infections caused by stagnant urine flow.

Endoscopic Internal Urethrotomy

While a true posterior obstruction may be present, it is thought to be rare.[15] However, the appearance of the posterior urethra is occasionally consistent with an obstructive process. Endoscopic internal urethrotomy has been advocated, with incision of the abnormal area with the hope of creating balanced voiding and decreased residual urine.[53–55] This procedure has been deemed effective, but long-term success has not been substantiated.[3, 4, 40]

Urinary Diversion

Urinary diversion may play a temporary role in the management of acute renal failure or urinary sepsis.[48] Children with true urethral atresia or obstruction will often have with a patent urachus effectively emptying their lower urinary tract and allowing for appropriate decompression of their upper urinary tracts. Vesicostomy may be beneficial in the compromised infant who does not have a patent urachus and is not a candidate for intermittent catheterization.[38] When vesicostomy is indicated, a standard Blocksom procedure, as described by Duckett, can be performed.[52] The stomal site is placed above the pubic symphysis and a rectangular wedge of fascia is excised. The vesicostomy is placed in the dome of the bladder with excision of the pseudodiverticulum when present.

Upper urinary tract diversion may be necessary in those few infants who show progressive renal insufficiency, urinary stasis, or recurrent urinary tract infections.[4] Proximal urinary diversion has been advocated to provide the most direct elimination of urine resulting in improved upper urinary tract decompression and preservation of renal function.[46, 56–58] However, because of the discrepancy between proximal and distal dilation, the renal pelvis and proximal ureter often are only minimally dilated, causing cutaneous pyelostomy or proximal loop ureterostomy to be technically difficult. In addition, temporary proximal ureteral diversion can complicate subsequent urinary reconstruction, particularly when ureteral tapering is necessary. When upper urinary tract decompression is required, low distal cutaneous ureterostomy has proven to be a better form of urinary drainage (Fig. 20.8).[48] The size of the ureter may lead to confusion between ureter and bowel. When in doubt, a no. 21 gauge needle can be inserted to aspirate lumenal contents and confirm the presence of urine. The large size of the ureter prevents postoperative stenosis and allows for a cutaneous end or loop ureteral stoma. When definitive reconstructive surgery is required, the proximal urinary system remains uncompromised, allowing for easier mobilization and greater flexibility if ureteral tailoring is warranted.[4]

Definitive Urinary Reconstruction

Although the combination of intermittent catheterization and prophylactic antibiotics has resulted in effective decompression of the lower and upper urinary tracts, improved function, and fewer episodes of urosepsis, selected children may benefit from a more aggressive management approach.[26, 57] When definitive urinary reconstruction is required, the approach to the ureter can be retroperitoneal. However, a transperitoneal approach is more practical because of the excessive tortuosity of the ureter and the associated abdominal wall reconstruction, which is frequently undertaken simultaneously. The ureter is isolated at the level of the bladder, and proximal dissection ensues. Dissection should be continued proximally through any transition zone between a dilated distal ureter and more normal-appearing proximal ureter. Care must be taken to prevent devascularization of the ureter. Ureteral length for a primary ureteroneocystostomy should not be a problem even with removal of all of the abnormal distal ureter.

The ability of the ureter to transmit urine into the bladder is inversely proportional to the dilation of the ureter. Ureteral tapering improves peristaltic activity and enhances urinary flow into the bladder. Various techniques have been described for ureteral tapering including ureteral imbrication and formal ureteral excision.[58–61] Ureteral imbrication is appropriate for marginally dilated ureters, but when massive ureteral dilation is present, formal excision is preferred to eliminate the bulky tissue that results from imbrication. Ureteral tapering should be performed over a no. 10 or no. 12 French catheter. The excised segment of ureter may

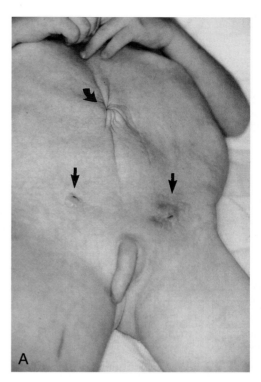

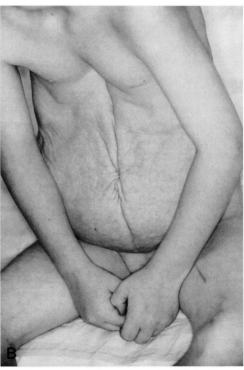

FIG. 20.8. A, Seven-year follow-up on the child in Figure 21.1. Straight arrows show sites of distal cutaneous ureterostomy. Note urine at site of right ureterostomy, left renal unit had insignificant renal function. Distal cutaneous ureterostomy totally decompressed left and right systems. Curved arrow indicates site of urachal membrane that ruptured as an infant and spontaneously closed over the next several years. B, Same child in sitting position.

take an unconventional course to preserve adequate ureteral blood supply. When a dilated renal pelvis and proximal ureter are encountered, appropriate tapering is also required of them with mandatory preservation of the proximal ureteral blood supply.[48]

Reduction Cystoplasty

Reduction cystoplasty appears to be a compelling component of urinary reconstruction. However, long-term follow-up of reduction cystoplasty has shown no objective advantage.[39, 42] With time the bladder regains its large size and loses its tone and this leads to inadequate emptying. Thus, reductive cystoplasty is not warranted as the sole reconstructive procedure. Intermittent catheterization would be a more appropriate form of management for the large, poorly contracting bladder. When formal urinary reconstruction includes ureteral tailoring, reductive cystoplasty can be performed simultaneously and may provide limited improvement of bladder emptying. When reduction cystoplasty is undertaken, it should incorporate the urachus, pseudodiverticulum and most of the dome (Fig. 20.9). The bladder is then closed in a pants-over-vest technique to reinforce the detrusor muscle.[48] A suprapubic tube should be placed at the time of closure and used for

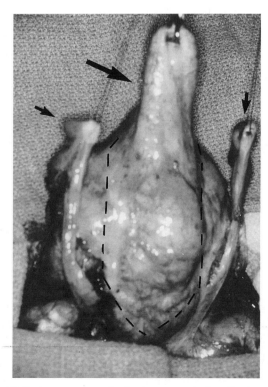

FIG. 20.9. Large arrow indicates pseudodiverticulum, urachal cap. Dotted line indicates portion to be removed. Small arrows show mobilized testes after transection of gonadal vessels.

postoperative assessment of the effectiveness of spontaneous bladder emptying. An appendicovesicostomy is a practical addition to urinary reconstruction, particularly for the child requiring intermittent catheterization.[48]

Abdominal Wall Reconstruction

The need for abdominal wall reconstruction is often cosmetic but should not be underestimated to provide for an appropriate self-image. Initially, elastic corsets were used with adequate results. Randolph popularized a procedure for abdominal wall reconstruction with excision of most of the abnormal portion of the lower abdominal wall, which preserved segmental motor nerves to the retained upper abdominal wall musculature.[62] While adequate, this procedure often resulted in persistent lateral bulging.

There is evidence showing that the muscular defect of the abdominal wall is more pronounced centrally and caudally. On that premise, Erhlich proposed a midline approach for abdominal wall reconstruction that incorporated a pants-over-vest fascial closure preserving the lateral fascia and muscles.[63] While this provided excellent lateral support, the umbilicus was sacrificed. Monfort refined the midline approach to abdominal wall reconstruction with preservation of a central fascial plate to retain the umbilicus.[64] His procedure has resulted in excellent operative exposure and postoperative cosmesis.[65]

Monfort's approach requires a midline incision through the skin from the tip of the xiphoid inferiorly, circumscribing the umbilicus and ending at the pubis. Full thickness skin and subcutaneous tissue flaps are created bilaterally (Fig. 20.10). The dissection is carried to the anterior axillary line. There is often variability and asymmetry of affected muscle and fascia and therefore care must be taken not to enter the peritoneum when mobilizing the flaps. An incision is made through the fascia entering the peritoneum. This incision should be made lateral to the superior epigastric artery. The incision is carried parallel to the artery from the costal margin to the symphysis pubis. The contralateral superior epigastric artery is then identified and a second parallel incision is made lateral to that artery. This leaves an intact central facial bridge with an umbilical island supported by both superior epigastric arteries. The two lateral incisions provide excellent exposure when major urinary reconstruction or orchidopexy is undertaken (Fig. 20.11).

The timing for abdominal wall reconstruction should be based on the need for other operative intervention. If the child will not require upper urinary tract reconfiguration, abdominal wall reconstruction can be undertaken at any time. If, however, there is a potential need for upper urinary tract remodeling, abdominal wall reconstruction should be deferred until that time.

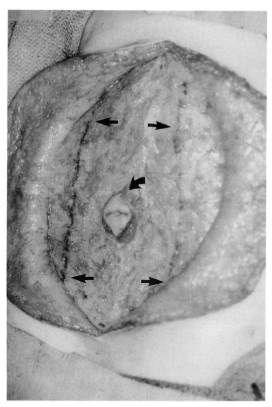

FIG. 20.10. Monfort abdominal wall reconstruction with re-flected skin flaps. Curved arrow shows presence of umbilicus. Straight arrows show a line to be used for entering the perito-neum, which is lateral to the superior upper epigastric artery.

Orchidopexy

The timing for orchidopexy is individualized based on the child's need for urinary reconstruction. If urinary tract reconstruction is required, orchidopexy should be performed simultaneously. If reconstructive surgery is not required, the timing for orchidopexy is variable. Placement of the testes in the scrotum is important for psychological and hormonal factors. Unfortunately, fer-tility does not appear to be affected. As indicated earlier, there is controversy regarding the potential for germ cell tumors.[34, 35]

Sacrifice of the gonadal artery may be required if the testicle is to be delivered into the scrotum as described by Fowler and Stephens.[66] However, if orchidopexy is undertaken within the first year of life, there is often adequate vascular length to deliver the testicle directly into the scrotum without transection of the testicular artery.

A staged approach using laparoscopic-assisted liga-tion of the gonadal artery followed by a 6-month delay before delivering the testicle into the scrotum has also been described.[67] This is an appealing alternative, partic-ularly for older boys who do not require urinary tract reconstruction or abdominal wall reconstruction.

The testes are often closely associated with dilated distal ureters. To determine whether the testicle can be delivered into the scrotum without sacrifice of the gonadal artery, the testis should be released from the ureter. Care should be taken not to disrupt the vascular

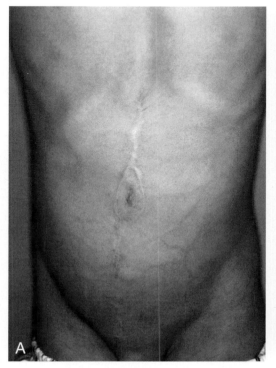

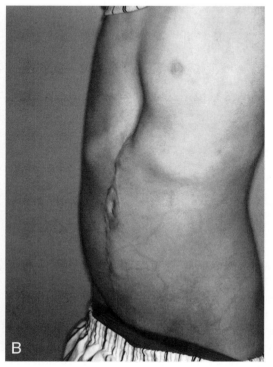

FIG. 20.11. Postoperative appearance after Monfort abdominal wall reconstruction.

supply of peritoneal pedicle running on both sides of the vas deferens. These vessels must be preserved if transection of the testicular artery is undertaken. Microvascular testicular autotransplantation has also been used successfully. The testicular artery is anastomosed to the inferior epigastric vessels.[68, 69] However, this procedure has not gained popularity because of the technical ease and effectiveness of the staged Fowler-Stephens orchidopexy.[67]

CONCLUSIONS

Children with TS have a variable but complex set of problems. The outlook remains poor for those children born with severe pulmonary and renal dysplasia. Children with minimal to marginal pulmonary dysplasia can do well regardless of renal dysplasia, provided appropriate urologic care is undertaken. Prophylactic antibiotics and intermittent catheterization may play a critical role in the management of these children. A select group of children benefit from aggressive urinary tract reconstruction. With current techniques, abdominal wall remodeling provides a satisfactory cosmetic result with preservation of the umbilicus. All boys benefit from bilateral orchidopexy. Early intervention may allow the testes to be brought into the scrotum without transection of the spermatic vessels.

MEGACYSTIS

Congenital megacystis unrelated to TS or a neurogenic bladder is rare. Megacystis megaureter syndrome secondary to vesicoureteral reflux has been reported.[70] The constant recycling of the urine from ureters to bladder because of reflux leads to progressive dilation of the bladder. The bladder though maintains normal detrusor function. After correction of the vesicoureteral reflux there is effective bladder emptying and improvement in the megacystis.

MEGACYSTIS MICROCOLON

Megacystis is associated with a rare condition of microcolon. This has been described as the megacystis microcolon intestinal hypoperistalsis syndrome (MMIHS).[71, 72] This condition has a female predilection and is characterized by hypoperistalsis, malrotation, dilated proximal ileum, narrowed distal ileum and colon, and bladder distention. MMIHS was originally described in 1976 by Berdon and since then there have been fewer than 100 reported cases.[73] MMIHS is an autosomal recessive problem. The pathogenesis is varied with possible associations with an abnormal autonomic nervous system,[74–77] degenerative smooth muscle disease,[78] imbalance of gut peptides,[79] pharmacologic interactions,[80, 81] and dysganglionosis or inflammation.[82]

Prognosis for MMIHS remains poor with death because of nutritional abnormality, sepsis, cardiac arrhythmia, complications of total peripheral nutrition, and renal failure.[71, 72] Pharmacologic agents and gastrointestinal hormones have been used unsuccessfully in regaining gastrointestinal peristalsis.[74]

Pathogenesis of the bladder distention is unknown. There is speculation that transmural-fibrosis of the bladder wall causes dyssynergic voiding with detrusor contractions occurring against a closed sphincter, ultimately resulting in bladder distention. The overly distended bladder may then interfere with the normal developmental rotation of the intestine.[71] Intermittent catheterization remains a necessary component for urinary drainage. It allows for stabilization of the bladder pathology and prevention of upper urinary tract deterioration.

BLADDER DIVERTICULUM

Primary

Bladder diverticula are most often secondary to posterior urethral valves, neurogenic bladder, or acquired secondary to outlet obstruction from bladder dysfunction.[83] Primary congenital diverticula are uncommon and occur more often in boys. They are usually solitary and located on the lateral bladder wall in the region of the ureteral hiatus. When the diverticulum arises superior to the ureteral orifice within the muscle meshwork contiguous with the ureteral orifice, protrusion can lead to incorporation of the ureteral orifice with subsequent vesicoureteral reflux (Fig. 20.12).[84]

When congenital diverticula of the bladder are noted after a urinary tract infection, diverticulectomy is the appropriate treatment. This can be performed without the need for ureteroneocystostomy if the ureteral orifice is uninvolved. When Hutch diverticula are encountered, excision of the diverticulum and reimplantation of the

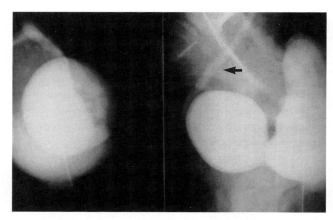

FIG. 20.12. Typical appearance of a Hutch diverticulum with associated vesicoureteral reflux (*arrow*).

ureter are required. Care must be taken to reconstitute the bladder base providing appropriate muscular support for the ureter.

Menkes Disease

Bladder diverticula are also noted in neurodegenerative disorders of childhood such as Menkes disease.[85] This is a progressive neurodegenerative condition inherited as a sex-linked recessive trait.[86] The gene abnormality is located on chromosome XQ12-Q13. Early manifestations are noted with hypothermia, hypotonia, and generalized myoclonic seizures. The faces of these children are distinctive with chubby, rosy cheeks, and their hair is kinky, colorless, and friable. Failure to thrive is often caused by feeding difficulties and associated severe mental retardation. Low serum copper and ceruloplasmin levels are present. If untreated, death usually occurs by the third year of life.[86] Because of the poor prognosis, a conservative approach is recommended for the bladder diverticula unless severe recurrent urinary tract infections are encountered.

Ehlers-Danlos

Ehlers-Danlos syndrome is a genetically heterogeneous connective tissue disorder. Children initially appear normal but skin hyperelasticity and joint hypermobility are soon encountered.[87] The defect is caused by a quantitative deficiency of collagen. The children often have urinary tract infections and poor bladder emptying. The diverticula are multifocal and variable in size (Fig. 20.13).[88] These children are at significant operative risk because of serious bleeding and poor wound healing. Thus, a conservative approach should be taken. Operative intervention is reserved for children with uncontrolled urinary tract infections and upper urinary tract deterioration.

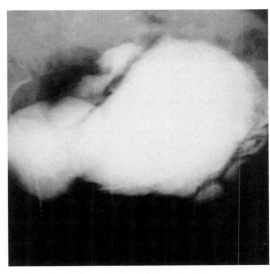

FIG. 20.13. Cystogram of a child with Ehlers-Danlos syndrome showing multifocal diverticula of various variable size.

REFERENCES

1. Parker RW. Absence of abdominal muscles in an infant. Lancet 1985;1:1252–1254.
2. Osler W. Congenital absence of the abdominal muscles with distended and hypertrophied urinary bladder. Bull Johns Hopkins Hosp 1901;12:331–333.
3. Skoog SJ. Prune belly syndrome. In: Kelalis PP, King LR, Belman AB, eds. Clinical Pediatric Urology. Philadelphia: WB Saunders, 1992;943–976.
4. Greskovich FJ, Nyberg LM. The prune belly syndrome: a review of its etiology, defects, treatment and prognosis. J Urol 1988; 140:707–711.
5. Wheatley JM, Stephens FD, Hutson JM. Prune belly syndrome: ongoing controversies regarding pathogenesis and management. Sem Pediatr Surgery 1996;5:95–106.
6. Rabinowitz R, Schillinger JF. Prune belly syndrome in the female subject. J Urol 1977;115:454.
7. Reinberg Y, Shapiro E, Manivel JC, et al. Prune belly syndrome in females: a triad of abdominal musculature deficiency and anomalies of the urinary and genital systems. J Pediatr 1991;118: 395–398.
8. Adeyokunnu AA, Familusi JB. Prune belly syndrome in two siblings and a first cousin. Am J Dis Child 1982;136:23–25.
9. Ives EJ. The abdominal muscle deficiency triad syndrome—experience with 10 cases. Birth Defects 1974;10:127–135.
10. Hoagland MH, Hutchins GM. Obstructive lesions of the lower urinary tract in the prune belly syndrome. Arch Pathol Lab Med 1987;111:154.
11. Amacker EA, Grass FS, Hickey DE, Hisley JC. An association of prune belly anomaly with trisomy 21. Am J Med Genet 1986;23:919.
12. Curry CJR, Jenson K, Holland J, et al. The Potter sequence: a clinical analysis of 80 cases. Am J Med Genet 1984;19:679.
13. Stumme EG. Ueber die symmetrischen kongenitalen Bauchmuskeldefekte und uber die Kombination derselben mit anderen Bildungsanomalien des Rumpfes. Mitt Grenzgebiete Med Chir 1903;11:548.
14. Beasley SW, Bettenay F, Hutson JM. The anterior urethra provides clues to the etiology of prune belly syndrome. Pediatr Surg Int 1988;3:169–172.
15. Stephens FD, Gupta D. Pathogenesis of the prune belly syndrome. J Urol 1994;152:2328–2331.
16. Stephens FD. Morphology and embryogenesis of the triad. In: Stephens FC, ed. Congenital malformation of the urinary tract. New York, NY: Praeger, 1983;485–451.
17. Mackie GG, Stephens FD. Duplex kidneys: a correlation of renal dysplasia with position of the ureteral orifice. J Urol 1975;114:274.
18. Nunn N, Stephens FD. The triad syndrome: a composite anomaly of the abdominal wall, urinary system and testes. J Urol 1961;86:782–794.
19. Wigger HJ, Blanc WA. The prune belly syndrome. Pathol Annu 1997;12:17–39.
20. Moerman P, Fryns J-P, Goddeeris P, et al. Pathogenesis of the prune belly syndrome: a functional urethral obstruction caused by prostatic hypoplasia. Pediatrics 1984;73:470–475.
21. Mininberg DT, Montoya F, Okada K, et al. Subcellular muscle studies in the prune belly syndrome. J Urol 1973;109:524–526.
22. Duckett JW Jr. Prune belly syndrome. In: Welch KJ, Randolph JG, Ravitch MM, et al., eds. Pediatric Surgery. Chicago: Year Book Medical Publishers, 1986;1193–1203.
23. Osathanondh V, Potter EL. Pathogenesis of polycystic kidneys. Arch Pathol 1964;77:510–513.
24. Manivel JC, Pettinato G, Reinberg Y, et al. Prune belly syndrome: clinocopathologic study of 29 cases. Pediatr Pathol 1989; 9:691–711.
25. Berdon WE, Baker DH, Wigger HJ, et al. The radiologic and pathologic spectrum of the prune belly syndrome. The importance

of urethral obstruction in prognosis. Radiol Clin North Am 1977;15:83–92.

26. Fallat ME, Skoog SJ, Belman AB, et al. The prune belly syndrome: a comprehensive approach to management. J Urol 1989;142:802.

27. Gearhart JP, Lee BR, Partin AW, et al. Quantitative histological evaluation of the dilated ureter of childhood, II: Ectopia, posterior urethral valves and the prune belly syndrome. J Urol 1995; 153:172–176.

28. Ehrlich RM, Brown WJ. Ultrastructural anatomic observations of the ureter in the prune belly syndrome. Birth Defects 1977;13:101.

29. Lattimer JK. Congenital deficiency of the abdominal musculature and associated genitourinary anomalies: a report of 22 cases. J Urol 1958;79:343–352.

30. Workman SJ, Kogan BA. Fetal bladder histology in posterior urethral valves and the prune belly syndrome. J Urol 1990; 144:337–339.

31. Deklerk DP, Scott WW. Prostatic maldevelopment in the prune belly syndrome: a defect in prostatic stromalepithelial interaction. J Urol 1978;120:341.

32. Sellers BB, McNeal R, Smith RV, et al. Congenital megalourethra associated with prune belly syndrome. J Urol 1976;116:814.

33. Orvis BR, Bottles K, Kogan BA. Testicular histology in fetuses with prune belly syndrome and posterior urethral valves. J Urol 1988;139:335.

34. Uehling DT, Zadina SP, Gilbert E. Testicular histology in triad syndrome. Urology 1984;23:364.

35. Massad CA, Cohen MB, Kogan BA, et al. Morphology and histochemistry of the infant testis in the prune belly syndrome. J Urol 1991;146:1598–1600.

36. Tayakkanonta K. The gubernaculum and its nerve supply. Aust N Z J Surg 1963;33:61.

37. Alford BA, Peoples WM, Resnick JS, L'Heureux PR. Pulmonary complications associated with the prune belly syndrome. Radiology 1978;129:401.

38. Teramoto R, Opas LM, Andrassy R. Splenic torsion with prune belly syndrome. J Pediatr 1981;98:91.

39. Kinahan TJ, Churchill BM, McLorie GA, et al. The efficiency of bladder emptying in the prune belly syndrome. J Urol 1992; 148:600–603.

40. Perlmutter AD. Reduction cystoplasty in prune belly syndrome. J Urol 1976;116:356.

41. Hannon MK. New concept in bladder remolding. Urology 1982; 19:6.

42. Bukowski TP, Perlmutter AD. Reduction cystoplasty in the prune belly syndrome: a long term follow-up. J Urol 1994;152: 2113–2116.

43. Woodhouse CRJ, Snyder H. Testicular and sexual function in adults with prune belly syndrome. J Urol 1985;133:607.

44. Elder JS. Intrauterine intervention for obstructive uropathy. Kidney 1990;22:19.

45. Nakayama DK, Harrison MR, Chinn DH, et al. The pathogenesis of prune belly. Am J Dis Child 1984;138:834–836.

46. Welsch KJ, Kearney GP. Abdominal musculature deficiency syndrome: Prune-belly. J Urol 1974;111:693–700.

47. Woodard JR, Parrott TS. Reconstruction of the urinary tract in prune belly uropathy. J Urol 1978b;119:824.

48. Joseph DB. Triad syndrome. In: Graham SD, Glenn JF, eds. Glenns Urologic Surgery. Philadelphia: Lippincott-Raven, 1998: 723–728.

49. Duckett JW. Prune belly syndrome. In: Welsch KJ, Randolph JG, Ravitch MM, et al., eds. Pediatric Surgery. Chicago, IL: Year Book, 1986;1193–1203.

50. Ransley PG. Prune, pseudo prune and other dysplastic uropathies. In: Whitaker RH, ed. Current Perspectives in Pediatric Urology. New York, NY: Springer Verlag, 1989.

51. McMullin ND, Hutson JM, Kelly JH. Minimal surgery in the prune-belly syndrome. Pediatr Surg Int 1988;3:51–54.

52. Duckett JW Jr. Cutaneous vesicostomy in childhood. Urol Clin North Am 1974;1:485.

53. Cukier J. Resection of the urethra with the prune belly syndrome. Birth Defects 1977;13:95.

54. Snyder HM, Harrison NW, Whitfield HN, Williams DI. Urodynamics in the prune belly syndrome. Br J Urol 1976;48:663.

55. Woodhouse CRJ, Kellett MJ, Williams DI. Minimal surgical interference in the prune belly syndrome. Br J Urol 1979;51:475.

56. Randolph JG. Total surgical reconstruction for patients with abdominal muscular deficiency ("prune belly") syndrome. J Pediatr Surg 1977;12:1033.

57. Wooddard JR, Trulock TS. Prune belly syndrome. In: Walsh PC, et al., eds. Campbell's Urology, 5th ed. Philadelphia: WB Saunders, 1986;2159–2167.

58. Hendren WH. Functional restoration of decompensated ureters in children. Am J Surg 1970;199:477.

59. Kalicinski ZH, Kansy J, Kotarbinska B, et al. Surgery of megaureters—modification of Hendren's operation. J Pediatr Surg 1977; 12:183.

60. Starr A. Ureteral plication: a new concept in ureteral tailoring for megaureter. Invest Urol 1979;17:153.

61. Ehrlich RM. The ureteral folding technique for megaureter surgery. J Urol 1985;134:668.

62. Randolph JG, Cavett C, Eng G. Abdominal wall reconstruction in the prune belly syndrome. J Pediatr Surg 1981a;16:960.

63. Ehrlich RM, Lesavoy MA, Fine RN. Total abdominal wall reconstruction in the prune belly syndrome. J Urol 1986;136:282.

64. Monfort G, Guys JM, Bocciardi A, Coquet M, Chevallier D. A novel technique for reconstruction of the abdominal wall in the prune belly syndrome. J Urol 1991;146:639–640.

65. Parrott TS, Woodard JR. The Monfort operation for abdominal wall reconstruction in the prune belly syndrome. J Urol 1992; 148:688–690.

66. Fowler R, Stephens FD. The role of testicular vascular anatomy in the salvage of high undescended testes. Aust N Z J Surg 1959;29:92.

67. Law GS, Pérez LM, Joseph DB. Two-stage Fowler-Stephens orchidopexy with laparoscopic clipping of the spermatic vessels. J Urol 1997;158:1205.

68. Wacksman J, Dinner M, Staffon RA. Technique of testicular autotransplantation using a microvascular anastomosis. Surg Gynecol Obstet 1980;150:399.

69. Woodard JR, Parrott TS. Orchidopexy in the prune belly syndrome. Br J Urol 1978a;50:348.

70. Gearhart JP. Bladder and urachal abnormalities: the exstrophy-epispadias complex. In: Kelalis PP, King LR, Belman AB, eds. Clinical Pediatric Urology. Philadelphia: WB Saunders, 1992; 579–619.

71. Srikanth MS, Ford EG, Isaacs H, Mahour GH. Megacystis microcolon intestinal hypoperistalsis syndrome: late sequelae and possible pathogenesis. J Pediatr Surg 1993;28:957–959.

72. Kupferman JC, Stewart CL, Schapfel DM, Kaskel FJ, Fine RN. Megacystis-microcolon-intestinal hypoperistalsis syndrome. Pediatr Nephrol 1995;9:626–627.

73. Berdon WE, Baker DH, Blanc WA, et al. Megacystis microcolon intestinal hypoperistalsis syndrome: a new cause of intestinal obstruction in the newborn. Report of radiologic findings in five newborn girls. Am J Roentgenol 1976;126:957–964.

74. Anneren G, Meurling S, Olsen L. Megacystis microcolon intestinal hypoperistalsis syndrome (MMIHS), an autosomal recessive disorder: clinical reports and review of the literature. Am J Med Genet 1991;41:251–254.

75. Jona JZ, Werlin SL. The megacystis microcolon intestinal hypoperistalsis syndrome: report of a case. J Pediatr Surg 1981; 16:749–751.

76. Kubota M, Ikeda K, Ito Y. Autonomic innervation of the intestine from a baby with megacystis microcolon intestinal hypoperistalsis syndrome: electrophysiological study. J Pediatr Surg 1989; 24:1267–1270.

77. Gillis DA, Grantmyre EB. Megacystis microcolon intestinal hypoperistalsis syndrome: survival of a male infant. J Pediatr Surg 1985;20:279–281.

78. Puri P, Lake BD, Gorman F, et al. Megacystis microcolon intestinal hypoperistalsis syndrome: a visceral myopathy. J Pediatr Surg 1983;18:64–68.

79. Hiroe R, Toyohara T. Autonomic innervation of the intestine from a baby with megacystis microcolon intestinal hypoperistalsis syndrome: immunohistochemical study. J Pediatr Surg 1989; 24:1264–1266.

80. Dogruyol H. Do certain drugs cause the megacystis microcolon

intestinal hypoperistalsis syndrome. Turk J Pediatr 1989;31: 253–256.

81. Kirtane J, Talwalker V, Dastur DK. Megacystis microcolon intestinal hypoperistalsis syndrome: possible pathogenesis. J Pediatr Surg 1984;19:206–208.

82. Srikant MS, Ford EG, Isaacs H Jr, Mahour GH. Megacystis microcolon intestinal hypoperistalsis syndrome: late sequelae and possible pathogenesis. J Pediatr Surg 1993;28:957–959.

83. Stage KH, Tank ES. Primary congenital bladder diverticula in boys. Urology 1992;40:536.

84. Stephens FD, Smith ED, Hutson JM. Congenital anomalies of the urinary and genital tracts. Oxford Isis Medical Media 1996.

85. Bankier A. Menkes disease. J Med Genet 1995;32(3):213–215.

86. Haslan RHA. Neurodegenerative disorders of childhood. In: Behrman RE, Kliegman RM, Arvin AM, eds. Nelson's Textbook of Pediatrics. Philadelphia: WB Saunders, 1996;1727–1728.

87. Darmstadt GL, Lane AT. The skin. In: Behrman RE, Kliegman RM, Arvin AM, eds. Nelson's Textbook of Pediatrics. Philadelphia: WB Saunders, 1996;1875–1876.

88. Bade JJ, Ypma AF, VanElk P, Mensink HJ. A pelvic mass: bladder diverticulum with haemorrhage in Ehlers-Danlos Scandinavia. J of Urology & Nephrology 1994;28:319–322.

CHAPTER 21

Bladder and Cloacal Exstrophy

John P. Gearhart

BLADDER EXSTROPHY

Exstrophy of the bladder is rare and the incidence of bladder extrophy is calculated to be from 1 per 30,000 to 50,000 live births with male to female ratio ranging from 1.5 to 5 to 1.[1,2] There is some evidence for genetic predisposition to exstrophy and epispadias. The risk for recurrence of exstrophy or epispadias in a given family is 1 of 275 births. The likelihood of an exstrophic parent producing a child with exstrophy or epispadias is increased to 1 of 70, or 500 times the risk of the general population.[3,4]

The exstrophy-epispadias complex represents one of the most difficult surgical challenges for the pediatric urologist. Although this is one of the most severe birth defects compatible with survival, contemporary management and appropriate reconstruction can provide patients with a normal life. The approach has evolved through decades of experience and consists of a staged approach.

It is crucial that proper reconstruction be successful with the initial attempt, which provides the best chance for obtaining an adequate bladder capacity and thereby urinary continence. Children who undergo two or more closures almost never achieve satisfactory continence because their bladders hardly ever achieve adequate capacity for bladder neck reconstruction alone without augmentation.[5] To this end, care of the patient with exstrophy should be undertaken only by a surgeon experienced with this condition, and only at those centers equipped and staffed for proper postoperative management.

The goals of exstrophy reconstruction are anatomic closure of the bladder and abdominal wall, preservation of renal function, urinary continence with volitional voiding, and functional and cosmetically satisfactory external genitalia. This chapter describes a method by which these goals usually are accomplished at the author's institution, and report his group's experience with more than 523 patients with exstrophy-epispadias observed at Johns Hopkins Hospital.

Prenatal Diagnosis

Exstrophy fo the bladder is rarely diagnosed prenatally. A retrospective reivew of 43 prenatal ultrasound studies from 25 pregnancies resulting in live delivery of an infant with classic bladder exstrophy identified five criteria associated with bladder exstrophy: 1) a bladder that was never demonstrated on ultrasound was found in 71% of the cases, 2) a lower abdominal bulge that represents the exstrophied bladder was found in 47% (Fig. 21.1), 3) a small penis with anteriorly displaced scrotum was found in 57% of the males, 4) a low set umbilical insertion was found in 29%, 5) abnormal widening of the iliac crests was found in 18%.[6] Because the fetal bladder can be seen on prenatal ultrasound after 14 weeks gestation, the prenatal diagnosis of bladder exstrophy should be entertained anytime the bladder is not demonstrated or if any of these factors or combination of factors are noted.[6]

The Newborn Period and Preoperative Considerations

Immediately after birth a complete physical examination is performed (Fig. 21.2). The umbilical cord is secured with a heavy silk suture, rather than a plastic clip, to prevent bladder mucosal trauma and damage. The bladder mucosa is best protected with clear plastic wrap and each time the diaper is changed the bladder surface should be irrigated with sterile saline and the plastic wrap replaced. Ultrasonography of the kidneys is performed to rule out hydronephrosis, the back and buttocks are carefully examined to rule out spinal abnormalities, and a neurologic examination is performed to evaluate lower urinary tract and lower extremity innervation. Spinal ultrasound and radiographs are performed when abnormalities are suspected, but the incidence of spinal cord anomalies is low.[7]

Intravenous antibiotics are started before surgery and maintained for 7 to 10 days after surgery. Oral prophylactic antibiotics are used thereafter until bladder neck reconstruction and ureteral reimplantation have

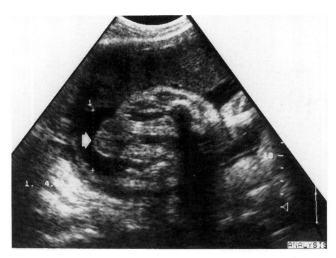

FIG. 21.1. A transverse view of the lower abdomen in the male fetus with bladder exstrophy. The bladder mass can be seen on the anterior aspect of the abdomen (*arrow*).

obviated vesicoureteral reflux. The anesthesiologist should be alerted to avoid the use of nitrous oxide, if possible, to minimize bowel distention and facilitate abdominal wall closure. In addition, a nasogastric tube is placed once anesthesia is initiated and left in place postoperatively until normal bowel function resumes. Products containing latex should be avoided to minimize catastrophic latex reactivity.

Initial Bladder Closure

Closure of the pelvic ring is important for the initial closure and for the eventual attainment of urinary continence. When the initial closure is carried out within the first 72 hours of life (while the newborn is still under the effect of the maternal hormone, relaxin) the pelvic ring can sometimes be closed effectively without the

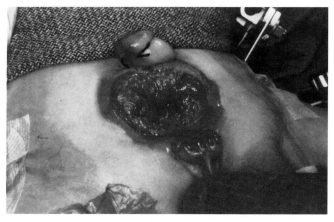

FIG. 21.2. Newborn male with bladder exstrophy. Note the large bladder template and the very short urethral groove with diminutive phallus.

need for osteotomies.[8] However, in the author's opinion, besides bringing the pelvic ring together, osteotomies allow for better approximation of the erectile bodies and elongation of the penis in the male and for the approximation of the clitoral bodies and creation of labia majora in the female. In addition, it moves the perineal structures more posteriorly and allows the bladder neck and posterior urethra to be displaced backward in a more normal position.

The choice of procedure should be made only on the basis of examination under general anesthesia. However, when the pubic separation is wide, the surgery is being performed on an older patient, or when an earlier closure has failed, osteotomy is essential to achieve good closure of the pelvic ring. The osteotomy should be performed at the same time of the bladder closure because it reduces tension on the abdominal wound and helps secure the closure. In addition, the osteotomy helps restore the pelvic anatomy and thus increases the chances of eventual continence and reduces the likelihood of later uterine prolapse.[9] The author's preference is the combined anterior innominate and vertical iliac osteotomy, which involves dividing the innominate bone above the acetabulum.[10] Formerly, only an anterior innominate osteotomy was used for failure or late closure of bladder exstrophy because results were superior to those of the older approach of posterior iliac osteotomy.[11] These results include elimination of the need to turn the patient intraoperatively, less blood loss, better apposition and mobility of the pubic rami at the time of closure, and allowing for secure external fixation in the child older than 6 months of age. However, the initial and long-term follow-up of a new combined osteotomy in more than 64 patients has led to its exclusive use in all of our patients with exstrophy.[10, 11]

In most cases, a combined anterior innominate and vertical iliac osteotomy is conducted within the periosteum through the same anterior skin incision for better pelvic correction (Fig. 21.3).[10] McKenna et al.[12] have proposed the diagonal mid-iliac osteotomy performed through the same incision of the exstrophy closure. However, the experience with this technique is limited and only short-term follow-up is available. In addition, there is a concern about the risk of infection because the incision is made next to the colonized bladder. Long-term follow-up and larger numbers will define the role of this approach. Osteotomy of the superior ramus of the pubis (pelvic osteotomy)[13, 14] is another technique that has been used recently. This approach, which was successfully used in neonates for primary closure, is insufficient for reclosure or for late closure of bladder exstrophy.

Patients undergoing closure without osteotomy and those who had only a posterior osteotomy are maintained in modified Bryant's traction for 4 weeks. If an anterior approach is used, the external fixator is left in

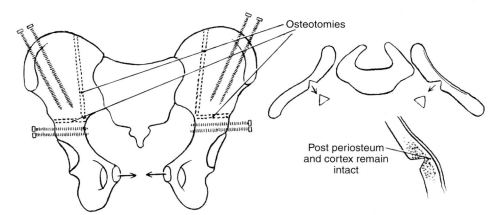

FIG. 21.3. The combined anterior innominate and posterior vertical osteotomies for closure of bladder exstrophy. Developed by Sponseller.

place for 4 to 6 weeks, (Fig. 21.4) and light Buck's traction is maintained with the legs supported on a pillow.

The bladder closure starts with dissection and excision of the umbilicus (Fig. 21.5*A–D*). The bladder muscle is freed from the rectus sheath on each side. The peritoneum is exposed above the bladder, and a careful extraperitoneal dissection reveals the retropubic space on each side (Fig. 21.5*E & F*). The wide band of fibers and muscle representing the urogenital diaphragm is detached subperiosteally from the pubis bilaterally down to the inferior ramus to allow the bladder neck and posterior urethra enough mobility to fall deep within the pelvic ring (Fig. 21.5*G & H*). The bladder is closed in the midline using running 3-0 polyglycolic acid sutures in the first layer and interrupted sutures in the second layer (Fig. 21.5*I & J*). The posterior urethra is also closed well onto the base of the penis proximally over a 14-French catheter. The posterior urethra and urethral

opening should allow enough resistance to stimulate bladder growth and prevent bladder prolapse, but not be so tight as to cause dilation of the upper tracts. The suture line should be covered with a second layer of local tissue, if possible.

The bladder is drained by a 10-French suprapubic malecot catheter for 4 weeks and with a 3.5-French ureteral stent for 2 weeks to avoid ureteral obstruction and hypertension. The urethra is not stented so as to avoid pressure necrosis and prevent accumulation of secretions, which could become infected and lead to wound disruption. After the bladder and urethra are closed and all drainage tubes are placed, the pelvis is closed by placing medial pressure on both greater trochanters. A no. 2 nylon horizontal mattress suture is placed in the pubis with the knot tied away from the neourethra (Fig. 21.5*K*). A simple umbilicoplasty is performed with a U-shaped skin flap, and the drainage tubes are brought out through this site. Then, midline closure of the rectus muscles and fascia is performed using interrupted figure-of-eight 2-0 polyglycolic acid sutures.

If the male urethral plate is too short to allow primary closure, it can be divided and elongated by using paraexstrophy skin flaps.[15] However, a review of 78 patients who had paraexstrophy skin flaps as part of their initial reconstruction showed a 40% complication rate, most commonly a urethral stricture.[16] Therefore, the author has reduced the use of this technique. If paraexstrophy flaps are necessary, it is important to follow plastic surgical principles to ensure viability of these rotational flaps. If paraexstrophy flaps are used, any drainage tubes exiting the urethra can cause ischemia of these flaps and stricture formation and thus they must be only brought out suprapubically.[16]

In the female, paraexstrophy skin flaps should never be used because the female urethra needs no lengthening, and their use is associated with a high complication rate, including urethro-vaginal fistula. Broad spectrum

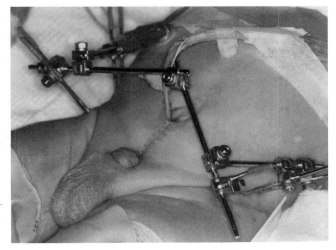

FIG. 21.4. Fixator pins and external fixating device, along with urinary drains used after bladder exstrophy closure.

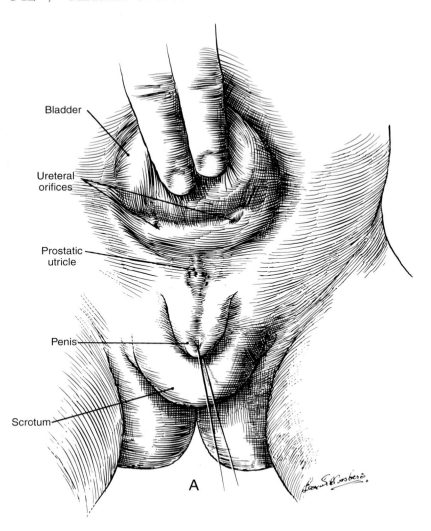

Bladder

Ureteral
orifices

Prostatic
utricle

Penis

Scrotum

A

FIG. 21.5. Steps in primary bladder closure with or without osteotomy. **A,** Exstrophy in newborn male. **B–D,** Incision around the umbilicus and bladder down to the urethral plate. **E–G,** Incision of paraexstrophy rotation flaps are needed to lengthen the posterior urethra. **H and I,** Development of the retropubic space from below the area of umbilical dissection to facilitate separation from the rectus sheath and muscle. **J,** Medial fan of the rectus muscle attaching behind the prostate to urogenital diaphragm. Urogenital diaphragm and anterior corpus are freed from the pubis in a periosteal plane. **K,** Urogenital diaphragm is incised. **L and M,** Ureteral stents and S-P tube are left to drain the bladder, and the bladder and the urethra are closed in two layers. **N,** Closures of the abdominal wall, the symphysis pubis and reconstruction of a new umbilicus.

antibiotics are administered before, during, and after the procedure to prevent contamination of the clean surgical wound from the colonized bladder exstrophy. Because of the high probability of inguinal hernia, bilateral inguinal exploration is performed through the same surgical incision and if hernias are found, they are repaired.[17]

Newborns are maintained in external fixation and modified Buck's traction for 4 weeks, until satisfactory healing is assessed radiographically. If an osteotomy is not performed, modified Bryant's traction is used to help maintain the pubic bones in apposition. Children who have had failed closure attempts undergo the same type of osteotomy as newborns and are maintained at bedrest, in external fixation and modified Buck's traction, for 6 to 8 weeks. "Mummy wrapping" is an insecure and unreliable method of maintaining pelvic ring closure.[5]

The postoperative management of the patient with exstrophy, especially after the initial bladder closure, is as important to the success of the operation as the procedure itself. Nurses experienced with patients with exstrophy should be charged with their daily care while the closure of the pelvis, bladder, and abdominal wall heal. These children should be kept comfortable and relaxed to prevent any abdominal straining or twisting. To this end, adequate analgesics, sedatives, and antispasmodics should be administered. Nasogastric suction is continued until there is evidence of bowel function, and then diet should be slowly advanced; if necessary, parenteral nutrition should be instituted. In addition, all possible measures should be taken to keep the wounds clean and free from infection, and strict attention to handwashing and dressing changes cannot be overemphasized. If an external fixation device is used, then proper care of the pin sites with peroxide-soaked cotton swabs must be performed at least three times daily.

The factors that are important for achieving successful primary closure have been well-documented. These include use of osteotomy, avoidance of urethral tubes and abdominal distention, use of postoperative antibiotics,

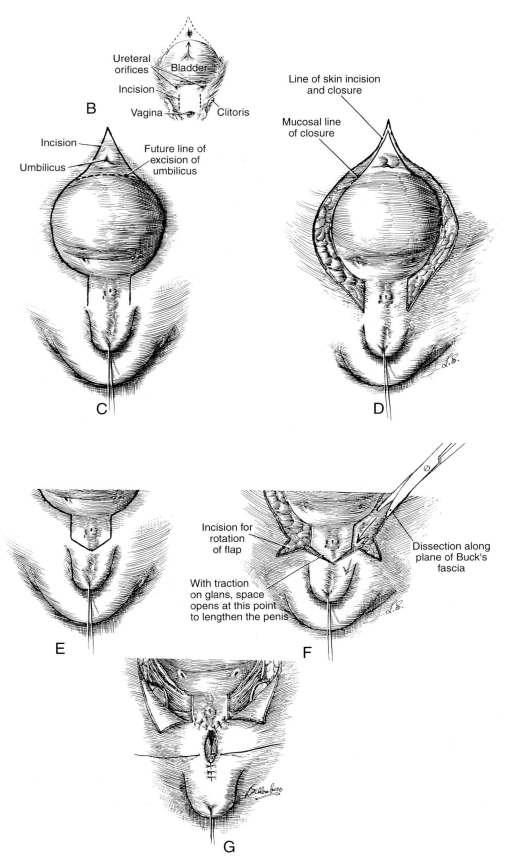

B

Ureteral orifices
Bladder
Incision
Vagina
Clitoris

C

Incision
Umbilicus
Future line of excision of umbilicus

D

Line of skin incision and closure
Mucosal line of closure

E

F

Incision for rotation of flap
With traction on glans, space opens at this point to lengthen the penis
Dissection along plane of Buck's fascia

G

FIG. 21.5. *Continued.*

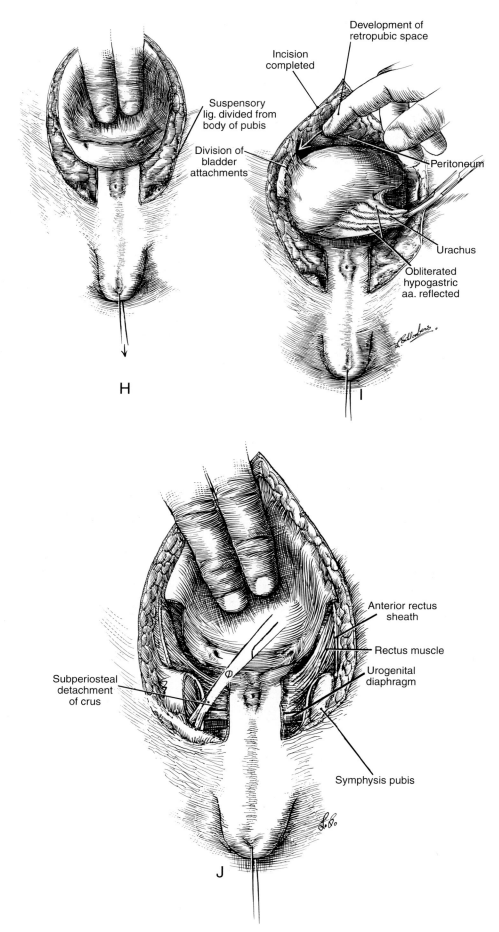

Suspensory lig. divided from body of pubis

Division of bladder attachments

Incision completed

Development of retropubic space

Peritoneum

Urachus

Obliterated hypogastric aa. reflected

H

I

Anterior rectus sheath

Rectus muscle

Urogenital diaphragm

Symphysis pubis

Subperiosteal detachment of crus

J

FIG. 21.5. *Continued.*

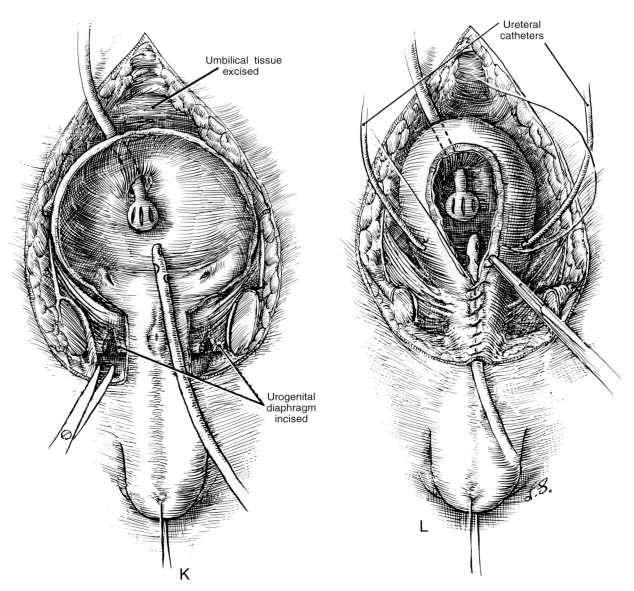

Umbilical tissue
excised

Urogenital
diaphragm
incised

Ureteral
catheters

K

L

FIG. 21.5. *Continued.*

pelvic immobilization and fixation, ureteral stenting catheters, and proper pain control.[18,19] The bladder outlet is calibrated with a sound 4 to 6 weeks after closure, and if adequate, the suprapubic tube is removed after a urine culture is obtained. An intravenous urogram or sonogram is obtained to assess the status of the upper urinary tracts before the patient leaves the hospital. If the initial studies show good drainage, the upper urinary tracts are evaluated by ultrasound at 6-month intervals. Prophylactic antibiotics are usually continued. In patients with upper urinary tract dilation and high residual urine, cystoscopy followed by urethral dilation or intermittent catheterization may be necessary. Occasionally patients will develop recurrent pyelonephritis without bladder outlet obstruction, and bilateral ureteral reim-

plantation will need to be performed as a separate stage before bladder neck reconstruction. If uncontrollable hydronephrosis develops, revision of the bladder outlet is performed. Rarely, a child will require urinary diversion, to a nonrefluxing colon conduit,[20] or a single-staged reconstruction with bladder augmentation and continent diversion to protect renal function.

Epispadias Repair

Epispadias repair is usually performed on children approximately 1 year of age because it has been shown that the epispadias repair can contribute significantly to the development of bladder capacity (Fig. 21.6*A* & *B*). A median increase in bladder capacity of 54.5 mL was

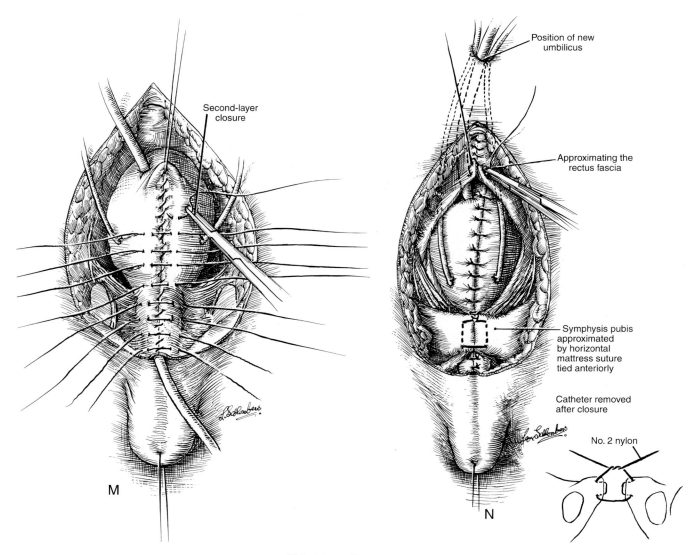

Second-layer closure

Position of new umbilicus

Approximating the rectus fascia

Symphysis pubis approximated by horizontal mattress suture tied anteriorly

Catheter removed after closure

No. 2 nylon

M

N

FIG. 21.5. *Continued.*

achieved within 22 months after primary epispadias repair in males with exstrophic bladders smaller than 60 mL.[21] Because boys with bladder exstrophy have a small penis with little extra penile skin, stimulation with intramuscular testosterone 2 mg/kg is used, 5 weeks and 2 weeks preceding the surgical repair.[22]

The goals of penile reconstruction in patients with exstrophy are to reconstruct the urethra and glans penis, release potential penile length, correct dorsal chordee, and achieve adequate skin coverage. There are several approaches to epispadias repair. The author's preference is the modified Cantwell-Ransley urethroplasty in which the urethral plate is tubularized and transferred to the ventral side of the corpora.[23, 24]

As mentioned earlier, the Cantwell-Ransley technique is preferred for epispadias repair (Fig. 21.6A–K).[22] It provides a straighter urethra, better correction of

chordee, a lower fistula rate, and a better cosmetic result than the modified Young technique that was previously used. Briefly, traction is placed on the penis with a nylon stitch through the glans. A Z-plasty incision is made at the base of the penis to permit exposure and division of the suspensory ligament and tethering scar tissue (Fig. 21.6A & B). An IPGAM procedure (reverse MAGPI) is performed at the distal urethral plate to allow the meatus to be advanced out onto the glans. Parallel incisions 18 mm apart are made on the long axis of the urethral plate from the tip of the glans to the prostatic urethra (Fig. 21.6A & B). Glandular wings are developed by excising triangular-shaped areas of skin adjacent to the distal urethra, and the skin lateral to the urethral plate is undermined and mobilized (Fig. 21.6C & D). The skin of the penis is degloved, and then the corpora cavernosa are separated from each other and from the

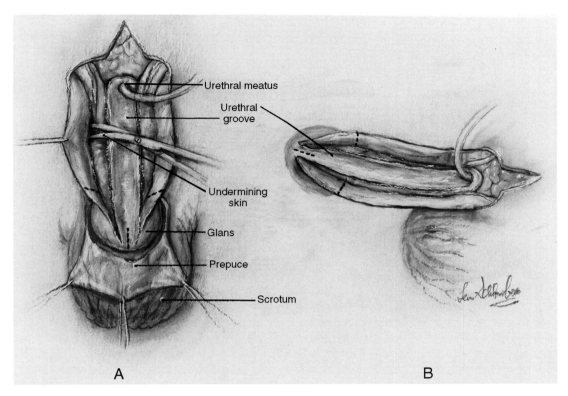

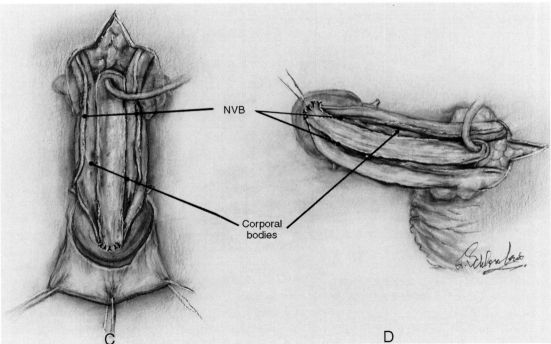

FIG. 21.6. Steps in Cantwell-Ransley epispadias repair. **A and B,** Incision of the urethral groove and mobilization of penile skin. **C and D,** Meatal advancement is performed and neurovascular bundles are identified and exposed. **E and F,** Separation of the urethral groove from the corporal bodies with dissection initially started from below. **G and H,** Mobilization of the neurovascular bundles from corporal bodies and incision in corporal bodies. Incision in corporal bodies. Closure of urethral groove to tip of penis, closure of corporal incision displacing the urethra ventrally. Further sutures placed distally to further bury the urethra under the corporal bodies. **I,** Corpora closed above the ventrally displaced urethra, and the glans is closed. **J and K,** Complete repair with the urethra below corporal bodies and skin closure of the penis.

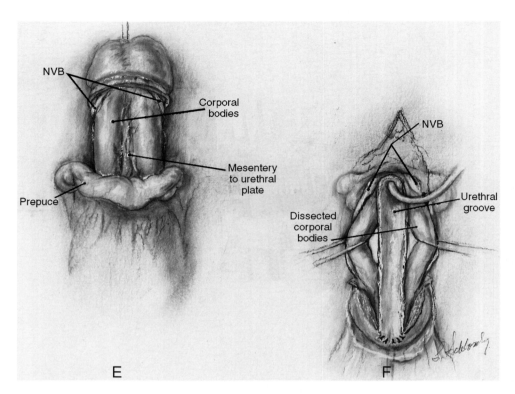

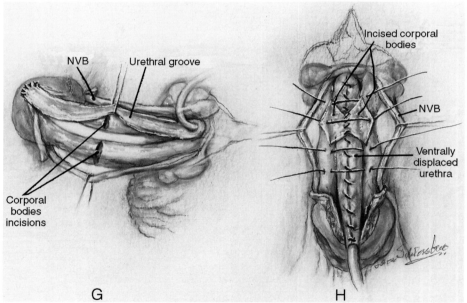

FIG. 21.6. *Continued.*

urethral plate (Fig. 21.6*E* & *F*). Care is taken to preserve the mesentary to the urethral plate, which arises proximally and courses between the corporal bodies. The neurovascular bundles are identified, dissected free of each corporal body, and isolated with vessel loops to prevent injury. The urethral plate is then closed linearly over an 8-French silicone stent with 6-zero polyglactin suture (Fig. 21.6*G*). The corpora are then transposed and rotated over the urethra and sutured together using 5-zero polydiaxanone, displacing the urethra ventrally while preserving the neurovascular bundles.

If correction of chordee is impossible with the described maneuvers, a cavernosocavernostomy is performed at the site of maximal angulation (Fig. 21.6*H*).[25]

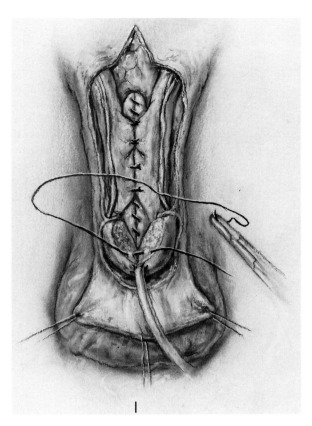

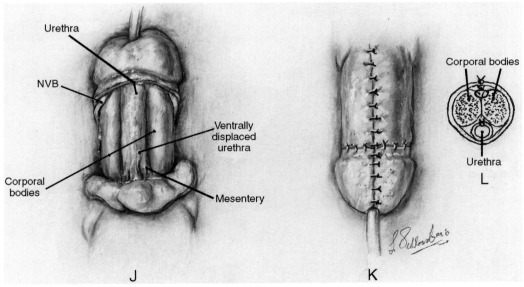

FIG. 21.6. *Continued.*

The glans wings are closed over the glandular urethra using subcuticular 5-zero polyglactin (Fig. 21.6*I*), the glans epithelium is closed with 6-zero polyglactin, and the skin is tailored and trimmed to cover the penis and closed with 5-zero polyglactin suture (Fig. 21.6*J & K*). The Z-plasty at the base of the penis is closed with interrupted 5-zero polyglactin sutures. The silicone stent is secured to the penis and left in the urethra to provide drainage for 10 to 12 days.

Combined Bladder Closure and Epispadias Repair

There has been recent interest in combined bladder exstrophy closure and epispadias repair. The author reviewed 16 patients who underwent combined repair after a prior failed closure. There were no instances of prolapse or dehiscence and all patients underwent an osteotomy at the time of closure. Continence rates and complications were the same as an age-matched group of patients with failed closures undergoing standard staged repair. This approach would be suitable for those patients undergoing late initial exstrophy closure or re-closure in select circumstances.[26]

Bladder Neck Reconstruction

Bladder neck reconstruction is usually performed when the child is 4- to 5-years of age and mature enough to cooperate with toilet training. The bladder capacity is measured under anesthesia. If the capacity is 60 mL or greater, bladder neck reconstruction can be considered. Because all patients with exstrophy have vesicoureteral reflux, an antireflux procedure is required at the time of bladder neck reconstruction. The bladder is exposed and opened using a midline or a lower transverse incision and the bladder neck is dissected completely free of surrounding structures (Fig. 21.7A). The intersymphseal bar can be incised to enhance visualization. After bilateral cross trigonal (Cohen) or cephalotrigonal[27] ureteral reimplantation is performed (Fig. 21.7B & C), a 15-mm wide mucosal strip extending from the midtrigone to the prostatic urethra in a length of 3 cm, is outlined

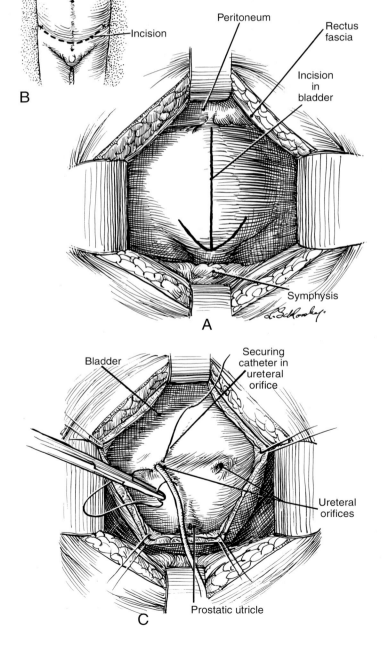

FIG. 21.7. Steps in Young-Dees Leadbetter reconstruction for continence. **A and B,** Midline incision of the bladder. **C–G,** Ureteral mobilization with transtrigonal or cephalotrigonal course for reimplantation. Mucosal strip of trigone forms the bladder neck and prostatic urethra. Lateral denuded muscle triangles are lengthened by several small incisions to allow tailoring of the bladder neck reconstruction. **H and I,** The denuded muscle is closed over the closed mucosal strip. **J,** Bladder neck suspension is performed, and the bladder neck and urethra are unstented. Drainage is by ureteral catheters and suprapubic tube. Bladder outlet resistance can be estimated by water manometer. (Drawings by Leon Schlossberg.)

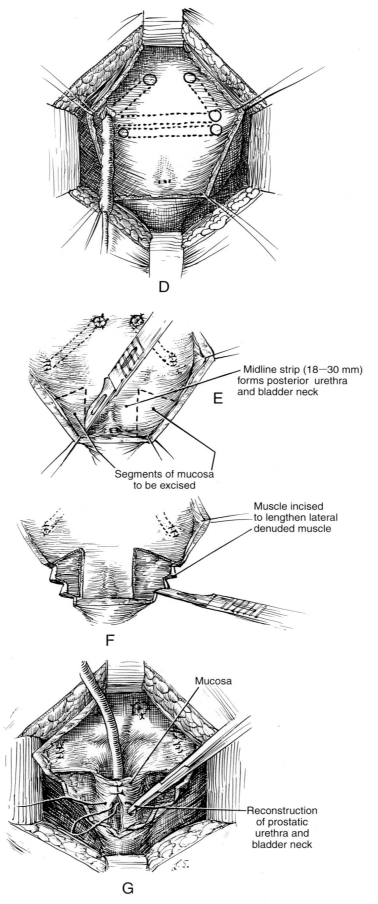

FIG. 21.7. *Continued.*

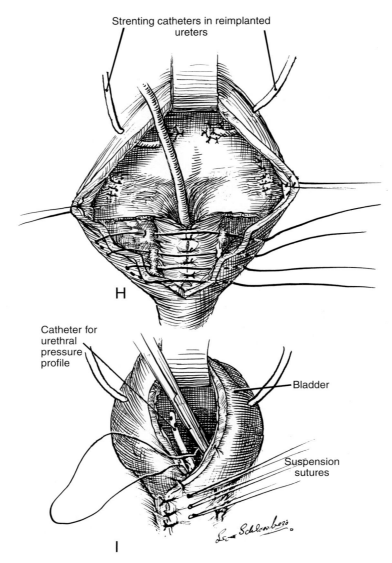

Strenting catheters in reimplanted
ureters

Catheter for
urethral
pressure
profile

Bladder

Suspension
sutures

FIG. 21.7. *Continued.*

(Fig. 21.7*D*). Then triangles of bladder wall lateral to this strip are denuded of mucosa (Fig. 21.7*E*). The mucosal strip is rolled into a tube over an 8-French urethral catheter, using interrupted 4-0 polyglycolic acid sutures (Fig. 21.7*F*). The denuded muscle flaps are overlapped and sutured in place with 3-0 polyglycolic acid sutures to reinforce the neobladder neck (Fig. 21.7*G* & *H*).

Intraoperative urodynamics may be helpful in assessing the adequacy of the reconstruction. Retrospective comparisons of the values of intraoperative urethral pressure profiles demonstrate correlation with eventual continence or incontinence. Closure pressures of 70 to 100 cm H_2O are required to prevent leakage when the bladder pressure is increased to 50 cm H_2O intraoperatively.[27] Suspension of the bladder neck and proximal urethra in the manner of Marshall et al. further enhances

the urodynamic parameters at the time of surgery.[28] At the end of the procedure the adequacy of the reconstruction is tested by a water manometer (Fig. 21.7*I*). There should be no leakage at 50 cm water pressure.

Complete urinary drainage is achieved with ureteral stents and a suprapubic cystostomy tube. Usually no tube is left through the bladder neck and the bladder is closed using continuous and interrupted 3-0 polyglactin sutures in two layers, respectively. Postoperative bladder spasm and pain can be prevented through the use of benzodiazepines, anticholinergic, nonsteroidal anti-inflammatory agents, or epidural analgesia. The stents are left in place for 2 to 3 weeks. Three weeks postoperatively a soft 8-French catheter is passed through the urethra to calibrate its size. Then the suprapubic tube is clamped before removal to assure adequate voiding.

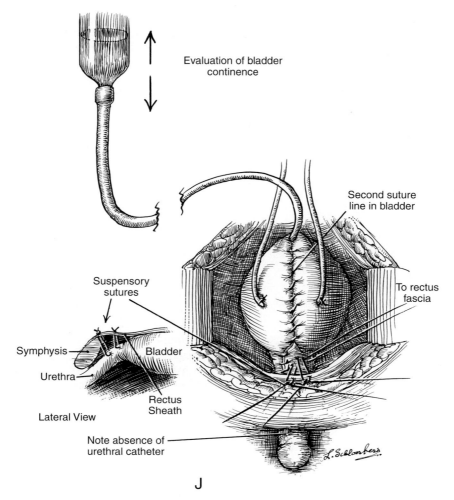

Evaluation of bladder continence

Second suture line in bladder

To rectus fascia

Suspensory sutures

Symphysis

Bladder

Urethra

Rectus Sheath

Lateral View

Note absence of urethral catheter

J

FIG. 21.7. *Continued.*

After removal of the suprapubic tube, it is expected that there will be a short dry interval. Initially, the bladder capacity is small and the patients are unfamiliar with the sensation of bladder filling or the need for voiding. Therefore, several months of readjustment often is required before a reasonable dry interval is achieved. Hints of initial success are an early dry interval of 15 minutes and the absence of stress incontinence or continuous urethral dribbling.

Results

The results of functional closure of bladder exstrophy can be expected to be as high as a 75 to 85% continence rate with preservation of renal function, as documented by several series.[2, 8, 9, 29, 30] The success of initial bladder closure impacts significantly on the eventual ability to achieve continence through spontaneous voiding without the use of clean intermittent catheterization.[9, 19, 32] In a recent review by Lakshmanan et al. of 88 consecutive patients with exstrophy treated from birth through all stages of reconstruction by only two senior surgeons, the continence rate exceeded 85%.[31] After one failure, the chances to achieve capacity for bladder neck reconstruction are reduced to 40%.[32] After more than two failed exstrophy closures, only 40% achieve enough bladder capacity for bladder neck reconstruction and only 50% achieve continence, so that only 20% are voiding spontaneously and are continent.[5] Thus, an initial bladder closure of an acceptable bladder template can be expected to be successful when performed at a center with much experience, with osteotomies when needed, and with appropriate pelvic fixation and immobilization for the prescribed time.[2, 32]

Recently, with the introduction of the Cantwell-Ransley epispadias repair, better results have been achieved than with the modified Young technique. The Cantwell-Ransley technique achieves a straighter urethra that is easier to catheterize, has less chordee, better cosmesis, and less chance of urethrocutaneous fistulae (<15%).[24]

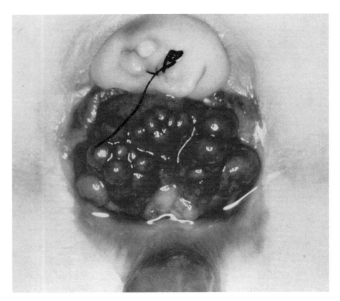

FIG. 21.8. Newborn male with small polypoid bladder template unsuitable for primary closure.

Alternatives to Primary Staged Closure

Rarely, the child with exstrophy is born with such a small bladder patch that the chance for it to function adequately, even after reconstruction, is essentially nil (Fig 21.8). Options include closing the bladder, no matter how small, to allow for later reassessment and use, or to provide urinary diversion, with or without cystectomy, early on. A tubularized bladder plate may ultimately serve as a urethra in an Arap procedure.[33] However, augmentation cystoplasty at the time of initial bladder closure may be counterproductive and should not be performed.

Whether the bladder is closed, a nonrefluxing sigmoid colon conduit can provide social dryness. Later, if a continent diversion is desired, the sigmoid conduit can be incorporated into the diversion and preclude the need to repeat ureteral reimplantation. Although ureterosigmoidostomy has the advantages of eliminating the need for catheterization and an abdominal stoma, and has been successful in some patients, it bears significant risks of upper urinary tract obstruction, infection, and colon carcinoma.[34–36] Therefore, use of an isolated colon segment and later continent urinary reservoir with an abdominal stoma has been the practice at this institution for the last decade.[37]

Major Complications and Their Management

Despite the most meticulous techniques and optimal management, complications can develop at any stage of the reconstruction. The most serious early complication with respect to the initial closure is wound dehiscence. If this occurs, it is important to resist the temptation to reclose the bladder for at least 6 months to allow for healing and improvement in tissue strength. Subsequent closures must include an osteotomy. In the past, temporary femoral nerve palsy was seen in two patients with an anterior osteotomy. However, because the authors have stopped tightening the external fixator until at least 1 week after the bladder closure, no cases have been seen.[10] If functional reconstruction is impossible or unsuccessful, the author recommends a colonic conduit in preparation for later continent urinary reservoir reconstruction.

Urethral stricture may develop after the initial closure of the urethra or at the time of epispadias repair, especially if paraexstrophy skin flaps are used.[15] This may require major reconstructive efforts or urinary diversion. The nylon suture used to approximate the pubic symphysis may develop a stitch abscess, urethral polyp, recurrent ITU, painful or difficult catheterization, or erosion into the urethra. The stitch can be removed cystoscopically or through a small suprapubic incision and is usually curative.

Urinary continence, defined as a 3-hour dry interval, is usually achieved within 1 year after bladder neck reconstruction. Previously, it was suggested that puberty may improve the urinary continence in these patients secondary to prostate growth.[38] However, a study of MRI evaluation of prostate size and configuration suggests that there is no anatomic basis for a significant contribution to the outlet resistance by the postpubertal enlarged prostate.[39] In the author's experience, those who do not achieve a 3-hour dry interval within 1 to 2 years after bladder neck reconstruction are unlikely to develop meaningful continence.

While incontinence after bladder neck reconstruction may improve with time, collagen in the urethra, revision of the bladder neck, or insertion of an artificial sphincter[40] may be of benefit. Collagen injection in the submucosa of the urethra can improve coaptation and increase outlet resistance. This can improve continence in approximately half the patients for whom it is used, while the other half may be expected to improve with additional surgery.[41] It may also be used before bladder neck reconstruction to increase outlet resistance and promote an increase in bladder capacity.[41] Some surgeons favor using the artificial urinary sphincter for persistent incontinence;[40] however, the author avoids this whenever possible because of the risks of erosion and mechanical failure that require revision. If an artificial sphincter is used, placement of tissue between the cuff and the urethra, such as omentum, may help prevent these problems.

After ureteral reimplantation, the upper urinary tract must be monitored for obstruction and treated accordingly if it develops. Urinary stones can form in these patients and usually occur in the bladder.[42] This appears to be a consequence of the surgical treatment of exstrophy, rather than any underlying predisposition. Risk factors for stone formation are created by the reconstruction and include foreign bodies, retained suture material, infection, immobilization, and urinary stasis.[42]

Summary

Despite the tremendous challenge of caring for exstrophy patients, a staged reconstruction with attention to details and meticulous techniques can provide these children with a functional urinary tract and a normal social life. The exstrophy surgeon must recognize that each patient is an individual and may require some variation in management to achieve this goal. The approach outlined here has been successful in most cases and should serve as a useful guideline in this endeavor.

CLOACAL EXSTROPHY

Cloacal exstrophy (also known as vesicointestinal fissure, ileovesical fissure, or splanchnic exstrophy) is the most severe defect that can occur in the formation of the ventral abdominal wall. This entity is rare, occurring 1 in 200,000 to 400,000 live births. Formerly, the incidence between sexes was thought to be similar; current reports indicate a 2:1 male/female ratio.[2] With newer techniques of prenatal ultrasound, this condition can reliably be diagnosed by the presence of sacral myelomeningocele (usually present in half of the patients), "rocker bottom" feet, splaying of the pubic rami, and a large cystic mass protruding from the infraumbilical anterior abdominal wall.[43] The mode of inheritance of this condition is unknown because people with this disorder have never produced offspring. With modern prenatal diagnosis, counseling can be undertaken and perinatal management improved.

Embryology and Anatomy

Two main theories on the embryology of cloacal exstrophy have been proposed.[2] Patten and Barry proposed that the paired primordia of the genital tubercles are displaced caudally. This permits persistence of the more cephalad cloacal membrane. Thus, if there is incomplete urorectal septal division and disintegration of the unstable cloacal membrane, then the exstrophied bladder and bowel would be on the ventral abdominal surface. The theory advanced by Marshall and Muecke suggests that the cloacal membrane is overly developed. This overdevelopment prevents migration of the mesenchymal layer between the inner endodermal and outer ectodermal layers. As previously mentioned, the unstable membrane ruptures, and if this occurs before fusion of the genital tubercles and before caudal movement of the urorectal septum, then the ventral abdominal defect arises.

Anatomically, there is exstrophy of the foreshortened hindgut or cecum, which displays its bulging mucosa between the two hemibladders. The orifices of the terminal ileum, the rudimentary tailgut, and a single or paired appendix are apparent on the surface of the everted cecum. The tailgut is blind ending, and the ileum is usually prolapsed (Figs. 21.9 and 21.10*A*).

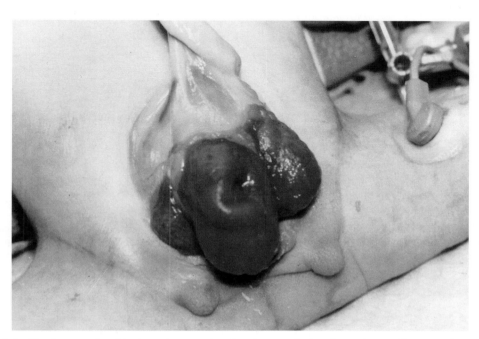

FIG. 21.9. Newborn male with cloacal exstrophy showing omphalocele, prolapsed ileum and symmetric bladder halves. Note the bifid penis.

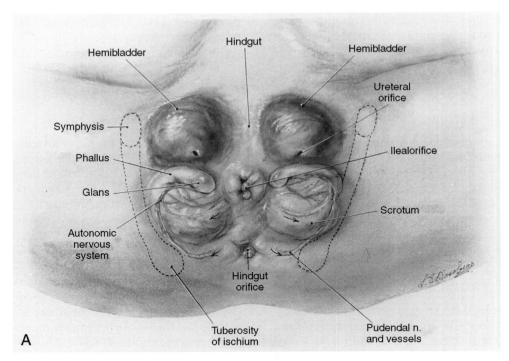

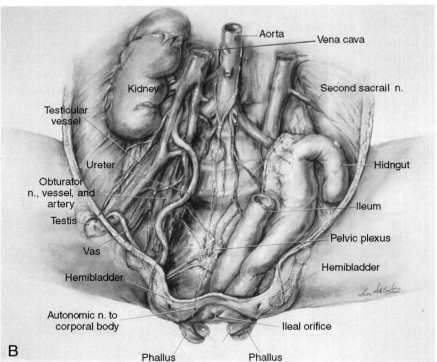

FIG. 21.10. A, Artist drawing of cloacal exstrophy with ileocecal valve reduced. **B,** Internal view of patient with cloacal exstrophy. Pudendal vessels, nerves, and other vessels and autonomic innervation to the corporal bodies are demonstrated. Internal structure of the pelvis along with duplication of the dissected specimen is also shown.

Formerly, the anatomy of the bony pelvis in cloacal exstrophy was generally described as a widened pubic symphysis with hips that are externally rotated and abducted. However, Sponseller and associates have recently described the markedly severe abnormalities of the bony pelvis associated with cloacal exstrophy.[44] Using CT scans of the pelvis in controls and patients with cloacal exstrophy, the interpubic diastasis was found to have a mean of 0.5 cm in controls and 8 cm in patients with cloacal exstrophy. The anterior segment length (distance from the triradiate cartilage to the pubis) was 37% shorter in patients with cloacal exstrophy than in controls. Also, the angle of the iliac wing was markedly increased at 45°, showing the amount of external rotation. Likewise, the ischiopubic angle was markedly increased in patients with cloacal exstrophy. Overall, patients with cloacal exstrophy have extreme abnormalities of the pelvis and asymmetry between the sides, sacroiliac joint malformations, and occasional hip malformations.

Schlegel and Gearhart first defined the neuroanatomy of the pelvis in the child born with cloacal exstrophy syndrome (Fig. 21.10*B*). The autonomic innervation to the bladder halves and corporal bodies arises from a pelvic plexus on the anterior surface of the sacrum. The nerves to the hemibladders travel along the midline on the posteroinferior surface of the pelvis and extend laterally to the hemibladders. The autonomic innervation of the phallic halves arises from the sacral pelvic plexus, travels in the midline, perforates the inferior portion of the pelvic floor, and courses medially to the hemibladder. Duplication of the vena cava is also seen.

The phallus is usually separated into a right and left half with adjacent scrotum or labia. Occasionally, the penis is together in the midline, but the structure is diminutive and the corporal bodies small, so that rearing the child as a girl is appropriate for many of these patients.[2] In their series, Husmann and colleagues found that all eight genotypic boys with cloacal exstrophy had phallic inadequacy; and of four who have reached puberty, two are impotent and three have required intense psychiatric counseling.[46] Sexual conversion should be considered as part of the treatment plan in all genotypic boys with the cloacal exstrophy syndrome. However, if the phallic halves are of adequate size and can be joined after osteotomy, rearing as male can be considered. Also, if one of the phallic halves is dominant, rearing as male can be considered.

Manzoni and associates have suggested a gridlike schema to describe cloacal exstrophy and to better delineate its variants.[47] In type I classic cloacal exstrophy, the hemibladders may be confluent cranial to the bowel patch, lateral to the bowel (most common), or confluent caudal to the bowel. Type IIA grids show variations of the bladder (covered bladder or hemibladder); type IIB

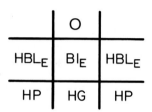

FIG. 21.11. Coding grid used to describe classic cloacal exstrophy and its variants. O, omphalocele; HBL, hemibladder; B1e, everted bowel; HP, hemiphallus; HG, hindgut. (Modified from Hurwitz RS, et al. J Urol 1987;138:1060.)

grids show variations of distal exstrophied bowel segments (duplications); and type IIC grids depicts the situation in which both bowel and bladder variations occur. The grid also describes the penis (hemi or united) and the clitoris and vaginal status (duplications). The authors have modified the grid concept to describe the status of the hindgut remnant (Fig. 21.11).

Associated Conditions

Although cloacal exstrophy is one of the most severe congenital anomalies compatible with life, these patients can be reconstructed and lead productive lives. These children face multiple problems, in part owing to the various associated anomalies, but with a multidisciplinary approach in a center with exstrophy experience, the results can be satisfactory.

Central Nervous System Anomalies

Of the anomalies associated with cloacal exstrophy, those involving spinal dysraphism associated with myelomeningocele are the most severe. Besides the neurosurgical management of this anomaly, it has important implications with regard to hydrocephalus, intellect, eventual ambulation, and bladder function in the patient with cloacal exstrophy.

The incidence of spina bifida in various series ranges from 29 to 86%, but these figures include patients with meningoceles and lipomeningoceles.[48] In the series by Howell and associates, the level of the myelomeningocele was 72% lumbar, 14% sacral, and 14% thoracic.[49] In the series by Ben-Chaim and colleagues, the levels were 80% lumbar, 10% sacral, and 10% thoracic.[50] Close consultation with a pediatric neurosurgeon must be established to determine the timing of spinal repair and a plan of treatment priorities.

Upper Urinary Tract Anomalies

Because the lower urinary tract is exstrophied, attention is often focused in this area. Several series have demonstrated, however, the common occurrence of upper tract anomalies.[48] The most common anomalies are those of pelvic kidney and renal agenesis, occurring in up to a third of the patients. Hydronephrosis and hydroureter were present in a third of the patients in Howell's series,[49] whereas in the series by Ben-Chaim and associates, this defect was found in only 1 of 22 patients.[50] Instances of the ureter draining into the vasa in boys and into the uterus, vagina, or fallopian tube in girls have also been reported.

Müllerian and Testis Anomalies

Duplication anomalies of the uterus and vagina are the most commonly found Müllerian anomalies. Hurwitz found duplication of the vagina in 43% of the patients,[51] whereas Tank and Lindenauer found this anomaly in 65%.[52] In addition, vaginal agenesis occurs in 25 to 43% of patients.[52] Partial or complete duplication of the uterus has been described in up to 95% of patients.[48] Normal ovarian tissue was found in six of seven female patients in Hurwitz's series.[51] Müllerian structures, however, should be preserved because these can be used in lower urinary tract reconstructive efforts later in life.

In the series by Hurwitz and colleagues[51] and Ricketts and colleagues,[53] the testis was undescended and was found in the groin or abdomen in most patients. Formerly, because nearly all patients were raised as females, little interest existed in testis anatomy. However, recent data by Mathews et al. have shown normal testis architecture and spermatocyte number in whole testis biopsy in this group of patients.[54]

Skeletal Anomalies

Skeletal system anomalies of the vertebral bodies and lower limb are commonly seen in patients with cloacal exstrophy. Vertebral anomalies have been reported in up to 80% of the patients.[2] Lower limb abnormalities are seen in 12 to 65% of patients.[48] These include club foot, congenital hip dislocation, agenesis, and severe deformity of the foot and leg.

Gastrointestinal System Anomalies

Because omphaloceles are so commonly associated with the cloacal exstrophy complex, most surgeons consider them an integral part of the disorder. Most series report an incidence of more than 85% in most cases.[55] The size of the omphalocele can vary, but immediate closure is required to prevent rupture of the omphalocele with its attendant problems. In the authors' experience, all omphalocele defects were closed primarily, and in no cases were prosthetic materials used. The use of a silicone silo has been reported when the omphalocele is extremely large. Although most attention has been

taken to the repair of the omphalocele defect, other serious anomalies of the gastrointestinal tract have been described, including malrotation, bowel duplication, duodenal atresia, and Meckel's diverticulum.[55] The short gut syndrome has been variously reported in 25 to 50% of the patients in most series.[53, 55] Importantly, this problem has been reported with normal small bowel length, suggesting absorptive dysfunction and emphasizing the absolute need to preserve as much large bowel as possible.

Cardiovascular and Pulmonary Anomalies

Life-threatening anomalies of the pulmonary and cardiovascular systems are rare. Cyanotic heart disease and aortic duplication have been described, as has duplication of the vena cava.[48] A bilobular lung and atretic upper lobe bronchus have been reported.[48]

Surgical Management

Steinbuchel described the first reported surgically reconstructed cloacal exstrophy.[56] The omphalocele was corrected at birth, and the atretic colon was pulled through to the perineum; however, the neonate died at 5 days of age. Formerly, surgical reconstruction of cloacal exstrophy was considered futile, and untreated neonates usually died from prematurity, sepsis, short bowel syndrome, or renal and central nervous system deficits. Remigailo and colleagues reported the most unusual case of a well-adjusted, 18-year-old patient with cloacal exstrophy who had never undergone surgical reconstruction.[57]

In the past, survival was the greatest challenge facing these patients. When the importance of separating the genitourinary tract from the gastrointestinal tract became apparent, survival increased. Rickham reported on the first patient with cloacal exstrophy to survive surgical reconstruction.[58] The omphalocele was repaired, the intestinal strip was separated from the hemibladders, and the blind-ending colon was pulled out through the perineum. The hemibladders were then reapproximated. An ileal conduit was constructed at age 18 months, and a cystectomy was subsequently performed. After early reconstructive efforts, the patient was left with two ostomies: one to collect urine and the other to collect stool. Because survival is no longer the major issue, achieving a good quality of life is now the greatest challenge facing these patients.[2]

Immediate Neonatal Assessment

The authors' approach to the reconstruction of cloacal exstrophy is by staged surgical reconstruction. In some cases, the infant's condition at birth may be critical, and attempts to reconstruct and repair the defect may be futile or morally or ethically unwise.[2] Often, the severity of cloacal exstrophy is enhanced by the nature and severity of the associated anomalies. The more robust infant will survive, and reparative surgery is initiated at birth.

Surgical management and preoperative assessment should be undertaken by a multidisciplinary team that includes surgeons who are familiar with all principles of exstrophy treatment, its options, and later reconstructive techniques. Also included in the team should be a neonatologist, a neurosurgeon, and an orthopedic surgeon familiar with the osteotomy techniques needed for a secure pelvic closure.

Surgical Options in the Newborn Period

The authors' preference is a one-stage closure when the infant is in excellent condition and has favorable anatomy with minimal associated anomalies. However, many of these infants are premature, are small for gestational age, and have such severe associated anomalies that it is difficult for them to undergo an extensive one-stage procedure in the newborn period. During either a one-stage or two-stage procedure, the omphalocele is excised, and the bowel is separated from the bladder halves. The lateral vesicointestinal fissure is closed in continuity, and a short colostomy is created from the end of the distal colon segment. The hemibladders then are reapproximated in the midline to create a single exstrophic bladder. If a one-stage procedure is selected, the entire bladder is closed completely after a bilateral anterior and vertical iliac innominate osteotomy has been performed. This osteotomy allows placement of pins for external fixation and is preferred when severe lumbosacral dysraphism is present. With a large omphalocele defect, bladder closure and osteotomy may be delayed until respiratory and gastrointestinal stability are achieved.[2]

Management of the Bowel in Cloacal Exstrophy

The management of the bowel in cloacal exstrophy must be closely integrated with the management of the urinary tract. The traditional approach that cloacal exstrophy is mainly an ileocecal exstrophy separating two hemibladders that is treated with a two-stomal diversion needs rethinking in light of modern reconstructive surgery. The grid coding system for cloacal exstrophy has previously been mentioned and ensures that a precise description of the bladder and bowel anomalies are undertaken, that variant patterns are identified, and that appropriate early decisions are made concerning the exstrophied bowel and hindgut.[2]

The principles guiding the management of the bowel in cloacal exstrophy are to conserve all bowel segments, to minimize fluid and electrolyte loss, and to make bowel available for later urinary tract reconstruction and for vaginal reconstruction in adolescence. Formerly, patients died from fluid and electrolyte loss with a short bowel and terminal ileostomy. The authors have instituted early total parenteral nutrition to help these infants grow so that the short gut syndrome becomes less of a problem as the patients get older. Careful preservation of the hindgut segment is important and its use initially as a fecal colostomy may help intestinal absorption and prevent fluid loss.[59] Also, the hindgut enlarges if used for a fecal colostomy and later can be used as a bladder augmentation or vaginal replacement. In the ideal situation, a long hindgut segment is apportioned to both the bladder and bowel. In this case, the exstrophied segment is left in situ with the bladder, the more distal hindgut is mobilized on its mesentery and anastomosed to the small bowel, and a terminal colostomy is fashioned.

Placement of the colostomy or ileostomy at a favorable location is of prime importance. It should be placed where it can easily be managed with an appliance. In the rare instance in which there is an adequate hindgut and no neurologic deficit, a colostomy can be created with a later posterior sagittal anorectoplasty to bring the colon to the perineum. Ricketts and associates have used this approach in two patients with success, although daily enemas are required.[53] Careful evaluation of neurologic status and magnetic resonance imaging studies of these patients must be accomplished before this approach is chosen. Finally, every effort must be expended to save both of the appendiceal structures for later continent stoma construction if needed.

Management of the Phallic Structures and Vagina

In boys with cloacal exstrophy, the penis is usually represented by two widely separated small phallic structures. Because these structures are rudimentary and wide apart, attempts at reconstruction have been generally unsatisfactory.[2] In an effort to reconstruct the genitation, the medial aspects of the bifid phallus are denuded of mucosa and skin and brought together in the midline. This is usually done at the time of bladder closure and osteotomy. If there is a single phallic structure in the midline (20% of patients), the urethral plate is dissected from the corporal bodies and dropped between them to the perineum for a urethra opening if a female sex of rearing is chosen. The corpora and glans are then recessed for a more appropriate female appearance, and labial folds are created from the scrotum by a posteriori Y-V plasty. If male sex of rearing is appropriate then the phallic halves are joined medially after an osteotomy is performed. If a dominant phallic half is present the diminutive half is removed and the dominant half moved to the midline with osteotomy (Fig. 21.12).

Genital anomalies in girls is usually corrected at the time of bladder closure and osteotomy. The medial aspect of the hemiclitoris is denuded of mucosa, and the halves are brought together with a 5-0 Vicryl for the subcutaneous layer and fine 6-0 Vicryl for the epithelial layer.[2]

Commonly, duplicate vaginas are far apart and on opposite sides of the pelvis. In the unusual case of the vaginas being close together, they should be joined in the midline and used for later reconstruction. The ostia of the vaginas may be difficult to find at the time of the initial closure, and the surgeon should be aware that the ostias can enter the posterior wall of the bladder. It is acceptable to leave the vaginas in situ, but further surgery will be needed to bring one of these to the perineum.

In the genotypic male patient raised as a girl, the vagina is usually created at the time of puberty. In the past, vaginas have been created by anatomic "scraps" such as portions of duplicated bowel, unneded dilated ureter, or a few centimeters of the distal colonic segment.[2] It is probably better to wait until puberty and construct a vagina from intestine or from a free full-thickness skin graft. There is a paucity of the literature regarding the construction of a neovagina in the patient with cloacal exstrophy, but as more of these patients reach puberty, experience with this entity will increase, and long-term information will be available.

Reconstruction of the Lower Urinary Tract

Bladder Closure

Whether the bladder is closed at initial operation or as a second procedure, care must be taken when the bowel is separated from the bladder halves to avoid damage to the blood supply of the bowel mesentery and to the autonomic vesical innervation, which becomes exposed at the medial aspect of the hemibladder.[45] The bladder closure is performed much as that of classic bladder exstrophy described earlier.[2] In girls, a double vagina may complicate closure of the urethra. If possible, the vaginas are joined and positioned posteriorly, and the tissue on the anteromedial aspect is tubularized to form a urethra. If this tissue is unavailable, then local tissues are used to form a urethral channel. As mentioned previously, in the genotypic male patient raised as a girl, the urethral plate is raised from the corpora, much as in the initial part of a Cantwell-Ransley repair, and then brought ventral to the corpora as a perineal urethra.

Drainage of the urinary tract is accomplished by ureteral stents and suprapubic catheter all exiting from the abdomen. No urethral stent or catheter is used. After bladder closure, free incontinent drainage of urine through the urethra is expected, but antibiotic suppression and close monitoring are necessary to avoid retention, infection, and reflux nephropathy.

Osteotomy is performed in all of the authors' patients with cloacal exstrophy based on success with this procedure for classic bladder exstrophy.[10, 50] The goal is to achieve tension-free approximation of the widely separated pubic bones and of the anterior abdominal wall. Anterior innominate osteotomy, combined with ventral iliac osteotomy, also provides large cancellous surfaces with good healing potential (Fig. 21.3). Furthermore, in cases of extreme pubic diastasis, combined anterior innominate and posterior iliac osteotomy may be done within the periosteum through the same skin incision for better correction after osteotomy. Recent work by Silver et al. has shown that an osteotomy can be performed before exstrophy closure and the extreme diastasis gradually reduced over a period of 2 to 3 weeks by medial tightening of the fixator device. At the time

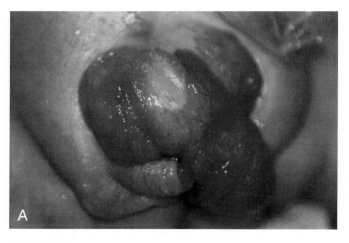
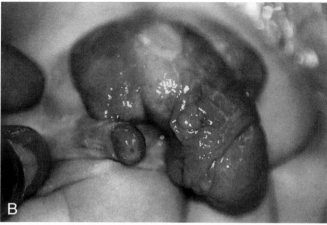

FIG. 21.12. A and B, Newborn male with cloacal exstrophy with dominant right hemiphallus and small left hemiphallus suitable for male sex of rearing.

of the exstrophy closure the additional 2 to 3 cm of diastasis are easily brought together and the external fixator continues to be tightened during the remainder of the hospitalization.[60] Immobilization is provided by an external fixator and modified Bryant traction or Buck traction for 4 to 6 weeks.

The importance of an osteotomy at the time of cloacal exstrophy closure has become more obvious during the past several years. In a series reported by Ben-Chaim and colleagues, nine patients were referred for further treatment after closure elsewhere without osteotomy.[50] Of these patients with cloacal exstrophy, six developed dehiscence, one a large ventral hernia, and one a major bladder prolapse. In contrast, of 12 of the authors' patients who underwent osteotomy at the time of cloacal exstrophy closure, there was one dehiscence and one minor prolapse. Therefore, it is clear that osteotomy has a significant role in the closure and success rates of cloacal exstrophy.

Management of Urinary Incontinence

Urinary incontinence is managed by diapering only during the early years. Intermittent catheterization is likely to be needed for emptying after any procedure to enhance outlet resistance. This may be due in part to spinal defects, which can cause a neurologic deficit in bladder function, or to a small bladder capacity, which may require augmentation. In both instances, bladder detrusor activity usually is impaired. Surgery to produce a continent reservoir should be delayed until the child is old enough to participate in self-care.[61] The choice between a catheterizable urethra or an abdominal stoma depends on the adequacy of the urethra and bladder outlet, the intellect and dexterity of the child, and the child's orthopedic status regarding the spine, hip joints, braces, and ambulation.

The time to initiate management of urinary incontinence is determined by the age at which the child can understand and manage the type of bladder emptying required. Social factors, intelligence, school support, and mobility are important considerations for this group.

Occasionally, hindgut is available for bladder enhancement, but ileum has traditionally been used. In an effort to avoid further loss of absorptive surface by preserving the hindgut and ileum, Adams and colleagues have used gastrocystoplasty with success.[62] Regardless of which bowel segment is chosen, bladder augmentation should be delayed until bowel function is mature and nutrition and acidosis are no longer a problem or their effects minimized.

Some patients have a functioning bladder and can void through a reconstructed bladder outlet. However, innovative methods may be needed to construct a continent outlet in patients without substantial native ure-

thral tissues.[2] These techniques include use of the vagina to form a urethra, with reimplantation of the vagina into the bladder for continence, or an ileal nipple, as described by Hendren.[63, 64]

Personal Experience With Achieving Continence in the Patient with Cloacal Exstrophy

The author's unit observes 25 patients with cloacal exstrophy, of whom 14 have undergone continence procedures. Four patients underwent Young-Dees bladder neck plasty only; one patient had bladder neck suspension; three had Young-Dees-Leadbetter urethroplasty and augmentation; four had Young-Dees-Leadbetter urethroplasty, augmentation, and continent abdominal

TABLE 21.1. *Management considerations in patients with cloacal exstropy*

Immediate neonatal assessment
Evaluate associated anomalies
Decide whether to proceed with reparative surgery

Functional bladder closure (soon after neonatal assessment)
One-stage repair (few associated anomalies)
Excision of omphalocele
Separation of cecal plate from bladder halves
Joining and closure of bladder halves
Bilateral anterior innominate and vertical iliac osteotomy
Gonadectomy in boys with duplicated or absent penis undergoing gender change
Joining phallic halves in those raised as males
Terminal ileostomy or colostomy
Genital revision if needed

Two-stage repair—first stage (newborn period)
Excision of omphalocele
Separation of cecal plate from bladder halves
Joining of bladder halves
Gonadectomy in boys with duplicated or absent penis
Terminal ileostomy or colostomy

Two-stage repair—second stage (4–6 months of age)
Closure of joined bladder halves
Joining phallic halves in those raised as males
Bilateral anterior innominate and vertical iliac osteotomy
Genital revision if needed

Anti-incontinence or reflux procedure (4–5 years of age)
Bladder capacity >60 mL minimum (small group of patients)
Young-Dees-Leadbetter bladder neck reconstruction
Bilateral Cohen ureteral reimplantations
Marshall-Marchetti bladder neck suspension

Bladder capacity <60 mL (most patients)
Young-Dees-Leadbetter bladder neck reconstruction
Bilateral Cohen ureteral reimplantations
Bowel segment used to augment bladder > or <
Continent diversion with abdominal or perineal stoma

Vaginal reconstruction
Vagina constructed or augmented using colon, ileum, or full-thickness skin graft

stoma; and two had closure of the bladder neck, augmentation, and creation of a continent abdominal stoma. The upper tracts remain normal in 21 patients. Two patients required revision of their continent stomas owing to catheterization difficulties. One patient required injection of collagen into the reconstructed bladder neck, and one patient who had bladder neck reconstruction and bladder augmentation underwent reoperation with bladder neck closure and ileal Mitrofanoff continent diversion because continence was not achieved. Overall, 12 patients (86%) experience diurnal continence, whereas 79% are dry at night. Twelve are on a CIC regimen, and two are voiding spontaneously.

Despite the complexity of this anomaly, a staged approach to lower tract reconstruction can produce urinary continence. An individualized approach is required to find the most suitable solution for each patient's bladder and bowel anatomy and function, according to the patient's intellectual and neurologic and orthopedic capabilities. Ricketts and associates have developed a scoring system to analyze bladder and bowel continence.[53] In the absence of multiple cases owing to the rarity of this condition, use of this scoring system may allow a collective experience to be analyzed and thus optimization of future management of this complex disorder. A summary of these multiple options in management is included in Table 21.1.

REFERENCES

1. Lancaster PAL. Epidemiology of bladder exstrophy and epispadias: a communication from the International Clearinghouse for Birth Defects Monitoring System. Teratology 1987;36:221.
2. Gearhart JP, Jeffs RD. Exstrophy-epispadias complex and bladder anomalies. In: Walsh PC, et al., eds. Campbell's Urology, 7th ed. Philadelphia: W.B. Saunders Company, 1997;2:1939.
3. Shapiro E, Lepor H, Jeffs RD. The inheritance of exstrophy/epispadias complex. J Urol 1980;132:308.
4. Ives E, Coffey R, Carter CO. A family study of bladder exstrophy. J Med Genet 1980;17:139.
5. Gearhart JP, Ben-Chaim J, Sciortino C, Peppas DS, Sponseller PD, Jeffs RD. The multiple failed exstrophy closure: strategy for management. Urology 1996;47:240.
6. Gearhart JP, Ben-Chaim J, Jeffs RD, Saunders R. Criteria for prenatal diagnosis of classic bladder exstrophy. Obstet Gynecol 1995;85(6):961.
7. Caddedu J, Silver RI, Ladkshamanan Y, Benson J, Jeffs RD, Gearhart JP. Spinal anomalies in cases of classic bladder exstrophy. Br J Urol 1997;79:975.
8. Gearhart JP, Jeffs RD. State of the art reconstructive surgery for bladder exstrophy at The Johns Hopkins Hospital. Am J Dis Child 1989;143:1475.
9. Oesterling JE, Jeffs RD. The importance of a successful initial bladder closure in the surgical management of classical bladder exstrophy: analysis of 144 patients treated at The Johns Hopkins Hospital between 1975 and 1985. J Urol 1987;137:258.
10. Gearhart JP, Forschner DC, Sponseller PD, Jeffs RD. A new combined vertical and horizontal pelvic osteotomy approach for the initial and secondary repair of bladder exstrophy. J Urol 1996;155:689.
11. Sponseller PD, Gearhart JP, Jeffs RD. Anterior innominate osteotomies for failure or last closure of bladder exstrophy. J Urol 1991;146:137.
12. McKenna PH, Khoury AE, McLorie GA, Churchill BM, Babyn PB, Wedge JH. Iliac osteotomy: a model to compare the options in bladder and cloacal exstrophy reconstruction. J Urol 1994;151:182.
13. Frey P, Cohen SJ. Anterior pelvic osteotomy, a new operative technique facilitating primary bladder exstrophy closure. Br J Urol 1989;64:641.
14. Schmidt AH, Keenen TL, Tank ES, Bird CB, Beals RK. Pelvic osteotomy for bladder exstrophy. J Pediatr Orthopedics 1993;13:214.
15. Duckett JW. Use of paraexstrophy skin pedicle grafts for correction of exstrophy and epispadias repair. Birth Defects 1977;13:175.
16. Gearhart JP, Peppas DS, Jeffs RD. Complications of paraexstrophy skin flaps in the reconstruction of classical bladder exstrophy. J Urol 1993;150:627.
17. Connolly JA, Peppas DS, Jeffs RD, Gearhart JP. Prevalence and repair of inguinal hernia in children with bladder exstrophy. J Urol 1995;154:1900.
18. Lowe FC, Jeffs RD. Wound dehiscence in bladder exstrophy: an examination of the etiologies and factors for initial failure and subsequent success. J Urol 1983;130:312.
19. Husmann DA, McLorie GA, Churchill BM. Closure of the exstrophic bladder: an evaluation of the factors leading to its success and its importance on urinary continence. J Urol 1989;142:522.
20. Hendren WH. Nonrefluxing colon conduit for temporary or permanent urinary diversion in children. J Pediatr Surg 1975;10:381.
21. Gearhart JP, Jeffs RD. Bladder exstrophy: increase in capacity following epispadias repair. J Urol 1989;142:525.
22. Gearhart JP, Jeffs RD. The use of parenteral testosterone therapy in genital reconstructive surgery. J Urol 1988;138:1077.
23. Gearhart JP, Sciortino C, Ben-Chaim J, Jeffs RD. The Cantwell-Ransley epispadias repair: lessons learned. Urology 1995;46(1):92.
24. Gearhart JP, Leonard MP, Burgers JK, Jeffs RD. The Cantwell-Ransley technique for repair of epispadias. J Urol 1992;148:851.
25. Ransley PG, Duffy PG, Wollin M. Bladder exstrophy closure and epispadias repair. In: Operative Surgery—Pediatric Surgery. Edinburgh: Butterworths, 1989;620.
26. Gearhart JP, Mathews RI, Taylor S, Jeffs RD. Combined bladder closure and epispadias repair in the reconstruction of bladder exstrophy. Presented at American Academy of Pediatrics, New Orleans, LA. November 2, 1997.
27. Canning DA, Gearhart JP, Peppas DS, Jeffs RD. The cephalotrigonal reimplant in bladder neck reconstruction for patients with exstrophy or epispadias. J Urol 1993;150:156.
28. Gearhart JP, Williams KA, Jeffs RD. Intraoperative urethral pressure profilometry as an adjunct to bladder neck reconstruction. J Urol 1986;136:1055.
29. Marshall VF, Marchetti AA, Krantz KE. The correction of stress urinary incontinence by simple vesicourethral suspension. Surg Gynecol Obstet 1949;88:509.
30. Mollard P, Basset T, Bringeon G. Results of bladder and urethra reconstruction for exstrophy. (French) Chir Pediatr 1986;27:27.
31. Connor JP, Hensle TW, Lattimer JK, Burbige KA. Long-term follow-up of 207 patients with bladder exstrophy: an evolution in treatment. J Urol 1989;142:793.
32. Lakshmanan Y, Peppas DS, Gearhart JP, Jeffs RD. Bladder exstrophy: a twenty-one year experience with functional reconstruction in 88 consecutive patients followed from birth. J Urol 1977. Accepted for publication.
33. Gearhart JP, Peppas DS, Jeffs RD. The failed exstrophy closure: strategy for management. Br J Urol 1993;71:217.
34. Arap S, Martins GA, Menezes DE, Goes G. Initial results of the complete reconstruction of bladder exstrophy. Urol Clin North Am 1980;7:477.
35. Stockle M, Becht E, Voges G, Reidmiller H, Hohenfellner R. Ureterosigmoidostomy: an outdated approach to bladder exstrophy? J Urol 1990;143:770.
36. Gittes RF. Carcinogenesis in ureterosigmoidostomy. Urol Clin North Am 1986;13:201.
37. Gearhart JP, Peppas DS, Jeffs RD. The application of continent urinary stomas to bladder augmentation or replacement in the failed exstrophy reconstruction. Br J Urol 1995;75:87.
38. Kramer SA, Kelalis PP. Assessment of urinary continence in epispadias review of 70 cases. J Urol 1982;128:290.

39. Gearhart JP, Yang A, Leonard MP, Jeffs RD, Zerhouni EA. Prostate size and configuration in adults with bladder exstrophy. J Urol 1993;149:308.
40. Decter RM, Roth DR, Fishman IJ, Shabsigh R, Scott FB, Gonzales ET. Use of the AS800 device in exstrophy and epispadias. J Urol 1988;140:1202.
41. Ben-Chaim J, Jeffs, RD, Peppas DS, Gearhart JP. Submucosal bladder neck injections of glutaraldehyde cross-linked bovine collagen for treatment of urinary incontinence, in patients with exstrophy/epispadias complex. J Urol 1995;154:862.
42. Silver RI, Gross DA, Jeffs RD, Gearhart JP. Urolithiasis in the exstrophy/epispadias complex. J Urol 1997;158:1322.
43. Langer JC, Brennan B, Lappalainen RE, et al. Cloacal exstrophy prenatal diagnosis before rupture of the cloacal membrane. J Pediatr Surg 1992;27:1352.
44. Sponseller PD, Bisson LS, Gearhart JP, et al. The anatomy of the pelvis in the exstrophy complex. Bone Joint Surg 1995;77:177.
45. Schlegel PN, Gearhart JP. Neuroanatomy of the pelvis in an infant with cloacal exstrophy: a detailed microdissection with histology. J Urol 1989;141:583.
46. Husmann DA, McLorie GA, Churchill BM. Phallic reconstruction in cloacal exstrophy. J Urol 1989;142:563.
47. Manzoni GA, Ransley PG, Hurwitz RS. Cloacal exstrophy and cloacal exstrophy variants: a proposed system of classification. J Urol 1987;138:1065.
48. Diamond DA. Management of cloacal exstrophy. Dial Pediatr Urol 1990;13:1.
49. Howell C, Caldamone A, Snyder H, et al. Optimal management of cloacal exstrophy. J Pediatr Surg 1983;18:365.
50. Ben-Chaim J, Peppas DA, Sponseller PD, et al. Applications of osteotomy in the cloacal exstrophy patient. J Urol 1995;154:865.
51. Hurwitz RS, Manzoni GA, Ransley PG, et al. Cloacal exstrophy: a report of 34 cases. J Urol 1987;138:1060.
52. Tank ES, Lindenauer SM. Principles of management of exstrophy of the cloaca. Am J Surg 1970;119:95.
53. Ricketts RR, Woodard JR, Swiren GT, et al. Modern treatment of cloacal exstrophy. J Pediatr Surg 1991;26:444.
54. Gearhart JP, Marsh D, Mathews R. Gonad morphology in cloacal exstrophy. Implications for gender assignment. 1st International Symposium on the Exstrophy-Epispadias Complex. Baltimore, MD. April 9–10, 1997.
55. Soper RT, Kilger K. Vesicointestinal fissure. J Urol 1964;92:490.
56. Steinbuchel W. Veber nabelschurbruch and blassenbauchspalte mit codken bildung von seiten des dunndormers. Arch Gynaeckol 1900;60:465.
57. Remigailo RV, Woodard JR, Andrews HG, et al. Cloacal exstrophy: 18 year survival of untreated case. J Urol 1976;116:811.
58. Rickham PP. Vesicointestinal fissure. Arch Dis Child 1960;35:97.
59. Husmann DA, McLorie GA, Churchill BM, et al. Management of the hindgut in cloacal exstrophy: terminal ileostomy versus colostomy. J Pediatr Surg 1988;23:1107.
60. Silver R, Gearhart JP, Sponseller P. Staged closure with preliminary osteotomy in the cloacal exstrophy patient. J Urol 1997 (submitted for publication).
61. Gearhart JP, Jeffs RD. Reconstruction of the lower urinary tract in cloacal exstrophy. Dial Pediatr Urol 1990;13:4.
62. Adams MC, Mitchell ME, Rink RC. Gastrocystoplasty: an alternative solution for the problem of urological reconstruction in the severely compromised patient. J Urol 1988;140:1152.
63. Gearhart JP, Jeffs RD. Techniques to create urinary continence in the cloacal exstrophy patient. J Urol 1991;146:616.
64. Hendren WH. Ileal nipple for continence in cloacal exstrophy. J Urol 1992;148:372.

CHAPTER 22

Pediatric Neurogenic Bladder: Etiology and Diagnostic Evaluation

Stephen R. Kraus and Timothy B. Boone

Disorders of voiding in children often are complex and difficult to diagnose because lower urinary tract symptoms may be indistinct and incapable of accurately indicating the underlying pathology. In the pediatric patient population, congenital abnormalities and abnormal development of the neuro-vesical axis may cause significant morbidity and psychosocial maldevelopment. The impact of voiding dysfunction on social well-being, and ultimately on continence and the upper urinary tract, warrants our attention to its detection and management.

Neurogenic voiding disorders have a variety of causes. This chapter outlines the normal physiology of the lower urinary tract and reviews pathologic conditions, clinical presentations, evaluation, and management of children with neurogenic bladder dysfunction.

NORMAL LOWER URINARY TRACT FUNCTION AND DEVELOPMENT

Normal lower urinary tract function allows for safe and continent storage of urine with elimination under volitional control, all while maintaining socially acceptable voiding behavior. The micturition cycle can be divided into two phases: the filling phase and the expulsion phase. Storage of urine occurs with the accommodation of increasing volumes of urine under low pressure. This permits continual drainage of urine in a nonrefluxing manner from the upper tracts by both ureters. As the bladder reaches its functional capacity, it begins to make the individual aware of lower tract activity through afferent neural signaling. This warning allows the individual to eliminate the stored urine in a socially acceptable manner. Throughout this cycle, the lower urinary tract provides passive and active continence.[1,2]

Lower urinary tract function is under the control of autonomic and somatic nervous systems.[2] The sympathetic component of the spinal micturition pathways originates from the thoracolumbar region of the spinal cord, namely T11 through L2. Efferent impulses, transmitted through the paravertebral chain, course mainly through the hypogastric nerve to supply the pelvic viscera, including the bladder and urethra. Parasympathetic control is generated from the sacral spinal cord, namely S2–S4 where the sacral parasympathetic nucleus is located. Efferent impulses are carried by the pelvic nerve through the pelvic plexus to the bladder. Voluntary somatic pathways originate from Onuf's nucleus, also located in the S2–S4 spinal segments. Transmission occurs through the pudendal nerve that innervates the pelvic musculature and the external urethral sphincter (rhabdosphincter).[1,3]

Coordination of the various nervous system components is mandatory for normal micturition to occur. During filling, sympathetic impulses assist in bladder volume accommodation and increase smooth muscle tone in the trigone and proximal urethral areas. This enables the bladder to expand under low pressure while assisting with continence by increasing outflow resistance. Somatic stimulation of the external sphincter maintains its closure, thus increasing outflow resistance. During voiding, parasympathetic stimulation causes bladder contractions while somatic stimulation of the external sphincter ceases, allowing it to relax.[1,3]

The normal infant bladder lacks inhibitory control from the higher neural centers. The micturition cycle occurs spontaneously as dictated by spinal cord reflex pathways responding to the bladder's increasing stretch during filling. As the bladder fills and exceeds its volume threshold, afferent impulses are generated that activate the sacral spinal reflex. A coordinated detrusor contraction with outlet relaxation occurs, allowing micturition to proceed. For this to occur, the pontine micturition center must be intact and in communication with the sacral micturition reflex center. Despite the lack of supraspinal control, reflexive voiding remains coordinated. As the child ages, supraspinal control over the reflex voiding pattern emerges. During this time, neural pathways are finally maturing. By the age of 2, most children are aware of and able to announce that their bladders are full and that they need to urinate. However, the ability to volitionally initiate voiding or void with less than a full bladder often is not yet mastered. From 18 months to 3 years of age, these behaviors have been attained and children also begin coordinating them with the conscious sensation of bladder fullness. During this period, functional bladder capacity increases allowing for a more practical voiding frequency. Spontaneous bladder activity ceases and an adult-like pattern of urinary control emerges. During the transition phase to this final goal, urinary control may be mixed. Continence may be maintained not by cortical suppression of detrusor activity but rather by volitional tightening of the external sphincter during uncontrolled detrusor contractions. This phase is probably experienced by most children, but the persistence of this uncoordinated voiding pattern may lead to dysfunctional voiding.[4] The development of normal urinary control involves a complex behavioral and neurophysiologic relationship.

The neuro-vesical axis can be conceptually divided into segments, based on the anatomic and physiologic relationships of the micturitional components. As can be seen in Figure 22.1, such a breakdown allows for the

TABLE 22.1. *Neurogenic bladder dysfunction evaluation*

History
  Bowel and bladder habits
  Pattern of incontinence
  Birth and development
Physical examination
  Abdomen
  Back and spine
  Genitalia
  Lower extremities
    Reflexes
    Muscle mass
    Gait
    Perineal sensation, tone, and reflexes
Laboratory
  Urine analysis and culture
  Urine specific gravity
  Serum creatinine level
  24-hour urine creatinine clearance
Radiography
  Renal and bladder sonography
  Nuclear renal scan
  Excretory urography
  Voiding cystourethrography
    *Can be combined with urodynamics
  Spine radiograph
  Magnetic resonance imaging
Urodynamics
  Flow rate
  Residual urine
  Cystometrogram with pressure/flow
  External urethral sphincter electromyography
  Dynamic urethral pressure profile

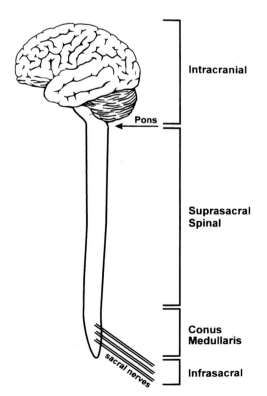

FIG. 22.1. Anatomic levels representing potential sites of neurologic injury or disease leading to voiding dysfunction. (Used with permission of Norris and Stashin. History, physical examination, and classification. Urol Clin North Am 1996;23(3):338.)

characterization of the neurogenic bladder based on the location of the underlying lesion and the predicted properties of the bladder dysfunction. Nevertheless, within the same disease groups, variability exists in urodynamic and clinical findings. This is especially true for patients with incomplete lesions, multiple level lesions, or injuries with mixed patterns. Thus, such an anatomic characterization is merely for conceptualization and prediction of the clinical outcome. By no means should such generalizations based on anatomic level preclude a full clinical workup.

DIAGNOSTIC EVALUATION

All patients exhibiting any type of neurologic disease should undergo a thorough clinical history and physical examination (Table 22.1). The history should include questions related to details of birth, developmental milestones, bowel habits, voiding habits and pattern, timing of incontinence, details of any known neurologic illnesses or injuries, and familial medical history. Careful attention should be directed to changes in voiding patterns, especially after a neurologic insult. When did the child become "potty trained"? Does the child void spontaneously or does the child strain or push to void? Are there periods of dryness or is there constant leakage? Do accidents occur with stress maneuvers such as laughing, coughing, or sneezing? Do accidents coincide with sensation of urgency or is there a lack of any sensation? Was the child initially continent only to have periods of leakage later? Does the child have frequent urinary tract infections? During the physical examination, a careful inspection of the child's back is important. Hemangiomas, hair tufts, and deep dimples and asymmetry of the gluteal cleft are cutaneous evidence of an underlying occult spinal dysraphism or sacral agenesis (Fig. 22.2). The genitals should be examined and the presence or absence of congenital anatomic anomalies noted. A careful neurologic evaluation is an essential component of the physical examination and should include an assessment of perianal and perineal sensation to pin prick and light touch, anal sphincter tone, presence or absence of a bulbocavernosus and cutaneous reflex (anal wink) (see Table 22.2). Gross motor and sensory functions of the lower extremities along with muscle mass and strength should be evaluated, especially in comparison

TABLE 22.2 *Sacral arc reflexes*

Digital anal reflex	The examining finger is inserted into the anus. A reflex contraction of the external sphincter is a positive indication.
Bulbocavernosus reflex	Brisk squeezing of the glans penis or clitoris elicits a contraction of the external sphincter around the examining finger in the anus.
Suprapubic tap reflex	Tapping over the suprapubic region may elicit a contraction of the external sphincter around the examining finger in the anus.
Catheter tug reflex	For patients with indwelling catheters, a brisk tug on the catheter elicits a contraction around the examining finger in the anus.
Anocutaneous reflex	Light pin-prick in perianal region results in "anal wink."

with the contralateral extremity and relative to the upper extremities. The presence or absence of deep tendon reflexes, as well as inspection of the child's gait, may also provide invaluable clues.[5–7]

Initial laboratory studies including a urinalysis and urine culture should be obtained. Remember that many patients with a neurogenic bladder will have bacteriuria as a result of intermittent catheterization. Though asymptomatic patients need not be treated with antibiotics, those initially presenting with pyuria and bacteriuria require full evaluation. Determination of serum urea nitrogen and creatinine can be used for an initial assessment of renal function, although a more detailed baseline evaluation may be obtained by measuring creatinine clearance or using nuclear renoscintography.[6]

Radiologic imaging of the entire urinary tract is mandatory in the workup of the child with neurogenic voiding dysfunction. This is especially true before initiation of any management scheme or before surgery is planned. Baseline evaluation, in concert with surveillance studies, ensures that the upper urinary tract (i.e., kidneys and ureters) is not damaged and the problem has not worsened despite therapy. The renal parenchyma and architecture and the proximal collecting system can be assessed satisfactorily by renal ultrasound. Ultrasound can often detect caliectasis, hydronephrosis, hydroureter, and parenchymal thinning. In the past, the excretory urogram often was used for initial and follow-up imaging, but its current use probably should be limited to initial evaluation or to situations in which fine anatomic detail is required, such as in surgical planning or stone localization. A voiding cystourethrogram (VCUG) also is obtained to evaluate bladder wall thickening, bladder diverticulum, and vesicoureteral reflux, and to identify any abnormalities of the bladder neck.[6, 8, 9] With the advent of videourodynamics, we recommend that, when available, the VCUG be obtained at the time of urodynamic evaluation. The use of real-time

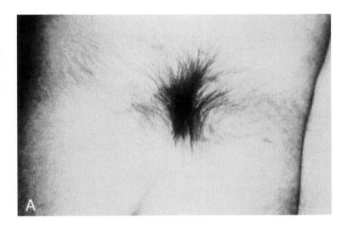
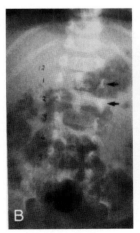
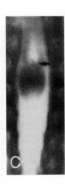
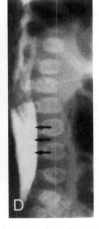

FIG. 22.2. A, Hair tuft just above gluteal crease in a 6-month-old girl, indicating potential underlying spinal dysraphism **(A). B–D,** Abnormal vertebrae and myelography consistent with diastematomyelia and tethering of the distal spinal cord. (Used with permission from Bauer S. In: Krane and Siroky, eds. Clinical Neurology, 2nd ed. Philadelphia: Lippincott. 1991;384.)

videourodynamics offers not only the static images that are obtained on routine VCUG, but also the opportunity to radiologically visualize the lower urinary tract while simultaneously obtaining urodynamic data and thus obtaining a clear and precise picture of what occurs when the patient stores and empties urine. Dynamic data obtained with videourodynamics often allow the urologist to identify subtle problems that may be missed on routine cystometry and pressure flow studies.[7, 9]

URODYNAMICS

Rationale

The main goal of urologic management in the child with neurogenic voiding dysfunction is the preservation of renal function. This is accomplished by the safe storage and evacuation of urine. Upper urinary tract function is directly impacted by lower tract function. Issues such as social continence, although often more important to the patient and family, should remain secondary to the safety of the upper urinary tracts. The goals of urodynamic evaluation are to reproduce what patients experience during their normal routine while simultaneously obtaining a radiologic and urodynamic depiction of what is occurring. To better conceptualize these events, it is often best to think in terms of storage and emptying phases (Table 22.3).

Problems of storage include alterations in detrusor function, inadequate outlet closure mechanism, or both. Impairment of detrusor function can include: 1) loss of compliance as a result of increased tone or loss of elasticity of the detrusor muscle or bladder wall fibrosis, and 2) overactivity manifested by uninhibited contractions, which can alter the functional detrusor storage capability. If the neurologic cause is known, this overactivity is termed detrusor hyperreflexia. Loss of bladder compliance during storage can cause severe damage to the upper urinary tracts if detrusor pressures become too high. In a classic study, McGuire and coworkers noted that detrusor pressures greater than 40 cm were associated with a higher risk of hydronephrosis, reflux, and renal deterioration.[10] Incontinence will occur when high detrusor pressures overcome the normal urethral outlet resistance. However, incontinence may also occur when the bladder neck, external sphincter, or both are unable to maintain adequate outlet resistance. Low resistance at the outlet may allow leakage during filling, even when filling is occurring at the normally low detrusor pressures. Loss of the proximal urethra's ability to respond to increases in abdominal pressures will also result in incontinence.

Problems with elimination of urine are also common. Inadequate detrusor contractions resulting in incomplete emptying or retention can be seen with a hypocontractile or areflexic bladder. Such conditions are often associated with neurologic abnormalities involving lower motor neurons, lesions at or below the level of the sacral micturition center, and damage to the peripheral innervation of the bladder (Fig. 22.3A & B).[11] Some lesions that involve the central nervous system above the sacral segments but below the pontine micturition center can result in discoordinated micturition when the normal synergy between detrusor and external sphincter no longer exists. The reflex relaxation of the external sphincter that normally precedes the detrusor contraction is lost, and in some instances the external sphincter contracts simultaneously.[11] In the neurologically mediated state referred to as detrusor-sphincter dyssynergia (DESD), detrusor pressures can become dangerously

TABLE 22.3 *Classification of voiding dysfunction*

Failure to store	Failure to empty
Because of the bladder	Because of the bladder
Detrusor hyperactivity	Detrusor areflexia
Involuntary contractions	Sacral neurologic disease and injury
Suprasacral neurologic disease	Peripheral nerve disease and injury
Bladder outlet obstruction	Primary myogenic disorder
Idiopathic	Idiopathic
Decreased compliance	Because of the outlet
Fibrosis	Anatomic obstruction
Idiopathic	Bladder neck fibrosis
Sensory urgency	Posterior urethral valve
Inflammatory	Urethral stricture
Infectious	Functional obstruction
Neurologic	Detrusor-sphincter dyssynergia
Psychological	Smooth sphincter
Idiopathic	Striated sphincter
Because of the outlet	Hinman-Allen syndrome
Stress incontinence	
Nonfunctional bladder neck-proximal urethra	

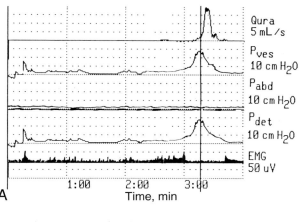

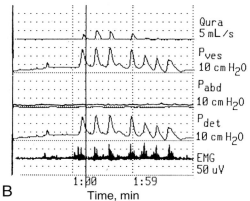

FIG. 22.3. A, Normal micturition with coordination of bladder contraction and external urethral sphincter relaxation. **B,** Detrusor-external sphincter dyssynergia showing the bladder and sphincter contracting against each other **(B).**

high as the contracting bladder tries to overcome an actively closed sphincter. Persistence of this functional obstruction will eventually result in detrusor hypertrophy, loss of compliance, and, finally, myogenic failure with high storage pressures.

Methods

The use of urodynamic testing in children has strengthened our understanding of the pathophysiology of pediatric voiding dysfunction (Table 22.4). Nevertheless, its value has been questioned because of the effort required in evaluating the awake child, a concern more valid in the past, when the information that was obtainable was very limited. Technologic advances and our

understanding of what to look for have significantly improved our diagnostic acumen.[12]

The main goal of urodynamic evaluation in the child is to identify neuro-vesical dysfunction that could potentially lead to renal and bladder damage as the individual ages. Once such conditions have been detected, simple urodynamic testing should be used for continuous follow-up to ensure that current management plans are successful. As the child matures, urodynamics will continue to play an important role by providing the data needed to devise a strategy for achieving continence. Serial urodynamic testing may also confirm the clinical suspicion of spinal cord tethering.[9]

Children with overt neurologic disease should be observed urodynamically from birth onward. Though older children who initially have late voiding dysfunction are less likely to need such formal evaluation of their lower urinary tract, a small subset of older children will have a significant neuro-vesical dysfunction and will require urodynamics testing. This group includes those with occult spinal dysraphism, Hinman-Allen syndrome (nonneurogenic-neurogenic bladder), and other spinal cord abnormalities such as lipoma of the cord, syrinx, cord cysts, tethering of the cord, and sacral agenesis.[9]

Uroflowmetry

Measurement of urinary flow rate is probably the most common urodynamic test performed. Various nomograms have been established in an attempt to standardize uroflow values in children. Mattson and Spangberg demonstrated that increasing flow rates seen in advancing age groups were a reflection of increased voided volume and not caused by age differences. They constructed nomograms for maximum and average flow rates based on voided volumes.[13] The Miskolc nomogram, established by Szabo and Fegyverneki, provides surface area adjusted flow rates for normal boys and girls.[14]

The use of such nomograms allows the urologist to better characterize normal and abnormal flow rates and should prove useful in the screening of children for voiding dysfunction.[12] However, uroflowmetry should not be solely relied on for the identification of children with voiding dysfunction. Although useful as a screening device, it provides no means for assessing detrusor function as evidenced by impaired detrusor compliance or high voiding pressures that cannot be detected by uro-

TABLE 22.4. *Predicted bladder and urethral function based on neurologic lesion location*

Neurologic lesion	Bladder effect	Internal sphincter effect	External sphincter effect
Infrasacral or conus medullaris	Areflexic or hypocontractile	Coordinated with bladder	Denervated
Suprasacral spinal cord	Hyperreflexic	Dyssynergia if T6 or higher	DESD
Suprapontine	Hyperreflexic	Coordinated with bladder	Coordinated with bladder

DESD, Detrusor-external sphincter dyssynergia.

flow measurements.[15] In addition, practical limitations of uroflowmetry restrict its use to cooperative children who are capable of voiding on command.

Cystometrogram (CMG)/Pressure-Flow Study

Invasive urodynamic testing requires that those working with children have both patience and expertise. However, age of the patient should not be a limiting factor. Urodynamic evaluation is possible whether the child is a newborn or an adolescent. Although the awake child is not always cooperative, the use of sedation or anesthesia should be avoided when possible. A successful and accurate study requires an active dialogue between the patient and evaluator, but occasionally, the use of oral midazolom may be considered. A supportive environment is important in helping the child feel less anxious and, hopefully, more cooperative. It is often helpful to have children tour the facility before the study so that they are familiar with what to expect. A parent routinely is present in the urodynamic room. Distractions such as toys, games, television, videotapes, music, conversation, and even food can often help decrease a child's level of anxiety.

A 7-French triple lumen catheter can be used to catheterize young children. A 5-French feeding tube with a three-way stopcock valve is an alternative for male infants. Use of a suprapubic catheter is rarely necessary. A small catheter with a balloon is inserted into the rectum for measurement of intra-abdominal pressures. The urethral catheter is zeroed to atmospheric pressure at the level of symphysis pubis. Next the catheter with all ports is advanced into the bladder. The urethral catheter is then slowly withdrawn so that the first or most proximal port is situated at the level of the external urethral sphincter. This is often achieved with fluoroscopic confirmation or by withdrawing the tube until the proximal channel reaches a maximum increase in urethral pressure recording (maximum urethral closure pressure). The location of this increase in pressure corresponds to the level of the external urethral sphincter. Patch electrodes are applied for electromyography (EMG) recording of striated external sphincter activity. Use of EMG has proven to be a helpful adjunct to the bladder and urethral pressure tracings and will often characterize sphincter activity and help distinguish between conditions such as DESD and nonneurogenic-neurogenic bladder. Latex products should be avoided in all patients undergoing urodynamic evaluation. Substitutes for latex products are used with all patients with spina bifida because of their increased risk of developing latex allergies.[9]

After proper calibration, the study is initiated by instilling room temperature normal saline or radiographic contrast material under gravity. The sterile fluid is instilled at a slow fill rate, usually from 5 to 50 mL/minute.

Estimation of the fill rate (in mL/min) can be made by dividing the age-estimated bladder capacity by 10.[9] It is important to slow the instillation rate in the presence of uncontrolled detrusor activity because fast rates can produce artifactual detrusor contractions.

During filling, infused volume and vesical (Pves) and abdominal (Pabd) pressures are measured. The detrusor pressure (Pdet) is then calculated by subtracting Pabd from Pves (Pdet = Pves − Pabd). Any uninhibited contractions are noted along with the volume at which they occurred. When possible, the child is asked to report any awareness regarding first sensation, first urge, severe urge, and impending void, and these are correlated to the volume infused at that time and to any urodynamic event that occurred. Compliance is a measure of the bladder's storage capability, specifically as it relates to bladder capacity. Compliance is defined as delta volume/delta pressure and can be calculated for any volume increment. Bladders with values less than 20 mL/cm H_2O are considered to have decreased compliance. This indicates poor storage characteristics because bladder filling is occurring under higher pressures. The Detrusor Leak Point Pressure (DLPP) is a measure of the intrinsic bladder pressure during filling at the time that urinary leakage occurs (Fig. 22.4). This is different from the Valsalva Leak Point Pressure (VLPP), which is a measurement of sphincteric competence during stress maneuvers such as cough or valsalva (Fig. 22.5).[16] DLPP is another means of characterizing bladder storage as McGuire noted that patients with high DLPP (>40) were at higher risk for renal damage (Fig. 22.6).[10]

The study is incomplete until the child voids. At this time, EMG activity is carefully monitored and a determination is carefully made of whether the sphincter relaxes before and during the void. Visualization of the individual pressure tracings will determine whether emptying was accomplished by a detrusor contraction or abdominal straining. Voided volume, flow rates, flow pattern, and postvoid residual are analyzed.

Video-Urodynamics

The urodynamics component of Video-Urodynamics is performed in a fashion identical to that of the CMG/PF study. It is done with the aid of simultaneous fluoroscopy using contrast medium for infusion. During the study, vesicoureteral reflux, if present, can be detected as well as the respective detrusor pressure at that time (Fig. 22.7). Imaging of the bladder may denote bladder wall hypertrophy, diverticula, and the presence of any filling defects. Visualization of the bladder neck during filling can provide insight regarding its degree of competency.[7] For example, patients with low level spinal lesions or lower motor neuron deficits (i.e., sacral agenesis or myelomeningocele) that affect the autonomic or somatic input to the bladder outlet may be seen to have

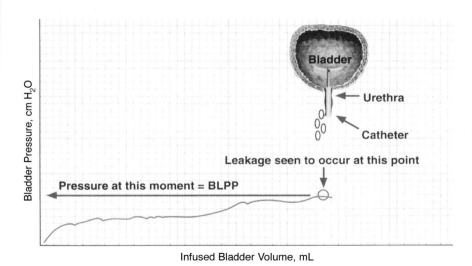

FIG. 22.4. Determining the BLPP. The BLPP is the intravesical pressure at the moment when fluid is first seen from the urethra around the catheter. (From War J. Leak point pressure testing. Contemp Urol 1998;10(4):14.)

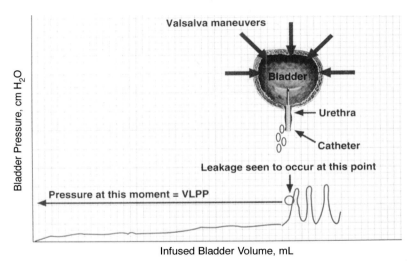

FIG. 22.5. Determining the VLPP. The VLPP is the pressure at which leakage occurs (or the peak pressure without leakage) as the patient performs a series of strong Valsalva maneuvers. (From War J. Leak point pressure testing. Contemp Urol 1998;10(4):19.)

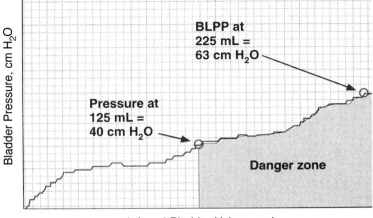

FIG. 22.6. The danger zone defines the storage pressure in the bladder from 125 to 225 mL when the pressure exceeds 40 cm H_2O and the upper tracts are at significant risk for damage. (From War J. Leak point pressure testing. Contemp Urol 1998;10(4):22.)

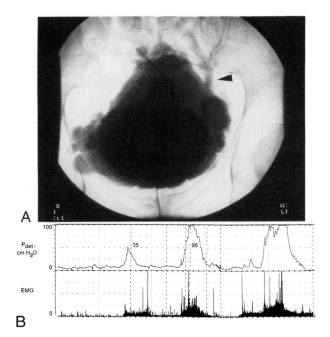

FIG. 22.7. A, Fluoroscopic image showing the videourodynamics of the bladder with a left vesicoureteral reflux (*arrow*) and severe trabeculation. **B,** CMG–EMG evidence of DESD with obstruction.

a wide open bladder neck and nonfunctioning sphincter. During voiding, simultaneous imaging of the bladder and urethra are helpful in identifying detrusor-sphincter dyssynergia.[17]

MYELODYSPLASIA

Etiology and Epidemiology

Spinal dysraphism is a group of abnormalities resulting from failure of the neural tube and bony elements of the spinal cord to fuse normally. The nervous system begins its development during the third week of embryogenesis. The neural groove, derived from the neural ectoderm, deepens and eventually forms the neural tube. Fusion of the neural tube begins in the center and proceeds cranially and caudally. Its completion is concomitant with the onset of the vertebral development, which begins in the fourth week. Normally, the vertebral arches fuse posteriorly to produce the spinous processes.[18, 19]

Myelodysplasia (also known as spina bifida) occurs when the caudal end of the neural tube and vertebral arches do not fuse normally. It occurs in approximately 1 per 1000 births in the United States and is the most common cause of neuropathic bladder dysfunction in children. However, its incidence has decreased, probably because of improved prenatal care, earlier detection, and termination of pregnancy. Etiologic factors that have been implicated include maternal exposure to vari-

ous teratogens or medications, maternal exposure to excessive heat, and, most recently, to a deficiency of folic acid.[19] Studies have shown that dietary supplementation of folic acid may decrease such defects by as much as sevenfold. A familial form of myelodysplasia has been implicated because the presence of one or two children with spina bifida increases the risk of subsequent children having the disease to 5% and 10%, respectively. Nevertheless, more than 90% of all myelodysplastic births have no family history.[18]

Early diagnosis of the disease has been made possible using maternal screening with serum alpha-fetoprotein. Although lacking in specificity, especially for samples obtained later in gestation, an elevated value obtained within 24 weeks gestation that is greater than three standard deviations from the norm carries a 70% risk. Sonography as a single modality for the assessment of spinal dysraphism is poor. However, when it is combined with an elevation of alphafetoprotein, there is 80% sensitivity and 99% specificity in detection of a spinal dysraphism. The early diagnosis of this disease allows for prenatal counseling and planning for the delivery. The mode of delivery may have a significant impact on the neurologic outcome.[18] Luthy et al. have shown that there is a lower rate of paralysis when Cesarean section is performed before the onset of labor.[20] In addition, early warning makes it possible to assemble the proper support staff including neurosurgery, pediatric urology, neonatology, specialized nursing, and social service.[19]

"Spina bifida occulta" refers to the failure of vertebral arch fusion. "Spina bifida cystica" is the term used to describe the protrusion of a sac through the vertebral arch defect. This sac can contain components of nerve tissue, meninges, spinal fluid, and fat. When the sac contains the meninges only, it is called a meningocele. A myelomeningocele, which exists in more than 90% of patients with spina bifida cystica, contains meninges and elements of the spinal cord within the sac. Lipomyelomeningocele describes the development of fatty tissue that becomes intricately involved in spinal cord structures with both components protruding into the sac. Myeloschisis, in which the spinal cord is completely exposed without any meningeal covering, represents the most severe form of spina bifida cystica.[18]

Myelodysplasia most commonly affects the lumbar region of the spinal cord. Incidence by level has been reported as follows: lumbosacral 47%, lumbar 26%, sacral 20%, thoracic 5%, and cervical 2%. Most meningoceles are directed posteriorly, although on rare occasion, the sac may protrude anteriorly, especially with sacral lesions.[18]

Initial management consists of neurosurgical evaluation and treatment. Closure of the spinal defect is usually performed within the first 24 to 48 hours. During the interval before closure, the patient is carefully examined for other associated abnormalities. The central nervous system is assessed sonographically and with CT scan to identify the presence of hydrocephalus and other cerebral abnormalities. Approximately 85% of neonates with myelodysplasia have Arnold Chiari syndrome in which the cerebral spinal fluid is obstructed by herniated cerebellar tonsils at the level of the fourth ventricle. Ventriculoperitoneal shunt is often required to alleviate the hydrocephalus. The newborn is also evaluated for GI and cardiac abnormalities. A higher incidence of genitourinary abnormalities is well-known, including renal fusion anomalies and cryptorchidism.[18, 19]

The neurologic deficits can vary considerably with regard to the level of the actual vertebral defect. There may be a discrepancy of as many as three vertebral levels in any direction between the neurologic lesion and the actual bony level of the spinal defect. In addition, one side of the body may be affected more than the other. Some children, especially those with higher level lesions, may have complete reconstitution of their spine in the sacral area with preservation of sacral reflex arc function.[5]

Once the infant is stable, especially after back closure has been performed, urologic evaluation may be undertaken. Laboratory studies usually include serum chemistries (including creatinine) and urinalysis. It is important to obtain serum chemistries at least 24 hours after delivery because initial values are reflective of the maternal levels rather than those of the newborn. Initial radiologic assessment, consisting of renal and bladder ultrasound, is performed. VCUG identifies the presence or absence of vesicoureteral reflux and surveys the entire lower urinary tract.[5, 18] Recently, the use of VCUG has been replaced with simultaneous cystometrography, perineal electromyography and voiding cystourethrography.[21]

Rationale and Findings

It has been estimated that approximately 95% of children with spina bifida have decreased urinary tract function.[19, 22] The main goal in the management of infants with myelodysplasia is the early detection of dysfunction and the preservation of renal function. Studies have shown that 10 to 30% of newborns with myelodysplasia have evidence of upper urinary tract pathology on initial radiologic assessment,[6, 23] and this percentage increases to approximately 50% by the age of 5.[24] In 1997, Wu et al. reported initial radiologic presentation of hydronephrosis and vesicoureteral reflux in 28% and 21%, respectively.[25] The identification of children who already have evidence of upper urinary tract deterioration, as well as those at risk for its future development, is critical so that otherwise preventable renal damage may be avoided. Furthermore, it is hoped that the prompt use of medical therapy will eliminate the need for more aggressive surgical intervention subsequently.

The goal of modern therapy is to achieve safe mechanical drainage for those with impaired emptying and pharmacologic reduction in filling pressures in those with loss of bladder compliance or elevated detrusor pressures. The introduction of clean intermittent catheterization has revolutionized our ability to drain the bladder safely while keeping infection rates down. Anticholinergics have been shown to help reduce bladder filling pressures with minimum side effects.

The use of clean intermittent catheterization (CIC) represents the single most significant advance in the management of children with myelodysplasia.[22] Since its introduction by Lapides in 1972,[26] it has proved to be a safe and reliable procedure that is easily learned. It provides an effective means for mechanical bladder emptying when normal and efficient bladder emptying cannot be achieved.[27] Although some clinicians believe that clean intermittent catheterization is an additional burden to an already overwhelmed family, many have shown that it is an easily learned technique that is well-tolerated by both sexes and without significant complications. Joseph et al. looked at CIC performed in 38 neonates and found no evidence of urethral injuries, false passage, stricture, epididymitis, meatal stenosis, or meatitis. Although 42% had chronic bacteriuria, only 5% developed a significant or febrile UTI. Furthermore, there was no evidence of increased stress reported by the families who were performing CIC.[22] The success of CIC with regard to continence and achieving independence was questioned by Purcell and Gregory who noted 30% had persistent incontinence despite CIC and only 24% were dry. Furthermore, fewer than a third of the children (mean age 9 years) could perform the procedure independently.[28] This sharply contradicts the high success rates that most have had with CIC. Lindehall et al. found that in teenagers and young adults performing long-term catheterization, the technique was accepted as a daily part of life. Even if complete dryness was not achieved, patients valued the smaller and fewer pads used and the decrease in overall leakage. Patients also felt that CIC allowed them to achieve improved personal relationships and a better quality of life.[29]

By blocking the action of acetyl choline at the postganglionic cholinergic receptor, anticholinergic medication reduces parasympathetic activity, which normally stimulates detrusor musculature and induces its contraction. This results in increasing detrusor compliance and decreasing detrusor filling and voiding pressures. Oxybutynin has anticholinergic and antispasmodic properties on the bladder and is associated with minimum side effects. Its effectiveness has been well-documented.[18, 30, 31]

The most serious problems in the newborn are related to problems of storage. Because of the potentially devastating consequences of renal damage, identification of these problems is necessary so that proper intervention can be promptly implemented. Blaivas et al. noted that no correlations could be derived between a patient's urinary symptoms, urodynamic findings, and the clinical neurologic level. They concluded that bladder characteristics could not be predicted based on the clinical neurologic examination and that urodynamic studies should be performed in all patients with a spinal dysraphism.[32] Urodynamic classification of the myelodysplastic neurogenic bladder is the first step in identifying detrusor dysfunction and in planning long-term lower urinary tract management. In addition, urodynamics is helpful in devising a strategy for achieving continence once the child is able and willing to do so.

Bauer et al. divided patients into three categories based on urodynamic characteristics and external urethral sphincter activity. Inclusion in the respective groups carried different risks for upper urinary tract deterioration. Fifty percent of all patients demonstrated DESD, which carried a 72% risk of upper tract deterioration. Twenty-five percent of all patients demonstrated complete absence of external urethral sphincter EMG activity. Of these patients, 11% developed upper urinary tract deterioration that was attributed to outlet obstruction caused by urethral fibrosis. Twenty-five percent of all patients had synergistic voiding that was associated with a 22% risk of upper urinary tract deterioration because some children converted from synergistic to dyssynergic voiding. Although Spindel et al. noted that 5 of 13 patients with synergistic voiding at birth progressed to a dyssynergic state within the first year, few studies have documented a shift from coordinated micturition to a dyssynergic pattern.[33]

McGuire and coworkers were able to correlate urodynamic findings with radiologic evidence of renal deterioration. They noted that of those patients with DLPP greater than 40 cm, 68% developed vesicoureteral reflux and 81% developed dilation of the upper tracts.[10] Others have attempted to improve our ability to identify those patients at risk for upper urinary tract deterioration. Bauer et al. confirmed that urodynamic studies could provide predictive information for determining the fate of the upper urinary tracts. They found that the presence or absence of DESD was the most important parameter for identifying those in the high risk group.[24] Galloway et al., also attempting to better identify high-risk children, developed a hostility score that incorporated DLPP, bladder compliance, detrusor contractility, reflux, and external urethral sphincter activity.[34] Realizing that bladder capacity and storage pressures should be taken into account, Landau et al. developed the concept of "pressure specific bladder volume," which is defined as the volume of urine that can be stored in a bladder at or below a specified pressure.[35] Despite the overwhelming evidence in support of urodynamics, there is no clearcut consensus regarding the proper timing of its use. Spindel and colleagues noted that 37% of newborns with myelodysplasia demonstrated changes in external urethral sphincter activity, mostly within the first year.[33] Roach et al. reported that patients with initially favorable urodynamic parameters who subsequently worsened, did so within the first 6 months.[36]

Patterns of Neurogenic Bladder Dysfunction in Myelodysplasia

McGuire reported that 83% of patients studied were areflexic with most (30 of 35) having decreased compliance. Most of the children were areflexic with a DLPP set by a degree of fixed resistance at the external urethral sphincter. Three of the seven patients who manifested detrusor activity did so in a dyssynergistic pattern.[10] Sidi et al., in a prospective study, divided their patients into two groups. Thirty percent were found to have decreased compliance or high bladder outlet pressures associated with DESD, whereas 70% were areflexic and had low pressures at the bladder outlet.[37] Bauer et al. noted that 41% of their patients with areflexic bladders also had decreased compliance.[24] In summary, areflexia is the most common pattern of neurogenic bladder dysfunction in patients with myelodysplasia. Loss of compliance is a significant problem in a large subgroup of these children.

Vesicoureteral Reflux

The neurogenic bladder of myelodysplasia is one of the most common causes of secondary vesicoureteral reflux. It is reported to occur in up to 27 to 30% of children with myelodysplasia. In the presence of urinary tract infection, vesicoureteral reflux can cause pyelonephritis, scarring, and loss of renal function.[38] Flood et al. noted a correlation between DLPP greater than 40 cm and the presence of reflux. No correlations were seen between DLPP and vesicoureteral reflux grade or between vesicoureteral reflux grade and rate of improvement or resolution. However, they noted that maintaining detrusor pressures less than 40 cm at typical capacity was associated with an 80% spontaneous resolution or improvement rate for vesicoureteral reflux.[39] Agarwal et al. demonstrated a 63% resolution rate of reflux with medical therapy by reducing the average DLPP from 50 cm to 30 cm.[40] Klose and colleagues reported that vesicoureteral reflux resolved in 90% after administration of intermittent catheterization and anticholinergic therapy.[41] These studies confirm that vesicoureteral reflux in the myelodysplastic neurogenic bladder is related to poor storage parameters and that it can be successfully treated in a nonoperative fashion with proper bladder management and surveillance.

Timing of Lower Urinary Tract Assessment

Determining when to initiate urologic workup or when to implement therapy is not a clear-cut decision. Some clinicians believe that not all infants with myelodysplasia will experience lower urinary tract dysfunction and renal deterioration. Furthermore, some are not convinced that such progression is irreversible and believe that prophylactic intervention may be unnecessary for many children. Chiaromonte proposed that hydronephrosis at onset may be a transient phenomenon secondary to the spinal shock of early back closure. Spontaneous resolution of such hydronephrosis may account for the high success rates achieved by those in favor of early intervention.[23] Klose et al. argue against the routine use of screening urodynamics, believing it will result in the overtreatment of many children who would otherwise have reversible upper urinary tract deterioration or none at all. This is based on their observation that most upper tract deterioration is reversible once CIC and anticholinergics have been initiated.[41] Teichman adds to this argument by reporting a low 5% rate of renal deterioration that urodynamics was unable to predict, in patients managed with "aggressive observation and prompt intervention." However, this study defined renal deterioration only as parenchymal loss or decreased renal function on nuclear scintiography.[42]

Though the arguments against the early use of urodynamics or early aggressive intervention are not without merit, it has been demonstrated that short- and long-term outcomes are dramatically improved when these screening modalities are used early. Kasabian compared expectant management versus early intervention in two groups of neonates with myelodysplasia. Upper urinary tract deterioration was seen in 48% of those expectantly managed and in fewer than 8% of those prophylactically managed.[30] Kaufman et al. radiologically observed 181 patients and found 79 who developed upper urinary tract damage; they were subsequently placed on CIC and anticholinergic therapy. Despite initiation of prompt treatment, overall outcomes were worse. Radiologic stabilization or improvement was seen in 69% of those with hydronephrosis or vesicoureteral reflux, but only 42% experienced an improvement in bladder compliance. It was concluded that late therapy may improve radiologic findings of the upper urinary tract, but the effects on bladder compliance were not readily reversible.[43] These findings were confirmed by Wu et al. who noted that although no difference was seen in the renal outcomes between patients treated early versus those treated later, an increase in noncompliance and a higher rate of augmentation cystoplasty was seen in the group treated later.[25] Thus, early intervention provides better

early and long-term outcomes. Furthermore, therapy after detection of renal deterioration still had a poorer outcome.

Continence in the Child with Myelodysplasia

Once the child with myelodysplasia reaches school age (4–5 years), the issue of urinary incontinence takes on a more significant role. At this point, the child is faced with social and psychological pressures to achieve acceptable continence. Left untreated, approximately 95% of children with myelodysplasia will be incontinent.[18] Uninhibited detrusor contractions, small bladder capacity, poor compliance, and denervation of the external urethral sphincter represent the major causes of incontinence in this patient population.

The approach undertaken should be determined by the cause of the urinary leakage. Voiding and catheterization diaries should be kept with attention paid to voided volumes, frequency of bladder emptying, number and time of any urinary accidents, and volume intake. Sometimes, simple manipulation of fluid intake or changing the scheduled time or frequency of catheterization may be all that is necessary to achieve continence. A bowel regimen is also important because severe constipation can interfere with attempts to stay dry.

Urodynamics plays a vital role in defining the type of incontinence that a child with myelodysplasia may be experiencing. The bladder outlet and urethral sphincter must be assessed for competency. It is not uncommon to find an open bladder neck and a nonfunctioning external sphincter in a child with myelodysplasia, especially one with the low level lesions. A low DLPP, although beneficial for preservation of the upper urinary tracts, will allow leakage, especially in the presence of decreased detrusor compliance. A low VLPP indicates sphincteric incompetence against increases in abdominal pressures such as those associated with coughing or valsalva maneuvers. The detection of uninhibited contractions heralds the diagnosis of detrusor hyperreflexia and may cause symptoms of urge incontinence. During voiding, visualization of an uncoordinated sphincter on fluroscopy or increased EMG activity indicates the presence of DESD. Leakage may occur in the setting of DESD when there is outlet obstruction associated with high pressure ineffective voiding or overflow incontinence. Overflow incontinence may also be seen in the areflexic bladder.

Defining the exact mechanism behind the urinary incontinence makes it possible to institute management directed at the specific problem. Detrusor overactivity and decreased compliance can be treated with the use of anticholinergic medications. Areflexia or other causes of ineffective emptying are managed with the use of intermittent catheterization. Alpha adrenergic agonists can be used for sphincter insufficiency.[44] The success rates for achieving continence by nonsurgical means are variable. Purcell reported a 41% dry rate in children placed on CIC.[28] Higher success rates have been reported by Lindehall, who reported dry or improved continence in 24 of 26 patients,[29] and Kaplan, who cited an 84% continence rate.[83]

OCCULT SPINAL DYSRAPHISM

"Occult spinal dysraphism" is the term applied to a group of concealed abnormalities in the formation of the spinal column. Although these lesions do not result in an open vertebral canal, they still affect the lower spinal cord or nerve roots.[2, 45] Spinal cord fixation may occur with any of these lesions resulting in a "tethered cord" syndrome with all of the associated neurologic sequela.[46] If the conus medullaris does not rise during growth, an ischemic injury to the cord may result.[47, 48] In addition, compression of the cauda equina or sacral nerve roots by an associated lipoma can occur.[49] This variation in the types of injuries that may be encountered, as well as in the neurologic consequences that each injury might evoke, leads to a wide range of neurologic findings in this patient population. It is not uncommon for urodynamic testing to be the only means of identifying whether occult spinal dysraphism has impacted on lower spinal cord function.[50, 51]

The incidence of occult dysraphism is approximately 1 in 4,000 births. More than 90% of afflicted children will have a cutaneous abnormality in the area of the lower midline spine manifested as a skin dimple, skin tag, hair tuft, vascular malformation, or subcutaneous lipoma. Lower extremity abnormalities also observed are high arched feet (*pes cavus*), digit malformations, asymmetrical muscle size or strength, uneven lower extremity length, and difficulties with gait.[45] If not suspected and examined for, these abnormalities can often be missed in the newborn. The neurologic manifestations often are unnoticed, only to be identified later when signs of neurogenic bladder dysfunction or lower extremity problems become evident. The infant may have continuous dribbling that goes unnoticed. As children get older, they may experience difficulties with toilet training, despite achieving some voluntary control.[52]

Lower urinary tract dysfunction has been reported in up to 40% of children with an occult spinal dysraphism.[53] Keating et al. examined children with occult spinal lesions and noted that a third of those children with normal neurologic examination results manifested abnormalities on urodynamic studies.[51] Urodynamic findings in the infant with occult dysraphism were characterized by Atala et al. who reported abnormalities in 36% with most patients having some form of a pure or mixed upper motor neuron lesion. DESD or detrusor hyperreflexia alone was found in 55%, and the remainder had

a combination of DESD or detrusor hyperreflexia and abnormal motor unit potentials. No infant demonstrated a pure lower motor neuron lesion or areflexia.[47] In looking at the difference between younger and older children, Keating noted that 92% of older children (average age 11 years) had abnormal urodynamic patterns. Of these patients, 55% had a mixed upper and lower type motor neuron lesion, whereas 27% had pure upper and 18% had pure lower type lesions.[51]

A policy of performing early elective correction of these lesions has been adopted by many neurosurgeons. As the urologic manifestations of occult spinal lesions are often the earliest and sometimes the only clinical signs and symptoms,[54] the impact of early compared to late neurosurgical intervention on the lower urinary tract has been examined. Keating compared urodynamic results before and after neurosurgical correction in infants (average age 8 months) and older children (average age 11 years). In the younger group, 60% with abnormal urodynamic studies reverted to normal while 30% improved and 10% worsened. The older group fared less well, as only 27% normalized, 27% improved, 27% remained stable, and 19% worsened.[51] Similar findings were seen by Atala et al. who noted 82% improvement in the lower urinary tract of infants compared to only 17% in older children (average age 10 years).[47] Satar et al. also reported poorer urodynamic outcomes after delayed neurosurgical correction (16% improved, 68% unchanged, and 26% worse) and concluded that the urologic and neurologic findings in older children with occult spinal lesions were more likely to be irreversible and that early diagnosis and intervention were imperative.[52]

The role of urodynamic testing in the child with occult spinal dysraphism is not limited to a functional assessment of the lower urinary tract. Satar reported on its use for the early detection of cord fixation in the patient with a previous correction, noting that even after surgical correction the spinal cord on MRI will often exhibit the appearance of being tethered. Satar concluded that urodynamic assessment offers a good method for monitoring damage to the spinal cord and that "EMG evaluation of external urethral sphincter is the most sensitive indicator of progressive deterioration."[55]

SACRAL AGENESIS

Agenesis of the sacrum is a rare congenital anomaly of the lower vertebral column that often produces neurogenic bladder dysfunction. It is defined as the absence of part or all of one or more sacral vertebral bodies. When the defect also involves the lumbar vertebrae and includes anomalies of the anorectal and urogenital systems, it is referred to as caudal regression syndrome.[56] The incidence of sacral agenesis ranges from 0.09 to 0.43%.[57] Although the exact etiology is unknown, it has been postulated that teratogenic factors play a role in its development. Insulin-dependent mothers carry a 1% risk of giving birth to a child with sacral agenesis, and 16% of children with this disorder have mothers who took insulin during pregnancy. Even mothers with only gestational diabetes are at significant risk for delivery of a child with sacral agenesis.[57, 58]

The sacral defect often goes undetected even though it usually is readily palpable. Careful physical examination may reveal flattening of the buttocks, abnormal pigmentation and hair distribution in the lumbosacral area, loss of the upper extent of the gluteal cleft, wide buttock dimples, palpation of a sacral groove-like defect or a soft sacral mass, and deformities of the lower extremities. Sacral agenesis may ultimately become clinically evident with the onset of symptomatic lower urinary tract dysfunction, frequent urinary tract infections, or disorders of the lower extremities.[57, 59] It is best confirmed by radiograph with the lateral view providing the most optimal imaging.[58] Reports of vesicoureteral reflux, hydronephrosis, pyelonephritis, renal parenchymal scarring, bladder diverticula, and renal deterioration have been attributed to a delay in the detection of the lower urinary tract dysfunction.[58, 60, 61] Mariani et al. noted vesicoureteral reflux in 91% of their patients who had sacral agenesis.[62]

The neurologic implications of sacral agenesis can be variable. Neurologic deficits do not correlate closely with the level of the osseous abnormality despite the fact that the conus comes to an abrupt ending at the level of the sacral deformity. The corresponding nerve roots from this deformed area may be distorted or absent. When present, the nerve roots are often imbedded in dense fibrous tissue. It has been theorized that this creates traction on the spinal cord with ischemia, producing a picture similar to the tethered cord syndrome.[57, 60]

The motor nerve deficit seen in sacral agenesis is more pronounced than the sensory deficit. Preservation of lower extremity or perianal sensation does not preclude a neurologic deficit and is a poor indicator of bladder and sphincteric function.[62] The high degree of variability of the neurologic deficits prohibits the accurate clinical assessment of the lower urinary tract without the use of urodynamic testing.[57, 58, 62]

Studies by Koff and Deridder did not demonstrate a specific neurourologic pattern. All 11 children who underwent cystometrograms were found to have evidence of various types of neurogenic bladder dysfunction. Three demonstrated detrusor hyperreflexia, four were areflexic, and four had mixed components of upper and lower motor neuron bladder dysfunction. Twelve patients underwent perineal electromyography with seven displaying evidence of denervation. Of the five patients with normal EMGS, four had neurogenic bladder dysfunction.[60] Saito et al. evaluated 15 patients and

demonstrated detrusor areflexia in 13, while 2 had normal lower urinary tracts. However, 10 of these "areflexic" patients demonstrated involuntary detrusor contractions during filling. Follow-up studies revealed that 80% remained areflexic with stable compliance patterns and that most no longer demonstrated any involuntary contractions.[59] Guzman et al. evaluated 16 patients with sacral agenesis and noted that 7 had areflexic bladders without any involuntary contractions, whereas the remaining 9 had detrusor hyperreflexia; 3 demonstrated DESD.[57] Gotoh et al. also found similar results with respect to the incidence of upper and lower motor neuron types of bladder dysfunction in 13 children observed urodynamically. Nine of these children demonstrated poor compliance (<10 mL/cm H_2O).[58]

Strategies for management of the lower urinary tract in sacral agenesis are similar to those of other neurogenic bladders. Saito and associates reported that all 15 of their patients were on CIC and that complete continence was achieved in 11 while the remaining 4 had socially acceptable continence.[59] Guzman noted an overall dry rate of 75%. In 16 patients, 7 were dry with CIC alone, 3 of 6 were dry with CIC and anticholinergic therapy, 2 were dry after placement of artificial sphincters, and 1 remained diverted.[57] Less favorable results were seen by Gotoh who reported a continence rate of only 50% with use of CIC combined with anticholinergic medication. However, his population of patients had a high rate of urethral abnormalities.[58]

IMPERFORATE ANUS

Imperforate anus may be associated with a multitude of urologic problems, which include structural anomalies of the urinary tract and vertebral abnormalities and their associated neurologic deficits. Vertebral involvement has been seen in up to 45% of these patients and the presence of an occult spinal dysraphism has been recognized as a cause of lower urinary tract dysfunction. In addition, definitive surgical correction of the imperforate anus may result in damage to the innervation of the lower urinary tract.[63, 64]

The presence of vertebral bony anomalies warrants a radiographic assessment of the spinal column. Early urodynamic evaluation is indicated in all patients with evidence of spinal cord involvement. In addition, it is thought that urodynamic studies should be performed before definitive surgical repair associated with high (supralevator) lesions.[65] With the advent of the Pena procedure, which uses a midline approach, the chance of traumatizing the laterally coursing pelvic floor nerves, such as the pudendal nerve, has been reduced. Urodynamic and perianal EMG studies are performed after surgical repair if fecal or urinary continence has not been obtained by a reasonable age or if new onset incontinence develops.[45]

Greenfield and Fera prospectively performed urodynamic studies in 14 patients with imperforate anus before any surgical intervention. DESD was seen in four (29%), three of whom had high lesions.[64] Kakizaki et al. evaluated 21 patients with imperforate anus in whom urodynamics revealed a normal lower urinary tract in 12 and DESD in 9. High lesions were seen in 22% of those with a normal lower urinary tract and in all of those with DESD. Seven of these 9 patients had vesicoureteral reflux. Renal deterioration was seen in three patients. All three had DESD and had previously demonstrated poor compliance and high grade vesicoureteral reflux at initial presentation. They concluded that urodynamic evaluation was warranted in all patients before undergoing anorectoplasty because of the high incidence of congenital neurogenic bladder dysfunction as opposed to surgically induced neural trauma to the innervation of the lower urinary tract.[65]

CEREBRAL PALSY

Cerebral palsy represents an injury to the brain that occurs in the perinatal period and has been attributed to a period of perinatal anoxia or infection. It carries an incidence of 1.5 per 1,000 births and is seen commonly in premature babies, although it may also occur after seizures, infections, or intracranial hemorrhage. The condition produces neuromuscular deficits attributed to the cerebral dysfunction. Afflicted children display delayed gross and fine motor development and other upper motor neuron types of dysfunction such as altered muscle tone and hyperactive reflexes.[45]

Most children with cerebral palsy achieve total urinary control. Often, the age at which continence is obtained is delayed. Although incontinence is seen in some children, the leakage is usually attributed to factors such as physical impairment that causes an inability to reach the bathroom in a timely fashion and severe mental retardation that makes voluntary continence control unattainable.[45,66] The actual incidence of neurogenic bladder dysfunction in cerebral palsy is unknown. McNeal et al. suggested that 36% of children with cerebral palsy have voiding symptoms suggestive of lower urinary tract dysfunction.[67]

Decter et al. studied 57 patients with cerebral palsy using urodynamic testing. Urinary incontinence was present in 86%. An upper motor neuron type of dysfunction seen as detrusor hyperreflexia was evident in 86% of the children. Eleven percent had EMG evidence of incomplete lower motor neuron involvement of the external urethral sphincter. Complete lower motor neuron dysfunction was never seen. It is thought that the uninhibited contractions from detrusor hyperreflexia make urinary continence difficult to obtain.[68] Drigo et al. noted detrusor hyperreflexia in all children with cerebral palsy

and DESD was present in 20%.[69] Similar findings were also noted by Reid and Borzyskowski.[70]

Most children with cognition sufficient for toilet training will eventually gain bladder control. Urodynamic evaluation of those children with cerebral palsy who do not achieve urinary continence is warranted to define the exact type of lower urinary tract dysfunction. The presence of DESD in patients with cerebral palsy remains a controversial issue. Because DESD occurs after disruption of the communication between the sacral spinal cord and the pontine micturition center, its presence implies a neurologic insult somewhere between the two areas. Although a concurrent anoxic injury to the spinal cord is possible, Mayo's theory of nonrelaxation of the external urethral sphincter, as seen in patients with Parkinson's, seems more plausible.[66,71] Therefore, we believe that the external urethral sphincter activity seen with detrusor contractions in this patient population represents pseudodyssynergia and not genuine DESD.

SPINAL CORD INJURY IN CHILDREN

Spinal cord injury in children is relatively uncommon. The incidence in children has been said to range from 0.65 to 9.6% of all spinal cord injuries. There is a higher incidence in male children in whom injuries are usually the result of motor vehicle accidents, falls from significant heights, sporting accidents, and diving injuries.[72] There is also an increased risk of injury to the spinal cord of the fetus with a breech presentation. It has been estimated that 20% of breech newborns with hyperextended necks that are delivered vaginally may sustain some form of spinal injury, usually at the level of the cervicothoracic junction.[73,74] Iatrogenic injuries to the spinal cord such as those occurring after surgery to correct scoliosis have also been described.[75]

Injuries to the spinal cord in children are intrinsically different from those in adults. These differences are attributable to the different mechanism of injuries seen in children and the differences in the development and structure of the spinal cord in children. Infants, because of the relative size and heaviness of their heads, are more predisposed to flexion type injuries of the cervical cord, typically between C2 and C3. As children grow, the level drops until it reaches the C5–C6 level often seen in adults. Thus, the likelihood of high cervical injury is greater in children. In addition, the poor development of the paraspinal support structures in children renders their spines hypermobile. This hypermobility predisposes children to ischemic injury of the spinal cord.[72]

The spinal cord of children may sustain injury without radiographic evidence of osseous trauma. Spinal cord injury without radiographic abnormality (SCIWORA), which occurs almost exclusively in children, is reported in 16 to 67% with a spinal cord injury. A latent period has been seen in children with SCIWORA in whom the neurologic deficit may not be manifest for as many as 4 days after the injury. However, the latent period does not indicate that the injury is any less serious.[72]

After initial stabilization, the child with a spinal cord injury is evaluated with a urine culture, baseline testing of renal function, imaging of the entire urinary tract, and urodynamic assessment. Ultrasound is an excellent initial imaging modality given its noninvasiveness and capability of accurately assessing renal parenchyma and the presence of hydronephrosis. Urodynamics should be performed after the period of initial spinal shock is gone. Videourodynamics is preferred because of its ability to detect vesicoureteral reflux and because it is highly accurate in identifying external sphincter dysfunction.

Management of the pediatric neurogenic bladder caused by spinal cord injury is similar to that of adults. When emptying is impaired, the bladder is drained mechanically, usually with intermittent catheterization. Detrusor hyperreflexia, which is most often seen with a higher level injury, is managed with anticholinergic drugs and intermittent catheterization. Detrusor sphincter dyssynergia can often be managed in a similar fashion. Urologic reconstruction with augmentation cystoplasty or use of a continent catheterizable abdominal stoma may be used if self-catheterization through the urethra is impossible. Moving the catheterization site to the abdominal wall often makes the process more manageable for the child who has limited hand function. Sphincterotomy is rarely indicated in the child.[72] Its irreversible outcome should be strongly considered before rendering children permanently incontinent and dependent on external catheter drainage for the rest of their lives.

NONNEUROGENIC-NEUROGENIC BLADDER (HINMAN-ALLEN SYNDROME)

Nonneurogenic neurogenic bladder is recognized as a syndrome of dysfunctional voiding in the absence of an identifiable neurologic or anatomic cause. It is an acquired syndrome of detrusor sphincter dyssynergia whereby active contraction of the external sphincter occurs in response to a detrusor contraction.[76] This dyssynergic sphincter contraction during voiding results in a functional outflow obstruction.

Hinman introduced the theory that dysfunctional voiding was caused by a functional discoordination between bladder and sphincter rather than by an occult isolated neurologic defect that manifested itself only through altered micturition.[77] This was supported by Allen who also widened the syndrome to include other dysfunctional states such as lazy bladder syndrome.[78] It was hypothesized that the normal infant bladder's reflexive voiding pattern underwent a transition to willful control by using the external sphincter to "hold back" urination during the time of detrusor contraction. This could be caused by the sphincter's ability to suppress detrusor activity through reflex inhibition. This behavior of the contracting external sphincter has been termed "the guarding reflex."[79] In addition, the infant may volitionally contract the sphincter to hold back emptying and keep the outlet closed until the detrusor contraction subsides. With time, detrusor capacity increases, detrusor hyperactivity decreases, and the central inhibition of the detrusor contraction takes over as the main determinant in volitional control. Hinman and Allen believed the syndrome represented a persistent state of this transitional period in which contraction of the external sphincter remained the major determinant for volitional control. McGuire postulated that children who learn to contract their sphincter in response to the urge from uninhibited contractions of infancy persist in this activity because it has become a response to the bladder's normal signal of fullness and the desire to void.[80]

The Hinman-Allen syndrome is characterized by recurrent urinary tract infection, infrequent voiding pattern, urge and stress urinary incontinence, and fecal soiling. Urine flow is intermittent and is usually associated with straining. Disruptive family dynamics is almost routinely present. Parental domineering is often found and alcoholism and divorce are also common. Wetting and delayed toilet training are perceived by the parents as characteristics of failure and immaturity. Children are punished for what the parents believe to be purposeful and defiant behavior. Children, confused and fearing further punishment, try to withhold urination and defecation by using their voluntary sphincter muscles. However, in many cases it is difficult to determine whether the family dynamics cause or are a result of the dysfunctional voiding.[81]

Histories should include questions about early toilet training, whether there were periods of continence and, if so, when the lapses developed. Records should indicate when wetting events occurred, the frequency and character of voiding, and whether there was any relation between urinary infections and bowel problems. Evaluation of the parent-child relationship is made throughout the visit, even before the child is actually seen by the physician. Physical examination may reveal damp pads, fecal soilage, squatting, or even the witnessing of the child using his or her heel pressed against the perineum to hold back urination (Vincent's curtsey). Neurologic assessment should be performed with special attention directed at perineal sensation, anal tone, anal contraction and lower extremity function. Laboratory tests should include urinalysis, urine culture, and serum chemistries, including creatinine and urea nitrogen evaluations.

Radiographic evaluation of these children often reveals hydronephrosis and renal scarring. Vesicoureteral reflux has been reported in up to 50% of patients and the bladder is usually grossly distended with severe trabeculation. Fecal impaction and chronic constipation also can be seen.[78]

Urodynamic studies demonstrate a bladder with significantly enlarged capacity, decreased compliance, and uninhibited detrusor contractions during filling. Emptying is characterized by high pressure voiding, the need for abdominal straining, and a nonrelaxing external sphincter. Urinary flow is often intermittent and slow, and the postvoid residual is elevated.

Management of children with the Hinman syndrome traditionally consisted of multiple urologic procedures in an attempt to correct reflux and improve emptying. Since the recognition of this psychological dysfunctional voiding syndrome, treatment has been focused on alleviating the stresses of the child, proper counseling, and helping the child empty more successfully.[81] Strategies such as timed voiding, behavioral modification, anticholinergic medication, intermittent catheterization, and adherence to a planned bowel regimen have been implemented with success. This includes diet adjustments and use of laxatives, stool softeners, enemas, and digital disimpaction. Antibiotic suppression should be instituted if vesicoureteral reflux or recurrent urinary tract infection is present. The use of biofeedback was introduced in 1979 and has played an important role in behavioral modification. External urethral sphincter activity is measured using perineal electromyelography and is recorded during urinary flow. The child learns to associate the relaxation of the sphincter with urination and maintaining the urinary flow.[77] Yang and Mayo reported their results in the management of children with Hinman's syndrome. They noted a 30% cure and 30% unchanged rate in 27 patients. The remaining 40% (11 patients) had significant morbidities related to the disease. Most patients required at least one major urologic surgery. Four patients in this group developed renal insufficiency and two of the four eventually underwent renal transplantation. Patients in the other two groups were managed with nonoperative measures. The eight patients who did not improve were reported as being noncompliant with treatment protocols.[76] Phillips and Uehling's report of unfavorable outcomes in children being treated for Hinman's syndrome further exemplifies that children with this syndrome are at significant risk for deterioration. King noted that despite attempts to initiate prompt treatment, successful outcomes often are not achieved. Poor compliance to treatment recommendation or total ignorance of the problem was seen, which he attributed to lack of family support.[82]

REFERENCES

1. Elbadawi A. Functional anatomy of the organs of micturition. Urol Clin North Am 1996;23(2):177.
2. Bauer SB. Neurogenic bladder dysfunction. Pediatr Clin North Am 1987;34(5):1121.
3. de Groat WC. Anatomy and physiology of the lower urinary tract. Urol Clin North Am 1993;20(3):383.
4. Klimberg I. The development of voiding control. AUA Update Series, V.7, Lesson 21 1988;162.
5. Bauer SB. Neuropathology of the lower urinary tract. In: Kelalis PP, King LR, Belman AB, eds. Clinical pediatric urology. Philadelphia: WB Saunders, 1992;399.
6. Bauer SB. Early evaluation and management of children with spina bifida. In: King LR, ed. Urologic surgery: Neonates and young infant. Philadelphia: WB Saunders, 1988;252.
7. Ewalt DH, Bauer SB. Pediatric neurourology. Urol Clin North Am 1996;23(3):501.
8. Bellinger M. "Myelomeningocele and neuropathic bladder. In: Gillenwater JY, Grayhack JT, Howards SS, Duckett JW, eds. Adult and pediatric urology. St. Louis: Mosby Yearbook, 1996; 2489.
9. Wan J, Greenfield SP. Pediatric urodynamics. In: Blavias J, Chancellor M, eds. Atlas of urodynamics. Baltimore: Williams and Wilkins, 1996;251.
10. McGuire EJ, Woodside JR, Borden TA, Weiss RM. Prognostic value of urodynamic testing in myelodysplastic patients. J Urol 1981;126:205.
11. Norris JP, Staskin DR. History, physical examination and classification of neurogenic voiding dysfunction. Urol Clin North Am 1996;23(3):337.
12. Boone TB. Urodynamic evaluation of the bladder in children. Curr Opin Urol 1996;6:296.
13. Mattsson S, Spangberg A. Urinary flow in healthy schoolchildren. Neurourology & Urodynamics 1994;13(3):281.
14. Szabo L, Fegyvereki S. Maximum and average urine flow rates in normal children—the Miskolc nomograms. Br J Urol 1995;76:16.
15. Jorgenson JB, Jensen KM. Uroflowmetry. Urol Clin North Am 1996;23(2):237.
16. Blaivas J, Chancellor M. Cystometry, ed. Atlas of Urodynamics. Baltimore: Williams and Wilkins, 1996;31.
17. McGuire EJ, Cespedes RD, Cross CA, O'Connell HE. Videourodynamic studies. Urol Clin North Am 1996;23(2):309.
18. Selzman AA, Elder JS, Mapstone TB. Urologic consequences of myelodysplasia and other congenital abnormalities of the spinal cord. Urol Clin North Am 1993;20(3):485.
19. Sutherland RS, Mevorach RA, Baskin LS, Kogan BA. Spinal dysraphism in children: An overview and an approach to prevent complications. Urology 1995;46:294.
20. Luthy DA, Wardinsky T, Shurtleff DB, Hollenbach KA, Hickok DE, Nyberg DA, Benedetti TJ. Cesarean section before the onset of labor and subsequent motor function in infants with meningomyelocele diagnosed antenatally. N Engl J Med 1991;324:662.
21. Hernandez RD, Hurwitz RS, Foote JE, Zimmern PE, Leach GE. Nonsurgical management of threatened upper urinary tracts and incontinence in children with myelomeningocele. J Urol 1994; 152:1582.
22. Joseph DB, Bauer SB, Colodny AH, Mandell J, Retik AB. Clean intermittent catheterization of infants with neurogenic bladder. Pediatrics 1989;84(1):78.
23. Chiaramonte RM, Horowitz EM, Kaplan GW, Brock WA. Implications of hydronephrosis in the newborn with myelodysplasia. J Urol 1986;136:427.
24. Bauer SB, Hallett M, Khoshbin S, et al. Predictive value of urodynamic evaluation in newborns with myelodysplasia. JAMA 1984; 252:650.
25. Wu HY, Baskin LS, Kogan BA. Neurogenic bladder dysfunction due to myelomeningocele: Neonatal versus childhood treatment. J Urol 1997;157:2295.
26. Lapides J, Diokno AC, Silber SJ, Lowe BS. Clean intermittent catheterization in the treatment of urinary tract disease. J Urol 1972;107:458.
27. Diokno AC, Sonda LP, Hollander JB, Lapides J. Fate of clean intermittent self-catheterization therapy 10 years ago. J Urol 1983; 129:1120.
28. Purcell MH, Gregory JG. Intermittent catheterization: Evaluation of complete dryness and independence in children with myelomeningocele. J Urol 1984;132:518.

29. Lindehall B, Moller A, Hjalmas K, Jodal U. Long-term intermittent catheterization: The experience of teenagers and young adults with myelomeningocele. J Urol 1994;152:187.

30. Kasabian NG, Bauer SB, Dyro FM, Colodny, AH, Mandell J, Retik AB. The prophylactic value of clean intermittent catheterization and anticholinergic medication in newborns and infants with myelodysplasia at risk of developing urinary tract deterioration. AJDC 1992;146:840.

31. Baskin LS, Kogan BA, Benard F. Treatment of infants with neurogenic bladder dysfunction using anticholineric drugs and intermittent catheterisation. Br J Urol 1990;66:532.

32. Blaivas JG, Labib KL, Bauer SB, Retik AB. Changing concepts in the urodynamic evaluation of children. J Urol 1977;117:778.

33. Spindel MR, Bauer SB, Dyro FM, et al. The changing neurologic lesion in myelodysplasia. JAMA 1987;258:1630.

34. Galloway NTM, Mekras JA, Helms M, Webster GD. An objective score to predict upper tract deterioration in myelodysplasia. J Urol 1991;145:535.

35. Landau EH, Churchill BM, Jayanthi VR, et al. The sensitivity of pressure specific bladder volume versus total bladder capacity as a measure of bladder storage dysfunction. J Urol 1994;152:1578.

36. Roach MB, Switters DM, Stone AR. The changing urodynamic pattern in infants with myelomeningocele. J Urol 1993;150:944.

37. Sidi AA, Dykstra DD, Gonzalez R. The value of urodynamic testing in the management of neonates with myelodysplasia: A prospective study. J Urol 1986;135:90.

38. Cohen RA, Rushton HG, Belman AB, Kass EJ, Majd M, Shaer C. Renal scarring and vesicoureteral reflux in children with myelodysplasia. J Urol 1990;144:541.

39. Flood HD, Ritchey ML, Bloom DA, Huang C, McGuire EJ. Outcome of reflux in children with myelodysplasia managed by bladder pressure monitoring. J Urol 1994;152:1574.

40. Agarwal SK, McLorie GA, Grewal D, Joyner BD, Bagli DJ, Khoury AE. Urodynamic correlates of resolution of reflux in meningomyelocele patients. J Urol 1997;158:580.

41. Klose AG, Sackett CK, Mesrobian HJ. Management of children with myelodysplasia: Urologic alternatives. J Urol 1990;144:1446.

42. Teichman JM, Scherz HC, Kim KD, Cho DH, Packer MG, Kaplan GW. An alternative approach to myelodysplasia management: Aggressive observation and prompt intervention. J Urol 1994;152:807.

43. Kaufman AM, Ritchey ML, Roberts AC, Rudy DC, McGuire EJ. Decreased bladder compliance in patients with myelomeningocele treated with radiological observation. J Urol 1996;156:2031.

44. Rudy DC, Woodside MD. The incontinent myelodysplastic patient. Urol Clin North Am 1991;18(2):295.

45. Bauer SB. Neurogenic dysfunction of the lower urinary tract in children. In: Walsh PC, Retik AB, Stamey TA, Vaughn ED, eds. Campbell's Urology. Philadelphia: WB Saunders, 1992;1634.

46. Perez LM, Barnes N, MacDiarmid SA, Oakes J, Webster GD. Urological dysfunction in patients with diastematomyelia. J Urol 1993;148:1503.

47. Atala A, Bauer SB, Dyro FM, et al. Bladder functional changes resulting from lipomyelomeningocele repair. J Urol 1992;148:592.

48. Yamda S, Zinke DE, Sanders D. Pathophysiology of tethered cord syndrome. J Neurosurg 1981;54:494.

49. Yamada S, Knierim D, Yonekura M, Schultz R, Maeda G. Tethered cord syndrome. J Am Paraplegia Soc 1983;6(suppl 3):58.

50. Khoury AE, Hendrick EB, McLorie GA, Kulkarni A, Churchill BM. Occult spinal dysraphism: Clinical and urodynamic outcome after division of the filum terminale. J Urol 1990;144:426.

51. Keating MA, Rink RC, Bauer SB. Neurourological implications of the changing approach in management of occult spinal lesions. J Urol 1988;140:1299.

52. Satar N, Bauer SB, Shefner J, Kelly MD, Darbey MM. The effects of delayed diagnosis and the treatment in patients with an occult spinal dysraphism. J Urol 1995;154:754.

53. Mandell J, Bauer SB, Hallett M, et al. Occult spinal dysraphism: A rare but detectable cause of voiding dysfunction. Urol Clin North Am 1980;7:349.

54. Kaplan WE, McLone DG, Richards I. The urological manifestations of the tethered spinal cord. J Urol 1988;140:1285.

55. Satar N, Bauer SB, Scott M, Shefner J, Kelly M, Darbey M. Late effects of early surgery on lipoma and lipomeningocele in children less than one year old. J Urol 1997;157:1434.

56. Boemers TM, van Gool JD, de Jong TP, Bax KM. Urodynamic evaluation of children with the caudal regression syndrome (caudal dysplasia sequence). J Urol 1994;151:1038.

57. Guzman L, Bauer SB, Hallett M, Khoshbin S, Colodny AH, Retik AB. Evaluation and management of children with sacral agenesis. Urology 1983;22:506.

58. Gotoh T, Shinno Y, Kobayashi S, Watarai Y, Koyanagi T. Diagnosis and management of sacral agenesis. Eur Urol 1991;20:287.

59. Saito M, Kondo A, Kato K, Diagnosis and treatment of neurogenic bladder due to partial sacral agenesis. Br J Urol 1991;67:472.

60. Koff SA, Deridder PA. Patterns of neurogenic bladder dysfunction in sacral agenesis. J Urol 1977;118:87.

61. Braren V, Jones WB. Sacral agenesis: Diagnosis, treatment and follow-up of urological complications. J Urol 1979;121:543.

62. Mariani AJ, Stern J, Khan AU, Cass AS. Sacral agenesis: An analysis of 11 cases and review of the literature. J Urol 1979;122:1284.

63. Steers WD, Barrett DM, Wein AJ. Voiding dysfunction: Diagnosis, classification and management. In: Gillenwater JY, Grayhack JT, Howards SS, Duckett JW, eds. Adult and pediatric urology. St. Louis: Mosby, 1996;1220.

64. Greenfield SP, Fera M. Urodynamic evaluation of the patient with an imperforate anus: A prospective study. J Urol 1991;146:539.

65. Kakizaki H, Nonomura K, Asano Y, Shinno Y, Ameda K, Koyanagi T. Preexisting neurogenic voiding dysfunction in children with imperforate anus: Problems in management. J Urol 1994;151:1041.

66. Boone TB. The bladder and genitourinary tract in the cerebral palsies. In: Miller G, Clark GD, eds. Cerebral palsies: Causes, consequences and management. Boston: Butterworth-Heinemann, 1998;299–307.

67. McNeal DM, Hawtrey CE, Wolraich ML, Mapel JR. Symptomatic neurogenic bladder in a cerebral-palsied population. Dev Med Child Neurol 1983;47:612.

68. Decter RM, Bauer SB, Khosbin S, et al. Urodynamic assessment of children with cerebral palsy. J Urol 1987;138:1110.

69. Drigo P, Seren F, Artibani W, Laverda AM, Battistella PA, Zacchello G. Neurogenic veiscourethral dysfunction in children with cerebral palsy. Ital J Neurol Sci 1988;9:151.

70. Reid CJD, Borzyskowski M. Lower urinary tract dysfunction in cerebral palsy. Arch Dis Child 1993;68:739.

71. Mayo ME. Lower urinary tract dysfunction in cerebral palsy. J Urol 1992;147:419.

72. Dector RM, Bauer SB. Urologic management of spinal cord injury in children. Urol Clin North Am 1993;20(3):475.

73. Abroms IF, Bresnan MJ, Zuckerman JE, et al. Cervical cord injuries secondary to hyperextension of the head in breech presentations. Obstet Gynecol 1973;41:369.

74. Leventhal HR. Birth injuries of the spinal cord. J Pediatrics 1960;56:447.

75. Fam B, Yalla SV. Vesicourethral dysfunction in spinal cord injury and its management. Semin Neurol 1988;8:150.

76. Yang CC, Mayo ME. Morbidity of dysfunctional voiding syndrome. Urology 1997;49:445.

77. Hinman F. Nonneurogenic neurogenic bladder (the Hinman syndrome) 15 years later. J Urol 1986;136:769.

78. Allen TD. The non-neurogenic neurogenic bladder. J Urol 1977;117:232.

79. Park JM, Bloom DA, McGuire EJ. The guarding reflex revisited. Br J Urol 1997;80:940.

80. McGuire EJ, Savastano JA. Urodynamic studies in enuresis and the nonneurogenic neurogenic bladder. J Urol 1984;132:299.

81. Phillips E, Uehling DT. Hinman syndrome: A vicious cycle. Urology 1993;42:317.

82. King L. Editorial comments. Urology 1993;42:319.

83. Kaplan WE. Management of myelomeningocele. Urol Clin North Am 1985;12(1):93.

CHAPTER 23

Nonsurgical Management of the Neurogenic Bladder

Ross M. Decter

INTRODUCTION

Neurogenic bladder dysfunction is caused by a variety of congenital or acquired lesions. Most children with neurogenic bladders are born with myelodysplasia, and many advances in the management of the neurogenic bladder have come about as a result of discoveries made by pediatric urologists caring for these patients. The lessons learned in the evaluation and management of the bladder dysfunction of these patients have been applied to patients with neurogenic bladders resulting from other causes. Therefore, a large proportion of this chapter will be devoted to reviewing nonsurgical modalities discovered and used in the management of children with spina bifida, but many of these approaches are equally applicable to the management of the neurogenic bladder from other causes.

It is only 25 years since E. Durham Smith summarized progress in the management of children with spina bifida.[1] He reported that when these children were left untreated, 58% of them developed structural changes in their urinary tract after the age of three. When they were treated with what was then current management, urinary diverison by ileal conduit or cutaneous ureterostomy, 90% of patients with normal IVPs prior to diversion retained normal studies at least two years after diversion. It was also recognized that early diverison led to a lower risk of long-term renal deterioration. Complications requiring reoperative surgery occurred often after urinary diversion; but, on balance, early diversion seemed the best hope for long-term renal preservation and socially acceptable continence. There was no reliable or readily performed technique for safely and predictably emptying the neurogenic bladder at that time. Within a few years, though, the advent of clean intermittent self-catheterization (CIC) championed by Lapides revolutionized the management of the neurogenic bladder.[2,3]

At about the time that CIC was introduced, several investigators recognized that although urinary diversion offered an excellent short-term solution to a difficult problem, it held a significant risk for subsequent operative interventions.[4,5,6] These observations, along with the greater application of CIC, lead to a new era in the management of the neurogenic bladder. By the mid 1970s, innovative pediatric urologic surgeons were taking down ileal conduits or other forms of diversion and creating bladders that could reliably store urine and could then be emptied by clean intermittent catherization.[7] This was an era of significant progress in the surgical management of the neurogenic bladder, but it also heralded the beginning of a period of advances and refinement in the nonsurgical management of the neurogenic bladder.

Preeminent among these advances was the establishment of the efficiency and safety of clean intermittent catheterization; but of nearly equal significance was a greater comprehension of the urodynamic consequences of the neurologically impaired bladder and the ability to predict which patients were most likely to suffer structural and functional urinary tract changes as a consequence of their lesions. Along with these advances came an expanded capacity to alter adverse bladder activity pharmacologically and to minimize its detrimental sequelae. In the current state of refinement of management, many investigators are now trying to determine how they can evaluate and manage patients with neurogenic bladders in a safe yet cost-efficient, manner.

The urodynamic evaluation of children with neurogenic bladders is the subject of chapter 22, but several points deserve reiteration to facilitate a clear understanding of the rationale for aspects of the nonsurgical management of these children. McGuire deserves credit for drawing attention to the predictive value of urodynamic testing.[8] He evaluated a group of children with myelodysplasia and found that storage of urine at high intravesical pressures portended the likelihood of upper urinary tract deterioration, either hydronephrosis or reflux. Specifically, he noted that if the bladder storage characteristics were such that urine leaked from the urethra when the intravesical pressure was greater than 40 cm H_2O, 68% of patients developed reflux and 81% manifested hydronephrosis. In contrast, if urine leaked at less than 40 cm H_2O, no child developed reflux and only 10% developed ureteral dilatation. This description of a critical bladder pressure that could distinguish those children with "safe" systems from those with "at-risk" systems is a conceptually simple concept that is relatively easy to measure, and it has been universally accepted as one important factor in predicting the outcome of children with neurogenic bladders. The intravesical pressure at the time that urethral leakage occurs is known as the detrusor leak point pressure (LPP), and values of 40 cm H_2O or greater are predictive of the risk of upper tract deterioration. Bauer has performed elegant urodynamic studies that include external sphincter EMG recordings in infants with myelodysplasia, and his group has described the significance of detrusor sphincter dyssynergia (DSD) in these infants.[9] Of a group of infants with myelodysplasia, these investigators diagnosed DSD in half the patients and noted that 72% of the group with DSD had or developed hydronephrosis, whereas only 22% of the children with synergic sphincters and 11% with absent sphincteric activity suffered this outcome. These studies pioneered the concept of the predictive value of urodynamic testing and led to the belief currently held by most investigators that storage of urine at pressures above 40 cm H_2O or the presence of DSD are potentially harmful to the upper urinary tracts. The concept of bladder pressure as a significant parameter in determining outcome has been assessed in other patient populations. Hackler evaluated bladder pressure and volume relationships in a group of spinal cord injury (SCI) patients. He found that a low compliance or high intravesical pressure at a given volume of bladder filling was predictive of outcome. Patients with low compliance manifested hydronephrosis in 64% of renal units and reflux in 46%, whereas in patients with normal compliance, only 21% of the renal units demonstrated hydronephrosis and 6% showed reflux.[10] The major goals in the management of the neurogenic bladder in children revolve around modifying bladder activity so that the storage phase will occur at safe pressures and intermittent emptying of the bladder will be complete and predictable.

NEUROMUSCULAR RELATIONS

An understanding of the normal neuroanatomic relations of the bladder and sphincter mechanisms is important in any discussion of the management of the neurogenic bladder as the clinical approach to drug management is predicted largely on the concept of mod-

ulating normally distributed and functioning nerves and muscles. It is important to understand that changes in the normal neuroanatomic relations after neurologic injury may be more complex than an analysis of the direct consequences of the injury would predict. Subtle neuromechanical alterations may occur after an injury. These changes may be a result of the plasticity of the nervous system, as exemplified by altered adrenergic innervation after decentralization,[11, 12, 13] altered intracellular factors such as modulation of receptor operated calcium channels,[14] or extracellular factors evidenced by changes in collagen types and distribution.[15] These changes are incompletely understood, but their occurrence indicates that the concept of pharmacologic manipulation based on presumed normal neuroanatomic relations may be partially flawed.

THE SMOOTH MUSCLE CELL

The contraction of a smooth muscle cell is a result of interactions between its contractile proteins or filaments. The contractile proteins of smooth muscle cells are myosin, actin, and tropomyosin. Myosin is the major component of the thick filaments; the other proteins compose the thin filaments.[14] One theory proposes that muscle cell contraction occurs when these filaments slide on each other. It is theorized that calcium derived from either an intracellular or extracellular source is complexed to calmodulin, a specific calcium-binding protein, and that this complex, by binding to a myosin light chain kinase, causes phosphorylation of the myosin.[16] Phosphorylated myosin then allows actin to activate a myosin MG2+-ATPase that releases the energy to cause cross-bridging between the thick and thin filaments and actual muscular contraction.[14] Calcium is a major determinant of muscular contraction and, therefore, drugs affecting calcium fluxes may impact on bladder function.

Bladder smooth muscle function is also influenced by potassium. There may be at least two types of potassium channels in bladder smooth muscle.[17] Opening of potassium channels results in hyperpolarization of the cell and muscular relaxation.[14, 18] Introduction of agents modulating potassium channels offers another possible technique to manipulate bladder activity.

MUSCULAR STRUCTURE OF THE BLADDER AND OUTLET

The bladder is described as consisting of three smooth muscle layers. However, these layers interlace and distinct separation is not possible. The smooth muscle cells of the bladder body are not unlike those observed in other muscular organs. The syncytial arrangement of the muscles functionally reduces all dimensions of the bladder lumen after contraction, thereby facilitating evacuation.

The bladder outlet consists of the bladder base, urethra, and external urethral sphincter.[14] A portion of the bladder base, in the region of the bladder neck, contains small-diameter smooth muscle cells that are different from those of the detrusor proper. Additionally, as the innervation to the bladder neck is different from that to the bladder body, it is usually considered as a separate functional unit.[19] In the male, the smooth muscle of the bladder neck forms a circular collar (part of the internal sphincter), and the fibers of the bladder neck extend distally to surround the preprostatic urethra. In the female, the bladder neck fibers do not form a circular collar but rather extend obliquely or longitudinally into the urethral wall.[19]

Gosling[20] considers the male urethra in four parts: the preprostatic, prostatic, membranous, and penile.[19] The preprostatic urethra extends from the bladder neck into the base of the prostate. The muscular fibers in this region are continuous with the bladder neck and extend into the capsule of the prostate. The combined bladder neck and preprostatic fibers form the preprostatic or internal sphincter. Anatomically, the bladder neck seems constructed to aid in continence and although its role of closure to prevent retrograde ejaculation is accepted, it is also clear that patients remain dry after transurethral resection of the bladder neck.

The membranous urethra consists of an inner layer of smooth muscle extending distally from the prostatic urethra surrounded by a circularly oriented striated muscle rhabdosphincter. The striated muscles of the rhabdosphincter are small slow-twitch fibers that are fatigue resistant.[20] This type of muscle fiber is ideal for maintenance of a continence zone.

Continence in the male after bladder neck resection has been attributed to urethral occlusion by the muscular components of the membranous urethra.[14] The levator ani or pelvic floor muscles are adjacent to, but separate from, the rhabdosphincter. The fibers of these periurethral muscles are composed of both the slow- and fast-twitch type. These muscles are suited to rapid augmentation of outlet resistance during increases in abdominal pressure. In the female, the rhabdosphincter is also composed of small slow-twitch striated fibers that surround an inner layer of smooth muscle extending down from the bladder neck. The female rhabdosphincter is thickest in the midurethra. The pelvic floor musculature is adjacent to, but separate from, the rhabdosphincter of the urethral wall as in the male.

NEUROLOGIC PATHWAYS TO THE BLADDER

The bladder and its outlet are innervated by the autonomic and somatic nervous systems. Both divisions of the autonomic system affect bladder function. The parasympathetic input to the bladder arises from the intermediolateral cells of the second, third, and fourth sacral cord segments. The preganglionic parasympathetic fibers travel in the pelvic nerve to ganglia located in the pelvic plexus and on the bladder surface. The neurotransmitter of the preganglionic and postganglionic parasympathetic fibers is acetylcholine. In addition to receiving stimulatory parasympathetic influences, the postganglionic parasympathetic fibers also receive inhibitory sympathetic (adrenergic) input. The cell bodies of the sympathetic nerves to the bladder are located in the intermediolateral grey matter of the cord from T10 to L2. Some preganglionic sympathetic fibers synapse in the paravertebral ganglia, while others continue through the ganglia without synapsing. Both preganglionic and postganglionic sympathetic fibers project peripherally as the hypogastric nerve. The hypogastric nerve and pelvic nerve meet and branch to form the pelvic plexus. The sympathetic preganglionic neurotransmitter is acetylcholine, and the sympathetic postganglionic neurotransmitter is noradrenaline. The striated muscles of the rhabdosphincter and the periurethral muscles are innervated by the pudendal nerve.[21] The cell bodies of the pudendal nerve lie in the intermediolateral columns of S2 to S4,[19] anterior to the parasympathetic cell bodies in a region called Onuf's nucleus.[14]

Neurotransmitters

Classically, acetylcholine is described as the preganglionic neurotransmitter in the autonomic nervous system. Acetylcholine acts on nicotinic receptors at the ganglia, and the excitatory input it engenders in the bladder can be abolished by nicotinic ganglionic blocking agents. Postganglionic parasympathetic nerve terminals, which can be detected as agranular vesicles on electron microscopy, also contain acetylcholine. Stimulation of the pelvic nerves produces a bladder contraction, an effect mediated by acetylcholine release at the postganglionic muscarinic receptors. The muscarinic antagonist atropine will inhibit this action to a variable degree depending upon the species studied. The fact that atropine does not completely block bladder contraction after pelvic nerve stimulation is known as atropine resistance. This phenomenon can be explained by postulating the function of more than one neurotransmitter at the postganglionic parasympathetic junction. In fact, numerous neurotransmitters are probably operating to modulate transmission at these junctions, and the concept of a single neurotransmitter at an individual junction is overly simplistic.[22] A listing of the classical and other putative neurotransmitters is shown in Table 23.1.

Autonomic Nerves and Receptors in the Bladder

Muscarinic receptors are abundantly distributed throughout the human detrusor, and are present at a lower density in the urethra.[23] The apparent alteration in the density of muscarinic receptors in some patients

TABLE 23.1. *Proposed transmitters in the autonomic nervous system*

Classical:
  Acetylcholine
  Noradrenaline
Purinergic:
  Adenosine triphosphate
Aminergic:
  5-Hydroxytryptamine
  γ-Aminobutyric acid
  Dopamine
Peptidergic:
  Enkephalin/Endorphin
  Vasoactive intestinal polypeptide/Peptide HI
  Substance P
  Gastrin-releasing peptide/Bombesin
  Somatostatin
  Neurotensin
  Luteinizing hormone–releasing hormone
  Cholecystokinin/Gastrin
  Neuropeptide Y/Pancreatic polypeptide
  Galanin
  Angiotensin
  Adrenocorticotrophic hormone
  Calcitonin gene-related peptide

(Adapted from Burnstock, G. Acta Physiol. Scand. 1986;126:67, with permission.)[12]

suffering neurologic injury[24] is an example of an unexpected consequence of injury and of the complexity of neuromuscular bladder function. In contrast to the rich cholinergic muscarinic receptor distribution, postganglionic sympathetic adrenergic receptors are sparsely distributed in the bladder body.[23] There is some controversy about the distribution of adrenergic nerves in the bladder neck and urethra. Ek[23] found a very scarce supply of adrenergic nerves in both the male and female urethra. He identified very few adrenergic nerves at the bladder body, but he noted a greater number in the region of the trigone.[23] Benson's[25] evaluations also detected few adrenergic nerve terminals in the bladder body. Gosling[26] found a sparse distribution of adrenergic nerves in the male and female bladder neck and female urethra, but he detected an increase in the density of adrenergic nerves at the male vesicourethral junction. In the preprostatic urethra these nerves were relatively numerous. Despite the paucity of adrenergic nerve fibers identified in the human detrusor, there is ample pharmacological data supporting the efficacy of agents directed toward the adrenergic system.[27, 28, 29] Alpha adrenergic receptors predominate in the bladder base,[27] and beta receptors are found in the bladder body.[30]

As noted earlier, a neurologic injury may have a more profound effect than the direct consequences of the actual lesion would suggest. After parasympathetic decentralization in cats, Sundin observed adrenergic sprouting and an increase in the number of adrenergic terminals in the detrusor muscle. The response to hypo-gastric nerve stimulation changed from brief contraction and subsequent relaxation to a sustained bladder contraction.[31] Studying an experimental model of parasympathetic decentralization by division of the S1 to S3 nerve roots, DeGroat deduced that reinnervation of the denervated cholinergic ganglia cells by ipsilateral sympathetic preganglionic nerves from the hypogastric nerves had occurred. The normal inhibitory effect of hypogastric nerve stimulation converted to a stimulatory bladder contraction mediated by acetylcholine release.[12] The altered response to hypogastric nerve stimulation is similar in these two models, but the proposed mechanism for that altered response is different.

Sundin[11] observed an increase in the size and number of adrenergic nerve terminals in the bladder body of patients who had suffered parasympathetic denervation. In vitro testing of muscle strips from these bladders and cystometrograms performed on these patients using α agonists and blockade revealed a functional correlate of this new innervation. In normal bladder body muscle strips there was no response to α agonists, whereas in the denervated specimens, a significant increase in muscle tension was observed. In addition, after α blockade, the cystometrogram of these patients showed a shift to the right.

The extrapolation that adrenergic hyperinnervation by intact pathways leads to poor bladder compliance has been questioned by Sislow and Mayo.[13] They observed poorer compliance in patients undergoing radical pelvic surgery when both the parasympathetic and sympathetic nerves were subjected to damage than in patients with a more purely parasympathetic decentralization resulting from a conal–cauda equina injury. On the basis of these findings, the authors question the role of adrenergic hyperinnervation by intact sympathetic pathways as a cause of poor compliance observed clinically after parasympathetic decentralization. With regard to drug therapy of the lower urinary tract, it is important to realize that a neurologic injury may cause unexpected changes in the innervation of the bladder and, therefore, preclude an anticipated drug effect. The experimental models and human experience are at times disparate, and our understanding of the plasticity of the nervous system in response to injury is in its infancy.

CLASSIFICATION

A management plan of any disorder generally relies on a pathophysiological understanding that allows one to characterize the problem and appropriately position it in an overall management scheme. A variety of classification systems have been devised to describe lower urinary tract dysfunction, and each has some merit.[32, 33, 34] We find the system of Krane and Siroky[35] that defines the relationship of the bladder and smooth and striated muscular sphincters to be the most clearly descriptive

TABLE 23.2. *Krane and Siroky classification of neurourologic disorders*

I. Detrusor hyperreflexia
   A. Coordinated sphincters
   B. Striated sphincter dyssynergia
   C. Smooth muscle sphincter dyssynergia
II. Detrusor areflexia
   A. Coordinated sphincters
   B. Nonrelaxing striated sphincter
   C. Denervated striated sphincter
   D. Nonrelaxing smooth muscle sphincter

(Adapted from Krane and Siroky, Clinical Neurourology, 1979 with permission.)[25]

TABLE 23.4. *Pharmacologic management of the bladder*

Drugs to facilitate bladder emptying

A. Increasing bladder contractility.
   1. Parasympathomimetic agents.
   2. Blockers of inhibition.
     a. α antagonists.
     b. Opioid antagonists.
B. Decreasing outlet resistance.
   1. At the smooth muscle sphincter.
     a. α antagonists.
   2. At the striated sphincter.
     a. Benzodiazopines.
     b. Baclofen.
     c. Dantrolene.

Drugs to facilitate bladder storage

A. Decreasing bladder contractility.
   1. Anticholinergics.
   2. Musculotropics.
   3. Tricyclic antidepressants.
   4. Calcium channel blockers.
   5. Potassium channel openers.
   6. Prostaglandin antagonists.
   7. β agonists.
B. Increasing outlet resistance.
   1. α agonists.
   2. Tricyclic antidepressants.

(Adapted from Wein, Campbell's Urology, 6th Edition, 1992 with permission.)[30]

(Table 23.2). A well-performed video urodynamic study is mandatory to classify a bladder by this system. In some instances, the precise definition of the bladder and sphincter relationships allowed by this system will affect a particular aspect of therapy. This assessment may be important, especially in those instances when the "expected" consequence of a neurologic lesion differs from the actual urodynamic outcome[36] (Table 23.2).

The practical approach to voiding dysfunction alluded to by Gibbon[33] and formalized by Wein[37] has appeal. Wein's system, which guides the thinking of the current generation of urologists,[38, 39] takes a simple approach to bladder dysfunction (Table 23.3).

The bladder functions either to store or evacuate urine, and all available therapies can be classified by their effect on storage or emptying. This approach is especially attractive when one considers the pharmacologic management of the bladder because available agents are conveniently divided into those same categories (Table 23.4). We will focus primarily on the agents currently in common use in children with neurogenic dysfunction. Wein's[37] classification system will serve as the framework for this discussion.

DRUGS TO FACILITATE BLADDER EMPTYING

These agents act either to increase bladder contractility or decrease the outlet resistance. They are used infrequently in children with neurogenic dysfunction because

TABLE 23.3. *Classification of bladder dysfunction*

Failure to empty:
   Due to the bladder
   Due to the outlet
Failure to store:
   Due to the bladder
   Due to the outlet

(Adapted from Wein, J Urol 1981;125:27, with permission.)[27]

the emptying afforded by clean intermittent catheterization (CIC) essentially obviates any of the benefits these agents might confer on bladder function.

Agents to Increase Bladder Contractility

The prototypical parasympathomimetic agent, bethanechol chloride (BC), acts to increase bladder contractility by its action at the postganglionic parasympathetic site. BC has a relatively selective action on the muscarinic receptors of the bowel and bladder. Although BC has been used for years to improve emptying in adults with both non-neurogenic and neurogenic disorders, its true efficacy is still not clearly defined.[40] Other agents proposed to increase bladder contractility include alpha adrenergic agonists, which may act by releasing an α-mediated inhibition of cholinergic transmission[41] and opioid antagonists.[42, 43] We have not seen reports documenting improved bladder emptying in response to these agents in children.

Agents to Decrease Outlet Resistance

Improved bladder emptying may result from manipulation of the outlet at either the smooth muscle or striated sphincter. Although most often we bypass disordered function at these levels by CIC,[44] there will be some patients in whom CIC is impractical or whose parents reject the concept of catheterization. There are a few patients with incomplete spinal cord injuries or myelodysplastic patients with minimal bladder dysfunction in whom pharmacologic manipulation of the outlet will facilitate self-voiding. The bladder neck and smooth muscle sphincter are responsive to sympathetic stimulation. Sympathetic nerve stimulation or α agonists will increase internal sphincter pressure while α blockade will decrease it.[28]

Phenoxybenzamine (POB) was the α blocker initially used to manipulate the smooth muscle sphincter. In patients with neurogenic bladder neck dysfunction who void spontaneously, POB has been shown to decrease residual urine and improve their voiding pattern,[28] with the only observed side effect being orthostatic hypotension. Patients with neurogenic bladders due to spinal cord injury (SCI) have benefitted from POB therapy. Scott achieved bladder "balance" using POB to alter the outlet resistance in patients with lower motor neuron (LMN) lesions, upper motor neuron (UMN) lesions with intact sympathetics (cord injury between L2 and S2), and upper motor neuron lesions that manifest autonomic dysreflexia.[45] Hachen[29] documented the efficacy of POB in another large group of SCI patients. The outcomes were better in patients with autonomous (lower motor neuron lesion) than automatic (upper motor neuron lesion) bladders. In the former category, he documented a decrease in postvoid residuals by 43%, reduction or disappearance of autonomous waves a third of the time, and improvement in bladder capacity over half of the time. Only 10% of these patients required bladder neck resection. Results were not as good in patients with UMN lesions, because POB does not overcome the problem of detrusor external sphincter dyssynergia. An analysis of this report suggests the effect of POB in the SCI bladder may not simply be the result of its lowering the outlet resistance. In patients with parasympathetic decentralization, increased adrenergic innervation can convert the β (relaxant) effect of sympathetic stimulation to an α (contractile) one.[11] POB has been shown to decrease filling pressure in decentralized primates[46] so, it may have a dual role, improving storage by increasing compliance as well as facilitating emptying by decreasing outlet resistance. POB has enjoyed less clinical application since reports of its inducing gastrointestinal tumors in rats[47] and peritoneal sarcomas in rats and mice. However, other more specific alpha blockers have been employed to achieve similar effects.

Prazosin is an antihypertensive drug with a specific action on the postsynaptic α-1 receptors. It blocks the contraction of human urethral smooth muscle produced by noradrenaline in vitro.[48] In patients with lower motor neuron and autonomous bladders, Andersson[48] demonstrated prazosin caused a reduction of the intraurethral pressure, decreased intravesical pressures during filling, and inhibited autonomous bladder contractions. One meningomyelocele patient in his series was able to void efficiently enough on prazosin so that she no longer required CIC.[48] Other α-1 blockers have been developed with similar effects on the lower urinary tract. Terazosin, another selective α-1 adrenergic blocker, has been used in patients with spinal cord injury. Swierzewsky and colleagues[49] used Terazosin in 12 spinal cord injury patients who had poor vesical compliance despite CIC and anticholinergic therapy. Detrusor compliance improved in all patients and, in spite of the theoretical risk of decreasing outlet resistance, patients reported less incontinence. The improved compliance may be due to blockade of altered detrusor adrenergic innervation seen after neurologic injury.[11] Alfuzosin is another potent α-1 blocker with urodynamic effects similar to Prazosin.[50]

There are three types of orally administered drugs that decrease outlet resistance by their action on striated muscle. Unfortunately, none of these agents is specific for the urethral striated sphincter. The benzodiazepines, prototypically diazepam (Valium), function through a central action on the neurotransmitter gamma-aminobutyric acid (GABA) to cause skeletal muscle relaxation. We have not seen any published reports of efficacy in children but suspect that sedation or alteration of cerebral function limit its applicability.

Baclofen (Lioresal) acts by a central alteration in GABA activity that is not completely understood. It has been useful in the treatment of skeletal muscle spasticity. Forante and colleagues[51] treated 25 SCI patients with baclofen and documented a decrease in urethral sphincter resistance with a significant reduction in residual urine in 73% of the patients. Reported side effects of baclofen include somnolence and upper extremity weakness.[51] Baclofen is excreted by the kidneys, so dose reduction is necessary in patients with renal insufficiency to prevent significant neurological side effects.[52] Dantrolene sodium (Dantrium) is a direct skeletal muscle relaxant that probably works by interfering with sarcoplasmic reticulum calcium fluxes. Murdock and colleagues[53] used dantrolene in a highly selected group of six patients with neurologic disorders who manifested urethral obstruction only at the level of the striated sphincter. During therapy, residual urine decreased and sphincter EMG activity during filling and voiding decreased.[53] Hackler and colleagues[54] used Dantrium in a group of 25 adults with complete SCI. Fifteen patients completed the study and eight of these benefitted from the drug with reduced residual urines. However, side effects of dizziness, weakness, fatigue, and malaise occurred frequently.[54] Fatal hepatotoxicity has been observed after Dantrium therapy. Overall, the side effect profiles of the agents that work on the striated sphincter tend to limit their use in children.

An alternative to the orally administered drugs to decrease outlet resistance is the local injection into the striated sphincter of Botulinum A toxin. Botulinum A toxin paralyzes skeletal muscle by a presynaptic blockage of neurotransmitter release. Skeletal muscles treated with Botulinum toxin show effects of denervation and, ultimately, muscle atrophy.[55] This agent has been injected into the external sphincter to treat detrusor sphincter dyssynergia in a limited number of adults with SCI.[56] Sphincteric paralysis caused by the toxin decreases urethral pressure, postvoid residual, and bladder pressures during voiding.[56] Use of Botulinum A toxin requires direct injection of the agent into the striated sphincter. There are no reports of its application in children with SCI, and its role remains to be defined.

DRUGS TO FACILITATE BLADDER STORAGE

Drugs which facilitate bladder storage act either to decrease bladder contractility or increase the outlet resistance. These groups of agents are used extensively in the management of the pediatric neurogenic bladder.

Agents to Decrease Bladder Contractility

The major physiological event which causes a bladder contraction is the release of acetylcholine at the postganglionic parasympathetic muscarinic receptors. Atropine, a muscarinic receptor blocker, depresses this action. In fact, atropine or other anticholinergic agents will decrease uninhibited contractions (UC) from any cause. The typical urodynamic consequences of an anticholinergic agent are an increase in the bladder capacity to the onset of the first uninhibited contraction, a decrease in the magnitude of those contractions, and an overall increase in bladder capacity.[57] Atropine increases compliance in the decentralized primate bladder,[46] but it does not affect compliance in patients who manifest only uninhibited contractions.

The side effects common to all anticholinergic agents include a dry mouth caused by inhibition of salivation, blurred vision resulting from blockade of the ciliary muscle of the eye, tachycardia, constipation, and drowsiness. These agents are contraindicated in patients with narrow-angle glaucoma, an extremely unusual condition in children. The orally administered dose of atropine required to achieve a desired effect on the bladder causes excess side effects, so it is seldom used as the anticholinergic agent of choice. In the last decade, intravesical drug administration in children on intermittent catheterization has been employed using a variety of agents. Glickman and colleagues[58] reported on the use of intravesical atropine in 12 SCI patients with detrusor hyperreflexia. In the seven patients who retained the solution, there was a significant reduction in the amplitude of the uninhibited contractions and an increase in bladder capacity prior to the onset of uninhibited contractions with no observed side effects.[58] Ekström and colleagues used intravesical atropine in a group of 12 patients with neurogenic bladders. Urodynamic evaluation revealed five of the 12 demonstrated an increase in their bladder capacity. Four of these five noted decreased leakage of urine and one became dry.[59] The role of intravesical atropine in children is unexplored.

There are a variety of anticholinergic agents available, all with similar effects on the bladder. Propantheline bromide (Pro-Banthine) is commonly used. Dosing usually starts at 7.5 mg three times a day in younger children and is titrated up to 30 mg four times a day to achieve the desired effect. Other antimuscarinic agents include glycopyrrolate (Robinul) and hyoscyamine sulfate (Levsin). The antimuscarinic efficacy of these agents is not superior to that of Pro-Banthine,[47] although the liquid formulations of Levsin facilitate its administration to younger children. Methantheline (Banthine) is active both as a ganglionic blocker and as an antimuscarinic agent, but it is no more effective than Pro-Banthine and has a similar side effect profile.[47]

There are three musculotropic or direct smooth muscle relaxants commonly used to modify bladder activity. Each of these agents has a triple action on the bladder. They function as direct smooth muscle relaxants (spasmolytics), anticholinergics, and local anesthetics. The relative contribution of each of these individual actions to their overall effect on bladder activity is not clearly defined.

Oxybutynin chloride (Ditropan), a tertiary amine, was first utilized in urologic practice in the early 1970s,[60] and it is the musculotropic drug most widely used in children. Ditropan has twice the local anesthetic effect of lidocaine.[61] In rabbit bladder studies, oxybutynin had a much weaker anticholinergic activity than Pro-Banthine and atropine, but its spasmolytic effect was twice that of Pro-Banthine and 10 times that of atropine.[62] In a double-blind study comparing Ditropan (5 mg TID) to placebo in patients with detrusor instability, Moisey found five of seven patients with instability from neurogenic cause subjectively improved. There was no response to the placebo in these patients. Overall, 17 of 30 patients in the study suffered side effects; a dry mouth was the side effect most frequently observed.[63] Kawabe administered Ditropan 4 mg three time a day to nine adults with neurogenic bladders. In a short-term study of 7 to 12 days, he observed clinical improvement with less frequency, urgency, and incontinence in seven of the nine patients.[64]

In pediatric practice, Ditropan has become the initial drug of choice for treating incontinence resulting from detrusor hypertonia and/or hyperreflexia. Over the past few years several of our myelomeningocele patients who had been totally dry on Ditropan and intermittent catheterization presented with new incontinence. At evaluation, their urine was sterile and the only change in their regime we discovered was a new "Ditropan" prescription filled with a generic "equivalent." When these patients resumed the non-generic form of oxybutynin, Ditropan, their wetting disappeared. It seems that not all generics are equally effective. The Physician's Reference enumerates a lengthy list of adverse reactions experienced by patients on Ditropan. In practice, side effects are observed quite frequently.[65] Many of our patients manifest cutaneous vasodilation causing flushing and a tendency to overheat due to decreased sweating, which can be quite problematic, especially in the summer. Other children frequently complain of dry mouth, visual alterations, and minor CNS mood disturbances.

An attempt to maximize the local effect of the drug on the bladder and minimize systemic side effects led to the evaluation of the intravesical route of administration. Brendler and colleagues[66] reported 10 of 11 patients using intravesical Ditropan noted subjective improvement, became continent, and experienced no side effects. In a group of children with neurogenic bladders, Greenfield reported clinical improvement in 80% of the patients with neither local nor systemic side effects. Urodynamic evaluations revealed significant increases in bladder capacity and decreases in maximum filling pressures.[67] In a follow-up report from the same institution[68] with a larger group of patients, the positive urodynamic improvements, persisted and 81% of the patients had improved continence. However, intolerable anticholinergic side effects experienced by 25% of the patients caused them to discontinue intravesically administered Ditropan.

A pharmacokinetic study comparing intravesically and orally administered Ditropan was undertaken to elucidate the reason for the infrequent occurrence of side effects in patients on intravesical Ditropan. Massad and associates found that both routes of administration led to high plasma levels. They concluded that the absence of side effects was not due simply to poor systemic absorption. They theorized that a hepatic metabolite might be responsible for side effects, thus explaining their occurrence after oral administration as the drug passed through the portal circulation. This concept was supported by the observation of side effects in two patients who had undergone bladder augmentation with bowel and experienced adverse reactions after receiving intravesical Ditropan.[69] Other studies have confirmed the low incidence of side effects and excellent efficacy of intravesical Ditropan,[70, 71] and an animal study detected no local deleterious effect of topical oxybutynin.[72] Overall, experience with intravesical Ditropan has been satisfactory, although a few patients have experienced typical side effects after this route of administration.

Because Ditropan and Pro-Banthine are among the agents most commonly employed to treat detrusor hyperreflexia and instability, their efficacy has been compared. Gajewski and Awad performed a prospective randomized study of Ditropan and Pro-Banthine in patients with hyperreflexia resulting from multiple sclerosis. Symptomatic response was good and fair in 80% of the patients on Ditropan and in 45% of those on Pro-Banthine. The mean increase in maximum cystometric capacity was significantly greater in the patients treated with Ditropan. Side effects of sufficient severity to dictate discontinuing use of the medication occurred with equal frequency with both drugs.[73]

Holmes et al. compared the efficacy of Ditropan to that of Pro-Banthine in a single blind cross-over trial in 23 women with detrusor instability who attended a gynecology clinic. Sympatomatic improvement was not statistically different between the two agents. The maximum cystometric capacity was statistically significantly greater when Ditropan was employed. These authors commented that they did not demonstrate a "clear difference between oxybutynin and propantheline,"[74] In a randomized, double-blind, placebo-controlled multicenter study Thüroff and colleagues[65] compared oxybutynin, propantheline, and a placebo in 69 patients with detrusor hyperactivity. Both the mean bladder volume at first involuntary contraction and the mean cystometric bladder capacity increases were significantly greater with oxybutynin than with the placebo. In both these parameters, the effect of oxybutynin was greater than that of propantheline but not to the levels of statistical significance. The majority of clinical studies suggest Ditropan is superior to Pro-Banthine. Ditropan is my initial drug of choice for decreasing bladder contractility. The combination of Ditropan and a pure anticholinergic should have an additive effect, and I use this combination at times.

The other musculotropic agents available are dicyclomine (Bentyl) and flavoxate hydrochloride (Urispas). Fischer and colleagues[75] reported on the use of Bentyl in 14 adult patients with uninhibited neurogenic bladders. All patients experienced a positive urodynamic response with increased bladder capacity, delay to first uninhibited contraction, and delay of the urge to void.[75] We find Bentyl a useful agent, especially in the children who do not tolerate oxybutynin. Its liquid formulation facilitates administration in younger children. Flavoxate (Urispas) and Pro-Banthine were administered by Bradley and Cazort in a double-blind fashion to 46 adults with a variety of disorders resulting in irritable bladder symptoms. Flavoxate was superior in providing symptomatic relief, although the differences were not statistically significant and none of the patients had neurogenic bladders.[76] Benson and colleagues[77] evaluated the effect of flavoxate on bethanechol chloride, and barium chloride-stimulated canine detrusor contractions. They found flavoxate minimally suppressed the detrusor contraction elicited by these agents. The authors postulated that the clinical effect of the drug could be a result of its local anesthetic action because they did not observe a significant anticholinergic or spasmolytic effect. Briggs and colleagues evaluated flavoxate in six elderly incontinent patients with detrusor instability and found no effect in the short term on incontinence.[78] We have not seen reports of flavoxate use in children with neurogenic bladders.

The tricyclic antidepressant imipramine hydrochloride (Tofranil) improves urine storage. Imipramine improves storge by a dual effect on the bladder: it depresses contractility while it augments bladder outlet resistance.[79, 80] Imipramine's mechanism of action is described as being threefold: an anticholinergic action, a role to block the reuptake of noradrenaline in the synaptic cleft, and a presumed central sedative action.[47] In addition, Benson and colleagues[77] demonstrated in the canine bladder a musculotropic relaxant action, which they found to be more potent than that of flavoxate. Labay and Boyarsky[81] also postulated a direct effect of imipramine on the smooth muscle beyond the muscarinic receptor. The anticholinergic and musculotropic actions of imipramine decrease bladder contractility, and the alteration of adrenergic activity augments the β effect on the bladder body to relax it and the α effect at the bladder outlet to contract it. Because mechanism of action of imipramine is not that of a simple anticholinergic agent, the probability exists of an additive effect with a pure anticholinergic. In fact, we often combine imipramine with Pro-Banthine (propantheline bromide) or Ditropan (oxybutynin hydrochloride) in myelodysplasic children using CIC, and have observed improved continence over each agent alone. One of the side effects of the tricyclics, especially with overdosage, is the possibility of cardiotoxicity. We warn parents to be sure their child's supply of imipramine is out of the reach of all children in the home to avoid accidental poisoning.

Bladder smooth muscle contraction is dependent on the entry of extracellular calcium via calcium channels. Agents which block those channels (such as nifedipine and verapamil) will reduce contractile activity, and it seems reasonable that they would be explored as agents to improve bladder storage. Gotoh and colleagues[82] studied in vitro and in vivo rabbit bladder responses to topical verapamil. They found that muscle bathed in verapamil showed reduced spontaneous contractile activity and diminution of the contractile response to direct electric stimulation and to acetylcholine exposure. Sixty minutes after intravesical administration of verapamil, the rise in intravesical pressure in response to pelvic nerve stimulation was less than 17% of control, and no effect on systemic blood pressure was observed. In an experimental rabbit model producing hyperreflexia, Levin and colleagues[83] used intravesical verapamil and nifedipine and demonstrated a dose-dependent decrease in the amplitude and frequency of uninhibited contractions. With increasing intravesical doses of the calcium blockers, there was a progressive decrease in the mean arterial blood pressure.

The prominent systemic cardiovascular effects limit the value of orally administered calcium blockers when they are used as agents to modify bladder activity, and they have not proven effective.[84]

The intravesical route has appeal as a mode of administration, because it increases the local effect and limits the systemic effects of these agents. Intravesical Verapamil was used in patients with detrusor hyperreflexia (DH) and detrusor instability by Mattiasson and colleagues.[88] They documented moderate but significant increases in bladder capacity only in the patients with DH.[88] I have seen no published data on the intravesical use of a calcium channel blocker in children with neurogenic bladders. In children on CIC this route of administration is attractive, and perhaps with refinements in dosing, calcium channel blockers will be used either alone or in a "cocktail" with other intravesical agents.

Potassium channel opening agents relax smooth muscle by increasing potassium efflux from the cell, causing hyperpolarization of the membrane. Membrane potential is primarily dependent on the potassium gradient, and hyperpolarization reduces the sensitivity of the cell to myogenic activity and increases the threshold for neurologically stimulated contractions.[89] Pinacidil and Cromakalim are vasodilators which act as K+ channel openers.[18, 90] In an evaluation of these agents on normal and hypertrophied rat bladders, Malmgren and colleagues[90] found that they depressed the contractile response to carbachol and electric field stimulation.

Fovaeus and colleagues[18] evaluated Pinacidil action on human detrusor strips and concluded that it functioned as a K+ channel opener, hyperpolarizing the bladder cells and thereby decreasing the contractile response to carbachol, low concentrations of potassium, and electrical stimulation. In their evaluation of the effect of intravesical pinacidil and cromakalim, Levin and colleagues,[83] in a rabbit model, recorded a dose-dependent decrease of contractile activity. Hedlund and colleagues[85] used pinacidil in a group of ten men with detrusor instability owing to bladder outlet obstruction. The authors could not document a positive effect of pinacidil on unstable detrusor contractions in these patients. Manipulations of the detrusor cell excitability potential with K+ channel openers remain a largely unexplored therapeutic avenue in children with neurogenic bladders.

To complete the discussion of drugs which may function to improve bladder storage by decreasing contractility, we will mention the prostaglandin inhibitors, β agonists, and capsaicin. Prostaglandins (PG) E_1, E_2, $F_{1\alpha}$, and F_2 produce contraction of human bladder muscle.[18] Flurbiprofen is a potent inhibitor of PG synthesis. Cardozo and colleagues[86] evaluated the effect of Flurbiprofen in 30 women with detrusor instability in a double blind crossover trial. Symptoms of instability were significantly decreased with the prostaglandin inhibitor.

β adrenergic receptors are predominantly distributed in the human bladder body[30] and they mediate bladder relaxation. Lindholm and Lose[87] used the β agonist terbutaline in 15 females with idiopathic urge incontinence. Fourteen noted subjective improvements and 12 became continent. Transient side effects (palpitations, tachycardia, and/or tremor) were noted frequently.[86] Not all reports on use of β agonists for detrusor instability have been favorable[87] and neither PG inhibitors nor β agonists have enjoyed much clinical use in pediatric practice.

Capsaicin is a neurotoxic agent with selective action on unmyelinated nerve fibers. It has been administered intravesically in an attempt to selectively destroy the afferent nerves that give rise to abnormal reflex detrusor contractions.[91] Fowler and colleagues[91] studied 12 patients with spinal cord disease treated with Capsaicin. Improved bladder function was recorded in nine patients after a single intravesical treatment. Complete continence was achieved in five of the nine. Urodynamic studies demonstrated an increase in bladder capacity and a decrease in the maximum detrusor pressure. Further studies will be required before clinical application in children is considered.

Agents to Increase Outlet Resistance

Storage of urine can be improved by pharmacological manipulation of the bladder outlet. The bladder base is innervated by adrenergic nerve fibers,[26] and the muscles of the outlet respond to alpha agonists by contraction.[27, 30, 92, 93] There is no response of the outlet to β stimulation.[27] α agonists, therefore, improve urine storage by increasing the outlet resistance. Ephedrine is a sympathomimetic agent which stimulates both α and β receptors by causing the release of noradrenaline from the adrenergic nerves and also by directly stimulating adrenergic receptors.[94]

Diokno and Taub[95] administered ephedrine sulfate to a group of 38 patients who were incontinent for a variety of reasons. Mildly to moderately affected patients with neurogenic lesions enjoyed improved continence, but three severely affected myelodysplastic patients were unchanged. The improvement observed was transient in some patients. In the patients with good responses, an increase in the pressure over the entire urethra was demonstrated by urethral pressure profilometry.[94] I have used ephedrine sulfate in patients with myelomeningocele with variable results. Recently my patients have had difficulty obtaining ephedrine from their pharmacies, so I now prescribe pseudoephedrine (Sudafed) which they can purchase over the counter. Phenylpropanolamine hydrochloride acts as an α agonist with less central stimulation.[38] It is a constituent of a variety of nasal decongestants and appetite suppressants, and may be used as an alternative to ephedrine.

Side effects of α agonists include hypertension, anxiety, insomnia, cardiac arrhythmias, and headaches. Anxiety and insomnia seem most problematic in children. My overall impression of the α agonists is that they more often improve than resolve neurogenic incontinence. There is no simple way of predicting which children with myelodysplasia will respond favorably to these agents, so they are used in many on a trial basis.

CLEAN INTERMITTENT CATHETERIZATION

The value of aseptic intermittent bladder catheterization in preventing early urinary tract infections in the spinal cord injury patient was clearly documented by Guttman and Frankel in 1966.[96] Their technique required that the catheter be passed by either a doctor or nurse using sterile technique. It was the general opinion that there was inadequate manpower in the United States to adopt this approach realistically. Intermittent self-catheterization using a clean technique was first proposed by Lapides and colleagues.[2, 3] In two papers, the authors described their initial experience with a 30-year-old female with multiple sclerosis who, in the early winter of 1970,[97] was taught clean intermittent self-catheterization as an alternative to urinary diversion. The patient readily learned and accepted the technique. As she did well, several other patients were introduced to the technique. By March of 1971, 14 patients were performing clean intermittent catheterization (CIC); 11 had neurogenic bladders and three had atonic bladders as a consequence of infrequent voiding. The authors noted that the patients were extremely happy with this technique of bladder management. Four of their patients had positive urine cultures, but only one of these had symptoms requiring treatment. The technique of CIC was easy to teach and, as it lent itself to practical everyday use, it was soon widely adopted.

Lapides and colleagues updated their experience in 1976, describing the outcomes in 218 patients started on CIC because of recurrent infections or incontinence.[98] Patients with neurogenic bladders comprised 168 of the 218 patients. Most of the neurogenic lesions were caused by spinal cord injury, myelodysplasia, multiple sclerosis, or spinal cord tumors. Forty-eight percent of their patients were free of infection and, although 52% had positive urine cultures, there was only one episode of pyelonephritis. That patient subsequently required ureteral reimplantation. Researchers noted two cases of urethritis and two attacks of epididymitis. There were no instances of upper urinary tract deterioration, and in nine of the 33 patients who had initially abnormal upper urinary tracts, hydronephrosis improved after the institution of clean intermittent catheterization. Another report from the same institution assessed the 10-year follow-up of the 60 patients started on intermittent self-catheterization prior to May 1972. Twenty-seven of the 60 patients still performed CIC, and 19 of them (70%) had neurogenic bladders. Intermittent bacteriuria was noted in 74% of these patients, but only two patients suffered attacks of pyelonephritis, and both of these required ureteral reimplantation. Subsequent to their ureteral reimplantation, they had no more episodes of pyelonephritis. The authors concluded that chronic bacteriuria seemed to have no adverse effect on the upper urinary tracts if the patient didn't have reflux. One patient with asymptomatic bacteriuria was recognized to have developed a bladder calculus on a pubic hair nidus. No urethral strictures, false passages, or renal deterioration were observed. Urinary incontinence was a major indication for CIC in 10 of the patients, and it was eliminated by CIC alone in four and with the aid of pharmacological manipulation of the bladder in the other six.[99]

These initial experiences with CIC raised concerns about its impact in several areas: What is the effect or significance of intermittent bacteriuria? Does CIC impact on reflux? and How effective is CIC at ameliorating incontinence? All investigators agree that bacteriuria occurs frequently in patients practicing CIC.[100, 101, 102, 103, 104] In infants and younger children started on CIC, the incidence of intermittent bacilluria is between 40 and 85%. It seems, when CIC is started in older children, the incidence of positive urine cultures may be higher.[105] Although bacilluria occurs frequently in these patients, more severe invasive infections are recorded infrequently.[103] Kass and colleagues, reviewing 255 children on CIC, documented bacilluria in 56% of their patients; but febrile urinary tract infections occurred in only 11%, and fresh renal damage in 2.5%. They noted that the occurrence of reflux was a strong predictor of febrile urinary tract infections in these children. Febrile UTI developed in 37% of the children with reflux, but in only 3% of the patients without reflux. The significance of bacilluria associated with reflux was affirmed by Joseph and colleagues. In a review of 38 babies with myelodysplasia started on CIC, they recorded intermittent bacteriuria in 42% of the children. Reflux was documented in 16 of the 38 babies and, among these, recurrent or symptomatic bacteriuria was treated readily in all except the three children with grade IV or V reflux. These three children all suffered breakthrough infections and upper urinary tract deterioration. Recently, Ottolini and colleagues[104] retrospectively reviewed 207 spina bifida patients treated with CIC. One hundred seventy-six (85%) had one or more episodes of asymptomatic bacteriuria and 72 (35%) had febrile episodes associated with a positive urine culture. New renal scars were detected in 42 patients. Logistic regression analysis revealed that factors associated with scarring were febrile infection, age more than 20 years, bladder trabeculation, and reflux. Asymptomatic bacteriuria was not associated with scarring. Positive cultures

are recorded less frequently if children undergoing CIC are receiving antibacterial medication.[106, 107] On the other hand, as intermittent bacteriuria seems to have an adverse effect only on children with high-grade reflux, it seems reasonable to question the use of long-term antibiotics in the children practicing CIC who do not have reflux.[101]

The parents of many patients undergoing CIC are concerned about their child's intermittently foul-smelling or cloudy urine. Although these urines are usually infected, in the children who do not have reflux, I recommend pushing oral fluids, increasing the frequency of catheterization, and ensuring complete emptying of the bladder at each catheterization. The abnormality of the urine often disappears with these measures. If the child becomes symptomatic with increased wetting, pain with catheterization, or fever, I will treat with culture-specific antibiotics. Although I reassure parents that asymptomatic bacteriuria is expected and seemingly of little significance for most children undergoing CIC, some parents assiduously strive to maintain sterile urine. It seems reasonable to assume that using a sterile catheter each time the bladder is emptied would decrease the likelihood of bladder contamination caused by the catheter and therefore decrease the incidence of bacilluria. It has been demonstrated that catheters can be sterilized before reuse by employing a standard kitchen microwave[108] or a variety of cleaning solutions.[109] Does the use of a sterile catheter prevent bacteriuria? Moore and colleagues cultured urines monthly in a cross-over study of 30 spina bifida patients undergoing CIC who were using either sterile single-use catheters or catheters washed in soap and water and air dried. Prophylactic antibiotics were used by about a third of the patients. Positive urine cultures were recorded 38% of the time in both the sterile and clean catheter arms of the study.[110] The authors concluded that use of a sterile catheter does not decrease the incidence of bacteriuria when compared to the use of a clean catheter technique.

There is a paucity of literature concerning bacteriuria in the intermittently catheterized SCI child. The experience recorded in SCI adults suggests that prophylaxis of infections (whether by intravesical antibiotics, oral antibiotics, urinary antiseptics, or a combination of these) will decrease the incidence of bacilluria in the acute phase immediately after injury when these patients are managed by intermittent catheterization using a sterile technique.[111, 112]

The role of CIC in children with spina bifida with reflux has been examined. Reflux was present in 16 of 38 infants at the time CIC was initiated in Joseph's study. Reflux resolved in seven of the 13 patients (53.8%) with grades I to III reflux, and was stable in the other six (46.1%) of this group. The three children with grade IV or V reflux suffered upper urinary tract deterioration and breakthrough infections.[102] Antireflux surgery in children undergoing CIC in the Kass series was required in 60% of patients with kidneys with grade III and 64% of those with grade IV or V reflux.[101] Researchers noted that only two of 15 (13%) patients with grades I and II reflux required surgery. In their series, the presence of bacteriuria did not adversely impact on the resolution of reflux. In patients with bacteriuria, reflux disappeared in 47% of kidneys with grades I and II reflux and 32% of grade III kidneys, but in none of the kidneys with grade IV or V reflux. Whereas, in the patients undergoing CIC with sterile urine, reflux disappeared in 50% of those with kidneys with grade I or II reflux, 34% with grade III reflux in kidneys, and none with grade IV or V reflux. In a recent series, Khoury and colleagues reviewed myelomeningocele patients born between 1978 and 1985 who were followed for ten years. They found 50 children who either presented with or developed reflux. Clean intermittent catheterization and pharmacologic bladder management led to resolution of reflux in 28 of 50 (56%) of the patients. Twenty-two patients (44%) required one or more surgical procedures. Scars developed in only five of 71 patients with kidneys at risk (7%).[113]

Considering that reflux is often improved by CIC, it might be expected that hydronephrosis would also be ameliorated by the effects of clean intermittent catheterization. In a group of 87 children using CIC for up to ten years, Lindehall and colleagues[114] reported that all 11 patients who had upper urinary tract dilatation unassociated with reflux at the initiation of CIC manifested resolution of their hydronephrosis. On the other hand, of the 13 patients initiating CIC who manifested dilatation with associated reflux, only seven (54%) showed resolution of the dilatation and three (23%) had resolution of reflux.

Kass and colleagues,[101] in a series reviewing 225 children undergoing CIC, observed 25 kidneys with hydronephrosis and/or scarring without reflux at the initiation of CIC. Seventeen of the hydronephrotic kidneys evidenced decreased hydronephrosis on treatment. Joseph and colleagues'[102] study of infants with myelodysplasia started on CIC reported that four of 120 children had hydronephrosis unassociated with reflux at the initiation of therapy. Three of these four infants suffered progressive hydronephrosis in spite of CIC, but no child on CIC developed hydronephrosis. The report of Cass and colleagues[106] noted eight of 154 units were dilated at the onset of CIC and only one of the eight (12.5%) improved, while 87.5% were unchanged. Reflux coexisted in three of eight (37.5%) units at the initiation of CIC. They also documented that only four of 138 (2.8%) normal renal units developed hydronephrosis while the patient was on CIC. The effect of clean intermittent catheterization on hydronephrosis is variable. Lack of improvement in hydronephrosis while the child is on CIC seems to relate to the presence of associated high-grade reflux and the age of the patient. Infants with hydronephrosis observed shortly after birth seem less likely to be improved by CIC alone, and high-grade reflux is a definite risk factor for upper tract deterioration. It appears unlikely that hydronephrosis will develop in infants with normal kidneys if the child is on CIC.

Continence is a major goal of the management of children with neurogenic dysfunction. CIC alone or combined with appropriate drug therapy allows many children to avoid the inconvenience and embarrassment of wetting. Cass and colleagues reviewed CIC use in 84 children with neurogenic bladders followed for up to three years and noted that 41 were totally dry (49%), 14 were slightly damp (17%), eight were frequently damp (9%), seven had wet and dry periods (8%), and 14 showed continuous wetness (17%). Almost all of these children were taking chemoprophylactic antibiotics. Seventy-five percent of the children were receiving some type of agent to modify bladder activity.[106] Hilwa and Perlmutter defined continence as dryness for at least two hours after catheterization, and noted that 22 of 24 (83%) of their patients were continent. Fifteen of 16 girls and eight of nine boys required adjunctive drug therapy to achieve this goal. Continence was rather liberally defined in that series. The authors also stated that only four of 25 (16%) of their patients at last review were dry at night and also dry for four to six hours after catheterization in the daytime.[115] Lindehall and colleagues interviewed a group of 26 teenagers with myelodysplasia who had all been undergoing CIC for at least five years. Twenty-four of the 26 described subjective decreases in wetting, and even those who were not totally dry valued the improved continence they experienced. None of the 26 wanted to go back to the technique of bladder emptying they had used before they had started CIC.[116] Our experience suggests that the majority of children on CIC require adjunctive drug therapy to achieve the desired degree of continence. Slightly less than half of the patients we see on CIC with associated drug therapy are totally dry between catheterizations and at night. Another 20 to 30% experience minor to tolerable degrees of wetting, readily managed by pads and acceptable to the patient. The remainder require other therapies to achieve continence.

CIC has become a routine part of the urologic methodology, utilized at all ages for bladder dysfunction due to a variety of etiologies. Considering how frequently CIC is performed, it is reassuring that direct complications of the technique occur infrequently and are usually minor.[117] Minor urethral trauma resulting in hematuria occurs occasionally, but more severe urethral lesions such as false passages[118] or strictures are seen infrequently. Even neonates have suffered no ill effects from CIC. Bladder stones have been recorded in some patients on CIC. These stones form on a pubic hair nidus which has been accidentally pushed into the bladder by the catheter.[117] Catheters may knot in the bladder,[119] and occasionally they are "lost" in the bladder when they are inadvertently pushed in too far.[120] Severe complications such as bladder perforation, necrosis, or vesicoenteric fistulas are rarely attributed to CIC.[121, 122] The safety and efficacy of CIC make the technique one of the major advances in urologic management of the last 25 years.

BLADDER STIMULATION

Another approach to the modulation of bladder activity is to more directly influence the nerves subserving bladder function. Some of these techniques utilize selective nerve root division[123] and others require implantation of stimulating devices combined with sectioning of nerve roots.[124, 125] As these are surgical approaches, they are beyond the scope of this chapter. However, transurethral electrical bladder stimulation is a non-surgical technique performed to stimulate bladder nerves.

The technique of intravesical transurethral bladder stimulation introduced in Hungary by Katona[126] was first used in 1984 in America by Kaplan and Richards[127] from Chicago. The technique delivers electrical stimulation to the interior of the bladder by means of a transurethral "electrocatheter." The initial objective of stimulation is to normalize bladder tone and stimulate the urge to void by exciting activity in the sensory limb of the reflex arc.[127] Stimulation is delivered in individual sessions lasting about one-and-a-half hours. Twenty to 30 sessions constitute a series of treatment, and the children have a rest period from three to six months before a second shorter series of treatments is initiated. The number of series of stimulation employed is variable depending on the patient's progress. The ultimate goal of bladder stimulation is to create conscious control of voiding.[127] Experience with the technique revealed that some patients enjoyed other urodynamic benefits, including increased bladder capacity[128] and lower bladder pressures.[129] Cheng and colleagues[129] reported a multi-center study of 568 patients from 11 institutions undergoing bladder stimulation. Three hundred and thirty-five patients had adequate urodynamic studies for evaluation. The authors noted that 53% of the patients experienced a 20% or greater increase in their bladder capacity after treatment, and among that subset of patients the expected bladder capacity increased from 66 to 86%. The beneficial effect of stimulation on bladder capacity was more evident when the patient's capacity prior to treatment was more severely compromised. In the same subset of patients who experienced a 20% or greater increase in their bladder capacity, bladder pressures were evaluated. Bladder pressure at capacity decreased by 25% or more in 16% of the patients, increased by 25% or more in 10% of the patients, and was unchanged in 74% of the patients. Although these effects of bladder stimulation on bladder pressure seem modest, the investigators[130] were able to avoid bladder augmentation in the short-term in a small group of patients with adverse urodynamic characteristics undergoing bladder stimulation.

Although these results are encouraging, other investigators have not shared equal success. Boone and colleagues,[131] in a short-term, randomized, sham-controlled and blinded clinical study, could not demonstrate any beneficial effects of bladder stimulation. Lyne and Bellinger[132] were able to record detrusor contractions during stimulation in all of their patients. Eight of 12 (67%) of their fully evaluable patients had a measurable increase in bladder capacity. However, in three of these eight, the effect was transient. Four of the 12 (33%) experienced a decrease in capacity during stimulation. No patient achieved volitional voiding. Nicholas and Eckstein[133] performed stimulation in 20 children following Katona's technique. Cystometrograms done after treatment failed to show normal bladder contractions in any patient. There was no change observed in the children's state of continence. Decter and colleagues[134, 135] described 18 patients undergoing serial stimulation; six (33%) demonstrated a greater than 20% increase in age, adjusted bladder capacity. Five (28%) of their patients had a clinically significant reduction in their end filling pressures. Despite these urodynamic gains, the authors did not regard the changes as sufficiently significant to materially alter the day-to-day bladder emptying regime of these children. Long-term studies will be required before a role is determined for intravesical transurethral bladder stimulation in the management of children with myelodysplasia.

AN OVERVIEW OF NON-SURGICAL MANAGEMENT

The goals of management of the neurogenic bladder are to preserve the upper urinary tracts and provide socially acceptable continence. Continence is not expected in infants and young children, and in this age group the focus is on preventing renal parenchymal loss. Many of the lessons learned in management of children with neurogenic dysfunction are drawn from the experience of the spina bifida population. Newborns with myelodysplasia are at high risk of upper urinary tract deterioration.[1] Although urodynamic evaluation provides some predictive parameters suggesting the likelihood of developing upper urinary tract problems,[8, 9, 10] agreement on the value of these parameters is not universal, and the urologic management of the child with myelodysplasia is controversial.

Management schemes are currently divided into two different approaches in the evaluation and treatment of these children. The prophylactic-intervention school suggests that predictors of a poor outcome can be based on urodynamic parameters and that appropriate interventions in children with these advese parameters will prevent upper urinary tract deterioration.[136–139] The aggressive, imaging, prompt-intervention school suggests that frequent radiographic evaluation provides early evidence of deterioration and that appropriate intervention can reverse that trend and frequently normalize it.[140, 141] All investigators agree that upper urinary tract deterioration in infants with spina bifida can occur and that careful follow-up is mandatory.

Teichman et al. reported on 283 patients managed by aggressive observation and prompt intervention and found that 18.8% of patients had progressive hydronephrosis, renal parenchymal scar or thinning, or elevated serum creatinine. However, only 5% had radiologic evidence of parenchymal dysfunction as seen on IVP, CT, or nuclear scan at follow-up after CIC with or without anticholinergics was instituted.[140] Edelstein et al. prospectively evaluated 56 newborns urodynamically.[138] Twenty of these patients were urodynamically defined as "at risk" for renal deterioration, and 36 patients were "not at risk". Renal deterioration in this report was defined by new or worsening hydronephrosis, reflux, or increasing postvoid residuals. These investigators prophylactically started the "at risk" group on CIC with or without anticholinergics, and those in the "not at risk" group were allowed to void on their own until follow-up studies indicated renal deterioration. Fifteen percent of the "at risk" group developed renal deterioration, and 11% of the "not at risk" group had deterioration. Although the term "renal deterioration" is variably defined by different authors, both prophylactic intervention predicted urodynamically and prompt intervention based on serial imaging seemed to yield comparable rates of "renal deterioration."

Other investigators have documented the efficacy of prompt intervention in reversing upper urinary tract changes. Klose et al. reported on 25 patients who manifested renal deterioration while being followed conservatively.[141] After institution of appropriate management, including CIC with or without anticholinergics, reflux resolved in sixty-seven percent of their patients and improved in 24%. Hydronephrosis unassociated with reflux occurred in four patients, and it resolved in all those treated with CIC with or without anticholinergics. Four of the 25 patients (16%) required surgical procedures including four vesicostomies, three ureteral reimplantations, and two bladder augmentations. Although these results validate the premise that CIC and drug therapy can reverse upper urinary tract deterioration if the changes are acted upon promptly, this approach does not obviate the need for surgical intervention.

As it appears that CIC and drug therapy instituted to reverse upper urinary tract changes are partly effective at ameliorating these changes, perhaps prophylactic CIC instituted because of adverse urodynamic parameters would be totally protective. Edelstein et al. reported a two-part study in which they followed a total of 127 patients with initially normal radiologic studies (series 1: 71 patients, series 2: 56 patients).[138] Twenty patients from series 2 were stratified urodynamically as high-risk and started on CIC with or without anticholinergics. In spite of prophylactic CIC, four surgical procedures with the intent of upper urinary tract preservation were required in three of these patients: three ureteral reimplantations, one bladder augmentation. The 71 patients from series 1 and the 36 patients from series 2 who had no adverse urodynamic parameters were followed with observation and prompt intervention if radiologic evidence of renal deterioration arose. Six surgical procedures with the objective of upper urinary tract preservation were performed on these patients including three vesicostomies, one ureteral reimplantation, and two bladder augmentations. Four other bladder augmentations were eventually performed to attempt to achieve continence. These data suggest that prophylactic CIC in patients with poor urodynamic parameters does not preclude surgical intervention. This probably reflects that bladders with poor urodynamic parameters are prone to complications, a fact that may not be totally averted by prophylactic intervention. However, the use of CIC in early childhood results in better adaptation to CIC as the child grows. Sometimes it is more difficult to start CIC in older children, primarily because it is something new for them to learn.[142]

These series suggest that close follow-up with prompt intervention and prophylactic intervention yield comparable rates of renal deterioration. We expect that further refinements based on urodynamic findings will allow investigators to categorize the patient population, identifying the group of children who won't respond to non-operative approaches. Early operative intervention in these children may ultimately lead to near-perfect preservation of the upper urinary tracts. In older children, the goals of management expand as continence becomes a consideration. The objective in these children is to modify bladder activity, creating a low-pressure reservoir that will hold urine and allowing it to be reliably and predictably emptied by CIC. The combination of drugs designed to decrease bladder contractility and increase outlet resistance with a well-performed CIC program achieves acceptable degrees of continence in the majority of patients. Patients with recalcitrant wetting in spite of sterile urine, multidrug manipulation of their bladder, and a consistently performed CIC program require repeat urodynamic studies to define the relative contribution of bladder and outlet factors to their incontinence. If further refinements in drug therapy suggested by the urodynamic study do not achieve continence, a discussion of the available surgical options are explored with the patient and parents.

REFERENCES

1. Smith ED. Urinary prognosis in spina bifida. J Urol 1972; 108:815.

2. Lapides J, Diokno AC, Silber SJ, Lowe BS. Clean, intermittent self-catheterization in the treatment of urinary tract disease. Trans Am Assoc of Genito-urinary Surg 1971;63:92.

3. Lapides J, Diokno AC, Silber SJ, Lowe BS. Clean, intermittent self-catheterization in the treatment of urinary tract disease. J Urol 1972;107:458.

4. Shapiro SR, Lebowitz R, Colodny AH. Fate of 90 children with ileal conduit urinary diversion a decade later: Analysis of complications, pyelography, renal function and bacteriology. J Urol 1975;114:289.

5. Schwarz GR, Jeffs RD. Ileal conduit urinary diversion in children: Computer analysis of followup from 2 to 16 years. J Urol 1975;114:285.

6. Pitts WR Jr, Muecke EC. A 20-year experience with ileal conduits: The fate of the kidneys. J Urol 1979;122:154.

7. Hendren H. Reconstruction of previously diverted urinary tracts in children. J Pediatr Surg 1973;8:135.

8. McGuire EJ, Woodside JR, Borden TA, Weiss RM. Prognostic value of urodynamic testing in myelodysplastic patients. J Urol 1981;126:205.

9. Bauer SB, Hallett M, Khoshbin S, Lebowitz RL, Winston KR, Gibson S, Colodny AH, Retik AB. Predictive value of urodynamic evaluation in newborns with myelodysplasia. JAMA 1984;252:650.

10. Hackler RH, Hall MK, Zampieri TA. Bladder hypocompliance in the spinal cord injury population. J Urol 1989;141:1390.

11. Sundin T, Dahlström A, Norlén L, Svedmyr N. The sympathetic innervation and adrenoreceptor function of the human lower urinary tract in the normal state and after parasympathetic denervation. Investig Urol 1977;14:322.

12. DeGroat WC, Kawatani M. Reorganization of sympathetic preganglionic connections in cat bladder ganglia following parasympathetic denervation. J Physiol 1989;409:431.

13. Sislow JG, Mayo ME. Reduction in human bladder wall compliance following decentralization. J Urol 1990;144:945.

14. Steers WD. Physiology of the urinary bladder. In: Campbell's urology. 6th edition, Walsh PC, Retik A, Stamey T, Vaughan ED Jr, eds. Philadelphia: WB Saunders Co., Chapter 5, 1992;142–176.

15. Ewalt DH. Extracellular matrix changes in the noncompliant neurogenic bladder. Dialogues in Ped Urol 1993;16:4.

16. Brading A. Physiology of bladder smooth muscle. In: The physiology of the lower urinary tract. Torrens M, Morrison JFB, eds. Springer-Verlag: Berlin Heidelberg, Chapter 6, 1987;161–191.

17. Fujii K, Foster CD, Brading AF, Parekh AB. Potassium channel blockers and the effects of cromakalim on the smooth muscle of the guinea-pig bladder. Br J Pharmacol 1990;99:779.

18. Fovaeus M, Andersson K-E, Iiedlund H. The action of pinacidil in the isolated human bladder. J Urol 1989;141:637.

19. Dixon J, Gosling J. Structure and innervation in the human. In: The physiology of the lower urinary tract. Torrens M, Morrison JFB, eds. Springer-Verlag: Berlin Heidelberg, Chapter 1, 1987; 3–22.

20. Gosling JA, Dixon JS, Critchley HOD, Thompson SA. A comparative study of the human external sphincter and periurethral levator ani muscles. Br J Urol 1981;53:35.

21. Juenemann KP, Lue TF, Schmidt RA, Tanagho EA. Clinical significance of sacral and pudendal nerve anatomy. J Urol 1988;139:74.

22. Burnstock G. The changing face of autonomic neurotransmission. Acta Physiol Scand 1986;126:67.

23. Ek A, Alm P, Andersson K-E, Persson CGA. Adrenergic and cholinergic nerves of the human urethra and urinary bladder. A histochemical study. Acta Physiol Scand 1977;99:345.

24. Lepor H, Gup D, Shapiro E, Baumann M. Muscarinic cholinergic receptors in the normal and neurogenic human bladder. J Urol 1989;142:869.

25. Benson GS, McConnell JA, Wood JG. Adrenergic innervation of the human bladder body. J Urol 1979;122:189.

26. Gosling JA, Dixon JS, Lendon RG. The autonomic innervation of the human male and female bladder neck and proximal urethra. J Urol 1977;118:302.

27. Benson GS, Wein AJ, Raezer DM, Corriere JN. Adrenergic and cholinergic stimulation and blockade of the human bladder base. J Urol 1976;116:174.

28. Krane RJ, Olsson CA. Phenoxybenzamine in neurogenic bladder dysfunction. II. Clinical considerations. J Urol 1973;110:653.

29. Hachen IIJ. Clinical and urodynamic assessment of alpha-adrenolytic therapy in patients with neurogenic bladder function. Paraplegia 1980;18:229.

30. Nergärdh A, Boréus LO. Autonomic receptor function in the lower urinary tract of man and cat. Scand J Urol Nephrol 1972;6:32.

31. Sundin T, Dahlström A. The sympathetic innervation of the urinary bladder and urethra in the normal state and after parasympathetic denervation at the spinal root level: An experimental study in cats. Scand J Urol Nephrol 1973;7:131.

32. Comarr AE. The practical urological management of the patient with spinal cord injury. Br J Urol 1959;31:1.

33. Gibbon NOK. Nomenclature of neurogenic bladder. Urology 1976;8:423.

34. Lapides J. Neuromuscular vesical and ureteral dysfunction. In: Urology. 3rd edition, Campbell MF, Harrison JII, eds. Philadelphia: WB Saunders Co., Chapter 33, 1970;1343–1379.

35. Krane RJ, Siroky MB. Classification of neuro-urologic disorders. In: Clinical neuro-urology. Boston: Little Brown and Co., 1979;143–158.

36. Kaplan SA, Chancellor MB, Blaivas JG. Bladder and sphincter behavior in patients with spinal cord lesions. J Urol 1991;146:113.

37. Wein AJ. Classification of neurogenic voiding dysfunction. J Urol 1981;125:605.

38. Wein AJ. Practical uropharmacology. Urol Clin North Am 1991;18:269.

39. Barrett DM, Wein AJ. Voiding dysfunction: Diagnosis, classification, and management. In: Adult and pediatric urology. Gillenwater JY, Grayhack JT, Howards SS, Duckett JW, eds. Chicago: Year Book Medical Publishers, Chapter 28, 1987;863–962.

40. Finkbeiner AE. Is bethanechol chloride clinically effective in promoting bladder emptying? A literature review. J Urol 1985;134:443.

41. Raz S, Smith RB. External sphincter spasticity syndrome in female patients. Urology 1976;115:443.

42. Vaidyanathan S, Rao MS, Chary KSN, Sharma PL, Das N. Enhancement of detrusor reflex activity by naloxone in patients with chronic neurogenic bladder dysfunction. Preliminary report. J Urol 1981;126:500.

43. Wheeler JS Jr., Robinson CJ, Culkin DJ, Nemchausky BA. Naloxone efficacy in bladder rehabilitation of spinal cord injury patients. J Urol 1987;137:1202.

44. Decter RM, Bauer SB. Urologic management of spinal cord injury in children. Urol Clin North Am 1993;20:475.

45. Scott MB, Morrow JW. Phenoxybenzamine in neurogenic bladder dysfunction after spinal cord injury. I. Voiding dysfunction. J Urol 1978;119:480.

46. McGuire EJ, Savastano J. Effect of alpha adrenergic blockage and anticholinergics on the decentralized primate bladder. Neurourol Urodyn 1985;4:139.

47. Wein A. Neuromuscular dysfunction of the lower urinary tract. In: Campbell's urology. 6th edition, Walsh PC, Retik A, Stamey T, Vaughan ED Jr., eds., Philadelphia: WB Saunders Co., Chapter 13, 1992;571–642.

48. Andersson KE, Ek A, Hedlund II, Mattiasson A. Effects of prazosin on isolated human urethra and in patients with lower motor neuron lesions. Investig Urol 1981;19:39.

49. Swierzewski SJ III, Gormley EA, Belville WD, Sweetser PM, Wan J, McGuire EJ. The effect of terazosin on bladder function in the spinal cord injured patient. J Urol 1994;151:951.

50. Delauche-Cavallier MC, Richard M, Buzelin JM, Perrigot M, Leriche A, Attali P, Jardin A. Alpha-blocker therapy with alfuzosin in neurogenic bladder disease. Neurourol Urodyn 1993; 12:343.

51. Forante J, Leyson J, Martin BF, Sporer A. Baclofen in the treatment of detrusor-sphincter dyssynergia in spinal cord injury patients. J Urol 1980;124:82.

52. Mery JP, Kenouch S. Letter to the editor. Am J Kidney Dis 1987;10:326.
53. Murdock MM, Sax D, Krane RJ. Use of dantrolene sodium in external sphincter spasm. Urology 1976;8:133.
54. Hackler RH, Broecker BH, Klein FA, Brady SM. A clinical experience with dantrolene sodium for external urinary sphincter hypertonicity in spinal cord injured patients. Urology 1980;124:78.
55. Dykstra DD, Sidi AA. Treatment of detrusor-sphincter dyssynergia with Botulinum A toxin: A double-blind study. Arch Phys Med Rehabil 1990;71:24.
56. Schurch B, Hauri D, Rodic B, Curt A, Meyer M, Rossier AB. Botulinum-A toxin as a treatment of detrusor-sphincter dyssynergia: A prospective study in 24 spinal cord injury patients. J Urol 1996;155:1023.
57. Jensen D Jr. Pharmacological studies of the uninhibited neurogenic bladder. The influence of cholinergic excitatory and inhibitory drugs on the cystometrogram of neurological patients with normal and uninhibited neurogenic bladder. Acta Neurol Scand 1981;64:175.
58. Glickman S, Tsokos N, Glass J, Bywater HJ, Weidle GC, Nauth-Misir RR, Shaw PJR. Intravesical atropine suppression of detrusor hyperreflexia. Neurourol Urodyn 1992;11:330.
59. Ekström B, Andersson KE, Mattiasson A. Urodynamic effects of intravesical instillation of atropine and phentolamine in patients with detrusor hyperactivity. J Urol 1993;149:155.
60. Diokno AC, Lapides J. Oxybutynin: A new drug with analgesic and anticholinergic properties. J Urol 1972;108:307.
61. Lish PM, Labudde JA, Peters EL, Robbins SI. Oxybutynin—A musculotropic antispasmodic drug with moderate anticholinergic action. Arch Int Pharmacodyn 1965;156:467.
62. Fredericks CM, Anderson GF, Kreulen DI. A study of the anticholinergic and antispasmodic activity of oxybutynin (Ditropan) on rabbit detrusor. Investig Urol 1975;12:317.
63. Moisey CU, Stephenson TP, Brendler CB. The urodynamic and subjective results of treatment of detrusor instability with oxybutynin chloride. Br J Urol 1980;52:472.
64. Kawabe K, Abe S, Kanda T, Tei K. Clinical reevaluation of the effect of oxybutynin chloride on uninhibited neurogenic and reflex neurogenic bladder. Urol Int 1986;41:16.
65. Thüroff JW, Bunke B, Ebner A, Faber P, de Geeter P, Hannappel J, Heidler H, Madersbacher H, Melchior H, Schäfer W, Schwenzer T, Stöckle M. Randomized, double-blind, multicenter trial on treatment of frequency, urgency and incontinence related to detrusor hyperactivity: Oxybutynin versus propantheline versus placebo. J Urol 1991;145:813.
66. Brendler CB, Radebaugh LC, Mohler JL. Topical oxybutynin chloride for relaxation of dysfunctional bladders. J Urol 1989;141:1350.
67. Greenfield SP, Fera M. The use of intravesical oxybutynin chloride in children with neurogenic bladder. J Urol 1991;146:532.
68. Kaplinsky R, Greenfield S, Wan J, Fera M. Expanded followup of intravesical oxybutynin chloride use in children with neurogenic bladder. J Urol 1996;156:753.
69. Massad CA, Kogan BA, Trigo-Rocha FE. The pharmacokinetics of intravesical and oral oxybutynin chloride. J Urol 1992;148:595.
70. Mohler JL. Use of intravesical oxybutynin chloride: Physiologic basis and efficacy. Dialogues in Ped Urol 1993;16:2.
71. Madersbacher H, Jilg G. Control of detrusor hyperreflexia by the intravesical instillation of oxybutynin hydrochloride. Paraplegia, 1991;29:84.
72. Bonney WM, Robinson RA, Theobald RJ Jr. Topical effect of intravesical oxybutynin. J Urol 1993;150:1522.
73. Gajewski JB, Awad SA. Oxybutynin versus propantheline in patients with multiple sclerosis and detrusor hyperreflexia. J Urol 1986;135:966.
74. Holmes DM, Montz FJ, Stanton SL: Oxybutinin versus propantheline in the management of detrusor instability. A patient regulated variable dose trial. Br J Obstet Gynaecol 1989;96:607.
75. Fischer CP, Diokno A, Lapides J. The anticholinergic effects of dicyclomine hydrochloride in uninhibited neurogenic bladder dysfunction. J Urol 1978;120:328.
76. Bradley DV, Cazort RJ. Relief of bladder spasm by flavoxate. A comparative study. J Clin Pharm 1970;Jan/Feb:65.
77. Benson GS, Sarshik SA, Raezer DM, Wein AJ. Bladder muscle contractility. Comparative effects and mechanisms of action of atropine, propantheline, flavoxate and imipramine. Urology 1977;9:31.
78. Briggs RS, Castleden CM, Asher MJ. The effect of flavoxate on uninhibited detrusor contractions and urinary incontinence in the elderly. J Urol 1980;123:665.
79. Mahony DT, Laferte RO, Mahoney JE. Part VI. Observations on sphincter-augmenting effect of imipramine in children with urinary incontinence. Urology 1973;1:317.
80. Tullock AGS, Creed KE. A comparison between propantheline and imipramine on bladder and salivary gland function. Br J Urol 1979;51:359.
81. Labay P, Boyarsky S. The action of imipramine on the bladder musculature. Urology 1973;109:385.
82. Gotoh M, Hassouna M, Mokhless I, Elhilali MM. Intravesical instillation of a calcium entry blocker and its effects on detrusor contractility: In vitro and vivo experiments. Urology 1986;135:1304.
83. Levin RM, Zderic SA, Wein AJ. Effect of intravesical administration of calcium channel inhibitors and potassium channel openers on experimental hyperreflexia. Dialogues in Ped Urol 1993;16:4.
84. Andersson K-E. Clinical relevance of some findings in neuroanatomy and neurophysiology of the lower urinary tract. Clin Sci 1986;70(suppl. 14):21s.
85. Hedlund H, Mattiasson A, Andersson KE. Effects of pinacidil on detrusor instability in men with bladder outlet obstruction. J Urol 1991;146:1345.
86. Cardozo LD, Stanton SL, Robinson H, Hole D. Evaluation of flurbiprofen in detrusor instability. BMJ 2 Feb 1980;281.
87. Lindholm P, Lose G; Terbutaline (Bricanyl) in the treatment of female urge incontinence. Urol Int 1986;41:158.
88. Mattiasson A, Ekström B, Andersson K-E. Effects of intravesical instillation of verapamil in patients with detrusor hyperactivity. J Urol 1989;141:174.
89. Cook NS. The pharmacology of potassium channels and their therapeutic potential. Trends Pharmacol Sci 1988;9:21.
90. Malmgren A, Andersson K-E, Andersson PO, Fovaeus M, Sjögren C. Effects of cromakalim (BRL 34915) and pinacidil on normal and hypertrophied rat detrusor in vitro. J Urol 1990;143:828.
91. Fowler CJ, Beck RO, Gerrard S, Betts CD, Fowler CG. Intravesical capasaicin for treatment of detrusor hyperreflexia. J Neurol Neurosurg Psych 1994;57:169.
92. Naglo AS, Nergårdh A, Boréus LO. Influence of atropine and isoprenaline on detrusor hyperactivity in children with neurogenic bladder. Scand J Urol Nephrol 1981;15:97.
93. Awad SA, Downie JW. The effect of adrenergic drugs and hypogastric nerve stimulation on the canine urethra. A radiologic and urethral pressure study. J Urol 1976;13:298.
94. Caine M, Raz S, Zeigler M. Adrenergic and cholinergic receptors in the human prostate, prostatic capsule and bladder neck. Br J Urol 1975;47:193.
95. Diokno AC, Taub M. Ephedrine in the treatment of urinary incontinence. Urology 1975;5:624.
96. Guttmann L, Frankel H. The value of intermittent catheterisation in the early management of traumatic paraplegia and tetraplegia. Paraplegia 1966;4:63.
97. Bloom DA, McGuire EJ, Lapides J. A brief history of urethral catheterization. J Urol 1994;151:317.
98. Lapides J, Diokno AC, Gould FR, Lowe BS. Further observations on self-catheterization. J Urol 1976;116:169.
99. Diokno AC, Sonda LP, Hollander JB, Lapides J. Fate of patients started on clean intermittent self-catheterization therapy 10 years ago. J Urol 1983;129:1120.
100. Kass EJ, McHugh T, Diokno AC. Intermittent catheterization in children less than 6 years old. J Urol 1979;121:792.
101. Kass EJ, Koff SA, Diokno AC, Lapides J. The significance of bacilluria in children on long-term intermittent catheterization. J Urol 1981;126:223.
102. Joseph DB, Bauer SB, Colodny AH, Mandell J, Retik AB. Clean, intermittent catheterization of infants with neurogenic bladder. Pediatrics 1989;84:78.

103. Schlager TA, Dilks S, Trudell J, Whittam TS, Hendley JO. Bacteriuria in children with neurogenic bladder treated with intermittent catheterization: Natural history. J Pediatr 1995;126:490.

104. Ottolini MC, Shaer CM, Rushton HG, Majd M, Gonzales EC, Patel KM. Relationship of asymptomatic bacteriuria and renal scarring in children with neuropathic bladders who are practicing clean intermittent catheterization. J Pediatr 1995;127:369.

105. De la Iiunt MN, Deegan S, Scott JES. Intermittent catheterisation for neuropathic urinary incontinence. Arch Dis Child 1989;64:821.

106. Cass AS, Luxenberg M, Gleich P, Johnson CF, Hagen S. Clean intermittent catheterization in the management of the neurogenic bladder in children. J Urol 1984;132:526.

107. Johnson W II, Anderson JD, Chambers GK, Arnold WJD, Irwin BJ, Brinton JR. A short-term study of nitrofurantoin prophylaxis in children managed with clean intermittent catheterization. Pediatrics 1994;93:752.

108. Silbar EC, Cicmanec JF, Burke BM, Bracken RB. Microwave sterilization: A method for home sterilization of urinary catheters. J Urol 1989;141:88.

109. Kurtz MJ, Van Zandt K, Burns JL. Comparison study of home catheter cleaning methods. Rehab Nursing 1995;20:212.

110. Moore KN, Kelm M, Sinclair O, Cadrain G. Bacteriuria in intermittent catheterization users: The effect of sterile versus clean reused catheters. Rehab Nursing 1993;18:306.

111. Anderson RU. Prophylaxis of bacteriuria during intermittent catheterization of the acute neurogenic bladder. J Urol 1980;123:364.

112. Krebs M, Halvorsen RB, Fishman IJ, Santos-Mendoza N. Prevention of urinary tract infection during intermittent catheterization. J Urol 1984;131:82.

113. Khoury AE, Abramson R, Churchill BM, McLorie GA. Management of vesicoureteric reflux in myelomeningocele (MMC) patients. Presented at the 1995 American Academy of Pediatrics Meeting, San Francisco, California, 10/16/95.

114. Lindehall B, Claesson I, Hjälmäs K, Jodal U. Effect of clean intermittent catheterisation on radiological appearance of the upper urinary tract in children with myelomeningocele. Br J Urol 1991;67:415.

115. Hilwa N, Perlmutter AD. The role of adjunctive drug therapy for intermittent catheterization and self-catheterization in children with vesical dysfunction. J Urol 1978;119:551.

116. Lindehall B, Möller A, Hjälmäs K, Jodal U. Long-term intermittent catheterization: The experience of teenagers and young adults with myclomeningocele J Urol 1994;152:187.

117. Klauber GT, Sant GR. Complications of intermittent catheterization. Urol Clin North Am 1983;10:557.

118. Koleilat N, Sidi AA, Gonzalez R. Urethral false passage as a complication of intermittent catheterization. J Urol 1989;142:1216.

119. Foster H, Ritchey M, Bloom D. Adventitious knots in urethral catheters: Report of 5 cases. J Urol 1992;148:1496.

120. Klein EA, Wood DP, Kay R. Retained straight catheter: Complication of clean intermittent catheterization. J Urol 1986;135:780.

121. Reisman EM, Preminger GM. Bladder perforation secondary to clean intermittent catheterization. J Urol 1989;142:1316.

122. Wolfson BJ. Acquired vesicocolonic fistula in a child: A complication in management of a neurogenic bladder. Urol Rad 1984;6:223.

123. Franco I, Storrs B, Firlit CF, Zebold K, Richards I, Kaplan WE. Selective sacral rhizotomy in children with high pressure neurogenic bladders: Preliminary results. J Urol 1992;148:648.

124. Tanagho EA, Schmidt RA, Orvis BR. Neural stimulation for control of voiding dysfunction: A preliminary report in 22 patients with serious neuropathic voiding disorders. J Urol 1989;142:340.

125. Brindley GS. The first 500 patients with sacral anterior root stimulator implants: General description. Paraplegia 1994;32:795.

126. Katona F, Berènyi M. Intravesical transurethral electrotherapy in meningomyelocele patients. Acta Paediatrica Academiae, Scientiarum Hungaricae, 1975;16(3–4):363.

127. Kaplan WE, Richards I. Intravesical transurethral electrotherapy for the neurogenic bladder. J Urol 1986;136:243.

128. Kaplan WE, Richards TW, Richards I. Intravesical transurethral bladder stimulation to increase bladder capacity. J Urol 1989;142:600.

129. Cheng EY, Richards I, Balcom A, Steinhardt G, Diamond M, Richard M, Donovan JM, Carr MC, Reinberg Y, Hurt G, Chandra M, Bauer SB, Kaplan WE. Bladder stimulation therapy improves bladder compliance: Results from a multi-institutional trial. Urology 1996;156:761.

130. Cheng EY, Richards I, Kaplan WE. Use of bladder stimulation in high risk patients. J Urol 1996;156:749.

131. Boone TB, Roehrborn CG, Hurt G. Transurethral intravesical electrotherapy for neurogenic bladder dysfunction in children with myelodysplasia: A prospective, randomized clinical trial. J Urol 1992;148:550.

132. Lyne CJ, Bellinger MF. Early experience with transurethral electrical bladder stimulation. J Urol 1993;150:697.

133. Nicholas JL, Eckstein HB. Endovesical electrotherapy in treatment of urinary incontinence in spina-bifida patients. Lancet 1975;2(7948):1276.

134. Decter RM, Snyder P, Rosvanis TK. Transurethral electrical bladder stimulation: Initial results. J Urol 1992;148:651.

135. Decter RM, Snyder P, Laudermilch C. Transurethral electrical bladder stimulation: A followup report. J Urol 1994;152:812.

136. Geraniotis E, Koff SA, Enrile B. The prophylactic use of clean intermittent catheterization in the treatment of infants and young children with myelomeningocele and neurogenic bladder dysfunction. J Urol 1988;139:85.

137. Kasabian NG, Bauer SB, Dyro FM, Colodny AH, Mandell J, Retik AB. The prophylactic value of clean intermittent catheterization and anticholinergic medication in newborns and infants with myelodysplasia at risk of developing urinary tract deterioration. AJDC 1992;146:841.

138. Edelstein RA, Bauer SB, Kelly MD, Darbey MM, Peters CA, Atala A, Mandell J, Colodny A II, Retik AB. The long-term urological response of neonates with myelodysplasia treated proactively with intermittent catheterization and anticholinergic therapy. J Urol 1995;154:1500.

139. Wang SC, McGuire EJ, Bloom DA. A bladder pressure management system for myclodysplasia–clinical outcome. J Urol 1988;140:1499.

140. Teichman JMH, Scherz HC, Kim KD, Cho DH, Packer MG, Kaplan GW. An alternative approach to myelodysplasia management: Aggressive observation and prompt intervention. J Urol 1994;152:807.

141. Klose AG, Sackett CK, Mesrobian GJ II. Management of children with myelodysplasia: Urological alternatives. J Urol 1990;144.

142. Joseph DB, Bauer SB, Colodny SH, Mandell J, Retich AB. Clean intermittent catheterization of infants with neurogenic bladder. Pediatrics 1989;84:78–82.

CHAPTER 24

Surgical Options in the Management of the Neurogenic Bladder

John C. Pope IV and Richard C. Rink

The physiology of normal bladder function and the etiology, evaluation, and nonsurgical management of neuropathic bladder dysfunction are discussed elsewhere in this text. The bladder has two critical functions: 1) the ability to store urine at low pressures, and 2) the ability to spontaneously empty. In the normal situation, the bladder acts as a compliant reservoir and has a dynamic sphincter mechanism. Unfortunately, in patients with neurologic abnormalities, the coordination between the sphincter and bladder and the behavior of these two components individually may be abnormal. Surgical intervention becomes necessary in the management of the neurogenic bladder when more conservative medical measures do not achieve continence and protect the upper urinary tract.

Continence requires the storage of urine in a compliant, low pressure bladder with adequate urethral resistance. A hyperactive or noncompliant detrusor, inadequate urethral resistance, or a combination of both lead to bladder pressures that exceed outlet resistance, resulting in incontinence. Upper urinary tract safety ultimately depends on bladder pressure, which in turn ultimately depends on urethral resistance. It is accepted that sustained bladder pressures higher than 40 cm H_2O are detrimental to the kidneys.[1] When urethral resistance is high (leak point pressures >40 cm H_2O), a noncompliant bladder leads to high intravesical pressures, which results in upper urinary tract deterioration. With low urethral resistance, even if the bladder is noncompliant, the upper urinary tracts are usually spared injury because the high bladder pressures are vented through the bladder outlet. Lack of coordination between the detrusor and sphincter can result in intermittent high intravesical pressures that, over time, may also cause injury to the upper urinary tract.

Pediatric patients generally have neurogenic bladder dysfunction resulting from spinal dysraphism. Others can have a combination of anatomic and neuropathic abnormalities, such as cloacal exstrophy. These patients have highly variable bladder and sphincter dysfunction and thus do not fit into any one particular category of management. Instead, we envision each patient lying somewhere along the spectrum of problems ranging from isolated abnormalities of urethral resistance to poor vesical compliance or hyperactivity, or a combination thereof. Therefore, urodynamic evaluation is an essential component in understanding the pathophysiology of bladder dysfunction and in deciding which problems predominate and require treatment. The surgical options for treating these patients will be divided into two broad sections: 1) treatment of poor vesical compliance or hyperactivity, and 2) treatment of low urethral resistance. Conservative efforts at medical management should be exhausted before proceeding with surgical treatment. Algorithms for the medical and surgical management of neurogenic bladder are shown in Figure 24.1*A* & *B*; however, our discussion will be limited to surgical management.

TREATMENT OF POOR VESICAL COMPLIANCE AND HYPERACTIVITY

Efforts should first be made to improve bladder compliance using anticholinergic or antispasmodic medications. Failure of medical management warrants a surgical approach. Augmentation cystoplasty is an attempt to improve the function of the urinary bladder as a compliant storage vessel. The goals of bladder augmentation are to improve capacity while decreasing pressure. The options for augmentation cystoplasty along with its inherent risks are discussed in this chapter. The surgeon and patient considering such a procedure must understand that bladder augmentation results in a decreased ability to empty the bladder spontaneously[2] and each patient must accept that long-term, even

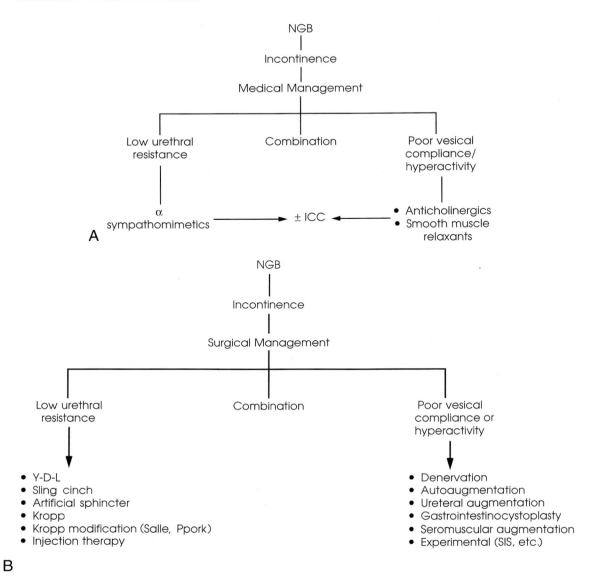

FIG. 24.1. A, The spectrum of etiology and medical management for neurogenic incontinence ranging from isolated abnormalities of urethral resistance to poor vesical compliance or hyperactivity, or a combination of the two. **B,** Same spectrum outlining surgical management.

permanent, intermittent catheterization may be necessary to empty the bladder.

Proper preoperative evaluation is essential. The patient's physiologic condition and psychosocial situation will influence the outcome of any surgical intervention. The patient and family must be made aware of the risks and benefits of the operative procedure. Renal function, liver function, concurrent abnormalities of the urinary tract (hydronephrosis, vesicoureteral reflux, and so on), bladder and sphincter dynamics, and the patient's ability to empty the bladder (spontaneously or with ICC) should be assessed before surgical treatment to ensure an optimal result. Assessment of urine output is critical, particularly if the patient has a concentrating defect. High urine volumes require creation of a larger storage

vessel. Although various options exist to augment the bladder without the use of the intestine, patients should undergo bowel preparation in case the preconceived plan proves impossible. A urine culture should be obtained and treated appropriately before surgery. Finally, preoperative cystoscopy is recommended to rule out any unexpected anatomic abnormality.

Once the patient has been thoroughly evaluated, educated, and prepared, there are several surgical options for treatment.

Bladder Denervation

Several authors have attempted to decrease bladder pressure by surgically interrupting the nerve supply to the bladder by performing selective sacral rhizotomy.[3–7] In theory, this would decrease or eliminate uninhibited detrusor contractions and result in a relatively flaccid, more compliant neurogenic bladder. The clinical success of this procedure has been sporadic, although more recent studies have shown that sacral rhizotomy performed at the same time as a procedure for untethering of the spinal cord can lead to remarkable improvements in bladder volume and pressure.[8] Further studies are needed to confirm long-term success, but these data suggest that there may be a role for rhizotomy in selected patients.

Autoaugmentation

Cartwright and Snow[9, 10] described an innovative procedure using native urothelial tissue to improve bladder compliance and capacity. This procedure, known as "autoaugmentation," involves excising only the detrusor muscle from the dome of the bladder, leaving the mucosa intact to protrude as a wide-mouthed diverticulum. Initially, a midline detrusor incision is made. Aided by having the bladder filled with saline, the muscle is excised laterally in either direction from the bulging mucosa (Fig. 24.2). The lateral edges of the detrusor muscle are secured to the psoas muscle bilaterally to prevent collapse of the diverticulum. Their early experience noted that compliance was improved in four of five patients, and that capacity increased in three of the five.[9]

This procedure has subsequently been modified by several surgeons, each providing a different name for the procedure depending on whether the detrusor muscle is simply incised to allow the mucosa to bulge or excised to create the diverticulum. No difference has been shown in the clinical success between vesicomyotomy (incision) and vesicomyectomy (excision).[11, 12] There are advantages to autoaugmentation. Because

native urothelial tissue is used, the excess mucus production, electrolyte changes, and possible tumor potential associated with enterocystoplasty is avoided. This is an extraperitoneal procedure, which eliminates the inherent risks of intra-abdominal surgery. It is compatible with intermittent catheterization and does not seem to complicate subsequent enterocystoplasty should failure occur. Complications from these procedures are generally uncommon and of little clinical significance. Perforation, a major concern after intestinocystoplasty, has not been reported.

The main disadvantage of autoaugmentation is that despite clinical improvement (improved continence or upper urinary tract changes) there is only a limited increase in capacity as measured by urodynamic studies.[13] The exact reasons for the clinical improvement are unknown; however, it has been suggested that an adequate preoperative volume may be the most important predictor of success. Landa et al. noted that if the maximum capacity and the volume of urine held at 40 cm H_2O are similar, the patient may be better served by intestinocystoplasty.[13] Finally, there is concern that any increase in capacity or compliance obtained with autoaugmentation may not be durable because of fibrosis of the diverticulum.[11]

Autoaugmentation and Demucosalized Gastrointestinal Segments

Because of concerns regarding fibrosis of the diverticulum in autoaugmentation and the inherent problems of the intestinocystoplasty, such as mucus production and electrolyte disturbances, some surgeons have recently elected to combine the two procedures. This is done by placing a demucosalized intestinal segment (sigmoid colon or stomach) on top of an autoaugmented bladder (Fig. 24.3). The reported early clinical success with this procedure has been good. Urodynamic compliance and capacity reportedly increased significantly in 88 to 100% of patients.[14–17] There have been no major complications reported, although Gonzalez reported two urodynamic failures that ultimately required ileocystoplasty, and two additional patients who developed significant hourglass deformities of the bladder.[15] Buson et al. noted that in the canine model, if the intestinal submucosa was removed with the mucosa, the intestinal patch contracted, but fibrosis did not occur when the submucosa was preserved.[18]

These procedures are associated with more blood loss, longer operative time, and are technically more demanding than simple augmentation or autoaugmentation, particularly those using the stomach. Although these seromuscular, urothelial-lined augmentations are theoretically attractive, the results reported have short-term follow-up at this time. The long-term effects on

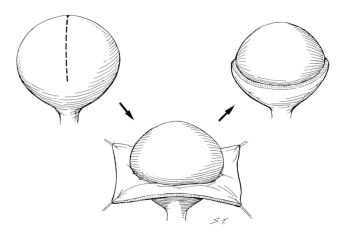

FIG. 24.2. Autoaugmentation. The bladder is incised in the midline as shown. The detrusor musculature is excised, leaving the mucosa protruding as a wide-mouthed diverticulum.

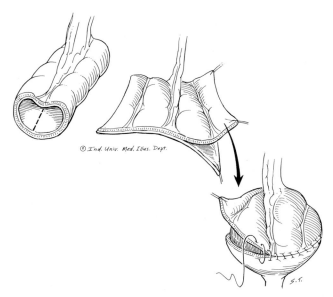

© Ind. Univ. Med. Illus. Dept.

FIG. 24.3. Autoaugmentation with demucosalized bowel segments. The mucosa is stripped from the intestine thus permitting urothelium to line the bowel segment.

the urothelium by the seromuscular segment or vice versa are unknown.

Ureterocystoplasty

In some clinical situations, massive ureteral dilation accompanies a small, noncompliant bladder (posterior urethral valves, exstrophic variants, and myelodysplasia). The dilated ureter is usually secondary to high-grade vesicoureteral reflux and typically drains a poorly functioning or nonfunctioning kidney. In such cases, these dilated ureters can be detubularized and reconfigured to serve as a urothelial-lined segment with muscle backing and used to augment the bladder.

Generally, ureterocystoplasty is performed through a midline, intraperitoneal incision after bowel preparation. This provides access to the intestine in case mobilization of the ureter for augmentation is unsuccessful. However, some authors have shown that this can be achieved through two incisions, remaining extraperitoneal (flank or posterior lumbotomy for nephrectomy and Pfannensteil for the augmentation).[19–21] In either situation, the technique is the same. A standard nephrectomy is performed throughout with great care to preserve the renal pelvic and upper ureteral blood supply. The renal pelvis and ureter are mobilized into the true pelvis to the bladder, which is then opened in the sagittal plane. Posteriorly, this incision is carried off center directly into the ureteral orifice of the ureter used for augmentation; thus, bivalving the bladder. The ureter is not detached from the bladder but is then opened longitudinally along its entire length taking care

to avoid its main blood supply (Fig. 24.4*A* & *B*). The ureter is folded on itself and the ureter-to-ureter and ureter-to-bladder anastomoses are performed with absorbable suture, creating a sphere (Fig. 24.4*C*). At times, it can be advantageous to leave a few centimeters of distal ureter intact.[22,23] We have had equally good results with both techniques and saving this distal ureter theoretically preserves the blood supply to the ureteral segment. Postoperatively, a suprapubic tube is left indwelling through the native bladder, and remains indwelling for 3 weeks, after which time intermittent clean catheterization (ICC) is started.

Nearly all patients in each series reported a significant increase in capacity, improved compliance, elimination of bladder instability, and improved or stable upper urinary tract.[21, 22, 24–26] Landau et al. compared age- and diagnosis-matched groups undergoing ureterocystoplasty and ileocystoplasty and found both groups had similar urodynamic results.[26] Complications have been uncommon with only rare episodes of early extravasation of urine being noted;[24] however, follow-up in these patients is not yet sufficient to prove ureterocystoplasty will stand the test of time.

This procedure using a megaureter for bladder augmentation has been universally successful in our hands.[27] There are no electrolyte or mucus problems created by the procedure because the lining is urothelium. The operation can be performed extraperitoneally and presumably has no increased malignant potential. The procedure has limited use because it is applicable only for those patients who have a nonfunctioning kidney that needs to be removed.

The main disadvantage is that most patients requiring augmentation cystoplasty do not have a dilated ureter available for use. The use of normal size ureters has been proposed;[28, 29] however, further experience will be required before their routine use can be advocated. Nonetheless, if a significantly dilated ureter is present in a child, a nephrectomy and ureteral augmentation would be our material of choice.

Gastrointestinal Cystoplasty

One of the major advances in pediatric urology during the past 20 years is the use of bowel segments for lower urinary tract reconstruction. Much knowledge has been gained about the physical and physiologic effects of interposing bowel in the urinary tract. Historically, many have recommended excision of the supra-trigonal bladder (in conditions such as tuberculosis) with the intestinal segment then anastomosed to the residual cuff of bladder. More recently, the bladder is generally preserved in patients with neurogenic dysfunction. A sagittal or stellate incision in the bladder is generally recommended provided it widely opens the bladder and prevents a narrow-mouthed anastomosis (Fig. 24.5). It

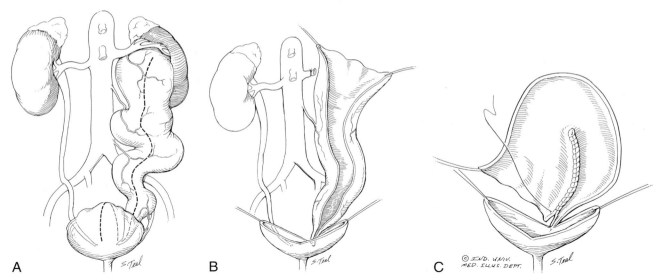

FIG. 24.4. A, Incision for detubularization of dilated ureter and pelvis and for bivalving of native bladder for ureteral cystoplasty. **B,** Ureteral cystoplasty. The nonfunctioning kidney is removed and the ureteral blood supply preserved. **C,** The ureter remains attached to the bladder, is reconfigured into a U-shaped patch that is anastomosed to the bladder.

is also known that any segment of bowel can be successfully used to augment the bladder provided it is detubularized and reconfigured into a sphere. This spherical shape provides several advantages, including maximizing the volume achieved for any given surface area of the bowel, blunting the native bowel contractility, and improving overall compliance.[30, 31] An example of an ileocystoplasty is shown in Fig. 24.6. In a similar fashion, this procedure can be performed with other sections of the gastrointestinal tract.

Each bowel segment has its own advantages and disadvantages (Table 24.1) and many factors are involved in deciding which segment will best serve each patient.

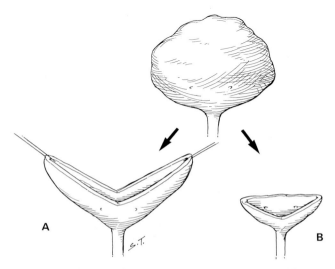

FIG. 24.5. The native bladder can be managed by: **(A)** making a sagittal incision to bivalve the bladder, or **(B)** performing a supratrigonal cystectomy.

Choice of Bowel Segment

In an effort to determine which intestinal segment is best for augmentation, we have reviewed our own institutional experience and the literature.[27, 32–34]

Ileum

When reconfigured, ileum provides the most compliant reservoir with the least risk of significant contraction. Mucus production, although greater than with a gastric augment, is less troublesome than with colonic segments and tends to decrease with time. Bacteriuria has occurred less often with ileum in some series, although that has not been the experience at our institution. Hyperchloremic acidosis is a risk with any bowel segment placed in contact with urine, but this risk appears less with ileum than with large bowel (colon, sigmoid) segments. There is usually an abundance of mobile ileum available if needed for a more extensive reconstruction (i.e., creating a catheterizable conduit if the appendix is absent, reaching a short ureter if ureteral length is a problem). It is difficult to create a submucosal tunnel for reimplantation of the ureter or appendix into an ileal segment. Occasionally, the mesentery may be short, making it difficult for the ileal segment to reach the pelvis. Diarrhea or vitamin B12 deficiency can occur but is rare when augmentation is done alone, especially if one preserves the distal 15 cm of ileum.

Cecum or Ileocecal Segment

Reconstructive urologists have used the ileocecal segment in numerous innovative procedures. There is a

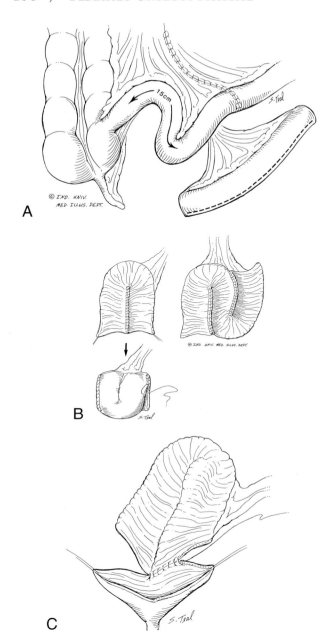

© IND. UNIV.
MED. ILLUS. DEPT.

A

© IND. UNIV. MED. ILLUS. DEPT.

B

C

FIG. 24.6. A, Beginning approximately 15 cm from the ileocecal valve, a 20- to 40-cm ileal segment is removed from the gastrointestinal tract and an ileoileostomy is performed. The proposed incision for detubularization of the ileal segment along the antimesenteric border is outlined. **B,** The detubularized segment is folded in half and the medial edges are anastomosed to form a U-shaped flap. The reconfiguration can be done in a U, S, or W type fashion or folded as a cup patch. **C,** The U-shaped flap is anastomosed to the bivalved bladder beginning in the midline posteriorly.

constant, reliable blood supply, and this segment of bowel is easy to mobilize and will easily reach into the pelvis in most cases. The cecum, because of its size, makes a large capacity reservoir, and the ileocecal valve can be used to provide a continence or antireflux mecha-

nism, if needed. Unfortunately, removal of 10% of patients with neurogenic bladder dysfunction have diarrhea.[35] As a general rule, we avoid removing this segment in this particular population. In patients with cloacal exstrophy, this segment may not be available and if so, removing it from the fecal stream can lead to problems within fluid and electrolyte balance. The ileocecal segment cytoplasty may result in hyperchloremic metabolic acidosis, and mucus production is problematic.

Sigmoid Colon

The sigmoid colon has been used extensively in children primarily because of its close anatomic proximity to the bladder. In those with neurogenic bladder dysfunction, it is often redundant making its use even more attractive. Submucosal tunnels are more reliably and easily performed in large bowel because of the much thicker wall and its more easily separated mucosa. Disadvantages include significant contractile activity despite detubularization and reconfiguration,[36] large amounts of mucus production, reportedly higher rates of bacteriuria, and at our institution, a higher rate of spontaneous perforation.[37] Hyperchloremic acidosis may occur and in some patients, bicarbonate therapy on a regular basis may be necessary.

Stomach

In pediatric reconstructive surgery, gastrocystoplasty has gained popularity during the past several years (Fig. 24.7A & B). The decreased incidence of infection, its location outside the field of pelvic radiation, the ease with which submucosal tunnels can be performed (similar to native bladder), the excellent muscle backing, and its net chloride excretion are advantages the stomach has over other bowel segments for urinary tract reconstruction. One major disadvantage is the development of the hematuria-dysuria syndrome in approximately a third of the patients,[38] particularly those with normal sensation. Patients who are incontinent or who have renal failure appear to be at increased risk for this problem probably because there is less urine in the bladder to dilute and buffer the gastric secretions. Another disadvantage is that frequent rhythmic contractions were noted commonly in all large series.[32] These contractions have been lessened by using a larger gastric patch. The most significant drawback appears to be profound hypochloremic metabolic alkalosis, which can be unresponsive to medication and in rare cases, has necessitated removal of the gastric segment. The gastric mucosa in the urinary bladder should always be bathed in urine. Buffering of the gastric segment output by urine appears to be necessary to prevent ulceration or even perforation.[39, 40] Thus, this segment should be avoided

TABLE 24.1. *Comparison of gastrointestinal segments in pediatric augmentation*

	Advantages	Disadvantages
Ileum	Most compliant Less mucus	Diarrhea Vitamin B_{12} deficiency Short mesentery Hyperchloremic acidosis Poor muscle backing
Sigmoid	Readily mobilized Easily implanted Good muscle backing	Unit contractions Lower compliance Mucus Hyperchloremic acidosis ? perforation risk
Ileocecal	Valve as antireflux/continence mechanism Good capacity reservoir Constant blood supply	Diarrhea Not always available Contractile
Stomach	Short gut/radiation Chloride pump Minimal mucus Fewer infections Ease of implantation Good muscle backing	Hypochloremic alkalosis Rhythmic contractions Hematuria/dysuria

in children who already have had or are likely to have bilateral nephectomy.

Medical Complications

Gastrointestinal. The removal of an enteric segment can result in significant metabolic problems. Secretory and osmotic diarrhea can occur after removal of large segments of ileum, the ileocecal valve, or colon.[41] The secretory diarrhea is caused by malabsorption of bile salts. When elevated bile salt load is presented to the colon, net excretion of water and electrolytes by colonic epithelium occurs, causing diarrhea. Decreased transit time may ensue, leading to osmotic diarrhea. This is especially pronounced in patients with neurogenic bladder dysfunction when the ileocecal valve is removed and thus we would avoid removal of this valve if at all possible.

The distal ileum is the site for vitamin B12 absorption. Removal of a significant portion of this bowel segment, therefore, may result in vitamin B12 deficiency and megaloblastic anemia. The terminal 15 to 20 cm of ileum should not be used for augmentation, although problems may arise even if that segment is preserved. Existing B12 stores in the body may last for several years before being depleted, resulting in a deficiency that may take several years to manifest itself.[42] This point should be kept in mind during long-term follow-up of these patients.

Metabolic. A rare but potentially serious complication when intestinal segments are used (excluding stomach) is hyperchloremic metabolic acidosis. Clinical signs and symptoms include lethargy, weakness, fatigue, anorexia, and polydipsia. The intestinal segment absorbs ammonia and chloride from the urine resulting in a state of chronic acid loading and removal of one of the body's natural acid-base control mechanisms.[43] It has been noted that nearly every patient has a decreased serum bicarbonate and an increased serum chloride level, although patients with normal renal function rarely develop acidosis.[44] The body excretes this increased acid load as titratable acid derived from bony buffers and this can ultimately lead to bone demineralization and growth retardation.[45] This metabolic acidosis is potentially lethal if unrecognized and all patients with frank acidosis should be treated appropriately with bicarbonate supplementation. Some question whether all patients undergoing intestinocystoplasty would benefit from bicarbonate therapy.

However, gastric mucosa acts as a barrier to chloride and acid absorption after being placed in the urinary tract and secretes hydrogen chloride. Serum chloride decreases and serum bicarbonate increases in these patients and rarely, they can develop hypochloremic, hypokalemic metabolic alkalosis requiring hospitalization. In our experience this severe metabolic derangement is usually seen after an acute gastrointestinal illness,[32] but others have noted that this may occur at any time in otherwise healthy patients. A gastric segment is an attractive alternative in patients with chronic renal insufficiency because their acidosis is in effect treated by the incorporation of stomach into the urinary tract. The stomach is also the obvious choice in those with short gut syndrome (e.g., cloacal exstrophy). Remember, for reasons previously discussed, a gastric segment is not an attractive alternative in patients who are anuric.

Urinary Tract Infections. Bacteriuria is a common sequalae after intestinocystoplasty, although patients

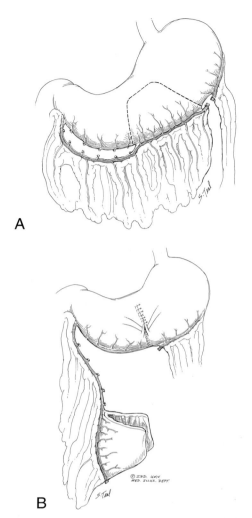

FIG. 24.7. A, A rhomboid-shaped stomach wedge is identified and resected from the greater curvature. **B,** The right gastroepiploic artery is used as the vascular pedicle and is ligated distal to the wedge so that the segment can easily be placed into the pelvis. The gastric wedge is then anastomosed to the bladder in the manner previously outlined for the ileal segment.

who can void spontaneously and empty a bowel bladder efficiently can generally maintain a sterile urine. Most patients, however, require ICC to empty their bladder after augmentation and these patients almost always experience bacteriuria at some time. Fortunately, this is rarely of clinical significance. We do not recommend the routine treatment of asymptomatic bacteriuria in this population; however, bacteriuria should be treated if symptoms such as new-onset incontinence, suprapubic pain, hematuria, malodorous urine, or markedly increased mucus production arise. Treatment is also recommended if the urine culture reveals urea-splitting organisms that may lead to eventual stone formation. Bacteriuria can be minimized by assuring complete bladder emptying with catheterization. Periodic bladder

irrigation is also helpful in keeping mucus collection to a minimum because mucus can interfere with catheter drainage leading to residual urine and subsequent infection. It should be noted that the incidence of pyelonephritis is no higher in patients with intestinocystoplasty than those with routine ileal conduit urinary diversion.[46] Also, comparison of different intestinal segments used for augmentation cystoplasty revealed significantly fewer symptomatic lower urinary tract infections in patients who had undergone gastrocystoplasty.[47] This was not true, however, for pyelonephritis.

Tumor Formation. It is known that carcinoma and polyp formation at the ureterocolonic anastomotic site is a reality in patients who have undergone ureterosigmoidostomy. These patients are at a 7,000-fold increased risk for tumor formation than age-matched controls.[48] This concern translates to patients who have undergone augmentation enterocystoplasty. Animal models have revealed tumor formation on or adjacent to the luminal surface of the augmented segment when using all intestinal segments.[49] Other experimental work done on rats has demonstrated hyperplastic growth in the augmented segment, with no segment showing any particular increased risk over another.[50, 51] The applicability of such findings to humans is unknown; however, it is important that patients and their families be made aware of such risks and overall management of these patients should include tumor surveillance.

Mucus Production. Once the urinary tract, gastrointestinal segments will continue to produce mucus, and in some patients, this can be a problem. It has been shown that the colon produces more mucus than does ileum, and that the stomach produces the least amount of all.[52] Mucus can cause impaired bladder drainage and can also serve as a nidus for stone formation or difficulty eradicating infection. We insist on daily bladder irrigations with saline to prevent mucus accumulation in hopes of avoiding these complications.

Surgical Complications

Bowel Obstruction. Postoperative bowel obstruction after augmentation is a rare occurrence with an incidence of approximately 3%.[34, 35] The incidence is low regardless of which bowel segment is used and this factor should not influence the surgeon's choice of a particular bowel segment.

Calculi. Bladder calculi have been reported to occur in 8 to 52% of patients after augmentation.[34, 53, 54] The reasons for these incongruous results are unclear; however, it is our belief that an aggressive approach to bladder irrigation and bladder emptying at our institution may account for a lower incidence of stones. Most stones are struvite in composition and bacteriuria is a significant risk factor. Infections with urea-splitting organisms should be treated aggressively and every attempt should be made to completely empty the bladder at frequent intervals to avoid urinary stasis. The bladder should be kept free of mucus to avoid inspissation, which can serve as a nidus for stone formation. Finally, foreign bodies in the bladder such as staples and nonabsorbable suture must be avoided.

Uninhibited Contractions. There is belief that detubularizing and reconfiguring a given bowel segment will prevent continued, rhythmic, sinusoidal contractions. While this is not always true, such contractions are generally not of clinical significance after detubularization. Occasionally they can lead to problems such as persistent incontinence, and vesicoureteral reflux, and may play a role in delayed perforation of the intestinal patch. In a series from our institution, 18 of 323 (6%) patients were identified who required a secondary patch augmentation of their previously augmented bladder.[55] Seven patients had continued incontinence after their initial augmentation, five had bladder perforation, two had incontinence and perforation, three had upper urinary tract deterioration, and one had incontinence and intractable pelvic pain. Preoperative urodynamic studies revealed detrusor pressures varying from 30 to 100 cm H_2O. All patients had adequate bladder outlet resistance. Original bowel segments used were: sigmoid (12/18), gastric (3/18), ileum (2/18), and cecum (1/20). Bowel segments used for re-augmentation were ileum (16) and sigmoid (3). Nine of the 10 patients with incontinence are now dry, and both patients with upper tract changes had resolution of their hydronephrosis. Examples of preoperative and postoperative urodynamics are shown in Figure 24.8. One difficult patient has had a subsequent bladder perforation and remains incontinent.

In summary, if the outcome of a bladder augmentation is less than optimal, it is important to reevaluate the patient's bladder uro-dynamics. In rare instances, these patients may continue to have high pressure contractions with a functionally small bladder capacity. In such situations re-augmentation with an additional bowel segment is a satisfactory alternative to supravesical diversion and provides good results in most cases. This treatment does not necessarily alleviate the contractions, but it increases the volume at which the contractions occur so they are no longer of clinical or functional significance.

Delayed Bladder Perforation. The potentially lethal complication of spontaneous, delayed bladder perforation is well-documented.[56–59] These perforations commonly occur within the bowel segment (not at the bowel/bladder anastomosis) and are thought to result from a problem with bladder overdistention. However, multiple factors, including blunt abdominal trauma, trauma from ICC, chronic urinary tract infection, local bowel wall ischemia, adhesions causing shearing of the bladder with filling and emptying, and the presence of high pressure contractions have been indicated as causes for perforation. There may not be any particular risk for perforation of one bowel segment over another. At Riley Children's Hospital, all patients who received a primary bladder augmentation or who presented with a perforated augmented bladder from 1978 to 1996 were reviewed.[37] They were categorized as to the type of intestinal segment used for augmentation and the occurrence of spontaneous perforation. In 323 patients who have undergone bladder augmentation at our institution, spontaneous perforation has occurred in 22 (7%). The perforation rate for sigmoid segments was 13/87 (15%), for gastric 2/39 (5.1%), for ileum 6/145 (4.1%), and for cecum (1/48 (2.0%). In our experience, multivariate analysis revealed that there is a significantly higher risk of perforation for sigmoid colon enterocystoplasty

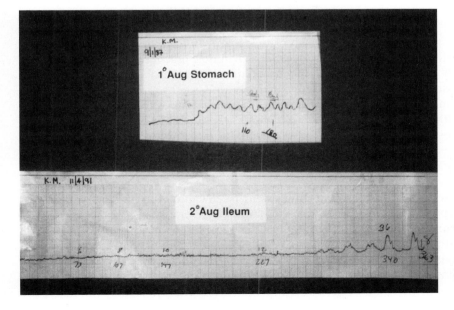

FIG. 24.8. Secondary bladder augmentation. Preoperative and postoperative UDS in a patient who had a primary gastrocystoplasty. The secondary augment was performed with an ileal segment. Note the unit contractions have been shifted to the right, now occurring at a clinically insignificant bladder volume.

($p < 0.05$). In a similar series from Boston Children's Hospital, the perforation rate was highest for ileal segments (9.3%), followed by ileocecal (4.3%), sigmoid (4.2%), and stomach (2.9%).[60] The difference in the results from these two studies may be related to a difference in our reconfiguration technique of sigmoid colon early in our series.

Patients with spontaneous bladder perforation typically are acutely ill with abdominal pain, distention, and fever, or occasionally with frank systemic septic shock. Patients with neurogenic abnormalities frequently have impaired abdominal sensation and often present late in the course of the illness. They may complain only of shoulder pain or have hiccupping from diaphragmatic irritation of the extravasated urine. Therefore, a high index of suspicion for the diagnosis is necessary. Contrast cystography is diagnostic in most cases, although some authors feel contrast computed tomography (CT) can improve diagnostic accuracy and that this procedure should be done on any child suspected of having a perforation if the initial cystogram is negative.[58, 59]

Patients who are in shock require immediate surgical attention. In the patients who are acutely ill but stable at the time of presentation, less invasive measures (i.e., percutaneous drainage and antibiotics)[61] can be tried initially. However, there should be a low threshold for surgical exploration in this group if nonoperative treatment does not lead to prompt improvement in the clinical picture.

Recently, we have discovered another way in which patients with bladder perforation can present—the silent urinoma. In a recent study,[37] three patients at routine follow-up had silent upper urinary tract changes or a palpable suprapubic mass found to be caused by a loculated fluid collection adjacent to the bladder. These patients were managed successfully with percutaneous drainage and antibiotics.

Summary

We use all segments of the gastrointestinal tract for lower urinary tract reconstruction. Each patient and clinical situation must be individually assessed before choosing a segment to use for augmentation. If a dilated, tortuous ureter is available associated with a nonfunctioning kidney, ureterocystoplasty is our first choice. We would only use autoaugmentation in the uncommon situation of poor bladder compliance but adequate bladder capacity. The short-term results of seromuscular cystoplasty preclude recommending its use. If a bowel segment is needed and compliance and capacity are the only concerns, our first choice of bowel segments would be ileum. If the patient has had significant pelvic radiation that affects the bowel, one should choose a segment that is outside the irradiated field, i.e., stomach or transverse colon. If ureteral reimplantation or a tunneled

Mitrofanoff conduit must be placed in the bowel segment, then colon or stomach may be a better choice. There is no perfect segment to use in all patients. Diagnosis, anatomy, renal function, and physical and mental capabilities differ in all children and as a result, the surgeon must understand and be able to use the segment that most appropriately meets the patient's needs.

Future Considerations

Given the known complications associated with intestinocystoplasty, the search continues to locate the ideal material for bladder replacement. Alloplastic materials such as acrylic molds, polyethylene, gelatin sponge, and paper have been used with limited success. Although problems such as infection, hydronephrosis, peritonitis, and bladder stones have occurred, one thing is clear: the bladder has a tremendous potential to regenerate given the proper scaffolding.

Recently, a biodegradable, collagen-rich material called porcine small intestinal submucosa (SIS) has been investigated as a bladder wall substitute in the rat and canine models. Initial studies revealed that complete regeneration of all three layers of the bladder (mucosa, smooth muscle, serosa) will occur without evidence of graft shrinkage or decreased bladder size.[62, 63] Urodynamic assessment in a long-term canine model demonstrated that SIS-regenerated bladders functioned normally without any associated morbidity.[64] In vitro contractility studies demonstrated that SIS-regenerated bladder is capable of receptor-mediated contraction and relaxation similar to normal bladders and that SIS-regenerated detrusor smooth muscle is reinnervated by afferent and efferent nerve fibers. In addition, in vitro compliance studies of SIS-regenerated bladders demonstrated similar stress and strain characteristics when compared to normal canine bladders.[65] Further histologic studies have revealed that neovascularization and smooth muscle and neural regeneration appear to occur through pannus ingrowth from the graft-native bladder interface. Smooth muscle regeneration appears to begin with the maturation of myofibroblasts that migrate into the graft as early as 2 weeks after augmentation and progresses to the formation of distinct smooth muscle bundles.[66]

Others are looking into the concept of bladder regeneration as well. The group at Boston Children's Hospital has approached this problem by harvesting native bladder cells (urothelial and bladder smooth muscle) and expanding them in cell culture on a biodegradable polymer matrix. These polymers seeded with cells are then used for bladder reconstruction in vivo.[28, 67] Results in this area of tissue engineering have been encouraging.

It is evident that bladder regeneration using one of several techniques is a potential option for urologic reconstruction. However, results are still preliminary, and much work must be done before this technology finds human applicability.

TREATMENT OF LOW BLADDER OUTLET RESISTANCE

Historically, reconstruction of the lower urinary tract in the neurogenic population was difficult and fraught with serious complications and failures. Two factors have emerged to change these results: 1) clean intermittent catheterization,[68] and 2) sophisticated urodynamic evaluation. The introduction of clean intermittent catheterization provided a way to efficiently empty any bladder; the goal of reconstruction then became the creation of a compliant storage vessel that would be continent and easily catheterizable. Accurate urodynamic evaluation gave objective information about bladder behavior, the status of the natural continence mechanism, and whether the patient could spontaneously empty his or her bladder readily. A compliant bladder with a low urethral resistance still results in a wet patient. However, high outlet resistance with a noncompliant bladder results in a high pressure system and eventual upper urinary tract deterioration. Therefore, the bladder and the bladder outlet must be addressed with the goal of producing a continent, low-pressure storage vessel for urine.

When urodynamic evaluation reveals a low leak point pressure, as a result of poor outlet resistance, medical therapy can be tried to improve urethral and bladder neck tone to achieve urinary continence (alpha sympathomimetic agents). If medical management fails, then there are several options for surgical correction of low outlet resistance. Before surgical reconstruction of the bladder neck is undertaken, the child must have a desire to be dry and be able to cooperate mentally and physically with all involved in his or her care.

Medical management for neurogenic incontinence is often unsuccessful, because of a fixed urethral resistance. When surgical therapy is contemplated, many options exist and each has its own advantages and disadvantages. In neurogenic population, it is important to know if the patient can empty to completion. If so, our choice would be to place an artificial urinary sphincter. If they cannot empty and will likely depend on clean intermittent catheterization, then we generally recommend one of the other bladder neck procedures.

Artificial Urinary Sphincter

The artificial urinary sphincter (AUS) (American Medical Systems) is a mechanical device consisting of a cuff that is placed around the bladder neck or bulbons urethra, in the male, a pressure regulating balloon usually placed beneath the abdominal fascia, and a pump/valve mechanism that is placed in the scrotum or labium

(Fig. 24.9). This device has an excellent long-term continence rate in the 80 to 90% range,[69–71] and it continues to be our procedure of choice if the patient can empty to completion. Also, it is the only option for treating low bladder outlet resistance, which allows the patient to potentially void independently without the need for CIC.

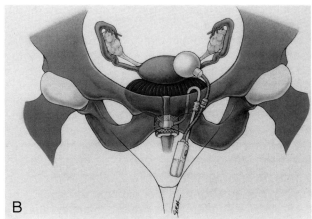

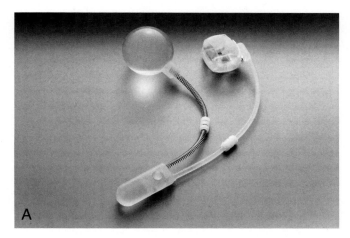

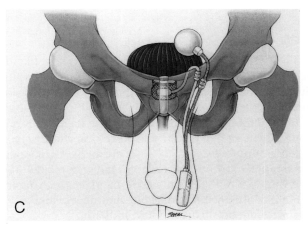

FIG. 24.9. A, AMS-800 artificial urinary sphincter. **B,** Around bladder neck in a female. **C,** Around bladder neck in male.

Disadvantages include a high rate of reoperation for device malfunction (12–15%), erosion (10–15%), and infection (2–4%), as well as the potential for silicone particle migration.[72] The relatively high rate of device revision is, in large part, a result of the fact that earlier models of the device were not as durable and had a shorter life span. With the newer AMS 800 model, it is anticipated that the mechanical complication rate will be lower. Erosions in the early series were felt to be caused by, in part, high balloon pressures (71–80 cm H_2O) leading to tissue atrophy with subsequent necrosis, and ultimately device erosion and infection. The lower pressure (61–70 cm H_2O) balloon commonly used may alleviate some of the erosion problems. Other authors state that erosions with the newer model device have occurred only in patients who had previously undergone surgery on the bladder neck. They recommend that the AUS should be considered the first choice of surgical treatment rather than a salvage operation.[73] Silicone particle migration has been reported in a small group of patients. We have had some males who had an AUS placed prepubertally who later lost the ability to empty to completion after the onset of puberty and ultimately required CIC. These patients have not been helped by the placement of a larger cuff[74] and they must be watched closely for upper urinary tract deterioration.

There have been several reports of bladder decompensation after placement of artificial urinary sphincter, resulting in a noncompliant, high pressure storage system.[75, 76] This change in bladder function can present as urinary infection, recurrent incontinence, vesicoureteral reflux, or deterioration of the upper urinary tract. There have even been reports of renal failure[70, 73] after sphincter placement. As a result, it is generally recommended that these patients undergo long-term surveillance with ultrasound and serum creatinine every 6 months, in addition to cystometrography every 2 years. Approximately a third of the patients receiving a primary AUS will ultimately require bladder augmentation.

Sling

The periurethral fascial or pubovaginal sling, like the AUS, produces a surgically created urethral obstruction. Success (continence) rates in females with neurogenic incontinence have ranged from 70 to 100%,[77–81] although patient numbers and time of follow-up have been relatively low. Optimal results appear to occur when simultaneous enterocystoplasty is performed.[82, 83] In males, slings appear to be less reliable and our results have been disappointing.[81] Only 25% of males with neurogenic incontinence had durable continence, and we do not recommend this procedure in them.

Similar to the AUS, bladder decompensation can occur after a sling procedure. Bladder dynamics must be

followed closely in these patients. As opposed to those patients with stress incontinence, individuals with neurogenic bladder dysfunction will require lifelong intermittent catheterization. Thus, intraoperative verification that the sling is not too tight and that a catheter can be passed easily into the bladder is an important technical point during the procedure.

Bladder Neck Reconstruction

Several procedures are available to reconstruct the bladder neck or urethra as a means for increasing outlet resistance. These procedures ultimately make the patient depend on ICC to empty. As with any procedure performed to increase bladder outlet resistance, close surveillance is necessary to detect bladder decompensation or upper urinary tract deterioration.

Young-Dees-Leadbetter Procedure

The Young-Dees-Leadbetter procedure has been used extensively in the exstrophy population but has had less applicability in the neuropathic group.[84–86] The continence rate with this procedure is high (90–95%), but it often takes multiple procedures and revisions to achieve these results. At our institution, 32% of patients with myelodysplastia who underwent a Young-Dees-Leadbetter procedure required a second operation and 11% required a third to achieve enough outlet resistance to become continent.[87]

Kropp Urethral Lengthening Procedure

The Kropp urethral lengthening procedure[88] has also been successful in patients with sphincteric insufficiency. A tubularized anterior bladder wall flap is tunneled underneath the submucosa to act as a one-way flap valve providing continence (Fig. 24.10). Continence rates ranging from 77 to 100% have been reported.[89–92] The major disadvantage, is that 26 to 100% of these patients have difficulty catheterizing their bladder after the procedure and many require reoperation.[89, 90, 93]

Kropp recently reported a consecutive series of 49 children who underwent the urethral lengthening and reimplantation procedure. Thirty-five patients (72%) never experienced any difficulty emptying their bladder by intermittent catheterization. Fourteen patients (28%) had difficulty with catheterization at some point after the procedure, in the early postoperative period, long after the surgery, or intermittently. Seven patients (14%) had the problem solved by simply placing an indwelling catheter for several weeks at a time. In five patients (10%), an obvious reason was ultimately identified requiring endoscopic correction. Only two patients (4%) required major surgical intervention to create an alternate access to the bladder.[93] In conclusion, most patients

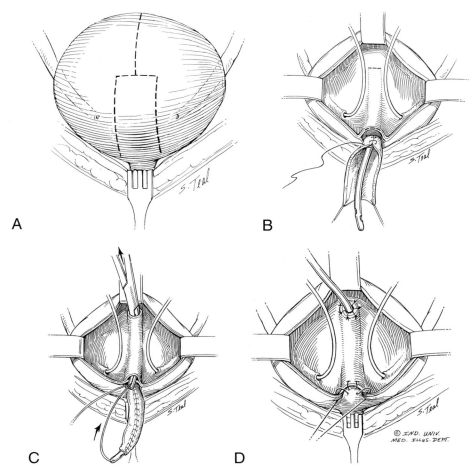

FIG. 24.10. A, Kropp urethral lengthening procedure. Proposed bladder incision outlining anterior bladder flap. **B,** Bladder flap is rolled into a tube over a catheter of appropriate size. **C,** Urethral tube is passed through a submucosal tunnel created between the two ureteral orifices that are stented for protection. **D,** Urethral tube is anchored and mucosal tunnel serves as continence mechanism.

who encountered difficulty in catheterization were managed successfully with minimally invasive methods and without compromising the goals of the original surgery.

Modifications of the Kropp Procedure

Modifications of the Kropp procedure have been reported in which the continence rate remained high but the catheterization difficulties appear to be reduced. Belman did not separate the urethral tube from the bladder and this modification has been adapted by Kropp.[91] The Salle modification lengthens the urethra using an onlay modification that maintains the posterior wall of the tube in situ.[90, 94] A full thickness anterior bladder wall flap based at the urethra is used as in the Kropp procedure; but in this case, it constitutes only the anterior wall of the neourethra (Fig. 24.11A). The flap is anastomosed to a longitudinal strip of the trigonal mucosa and musculature thus creating a complete tube (Fig. 24.11B–C). This tube is then covered by lateral posterior wall urothelium creating a compressible flap mechanism that occludes with bladder filling (Fig. 24.11D). Continence rates are slightly inferior to the Kropp procedure, but no catheterization problems have occurred although follow-up is still relatively short.

Injection Therapy

Injection therapy for incontinence is not a new concept, but the initial experiences were less than ideal because of side effects resulting from the substance injected. The most notorious of these is Teflon, whose use has been largely abandoned in the United States once it was found to migrate to locations distant to the injection site (brain, lung, spleen, and so on). Gluteraldehyde cross-linked collagen is the injectable agent available.

While early results have shown injectable collagen to be relatively successful in treating female intrinsic sphincter deficiency, its success in treating neurogenic

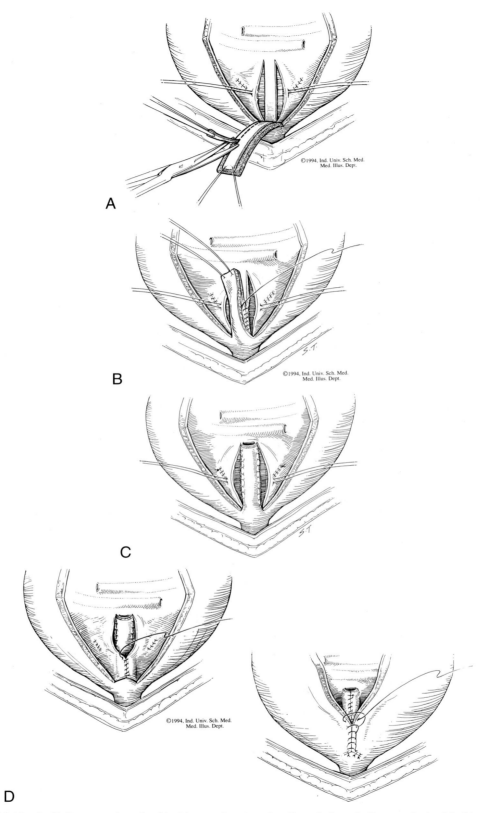

FIG. 24.11. A, Salle procedure for bladder neck reconstruction. A 1 × 4–5 cm anterior bladder wall flap similar to the Kropp procedure is used. Two parallel incisions are made through mucosa only. Mucosa is elevated lateral to these incisions while the midline mucosal strip remains intact. Note the ureters are reimplanted above the proposed incisions. **B,** The mucosa of flap is anastomosed to the posterior bladder mucosa over an 8-French catheter. **C,** The anterior flap musculature is approximated to the exposed trigonal musculature. **D,** Mucosa lateral to new urethra is approximated over the urethral tube. The anterior bladder wall is secured at the base of the neourethra and then the bladder is closed anteriorly.

incontinence in children has been less encouraging, with continence rates ranging from 35 to 64%.[95–99] Long-term durability of the procedure is also still questionable. The advantages are that this procedure can be done endoscopically as an outpatient with low morbidity. Patients in whom a previous bladder neck procedure has been unsuccessful may also derive significant benefit from treatment with a secondary injection of collagen.[98, 99] Even though success is limited, given the advantages, injection therapy with cross-linked collagen has a definite role in the treatment of neurogenic incontinence. Proper preoperative counseling must be given with realistic expectations.

There are other substances being evaluated for use as injectable agents (autologous fat, bladder muscle, small intestinal submucosa, and other polymers). There are also efforts ongoing to determine the best and easiest injection techniques and the ideal postoperative management. Until these issues are better refined, the clinical use of injection therapy for neurogenic incontinence will remain limited.

CATHETERIZABLE ABDOMINAL WALL STOMAS

Appendicovesicostomy

Clean intermittent catheterization is a mainstay in virtually all patients with a neuropathic bladder. These patients usually require catheterization for complete emptying and to achieve continence, especially in the presence of a bladder augmentation. Many of these patients ultimately develop difficulty catheterizing whether as a result of an anatomic problem (abnormal bladder neck or urethra) or a limiting physical condition. In these situations, alternative access to the bladder is often necessary. In 1980, Mitrofanoff described the use of the appendix as a continent vesicostomy for self-catheteriation (Fig. 24.12). The appendix is taken with its mesentery and reimplanted in the bladder in an anti-refluxing fashion. The other end of the appendix is brought out to the skin as a catheterizable stoma.[100] This stoma is commonly located at the umbilicus for a cosmetically superior result. Since this landmark article, Mitrofanoff and others have described their results and variations on the procedure.

When properly constructed, the appendicovesicostomy is rarely incontinent. Continence rates with intermittent catheterization ranging from 90 to 100% have been reported.[100–105] Most of these conduits are easily catheterized with a 10- to 12-French catheter. Complications, while rare, are usually related to stenosis of the stoma (5–7%).[102, 105] This problem can usually be corrected with simple revision of the stoma with or without periodic dilation. Other conduit problems have been reported much less commonly and include appendiceal

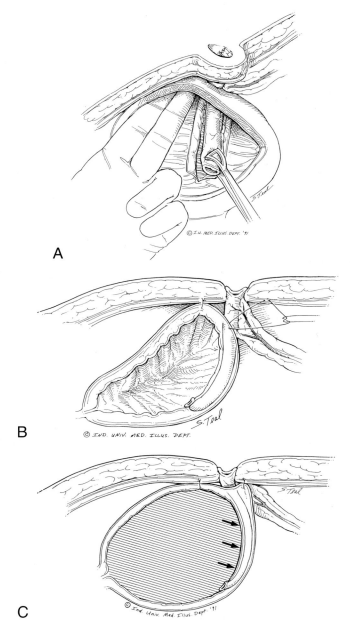

FIG. 24.12. A, Appendicovesicostomy. The appendix is brought through a hiatus in the bladder wall then reimplanted to the bladder. **B,** Sagittal view showing tunneled appendix giving access to bladder as a catheterizable stoma. **C,** A flap valve continence mechanism compresses the appendix against muscular backing as the bladder fills.

loss caused by necrosis,[105] stomal prolapse,[102] and inability to catheterize because of kinking or angulation of the conduit.[104] Stone formation in the augmented urinary bladders of patients with appendicovesicostomies ranges from 12 to 32%.[101, 105] The patients at our institution are taught the importance of complete emptying, and in addition, they are placed on an aggressive schedule of weekly bladder irrigations.

If the appendix has been removed or is unsuitable for use as a catheterizable stoma, several other options may be used instead. The distal ureter can be brought to the skin as a catheterizable ureterostomy (in a situation in which the kidney is removed or a proximal transureteroureterostomy is performed). Continence rates with this are good; however, higher rate of stomal stenosis and structure formation likely are caused by the ureter's less consistent blood supply. The bladder itself can be used by tubularizing a portion of it and bringing the neotube to the skin.[106, 107] We have been successful with this. A segment of tapered ileum can also be fashioned, tunneled into the bladder, or brought to the skin as a stoma, similar to the catheterizable limb of an Indiana pouch. Use of the fallopian tube as a catheterizable channel in a postpubertal woman has also been reported.[101]

Regardless of the segment used, the Mitrofanoff principle has revolutionized reconstruction of the lower urinary tract. The technique is relatively easy to learn and achieves a high rate of continence. Difficulty catheterizing is unusual and the ability to hide the stoma in the umbilicus is desirable. The appendicovesicostomy and its variants offer significant lifestyle advantages to patients and their families; however, it should be emphasized to them that lifelong follow-up is mandatory.

Antegrade Colonic Enema

Patients with neurologic abnormalities, either congenital or acquired, may have neuropathic bowel in addition to an abnormal lower urinary tract. Recent surveys have shown that 50 to 84% of patients with spina bifida who have a neuropathic bladder also have problems with bowel management.[108–110] Fecal incontinence or intractable constipation can be a serious problem in these children. Management of neuropathic bowel has historically consisted of diet manipulation (fiber, fluids, nonconstipating foods), enemas, stool softeners, laxatives, and suppositories. If these options were unsuccessful, the only realistic surgical option available was a permanent colostomy.

In 1990, Malone et al. described a novel technique called the ACE procedure (antegrade continence enema).[111] The ACE procedure is an adaptation of the Mitrofanoff principle and produces a catheterizable appendicocecostomy through which antegrade enemas can be given (Fig. 24.13). These enemas produce complete colonic emptying, thus alleviating constipation and virtually eliminating fecal soiling.

The procedure, as initially described, involves amputating the appendix, reversing it, and then reimplanting it into the cecum with a submucosal tunnel to ensure that it does not leak fecal material. The other end is then brought to the skin as an abdominal wall stoma.[111] More recently, others have described a more simple,

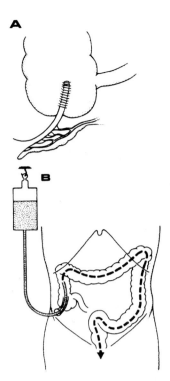

FIG. 24.13. Antegrade continence enema. Nonrefluxing appendicocecostomy **(A)** and the ACE principle **(B)**.

orthotopic appendicocecostomy, in which the cecum is imbricated around the base of the appendix to form the antireflux mechanism.[112, 113] When appendix is unavailable or is to be used for another type of reconstructive procedure (i.e., appendicovesicostomy), a tubularized enteric conduit can be formed from the ileum or cecum.

Success in terms of fecal continence ranges from 70 to 95%, with patients having neuropathic causes of incontinence achieving the best results.[113–115] In most patients, quality of life is significantly improved. Complications, while usually minor, are common, ranging from 30 to 60%. Most complications involve cutaneous stomal stenosis (8–25%). Other complications include appendicocecal obstruction, appendiceal necrosis, severe pain with enemas, and hyperphosphatemia. Fecal leak from the stoma site has only been a problem in patients who had an orthotopic appendicocecostomy with no cecal imbrication.[113]

Postoperatively, a 12-French catheter is typically left in place through the conduit for 3 weeks; however, enema instillation can begin as soon as the patient is tolerating a full oral diet. Irrigations are generally started with 50 mL of tap water and then increased by 50 mL increments every 2 to 3 days until adequate fecal evacuation occurs. Various other enema solutions have been reported including phosphate (Fleet's) (with or without a saline slush), saline, and soap-suds. All seem to work equally well; however, a period of trial and error is required to accurately determine each patient's needs in terms of enema solution, volume, and frequency. The enema solution can be absorbed, thus conditions such as phosphate poisoning, while rare, are possible.[113–115]

The ACE procedure can easily be performed in conjunction with a urologic procedure and adds little to the operative time or hospital stay. While complications are relatively frequent, this procedure remains an effective treatment alternative for patients with intractable constipation and fecal incontinence in whom standard medical therapies have been unsuccessful.

SUMMARY

The treatment goal in patients with neuropathic dysfunction of the lower urinary tract is to produce a continent, low pressure, compliant reservoir that can be emptied to completion. The bladder and sphincter mechanisms must be addressed individually with thorough radiographic and urodynamic evaluation and treated in conjunction with one another. Nonoperative management is tried initially with ICC and anticholinergic agents to treat the noncompliant or hyperactive bladder and alpha-adrenergic drugs used to tighten the incompetent bladder neck and urethra. If these conservative measures are unsuccessful, surgical options are available.

Augmentation enterocystoplasty remains the gold standard for the treatment of the small, noncompliant neurogenic bladder. We usually use ileum; however, any bowel segment can be used with similar success. There are inherent risks with interposing bowel into the urinary tract. Even though these risks are relatively low, better alternatives are being sought for use in bladder reconstruction. Certain patients may be candidates for sacral rhizotomy, ureterocystoplasty, autoaugmentation, and, in the future, bladder regeneration may play a role.

The therapeutic surgical options for the treatment of neurogenic sphincter incompetence are equally numerous. These include the artificial urinary sphincter, fascial and pubovaginal slings, numerous variations of bladder neck reconstruction, and the periurethral injection of various bulking agents (Teflon, collagen). While none of these options are ideal, it is the responsibility of the pediatric urologist to be familiar with them to provide the best possible solution for each patient.

It is of little benefit to the child and his or her family to attain urinary continence yet remain fecally incontinent. If conservative measures do not control the fecal stream and the child is undergoing surgery for urinary incontinence, an ACE procedure should be strongly considered.

REFERENCES

1. McGuire EJ, Woodside JR, Borden TA, Weiss RM. Prognostic value of urodynamic testing in myelodysplastic patients. J Urol 1981;126:205.
2. Gleason DM, Gittes RF, Bottaccini MR, Byen JC. Energy balance of voiding after cecal cystoplasty. J Urol 1972;108:259.
3. Franco I, Storrs BB, Firlit CF, Zebold K, Richards I, Kaplan WE. Selective sacral rhizotomy in children with high pressure neurogenic bladders: preliminary results. J Urol 1992;148:648.
4. Kaplan WE, McLone DG, Richards I. The urological manifestations of the tethered spinal cord. J Urol 1988;140:1285.
5. Rockswold GL, Bradley WE, Chou SN. Differential sacral rhizotomy in the treatment neurologic bladder dysfunction. Preliminary report of six cases. J Neurosurg 1973;38:748.
6. Rockswold GL, Chou SN, Bradley WE. Re-evaluation of differential scacral rhizotomy for neurological bladder disease. J Neurosurg 1978;48:773.
7. Storrs BB. Selective posterior rhizotomy for treatment of progressive spasticity in patients with myelomeningocele. Pediatr Neurosci 1987;13:135.
8. Schneidau T, Franco I, Zebold K, Kaplan WE. Selective sacral rhizotomy for the management of neurogenic bladders in spina bifida patients: long-term follow-up. J Urol 1995;154:766.
9. Cartwright PC, Snow BW. Bladder autoaugmentation: early clinical experience. J Urol 1989;142:505.
10. Cartwright PC, Snow BW. Bladder autoaugmentation: partial detrusor excision to augment the bladder without the use of bowel. J Urol 1989;142:1050.
11. Johnson HW, Nigro MK, Stothers L, Tearle H, Arnold WJ. Laboratory variables of bladder autoaugmentation in an animal model. Urology 1994;44:260.
12. Stothers L, Johnson H, Arnold W, Coleman G, Tearle H. Bladder autoaugmentation by vesicomyotomy in the pediatric neurogenic bladder. Urology 1994;44:110.
13. Landa HM, Moorhead JD. Detrusorectomy. Prob Pediatr Urol 1994;8:404.
14. Dewan PA, Stefanek W. Autoaugmentation gastrocystoplasty: early clinical results. Br J Urol 1994;74:460.
15. Gonzalez R, Buson H, Reid C, Reinberg Y. Seromuscular colocystoplasty lines with urothelium: experience with 16 patients. Urology 1994;45:124.
16. Horowitz M, Mitchell ME, Nguyen DH. The DAWG procedure: gastrocystoplasty made better. J Urol 1994;151:503.
17. Robinson RG, Delahunt B, Pringle KC. Autoaugmentation cystoplasty. J Urol 1994;151:500.
18. Buson H, Maivel JC, Dayanc M, Long R, Gonzalez R. Seromuscular colocystoplasty lined with urothelium: experimental study. Urology 1994;44:743.
19. Bellinger MF. Ureterocystoplasty. Curr Surg Tech Urol 1995;8:2.
20. Dewan PA, Nicholls EA, Goh DW. Ureterocystoplasty: an extraperitoneal urothelial bladder augmentation technique. Eur Urol 1994;26:85.
21. Reinberg Y, Allen RC, Vaughn M. Nephrectomy combined with lower abdominal extraperitoneal ureteral augmentation in the treatment of children with the vesicoureteral reflux dysplasia syndrome. J Urol 1995;153:177.
22. Wolf JS, Turzan C. Augmentation ureterocystoplasty. J Urol 1993;149:1095.
23. Adams MC, Brock JW III, Pope JC IV, Rink RC. Ureterocystoplasty: is it necessary to detubularize the distal ureter? American Urological Association Meeting, New Orleans, LA, 1997.
24. Churchill BM, Aliabadi H, Landau EH. Ureteral bladder augmentation. J Urol 1993;150:716.
25. Hitchcock RJI, Duffy PG, Malone PS. Ureterocystoplasty: the bladder "augmentation" of choice. Br J Urol 1994;73:575.
26. Landau EH, Jayanthi VR, Khoury AE, et al. Bladder augmentation: ureterocystoplasty vs. ileocystoplasty. J Urol 1994;152:712.
27. Rink RC, Adams MC. Augmentation cystoplasty. In: Walsh PC, Retik AB, Stamey TA, Vaughn ED Jr, eds. Campbell's Urology, 6th ed. Philadelphia: WB Saunders, 1997:3167.
28. Atala A, Lailas NG, Cilento BG, Retik AB. Progressive ureteral dilation for subsequent ureterocystoplasty. American Academy of Pediatrics Section on Urology Meeting, Dallas, TX, 1994.
29. McKenna PH, Bauer SB. Bladder augmentation with ureter. Dialog Pediatr Urol 1995;18:4.
30. Hinman F Jr. Selection of intestinal segments for bladder substi-

tution: physical and physiological characteristics. J Urol 1988;139:519.

31. Koff SA. Guidelines to determine the size and shape of intestinal segments used for reconstruction. J Urol 1988;140:1150.

32. Adams MC, Bihrle R, Rink RC. The use of stomach in urologic reconstruction. Am Urol Assoc Update Series 1995;14:218.

33. Rink RC, McLaughlin KP. Indication for enterocystoplasty and choice of bowel segment. Probl Urol 1994;8:389.

34. Rink RC, Hollensbe D, Adams MC. Complications of bladder augmentation in children and comparison of gastrointestinal segments. Am Urol Assoc Update Series 1995;14:122.

35. King LR. Protection of the upper tracts in children. In: King LR, Stone AR, Webster GD, eds. Chicago: Year Book Publishers, 1987;127.

36. Goldwasser B, Webster GD. Augmentation and substitution enterocystoplasty. J Urol 1986;135:215.

37. Pope JC IV, Casale AJ, Adams MC, Keating MA, Mitchell ME, Rink RC. Spontaneous perforation of the augmented bladder: from silence to chaos. American Urological Association Meeting, New Orleans, LA, 1997.

38. Nguyen DH, Bain MA, Salmonson KL, et al. The syndrome of dysuria and hematuria in pediatric urinary reconstruction with stomach. J Urol 1993;150:70.

39. Castro-Diaz D, Froemming C, Manivel JC, et al. The influence of urinary diversion on experimental gastrocystoplasty. J Urol 1992;148:571.

40. Reinberg Y, Manivel JC, Froemming C, et al. Perforation of the gastric segment of an augmented bladder secondary to peptic ulcer disease. J Urol 1992;148:369.

41. Steiner MS, Morton RA. Nutritional and gastrointestinal complications of the use of bowel segments in the lower urinary tract. Urol Clinics North Am 1991;18:743.

42. Steiner MS, Morton RA, Marshall FF. Vitamin B_{12} deficiency in patients with ileocolic neobladders. J Urol 1993;149:255.

43. Koch MO, McDougal WS. The pathophysiology of hyperchloremic metabolic acidosis after urinary diversion through intestinal segments. Surgery 1985;98:561.

44. Mitchell ME, Piser JA. Intestinocystoplasty and total bladder replacement in children and young adults: follow-up in 129 cases. J Urol 1987;138:579.

45. Hall MC, Koch MO, McDougal WS. Metabolic consequences of urinary diversion through intestinal segments. Urol Clin North Am 1991;18:725.

46. McDougal WS. Use of intestinal segments in the urinary tract: basic principles. In: Walsh PC, Retik AB, Stamey TA, eds. Campbell's Urology, 6th ed. Philadelphia: WB Saunders, 1992;2595.

47. Hollensbe DE, Adams MC, Rink RC, Keating MA. Comparison of different gastrointestinal segments for bladder augmentation. American Urological Association Meeting, Washington, DC, 1992.

48. Eraklus AJ, Folkman MJ. Adenocarcinoma at the site of ureterosigmoidostomies for exstrophy of the bladder. J Pediatr Surg 1978;13:730.

49. Little JS, Klee LW, Hoover DM, Rink RC. Long-term histopathologic changes observed in rats subjected to augmentation cystoplasty. J Urol 1994;152:720.

50. Buson H, Diaz DC, Manivel JC, Jessurun J, Dayanc M, Gonzalez R. The development of tumors in experimental gastroenterocystoplasty. J Urol 1993;150:730.

51. Klee LW, Hoover DM, Mitchell ME, Rink RC. Long term effects of gastrocystoplasty in rats. J Urol 1990;144:1283.

52. Kulb TC, Mitchell ME, Rink RC. Gastrocystoplasty in azotemic canines. North Central Section of the American Urological Association Meeting, Palm Springs, CA, 1992.

53. Blyth B, Ewalt DH, Duckett JW, Snyder HM. Lithogenic properties of enterocystoplasty. J Urol 1992;148:575.

54. Palmer LS, Franco I, Kogan SJ, Reda E, Gill B, Levitt SB. Urolithiasis in children following augmentation cystoplasty. J Urol 1993;150:726.

55. Pope JC IV, Keating MA, Casale AJ, Rink RC. Augmenting the augmented bladder: treatment of the contractile bowel segment. American Urological Association Meeting, New Orleans, LA, 1997.

56. Elder JS, Snyder HM, Hulbert WC, Duckett JW. Perforation of the augmented bladder in patients undergoing clean intermittent catheterization. J Urol 1988;140:1159.

57. Rink RC, Woodbury PW, Mitchell ME. Bladder perforation following enterocystoplasty. J Urol 1988;139:234.

58. Rushton HG, Woodard JR, Parrott TS, Jeffs RD, Gearhart JP. Delayed bladder rupture after augmentation enterocystoplasty. J Urol 1988;140:344.

59. Sheiner JR, Kaplan GW. Spontaneous bladder rupture following enterocystoplasty. J Urol 1988;140:1157.

60. Bauer SB, Hendren WH, Kozakewich H, et al. Perforation of the augmented bladder. J Urol 1992;148:699.

61. Slaton JW, Kropp KA. Conservative management of suspected bladder rupture after augmentation enterocystoplasty. J Urol 1994;152:713.

62. Kropp BP, Eppley BL, Prevel CD, et al. Experimental assessment of small intestine submucosa as a bladder wall substitute. Urology 1995;46:396.

63. Vaught JD, Kropp BP, Sawyer BD, Shannon HE, Thor KB. Detrusor regeneration in the rat using porcine small intestinal submucosal grafts: functional innervation and receptor expression. J Urol 1996;155:374.

64. Kropp BP, Rippy M, Badylak SF, et al. Regenerative urinary bladder augmentation using small intestinal submucosa: urodynamic and histopathologic assessment in long-term canine bladder augmentations. J Urol 1996;155:2098.

65. Kropp BP, Sawyer BD, Shannon HE, et al. Characterization of small intestinal submucosa regenerated canine detrusor: assessment of reinnervation, in vitro complance and contractility. J Urol 1996;156:599.

66. Pope JC IV, Davis MM, Smith ER Jr, Walsh MJ, Rink RC, Kropp BP. The ontogeny of canine SIS-regenerated urinary bladder. J Urol 1997;158:1105–1110.

67. Atala A, Vacanti JP, Peters CA, Mandell J, Retik AB, Freeman MR. Formation of urothelial structures in vivo from disassociated cells attached to biodegradable polymer scaffolds. J Urol 1992;148:658.

68. Lapides J, Diokno AC, Silber SJ, Lowe BS. Clean intermittent self-catheterization in the treatment of urinary tract disease. J Urol 1972;107:458.

69. Adams MC, Mitchell ME, Rink RC. Long-term results with artificial urinary sphincters in the pediatric population. American Urological Association Meeting, Dallas, TX, 1989.

70. Levesque PE, Bauer SB, Atala A, et al. Ten-year experience with the artificial urinary sphincter in children. J Urol 1996;156:625.

71. Gonzalez R, Koleilat N, Austin C, Sidi AA. The artificial sphincter AS800 in congenital urinary incontinence. J Urol 1989; 142:512.

72. Reinberg Y, Manivel JC, Gonzalez R. Silicone shedding from artificial urinary sphincter in children. J Urol 1993;150:694.

73. Gonzalez R, Merino FG, Vaughn M. Long-term results of the artificial urinary sphincter in male patients with neurogenic bladder. J Urol 1995;154:769.

74. Kaefer M, McLaughlin KP, Rink RC, Adams MC, Keating MA. A cuff above: upsizing artificial sphincter cuffs to facilitate voiding. Urology 1997.

75. Light JK, Pietro T. Alteration of detrusor behavior and the effect on renal function following insertion of the artificial sphincter. J Urol 1986;136:632.

76. Bauer SB, Reda EF, Colodny AC, Retik AB. Detrusor instability: a delayed complication in association with the artificial sphincter. J Urol 1986;135:1212.

77. McGuire EJ, Wang C, Usitalo H, Savastano J. Modified pubovaginal slings in girls with myelodysplasia. J Urol 1986;135:94.

78. Raz S, Ehrilch RM, Zeidman EJ, Alarcon A, McLaughlin S. Surgical treatment of the incontinent female patient with myelomeningocele. J Urol 1988;139:524.

79. Peters CA, Bauer SB. Urethral suspension procedures. Dialog Pediatr Urol 1989;12:3.

80. Elder JS. Pubovaginal and puboprostatic sling repair. Dialog Pediatr Urol 1989;12:5.

81. Ludlow JK, Keating MA, Wahle GR, McLaughlin KP, Adams MC, Rink RC. Fascial slings in incontinent children—the gender gap. American Urological Association Meeting, Las Vegas, NV, 1995.

82. Perez LM, Smith EA, Broecker BH, Massad CA, Parrott TS, Woodard JR. Outcome of sling cystourethropexy in the pediatric population: a critical review. J Urol 1996;156:642.
83. Decter RM. Use of the fascial sling for neurogenic incontinence: lessons learned. J Urol 1993;150:683.
84. Sidi AA, Reinberg Y, Gonzalez R. Comparison of artificial sphincter implantation and bladder neck reconstruction in patients with neurogenic urinary incontinence. J Urol 1987;138:1120.
85. Bauer SB, Peters CA, Colodny AH, Mandell J, Retik AB. The use of rectus fascia to manage urinary incontinence. J Urol 1989;142:516.
86. Lepor H, Jeffs RD. Primary bladder closure and bladder neck reconstruction in classic bladder exstrophy. J Urol 1983;130:1142.
87. Rink RC, Mitchell ME. Bladder neck/urethral reconstruction in the neuropathic bladder. Dialog Pediatr Urol 1987;10:5.
88. Kropp KA, Angwafo FF. Urethral lengthening and reimplantation for neurogenic incontinence in children. J Urol 1986;135:533.
89. Nill TG, Peller PA, Kropp KA. Management of urinary incontinence by bladder tube urethral lengthening and submucosal reimplantation. J Urol 1990;144:559.
90. Rink RC, Adams MC, Keating MA. The flip-flap technique to lengthen the urethra (Salle procedure) for treatment of neurogenic urinary incontinence. J Urol 1994;152:799.
91. Belman AB, Kaplan GW. Experience with the Kropp antiincontinence procedure. J Urol 1989;141:1160.
92. Mollard P, Mouriquand P, Joubert P. Urethral lengthening for neurogenic urinary incontinence (Kropp's procedure): results of 16 cases. J Urol 1990;143:95.
93. Waters PR, Chehade NC, Kropp KA. Urethral lengthening and reimplantation: management of catheterization problems. J Urol 1997;158:1053.
94. Salle, JLP. Urethral lengthening with anterior bladder wall flap for urinary incontinence. Presented at the 7th International Congress of Pediatric Surgery, Hamburg, Germany, 1992.
95. Wan J, McGuire EJ, Bloom DA, Ritchey ML. The treatment of urinary incontinence in children using glutaraldehyde cross-linked collagen. J Urol 1992;148:127.
96. Caione N, Lais A, de Gennaro M, Capozza N. Glutaraldehyde cross-linked bovine collagen in exstrophy/epispadias complex. J Urol 1993;150:631.
97. Capozza N, Caione P, de Gennaro M, Nappo S, Patricolo M. Endoscopic treatment of vesico-ureteric reflux and urinary incontinence: technical problems in the paediatric patient. Br J Urol 1995;75:538.
98. Leonard MP, Decter A, Mix LW, Johnson HW, Coleman GU. Treatment of urinary incontinence in children by endoscopically directed bladder neck injection of collagen. J Urol 1996;156:637.
99. Perez LM, Smith EA, Parrott TS, Broecker BH, Massad CA, Woodard JR. Submucosal bladder neck injection of bovine dermal collagen for urinary incontinence in the pediatric population. J Urol 1996;156:633.
100. Mitrofanoff P. Cystostomie continente transappendiculaire dans le traitement des vessies neurologiques. Chir Pediatr 1980;21:297.
101. Woodhouse CRJ. The Mitrofanoff Principle for continent urinary diversion. In: Webster G, Kirby R, King L, Goldwasser B, eds. Reconstructive Urology. Boston. Blackwell Scientific Publications, 1993;539.
102. Keating MA, Rink RC, Adams MC. Appendicovesicostomy: a useful adjunct to continent reconstruction of the bladder. J Urol 1993;149:1091.
103. Sumfest JM, Burns MW, Mitchell ME. The Mitrofanoff principle in urinary reconstruction. J Urol 1993;150:1875.
104. Duckett JW, Snyder HM. Continent urinary diversion: variations on the Mitrofanoff principle. J Urol 1986;136:58.
105. Duckett JW, Abdel-Hamid L. Appendicovesicostomy (and variations) in bladder reconstruction. J Urol 1993;149:567.
106. Casale AJ. Continent vesicostomy: a new method utilizing only bladder tissue. American Academy of Pediatrics Section on Urology, New Orleans, LA, 1991.
107. Rink RC, McLaughlin KP, Adams MC, Keating MA. Modification of the Casale Vesicostomy: continent diversion without the use of bowel. American Urological Association Meeting, Las Vegas, NV, 1995.
108. Lie HR, Lagergren J, Rasmussen F, Lagerkvist B, Hagelsteen J, Borjeson MC, Muttilainen M, Taudorf K. Bowel and bladder control of children with myelomeningocele: a Nordic study. Dev Med Child Neurology 1991;33:1053.
109. Malone PS. The management of bowel problems in children with urological disease. Br J Urol 1995;76:220.
110. Roberts JP, Moon S, Malone PS. Treatment of neuropathic urinary and faecal incontinence with synchronous bladder reconstruction and the antegrade continence enema procedure. Br J Urol 1995;75:386.
111. Malone PS, Ransley PG, Kiely EM. Preliminary report: the antegrade continence enema. Lancet 1990;336:1217.
112. Squire R, Kiely EM, Carr B, Ransley PG, Duffy PG. The clinical application of the Malone antegrade colonic enema. J Pediatr Surg 1993;28:1012.
113. Koyle MA, Kaji DM, Duque M, Wild J, Galansky SH. The Malone antegrade continence enema for neurogenic and structural fecal incontinence and constipation. J Urol 1995;154:759.
114. Griffiths DM, Malone PS. The Malone antegrade continence enema. J Pediatr Surg 1995;30:68.
115. Ellsworth PI, Webb HW, Crump JM, Barraza MA, Stevens PS, Mesrobian HGJ. The Malone antegrade colonic enema enhances the quality of life in children undergoing urological incontinence procedures. J Urol 1996;155:1416.

CHAPTER 25

Physiology of Micturition and Dysfunctional Voiding

Saul P. Greenfield and Julian Wan

The physiology of bladder function continues to be an area of research and discovery. It is of great interest to pediatric urologists because children have pathologic bladder behavior secondary to congenital and acquired abnormalities of innervation and bladder outlet obstruction. In vivo and in vitro studies of human tissue, along with animal models, have contributed a great deal to our understanding of bladder function. Differences among animal models, between animal models and humans, and between humans of different ages and sexes have also contributed contradiction and controversy. This chapter reviews the state of understanding of bladder function as it may apply to clinical pediatric urology.

INNERVATION OF THE LOWER URINARY TRACT

Gross Peripheral Neuroanatomy

Control of bladder function originates in the higher cortical centers and is mediated through spinal cord nuclei to efferent and afferent peripheral pathways. The posterior spinal cord roots receive afferent nerves, whereas the anterior roots transmit efferent impulses to the target organs. The smooth muscle of the bladder and urethra is autonomically innervated by sympathetic, parasympathetic, and purinergic systems, while the striated periurethral sphincter is thought to be "triple innervated" by autonomic and somatic nerves. This discussion confines itself to what is known about peripheral innervation of the bladder and sphincter.

The smooth muscle of the bladder and urethral sphincter are innervated by the autonomic nervous system.[1,2] Autonomic innervation is predominantly sympathetic and parasympathetic (Figs. 25.1 and 25.2). The efferent sympathetic nerves originate from T11 to L2. These nerves progress from the cord to the lumbar chain ganglia and then to the superior hypogastric plexus.

Nerves from this plexus form the right and left hypogastric nerve. The efferent parasympathetic nerves originate in the upper and middle sacral cord—S2 to S4—and progress from the cord to the pelvic nerve. The pelvic and hypograstric nerves meet to form the inferior hypogastric plexus. Nerves from this plexus then proceed to the lower ureter, bladder, and urethra. Many of the nerves from the hypogastric plexuses are preganglionic and ramify within intramural ganglia close to the target organ. Postganglionic nerves from the intramural ganglia then procede to directly innervate the smooth muscle. These ganglia and nerves comprise the "urogenital short neuron system." Intramural ganglia are found in the adventitia, muscularis, and suburothelium of the bladder and urethra.[2,3]

Afferent nerves travel from the urogenital smooth muscle to the hypogastric plexus and from there to the lumbar and sacral dorsal root ganglia through the hypogastric and pelvic nerves. In addition there are afferent sensory nerves that travel through the pudendal nerve to the sacral plexus and then to the sacral spinal cord. In some species, ventral and dorsal sacral nerve roots contain afferent nerve fibers. Sensory nerves are located within the bladder muscle and suburothelium and enable the individual to sense fullness, pain, and flow.[2] Afferent sensory nerves also play a crucial role in the reflex control of filling and voiding.[4,5]

The periurethral striated muscle or rhabdosphincter is somatically innervated from the anterior sacral cord (Onuf's nucleus) (Fig. 25.3). The rhabdosphincter is under voluntary control from higher cortical centers. Nerves progress directly from the cord to the striated muscle through the pudendal nerve.[6] In addition, there are autonomic nerve fibers, perhaps from the pelvic plexus, which have been documented in the striated sphincters of animal models.[7,8] This "triple innervation" (somatic, sympathetic, parasympathetic) theory is based on histochemical studies in the cat.[9] The adrenergic sym-

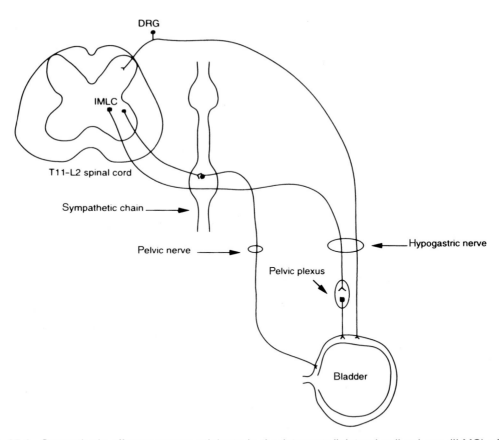

FIG. 25.1. Sympathetic efferent nerves originate in the interomediolateral cell column (ILMC) of the T11-L2 spinal cord. Some preganglionic nerves from this region of the spinal cord may synapse on postganglionic nerves in sympathetic chain ganglia or the pelvic plexus. Afferent sympathetic nerve signals are received in the dorsal root ganglia (DRG) located in T11-L2. The hypogastric nerve contains sympathetic afferent and efferent nerve fibers, while the pelvic nerve contains sympathetic fibers from the chain ganglia. (From Chai TC, Steer WD. Neurophysiology of micturition and incontinence. Urol Clin North Am 1996;23:223, reprinted with permission of W.B. Saunders Co.)

pathetic component alone has been corroborated in man.[7,10,11] The exact functional significance of autonomic participation in the striated muscle sphincter in man remains unknown. However, biopsy specimens of striated sphincter in patients with lower motor neuron lesions reveal adrenergic nerves, whereas biopsy speci-

mens from patients with functional detrusor-sphincter dyssynergia do not identify any adrenergic nerves.[10] This finding suggests that autonomic innervation of the striated sphincter may be compensatory at times and not uniformly present in normal individuals. Afferent innervation from the striated muscular sphincter

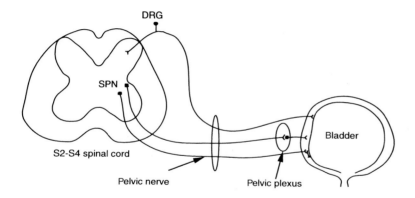

FIG. 25.2. Parasympathetic innervation of the bladder or urethra originates in the sacral parasympathetic nucleus (SPN) of the S2–S4 spinal cord. These efferent nerves synapse in the pelvic plexus or directly within the bladder or urethra. The dorsal root ganglia (DRG) of S2–S4 receive afferent signals from the target organs. Both afferent and efferent parasympathetic nerves travel through the pelvic nerve. (From Chai TC, Steer WD. Neurophysiology of micturition and incontinence. Urol Clin of North Am 1996;23:222, reprinted with permission of W.B. Saunders Co.)

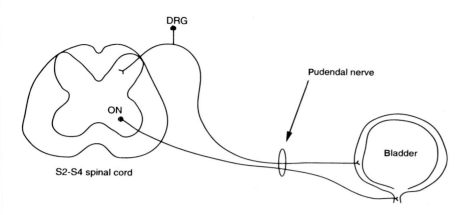

FIG. 25.3. Somatic innervation of the periurethral striated sphincter and bladder originates in Onuf's nucleus (ON) located in the S2–S4 spinal cord. Afferent signals are received by the dorsal root ganglia (DRG) located in the dorsal horns of S2–S4. The pudendal nerve contains these efferent and afferent nerve fibers. Autonomic innervation of the striated sphincter is not shown. (From Chai TC, Steer WD. Neurophysiology of micturition and incontinence. Urol Clin of North Am 1996;23: 223, reprinted with permission of W.B. Saunders Co.)

back to the sacral cord has not been documented in humans.[4]

Adrenergic, Cholinergic, and Purinergic Neurotransmitters

The sympathetic nerves are adrenergic and use norepinephrine as a neurotransmitter in postganglionic nerve endings. Preganglionic sympathetic nerves and all parasympathetic nerves are cholinergic and contain acetylcholine. A third and as yet incompletely understood autonomic system has been identified—the purinergic or peptidonergic system. Other neurotransmitters, such as vasoactive intestinal polypeptide (VIP), neuropeptide-Y, ATP, substance P, somatostatin, and calcitonin gene-related peptide, have been found in animal models and humans representing this system.[2, 4, 5, 12, 13] This system is thought to act as a modulator of overall autonomic activity.[4, 5] Neuropeptides have been found throughout the smooth and striated muscle of the lower urinary tract. In addition, in pathologic states of autonomic denervation, the effects of these neurotransmitters are thought to be exaggerated and to become clinically more significant.[5]

Existence of a third autonomic system was suspected when muscarinic blockade with atropine did not completely ablate in vitro bladder muscle contraction.[3, 14, 15] Furthermore, atropine has been shown to block contraction less in muscle specimens from patients with neurogenic bladders, suggesting that there is an enhanced purinergic factor in these abnormal bladders. VIP has been shown to have a relaxing effect on human detrusor muscle.[13, 16] VIP lowers basal tone in isolated muscle strips and inhibits spontaneous contraction.[17, 12] Substance P causes bladder muscle contraction in vitro.[13] Somatostatin serves to elevate basal tone and neuropeptide Y has been localized in the intramural ganglionic cells of the short neuron system.[13] Many of these neurotransmitters also cause changes in vascular smooth muscle and may help control local blood flow in the urogenital tract.

VIP concentrations have been found to be lower than normal in biopsy specimens of hypercontractile bladders.[13, 18] Histochemical studies of VIP and neuropeptide Y in the urethras of patients with spinal cord injury identified changes in concentration related to the level of the injury, again suggesting a compensatory role in pathologic states.[12, 19] In addition, ATP levels have been found to be higher than normal in the bladder muscle of myelomeningocele patients. ATP has been implicated in the initial phase of normal voiding in an animal model, when there is a rapid increase in bladder pressure.[20] Therefore, it has been suggested by some that hyperactivity in obstructed and neurogenic bladders may result from abnormal purinergic influence, mediated by ATP, VIP, and other purinergic neurotransmitters.[21]

Muscarinic cholinergic receptors are found throughout the smooth muscle of the lower urinary tract, but are more numerous in the bladder fundus.[4, 5, 14, 22] The preganglionic cholinergic receptors in the sympathetic and parasympathetic ganglia are nicotinic, as are the cholinergic receptors in the rhabdosphincter. Therefore, nicotinic-blocking agents such as botulinum toxin or pancuronium may be used to paralyze the striated sphincter, but do not result in complete incontinence because the smooth muscle sphincter remains unaffected.[3] Alpha-adrenergic receptors are more numerous in the smooth muscle of the posterior urethra and bladder base.[4, 14, 22] There are more alpha-adrenergic receptors found in the bladder neck in males than females and this is thought to be necessary to effect bladder neck closure during ejaculation.[23] Sparse populations of beta-adrenergic receptors are found in the bladder dome and these serve to relax the bladder during filling.[24] Studies of human fetal bladder have shown that beta-adrenergic and cholinergic receptors appear in fetal tissue after 3 months gestation.[25] Alpha-adrenergic receptors appear in the bladder base and urethra after 6 months gestation. Studies of autonomic activity in fetal sheep have also revealed sensitivity to beta-adrenergic and cholinergic agonists and blockade during gestation.[26]

Autonomic Coordination During Micturition

Micturition is voluntarily controlled by higher centers above the brainstem.[1,2,4,5] During bladder filling and storage the parasympathetic system is suppressed in the bladder fundus and trigone. This enables the bladder to fill at low pressures and the ureterovesical junctions to remain open. There is concomitant excitatory sympathetic activity through norepinephrine and alpha-adrenergic receptors to keep the bladder outlet closed, while beta-adrenergic receptors in the dome act to relax the detrusor. The rhabdosphincter is also tonically contracted. During voiding there is excitatory parasympathetic discharge. Acetylcholine acts on muscarinic receptors to cause the bladder to contract and the ureterovesical junctions to close. The bladder outlet opens and "funnels" because of suppression of sympathetic alpha-adrenergic transmission. Immediately before these events, the rhabdosphincter becomes suppressed and relaxes. This is seen as a drop in the maximal urethral pressure and the quiescence of the EMG readings during multichannel urodynamic recordings.

MUSCULAR ANATOMY AND FUNCTION

Although the smooth muscle of the bladder and urethra is structurally one anatomic unit, it has two distinct functional regions, described as the body and base (Fig. 25.4).[4,5] These two units roughly coincide to the areas above and below the trigone. Their differing functions are derived from the differences in autonomic innervation described earlier.[20] The body acts as a reservoir and pump, while the base remains flat during bladder filling and funnels during voiding to facilitate low pressure emptying. In addition, the smooth muscle action of Waldeyer's sheath allows for low pressure egress of urine out of the ureteral orifices during bladder filling and

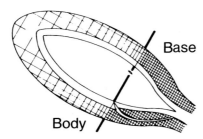

FIG. 25.4. The bladder body and base roughly coincide with the differences in autonomic innervation. The body functions as a reservoir and pump, while the base remains flat during bladder filling and funnels during voiding to facilitate low-pressure emptying. Contraction and relaxation of the smooth muscle of Waldeyer's sheath, surrounding the ureters, is also coordinated with bladder filling and emptying. (From Elbadawi A. Functional anatomy of the organs of micturition. Urol Clin North Am 1996;23:179, reprinted with permission of W.B. Saunders Co.)

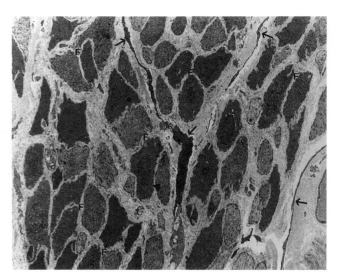

FIG. 25.5. This electron micrograph illustrates the bundle/fascicle organization of the detrusor (magnification ×3,800). The fascicles (F) are within bundles, which are separated by thick macrosepta (*arrows*) containing fibroblasts. The individual muscle cells are separated by thin macrosepta which contain collagen fibrils. (From Elbadawi A. Functional anatomy of the organs of micturition. Urol Clin North Am 1996;23:185, reprinted with permission of W.B. Saunders Co.)

conversely helps prevent vesicoureteral reflux during the high pressures of voiding.

Muscular Ultrastructure

The ultrastructural organization of the detrusor is important for proper function.[27] The smooth muscle cells are organized in fascicles that consist of four to twelve cells (Fig. 25.5). Each fascicle is surrounded by extracellular matrix (ECM) consisting of collagen, elastin, and rare fibroblasts.[4] Several fascicles are grouped into bundles that are also surrounded by ECM. These muscle bundles are longitudinal or circular throughout the bladder and proximal urethra. There are no discrete layers; the muscle bundles appear to be interwoven.[5] In males, smooth muscle forms part of the prostatic capsule and is a factor in bladder base function.[2,3]

The rhabdosphincter consists of circular fibers of striated muscle that surround the smooth muscle from the bladder base to the urogenital diaphragm.[8,28] There has been considerable debate as to which striated muscle functions as the so-called "striated muscle sphincter." It's apparent that the periurethral striated sphincter is separate and distinct from the urogenital diaphragm and the various pelvic supporting striated muscles in the male and female.[14,28,29,30] The periurethral striated sphincter is also distinct from the bulbocavernosus muscles. The urogenital diaphragmatic muscles play a role in continence, but are superficial to the periurethral striated muscle, which is closely applied to the smooth muscle layer.

The striated muscle cells consist of slow and fast twitch fibers that are under voluntary somatic control (Fig. 25.6). The corresponding fast and slow twitch myosin isoenzymes have been identified in the rhabdosphincter.[31] The slow twitch, fatigue-resistant fibers are tonically contracted during bladder filling. The fast twitch, easily fatigued fibers are used during voluntary attempts to stop micturition or during the willful holding of urine.[2] The rhabdosphincter may also play a role in the initiation of voiding by pulling down on the bladder neck, aiding in the change of the bladder outlet to a more funneled shape during voiding.[6] Studies of the levator ani muscles have also revealed fast and slow twitch fibers.[30] It has been suggested that the levator ani and other pelvic floor striated muscles acutely assist in voluntary urethral closure and may also play a role in maintaining continence during rapid shifts in intra-abdominal pressure. Beyond the middle third of the urethra in females and the bulbous urethra in males, the urethra serves merely as a urinary conduit.[28] However, normal ejaculation in males depends on the muscular propulsion of semen by properly innervated musculature in the bulbous urethra.

In humans there is thought not to be a one to one ratio of nerve endings to individual muscular cells, although there is some controversy on this point.[1, 4, 5] Only a subset of cells in a given fascicle may be directly innervated by a neuron. Electron microscope studies have revealed that normal muscle cells are 0.2 nm from each other, without intercellular links.[4] Thus, there is no electrical cell-to-cell excitation.[5] Efficient and coordinated detrusor contraction depends on electromechanical coupling, so that many individual muscle cell contractions begin when an adjacent cell pulls on its neighbor, not by direct neuronal excitation.[4, 5] These observations are significant in that pathologic behavior of obstructed or neurogenic bladders is derived in part by changes in ultrastructure, which result in altered coupling and muscular function. These ultrastructural changes are muscular cell hypertrophy and alterations of the extracellular matrix, which is between individual muscle cells and between fascicles.

EXTRACELLULAR MATRIX

The normal bladder is compliant and must have certain viscoelastic properties to function properly.[4, 5, 20] Compliance is defined as the change in volume divided by the change in pressure. Elasticity refers to the ability of the bladder to deform its shape under the stress of filling and voiding and then to resume its original shape when relatively empty and at rest. Viscosity refers to the bladder's ability to delay deformation by stress and this is in large part a property of the smooth muscle in the normal bladder, which relaxes during filling. The viscoelastic properties are influenced by the mechanical properties of the extracellular matrix (ECM). In the normal bladder much of this viscoelasticity derives from the ECM located in the suburothelial lamina propria.[32, 33] In pathologic states there are changes in the extracellular matix in the detrusor muscle layer and this is responsible for changes in mechanical function of the bladder.[32] The lamina propria, therefore, becomes less contributory to overall bladder viscoelastic behavior in abnormal bladders. This underlying mechanical dysfunction exacerbates the difficulties of patients who also may have abnormalities of neurologic control and who may also have muscular hypertrophy.

Recent studies of the extracellular matrix in children have revealed that there are subtypes of collagen that have different mechanical properties.[30, 34] Type I and type III predominate in the extracellular matrix of the lower urinary tract. Type I collagen has thicker fibers and is stiffer, whereas type III is thinner and more pli-

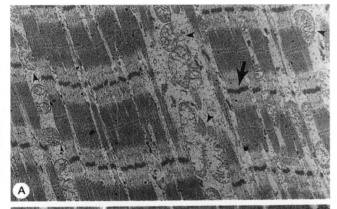

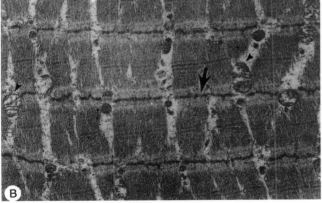

FIG. 25.6. Both slow and fast twitch myofibers are seen in these electron micrographs of periurethral striated muscle. **A,** (magnification ×10,940) slow twitch fibers. **B,** (magnification ×10,930) fast twitch fibers. The mitochondria (*small arrows*) are more abundant and the Z-discs (*large arrows*) are thicker in the slow twitch myofibers. (From Elbadawi A. Functional anatomy of the organs of micturition. Urol Clin North Am 1996;23:187, reprinted with permission of W.B. Saunders Co.)

able. Studies of human fetal collagen subtypes in the lower urinary tract reveal that as the normal fetus ages, the I : III ratio decreases with a concomitant increase in bladder compliance.[34] Elastin also increases with fetal age. A normal fetal bladder, therefore, becomes more compliant as gestation progresses.

Fibroblasts in the interstitium are thought to be the source of most of the connective tissue.[5] In the normal bladder there is little production or degradation and therefore little fibroblast activity. As will be discussed later, there are changes in extracellular matrix in obstructed and neurogenic bladders. Denervation experiments have suggested that the increase in ECM may in part derive from a slow down of collagen degradation caused by decreased function of endogenous proteases.[2] It has also been shown that the increase in extracellular matrix not only comes from the fibroblasts already present, but also from the smooth muscle cells themselves.[5] There appears to be dedifferentiation of smooth muscle cells under stress leading to the elaboration of collagen and elastin in the interstitium.[32] This is similar to what appears to occur to smooth muscle cells in vessel walls.[35] Stress in the form of increased wall tension caused by outlet obstruction or neurogenic hypercontractility may trigger this dedifferentiation in the bladder.

ULTRASTRUCTURE IN THE ABNORMAL BLADDER

Ultrastructural Changes in Adults

Changes in bladder ultrastructure have been studied in the aging male and female human bladder, in the congenitally obstructed bladder of children, in the neurogenic bladders of children with myelodysplasia, in adults with spinal cord injury, and in fetal and adult animal models of obstruction. While there are clear differences between all of these entities, there are many similarities. Specifically, pediatric bladder dysfunction may be better understood in light of what has been learned about ultrastructural changes in the abnormal adult bladder. Various ultrastructural changes are seen in the aging bladder and these depend on the sex of the individual and whether there is outlet obstruction in the male.

Bladder wall trabeculation may be caused by outlet obstruction or can occur in the absence of obstruction. Hypercontractility can be associated with trabeculation in adults and children.[4] It can be difficult to determine whether gross bladder wall hypertrophy is from individual muscle cell hypertrophy or hyperplasia.[20, 36] Electron microscopic observations and analysis of DNA content suggest that individual muscle cell hypertrophy is what occurs for the most part, although this may differ in differing animal models at different ages.[5] There is also an increase in extracellular matrix in trabeculated bladders.

In the absence of obstruction the aging detrusor in males and females may exhibit hypercontractility, which contributes to the symptoms of urgency, frequency, and incontinence. It has been observed in these aging, unobstructed bladders that there is a marked reduction in the distances between muscle cells resulting in direct cell to cell abutment.[4, 5] These abnormal abutments may serve as low resistance pathways for electrical coupling normally not present in younger bladders. This allows for an abnormally easy propagation of individual muscular contractions. The observed hyperreflexia, therefore, may be myogenic and neurogenic.[20] Aging can also result in degeneration of individual muscle cells, so that hypercontractility from abnormal coupling may be associated clinically with impaired contractility and poor emptying.[5] Abnormalities of electrical conduction in the detrusor muscle have been studied in the obstructed guinea pig and changes in sodium, potassium, and chloride cell membrane permeabilities have been demonstrated.[37] This may account for some of the instability seen in obstructed bladders.

The obstructed adult detrusor exhibits muscular hypertrophy along with an increase in the extracellular matrix.[4] The more abundant extracellular matrix in the aging adult bladder with outlet obstruction has proportionally more collagen than elastin and so is less compliant. A pathologic increase in ECM also results in less efficient mechanical coupling between individual cells and fascicles because there are widened spaces between cells and fascicles.[4, 5, 27] This may also inhibit the coordinated spread of a detrusor contraction.

Hypertrophic muscle cells cannot shorten fully,[5, 27] possibly because of the simple increase in cell size or a change in intracellular function. Animal experiments have demonstrated that outlet obstruction and smooth muscle hypertrophy are associated with changes in intracellular myosin fibers that may result in less force generated by an individual cell.[2, 38] Thus, the changes in the ECM and within individual muscle cells result in less efficient detrusor function in the obstructed adult bladder.

The obstructed bladder may also undergo alterations of innervation. Decreases in the amount of autonomic innervation to the obstructed detrusor muscle have been observed in animal models and humans.[5, 36, 39] Postjunctional denervation supersensitivity, typical of partial denervation, has been observed in an obstructed pig model.[36] These bladders were more sensitive to exogenous agonists, such as bethanechol, suggesting that this denervation response may play a role in the instability often associated with bladder outlet obstruction. The obstructed aging male bladder may also possess some of the other qualities described in aging bladders generally. Therefore, there may be areas of excessively close cellular abutment leading to foci of hyperactivity, in addition to impaired overall emptying. This corresponds to the clinical picture of urgency and frequency, along with varying degrees of urinary retention.

Studies in animal models have also demonstrated differences in the response to obstruction between old and young guinea pigs.[38, 40] Young animals appear capable of more smooth muscle cell growth than older animals, as judged by DNA synthesis activity, when the cells are stretched. Therefore, while children may be subject to the same stresses as adults (e.g., obstruction or neurogenic insult), the responses of the detrusor may differ qualitatively.

Ultrastructural Changes in the Fetus and Child

Studies of the fetal and infantile bladder in animal models and children have helped explain clinical observations in pediatric patients with functional abnormalities. The obstructed adult rabbit bladder may develop low capacity and low compliance within 14 days of obstruction.[41] These bladders rapidly increase in weight and develop grossly thickened bladder walls. There is muscular cell hypertrophy and an increase in extracellular matrix. There is a decrease in muscarinic receptor density resulting in decreased propagation of action potentials. Therefore, the number of motor end plates is fixed in the mature animal. Experiments on obstructed fetal sheep bladders have shown that there is increased smooth muscle mass caused by cellular hypertrophy and hyperplasia.[42] Hyperplasia was inferred because of the increase in DNA, although some investigators have shown that increases in DNA may also occur because of an increase in nuclear mass in each cell.[43] Thus, it is possible that increases in DNA may represent hypertrophy and not hyperplasia. It has also been shown that there is an increase in protooncogene expression, in part explaining the cellular growth seen in response to obstruction.[42, 43] Muscarinic receptors increase, but not in relation to myosin content, suggesting that in utero obstruction in this model may result in an increase in motor end plate number or size.[42] There were also changes in myosin heavy chain isoforms, suggesting that obstruction in the fetus, as in the adult, causes a change in intracellular muscle structure and function. There was overall reduced compliance.

Studies of normal fetal human bladders have revealed that there is no gender difference in extracellular matrix.[34] Type I (thick) collagen is the major fiber present overall, although type III (thin) are seen more within muscular bundle. The ratio of I:III increased with age of the fetus and elastin increased with age, as mentioned earlier. Similar studies in fetuses with congenital obstruction have revealed that there is a marked increase in the ratio of I:III compared to normal fetuses, and this may play a role in the diminished compliance noted in these bladders.[44] There was also increased elastin, although the elastin fibers were thicker. Muscular hyper-

trophy was also observed in these bladders. Increased collagen content has been documented in the bladder wall of neurologically normal children with enuresis and trabeculation.[45] These children had hypercontractility documented on urodynamic studies.

The bladders of children with myelodysplasia may also be less compliant and abnormally hypercontractile. Ultrastructural observations in specimens from these bladders have shown a relative paucity of muscle bundles with diminished size of individual muscle bundles.[46] There is a marked increase in extracellular matrix between fascicles and individual muscle cells, almost suggesting a compressive effect of the ECM on detrusor muscle. There is decreased muscarinic cholinergic receptor density that corresponds to the observation that there is less muscle overall in these bladders.[46, 47] Investigators have shown that these bladders may or may not demonstrate denervation supersensitivity to cholinergic agents.[5, 21, 47] This is not surprising, because no two individuals will have the same abnormalities of innervation, despite some urodynamic or functional similarities.

Furthermore, the observed hypercontractility in myelomeningocele bladders may be caused by various factors. These factors may be ultrastructural—such as excessively close muscular cell contact—or neurogenic.[48] The neurogenic factor may be abnormal parasympathetic excitation or excessive purinergic influence, as described earlier. Finally, urodynamic studies of newborns with myelodysplasia have confirmed that functional and gross structural changes can occur in utero in these bladders.[49] These changes are presumably secondary to the effects of voiding with higher than normal pressures or neurogenic hypercontractility, which starts in utero.

THE LOWER URINARY TRACT AND ARTIFICIAL NEURONAL MODULATION

There are ongoing efforts to replicate normal lower urinary tract innervation in the neurologically impaired individual by artificial means. The goal is to restore the normal functions of storage and emptying, rendering the patient continent with the ability to voluntarily void. These efforts have met with only partial success because of the difficulties inherent in artificially replicating neuronal function, and because the restoration of normal innervation may not altogether overcome the pathologic ultrastructural changes in the detrusor described earlier.

Neural modulation surgery has been carried out in adult patients with spinal cord injury or lesions.[50–56] Complete or selective posterior sacral root rhizotomy was first performed to ablate reflex voiding. This was then followed by anterior sacral nerve root stimulation using implanted electrodes. These patients have achieved increases in bladder capacity, voluntary emptying, and improvement in the symptoms of autonomic dysreflexia.[50, 51] Furthermore, in some individuals bladder trabeculation, vesicoureteral reflux, and hydronephrosis have improved or resolved.[52, 56] Selective sacral rhizotomy, without anterior root stimulation, has also been attempted in children with myelomeningocele and adults with spinal cord injury to increase bladder capacity and diminish uninhibited bladder contractions.[54] This has also met with partial success.

Recently, there have been attempts to further refine the artificial modulation of voiding by adding selective peripheral somatic denervation of the rhabdosphincter.[57, 58] By blocking the pudendal nerve, a further decrease in detrusor hypercontractility and an increase in bladder capacity has been observed in selected patients. Ablation of abnormal striated sphincter and pelvic floor activity has the theoretical advantage of preventing voiding with external sphincter dyssynergia.[59] In children, the best results after attempts at artificial neuronal modulation have been achieved in individuals with the least structural changes in the bladder wall.[53] Complications of these procedures include cerebrospinal fluid leak, infection around nerve roots with artificial stimulators, and the loss of erectile ability in males.

URODYNAMICS AND THE ASSESSMENT OF LOWER URINARY TRACT PHYSIOLOGY

Urodynamic testing allows the clinician to evaluate the summation of the previously discussed physiologic mechanisms. A complete description of urodynamic testing with normal and abnormal parameters is provided in Chapter 25. Normal voiding is complex and depends on the proper relationship between mechanical and neurologic systems. Urodynamic testing cannot often pinpoint the cause of dysfunctional voiding, but can enable the clinician to first diagnose that there is a problem and then help elucidate the cause.

The Cystometrogram and Detrusor Physiology

The cystometrogram (CMG) provides direct pressure and volume measurements from within the bladder lumen. Studies of normal children and adults reveal that during filling at rest, 99% of individuals store urine at pressures less than 30 cm H_2O.[60] Normal voiding pressures are varied, but are usually less than 80 cm H_2O. Formulas exist for the prediction of bladder capacity for different ages. Maizels proposed the formula: capacity (mL) = (age[years] + 2) × 30.[61] Houle's formula is: capacity (mL) = 16 × age (years) + 70.[60] These age-related formulas are derived from normal people of normal size and development, which may not be wholly applicable to patients with congenital abnormalities such as spina bifida. In a study of children with high pressure, small capacity bladders about to undergo bladder augmentation, the concept of pressure-specific bladder volume (PSBV) was developed.[62] This is the volume at which the bladder pressures are less than 20 or 30 cm H_2O, which is considered safe for upper urinary tract integrity (see later). A normal cystometrogram will not show any bladder contractions before voiding. The voiding contraction should be a single smooth increase and then decrement in bladder pressure and volume.

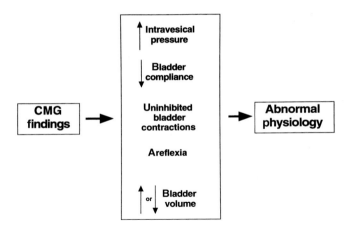

FIG. 25.7. The cystometrogram detects abnormal physiology, but will not always specifically pinpoint the underlying neuromuscular etiology.

The cystometrogram provides inferences regarding bladder innervation and ultrastructure. Abnormally high pressures or poor compliances, early contractions before voiding, absence of contraction, and abnormal volumes (large or small) suggest abnormal bladder physiology (Fig. 25.7). These abnormal CMG findings are unspecific for neurologic or myogenic causes and must be placed in context with the clinical history and radiographic findings. While an excellent clinical tool, the CMG can only approximate the nature of the underlying cause of dysfunction.

Assessing the Sphincter

Assessment of sphincteric function using urodynamics is similarly problematic. The direct measurement of urethral luminal pressure reflects the activity of the urethral smooth muscle, periurethral striated sphincter, and possibly the striated muscle of the pelvic floor. These factors cannot be dissected from one another with this measurement. Furthermore, in children the measurement of static midurethral pressures have not proved clinically useful, and therefore, a urethral pressure profile is rarely performed.[63] Of more interest is the dynamic behavior of the sphincter during bladder filling and voiding.

Leak Point Pressure

In the child who doesn't void, the question asked is what sort of resistance does the sphincter provide during bladder filling or contraction and during changes in transmitted abdominovesical pressure. Sphincteric function can be inferred by the intravesical pressures of voiding or the so-called "leak point pressure" (LPP) in the nonvoiding patient.[64–66] The LPP is the bladder pressure at which passive leakage occurs during the performance of a CMG. This measurement also reflects bladder wall compliance to some degree and thus does not purely assess the sphincter. If the LPP is low, it suggests that sphincter function is diminished. This does not necessarily mean that continence is diminished because the LPP also depends on bladder wall compliance and pressures at varying volumes. A patient with a low LPP may remain dry with the activities of daily life as long as bladder wall compliance allows the bladder pressures to remain low.

In the voiding patient, intraurethral pressure measurements should diminish immediately before the observed bladder contraction. As it drops it should equilibrate and become isobaric with intravesical pressures during voiding (Fig. 25.8). Failure of intraurethral pressure to diminish implies sphincteric malfunction. This failure to diminish may arise from nonreactivity of the smooth muscle sphincter or so-called dyssynergia of the rhabdosphincter.[59] The urodynamic pressure measurements cannot distinguish between the two, but this may not be clinically relevant in children with neurogenic bladder.[49] It can further be inferred that voiding with

extraordinarily high pressures (greater than 100 cm H_2O) may be caused by incomplete sphincteric relaxation, although bladder wall changes and abnormalities of detrusor innervation may also contribute to high voiding pressure, independent of sphincteric function.

In the nonvoiding child, the bladder is slowly filled and the urethral orifice is observed. The pressure in the urethral outlet at which leakage occurs is recorded. Leak point pressures of greater than 40 cm H_2O have been associated with deleterious lower and upper urinary tract changes.[64, 65] Children and adolescents with abnormally high leak point pressures may develop upper urinary tract changes severe enough to result in renal insufficiency. Bladder pressures in excess of 40 cm H_2O will overcome normal ureteral peristaltic pressures. This leads to hydronephrosis with or without vesicoureteral reflux. These changes in turn may lead to recurrent urinary tract infection, pyelonephritis, stones, and renal parenchymal damage.

Valsalva (Stress) Leak Point Pressure

Continence can be lost because of a variety of lower urinary tract factors: high bladder storage pressures, poor function of the sphincteric region, poor pelvic muscular support, or a combination thereof. The concept of the Valsalva leak point pressure (VLPP) or stress leak point pressure (SLPP) has been used to segregate these different causes in women with stress urinary incontinence and children with incontinence and neurogenic bladder.[67] This measurement attempts to show what happens when increases of intra-abdominal pressure are transmitted to the bladder. In children with neurogenic bladder dysfunction and incontinence, this measurement helps to distinguish those who may require medical or surgical facilitation of sphincteric function to achieve continence. Individuals with abnormal innervation are often wet not only because they lack adequate sphincteric resistance at rest, but also because their sphincter is poorly sealed, nonreactive, and cannot adjust to sudden changes in bladder pressure. Valsalva or coughing maneuvers recreate these shifts. To perform this test, the bladder is filled and abdominal pressure is increased by the Credé method or the patient is asked to cough or valsalva. The bladder pressures and urethral meatus are observed. The pressure at which leakage occurs is recorded. VLPPs of less than 60 cm H_2O imply that the observed incontinence is at least, in part, caused by sphincteric inadequacy. This test will not distinguish between smooth and striated muscular insufficiency.

Sphincter Electromyography

Electromyographic studies of the striated muscle sphincter may be performed.[68] These involve placing a needle electrode periurethrally directly into the sphinc-

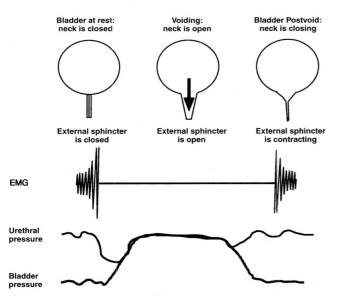

FIG. 25.8. As the bladder fills, urethral pressure is greater than vesical pressure. EMG shows contractile activity of external sphincter. During voiding, the urethral pressure initially drops just before the bladder begins to contract. The bladder pressure rises and the urethral pressure becomes isobaric. The EMG during this time becomes quiet reflecting the relaxation of the ext. sphincter. When micturition is completed the EMG shows increasing activity, and the urethral pressure rises. The bladder pressure falls to normal resting pressure.

ter or by using perianal patch electrodes. As should be evident from the previous discussion, these measurements probably do not reflect innervation of the smooth muscle bladder base and urethra. They cannot distinguish between adrenergic, cholinergic, or purinergic abnormalities of autonomic innervation. Furthermore, perianal patch electrodes record pelvic floor and perianal striated muscle innervation and not the rhabdosphincter exclusively.

These EMG recordings can document detrusor-external (striated) sphincter dyssynergia (DSD). DSD in myelodysplastic children is associated with the same upper urinary tract changes seen in those who have elevated LPPs and they often corroborate each other.[49, 69] Electromyographic recordings of sphincteric activity may have their greatest utility in voluntarily voiding children and young adults with nonneurogenic, neurogenic bladder syndrome. These individuals may have DSD of the rhabdosphincter for no known reason.[68, 70] Bladder pressure measurements and leak point and stress leak point pressure measurements are more clinically useful in nonvoiding children with structural neurologic disease.

CONCLUSION

As investigations continue in animal models and humans, it is hoped that further understanding of underlying physiologic mechanisms will result in improved therapies for dysfunctional voiding in children. Pharmacologic and surgical intervention is limited by ultrastructural changes that become permanent. There are no clinically useful therapies that have emerged so far from our incomplete understanding of the purinergic autonomic system. Artificial neuronal modulation, as discussed earlier, offers hope for some, but is not in wide use in children. Additional long-term studies are necessary. Early intervention, either prenatally or in infancy, for children with congenital bladder outlet obstruction offers some chance of forestalling ultrastructural changes in the detrusor.[71] Finally, studies of the aging bladder complement those of the fetal and infantile bladder. Better understanding of developmental physiology of the detrusor in normal and abnormal children may lead to improved treatments in the larger populations of elderly men and women with bladder outlet obstruction and urinary incontinence.

REFERENCES

1. Elbadawi A. Neuromorphologic basis of vesicourethral function, I: Histochemistry, ultrastructure, and function of intrinsic nerves of the bladder and urethra. Neuro Urodyn 1982;1:3–50.
2. Elbadawi A. Functional anatomy of the organs of micturition. Urol Clin North Am 1996;23:177–210.
3. Crowe R, Burnstock G, Light JK. Intramural ganglia in the human urethra. J Urol 1988;140:183–187.
4. Elbadawi A. Pathology and pathophysiology of detrusor in incontinence. Urol Clin North Am 1995;22:499–512.
5. Elbadawi A. Functional pathology of urinary bladder muscularis: the new frontier in diagnostic uropathology. Sem Diag Pathol 1993;10:314–354.
6. Hutch JA, Rambo OH Jr. A new theory of the anatomy of the internal urethral sphincter and the physiology of micturition, III: Anatomy of the urethra. J Urol 1967;97:696–704.
7. Elbadawi A. Ultrastructure of vesicourethral innervation, I: Neuroeffector and cell junctions in the male internal urethral sphincter. J Urol 1982;128:180–188.
8. Benoit G, Quillard J, Jardin A. Anatomic study of the inframontanal urethra in man. J Urol 1988;139:866–868.
9. Elbadawi A, Schenck EA. A new theory of the innervation of the bladder musculature. Innervation of the vesicourethral junction and external sphincter. J Urol 1974;111(pt. 4):613–615.
10. Crowe R, Burnstock G, Light JK. Adrenergic innervation of the striated muscle of the intrinsic external urethral sphincter from patients with lower motor spinal cord lesion. J Urol 1989;141:47–49.
11. Kumagai A, Koyanagi T, Takahashi Y. The innervation of the external urethral sphincter; an ultrastructural study in male human subjects. Urol Res 1987;15:39–43.
12. Milner P, Crowe R, Burnstock G, Light JK. Neuropeptide Y- and vasoactive intestinal polypeptide containing nerves in the intrinsic external urethral sphincter in the areflexic bladder compared to detrusor-sphincter dyssynergia in patients with spinal cord injury. J Urol 1987;135:888–892.
13. Klarskov P, Gerstenberg T, Hald T. Vasoactive intestinal polypeptide influence on lower urinary tract smooth muscle from human and pig. J Urol 1984;131:1000–1004.
14. Saito M, Kondo A, Kato T, Levin RM. Response of isolated human neurogenic detrusor smooth muscle to intramural nerve stimulation. Br J Urol 1993;72:723–727.
15. Andersson K-E, Sjorgen C. Aspects on the physiology and pharmacology of the bladder and urethra. Prog Neurobiol 1982;19:71–89.
16. Crowe R, Moss HE, Chapple CR, Light JK, Burnstock G. Patients with lower motor spinal cord lesion: a decrease of vasoactive intestinal polypeptide, calcitonin gene related peptide and substance P, but not neuropeptide Y and somatostatin-immunoreactive nerves in the detrusor muscle of the bladder. J Urol 1991;145:600–604.
17. Kinder RB, Mundy AR. Inhibition of spontaneous contractile activity in isolated human detrusor muscle strips by vasoactive intestinal polypeptide. Br J Urol 1985;57:20–23.
18. Gu JM, Restorick JM, Blank MA, et al. Vasoactive intestinal polypeptide in the normal and unstable bladder. Br J Urol 1983;55:645–647.
19. Crowe R, Burnstock G, Light JK. Spinal cord lesions at different levels affect either the adrenergic or vasoactive intestinal polypeptide-immunoreactive nerves in the human urethra. J Urol 1988;140:1412–1414.
20. Levin RM, Longhurst PA, Monson FC, Kato K, Wein A. Effect of bladder outlet obstruction on the morphology, physiology, and pharmacology of the bladder. Prostate 1990;S-3:9–26.
21. Saito M, Kondo A, Kato T, Hasegawa S, Miyake K. Response of the human neurogenic bladder to KCL, carbachol, ATP, and CaCl₂. Br J Urol 1993;72:298–302.
22. Ek A, Alm P, Andersson K-E, Persson CGA. Adrenergic and cholinergic nerves to the human urethra and urinary bladder. A histochemical study. Acta Physiol Scand 1977;99:345–352.
23. Gosling JA, Dixon JS, Lendon RG. The autonomic innervation of the human male and female bladder neck and proximal urethra. J Urol 1977;118:302–305.
24. Benson G, McConnell JA, Wood JG. Adrenergic innervation of the human bladder body. J Urol 1979;122:189–191.
25. Mitolo-Chieppa D, Schonauer S, Grasso G, Cicinelli E, Carratu MR. Ontogenesis of autonomic receptors in detrusor muscle and bladder sphincter of human fetus. Urology 1983;221:599–603.
26. Kogan B, Iwamoto HS. Lower urinary tract function in the sheep fetus: studies of autonomic control and pharmacologic responses of the fetal bladder. J Urol 1989;141:1019–1024.
27. Elbadawi A. Microstructural basis of detrusor contractility: the MIN approach to its understanding and study. Neurourol Urodyn 1991;10:77–85.

28. DeLancey JOL. Correlative study of paraurethral anatomy. Obstet Gynecol 1986;68:91–97.
29. DeLancey JOL. Pubovesical ligament: a separate structure from the urethral supports ("pubo-urethral ligaments"). Neurourol Urodyn 1989;8:53–61.
30. Gosling JA, Dixon JS, Critchley HOD, Thompson SA. A comparative study of the human external sphincter and periurethral levator ani muscles. Br J Urol 1981;53:35–41.
31. Tokunaka S, Murakami U, Fujii H, et al. Coexistence of fast and slow myosin isozymes in human external urethral sphincter. A preliminary report. J Urol 1987;138:659–662.
32. Ewalt DH, Howard PS, Blyth B, et al. Is lamina propria matrix responsible for normal bladder compliance? J Urol 1992;148:544–549.
33. Susset JG, Regnier CH. Viscoelastic properties of bladder strips-standardization of a technique. Invest Urol 1981;18:445–450.
34. Kim KM, Kogan BA, Massad CA, Huang Yi-C. Collagen and elastin in the normal fetal bladder. J Urol 1991;146:524–527.
35. Inoue T. The three dimensional ultrastructure of intracellular organization of smooth muscle cells by screening electron microscopy. In: Motta PM, ed. Ultrastructure of Smooth Muscle. Boston, MA: Kluwer, 1990, 63–67.
36. Speakman MJ, Brading AF, Gilpin CJ, Dixon JS, Gosling JA. Bladder outflow obstruction—a cause of denervation supersensitivity. J Urol 1987;138:1461–1466.
37. Seki N, Karim OMA, Mostwin JL. Changes in electrical properties of guinea pig smooth muscle membrane by experimental bladder outflow obstruction. Am J Physiol 1992;31:F885–F891.
38. Karim OMA, Seki N, Pienta KJ, Mostwin JL. The effect of age on the response of the detrusor to intracellular mechanical stimulus: DNA replication and cell actin matrix. J Cell Biochem 1992;48:373–378.
39. Gosling JA, Gilpin SA, Dixon JS, Gilpin CJ. Decrease in the autonomic innervation of human detrusor muscle in outflow obstruction. J Urol 1986;136:501–504.
40. Seki N, Karim OMA, Mostwin JL. Membrane electrical properties of guinea pig smooth muscle with growth. Neurourol Urodyn 1992;11:245–252.
41. Malkowitz SB, Wein AJ, Elbadawi A, Arsdalen KV, Ruggieri MR, Levin RM. Acute biochemical and functional alterations in the partially obstructed rabbit urinary bladder. J Urol 1986;136:1324–1329.
42. Peters CA, Vasavada S, Dator D, et al. The effect of obstruction on the developing bladder. J Urol 1992;148:491–496.
43. Cendron M, Karim OMA, Mostwin JL, Gearhart JP. In utero partial changes seen in the developing bladder. J Urol 1992;147:225A.
44. Kim KM, Kogan BA, Massad CA, Huang YI-C. Collagen and elastin in the obstructed fetal bladder. J Urol 1991;146:528–531.
45. Booth CM, Gosling JA. Histological and urodynamic study of the bladder in enuretic children. Br J Urol 1983;55:367–370.
46. Shapiro E, Becich MJ, Perlman E, Lepor H. Bladder wall abnormalities in myelodysplastic children: a computer assisted morphometric analysis. J Urol 1991;145:1024–1029.
47. Gup DI, Baumann M, Lepor H, Shapiro E. Muscarinic cholinergic receptors in normal pediatric and myelodysplastic bladders. J Urol 1989;142:595–599.
48. German K, Bedwan J, Davies J, Brading AF, Stephenson TP. An assessment of the contribution of viscoelastic factors in the aetiology of poor compliance in the human neuropathic bladder. Br J Urol 1994;74:744–748.
49. Kopp C, Greenfield SP. Effects of neurogenic bladder dysfunction in utero in neonates with myelodysplasia. Br J Urol 1993;71:739–742.
50. Van Kerrebroeck PEV, Koldwein EL, Rosier PFWM, Wijktsra H, Debruyne FMJ. Results of the treatment of neurogenic bladder dysfunction in spinal cord injury by sacral posterior root rhizotomy and anterior sacral root stimulation. J Urol 1996;155:1378–1381.
51. Franco I, Storrs B, Firlit CF, Zebold K, Richards I, Kaplan WE. Selective sacral rhizotomy in children with high pressure neurogenic bladders: preliminary results. J Urol 1992;148:648–650.
52. Koldewijn EL, Van Kerrebroeck PEV, Rosier PFWM, Wijkstra H, Debruyn FMJ. Bladder compliance after posterior sacral root rhizotomies and anterior sacral root stimulation. J Urol 1994;151:955–960.
53. Schneidau T, Franco I, Zebold K, Kaplan W. Selective sacral rhizotomy for the management of neurogenic bladders in spina bifida patients: long-term follow-up. J Urol 1995;154:766–768.
54. Gasparini ME, Schmidt RA, Tanagho EA. Selective sacral rhizotomy in the management of the reflex neuropathic bladder: a report on 17 patients with long-term follow-up. J Urol 1992;148:1207–1210.
55. McGuire EJ, Savastino JA. Urodynamic findings and clinical status following denervation procedures for control of incontinence. J Urol 1984;132:87–88.
56. Brindley GS, Polkey CE, Rushton DN, Cardozo L. Sacral anterior root stimulators for bladder control in paraplegia: the first 50 cases. J Neurol Neurosurg Psych 1986;49:1104–1114.
57. Tanagho EA. Neuromodulation in the management of voiding dysfunction in children. J Urol 1992;148:655–657.
58. Tanagho EA, Schmidt RA, Orvis BR. Neural stimulation for control of voiding dysfunction: a preliminary report in 22 patients with serious neuropathic voiding disorders. J Urol 1989;142:340–345.
59. Blaivis JG, Sinha HP, Zayed AAH, Labib KB. Detrusor-external sphincter dyssynergia: a detailed electromyographic study. J Urol 1981;125:545–548.
60. Houle A-M, Gilmour RF, Churchill BM, Gaumond M, Bissonnette B. What volume can a child normally store in the bladder at a safe pressure? J Urol 1993;149:561–564.
61. Berger RM, Maizels M, Moran GC, Conway JJ, Firlit CF. Bladder capacity (ounces) equals age (years) plus 2 predicts normal bladder capacity and aids in the diagnosis of abnormal voiding patterns. J Urol 1983;129:347.
62. Landau EZ, Churchill BM, Jayanthi V, et al. The sensitivity of pressure specific bladder volume versus total bladder capacity as a measure of bladder storage dysfunction. J Urol 1994;152:1578–1581.
63. Wan J, Greenfield SP. Pediatric urodynamics. In: Blaivis J, Chancellor M, eds. Atlas of Urodynamics. Baltimore: Williams & Wilkins, 1996;251–270.
64. Wang SC, McGuire EJ, Bloom DA. A bladder pressure management system for myelodysplasia: clinical outcome. J Urol 1988;140:1499.
65. McGuire EJ, Woodside JR, Borden TA. The prognostic value of urodynamic testing in myelodysplastic patients. J Urol 1981;126:205.
66. McGuire EJ, Fitzpatrick CC, Wan J. Clinical assessment of urethral spincter function. J Urol 1993;150:1452.
67. Wan J, McGuire EJ, Bloom DA, Ritchey ML. Stress leak point pressure: a diagnostic tool for incontinent children. J Urol 1993;150:700.
68. Bauer SB. Neuropathology of the lower urinary tract. In: Kelalis PP, et al., eds. Clinical Pediatric Urology. Philadelphia: W.B. Saunders, 1992;399–440.
69. Bauer SB, Hallett M, Khoshbin S. The prognostic value of urodynamic testing in myelodysplastic patients. J Urol 1981;126:205.
70. Hinman F. Urinary tract damage in children who wet. Pediatrics 1974;54:143–150.
71. Greenfield SP. Posterior urethral valves: new concepts. J Urol 1997;157:996.

CHAPTER 26

Urinary Infection in Children: Pathogenesis, Bacterial Virulence, and Host Resistance

William R. Strand

Bacterial infection, which is the most common malady of the urinary tract in children, may be defined by a spectrum of disease ranging from asymptomatic bacteriuria (ABU) to acute pyelonephritis. Although anatomic abnormalities are often presumed to be responsible for urinary infection in children, it has become clear that most infections occur in otherwise healthy children with anatomically normal urinary tracts. Bacterial isolates from children with acute pyelonephritis and anatomic abnormalities such as obstruction, vesicoureteral reflux (VUR), or indwelling urinary catheters are frequently indistinguishable from commensal fecal isolates. In the absence of these abnormalities, bacterial isolates often possess genes and their products that confer special virulence not found in fecal strains. The urinary tract has effective mechanisms to protect against infection, but these uropathogenic bacteria have evolved urovirulence factors able to circumvent these defenses. Bacteria expressing combinations of these urovirulence factors, including specific fimbriae, hemolysin, aerobactin, and capsular or lipopolysaccharide (LPS) antigens generally incite more severe inflammation, and are more likely to cause significant renal scarring.[1] Although classification of specific bacterial urovirulence factors and host defenses oversimplifies the complex interplay between bacteria and the colonized host, this approach may allow us to more easily understand the pathogenesis of urinary infection.

For ascending urinary infection to occur, bacteria must first spread from the periurethral area to the bladder, resist being washed away in the urine, and then multiply and travel to the kidney through the ureter. Bacterial adherence is the first critical step for infection to become established. Initial loose contact achieved by attachment of fimbriae with the uroepithelial cell surface is likely followed by tighter binding mediated by other bacterial surface proteins (afimbrial adhesins) at distinct sites. Bacteria growing in the urine are con-

stantly losing and reforming fimbriae, and are also capable of altering fimbrial expression in response to changes in their microenvironment (phase variation), including host production of specific antibodies for the fimbrial tip adhesin.

Bacteria that overcome host resistance to reach the upper urinary tract encounter an array of defenses designed to clear invading organisms from urine, tissue, and blood. Uropathogenic bacteria that resist the initial killing effect of this resistance initiate a host response that may lead to considerable collateral renal damage. This inflammatory response, triggered by adherence-mediated cytokine induction, is characterized by polymorphonuclear leukocyte (neutrophil) infiltration, with subsequent release of toxic lysosomal enzymes. Production of reactive oxygen species (ROS) ensues from release of lysosomal enzymes and from renal ischemia and reperfusion associated with neutrophil aggregation. Most renal damage from acute pyelonephritis is caused by host defenses trying to clear bacteria, rather than by any direct action of the bacteria themselves.

Escherichia coli (E. coli) is the most common urinary tract pathogen, responsible for these infections in more than 80% of cases.[2,3] The remainder of urinary infections are caused by few species, including *Proteus mirabilis, Klebsiella pneumonia, Pseudomonas aeruginosa,* and the *Enterococci*. This predilection for certain strains of bacteria to invade the urinary tract is termed bacterial tropism.[4,5] Although adherence of bacteria promotes colonization and inflammation of the urinary tract, other urovirulence factors, including hemolysin and cytotoxic necrotizing factor, are specifically able to damage uroepithelial cells.[6–8] Some of these urovirulence factors have been shown to be genetically linked on transmissible "pathogenicity islands," which are able to convey enhanced invasiveness.[8,9]

The legacy of acute pyelonephritis for some children is renal parenchymal scarring, which may lead to hypertension, proteinuria, and renal insufficiency. Other children may be spared these consequences despite apparently significant urinary infection. Host susceptibility may be variable and related to hereditary and familial factors, including blood group secretor status, the presence of anatomic abnormalities (VUR or ureteral duplication), or the familial preference for circumcision or breast feeding. Voiding dysfunction and constipation are more likely social and environmental contributions. Specific interactions between the host and invading bacteria, modulated by the timeliness of clinical diagnosis and antibiotic therapy, accounts for variation in severity of the inflammatory response during acute pyelonephritis.

Although great strides have been made in understanding the pathogenesis of urinary tract infections through application of molecular techniques, this information has changed clinical practice relatively little. However, these advances reveal how bacteria establish urinary infection by exploiting host cell features for their own benefit. Circumcision remains the most explicit clinical intervention available to diminish the risk of periurethral bacterial adherence leading to urinary infection. However, recognition and rectification of functional elimination disorders, including dysfunctional voiding and fecal retention, provides the most effective method for controlling factors responsible for urinary infection. It is hoped that perturbation of other factors involved in urinary infection may help to tip the balance in favor of renal preservation and resolution of bacterial growth for all children. Further work is underway to design effective vaccines based on specific determinants of urovirulence factors.

CLINICAL ASPECTS OF URINARY INFECTION

Approximately 1% of boys and 3% of girls have at least one symptomatic urinary tract infection during their first 10 years of life. In boys, the highest incidence occurs during the first month of life, and is generally associated with fever.[10, 11] Recurrent urinary infections occur in approximately 25% of boys and 40% of girls, usually within a year of the initial infection.[10, 11] Uncircumcised male infants have a 10-fold increase in the incidence of urinary infection compared to circumcised boys,[12–14] which is associated with enhanced preputial bacterial adherence.[15, 16] Although girls have fewer urinary infections as infants, they are more likely to have multiple recurrent infections.[10, 11] Increased periurethral colonization, demonstrated by culture[17] or by enhanced bacterial adherence to uroepithelial cells in urinary sediment,[18–20] usually precedes the onset of urinary infection in girls, and often changes clonal composition in recurrent infection.[21] Although heavy bacterial colonization is often present in healthy neonates, periurethral coloni-

zation generally declines rapidly in the first year of life and is rare after the age of 5.[17]

Development of urinary infection depends on the susceptibility of the host and the virulence of the invading bacteria, with most infections following an ascending route initiated by periurethral colonization by uropathogenic bacteria. Urinary infections are classified as complicated when an anatomic abnormality exists. Although urinary tract obstruction (posterior urethral valves, ureteropelvic or ureterovesical junction obstruction or ureterocele) is less commonly found in children with infection, the potential for renal damage is much greater when infection occurs.[22] Approximately half of all children with urinary infection have demonstrable VUR.[11, 23, 24] Because VUR provides effective transport of bacteria to the kidney, uroepithelial adherence becomes less important in perpetuation of urinary infection. Bacterial strains isolated from children with VUR are less often associated with P fimbriae,[25] but they continue to express type 1 fimbriae, which incite the inflammatory response.[26–28] Although VUR does not specifically cause urinary infection or inflammation, higher-grade reflux is more often associated with severe renal scarring.[29, 30]

Urinary infection may be further classified as ABU, cystitis, or acute pyelonephritis based on local or systemic symptoms. ABU indicates attenuation of uropathogenic bacteria by the host, or colonization of the bladder by nonvirulent bacteria incapable of activating a symptomatic response. Cystitis may represent early recognition of an infection destined to become pyelonephritis, or bacterial growth controlled by a balance of bacterial virulence and host response. Pyelonephritis, which is associated with fever and activation of the inflammatory response, leads to renal scarring in approximately a third of affected children.[24, 31] Although the incidence of renal scarring is commonly considered to be highest within the first year of life,[32] several recent studies suggest that this risk remains high in young children independent of age.[29, 33] In 157 children younger than 6 years treated for acute pyelonephritis, renal scarring was detected on nuclear renography in 36% of children younger than 1 year, and in 43% of those older than 1 year.[29] Children with renal scarring from pyelonephritis are recognized to be at increased risk for hypertension and renal failure, but these effects may not be apparent for decades.[10, 31, 34] This progression most often correlates with the renal cortical loss present on initial radiographic evaluation.[30]

Circumcision Status

In 1974, Winberg et al. concluded that the more rapid decline in the incidence of urinary tract infection with age in boys than in girls could be caused by earlier disappearance of a predisposing factor in males.[11] Then in 1982, Ginsberg and McCracken were the first to report that most male infants with urinary infections were uncircumcised (95%).[14] Wiswell et al. subsequently found the overall incidence of urinary infections in infants to be 0.43%, with uncircumcised males accounting for the highest percentage (1.12% uncircumcised males, 0.11% circumcised males, 0.57% females).[12] Although the highest risk for urinary infection in uncircumcised males is thought to be limited to the first year of life,[11] Craig et al. recently reported a fivefold decreased risk of symptomatic urinary infection in circumcised boys younger than 5 years old, independent of age.[35]

Circumcision limits the risk of urinary infection by radically changing bacterial adherence in the periurethral area. Without circumcision, gradual retraction of the prepuce also aids resistance from urinary infection by limiting proximity of colonizing bacteria to the urethral meatus.[5] An adherent prepuce covering the glans decreases to 50% by 1 year of age, and to only 10% by 3 years of age. In a prospective study of urethral cultures in male infants, a rapid decrease in urethral colonization followed circumcision, with an early increase and slow decline in colonization reported without circumcision.[36] Although P-fimbriated strains of *E. coli* bind to the inner preputial layer and promote colonization of the urinary tract,[16] renal inflammation and scarring is generally not caused by strains possessing only P fimbriae.[37] Type 1 fimbriae, which adhere only poorly to the prepuce and bladder urothelium,[4] bind more readily to uroepithelial cells in the ureter and kidney,[38] and best to neutrophils, thereby eliciting the inflammatory response associated with acute pyelonephritis.[39] Delivery of bacteria with type 1 fimbriae to the kidneys must be facilitated by vesicoureteral reflux or by the coincident expression of P fimbriae.[37] The presence of an anatomic risk factor, such as vesicoureteral reflux, allows pyelonephritis to occur with less virulent strains of bacteria (strains without P fimbriae).[25] Circumcision remains one method to limit the effect of another anatomic risk factor. The significant morbidity associated with acute pyelonephritis in infants[10,32] supports efforts directed at reducing risk whenever possible, but because the prevalence of urinary infection in boys is low, only 1 to 2% of boys undergoing circumcision to prevent pyelonephritis will realize this benefit from their surgery.

Voiding Dysfunction

An infrequent or inefficient urinary voiding pattern is commonly associated with diurnal enuresis and urinary infection,[40–43] and likely represents a bad habit that is reinforced inadvertently by parents or other caregivers. Frequently, these children are described as being good at holding their urine, but will often exhibit urinary urgency and occasional diurnal enuresis. This delayed voiding behavior is akin to pressing the snooze alarm repeatedly on an alarm clock, and ultimately being late

for school. Diurnal enuresis occurring even as seldom as once weekly is associated with an increased risk for urinary infection.[44]

An infrequent or inefficient voiding pattern is initially associated with bladder capacities larger than would be predicted for age. However, increased bladder storage pressures resultant from this functional urinary tract obstruction ultimately leads to progressive bladder trabeculation with bladder wall thickening and diminished storage capacity. Bladder trabeculation was noted radiographically or cystoscopically in up to 20% of girls with bacteriuria noted on screening urinalysis.[45, 46] The caliber of the urethra on voiding cystourethrogram (VCUG) is typically greater in dysfunctional voiders with recurrent urinary infections,[47] but represents an effect of voiding dysfunction rather than a cause. This "spinning top" urethral configuration leads to turbulent rather than laminar urine flow, and the vortex created promotes vaginal filling during voiding, and likely retrograde flow of urine into the bladder (Fig. 26.1). The presence of residual bladder urine correlates directly with the presence of bacteriuria and with its recurrence following treatment.[48] Effective treatment is directed toward complete and regular emptying of bladder urine by establishing a scheduled voiding regimen, and has

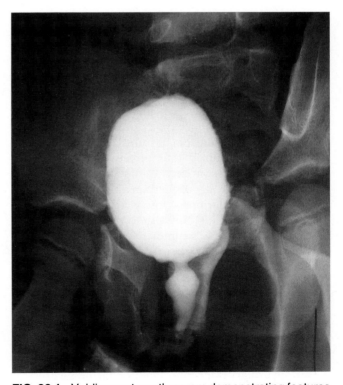

FIG. 26.1. Voiding cystourethrogram demonstrating features commonly found in girls with voiding dysfunction. High intravesical pressure from dysfunctional voiding leads to a "spinning top" urethral configuration and increased voided velocity. Turbulent flow and increased voided velocity creates a vortex, which promotes vaginal filling.

been shown to reduce the incidence of recurrent infection.[42] In contrast, bacteriuria has commonly been recognized to persist in girls treated with cystoscopic urethral dilation for presumed anatomic urethral stenosis.[49, 50]

Incomplete voiding also results from inadequate sphincter relaxation during detrusor contraction, and may follow attempts to push urine out quickly. Urodynamic evaluation in neurologically normal children with enuresis often demonstrates increased intravesical filling pressures and uninhibited bladder contractions. Interrupted voiding and incomplete bladder emptying are linked to increased pelvic floor activity during voiding.[51, 52] Lapides evaluated girls younger than 16 years with urinary infection and found detrusor instability in 61%, infrequent voiding in 30%, and true neurogenic bladder in only 6%.[53] The inflammatory reaction associated with urinary tract infection is thought to cause detrusor and sphincter hyperactivity, which perpetuates voiding dysfunction.

High intravesical pressures and bladder distension found in dysfunctional voiders[54] could also promote urinary infection by causing bladder ischemia.[43] Vesical blood flow was shown to decrease by more than 25% in dogs after 2 hours of bladder distension.[55] Urethral obstruction in mice, causing increased intravesical pressure, allowed nonpathogenic *E. coli* strains to cause pyelonephritis, and intensified the inflammatory damage caused by uropathogenic *E. coli* strains.[56]

Voiding dysfunction may be one part of an elimination disorder, which also includes constipation and encopresis.[57] Fecal retention and impaired sensation on rectal manometry are common, yet most of these children and families deny constipation.[57] Successful control of constipation decreases the incidence of diurnal enuresis[58] and recurrent urinary tract infection.[51, 52, 57–59] Medical management often remains unsuccessful until fecal retention is recognized and effectively treated. Although fecal retention and dysfunctional voiding are generally expected only in children after the age of toilet training, some children as young as 12 to 18 months manifest this behavior. Barriers to recognition include inattention to the child's elimination pattern (by parents and physicians), and lack of recognition that fecal retention may occur despite regular passage of stool. In effect, this approximates failure to recognize that a traffic snarl exists on the freeway because some cars are seen intermittently travelling down the exit ramp.

Familial Factors

Certain urinary tract abnormalities, including ureteral duplication and vesicoureteral reflux, are familial and predispose to urinary infection. The urothelial density of blood group antigens is also hereditary, and nonsecretors of the urothelial antigens are known to be more susceptible to developing urinary infection, presumably through enhanced binding by P fimbriae to the more exposed and accessible P blood group urothelial antigens. Choices regarding breast-feeding may be swayed by familial preferences. Other factors, including voiding dysfunction or fecal retention, are not specifically heritable but often are present in multiple family members.

Imaging in Urinary Infection

Children with well-documented urinary infection should be evaluated by renal (and bladder) ultrasonography and cystography, regardless of their age and symptoms. A contrast VCUG should be used for all boys to assess for possible posterior urethral valves, but a nuclear cystogram may be substituted for girls. Nuclear renography is best delayed at least 1 month to detect renal scarring, rather than to merely document renal inflammation. However, immediate nuclear renography is sometimes useful in cases in which an appropriate urine culture has not been obtained before antibiotic administration.

A VCUG (rather than a nuclear cystogram) may also be helpful in older girls, especially those with recurrent infections. The anatomic detail provided by the VCUG clarifies detection of significant fecal retention, bladder trabeculation, the "spinning-top" urethral deformity, and paraureteral diverticuli associated with elimination disorders. Specific attention should be addressed to the bladder capacity on cystography, and to the functional bladder capacity noted on any voiding diary records available. Diagnosis and treatment of underlying voiding dysfunction and fecal retention is an essential component of the successful management of urinary infection in children. Children with urinary infection should be maintained on low-dose antibiotic prophylaxis until their radiographic evaluation is completed, which should then be continued in children found to have VUR or significant voiding dysfunction until these risk factors are resolved.

More than half of all children with symptomatic urinary infections have anatomically normal urinary tracts, without hydronephrosis or VUR.[11, 23, 24] Although renal ultrasonography remains an integral part of recommended radiographic evaluation after urinary infection, it identifies renal scarring in only 40% of children with defects on nuclear renography,[60, 61] and in only 10% of the less severe cases.[24] Hyperechogenicity or effacement of the renal parenchyma in one or multiple areas indicates significant renal scarring. Use of color Doppler sonography to detect focal renal perfusion abnormalities (in a cooperative child) may enhance overall detection of acute pyelonephritis.[62] The search for a less distressing radiographic evaluation has led some to rely on renal imaging alone, arguing that only children with evidence for pyelonephritogenic scarring are at risk for progressive renal injury.[63] This ignores the significant risk posed by recurrent urinary infections linked to VUR or dysfunctional voiding. Assessment for renal scarring may be particularly important in children with VUR because it promotes direct inoculation of the renal parenchyma, and allows inflammatory renal damage to result from urinary infection with relatively less virulent uropathogenic bacteria.[25]

Nuclear Renography

In children with febrile urinary infections, technetium[99m] dimercaptosuccinic acid (DMSA) renography has emerged as the preferred imaging method for evaluation of acute pyelonephritis and renal cortical scarring.[64] Areas of reduced radiotracer uptake often represent reversible renal ischemia on an acute study, but correlate closely with parenchymal scarring on imaging after the acute infection has resolved.[24, 64, 65] Approximately two thirds of children with a febrile urinary infection have an abnormality on nuclear renography diagnostic for renal parenchymal infection,[24, 61] and 40% of these patients are recognized to develop resultant permanent scarring.[24, 32] In children with acute pyelonephritis, most kidneys recover without scarring when antibiotic therapy has been promptly and appropriately administered.[64]

Of the scars demonstrated by DMSA renography, more than 90% will be detected by intravenous pyelography (IVP).[60] IVP examinations are also less expensive and provide better anatomic detail. Thus, IVP is often more useful when a duplex collecting system is suspected by ultrasonography. In comparison, DMSA renal scan images are unaffected by bowel gas, and the risk of allergic reaction to the radiotracer is negligible. Because 60% of the administered dose of DMSA is tightly bound to proximal tubular cells, with only a small amount slowly excreted in the urine, DMSA allows precise visualization of the renal parenchyma, without interference from retained tracer in the collecting system.[61] Neither IVP nor nuclear renography is capable of distinguishing an old renal scar from focal infection. Although significant variability in interpretation of DMSA renal scans is common, using the pinhole collimator may enhance detection of renal scars with standard planar imaging. The overall accuracy of this method (92%) was roughly equivalent to single photon emission computed tomography (SPECT) imaging (96%) in a histologically correlated experimental study of pyelonephritis in piglets.[66]

In contrast to DMSA, technetium[99m] glucoheptonate (GH) is cleared by glomerular filtration, causing most of the administered dose to be excreted in the urine, which allows moderately good visualization of the collecting systems on early images. Approximately 20% of the administered dose of GH is firmly bound to proximal tubular cells, which also provides visualization of the renal cortex on delayed images.[61] Although GH is often more readily available than DMSA, the image quality and discrimination of renal scarring is generally inferior.

The relative risk for progressive renal deterioration may best be stratified using a combination of radiographic imaging studies, including nuclear renography. A long-term review of more than 3,600 children with prior urinary infections revealed that any single imaging test (renal ultrasonography, either contrast or nuclear cystography and nuclear renography) missed approximately half of the cases that developed progressive renal scarring.[31] No child with normal results in all three studies had progressive scarring. VUR was observed at presentation in 20 of 29 kidneys (70%) in which progressive damage developed, but also in 660 kidneys without renal damage. Renal scarring and VUR were the most important risk factors in infant boys and girls, respectively. In older children, VUR and renal scarring had similar predictive values, with the significance of recurrent infection only slightly less. Requiring results of two of these three imaging tests to be abnormal identified a group with a 17-fold increased risk of progressive renal damage. The three most important associations with subsequent deterioration were renal scarring (relative risk 6.94), VUR (relative risk 4.66) and recurrent urinary infection (relative risk 2.61).[31]

PATHOGENESIS OF PYELONEPHRITIS

Uropathogenic strains of E. coli can first be established in the colon by binding to mucosal receptors expressed by the host, exploiting the same adherence mechanisms that grant virulence within the urinary tract. Bacterial proliferation and adherence then permit movement from the gut to allow colonization of the periurethral mucosa.[12, 67] Although periurethral colonization by uropathogenic bacteria is considered to be the incipient step leading to pyelonephritis, mere expression of virulence factors by periurethral E. coli is not enough to predict subsequent infection of the urinary tract.[68] Vaginal filling secondary to high voided velocities and turbulent urine flow is often demonstrated on VCUG in girls with a dysfunctional voiding pattern. Creation of such a vortex leads to bacterial contamination of voided urine samples, and may promote passage of bacteria into the bladder at the termination of voiding.

To multiply, bacteria that reach the urinary tract must continually overcome the tendency to be washed away by urine flow and bladder voiding. They generally bind poorly to human uroepithelial cells, but demonstrate enhanced binding to Tamm-Horsfall protein (THP). Mannose and sialic acid residues in the carbohydrate chain of THP act as receptors for type 1 and S fimbriae, respectively.[69, 70] Bacterial binding to these residues allows THP to effectively trap type-1 and S-fimbriated bacteria, which enhances their tendency to be cleared from the bladder.[70] Although binding of bacteria to the oligosaccharides in the urothelial slime layer acts primarily as a natural barrier against infection, it also represents an initial site of colonization offering a platform for access to the urothelium.[69] Bacterial proliferation is aided by rapid generation times (as short as 33 minutes for some strains of *E. coli*) and by an exponential growth pattern.[71] A mathematical model of bladder filling and emptying suggests that bacterial strains with doubling times of less than 50 minutes are capable of maintaining critical concentrations without requiring bacterial adherence.[72] A prolonged voiding interval, increased storage pressure, or significant residual urine volume tips the balance in favor of uninterrupted growth of bacteria, allowing even relatively nonpathogenic bacteria to cause significant urinary infection.[56]

Binding of *E. coli* in proximity to the ureteral orifice exposes the urothelium to the effects of bacterial endotoxin, and leads to decreased ureteral tone and inefficient ureteral peristalsis.[73-75] The resulting relative ureteral obstruction produces ureteral dilation, allowing bacteria to bypass the ureteral orifice and to colonize the ureter in the absence of extant VUR.[74,75] Experimental studies of upper urinary tract infection in the monkey model suggested that stasis of urine caused by depressed ureteral peristalsis allows retrograde ureteral flow and propagation of infection.[75] Variable expression of uroepithelial adherence by bacteria (phase variation) is also thought to promote ascending infection by permitting migration of nonadherent organisms, which later lead to adherent progeny.[76] In effect, this allows bacteria to climb the ureteral ladder one rung at a time, except that each release and grasp of the ladder is performed by successive generations.

Intrarenal reflux of bacteria into the collecting ducts occurs as the shape of the renal papilla becomes altered with higher renal pelvic pressures.[75] In the primate model, intrarenal reflux can occur at relatively low pressures (32 mm Hg), particularly in the compound papillae found in the polar regions.[77] Experimental pyelonephritis produced in primates by causing pyelotubular backflow with contrast medium containing bacterial inoculum leads to a distribution of renal scarring identical to that of the intrarenal reflux.[75,77] Intrarenal reflux has also been demonstrated to occur in children in areas corresponding to subsequent renal scarring.[78]

Induction of the Inflammatory Response

Receptors for P-fimbriated *E. coli* are present in the collecting ducts and proximal tubules.[79] Bacterial proliferation typically leads to binding within the proximal tubules, which allows these bacteria to undergo endocytosis and internalization within the proximal tubular cells.[80] Bacterial surface proteins called invasins provoke uroepithelial ingestion of bacteria by causing changes in the host cell cytoskeleton, which allow engulfment of adherent bacteria.[81] P-fimbriated *E. coli* can be demonstrated within the renal tubules on ultrastructural studies after intrarenal reflux.[82] Exposure to endotoxin on the outer membrane of gram-negative bacteria causes release of cytokines from monocytes, macrophages, and uroepithelial and endothelial cells,[83] and elicits a combination of complement activation and phagocytic attack.[39] Although this inflammatory response is capable of eliminating most bacteria, there is also great potential for renal damage caused by nonspecific actions of the unleashed bactericidal agents.

Endotoxin is a mixture of lipopolysaccharide (LPS), lipoprotein, and phospholipid. The outer membrane,

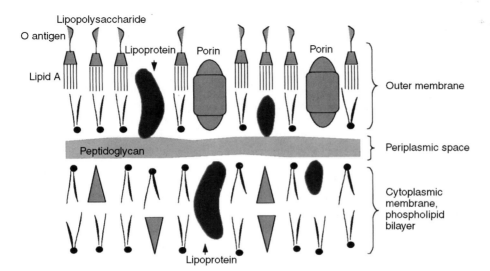

FIG. 26.2. Structure of gram-negative bacterial cell surface. Exposed O antigenic side chains of lipopolysaccharide are anchored to the outer membrane by lipid A. Phospholipids are confined mainly to the inner aspect of the outer membrane, and form a bilayer in the cytoplasmic membrane. The outer membrane is bound to the thin peptidoglycan by lipoproteins.[39]

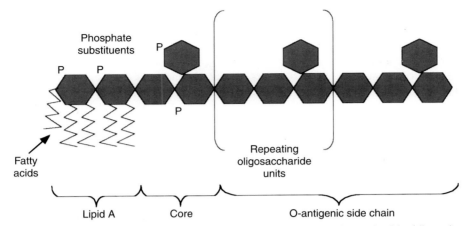

FIG. 26.3. Lipopolysaccharide structure. The lipid A portion of lipopolysaccharide (disaccharide with fatty acid and phosphate [P] substituents) is attached to an O antigenic side chain by a bridging oligosaccharide core region. Length of the O antigenic side chains is variable, and depends on the number of repeating oligosaccharide units incorporated into the chain.[39]

which primarily has phospholipids on its inner and LPS on its outer aspects, is covalently bound to the peptidoglycan by lipoproteins (Fig. 26.2). The lipid A portion of LPS is imbedded in the outer membrane, leaving its O antigenic polysaccharide portion exposed on the cell surface. LPS may be present in several forms because of variation in the length of the O-antigenic side chain[39] (Fig. 26.3). LPS released by lysing gram-negative bacteria is first bound by LPS-binding proteins (LBP), which then allows this LPS-LBP complex to interact with glycoprotein CD14 receptors on monocytes and macrophages, and with receptors on endothelial cells.[39, 84] The β_2-integrin CD11c/CD18 has also been identified as a second phagocyte receptor capable of activating neutrophils after binding to LPS.[85]

Exposure of uroepithelial cells to *E. coli* in tissue culture[86] in monkeys[87, 88] and in humans[89] leads to elevated cytokine levels (IL-6, IL-8). The *Lps* genotype expressed on chromosome 4 in the mouse is thought to control the uroepithelial cytokine response after *E. coli* infection, which ranges from a marked increase in urinary IL-6 (in *Lps^n/Lps^n* C3H/HeN mice) to no response (in *Lps^d/Lps^d* C3H/HeJ mice).[90] Because uroepithelial cells lack CD14, LPS alone provokes only a limited uroepithelial cytokine response.[86, 91] However, contact with P-fimbriated *E. coli* has been shown to upregulate expression of the intercellular adhesion molecule ICAM-1 on the uroepithelial surface, which is then capable of binding to β_2-integrins present on all neutrophils.[91–93] Elevated serum ICAM-1 levels have been clinically associated with renal scarring in children with vesicoureteral reflux.[94] Circulating CD14 can also bind to the LPS-LBP complex, facilitating activation of cells lacking membrane CD14.[39] Type 1-fimbriated bacteria

are capable of binding directly to β_2-integrins on neutrophils[39] and initiating the inflammatory response.[28]

LPS may also induce cytokine production by mimicking the action of ceramide, a second messenger in the sphingomyelin signal transduction pathway. Ceramide, known to enhance the synthesis and secretion of cytokines, has structural homology with a portion of lipid A.[95] Adherence by P-fimbriated *E. coli* augments IL-6 release from uroepithelial cells,[91] possibly by liberation of ceramide bound to uroepithelial glycolipid receptors for P fimbriae. LPS action may be blocked by bactericidal/permeability-increasing protein, which is a structural homologue of LBP produced by neutrophils.[39] *E. coli* O and K antigens can also directly stimulate neutrophils.[96] Variation in LPS responsiveness and subsequent cytokine production are suspected to play a role in the inconstant elaboration of renal inflammation and scarring exhibited in children with pyelonephritis.

Cytokines

Cytokines are protein mediators, produced at the site of injury and by immune cells throughout the body, that are capable of eliciting a significant tissue response at low concentrations.[39, 83] Although disturbance of the cytokine network is responsible for the inappropriate host defense associated with septic shock,[83] cellular release of cytokines also contributes to the local eradication of pathogens during localized bacterial infections. The proinflammatory cytokines IL-1, IL-6, IL-8, and TNF are considered the prime initiators of the immune response in pyelonephritis, but enhanced expression of anti-inflammatory cytokines (IL-10, TGF-β) is also found during acute pyelonephritis.[39, 97]

Both IL-1 and TNF knockout mice do not respond to LPS, and sustain proliferation of uropathogenic bacteria.[98-100] Knockouts of anti-inflammatory cytokines, IL-2 and IL-10, allow an inappropriate inflammatory response to commensal colonic bacteria.[101, 102] Transfection of the human IL-10 gene into mice decreases the local inflammatory response, and reduces mortality associated with experimental lethal endotoxemia.[103] Increased expression of TGF-β is also important in initiation and termination of tissue repair.[104]

IL-6 is an endogenous pyrogen produced by macrophages, monocytes, fibroblasts, endothelial cells, and renal tubular urothelium.[83, 105] IL-6 stimulates T- and B-lymphocytes and activates immunoglobulin synthesis. Initiation of acute-phase protein synthesis (C-reactive protein, serum amyloid A, and mannose-binding protein) by IL-6 also promotes opsonization of bacterial pathogens.[39, 106] In a mouse model of ascending urinary infection, bacterial LPS induces uroepithelial cells to secrete IL-6 into urine and serum, with the level of local and systemic response directly related to the degree of infection produced.[90] Formalin-killed *E. coli* also trigger an IL-6 response of shorter duration than live bacteria. Clinically, urinary IL-6 levels are often elevated in patients with bacteriuria and decline with successful treatment of urinary infection.[107] In children, elevation of urinary IL-6 has been reported to be independent[107] or depend[108] on the severity of urinary infection, but serum IL-6 levels are only elevated during pyelonephritis.[107] Detectable levels of urinary IL-6 during acute pyelonephritis in children carries a significant risk for renal scarring when studied by DMSA renal scan acutely and 1 year later.[109]

Neutrophil recruitment to the urinary tract follows a chemotactic gradient of IL-8 created between the tubular lumen and the vascular endothelium.[83] Urinary IL-8, secreted by the urothelium after exposure to adhering *E. coli*,[86] acts as a neutrophil chemoattractant in a manner that can be inhibited by anti-IL-8 antibodies.[110] After migration into the tubular lumen, neutrophils in turn produce large amounts of IL-8 after stimulation with *E. coli*, which further perpetuates the influx of neutrophils.[91] In clinical studies of urinary infection, urinary IL-8 levels are elevated significantly in patients with pyuria,[110] whereas serum IL-8 levels are not.[91] In a series of women with pyelonephritis, high concentrations of urinary IL-8 during acute infection correlated with lower glomerular filtration rates at follow-up evaluation.[105]

High affinity binding between vascular cell adhesion molecules and β_2-integrins expressed on all circulating leukocytes, halts neutrophils and promotes their extravasation into the connective tissue surrounding the blood vessel.[111] β_2-integrins express one of three possible different surface receptors, each made of one α subunit (CD11a, CD11b, or CD11c) associated with the same β subunit (CD18). These surface receptors exist in an inactive state on circulating phagocytes, but can be switched rapidly to an active form by IL-8 or TNF.[111] Other IL-8-related chemokines include neutrophil-activating peptide-2, macrophage inflammatory protein-2, and cytokine-induced neutrophil chemoattractant (CINC-1, CINC-2).[112] Interaction with interferon-γ causes monocytes attracted to the site of infection to become activated macrophages, thereby enhancing bactericidal capacity. Release of circulating IL-6 by recruited phagocytes stimulates hepatic synthesis of mannose-binding protein. Binding of this acute-phase protein to the mannose molecules commonly found on bacterial surfaces alters its structural conformation, and causes activation of the complement cascade.[113]

Complement Activation

The two pathways of complement activation differ in their initial activation steps, but then continue with an identical terminal sequence called the membrane attack pathway.[114] The alternative pathway is triggered by direct interaction between bacterial surface components and complement component C3.[114] Because this pathway is active before an antibody response has been mounted against invading pathogens, it is generally more important in the pathogenesis of urinary infection. The classical pathway, in contrast, is triggered by antibody binding to an antigen, but can also be triggered by bacterial LPS in the absence of antibody.[113, 114]

Cleavage products of component C3 (C3a, C3b) are normally present at low levels in blood, forming inactive complexes on interaction with serum control proteins (protein H). When C3b binds to LPS on bacterial surfaces, interaction with other serum proteins (proteins B, D, and properdin) forms an enzymatically active C3bBb complex called C3 convertase, which is responsible for further cleavage of C3. This interaction leads to a dramatic increase in C3b production near the bacterial surface, which promotes coating of bacteria with C3b fragments (opsonization).[114] Because phagocytes have receptors for active and inactive forms of C3b on their surfaces, opsonization empowers them to bind and ingest bacteria.[115] Although C3b may also attach to renal tubular cells provoking phagocytes to attack them, host cells are usually covered with abundant sialic acid residues affording protection from C3b binding.[113]

C5 convertase, which cleaves C5 into C5a and C5b, is formed when the C3 convertase complex binds to another molecule of C3b. The membrane attack complex (MAC), formed on the bacterial surface from components C5b, C6, C7, C8, and C9, attaches to the O side chains of bacterial LPS. The MAC is capable of bacterial killing in the absence of phagocytes by forming pores extending through the cytoplasmic membrane. Susceptibility to MAC (serum sensitivity) may be related to

$$\text{NADPH} + O_2 \xrightarrow{\text{NADPH oxidase}} \underset{\text{superoxide}}{O_2^{\cdot-}} + \text{NADP}^+ + \text{H}^+$$

$$O_2^{\cdot-} + O_2^{\cdot-} + 2\text{H}^+ \xrightarrow{\text{superoxide dismutase}} \underset{\substack{\text{hydrogen} \\ \text{peroxide}}}{\text{H}_2\text{O}_2} + O_2$$

$$\text{H}_2\text{O}_2 + \text{Cl}^- \xrightarrow{\text{myeloperoxidase}} \text{H}_2\text{O} + \underset{\substack{\text{hypochlorous} \\ \text{acid}}}{\text{ClO}^-}$$

FIG. 26.4. Series of reactions occurring in the phagolysosome. Enzymatic production of toxic reactive oxygen species is known as the respiratory burst because of the marked increase in associated oxygen consumption.[118]

shorter O side chains, which places killing activity closer to the bacterial surface.[113]

After diffusing away from the site of complement activation, C3a and C5a bind to specific receptors on circulating neutrophils and monocytes, causing cellular activation and enhanced killing capacity.[114] Neutrophil adherence to the vascular endothelium is then followed by migration along the C5a chemotactic gradient into renal tubules by diapedesis.[116] C3a produces vasodilatation, which further encourages extravasation of phagocytes into renal tubules. Aggregation of phagocytes along this gradient extending from the renal tubules to

the vascular endothelium also causes capillary obstruction, and eventually leads to renal ischemia.[117]

Renal Tubular Damage

Bacteria are killed after they are engulfed by endocytosis into the phagosome of the activated phagocyte. Fusion with lysosomes produces phagolysosomes and releases toxic enzymes capable of killing most bacteria (Fig. 26.4).[118] Debris from degraded bacteria (including LPS) is released by exocytosis, further stimulating the inflammatory response. Lysosomes may also fuse with the phagocyte membrane, which then releases toxic enzymes on the surface of the phagocyte, and allows damage of phagocytes and adjoining renal tubular cells.[119] Resultant cellular destruction provides nutrients required for continued bacterial growth.

Hydrolytic enzymes (lysozyme, proteases) released from lysosomes act directly by destroying peptidoglycan and bacterial membrane phospholipids. Bactericidal- and permeability-increasing protein, also released from lysosomes,[120] enhances action of these enzymes. Other enzymes work in combination to form toxic intermediates. Myeloperoxidase (found in the lysosome) and NADPH oxidase (located in the phagosome membrane) together produce reactive forms of oxygen (superoxide radical, hydroxyl radical, hydrogen peroxide, and singlet oxygen) during the respiratory burst of phagocytosis. These ROS cause cell injury primarily by lipid peroxida-

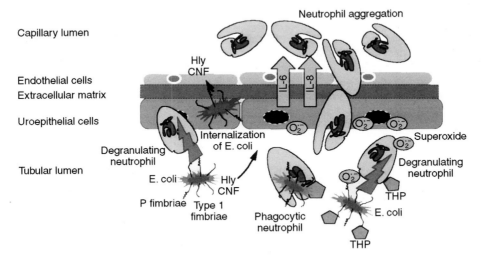

FIG. 26.5. Schematic representation of events that occur during the acute inflammatory response of pyelonephritis. Bacterial binding to uroepithelial cells leads to endocytosis and internalization of the bacteria within the proximal tubular cells. Bacterial lipopolysaccharide induces cytokine (IL-6 and IL-8) production by uroepithelial cells, which initiates the immune response and promotes chemotaxis of phagocytes. Neutrophils enter the tubular lumen and engage in bacterial killing by phagocytosis, with consequent release of toxic enzymes and reactive oxygen species. Damage to uroepithelial cells results from a combination of these toxic substances released by neutrophils, from exotoxins released by bacteria (hemolysin and cytotoxic necrotizing factor), and from ischemia resulting from neutrophil aggregation in the capillaries. This damage is compounded further by production of a burst of reactive oxygen species during reperfusion. THP, Tamm-Horsfall protein; Hly, hemolysin; CNF, cytotoxic necrotizing factor.

tion of cell membranes, but may also cause cleavage of DNA.[121] Cellular damage far distant from the initial site of free radical generation can occur once the autocatalytic chain reaction of lipid peroxidation begins.[122] Further reaction of ROS with chlorine atoms (catalyzed by myeloperoxidase) creates hypochlorous acid and other chlorine intermediates that are toxic to bacteria.[120] Although toxic nitric oxide (formed from L-arginine by nitric oxide synthase) may also be released into the renal tubules during this respiratory burst,[123] it has been suggested that this mechanism is inactive in human phagocytes.[124] Small, cationic peptides called defensins are also abundant in lysosomes, becoming bactericidal on release.[120] Action of these toxic products is nonspecific, damaging bacteria and renal tubular cells alike.

Release of ROS can also stimulate fibroblast proliferation,[125] thereby promoting fibrosis and renal scar formation. Bacterial strains with type 1 fimbriae causing renal scarring in rats stimulate a much greater production of superoxide from rat phagocytes, than nonfimbriated or P-fimbriated strains do.[27] Nonscarring strains of *E. coli* stimulate human phagocytes to release ROS primarily within the phagolysosome. In contrast, uropathogenic strains associated with renal scarring cause more active release of ROS from the surface of the phagocyte.[126] Greater exposure to ROS may account for enhanced renal tubular damage. Proximal tubular cells are generally more susceptible to injury from ROS in vitro when compared to cells of distal tubular origin (Fig. 26.5).[127]

Aerobic cells have developed antioxidant systems for protection from ROS damage. Nonenzymatic antioxidants include α-tocopherol, ascorbic acid and thiol-containing proteins. Lipophilic α-tocopherol is located primarily in membranes where it reacts with free radicals and protects against lipid peroxidation. Ascorbic

acid is water soluble and likely scavenges free radicals in solution. Thiol-containing compounds like cysteine and glutathione stop free radical reactions by donating electrons from their sulfhydryl groups.[128] The enzyme copper-zinc superoxide dismutase (CuZn SOD) is located in the proximal tubular cell cytoplasm[129] where it catalyzes conversion of superoxide to hydrogen peroxide. Two other cytoplasmic enzymes, glutathione peroxidase and catalase, further metabolize hydrogen peroxide safely to water.[128] Phagocytes, which lack CuZn SOD,[130] may be more readily damaged as ROS act unopposed on their surface. CuZn SOD can also be immunolocalized to uroepithelial surfaces during pyelonephritis,[129] presumably by release from damaged proximal tubular cells into the extracellular fluid and urine.

Further damage to renal tubular cells may result from ischemia and additional ROS released during reperfusion. The extent of ischemic tissue injury is directly related to the duration and degree of hypoxia; therefore, reperfusion injury is most significant during less severe episodes of ischemia (as occurs in pyelonephritis). Although reperfusion injury results to a great degree from neutrophil-mediated release of ROS,[131] ROS are also generated by a neutrophil-independent mechanism by renal tubular cells after warm ischemia in the kidney[132] and in cell culture.[133] During ischemia, an excess of hypoxanthine accumulates because high-energy phosphate compounds starting with adenosine triphosphate (ATP) are degraded sequentially, being used as the primary anoxic energy source. This buildup of substrate for xanthine oxidase primes the renal tubular cell for rapid formation of the superoxide anion during reperfusion (Fig. 26.6).[134] Because conversion of xanthine dehydrogenase to xanthine oxidase is favored during ischemia, a generous supply of enzyme is also ensured.[135] A sudden

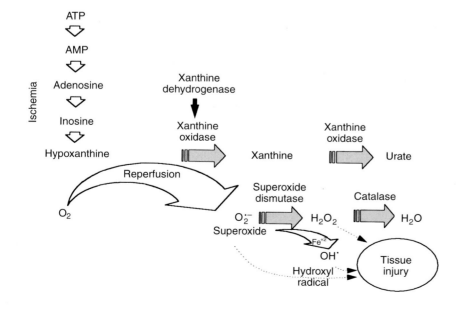

FIG. 26.6. Generation of reactive oxygen species in ischemic tissue during reperfusion. An excess of hypoxanthine substrate and xanthine oxidase enzyme accumulates during ischemia. Hypoxanthine is then rapidly converted to xanthine and urate when molecular oxygen becomes available, forming the superoxide anion as a transient and toxic intermediate. Next, superoxide is converted into hydrogen peroxide by superoxide dismutase present in uroepithelial cells. Tissue injury can result from brief exposure to superoxide, hydrogen peroxide, and the hydroxyl radical.[134]

excess of reducible molecular oxygen provided by reperfusion creates a burst of superoxide production. Accumulation of superoxide is further enhanced by reduction in CuZn SOD expression during ischemia.[135]

Modulation of the Inflammatory Response

Renal injury during pyelonephritis results primarily from the inflammatory response generated after bacteria reach the tubular lumen[88, 136, 137] and correlates directly with the number of neutrophils present.[138] Infiltration of phagocytes into the tubular lumen, and release of toxic products are the two main factors leading to renal injury.[75, 88] Although influx of phagocytes may be transiently prevented in the rat[139] and the monkey[140] by decomplementation with cobra venom factor, renal bacterial counts are significantly higher when compared to control animals. Such delayed initiation of the inflammatory response does not protect the kidney from scarring. Corticosteroid treatment reduces renal swelling during acute pyelonephritis, apparently by reducing plasma exudation rather than by limiting phagocyte infiltration.

Inflammatory renal damage can be diminished by prevention of ROS production during the reperfusion phase. Administration of CuZn SOD has been shown to prevent renal damage during acute pyelonephritis in the rat[27] and in the monkey.[141] CuZn SOD infused before ischemia and again at reperfusion protects against functional (reduction in glomerular filtration rate) and histologic (cellular necrosis and tubular obstruction) injury.[135] Administration of allopurinol with[137] or without[142] antibiotic therapy also granted protection from injury. Allopurinol inhibits the formation of active xanthine oxidase and the action of this enzyme. Scavengers of the hydroxyl radical (dimethylsulfoxide, reduced glutathione) and iron chelators (desferroxamine) also protect against renal ischemic injury.[135]

HISTORICAL PERSPECTIVE ON BACTERIAL VIRULENCE

Guyot[143] first reported bacteriologically mediated hemagglutination in 1908. In 1917, Lyon reported that isolates of *E. coli* from the urine of patients with cystitis were hemolytic more frequently than strains cultured from feces.[144] Visualization of nonflagellar filamentous appendages by electron microscopy, and their association with hemagglutination was first reported by Duguid et al. in 1955.[145] Bacteria covered with these fimbriae (from the Latin word for fringe) were noted to be good agglutinators of erythrocytes, and those without appendages did not agglutinate. They also showed that fimbrial expression *by E. coli* was variable, changing from a fimbriated to a nonfimbriated phase.[145] The genetic mechanism for this "on-off" switch was explained

for type 1 fimbriated strains by Abraham[146] 30 years after the presence of fimbriae was initially recognized.

Fimbriae were originally classified as mannose resistant (MR) or mannose sensitive (MS) depending on their ability to direct hemagglutination in the presence of mannosides, which are commonly found on the surfaces of bacteria (but not on human cells).[145, 147, 148] In 1977, Salit and Gotschlich demonstrated that type 1-fimbriated *E. coli* and purified type 1 fimbriae bind to monkey kidney cells in an MS fashion.[149] Increased adherence of uropathogenic *E. coli* strains to uroepithelial cells was first reported in 1976 by Svanborg-Edén et al.[19] Urinary infection in women was recognized to be preceded by introital colonization,[67] and periurethral and preputial colonization was recognized in children susceptible to urinary infections.[17] MR agglutination of human erythrocytes was later correlated with bacterial adhesion in patients with nonobstructive pyelonephritis.[150, 151] In 1980, the urothelial receptor for the MR bacterial fimbriae was identified as the P-blood group antigen.[152, 153] Many studies then confirmed that *E. coli* strains isolated from patients with pyelonephritis more commonly produce or have the genes for P fimbriae (approximately 80%) than do strains isolated from the feces of healthy controls.[2, 3, 25, 26, 154–157]

Lund et al.[158, 159] first demonstrated that the PapG protein in the P fimbriae system is the Galα(1-4)Gal adhesin that determines the specificity of binding. The operon responsible for the expression of this "*pyelonephritis-associated pilus*" (*pap*) was later cloned from the human urinary tract isolate J96.[160] The DNA sequence of the *pap* gene cluster was shown to encode 11 genes,[161, 162] with the *papG* gene product forming the adhesive PapG tip fibrillum located on the distal aspect of the P fimbriae (Fig. 26.7).[163] Three different PapG alleles (class I, II, and III) were recognized to bind to specific digalactose isoreceptor, permitting a diversity of adherence to different tissue types (tissue tropism).[164]

Bacterial Clones

E. coli can cause a variety of illnesses (diarrhea, dysentery, hemolytic uremic syndrome, septicemia, pneumonia, meningitis, and urinary infection), but each pathogenic strains is most commonly associated with only one disease. Before molecular techniques became available to categorize virulence factors, pathogenic bacteria were identified by their expression of three main bacterial surface antigens: the O polysaccharide antigen, the K (capsular) antigen, and the H (flagellar) antigen.[165] The O antigen, which defines the serogroup, is part of the LPS in the outer membrane that initiates the inflammatory response to bacteria. Although the O and K antigens aid resistance to phagocytosis, the H antigen is generally unrelated to urovirulence. Serotype refers to all three antigens. Uropathogenic bacterial

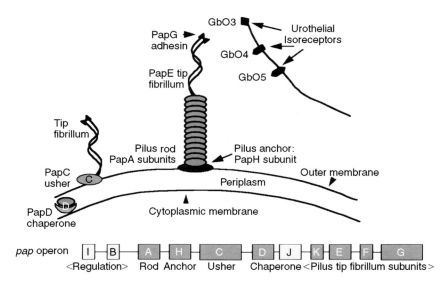

FIG. 26.7. P fimbriae construction regulated by the *pap* operon. The adhesive tip fibrillum of P fimbriae (consisting of PapE, PapF, and PapG subunits) is assembled and extruded from the outer membrane first. Addition of PapA subunits forms the thick, cylindrical pilus rod. PapD is a chaperone protein that prevents premature folding of the components of the fimbriae before they are assembled by the outer membrane usher, PapC. PapH halts construction and anchors the pilus rod to the outer membrane. Uroepithelial binding specificity is determined by the class of PapG tip adhesin expressed.[163]

clones possess similar characteristics, but cannot be predictably isolated as a homogeneous group by O:K:H serotyping (Table 26.1).

More recent classification schemes are based on expression of specific bacterial virulence factors. Although *E. coli* has more than 170 different O antigens, more than 80 different K antigens, and more than 50 different H antigens, only a small percentage of the 50,000 possible combinations cause urinary infection. This subset of uropathogenic *E. coli* express urovirulence factors, including adhesins, exotoxins, and aerobactin production, which provide a competitive advantage for growth, and empower uropathogenic strains to colonize or damage the urinary tract.[155] Expression of multiple urovirulence factors increases the likelihood that a particular strain will cause urinary infection, and influences the severity of the inflammatory response (Table 26.2). Most *E. coli* strains are avirulent because they lack these additional virulence factors.

Genes encoding bacterial adhesins and exotoxins occur in clusters on the chromosome, and in some cases, effective combinations of these clusters form contiguous virulence gene blocks capable of conveying enhanced invasiveness. Among *E. coli* strains causing urosepsis, specific O serotypes (O1, O2, O4, O6, O7, O18, O75)

usually express P fimbriae, and often express hemolysin and produce aerobactin.[155, 165] In a mouse model for ascending urinary infection, *E. coli* strains producing P fimbriae and hemolysin colonized the bladder and kidney, and killed nearly two thirds of the mice tested. Strains that produced only P fimbriae colonized the urinary tract but did not cause kidney damage or death. Strains lacking P fimbriae and hemolysin did not even colonize.[37] Adhesive fimbriae and hemolysin production were also found more frequently in virulent serogroups of *E. coli* isolated from girls with recurrent nonreflux pyelonephritis.[25]

The genes for synthesis and assembly of P fimbriae (*pap*) are recognized to be linked closely to genes for synthesis and excretion of hemolysin (*hly*).[166] The chromosomal location of genes responsible for aerobactin production are yet unknown. These linked operons for P fimbriae and hemolysin can be lost from uropathogenic strains by large spontaneous chromosomal deletions.[167]

Pathogenicity Islands

Certain groups of virulence genes located on the bacterial chromosome have been recognized to behave as distinct molecular and functional units. The term, patho-

TABLE 26.1. *Association of Escherichia coli serogroups with urinary infection*

Authors	Study group	Control group	Common serogroups (in study group)
Lomberg et al.[25]	Children without VUR with AP	Children with VUR with AP	O1, O2, O4, O6, O7, O8, O16, O18, O25, O75
Israele et al.[262]	Infants with AP and cystitis	Fecal isolates from infants	O1, O2, O4, O6, O18, O25, O75
Lindberg et al.[48]	Girls with AP or cystitis	Girls with ABU	O1, O2, O4, O6, O7, O16, O18, O75

AP, acute pyelonephritis; ABU, asymptomatic bacteriuria; VUR, vesicoureteral reflux.

TABLE 26.2. *Association of virulence factors among Escherichia coli clinical isolates*[155]

Virulence factor	Proportion of *Escherichia coli* strains (%)			
	Pyelonephritis	Cystitis	Bacteriuria	Fecal
O antigen	74	64	38	38
P-fimbriae	70	36	24	19
Type 1 fimbriae	60	71	58	60
K$_1$ capsular antigen	32	14	22	23
Serum resistance	61	63	25	52
Aerobactin	73	49	38	41
Hemolysin	49	40	20	12

Summarized from Johnson.[155]

genicity island (PAI), has been applied because they act as an island within the bacterial chromosome.[167, 168] These large, unstable regions of the chromosome can transfer between bacteria, conferring complex virulence properties to the recipient.[168] PAIs can also be lost at low frequency by spontaneous deletion.[9]

Two distinct PAIs (PAI-I, PAI-II) that vary in size and chromosomal location have been identified to occur in uropathogenic *E. coli.*[168] Both PAIs encode several virulence genes, and loss of these PAIs reduces hemolytic activity, serum resistance, MR hemagglutination, uroepithelial binding, and mouse lethality.[168, 169]

The locus of enterocyte effacement (LEE) is another recently recognized PAI, which encodes many genes required for *E. coli* to degrade the apical structure of enterocytes and cause diarrhea.[170] Although PAI-I and LEE encode completely different virulence genes, they share two remarkable similarities: insertion at precisely the same site in the *E. coli* genome, and identical DNA sequences at their 3′ ends.[168] The guanine-cytosine (GC) content of the LEE PAI (39%) differs significantly from the adjacent bacterial chromosome (51%).[168] Recognition that PAI-I and LEE insert at a specific site where prophages are also known to integrate has led to speculation that they actually represent segments of foreign DNA acquired during bacterial evolution.[9, 168, 170] The PAI-I region may once have been a mobile genetic element, which has been preserved by *E. coli* because it provides recipient bacteria with the competitive advantage of bacterial adherence and enhanced cytotoxicity.

UROVIRULENCE FACTORS THAT PROMOTE COLONIZATION

Bacterial Adhesins

Most uropathogenic *E. coli* strains produce fimbrial adhesins, with wild-type strains carrying approximately 500 fimbriae on their surface.[171] Fimbrial adhesins contain approximately 1,000 protein subunits, and typically consist of two distinct subassemblies: a thick pilus rod arranged in a helical cylinder, joined linearly to a thin, open helical tip fiber (tip fibrillum).[162, 171, 172] This config-

uration is reminiscent of a tower and a vertical antenna. The tip fibrillum generally mediates bacterial adherence by binding to specific carbohydrate residues of glycoproteins or glycolipids present on the host cell surface. Although the bacterial radius is small (approximately 250 nm), significant repulsive forces exist between the bacterial and host cell surfaces that normally limit bacterial adherence. These repulsive forces may be overcome when fimbriae (radius 2 to 10 nm) provide initial attachment of the bacteria to host cells.[74, 173, 174]

Other bacterial adhesins that cannot be visualized by electron microscopy are called afimbrial adhesins. Although the architecture of these afimbrial adhesins is not as well-known, they also bind selectively to uroepithelial receptor structures (portions of the Dr blood group antigen).[163] Outer membrane proteins (porins) that allow small molecules to enter the bacterial cell, may also act as afimbrial adhesins. This additional afimbrial binding reinforces initial, loose fimbrial attachment. Strongly adherent bacteria more effectively resist being washed away by urine flow, and may promote a more significant inflammatory response by enhanced delivery of toxins to uroepithelial cells.

P Fimbriae

P-fimbriated *E. coli* demonstrate specific binding to the globoseries of glycolipids (P blood group antigens) that are distributed in epithelial and nonepithelial tissues throughout the urinary tract in most humans.[26, 153, 175] These cell surface receptors are also shared by cynomolgus monkeys and the BALB/c mouse.[37, 176] P-fimbriated *E. coli* attach poorly to uroepithelial cells from the rare individuals with the p blood group phenotype who do not synthesize these receptors.[153, 177] Adherence to uroepithelial receptors promotes bacterial proliferation and facilitates ascending urinary infection. Although the proportion of P-fimbriated *E. coli* strains isolated from children with acute cystitis (19%) and ABU (14%) is similar to that of fecal isolates from control subjects (7%), most pyelonephritogenic isolates express P fimbriae (94 to 100%).[2, 3, 26] P fimbriae are found less often in pyelonephritogenic strains isolated from children with

VUR (36%).[25] The *pap* operon (*papA* through *papK*) encoding P fimbriae[161, 162] is detected in the bacterial chromosome in more than 90% of *E. coli* strains isolated from the urinary tract of children with acute pyelonephritis.[178–180] The *prs* (*P-related sequence*) operon is another P fimbrial gene cluster encoding fimbriae with somewhat different binding specificity, which is found more often in human cystitis isolates.[181]

P-fimbriated *E. coli* also adhere to human colonic epithelial cells,[175] which allows these uropathogenic strains to persist longer in the large intestine of children prone to urinary infection.[182] This binding (especially when combined with fecal retention) increases susceptibility to recurrent urinary infection by permitting the large intestine to serve as a repository for urovirulent bacteria between episodes. Children with acute pyelonephritis are known to carry P-fimbriated *E. coli* in their fecal flora more often than healthy controls do, both during and after treatment of infection.[182] P-fimbriated *E. coli* are also found more commonly in the fecal flora of children with ABU, with spontaneous clearance of ABU often linked to resolution of intestinal carriage of these strains.[182]

P fimbriae consists of repeating PapA protein subunits, which forms a thick, cylindrical rod that accounts for more than 99% of the fimbrial proteins.[163] The tip fibrillum is a composite of mainly repeating PapE protein subunits, with the PapG adhesin located at the distal end (Fig. 26.7).[162, 163] The assembly of fimbriae is a complex process that begins when PapA and four specialized tip proteins (PapK, PapE, PapF, and PapG) are secreted across the inner bacterial membrane into the periplasmic space. There, special chaperone proteins (PapD and PapJ) prevent these fimbrial proteins from folding into their final configurations. These chaperones also convey fimbrial proteins to the outer membrane usher PapC, which regulates fimbrial assembly.[163, 183] The tip fibrillum is assembled and extruded first, followed by sequential addition of PapA subunits, which pushes the tip structure outward from the bacterial surface.[158, 162, 184] The periplasmic protein PapH halts the extrusion process and anchors the fimbriae to the outer cell membrane.[163, 185] PapF (fibrillum initiator) and PapK (fibrillum terminator) are crucial to ensure that assembly of the adhesive tip fibrillum precedes that of the pilus rod, and that these subassemblies are firmly connected.[184] PapB and PapI are regulatory proteins, which participate in switching fimbrial production "on" and "off" (phase variation).[186, 187]

The PapG protein of the tip fibrillum is the adhesin that determines the specificity of P fimbrial binding to cell surface receptors.[158, 159] A *papG* mutant strain with deletion of the tip adhesin can express morphologically normal fimbriae but is incapable of adhesin.[163] Replacement of the *papG* gene in a pyelonephritogenic *E. coli* isolate with a *papG* allele containing a single base pair

deletion yields a truncated adhesin, and produces P fimbriae incapable of binding to digalactose receptors.[173] The mutant strain produced does not react with PapG-specific monoclonal antibody, and does not bind to tissue sections of cynomolgus monkey kidney.[173]

Three classes of PapG adhesins are known to direct high-affinity attachment to three corresponding host cell surface isoreceptors, which all contain the Galα(1-4)Gal disaccharide sequence.[152, 153, 188, 189] This digalactose receptor is linked by a β-glucose residue to a ceramide group that anchors the receptor in the lipid bilayer of the outer cell membrane.[155, 190] Reduction in bacterial adherence and urinary infection severity is observed when globotetraose, a digalactose receptor analog, is mixed with P-fimbriated *E. coli* before inoculation into mice bladders.[191]

The three classes of PapG isoreceptors differ in their composition of sugar residues distal to the Galα(1-4)Gal disaccharide. Class-I PapG adheres to globotriaosylceramide (GbO3 isoreceptor), class-II PapG to globotetraosylceramide (GbO4 isoreceptor), and class-III PapG (PrsG) to globopentaosylceramide (GbO5 isoreceptor, which is also called the Forssman antigen).[188, 189] Addition of these sugar residues causes shifts in the isoreceptors preferred conformation, thereby altering accessibility of the digalactose receptor.[163, 188] When isoreceptor folding is controlled by immobilizing these glycolipids in microtiter wells, class I and II PapG adhesins bind efficiently to all three globoseries isoreceptors. In contrast, class III PrsG adhesins, which require an additional sugar (GalNAcβ) distal to the Galα(1-4)Gal disaccharide for effective adherence, maintain their binding specificity.[188, 189] This combination of GalNAcβ and Galα(1-4)Gal moieties is found in globo-A glycolipids (blood group A determinant), and in the Forssman antigen.

E. coli may express multiple, antigenically distinct P fimbriae,[192] with various P fimbrial types exhibiting different tissue binding specificities.[193] Most pyelonephritogenic isolates in humans express class II PapG adhesins recognizing GbO4, which is the major digalactose isoreceptor in the human kidney.[181] Renal binding occurs predominantly in the luminal cells of the collecting ducts and renal tubules.[194] Although diminished binding affinity is detected in the uroepithelium of the bladder, stronger binding is detected in the muscular layers and endothelium of the bladder wall.[193–195] The PapE and PapF tip fibrillum components of P fimbriae also promote adherence to fibronectin within the bladder wall.[196, 197]

Pyelonephritogenic isolates in dogs generally express class III PrsG adhesins recognizing the Forssman antigen, which is the dominant canine isoreceptor.[164, 181] These class III PrsG adhesins exhibit enhanced binding to Bowman's capsule in humans.[194, 198] The renal receptor responsible for this attachment is thought to be the P blood group-related stage-specific embryonic antigen 4 (SSEA-4), which contains GalNAcβ and Galα(1-4)Gal within its long internal structure.[199] Isolation of class III PrsG adhesins in pyelonephritogenic *E. coli* strains and identification of the Forssman antigen are uncommon in humans[200] and in cynomolgus monkeys.[201] However, individuals who are blood group A$_1$ secretors express globo-A glycolipid determinants (isoreceptors for PrsG adhesins), and comprise the dominant population from which *E. coli* strains expressing PrsG adhesins can be isolated.[164, 181, 201] Strong binding affinity is detected in the uroepithelial and muscular layers of the bladder and ureter in these individuals.[195]

P fimbriae from clinical isolates may also display combined tissue binding specificities of PapG and PrsG adhesins.[193, 195] Purified P fimbriae from the *E. coli* KS71A strain exhibited binding to Bowman's capsule and to the vascular endothelium in the renal interstitium and glomeruli, as well as to the luminal aspects of the proximal and distal tubules and collecting ducts in the human kidney.[193]

Although P-fimbriated *E. coli* play an important role in establishing ascending pyelonephritis, their presence does not necessarily produce renal parenchymal inflammation.[24, 37, 202] Because human neutrophils lack a receptor for the PapG adhesin,[203] P-fimbriated *E. coli* do not bind to and are not killed by neutrophils unless they are opsonized. The strong negative electrostatic charge of the PapG protein also augments the repulsive force present between the bacterial surface and the neutrophil, both of which also carry a net negative charge.[163, 204] A consequent delay in initiation of the inflammatory response allowing bacterial proliferation may account for the high proportion of P-fimbriated *E. coli* strains in urosepsis isolates.[205] However, most P-fimbriated strains also express type 1 fimbriae, which are capable of inciting the inflammatory response by binding to neutrophils directly. Neutrophils are also recruited locally by IL-6 release, which results from P fimbrial binding to uroepithelial cells.[91]

Tropism

Bacterial cultures generally contain different subsets of organisms capable of interacting with different segments of the urinary tract. Because fimbrial binding is specific, the availability of suitable receptors often determines what body site is infected by which particular bacterial strains (Table 26.3). Tropism refers to the orderly restriction of commensal and pathogenic bacteria to certain hosts, tissues, and cell types.[5] Human erythrocytes, kidney, and bladder are rich in GbO3 and GbO4, but generally lack GbO5. In contrast, sheep erythrocytes and canine kidneys are rich in GbO5 and express only minute amounts of GbO3 and GbO4.[164] Although 50% of canine fecal and urinary *E. coli* isolates carry a class

III PrsG adhesin (corresponding to the dominant isoreceptor in dog kidneys), expression of the class II PapG adhesin is not found in canine fecal flora or as a cause of urinary infection in dogs.[163] In humans, class II PapG or class III PrsG adhesins can be found among fecal and urinary isolates, but most pyelonephritogenic *E. coli* strains express P fimbriae with the class II PapG adhesin (corresponding to the dominant isoreceptor in the human kidney). P fimbriated *E. coli* with the class III PrsG adhesin are more often selected in acute cystitis, especially in blood group A$_1$ secretors (corresponding to expression of the globo-A glycolipid isoreceptor in the bladder).[163, 164, 181, 201] Replacement of the class II PapG tip adhesin in a pyelonephritogenic *E. coli* strain with a class III PrsG adhesin by allelic exchange transformed the resulting mutant's binding specificity to favor the Forssman antigen, and abrogated its ability to cause prolonged bacteriuria and ascending pyelonephritis.[201]

Type 1 Fimbriae

The genes encoding type 1 fimbriae, which are common among the *Enterobacteriaceae,* are present in most uropathogenic *E. coli.*[147, 195, 206] Type 1 fimbriae are called MS because D-mannose blocks hemagglutination and attachment to target cells.[160] Proposed receptors for type 1 fimbriae include a variety of mannose-containing surface structures.[148, 195] Competitive binding by THP, which contains abundant mannose residues, inhibits attachment of type 1-fimbriated *E. coli* to uroepithelial cells.[69, 207] Binding to THP in this manner tends to enhance clearance of type 1-fimbriated strains and limits their virulence. Both MS and MR fimbrial adhesins adhere to constituents of cranberry and blueberry juices, which may further enhance clearance of urovirulent bacteria from bowel and bladder when compounds in these juices are ingested.[208] Type 1 fimbriae are expressed in approximately half of pyelonephritogenic *E. coli* strains (equivalent to percentage found in fecal isolates from normal controls) and in most cystitis isolates.[2, 26, 151, 209, 210] Type 1 fimbriae are also more likely to be expressed by strains isolated from patients with indwelling urinary catheters for a prolonged interval.[211]

The *fim* operon encoding type 1 fimbriae is organizationally similar to the *pap* operon encoding P fimbriae.[171, 212] Type 1 fimbriae also consist of a cylindrical pilus rod and a tip fibrillum.[162, 172] The type 1 tip fibrillum is relatively shorter than its P fimbrial counterpart and is composed of only three minor pilins (FimF, FimG, and FimH).[172] The FimH tip adhesin is analogous to PapG in that it mediates MS receptor binding.[195] Unlike P fimbriae, the type 1 tip fibrillum itself appears to form the helical cylinder forming the pilus rod, with the FimH adhesin intercalated along the pilus rod at potential breakpoints.[172] Mechanical shear forces on type 1-fimbriated bacteria may cause these fimbriae to unravel[213] or to break and expose new FimH adhesins.[214] FimF (initiator) and FimG (terminator) are important components in orderly fimbrial synthesis.[215] Phase variation for type 1 fimbriae is controlled by FimB and FimE.[146, 216, 217]

Expression of fimbriae by *E. coli* depends on growing conditions.[171, 211, 218] Bacteria grown in broth medium demonstrate enhanced type 1 fimbriae expression and suppressed P fimbriae expression. Growth on agar has the opposite effect.[219] Bladder colonization is more likely obtained with broth-grown (type 1-enhanced) cultures than with agar-grown (type 1-suppressed) cultures.[219] After intraurethral inoculation of a type 1-fimbriated *E. coli* strain, bacteria colonizing the mouse bladder continued to express type 1 fimbriae in contrast to bacteria isolated from the kidneys.[220]

Type 1 fimbriae display a binding pattern different from P fimbriae that is less conducive to establishing ascending urinary infection. Bladder uroepithelial binding does not occur, and only weak binding occurs in the renal tubules.[221] Nonetheless, inoculation of type 1-fimbriated *E. coli* into the murine bladder results in effective colonization that can be blocked by mannose or by anti-type 1 fimbrial antibody.[151, 219] The muscular layer of the bladder and the ureteral lumen provide strong binding sites for type 1 fimbriae.[4, 38, 171, 221] Bladder adherence may be further facilitated by binding of type 1 fimbriae to fibronectin exposed during exfoliation of uroepithelial cells.[201, 222, 223] Although distal tubular uroepithelial cells secrete THP, enhance type 1 fimbrial binding to the distal nephron is not observed.[195, 224] Identification of an immunologically related subtype of type 1 fimbriae (type 1C) that demonstrates enhanced binding to the renal tubules and collecting ducts,[221] suggests that binding to the distal nephron by type 1C fimbriae may contribute to the critical initial steps in establishment of renal inflammation and invasion.[195] Although P and type 1C fimbriae are not expressed on the same bacterial cells, there is a rapid phase switch between these two fimbrial types.[225]

Binding of type 1-fimbriated *E. coli* to β_2-integrins on the neutrophil surface leads to bacterial engulfment and elicits the inflammatory response.[85, 226–230] Nonfimbriated strains do not provoke this effect.[231] Although the respiratory burst is triggered by this binding, type 1-fimbriated *E. coli* appear to be somewhat resistant to phagocytic killing, possibly because protection is granted by the fimbriae themselves, which serve to separate the bacterial and phagocytic surfaces.[229, 232] It is likely that neutrophil stimulation by the FimH adhesin is responsible for initiation of the inflammatory response. When exposed to purified FimH coated on inert beads, neutrophils bind avidly to and internalize the beads, with coincident release of ROS.[232] FimH stimulation of B lymphocytes leads to immunoglobulin secretion.[233]

Phase Variation

Uropathogenic *E. coli* usually produce multiple adhesins, either combinations of different fimbriae or combinations of different serotypes of the same fimbriae.[180, 234] Expression of fimbriae, which requires a relatively high level of metabolic activity, is not continuous. Rather, regulated expression of various adhesins occurs in response to external signals, including temperature, and concentration of glucose and certain amino acids.[76, 218, 235] Bacteria that regularly express adhesins produce progeny at low frequency that lack adhesins. These, in turn, give rise at low frequency to bacteria expressing adhesins.[216, 218, 236, 237] Phase variation enables bacteria to react to different growth conditions, aiding evasion of host resistance.

Fimbriated phase variants have a selective advantage in liquid media when compared to agar plates. When P or type 1-fimbriated *E. coli* are grown at room temperature, fimbriae are not expressed.[237] After transfer to static broth medium at 37°C, hourly monitoring of cultures showed a progression of fimbrial expression. Only

TABLE 26.3. *Fimbrial and afimbrial adhesins associated with uropathogenic Escherichia coli*

Structure	Level of infection	Adhesin	Receptor
Fimbriae			
P fimbriae	Pyelonephritis/cystitis	PapG (adhesin class)	Galα(1-4)Gal moiety (isoreceptor)
		PapG-I	GbO3[a] (human bladder)
		PapG-II	GbO4[b] (human kidney)
		PapG-III	GbO5[c] (canine kidney)
Prs fimbriae	Cystitis	PrsG	GalNAcβ + Galα(1-4)Gal moiety
Type 1 fimbriae	Cystitis	FimH	Mannose oligosaccharides
S fimbriae	Cystitis	SfaS	NeuAc(α2-3)Gal(β1-4)GlcNAc
Afimbrial Adhesins			
Afa-1	Pyelonephritis	Afa1E	Decay-accelerating factor
Dr/Afa-111	Cystitis	DraA	Dr blood group marker

[a]GbO3, globotriaosylceramide.
[b]GbO4, globotetraosylceramide.
[c]GbO5, globopentaosylceramide.

24% of cells were nonfimbriated at 4 hours. Type 1C-fimbriated cells were detected first at 1 hour and were reported in 68% of cultures by 4 hours. P-fimbriated cells followed, becoming detectable at 2 hours, and involving 21% of cultures by 8 hours. Type 1-fimbriated cells were not found until 9 hours, but became apparent in 21% of cultures by 20 hours.[218]

The promoter region of the *pap* operon contains two sites that determine whether binding of critical activators occur, and thus whether the region is in the "on" or "off" configuration. Deoxyadenosine methylase (Dam)-mediated methylation adds methyl groups to the A residue in GATC sequences, and thereby protect these sites from cleavage by restriction enzymes.[238, 239] Although all GATC sites in *E. coli* are generally methylated, there is a brief period after DNA replication when one or both of the regulatory sites (GATC[1028] and GATC[1130]) may not yet be methylated.[186] Specific methylation patterns at these two sites lead to Pap fimbrial phase variation. The GATC[1028] site is nonmethylated in the "on" configuration, but methylated when "off," whereas the converse is true for the GATC[1130] site.[186] Methylation of the GATC[1028] site inhibits binding of the *leucine response protein* (Lrp) and PapI regulatory proteins near that site (both of which are required for pap transcription) and blocks formation of the "on" complex.[187] Methylation of the GATC[1130] site, required in the "on" complex, inhibits binding of Lrp to sites overlapping the promoter region and prevents repression of *pap* transcription.[187]

Although expression of type 1 fimbriae is also phase variable and controlled by Lrp, the mechanism is different and involves inversion of a 314 bp DNA fragment (*fim* switch), which contains the *fim* promoter.[146] The *fimB* and *fimE* genes, which are located adjacent to the *fim* switch, control phase variation.[146, 216, 217] The *fim* switch directs transcription of *fimA* (the major fimbrial subunit gene) when in the "on" orientation, but transcription is "off" when the *fim* switch is inverted.[240] Inversion occurs spontaneously at a rate of approximately 10^{-3} to 10^{-4}/cell per generation.[146, 216]

S Fimbriae

S-fimbriated *E. coli* bind to globoseries glycolipids in the urinary tract by recognizing sialic acid residues contained in the NeuAc(α2-3)Gal(β1-4)GlcNAc sequence as receptors.[70] S-fimbriated *E. coli* strains can be cultured from children with urinary infection, but this fimbrial type is more commonly associated with neonatal sepsis and meningitis.[79, 241] Although P and S-fimbriated strains of *E. coli* share the ability to bind to similar uroepithelial tissues, S-fimbriated strains are rarely found in pyelonephritis isolates.[193, 221] This likely occurs because uroepithelial attachment is effectively prevented by soluble THP, which contains abundant

sialic acid residues.[70] P fimbriae do not bind to THP.[193, 221]

Organization of the *sfa* operon (encoding S fimbriae) is similar to the *pap* and *fim* operons.[171, 212, 242] S fimbriae contain a thick pilus rod, connected to a helical tip fibrillum with the SfaS adhesin located at its distal aspect.[242] Two S fimbrial operons, which determine different major pilin structures, have been cloned from urinary infection (*sfa* I) and meningitis (*sfa* II) isolates.[243] The S-fimbrial family also consists of F1C fimbriae (encoded by the *foc* operon)[244] and S/F1C-related fimbriae (encoded by the *sfr* operon).[245] F1C fimbriae are significantly more common among children with pyelonephritis than among controls;[246] however, these strains often also contain P or P-related fimbriae.[234, 247, 248]

Purified S fimbriae exhibit binding to bladder uroepithelium,[221] the renal tubules, glomerulus, and Bowman's capsule.[249] Binding specificities for F1C fimbriae and S fimbriae are similar.[4, 250] S fimbriae also bind to laminin in the extracellular matrix of the bladder.[251] Binding by S-fimbriated bacteria to the renal tubules does not enhance expression of ICAM-1 and elicits only a limited inflammatory response.[92]

Dr Adhesins

Members of the Dr family of adhesins include the Dr hemagglutinin and afimbrial adhesins AFA-I and AFA-III.[252] The decay-accelerating factor (DAF), which is a regulatory protein that protects host tissues from cytotoxic activity during complement activation, acts as a common receptor for this family of adhesins.[252] Various Dr adhesins bind to similar but functionally distinct sites on this receptor.[252, 253] Type IV collagen also acts as a receptor for the Dr hemagglutinin.[196]

The Dr hemagglutinin forms a fibrillar coil structure,[254, 255] but the other Dr adhesin family members exhibit no detectable fimbrial structures.[256] Although the prevalence of Dr adhesins is similar in pyelonephritogenic and fecal isolates, these adhesins are more common among cystitis isolates then fecal strains.[257] *E. coli* strains bearing the Dr hemagglutinin bind to renal tubules and glomerular basement membranes, at sites distinct from those recognized by P fimbriae.[4, 79] Dr hemagglutinin binding to neutrophils does not provoke a significant inflammatory response or bacterial killing.[258]

Protective Capsule

The presence of a protective capsule minimizes complement activation and prevents ingestion of bacteria by phagocytes. Sialic acid residues incorporated into the capsule help to present the invading organism as "self," thereby limiting the inflammatory response initiated by the host. Capsular polysaccharides also coat the bacterial surface, interfering with detection of the O antigens.[259, 260] Although five of the K antigens (K_1, K_2, K_3, K_{12}, K_{13}) account for 70% of isolates from young girls with pyelonephritis,[261] encapsulated strains are no more common among urinary infection isolates than among fecal isolates from normal controls.[262] The amount of capsular polysaccharide (particularly K_1) correlates with bladder and kidney colonization, renal inflammation, and lethality in rats[263] and humans.[261]

By preventing C3 convertase from forming on their surfaces during complement activation, encapsulated bacteria also limit opsonization and phagocytosis. Because less C5b is also produced, the MAC is less likely to form on the bacterial surface. The K_1, K_5, and K_{54} capsules confer serum resistance.[259, 264]

Serum Resistance

Bacterial killing by fresh human serum depends on activation of complement, either through the classic or alternative pathways. Bacteria that are not killed by the MAC are called serum resistant. Longer LPS O antigenic side chains prevent effective MAC formation, possibly because the MAC forms too far from the outer membrane to exert a bactericidal effect. Serum-resistant E. coli strains are found more commonly in bacteremia, or pyelonephritis isolates than can be accounted for by their abundance in stool.[155, 265] Serum resistance is also more common in children with nonreflux pyelonephritis than in children with pyelonephritis associated with VUR.[25] Serum resistance in pyelonephritis isolates does not correlate with renal scarring[157] or with other bacterial virulence factors.[265]

Aerobactin

Aerobactin is a small molecule formed by the condensation of two lysine molecules and one citrate, which extracts iron from host iron-binding proteins and allows enhanced bacterial growth kinetics.[266] Aerobactin production is more commonly found in E. coli pyelonephritis isolates (70%) than in cystitis isolates (40%) or fecal controls (34%). Six urovirulent E. coli serotypes frequently possess aerobactin (O1:K1:H7; O2:K1:H4; O4:K12:H5; O7:K1:H-; O16:K1:H-; and O75:K5:H-).[267] Bacteria can also acquire iron by producing siderophores, which are excreted into urine and then taken up by special siderophore receptors on the bacterial surface. The internalized iron-siderophore complex is cleaved to release the iron molecule inside the bacteria. Other surface proteins (transferrin or lactoferrin) remove iron directly from host-binding proteins. Binding of P-fimbriated E. coli strains to uroepithelium may activate a regulatory gene, which controls iron acquisition.[268]

UROVIRULENCE FACTORS THAT DAMAGE THE HOST

Hemolysin

E. coli hemolysin is a calcium-bound, acetylated protein that is secreted extracellularly.[269] The cytolytic activity of hemolysin, primarily directed at phagocytes and renal tubular cells, results from the formation of membrane lesions (less than 2 nm in diameter) followed by rapid intracellular influx of fluid and cell rupture.[7, 270–272] Hemolysin also stimulates IL-1 release and impairs neutrophil chemotaxis and phagocytosis. Hemolysin production is found in approximately 50% of pyelonephritogenic strains, compared to only 12% of fecal strains.[1, 155] The genes for hemolysin production (hlyCABD) are linked to pap and prs operons in PAI-I.[166, 167, 273] Hemolytic strains of E. coli demonstrate enhanced hemolysin expression under low-osmolarity conditions, which may account for some of the variability observed in clinical populations with pyelonephritis.[274]

Destruction of the renal tubular epithelium by hemolysin promotes bacterial invasion of interstitial tissues.[7, 272] Mice challenged with a nonhemolytic, P-fimbriated E. coli strain developed renal colonization with mild focal inflammation, and all survived. After this strain was transformed with a hemolysin recombinant plasmid, 63% of mice challenged died, and renal segmental inflammation and abscess formation was detected in all survivors.[275] Immunization with hemolysin before challenge with this virulent strain nearly eliminated the renal inflammation, but did not change renal colonization.[275]

CNF1

Cytotoxic necrotizing factor1 (CNF1) is a protein toxin associated with E. coli strains causing urinary infection.[6] The CNF1 was found in 37% of urinary infection isolates, compared to 3% of normal fecal isolates.[6] Genes encoding CNF1 and hemolysin are linked within a PAI also containing the prs operon.[8]

OTHER UROPATHOGENIC BACTERIA

Enterococcus Faecalis

Most urinary infections with Enterococcus faecalis are catheter related and tend to resolve promptly when catheters are removed. Adherence to porcine renal tubular cell lines is enhanced in strains expressing a surface protein called aggregation substance.[276] This protein, which causes clumping of donor and recipient cells, is important in conjugative transfer of plasmids encoding for bacterial toxins.[277] Enterococci may also increase the virulence of the Enterobacteriaceae in mixed urinary infection.[278]

Pseudomonas Aeruginosa

Pseudomonas aeruginosa is normally found in soil and water, but its occurrence in human disease is closely related to the selective pressure of antibiotics used in anatomically or immunocompromised patients. *P. aeruginosa* grows well in urine and is a common cause of catheter-associated urinary infection, which may persist despite removal of drainage catheters. Production of an alginate polysaccharide bacterial coating, which forms a viscous gel around the bacteria able to resist phagocytosis, is regulated by a genetic switch (*algS* or *algT*) that allows bacteria to manifest mucoid or nonmucoid form.[279] LPS structure is also different in these two cell surface presentations. Mucoid strains exhibit a neutral charge and short O antigen chains (A form), whereas nonmucoid strains exhibit a negative charge and longer O antigen chains (B form). Aminoglycoside efficacy, which depends on the negative charge of the LPS layer, is likely inhibited by a shift from the negatively charged B form of LPS to the neutral A form. This phase variation is modulated by osmolarity and nitrogen concentration.[280]

Most *Pseudomonas* species are motile and possess one or more polar flagella. *P. aeruginosa* produce type 4 fimbriae (similar to *Neisseria gonorrhoeae*) and two forms of afimbrial adhesins (binding to mucin and epithelial cells, or to mucin alone). *P. aeruginosa* also produce neuraminidase, which removes sialic acid residues from uroepithelial cell and promotes type 4 fimbrial binding.[281] Other virulence factors include proteases, hemolysin, phospholipase C, and exotoxins capable of causing tissue damage and inhibiting phagocyte activity (ExoS and ExoA).[282] Although pyoverdin is an iron siderophore essential for growth, no role in virulence has been specifically identified. However, pyochelin and pyocyanin are important in production of ROS.[283]

Klebsiella Pneumonia

Klebsiella pneumoniae are nonmotile, encapsulated gram-negative rods. Individual strains can be characterized by more than 70 different capsular (K antigen) serotypes and by type 1 and type 3 fimbriae. Most *K. pneumoniae* strains have a well-defined capsule composed of two distinct layers[284] and express type 3 fimbriae on their surfaces.[285] Type 3 fimbriae mediate attachment to the renal tubular basement membranes, Bowman's capsule, and interstitial connective tissue,[286] and adhere strongly to urinary catheters.[287] Other virulence factors include iron-scavenging systems and urease production, which catalyzes the hydrolysis of urea to yield ammonia and carbamate. Bacterial adherence to bladder uroepithelium is enhanced by ammonia produced through urease activity.[288]

Proteus Mirabilis

Proteus mirabilis strains bind only to squamous epithelial cells and rarely account for symptomatic urinary infection in noncompromised hosts. Although *P. mirabilis* can colonize the vaginal and periurethral areas as efficiently as uropathogenic *E. coli* strains, they tend to be eliminated from the bladder more easily during normal voiding.[289, 290] Pathogenicity is also linked to the production of urease, which results in an increased urinary pH and precipitation of struvite crystals. Although *P. mirabilis* accounts for only a small proportion of urinary infections, it has a special predilection to cause ascending pyelonephritis. Four distinct fimbriae have been identified on *P. mirabilis*: MR/P, PMF (*P. mirabilis* fimbriae), ATF (ambient-temperature fimbriae), and NAF (nonagglutinating fimbriae). Virulence factors also include capsule polymers that enhance formation of stones, cytotoxic hemolysin (HpmA), and IgA-degrading metalloproteinase.

P. mirabilis may exist in two morphologically distinct forms[291, 292] depending on whether it is grown in liquid (swimmer cell) or solid (swarmer cell) culture medium. Swimmer cells are short fimbriated rods with fewer than 10 flagella, whereas swarmer cells are greatly elongated, nonseptated multinuclear rods expressing thousands of flagella. Urinary infection is suspected to be initiated by attachment to the bladder uroepithelium by PMF, with rapid transport to the kidney by highly flagellated swarmer cells, followed by specific binding to the renal epithelium.[292] Renal tissues are damaged by ammonia and hemolysin, and the bacteria are internalized by renal tubular uroepithelial cells, which further enhances the inflammatory response to infection.

HOST RESISTANCE

The frequency of urinary infection in children varies with age and gender. Some children never have a urinary infection, whereas others suffer from recurrent episodes. The clinical presentation of urinary infection is further influenced by access to medical care, including timely treatment of urinary infection and antenatal evaluation and management. A vast range of outcomes after urinary infection is also apparent, with some children developing significant renal scarring and progressive renal insufficiency, whereas others seem to have no sequelae. Host risk factors play a relatively limited role in determining the frequency of recurrence and the degree of inflammatory response found in children with urinary infection.

Periurethral Colonization

The large intestine, vaginal introitus, and periurethral areas serve as reservoirs for uropathogenic bacteria.[17]

Although periurethral colonization is relatively common in healthy infants to both gender, it decreases rapidly during the first year of life and becomes unusual after 5 years of age.[293] Persistence of bacterial strains within the kidney and bladder requires enhanced adherence to uroepithelial cells.[209] E. coli strains from girls and women with acute pyelonephritis or acute cystitis adhere to uroepithelial cells better than strains from subjects with ABU or from fecal flora in normal controls.[19, 294] Children with acute pyelonephritis, cystitis, and ABU carry P-fimbriated E. coli in their fecal flora more often than healthy controls,[182] which increases their susceptibility to recurrent urinary infection.

Vaginal pH

The vaginal environment in prepubertal girls with little vaginal estrogen and low epithelial glycogen content is usually neutral (mean pH 7.0), becoming more acidic with menarche (mean pH 4.9).[295] Vaginal estrogen increases the glycogen content of the vaginal epithelial cells and lowers the pH. This environment favors the growth of acid-tolerant lactobacilli, which interfere with the growth of uropathogenic bacteria and further generate lactic acid (maintaining a low vaginal pH).[295] Vaginal adherence by uropathogenic E. coli strains is significantly greater than vaginal adherence by strains that do not cause bacteriuria.[296] Premenarchal girls that develop urinary infection typically have heavy periurethral colonization preceding episodes of bacteriuria, in contrast to girls without urinary infection.[293]

Secreted Urinary Inhibitors

Bladder urothelium is capable of killing adherent bacteria[297] likely through binding by afimbrial adhesins, which stimulate cytokine production and promote a local inflammatory response.[298] Disruption of the bladder mucous layer increases susceptibility to infection and delays clearance of bacteria from the bladder.[299] A low molecular weight, hydrophilic antibacterial polyamine (capable of killing fecal strains of E. coli), has been isolated from urine. Variable concentrations of this component in the urinary tracts of different hosts is suspected to contribute to clinically observed differences in susceptibility to urinary infection.[91] Extracellular-superoxide dismutase (EC-SOD), the major SOD isozyme in serum and urine, offers protective activity similar to intracytoplasmic CuZn SOD from ROS released during urinary infection.[300, 301]

Although urine supports the growth of E. coli, variability in pH, osmolarity, urea, and organic acids may limit the importance of urovirulence factors. Bacterial growth is inhibited at high osmolarity (1,200 mosmol/kg) by high levels of urea and high concentrations of sodium and potassium salts. Dilute urine ($\leq$200 mosmol/kg) also inhibits bacterial growth, probably because of low nutrient content of urine. The renal medulla is more susceptible to infection than is the cortex because its relatively poor vascular supply leads to a delay in mobilization of leukocytes, and because hypertonicity and low pH impairs phagocytosis. Medullary renal tubular cells accumulate increased levels of glycine betaine to counteract the osmotic forces of the urine.[302] E. coli can also actively accumulate glycine betaine, which protects them against dehydration.[303] Expression of the outer membrane porin, protein F, is increased under conditions of low osmolarity and suppressed by high osmolarity, effectively modulating passive diffusion of urea into the cell under extreme conditions.[304] This effect decreases the susceptibility of E. coli to β-lactam antibiotics (which pass through porin channels) in hypertonic urine.[305]

THP, produced in the luminal cells of the thick ascending loop of Henle, is the most abundant protein in normal human urine.[91] Binding of type 1 and S-fimbriated bacteria to soluble THP promotes clearance of these strains from the urinary tract and limits their virulence. Although urinary excretion of THP is decreased in infants with urinary infection compared to controls,[262] this may indicate that THP is consumed by bacteria during infection[306] rather than representing a relative risk factor. Low molecular weight oligosaccharides (α-mannosides) found in urine also likely inhibit uroepithelial binding by type 1-fimbriated strains of E. coli.[70]

Secretory IgA and IgA myeloma proteins are secreted into the urine during urinary infection. These antibodies, which may be specific for the O and K antigens or the fimbriae of the invading bacterial strain, also contains terminal mannose residues capable of binding type 1-fimbriated E. coli.[91] Such competitive mannose binding presumably explains how myeloma IgA$_2$ proteins lacking anti-E. coli antibody activity are capable of inhibiting attachment of type 1-fimbriated E. coli to uroepithelial cells.[307] Mannose residues found on secretory IgA in human breast milk may also prevent colonization of the gut with type 1-fimbriated bacteria.[308, 309]

P Blood Group Phenotypes

The globoseries glycolipids of the P blood group system (P, P$_1$, and P^k) function as receptors for P fimbriae and mediate the adherence of P-fimbriated E. coli to colonic and uroepithelial cells.[310] Although there are five phenotypes for the P blood group system, essentially all humans express P$_1$ or P$_2$. Approximately two thirds of individuals have the P$_1$ phenotype and the three antigens (P, P$_1$, and P^k) expressed on their erythrocytes. A third of individuals have the P$_2$ phenotype, lack the P$_1$ antigen, and may have diminished P^k antigen on their cells.[311] Rare individuals of the P blood group phenotype do not synthesize functional digalactose containing glycolipids, causing their urothelial cells to lack functional receptors for P-fimbriated *E. coli*.[153] Clinical evidence of this theoretical protective state has not been demonstrated in humans, likely because of the low frequency of the p phenotype.

Girls with recurrent pyelonephritis and without VUR are more likely to possess the P_1 blood group phenotype (97%) than are age-matched children without urinary infection (75%) or girls with recurrent pyelonephritis and with VUR (84%).[156] The risk of having recurrent pyelonephritis was more than threefold greater for Japanese girls with the P_1 phenotype when compared with those having the P_2 phenotype.[312] An explanation for these observations remains elusive. Although *E. coli* adherence to voided uroepithelial cells from P_1 and P_2 subjects is identical,[289] anti-P_1 antibodies (found in individuals with the P_2 phenotype) have been suspected to inhibit bacterial binding to target cells and interfere with urinary infection.[312] Individuals with the P_1 phenotype have an increased tendency to carry P-fimbriated *E. coli* strains in their fecal flora, suggesting that they may express more or better receptors for P-fimbriated *E. coli* in their large intestine than do individuals with the P_2 phenotype.[182]

Secretor Status

Globoseries glycolipids on uroepithelial cells serve as receptors for P fimbrial adhesins.[153, 164] The carbohydrate compositions of globoseries and other cell surface glycolipids (ABH, P, Lewis antigens) are determined by the synthetic activities of genetically controlled glycosyltransferases.[313] The secretor gene also encodes a glycosyltransferase, and inheritance of this gene influences the cell surface glycolipid composition in tissues.[313] Nonsecretors possess exposed sialosyl gal-globosides on their uroepithelium, which allow binding by P-fimbriated uropathogenic *E. coli*.[314] These sites are fucosylated and processed to ABH cell surface antigens in secretors.[289, 314] Bathing of the uroepithelium with cell secretions further diminishes available fimbrial binding sites in secretors. Women and children with a history of recurrent urinary infection are more likely to be nonsecretors of blood group antigens than are control subjects.[315, 316] Children with Lewis (a-b-) phenotype had a threefold greater risk of urinary infection.[316] Nonsecretors are more likely to be colonized with fimbriated strains of *E. coli*[317] and to have a significant inflammatory response with urinary infection.[318]

PREVENTION OF RENAL SCARRING

Antibiotic Therapy

Early antibiotic treatment is the most effective method to limit the degree of renal inflammation and scarring.[22] In a recent review of 52 children who had symptomatic urinary infection associated with bilateral reflux and renal scarring, Smellie et al. noted a delay in diagnosis or effective treatment of infection in 96%. The incidence of renal scarring was much lower in cases with prompt diagnosis and treatment compared to those with delay.[319] In the monkey, leukocytosis in pyelonephritis is maximal by 24 hours, but ultrastructural studies showed no renal damage until 48 hours after bacterial inoculation.[82] Without treatment, there is a loss of up to 30% of renal function by 48 hours.[137] Renal damage could not be totally prevented when antibiotic therapy was delayed until 72 hours after infection.[137]

Fimbrial expression of periurethral bacterial isolates is influenced by antibiotic therapy. Amoxicillin given to girls with respiratory infection decreases the normal anaerobic vaginal flora and encourages aerobic gram-negative periurethral bacterial growth.[320] Periurethral flora normalized within 3 weeks of therapy. Girls given trimethoprim-sulfamethoxazole had no change in their periurethral microflora during or after therapy.[320] Co-trimoxazole has also been shown to diminish bacterial fimbrial expression for up to a week after cessation of antimicrobial therapy. Treatment with co-trimoxazole is, therefore, capable of sterilizing the urine and limiting the risk for recurrent infection.[321] In a study of adult female cynomolgus monkeys carrying the digalactose receptor for P fimbriae, persistent urinary colonization could be obtained in only 17% when the vagina was washed with a suspension of P-fimbriated *E. coli*, but was present in 100% after intravaginal amoxicillin administration.[322]

Bacterial Vaccines

Within the last decade, accumulated knowledge of specific bacterial virulence factors and the pathogenesis of urinary infection at a molecular level has allowed progress in creating vaccines that could be effective in preventing pyelonephritis caused by *E. coli* strains in children with normal urinary tract anatomy. However, it is not yet feasible to develop broadly cross-reactive urovirulence vaccines to prevent all types of infections for every patient population. There are no vaccines for any type of urinary infection approved by the U.S. Food and Drug Administration (FDA). There are two complex vaccines available in Europe, one of which (SolcoUrovac) has recently been tested by intravaginal instillation in a phase I trial in the United States.[323] Heat-killed uropathogenic isolates from six strains of *E. coli*, as well as from *P. mirabilis, Morganella morganii, Streptococcus faecalis,* and *K. pneumoniae* are included in this vaccine.[324] The other vaccine (Uro-Vaxom) consists of lyophilized membrane glycolipoproteins from selected strains of *E. coli*.[325]

Vaccination with heat-killed or formalin-killed *E. coli*

was recognized to prevent pyelonephritis in rats in 1974.[326] Immunization with whole bacteria was then noted to offer O-serotype-specific protection in rats.[327] However, the effectiveness and safety of this approach is limited by considerable variability in O antigens expressed by uropathogenic bacteria and significant risk for adverse reactions on immunization with LPS. K antigens have less variability than O antigens, but are only weakly immunogenic.[261] Anticapsular immunity to K_1, K_2, K_6, and K_{13} polysaccharides protects rats and rabbits from experimental ascending pyelonephritis when they are subsequently challenged by *E. coli* expressing a homologous K serotype.[328] Capsular resistance to phagocytosis and complement activation is thought to be negated by specific IgG binding. Parenteral immunization with outer membrane proteins of *P. mirabilis* prevent pyelonephritis by a homologous challenge strain in mice[329] and may be protective against other *Enterobacteriaceae*.

Parenteral immunization with homologous and heterologous purified P-fimbriae protected against development of ascending pyelonephritis in the BALB/c mouse (bladder inoculation)[37, 275, 330] and the cynomolgus monkey (intraureteral inoculation) models of ascending pyelonephritis.[331] Protection correlated with the presence of specific IgG antibodies to PapA (and not to PapG) in urine and serum, likely because PapA is consistently more highly immunogenic than PapG, and because there is a high degree of conservation among PapA pilins at genetic and protein levels.[155, 332] Parenteral immunization with a hemolysin vaccine affords additional protection from renal damage in the BALB/c mouse pyelonephritis model.[275] Synthetic PapA fimbrial vaccines recognizing protective epitopes in two separate regions of PapA also elicits cross-protection against heterologous fimbriated *E. coli* strains in BALB/c mice.[333] Systemic immunization with FimH in a murine cystitis model reduced bladder uroepithelial colonization by more than 99%, and anti-FimH IgG was detected in urine samples from protected mice.[334] Sera from vaccinated mice also inhibited binding of uropathogenic *E. coli* to human bladder cells on tissue section.[334]

REFERENCES

1. Tullus K, Jacobson SH, Katouli M, Brauner A. Relative importance of eight virulence characteristics of pyelonephritogenic *Escherichia coli* strains assessed by multivariate statistical analysis. J Urol 1991;146:1153.
2. Elo J, Tallgren LG, Väisänen V, Korhonen TK, Mäkela PH. Association of P and other fimbriae with clinical pyelonephritis in children. Scand J Urol Nephrol 1985;19:281.
3. Källenius G, Mollby R, Svenson SB, et al. Occurrence of P-fimbriated *Escherichia coli* in urinary tract infections. Lancet 1981;2:1369.
4. Korhonen TK, Virkola R, Westurlund B, Holthofer H, Parkkinen J. Tissue tropism of *Escherichia coli* adhesins in human extraintestinal infections. Curr Top Microbiol Immunol 1990; 151:115.
5. Roberts JA. Tropism in bacterial infections: urinary tract infections. J Urol 1996;156:1552.
6. Caprioli A, Falbo V, Ruggeri FM, Minelli F, Ørskov I, Donelli G. Relationship between cytotoxic necrotizing factor production and serotype in hemolytic *Escherichia coli*. J Clin Microbiol 1989;27:758.
7. Trifillis AL, Donnenberg MS, Cui X, et al. Binding to and killing of human renal epithelial cells by hemolytic P-fimbriated *E. coli*. Kidney Int 1994;46:1083.
8. Blum G, Falbo V, Caprioli A, Hacker J. Gene clusters encoding the cytotoxic necrotizing factor type 1, Prs-fimbriae and alpha-hemolysin form the pathogenicity island II of uropathogenic *Escherichia coli* strain J96. FEMS Microbiol Lett 1995;126:189.
9. Blum G, Ott M, Lischewski A, et al. Excision of large DNA regions termed pathogenicity islands from tRNA-specific loci in the chromosome of an *Escherichia coli* wild-type pathogen. Infect Immunol 1994;62:606.
10. Jodal U. The natural history of bacteriuria in childhood. Infect Dis Clin North Am 1987;1:713.
11. Winberg J, Andersen HJ, Bergström T, Jacobsson B, Larson H, Lincoln K. Epidemiology of symptomatic urinary infection in childhood. Acta Paediatr Scand 1974;252(Suppl):3.
12. Wiswell TE, Smith FR, Bass JW. Decreased incidence of urinary tract infections in circumcised male infants. Pediatrics 1985; 75:901.
13. Wiswell TE, Roscelli JD. Corroborative evidence for the decreasing incidence of urinary tract infections in circumcised male infants. Pediatrics 1986;78:96.
14. Ginsburg CM, McCracken GH Jr. Urinary tract infections in young infants. Pediatrics 1982;69:409.
15. Lincoln K, Winberg J. Studies of urinary tract infections in infancy and childhood, II: Quantitative estimation of bacteriuria in unselected neonates with special reference to the occurrence of asymptomatic infections. Acta Paediatr 1964;53:307.
16. Fussell EN, Kaack MB, Cherry R, Roberts JA. Adherence of bacteria to human foreskins. J Urol 1988;140:997.
17. Bollgren I, Winberg J. The periurethral aerobic bacterial flora in healthy boys and girls. Acta Paediatr Scand 1976;65:74.
18. Källenius G, Winberg J. Bacterial adherence to periurethral epithelial cells in girls prone to urinary tract infections. Lancet 1978;2:540.
19. Svanborg-Edén C, Jodal U, Hanson LÅ, Lindberg U, Åkerlund AS. Variable adherence to normal human urinary-tract epithelial cells of *Escherichia coli* strains associated with various forms of urinary-tract infection. Lancet 1976;2:490.
20. Svanborg-Edén C, Jodal U. Attachment of *Escherichia coli* to urinary sediment epithelial cells from urinary tract infection-prone and healthy children. Infect Immunol 1979;26:837.
21. Schlager TA, Hendley JO, Lohr JA, Whittam TS. Effect of periurethral colonization on the risk of urinary infection in healthy girls after their first urinary tract infection. Pediatr Infect Dis J 1993;12:988.
22. Ransley PG, Risdon RA. Reflux nephropathy: effects of antimicrobial therapy on the evolution of the early pyelonephritis scar. Kidney Int 1981;20:733.
23. Winter AL, Hardy BE, Alton DJ, Arubs GS, Churchill BM. Acquired renal scars in children. J Urol 1983;129:1190.
24. Rushton HG, Majd M, Jantausch B, Wiedermann BL, Belman AB. Renal scarring following reflux and nonreflux pyelonephritis in children: evaluation with ^{99m}technetium-dimercaptosuccinic acid scintigraphy. J Urol 1992;147:1327.
25. Lomberg H, Hellström M, Jodal U, Leffler H, Lincoln K, Svanborg-Edén C. Virulence-associated traits in *Escherichia coli* causing first and recurrent episodes of urinary tract infection in children with and without vesicoureteral reflux. J Infect Dis 1984; 150:561.
26. O'Hanley P, Low D, Romero I, et al. Gal-Gal binding and hemolysin phenotypes and genotypes associated with uropathogenic *Escherichia coli*. N Engl J Med 1985;313:414.
27. Matsumoto T, Mizunoe Y, Ogata N, Tanaka M, Kumazawa J. Role of superoxide in renal scarring following infection by mannose-sensitive piliated bacteria. Urol Res 1991;19:229.
28. Topley N, Steadman R, Mackenzie R, Knowlden JM, Williams

JD. Type 1 fimbriated strains of *Escherichia coli* initiate renal parenchymal scarring. Kidney Int 1989;36:609.

29. Stokland E, Hellström M, Jacobsson B, Jodal U, Lundgren P, Sixt R. Early ^{99m}Tc dimercaptosuccinic acid (DMSA) scintigraphy in symptomatic first-time urinary tract infection. Acta Paediatr 1996;85:430.

30. Merrick MV, Notghi A, Chalmers N, Wilkinson AG, Uttley WS. Long term follow up to determine the prognostic value of imaging after urinary tract infections. Part 2: Scarring. Arch Dis Child 1995;72:393.

31. Jakobsson B, Berg U, Svensson L. Renal scarring after acute pyelonephritis. Arch Dis Child 1994;70:111.

32. Winberg J, Bollgren I, Källenius G, Möllby R, Svenson SB. Clinical pyelonephritis and focal renal scarring. A selected review of pathogenesis, prevention, and prognosis. Pediatr Clin North Am 1982;29:801.

33. Benador D, Benador N, Slosman D, Mermillod B, Girardin E. Are younger children at highest risk of renal sequelae after pyelonephritis? Lancet 1997;349:17.

34. Winberg J. Commentary: progressive renal damage from infection with or without reflux. J Urol 1992;148:1733.

35. Craig JC, Knight JF, Sureshkumar P, Mantz E, Roy LP. Effect of circumcision on incidence of urinary tract infection in preschool boys. J Pediatr 1996;128:23.

36. Wiswell TE, Miller GM, Gelston HM Jr, Jones SK, Clemmings AF. The effect of circumcision status on periurethral bacterial flora during the first year of life. J Pediatr 1988;113:442.

37. O'Hanley P, Lark D, Falkow S, Schoolnik G. Molecular basis of *Escherichia coli* colonization of the upper urinary tract in BALB/c mice: Gal-Gal pili immunization prevents *E. coli* pyelonephritis in the BALB/c mouse and model of human pyelonephritis. J Clin Invest 1985;75:347.

38. Fujita K, Yamamoto T, Yokota T, Kitagawa R. In vitro adherence of type 1-fimbriated uropathogenic *Escherichia coli* to human ureteral mucosa. Infect Immunol 1989;57:2574.

39. Henderson B, Poole S, Wilson M. Bacterial modulins: a novel class of virulence factors which cause host tissue pathology by inducing cytokine synthesis. Microbiol Rev 1996;60:316.

40. Allen TD. The non-neurogenic neurogenic bladder. J Urol 1977;117:232.

41. Hinman F. Urinary tract damage in children who wet. Pediatrics 1974;54:142.

42. Koff SA. Bladder-sphincter dysfunction in childhood. Urology 1982;19:457.

43. Lapides J. Mechanisms of urinary tract infection. Urology 1979;14:217.

44. Hansson S. Urinary incontinence in children and associated problems. Scand J Urol Nephrol 1992;141:47.

45. McLachlan MSF, Meller ST, Verrier-Jones ER, et al. Urinary tract in schoolgirls with covert bacteriuria. Arch Dis Child 1975;50:253.

46. Newcastle Asymptomatic Bacteriuria Research Group: Asymptomatic bacteriuria in schoolchildren in Newcastle-upon-Tyne. Arch Dis Child 1975;50:90.

47. Immergut MA, Wahman GE. The urethral caliber of female children with recurrent urinary tract infections. J Urol 1968;99:189.

48. Lindberg U, Bjure J, Haugstvedt S, Jodal U. Asymptomatic bacteriuria in schoolgirls, III: Relation between residual urine volume and recurrence. Acta Paediatr Scand 1975;64:437.

49. Busch R, Huland H, Kollermann MW, Scherf H. Does internal urethrotomy influence susceptibility to recurrent urinary tract infection? Urology 1982;20:134.

50. Kaplan GW, Sammons TA, King LR. A blind comparison to dilatation, urethrotomy and medication alone in the treatment of urinary tract infection in girls. J Urol 1973;109:917.

51. Bauer SB, Retik AB, Colodny AH, Hallett M, Khoshbin S, Dyro FM. The unstable bladder of childhood. Urol Clin North Am 1980;7:321.

52. Kjølseth D, Knudsen LM, Madsen B, Nørgaard JP, Djurhuus JC. Urodynamic biofeedback training for children with bladder-sphincter dyscoordination during voiding. Neurourology Urodynamics 1993;12:211.

53. Lapides J, Diokno AC. Persistence of the infant bladder as a cause for urinary infection in girls. J Urol 1970;103:243.

54. Allen TD, Bright TC III. Urodynamic patterns in children with dysfunctional voiding problems. J Urol 1978;119:247.

55. Finkbeiner A, Lapides J. Effect of distension on blood flow in dog's urinary bladder. J Urol 1974;12:210.

56. Johnson DE, Russell RG, Lockatell CV, Zulty JC, Warren JW. Urethral obstruction of 6 hours or less causes bacteriuria, bacteremia, and pyelonephritis in mice challenged with "nonpathogenic" *Escherichia coli*. Infect Immunol 1993;61:3422.

57. O'Reagan S, Yazbeck S, Schick E. Constipation, bladder instability, urinary tract infection syndrome. Clin Nephrol 1985;23:152.

58. Loening-Baucke V. Urinary incontinence and urinary tract infection and their resolution with treatment of chronic constipation of childhood. Pediatrics 1997;100:228.

59. Neumann PZ, de Domenico IJ, Nogrady MB. Constipation and urinary tract infection. Pediatrics 1973;52:241.

60. Smellie JM, Rigden SPA, Prescod NP. Urinary tract infection: a comparison of four methods of investigation. Arch Dis Child 1995;72:247.

61. Björgvinsson E, Majd M, Eggli KD. Diagnosis of acute pyelonephritis in children: comparison of sonography and ^{99m}TC-DMSA scintigraphy. AJR 1991;157:539.

62. Eggli KD, Eggli D. Color Doppler sonography in pyelonephritis. Pediatr Radiol 1992;22:422.

63. Verrier Jones K. Commentary. Arch Dis Child 1995;72:255.

64. Rushton HG. The evaluation of acute pyelonephritis and renal scarring with technetium ^{99}m-dimercaptosuccinic acid renal scintigraphy: evolving concepts and future directions. Pediatr Nephrol 1997;11:108.

65. Rushton HG, Majd M, Chandra R, Yim D. Evaluation of ^{99m}technetium-dimercapto-succinic acid renal scans in experimental acute pyelonephritis in piglets. J Urol 1988;140:1169.

66. Majd M, Rushton HG, Chandra R, Andrich MP, Tardif CP, Rashti F. Technetium-99m-DMSA renal cortical scintigraphy to detect experimental acute pyelonephritis in piglets: comparison of planar (pinhole) and SPECT imaging. J Nucl Med 1996;37:1731.

67. Fowler JE Jr, Stamey TA. Studies of introital colonization in women with recurrent urinary infection, VII: The role of bacterial adherence. J Urol 1977;117:472.

68. Schlager TA, Whittam TS, Hendley JO, et al. Comparison of expression of virulence factors by *Escherichia coli* causing cystitis and *E. coli* colonizing the periurethra of healthy girls. J Infect Dis 1995;172:772.

69. Duncan JL. Differential effects of Tamm-Horsfall protein on adherence of *Escherichia coli* to transitional epithelial cells. J Infect Dis 1988;158:1379.

70. Parkkinen J, Virkola R, Korhonen TK. Identification of factors in human urine that inhibit the binding of *Escherichia coli* adhesins. Infect Immunol 1988;56:2623.

71. Hooke AM, Sordelli DO, Erguetti MC, Vogt AJ. Quantitative determination of bacterial replication in vivo. Infect Immunol 1985;49:424.

72. Gordon DM, Riley MA. A theoretical and experimental analysis of bacterial growth in the bladder. Mol Microbiol 1992;6:555.

73. Roberts JA. Experimental pyelonephritis in the monkey, III: Pathophysiology of ureteral malfunction induced by bacteria. Invest Urol 1975;13:117.

74. Roberts JA, Suarez GM, Kaack MB, Källenius G, Svenson SB. Experimental pyelonephritis in the monkey, VII: Ascending pyelonephritis in the absence of vesicoureteral reflux. J Urol 1985;133:1068.

75. Roberts JA. Etiology and pathophysiology of pyelonephritis. Am J Kidney Dis 1991;17:1.

76. Hacker J. Role of fimbrial adhesins in the pathogenesis of *Escherichia coli* infections. Can J Microbiol 1992;38:720.

77. Angel JR, Smith TW Jr, Roberts JA. The hydrodynamics of pyelorenal reflux. J Urol 1979;122:20.

78. Rolleston GL, Maling TMJ, Hodson CJ. Intrarenal reflux and the scarred kidney. Arch Dis Child 1974;49:531.

79. Nowicki B, Holthofer H, Saraneva T, Rhen M, Väisänen-Rhen V, Korhonen TK. Location of adhesion sites for P-fimbriated

and for 075X-positive *Escherichia coli* in the human kidney. Microbiol Pathogen 1986;1:169.

80. Chippendale GR, Warren JW, Trifillis AL. Internalization of *Proteus mirabilis* by human renal epithelial cells. Infect Immunol 1994;62:3115.

81. Isberg R. Discrimination between intracellular uptake and surface adhesion of bacterial pathogens. Science 1991;252:934.

82. Fussell EN, Roberts JA. The ultrastructure of acute pyelonephritis in the monkey. J Urol 1984;133:179.

83. Billiau A, Vandekerckhove F. Cytokines and their interactions with other inflammatory mediators in the pathogenesis of sepsis and septic shock. Eur J Clin Invest 1991;21:559.

84. Schumann RR, Leong SR, Flaggs GW, et al. Structure and function of lipopolysaccharide binding protein. Science 1990; 249:1429.

85. Ingalls RR, Golenbock DT. CD11c/CD18, a transmembrane signalling receptor for lipopolysaccharide. J Exp Med 1995; 181:1473.

86. Agace W, Hedges S, Andersson U, Andersson J, Ceska M, Svanborg C. Selective cytokine production by epithelial cells following exposure to *Escherichia coli*. Infect Immunol 1993; 61:602.

87. Roberts JA, Kaack MB, Baskin G, Martin LN. Events leading to septic death from experimental acute pyelonephritis in the monkey. J Urol 1993;150:1030.

88. Roberts JA, Kaack MB, Martin LN. Cytokine and lymphocyte activation during experimental acute pyelonephritis. Urol Res 1995;23:33.

89. Hedges S, Anderson P, Lidin-Janson G, Svanborg C. Interleukin-6 response to deliberate gram-negative colonization of the human urinary tract. Infect Immunol 1991;59:421.

90. de Man P, van Kooten C, Aarden L. Interleukin-6 induced at mucosal surfaces by gram-negative bacterial infection. Infect Immunol 1989;57:3383.

91. Agace W, Connell H, Svanborg C. Host resistance to urinary tract infection. In: Mobley HLT, Warren JW, eds. Urinary Tract Infections: Molecular Pathogenesis and Clinical Management. Washington, DC: ASM Press, 1996:221–243.

92. Kreft B, Placzek M, Doehn C, et al. S fimbriae of uropathogenic *Escherichia coli* bind to primary human renal proximal tubular epithelial cells but do not induce expression of intercellular adhesion molecule 1. Infect Immunol 1995;63:3235.

93. Agace WW, Patarroyo M, Svensson M, Carlemalm E, Svanborg C. *Escherichia coli* induces transuroepithelial neutrophil migration by an intercellular adhesion molecule-1-dependent mechanism. Infect Immunol 1995;63:4054.

94. Miyakita H, Puri P, Surana R, Kobayashi H, Reen DJ. Serum intercellular adhesion molecule (ICAM-1), a marker of renal scarring in infants with vesico-ureteric reflux. Br J Urol 1995;76:249.

95. Joseph CK, Wright SD, Bornmann JG, et al. Bacterial lipopolysaccharide has structural similarity to ceramide and stimulates ceramide-activated protein kinase in myeloid cells. J Biol Chem 1994;269:1706.

96. Miyata H, Moriguchi N, Kinoshita T, Kataoka S, Kanazaki M, Maki S. The chemiluminescence response of human polymorphonuclear leukocytes to *Escherichia coli* O and K antigens. Acta Pediatr 1993;82:132.

97. Khalil A, Brauner A, Bakhiet M, et al. Cytokine gene expression during experimental *Escherichia coli* pyelonephritis in mice. J Urol 1997;158:1576.

98. Taverne J. Transgenic mice in the study of cytokine function. Int J Exp Pathol 1993;74:525.

99. Rothe J, Lesslauer W, Lotscher H, et al. Mice lacking the tumour necrosis factor receptor 1 are resistant to TNF-mediated toxicity but highly susceptible to infection by *Listeria monocytogenes*. Nature (London) 1993;364:798.

100. Li P, Allen H, Banerjee S, et al. Mice deficient in IL-1β converting enzyme are defective in production of mature IL-1β and resistant to endotoxic shock. Cell 1995;80:401.

101. Sadlack B, Merz H, Schorle H, Schimpl A, Feller AC, Horak I. Ulcerative colitis-like disease in mice with a disrupted interleukin-2 gene. Cell 1993;75:253.

102. Kuhn R, Lohler J, Rennick D, Rajewsky K, Muller W. Interleukin 10-deficient mice develop chronic enterocolitis. Cell 1993;75:263.

103. Rogy MA, Auffenberg T, Espat NJ, et al. Human tumor necrosis factor receptor (p55) and interleukin-10 gene transfer in the mouse reduces mortality to lethal endotoxemia and also attenuates local inflammatory responses. J Exp Med 1995;181:2289.

104. Border WA, Noble NA. Transforming growth factor β in tissue fibrosis. N Engl J Med 1994;331:1286.

105. Jacobson SH, Hylander B, Wretland B, Brauner A. Interleukin-6 and interleukin-8 in serum and urine in patients with acute pyelonephritis in relation to bacterial-virulence-associated traits and renal function. Nephron 1994;67:172.

106. Van Snick J. Interleukin-6: an overview. Ann Rev Immunol 1990;8:253.

107. Hedges S, Stenqvist K, Lidin-Janson G, Martinell J, Sandberg T, Svanborg C. Comparison of urine and serum concentrations of interleukin-6 in women with acute pyelonephritis or asymptomatic bacteriuria. J Infect Dis 1992;166:653.

108. Benson M, Andreasson A, Jodal U, Karlsson Å, Rydberg J, Svanborg C. Interleukin 6 in childhood urinary tract infection. Pediatr Infect Dis J 1994;13:612.

109. Tullus K, Fituri O, Linné T, et al. Urine interleukin-6 and interleukin-8 in children with acute pyelonephritis in relation to DMSA-scintigraphy in the acute phase and at one year follow-up. Pediatr Radiol 1994;24:513.

110. Ko YC, Mukaida N, Ishiyama S, et al. Elevated interleukin-8 levels in the urine of patients with urinary tract infections. Infect Immunol 1993;61:1307.

111. Arnaout MA. Cell adhesion molecules in inflammation and thrombosis: status and prospects. Am J Kidney Dis 1993;21:72.

112. Shibata F, Kato H, Konishi K, et al. Differential changes in the concentrations of cytokine-induced neutrophil chemoattractant (CINC)-1 and CINC-2 in exudate during rat lipopolysaccharide-induced inflammation. Cytokine 1996;8:222.

113. Frank MM. Complement in host defense against bacterial infections. In: Ayoub EM, Cassell GH, Branche WC Jr, Henry PJ, eds. Microbial determinants of virulence and host response. Washington, DC: ASM Press, 1990;305–317.

114. Cooper NR. Complement and infectious agents. Rev Infect Dis 1988;10:S447.

115. Meylan PR, Glauser MP. Role of complement-derived and bacterial formylpeptide chemotactic factors in the in vivo migration of neutrophils in experimental *Escherichia coli* pyelonephritis in rats. J Infect Dis 1989;159:959.

116. Huston DP. The biology of the immune system. JAMA 1997;278:1804.

117. Kaack MB, Dowling KJ, Patterson GM, Roberts JA. Immunology of pyelonephritis, VIII: E. coli causes granulocytic aggregation and renal ischemia. J Urol 1986;136:1117.

118. Moslen MT. Reactive oxygen species in normal physiology, cell injury and phagocytosis. In: Armstrong D, ed. Free Radicals in Diagnostic Medicine. NY: Plenum Press, 1994:17–27.

119. Weiss S. Tissue destruction by neutrophils. N Engl J Med 1989;320:365.

120. Thomas EL, Lehrer RI, Rest RF. Human neutrophil antimicrobial activity. Rev Infect Dis 1988;10:S450.

121. Winrow VR, Winyard PG, Morris CJ, Blake DR. Free radicals in inflammation: second messengers and mediators of tissue destruction. Br Med Bull 1993;49:506.

122. Wispé JR, Roberts RJ. Molecular basis of pulmonary oxygen toxicity. Clin Perinatol 1987;14:651.

123. Bevilacqua MP, Pober JS, Wheeler ME, Cotran RS, Gimbone MA Jr. Interleukin 1 acts on cultured human vascular endothelium to increase the adhesion of polymorphonuclear leukocytes, monocytes, and related leukocyte cell lines. J Clin Invest 1985;76:2003.

124. Schneeman M, Schoedon G, Hofer S, Blau N, Guerrero L, Schaffer A. Nitric acid synthase is not a constituent of the antimicrobial armature of human mononuclear phagocytes. J Infect Dis 1993;167:1358.

125. Murrell GAC, Francis MJO, Bromley L. Modulation of fibroblast proliferation by oxygen free radicals. Biochem J 1990;265:659.

126. Mundi H, Bjorksten B, Svanborg C, Ohman L, Dahlgren C. Extracellular release of reactive oxygen species from human

neutrophils upon interaction with *Escherichia coli* strains causing renal scarring. Infect Immunol 1991;59:4168.

127. Andreoli SP, McAteer JA. Reactive oxygen molecule-mediated injury in endothelial and renal tubular epithelial cells in vitro. Kidney Int 1990;38:785.

128. Warner BB, Wispé JR. Free radical-mediated diseases in pediatrics. Sem Perinatol 1992;16:47.

129. Strand WR, Sesterhenn I, Rushton HG. Role of superoxide dismutase in the pathogenesis of pyelonephritis: immunological localization of superoxide dismutase in human renal tissues. J Urol 1989;142:616.

130. Fridovich I. Superoxide radical: an endogenous toxicant. Annu Rev Pharmacol Toxicol 1983;23:239.

131. Grisham MB, Hernandez LA, Granger DN. Xanthine oxidase and neutrophil infiltration in intestinal ischemia. Am J Physiol 1986;251:G567.

132. Paller MS. Effect of neutrophil depletion on ischemic renal injury in the rat. J Lab Clin Med 1989;113:379.

133. Paller MS, Neumann TV, Knobloch E, Patten M. Reactive oxygen species and rat renal epithelial cells during hypoxia and reoxygenation. Kidney Int 1991;40:1041.

134. Granger DN, Rutili G, McCord J. Superoxide radicals in feline intestinal ischemia. Gastroenterology 1981;81:22.

135. Greene EL, Paller MS. Oxygen free radicals in acute renal failure. Miner Electrolyte Metab 1991;17:124.

136. Glauser M, Lyons JM, Braude AI. Prevention of chronic pyelonephritis by suppression of acute suppuration. J Clin Invest 1978;61:403.

137. Roberts JA, Kaack MB, Baskin G. Treatment of experimental pyelonephritis in the monkey. J Urol 1990;143:150.

138. Ormrod D, Cawley S, Miller T. Neutrophil-mediated tissue destruction in experimental pyelonephritis. In: Kass EH, Svanborg-Edén CS, eds. Host-Parasite Interactions in Urinary Tract Infections. Chicago: University of Chicago, 1986;365–368.

139. Sullivan MJ, Harvey RA, Shimamura T. The effects of cobra venom factor, an inhibitor of the complement system, on the sequence of morphological events in the rat kidney in experimental pyelonephritis. Yale J Biol Med 1977;50:267.

140. Roberts JA, Roth JK Jr, Domingue G, Lewis RW, Kaack B, Baskin GB. Immunology of pyelonephritis in the primate model, VI: Effect of complement depletion. J Urol 1983;129:193.

141. Roberts JA, Roth JK Jr, Domingue G, Lewis RW, Kaack B, Baskin G. Immunology of pyelonephritis in the primate model, V: Effect of superoxide dismutase. J Urol 1982;128:1394.

142. Roberts JA, Kaack MB, Fussell EF, Baskin G. Immunology of pyelonephritis, VII: Effect of allopurinol. J Urol 1986;136:960.

143. Guyot G. Uber die bakterielle Haemagglutination (Bacterio-Haemagglutination). Zentralbl Bakteriol Parasitenkd Infektionskr Hyg Abt 1 Orig 1908;47:640.

144. Lyon MW Jr. A case of cystitis caused by *Bacillus coli-hemolyticus*. JAMA 1917;69:353.

145. Duguid JP, Smith IW, Dempster G, Edmunds PN. Non-flagellar filamentous appendages ("fimbriae") and hemagglutinating activity in *bacterium coli*. J Pathol Bacteriol 1955;70:335.

146. Abraham JM, Freitag CS, Clements JR, Eisenstein BI. An invertible element of DNA controls phase variation of type 1 fimbriae of *Escherichia coli*. Proc Natl Acad Sci USA 1985;82:5724.

147. Duguid JP, Clegg S, Wilson MI. The fimbrial and non-fimbrial haemagglutinins of *Escherichia coli*. J Med Microbiol 1979;12:213.

148. Old DC. Inhibition of the interaction between fimbrial hemagglutinins and erythrocytes by D-mannose and other carbohydrates. J Gen Microbiol 1972;71:149.

149. Salit IE, Gottschlich EC. Type 1 *Escherichia coli* pili: characterization of binding to monkey kidney cells. J Exp Med 1977;146:1182.

150. Källenius G, Mollby R. Adhesion of *Escherichia coli* to human periurethral cells correlated to mannose-resistant agglutination of human erythrocytes. FEMS Microbiol Lett 1979;5:295.

151. Hagberg L, Jodal U, Korhonen TK, Lidin-Janson G, Lindberg U, Svanborg-Edén C. Adhesion, hemagglutination, and virulence of *Escherichia coli* causing urinary tract infections. Infect Immunol 1981;31:564.

152. Källenius G, Mollby R, Svenson SB, Winberg J, Hultberg H.

153. Leffler H, Svanborg-Edén CS. Chemical identification of a glycosphingolipid receptor for *Escherichia coli* attaching to human urinary tract epithelial cells and agglutinating human erythrocytes. FEMS Microbiol Lett 1980;8:127.

154. Jacobson SH. A five-year prospective follow-up of women with nonobstructive pyelonephritis and renal scarring. Scand J Urol Nephrol 1991;25:51.

155. Johnson JR. Virulence factors in urinary tract infection. Clin Microbiol Rev 1991;4:80.

156. Lonberg H, Hanson LÅ, Jacobsson B, Jodal U, Leffler H, Svanborg-Edén CS. Correlation of P blood group, vesicoureteral reflux, and bacterial attachment in patients with recurrent pyelonephritis. N Engl J Med 1983;308:1189.

157. Lomberg H, Hellström M, Jodal U, Ørskov I, Svanborg-Edén C. Properties of *Escherichia coli* in patients with renal scarring. J Infect Dis 1989;159:579.

158. Lund B, Lindberg F, Marklund B-I, Normark S. The PapG protein is the alpha-D-galactopyranosyl (1-4) beta-D-galactopyranose-binding adhesin of uropathogenic *Escherichia coli*. Proc Natl Acad Sci USA 1987;84:5898.

159. Lund B, Marklund B-I, Strömberg N, Lindberg F, Karlsson K-A, Normark S. Uropathogenic *Escherichia coli* can express serologically identical pili of different receptor binding specificities. Mol Microbiol 1988;2:255.

160. Hull RA, Gill RE, Hsu P, Minshaw BH, Falkow S. Construction and expression of recombinant plasmids encoding type 1 and D-mannose-resistant pili from urinary tract infection *Escherichia coli* isolate. Infect Immunol 1981;33:933.

161. Lindberg F, Lund B, Johansson L, Normark S. Localization of the receptor-binding protein adhesin at the tip of the bacterial pilus. Nature 1987;328:84.

162. Kuehn MJ, Heuser J, Normark S, Hultgren SJ. P pili in uropathogenic *E. coli* are composite fibers with distinct fibrillar adhesive tips. Nature (London) 1992;356:252.

163. Hultgren SJ, Abraham S, Caparon M, Falk P, St Geme JW III, Normark S. Pilus and nonpilus bacterial adhesins: assembly and function in cell recognition. Cell 1993;73:887.

164. Stromberg N, Marklund B-I, Lund B, et al. Host-specificity of uropathogenic *Escherichia coli* depends on differences in binding specificity to Galα1-4 Gal-containing isoreceptors. EMBO J 1990;9:2001.

165. Johnson J, Ørskov I, Ørskov F, et al. O, K, and H antigens predict virulence factors, carboxylesterase B pattern, antimicrobial resistance, and host compromise among *Escherichia coli* strains causing urosepsis. J Infect Dis 1994;169:119.

166. Low D, David V, Lark G, Schoolnik G, Falkow S. Gene clusters governing the production of hemolysin and mannose-resistant hemagglutination are closely linked in *Escherichia coli* serotype O4 and O6 isolates from urinary tract infections. Infect Immunol 1984;43:353.

167. Hacker J, Bender L, Ott M, et al. Deletions of chromosomal regions coding for fimbriae and hemolysins occur *in vitro* and *in vivo* in various extraintestinal *Escherichia coli* isolates. Microbiol Pathog 1990;8:213.

168. Lee CA. Pathogenicity islands and the evolution of bacterial pathogens. Infect Agent Dis 1996;5:1.

169. Knapp S, Hacker J, Jarchau T, Goebel W. Large, unstable inserts in the chromosome affect virulence properties of uropathogenic *Escherichia coli* O6 strain 536. J Bacteriol 1986;168:22.

170. McDaniel TK, Jarvis KG, Donnenberg MS, Kaper JB. A genetic locus of enterocyte effacement conserved among diverse enterobacterial pathogens. Proc Natl Acad Sci USA 1995;92:1664.

171. Klemm P. Fimbrial adhesins of *Escherichia coli*. Rev Infect Dis 1985;7:321.

172. Jones CH, Pinkner JS, Roth R, et al. FimH adhesin of type 1 pili is assembled into a fibrillar tip structure in the *Enterobacteriaceae*. Proc Natl Acad Sci USA 1995;92:2081.

173. Roberts JA, Marklund B-I, Ilver D, et al. The Galα(1-4)Gal-specific tip adhesin of *Escherichia coli* P-fimbriae is needed for pyelonephritis to occur in the normal urinary tract. Proc Natl Acad Sci USA 1994;91:11889.

Identification of a carbohydrate receptor recognized by uropathogenic *Escherichia coli*. Infection 1980;8(suppl 3):288.

174. Roberts JA. Bacterial adherence and urinary tract infection. South Med J 1987;80:347.

175. Wold AE, Thorssén M, Hull S, Svanborg-Edén C. Attachment of *Escherichia coli* via mannose- or Galα1-4Galβ-containing receptors to human colonic epithelial cells. Infect Immunol 1988;56:2531.

176. Roberts JA, Kaack B, Källenius G, Möllby R, Winberg J, Svenson SB. Receptors for pyelonephritogenic *Escherichia coli* in primates. J Urol 1984;131:163.

177. Källenius G, Mollby R, Svenson SB, et al. The p^k antigen as receptor for the haemagglutinin of pyelonephritogenic *Escherichia coli*. FEMS Microbiol Lett 1980;8:297.

178. Hull RA, Hull SI, Falkow S. Frequency of gene sequences necessary for pyelonephritis-associated pili expression among isolates of *Enterobacteriaceae* from human extraintestinal infections. Infect Immunol 1984;43:1064.

179. Marklund B-I, Tennant JM, Garcia E, et al. Horizontal gene transfer of the *Escherichia coli* *pap* and *prs* pili operons as a mechanism for the development of tissue-specific adhesive properties. Mol Microbiol 1992;6:2225.

180. Plos K, Carter T, Hull S, Hull R, Svanborg-Edén C. Frequency and organization of pap homologous DNA in relation to clinical origin of uropathogenic *Escherichia coli*. J Infect Dis 1990;161:518.

181. Lindstedt R, Larsson S, Falk P, Leffler H, Svanborg C. The receptor repertoire defines the host range for attaching *Escherichia coli* strains that recognize globo-A. Infect Immunol 1991;59:1086.

182. Plos K, Connell H, Jodal U, et al. Intestinal carriage of P fimbriated *Escherichia coli* and the susceptibility to urinary tract infection in young children. J Infect Dis 1995;171:625.

183. Dodson KW, Jacob-Dubuisson F, Striker RT, Hultgren SJ. Outer membrane PapC usher discriminately recognizes periplasmic chaperone-pilus subunit complexes. Proc Natl Acad Sci USA 1993;90:3670.

184. Jacob-Dubuisson F, Heuser J, Dodson K, Normark S, Hultgren S. Initiation of assembly and association of the structural elements of a bacterial pilus depends on two specialized tip proteins. EMBO J 1993;12:837.

185. Baga M, Norgren M, Normark S. Biogenesis of *E. coli* Pap pili: PapH, a minor pilin subunit involved in cell anchoring and length modulation. Cell 1987;49:241.

186. Blyn LB, Braaten BA, Low DA. Regulation of *pap* pilin phase variation by a mechanism involving differential Dam methylation states. EMBO J 1990;9:4045.

187. Braaten BA, Nou X, Kaltenbach LS, Low DA. Methylation patterns in *pap* regulatory DNA control pyelonephritis-associated pili phase variation in *E. coli*. Cell 1994;76:577.

188. Stromberg N, Nyholm PG, Pascher I, Normark S. Saccharide orientation at the cell surface affects glycolipid receptor function. Proc Natl Acad Sci USA 1991;88:9340.

189. Johanson I, Lindstedt R, Svanborg C. Roles of the *pap*- and *prs* encoded adhesins in *Escherichia coli* adherence to human uroepithelial cells. Infect Immunol 1992;60:3416.

190. Hakomori S-I. Bifunctional role of glycosphingolipids: modulators for transmembrane signaling and mediators for cellular interactions. J Biol Chem 1990;265:18713.

191. Svanborg-Edén C, Freter R, Hagberg L, et al. Inhibition of experimental ascending urinary tract infection by a receptor analogue. Nature (London) 1982;298:560.

192. Hull S, Clegg S, Svanborg-Edén C, Hull R. Multiple forms of genes in pyelonephritogenic *Escherichia coli* encoding adhesins binding globoseries glycolipid receptors. Infect Immunol 1985;47:80.

193. Korhonen TK, Virkola R, Holthöfer H. Localization of binding sites for purified *Escherichia coli* P fimbriae in the human kidney. Infect Immunol 1986;54:328.

194. Karr JF, Nowicki B, Truong LD, Hull RA, Hull SI. Purified P fimbriae from two cloned gene clusters of a single pyelonephritogenic strain adhere to unique structures in the human kidney. Infect Immunol 1989;57:3594.

195. Nowicki BJ. In vitro models for the study of uropathogens. In: Mobley HLT, Warren JW, eds. Urinary Tract Infections: Molecular Pathogenesis and Clinical Management. Washington, DC. ASM Press, 1996:341–376.

196. Westerlund B, Kuusela P, Vartio T, Van Die I, Korhonen TK. A novel lectin-independent interaction of P fimbriae of *Escherichia coli* with immobilized fibronectin. FEBS Lett 1989;243:199.

197. Westerlund B, Korhonen TK. Bacterial proteins binding to the mammalian extracellular matrix. Mol Microbiol 1993;9:687.

198. Karr JF, Nowicki BJ, Truong LD, Hull RA, Moulds JJ, Hull SI. *pap*-2-encoded fimbriae adhere to the P blood group-related glycosphingolipid stage-specific embryonic antigen 4 in the human kidney. Infect Immunol 1990;58:4055.

199. Tippett P, Andrews PW, Knowles BB, Solter D, Goodfellow PN. Red cell antigens P (globoside) and Luke: identification by monoclonal antibodies defining murine stage-specific embryonic antigens -3 and -4 (SSEA-3 and SSEA-4). Vox Sang 1986;51:53.

200. Breimer ME. Chemical and immunological identification of the Forssman pentaglycosylceramide in human kidneys. Glycoconjugate 1985;2:375.

201. Roberts JA, Kaack MB, Baskin G, Marklund B-I, Normark S. Epitopes of the P-fimbrial adhesin of *E. coli* cause different urinary tract infections. J Urol 1997;158:1610.

202. Plos K, Lomberg H, Hull S, Johansson I, Svanborg-Edén C. *Escherichia coli* in patients with renal scarring: genotype and phenotype of Gal α1-4Galβ-Forssman- and mannose-specific adhesins. Pediatr Infect Dis J 1991;10:15.

203. Svanborg-Edén C, Bjursten LM, Hull R, et al. Influence of adhesins on the interactions of *E. coli* with human phagocytes. Infect Immunol 1984;44:672.

204. Tewari R, Ikeda T, Malaviya R, et al. The PapG tip adhesin of P fimbriae protects *Escherichia coli* from neutrophil bactericidal activity. Infect Immunol 1994;62:5296.

205. Tullus K, Brauner A, Fryklund B, et al. Host factors versus virulence-associated bacterial characteristics in neonatal and infantile bacteremia and meningitis caused by *Escherichia coli*. J Med Microbiol 1992;36:203.

206. Buchanan K, Falkow S, Hull RA, Hull SI. Frequency among *Enterobacteriaceae* of the DNA sequences encoding type 1 pili. J Bacteriol 1985;152:799.

207. Ørskov F, Ørskov I, Jann B, Jann K. Tamm-Horsfall protein or uromucoid is the normal urinary slime that traps type 1 fimbriated *Escherichia coli*. Lancet 1983;i:8173.

208. Ofek I, Goldman J, Zafriri D, Lis H, Adar R, Sharon N. Anti-*Escherichia coli* adhesin activity of cranberry and blueberry juices. N Engl J Med 1991;324:1599.

209. Hagberg L, Hull R, Hull S, Falkow S, Freter R, Svanborg C. Contribution of adhesion to bacterial persistence in the mouse urinary tract. Infect Immunol 1983;40:265.

210. Johnson JR, Moseley SL, Roberts PL, Stamm WE. Aerobactin and other virulence factor genes among strains of *Escherichia coli* causing urosepsis: association with patient characteristics. Infect Immunol 1988;56:405.

211. Mobley HLT, Chippendale GR, Tenney JH, Hull RA, Warren JW. Expression of type 1 fimbriae may be required for persistence of *Escherichia coli* in the catheterized urinary tract. J Clin Mibrobiol 1987;25:2253.

212. Hacker J, Schmidt G, Hughes C, Knapp S, Marget M, Goebel W. Cloning and characterization of genes involved in production of mannose-resistant neuraminidase-susceptible (X) fimbriae from a uropathogenic O6:K15:H31 *Escherichia coli* strain. Infect Immunol 1985;47:434.

213. Abraham SN, Land M, Ponniah S, Endres R, Hasty DL, Babu JP. Glycerol-induced unraveling of the tight helical conformation of *Escherichia coli* type 1 fimbriae. J Bacteriol 1992;174:5145.

214. Ponniah S, Endres RO, Hasty DL, Abrham SN. Fragmentation of *Escherichia coli* type 1 fimbriae exposes cryptic D-mannose-binding sites. J Bacteriol 1991;173:4195.

215. Russell PW, Orndorff PE. Lesions in two *Escherichia coli* type 1 pilus genes alter pilus number and length without affecting receptor binding. J Bacteriol 1992;174:5923.

216. Eisenstein BI. Phase variation of type 1 fimbriae in *Escherichia coli* is under transcriptional control. Science 1981;214:337.

217. Klemm P. Two regulatory *fim* genes, *fimB* and *fimE*, control the phase variation of type 1 fimbriae in *Escherichia coli*. EMBO J 1986;5:1389.

218. Nowicki B, Rhen M, Väisänen-Rhen V, Pere A, Korhonen TK. Immunofluorescence study of fimbrial phase variation in *Escherichia coli* KS71. J Bacteriol 1984;160:691.

219. Hultgren SJ, Portner TN, Schaeffer AJ, Duncan JL. Role of type 1 pili and effects of phase variation on lower urinary tract infections produced by *Escherichia coli*. Infect Immunol 1985;50:370.

220. Schaeffer AJ, Schwan WR, Hultgren SJ, Duncan JL. Relationship of type 1 pilus expression in *Escherichia coli* to ascending urinary tract infection in mice. Infect Immunol 1987;55:373.

221. Virkola R, Westerlund B, Holthöfer H, Parkkinen J, Kelomaki M, Korhonen TK. Binding characteristics of *Escherichia coli* adhesins in human urinary bladder. Infect Immunol 1988;56:2615.

222. Westerlund B, Kuusela P, Risteli J, et al. The 075X adhesin of uropathogenic *Escherichia coli* is a type IV collagen-binding protein. Mol Microbiol 1989;3:329.

223. Sokurenko EV, Courtney HS, Abraham SN, Klemm P, Hasty DL. Functional heterogeneity of type 1 fimbriae of *Escherichia coli*. Infect Immunol 1992;60:4709.

224. Virkola R. Binding characteristics of *Escherichia coli* type 1 fimbriae in the human kidney. FEMS Microbiol Lett 1987;40:257.

225. Rhen M, Mäkelä PH, Korhonen TK. P fimbriae of *Escherichia coli* are subject to phase variation. FEMS Microbiol Lett 1983;19:267.

226. Goetz MB, Silverblatt FJ. Stimulation of human polymorphonuclear leukocyte oxidative metabolism by type 1 pili from *Escherichia coli*. Infect Immunol 1987;55:534.

227. Ofek I, Sharon N. Lectino-phagocytosis: a molecular mechanism of recognition between cell surface sugars and lectins in the phagocytosis of bacteria. Infect Immunol 1988;56:539.

228. Baddour LM, Christensen GD, Simpson WA, Beachey EH. Microbial adherence. In: Mandell GL, Dangler RG, Bennett JE, eds. Principles and Practice of Infectious Disease, Vol 2. NY: Churchill Livingstone, 1989:9–25.

229. Keith BR, Harris SL, Russell PW, Orndorff PE. Effect of type 1 piliation on *in vitro* killing of *Escherichia coli* by mouse peritoneal macrophages. Infect Immunol 1990;58:3448.

230. Gbarah A, Gahmberg CG, Ofek I, Jacobi U, Sharon N. Identification of the leukocyte adhesion molecules CD/11CD18 as receptors for type 1 fimbriated (mannose specific) *Escherichia coli*. Infect Immunol 1991;59:4524.

231. Malaviya R, Ikeda T, Ross E, Abraham SN. Mast cell modulation of neutrophil influx and bacterial clearance at sites of infection through TNF-alpha. Nature 1996;381:77.

232. Tewari R, MacGregor JI, Ikeda T, Little JR, Hultgren SJ, Abraham SN. Neutrophil activation by nascent *fimH* subunits of type 1 fimbriae purified from the periplasm of *Escherichia coli*. J Biol Chem 1993;268:3009.

233. Ponniah S, Abraham SN, Endres RO. T-cell-independent stimulation of immunoglobulin secretion in resting human B lymphocytes by the mannose-specific adhesion of *Escherichia coli* type 1 fimbriae. Infect Immunol 1992;60:5197.

234. Mobley HLT, Jarvis KG, Elwood JP, et al. Isogenic P-fimbrial deletion mutants of pyelonephritogenic *Escherichia coli*: the role of αGal(1-4)βGal binding in virulence of a wild type strain. Mol Microbiol 1993;10:143.

235. Gally DL, Bogan JA, Eisenstein BI, Blomfield IC. Environmental regulation of the *fim* switch controlling type 1 fimbrial phase variation in *Escherichia coli* K-12: effects of temperature and media. J Bacteriol 1993;175:6186.

236. Schaeffer A, Jones J, Dunn J. Association of an in vitro *Escherichia coli* adherence to vaginal and buccal epithelial cells with susceptibility of women to recurrent urinary tract infection. N Engl J Med 1981;304:1062.

237. Van der Woude MW, Braaten BA, Low DA. Evidence for global regulatory control of pilus expression in *Escherichia coli* by Lrp and DNA methylation: model building based on analysis of pap. Mol Microbiol 1992;6:2429.

238. Bakker A, Smith DW. Methylation of GATC sites is required for precise timing between rounds of DNA replication of *E. coli*. J Bacteriol 1989;171:5738.

239. Modrich P. Methyl-directed DNA mismatch repair. J Biol Chem 1989;264:6597.

240. Gally DL, Rucker TJ, Blomfield IC. The leucine-responsive regulatory protein binds to the *fim* switch to control phase variation of type 1 fimbrial expression *Escherichia coli* K-12. J Bacteriol 1994;176:5665.

241. Korhonen TK, Valtonen MV, Parkkinen J, et al. Serotypes, hemolysin production, and receptor recognition of *Escherichia coli* strains associated with neonatal sepsis and meningitis. Infect Immunol 1985;48:486.

242. Schmoll T, Morschhauser J, Ott M, Van Die I, Hacker J. Complete genetic organization and functional aspects of the *Escherichia coli* S fimbrial adhesin determinant: nucleotide sequence of the genes sfa B, C, D, E, F. Microbiol Pathog 1990;9:331.

243. Hacker J, Kestler H, Hoschutzky H, Jann K, Lottspeich F, Korhonen TK. Cloning and characterization of the S fimbrial adhesin II complex of an *Escherichia coli* causing urinary tract infections. Infect Immunol 1993;61:544.

244. Riegman N, Kusters R, Van Vegel H, et al. F1C fimbriae of a uropathogenic *Escherichia coli* strain: genetic and functional organization of the *foc* gene cluster and identification of minor subunits. J Bacteriol 1990;172:1114.

245. Pawelzik M, Heeseman J, Hacker J, Opferkuch W. Cloning and characterization of a new type of fimbriae (S/FIC-related fimbriae) expressed by an *Escherichia coli* O75 : K1 : H7 culture isolate. Infect Immunol 1988;56:2918.

246. Pere A, Leinonen M, Väisänen-Rhen V, Rhen M, Korhonen TK. Occurrence of type-1C fimbriae on *Escherichia coli* strains isolated from human extraintestinal infections. J Gen Microbiol 1985;131:1705.

247. High NJ, Hales BA, Jann K, Boulnois J. A block of urovirulence genes encoding multiple fimbriae and hemolysin in *Escherichia coli* O4 : K12 : H-. Infect Immunol 1988;56:513.

248. Siitonen A, Martikainen R, Ikaheimo R, Palmgren J, Makela PH. Virulence-associated characteristics of *Escherichia coli* in urinary tract infections: a statistical analysis with special attention to type 1C fimbriation. Microbiol Pathog 1993;15:65.

249. Korhonen TK, Parkkinen J, Hacker J, et al. Binding of *Escherichia coli* S fimbriae to human kidney epithelium. Infect Immunol 1986;54:322.

250. Marre R, Kreft B, Hacker J. Genetically engineered S and F1C fimbriae differ in their contribution to adherence of *Escherichia coli* to cultured renal tubular cells. Infect Immunol 1990;58:3434.

251. Virkola R, Parkkinen J, Hacker J, Korhonen TK. Sialyloligosaccharide chain laminin as an extracellular matrix target for S fimbriae of *Escherichia coli*. Infect Immunol 1993;61:4480.

252. Nowicki B, Labigne A, Moseley S, Hull R, Hull S, Moulds J. The Dr hemagglutinin, afimbrial adhesin AFA-I and AFA-III, and F1845 fimbriae of uropathogenic and diarrhea-associated *Escherichia coli* belong to a family of hemagglutinins with Dr receptor recognition. Infect Immunol 1990;58:279.

253. Nowicki B, Hart A, Coyne KE, Lublin DM, Nowicki S. Short consensus repeat-3 domain of recombinant decay-accelerating factor is recognized by *Escherichia coli* recombinant Dr adhesin in a model of cell-cell interaction. J Exp Med 1993;178:2115.

254. Nowicki B, Barrish JP, Korhonen T, Hull RA, Hull SI. Molecular cloning of the *Escherichia coli* O75X adhesin. Infect Immunol 1987;55:3168.

255. Väisänen-Rhen V. Fimbriae-like hemagglutinin of *Escherichia coli* O75 strains. Infect Immunol 1989;46:401.

256. Labigne-Roussel AF, Lark D, Schoolnik G, Falkow S. Cloning and expression of an afimbrial adhesin (AFA-I) responsible for P blood group-independent, mannose-resistant hemagglutination from a pyelonephritis *Escherichia coli* strain. Infect Immunol 1984;46:251.

257. Nowicki B, Svanborg-Edén C, Hull R, Hull S. Molecular analysis and epidemiology of the Dr hemagglutinin of uropathogenic *Escherichia coli*. Infect Immunol 1989;57:446.

258. Johnson JR, Skubitz KM, Nowicki BJ, Jacques-Palaz K, Rakita RM. Nonlethal adherence to human neutrophils mediated by Dr antigen-specific adhesins of *Escherichia coli*. Infect Immunol 1995;63:309.

259. Cross AS, Kim KS, Wright DC, Sadoff JC, Gemski P. Role of lipopolysaccharide and capsule in the serum resistance of bacteremic strains of *Escherichia coli*. J Infect Dis 1986;154:497.

260. Weiser JN, Gotschlich EC. Outer membrane protein A (OmpA)

contributes to serum resistance and pathogenicity of *Escherichia coli* K-1. Infect Immunol 1991;59:2252.

261. Kaijser B. Immunology of *Escherichia coli:* K antigen and its relation to urinary-tract infection. J Infect Dis 1973;131:6.

262. Israele V, Darabi A, McCracken GJ Jr. The role of bacterial virulence factors and Tamm-Horsfall protein in the pathogenesis of *Escherichia coli* urinary tract infections in infants. Am J Dis Child 1987;141:1230.

263. Kaijser B, Larsson P, Olling S, Schneerson R. Protection against acute ascending pyelonephritis caused by *Escherichia coli* in rats, using isolated capsular antigen conjugated to bovine serum albumin. Infect Immunol 1983;39:142.

264. Russo TA, Moffitt MC, Hammer CH, Frank MM. Tn*pho*A-mediated disruption of K54 capsular polysaccharide genes in *Escherichia coli* confers serum sensitivity. Infect Immunol 1993;61:3578.

265. Jacobson SH, Östenson C-G, Tullus K, Brauner A. Serum resistance in *Escherichia coli* strains causing acute pyelonephritis and bacteraemia. APMIS 1992;100:147.

266. Montgomerie JZ, Bindereif A, Neilands JB, Kalmanson GM, Guze LB. Association of hydroxamate siderophore (aerobactin) with *Escherichia coli* isolated from patients with bacteremia. Infect Immunol 1984;46:835.

267. Ørskov I, Svanborg-Edén C, Ørskov F. Aerobactin production of serotyped *Escherichia coli* from urinary tract infection. Med Microbiol Immunol 1988;177:9.

268. Zhang JP, Normark S. Induction of gene expression in *Escherichia coli* after Pilus-mediated adherence. Science 1996; 273:1234.

269. Boehm DF, Welch RA, Snyder IS. Domains of *Escherichia coli* hemolysin (HlyA) involved in binding of calcium and erythrocyte membranes. Infect Immunol 1990;58:1959.

270. Mobley HLT, Green DM, Trifillis AL, et al. Pyelonephritogenic *Escherichia coli* and killing of cultured human renal proximal tubular epithelial cells: role of hemolysin in some strains. Infect Immunol 1990;58:1281.

271. Moayeri M, Welch R. Effects of temperature, time and toxin concentration of lesion formation by the *Escherichia coli* hemolysin. Infect Immunol 1994;62:4124.

272. Warren J, Mobley H, Hebel J, Trifillis A. Cytolethality of hemolytic *Escherichia coli* to primary human renal proximal tubular cell cultures obtained from different donors. Urology 1995; 45:706.

273. Welch RA, Pellett S. Transcriptional organization of the *Escherichia coli* hemolysin. J Bacteriol 1988;170:1622.

274. Carmona M, Balsalobre C, Munoa F, et al. *Escherichia coli* hha mutants, DNA supercoiling and expression of the haemolysin genes from the recombinant plasmid pANN202-312. Mol Microbiol 1993;9:1011.

275. O'Hanley P, Lalonde G, Ji G. Alpha-hemolysin contributes to the pathogenicity of piliated digalactoside-binding *Escherichia coli* in the kidney: efficacy of an alpha-hemolysin vaccine in preventing renal injury in the BALB/c mouse model of pyelonephritis. Infect Immunol 1991;59:1153.

276. Kreft B, Marre R, Schramm U, Wirth R. Aggregation substance of *Enterococcus faecalis* mediates adhesion to cultured renal tubular cells. Infect Immunol 1992;60:25.

277. Wirth R. The sex phermone system of *Enterococcus faecalis:* more than just a plasmid-collection mechanism? Eur J Biochem 1994;222:235.

278. Tsuchimori N, Hayashi R, Shino A, Yamazaki T, Okonogi K. *Enterococcus faecalis* aggravates pyelonephritis caused by *Pseudomonas aeruginosa* in experimental ascending mixed urinary tract infection in mice. Infect Immunol 1994;62:4534.

279. Roychoudhury S, Zielinski NA, Ninfa AJ, et al. Inhibitors of two-component signal transduction systems: inhibition of alginate gene activation in *Pseudomonas aeruginosa*. Proc Natl Acad Sci USA 1993;90:965.

280. Kadurugamuwa J, Lam J, Beveridge T. Interaction of gentamicin with the A band and B band lipopolysaccharides of *Pseudomonas aeruginosa* and its possible lethal effects. Antimicrob Agents Chemother 1993;37:715.

281. Strom MS, Lory S. Structure-function and biogenesis of the type IV pili. Annu Rev Microbiol 1993;47:565.

282. Coburn J. *Pseudomonas aeruginosa* exoenzymes S. Curr Top Microbiol Immunol 1992;175:133.

283. Britigan BE, Roeder TE, Rasmussen GT, Shasby DM, McCormick ML, Cox CD. Interaction of the *Pseudomonas aeruginosa* secretory products pyocyanin and pyochelin generates hydroxyl radical and causes synergistic damage to endothelial cells. J Clin Invest 1992;90:2187.

284. Amako K, Meno Y, Takade A. Fine structures of the capsules of *Klebsiella pneumonia* and *Escherichia coli* K1. J Bacteriol 1988;170:4960.

285. Tarkkanen A-M, Allen BL, Williams PH, et al. Fimbriation, capsulation, and iron-scavenging systems of *Klebsiella* strains associated with human urinary tract infection. Infect Immunol 1992;60:1187.

286. Tarkkanen A-M, Allen BL, Westerlund B, et al. Type V collagen as the target for type 3 fimbriae, enterobacterial adherence organelles. Mol Microbiol 1990;4:1353.

287. Mobley HLT, Chippendale GR, Tenney JH, et al. MR/K hemagglutination of *Providentia stuartii* correlates with adherence to catheters and with persistence in catheter-associated bacteriuria. J Infect Dis 1988;157:264.

288. Parsons CL, Stauffer C, Mulholland SG, Griffith DP. Effect of ammonium on bacterial adherence to bladder transitional epithelium. J Urol 1984;132:365.

289. Lomberg H, Cedergren B, Leffler H, Nilsson B, Carlström A-S, Svanborg-Edén C. Influence of blood group on the availability of receptors for attachment of uropathogenic *Escherichia coli*. Infect Immunol 1986;51:919.

290. Svanborg-Edén C, Larsson P, Lomberg H. Attachment *of Proteus mirabilis* to human urinary sediment epithelial cells in vitro is different from that for *Escherichia coli*. Infect Immunol 1980;28:804.

291. Belas R. Expression of multiple flagellin-encoding genes of *Proteus mirabilis*. J Bacteriol 1994;176:7169.

292. Mobley HLT. Virulence of *Proteus mirabilis*. In: Mobley HLT, Warren JW, eds. Urinary tract infections: molecular pathogenesis and clinical management. Washington, DC. ASM Press, 1996:245–269.

293. Bollgren I, Winberg J. The periurethral aerobic flora in girls highly susceptible to urinary infections. Acta Paediatr Scand 1976;65:81.

294. Svanborg-Edén C, Lidin-Janson G, Lindberg U. Adhesiveness to urinary tract epithelial cells of fecal and urinary *Escherichia coli* isolates from patients with symptomatic urinary tract infection or asymptomatic bacteriuria of varying duration. J Urol 1979;122:185.

295. Redondo-Lopez V, Cook RL, Sobel JD. Emerging role of lactobacilli in the control and maintenance of the vaginal bacterial microflora. Rev Infect Dis 1990;12:856.

296. Schaeffer AJ, Jones JM, Falkowski WS, Duncan JL, Chmiel JS, Plotkin BJ. Variable adherence of uropathogenic *Escherichia coli* to epithelial cells from women with recurrent urinary tract infection. J Urol 1982;128:1227.

297. Norden C, Green G, Kass E. Antibacterial mechanisms of the urinary bladder. J Clin Invest 1968;47:2689.

298. Mannhardt W, Becker A, Putzer M, et al. Host defense within the urinary tract, I: bacterial adhesion initiates an uroepithelial defense mechanism. Pediatr Nephrol 1996;10:568.

299. Mostafavi M, Stein PC, Parsons L. Production of soluble virulence factor by *Escherichia coli*. J Urol 1995;153:1441.

300. Adachi T, Ohta H, Yamada H, Futenma A, Kato K, Hirano K. Quantitative analysis of extracellular-superoxide dismutase in serum and urine by ELISA with monoclonal antibody. Clinica Chimica Acta 1992;212:89.

301. Hjalmarsson K, Marklund SL, Engström Å, Edlund T. Isolation and sequence of complementary DNA encoding human extracellular superoxide dismutase. Proc Natl Acad Sci USA 1987;84:6340.

302. Chambers ST, Kunin CM. Osmoprotective activity for *Escherichia coli* in mammalian renal papilla and urine: correlation of glycine and proline betaines and sorbitol with response to osmotic stress. J Clin Invest 1987;80:1255.

303. Kunin CM, Tong HH, White LVA, Villarejo M. Growth of

Escherichia coli in human urine: role of salt tolerance and accumulation of glycine betaine. J Infect Dis 1992;166:1311.

304. Robledo JA, Serrano A, Domingue GL. Outer membrane proteins of E. coli in host-pathogen interaction in urinary tract infection. J Urol 1990;143:386.

305. Malouin F, Chamberland S, Brochu N, Parr TR Jr. Influence of growth media on *Escherichia coli* cell composition and ceftazidime susceptibility. Antimicrob Agents Chemother 1991;35:477.

306. Reinhart HH, Obedeanu N, Robinson R, Korzeniowski O, Kaye D, Sobel JD. Urinary excretion of Tamm-Horsfall protein in elderly women. J Urol 1991;146:806.

307. Wold AE, Mestechy J, Svanborg EC. Agglutination of *Escherichia coli* by secretory IgA: a result of interaction between bacterial mannose-specific adhesins and immunoglobulin carbohydrate. Monogr Allergy 1988;24:307.

308. Coppa GV, Gabrielli O, Giorgi P, et al. Preliminary study of breast feeding and bacterial adhesion to uroepithelial cells. Lancet 1990;335:569.

309. Pisacane A, Graziano L, Mazzarella G, Scarpellino B, Zona G. Breast-feeding and urinary tract infection. J Pediatr 1992; 120:87.

310. Svanborg C. Resistance to urinary tract infection. N Engl J Med 1993;329:802.

311. Fletcher KS, Bremer EG, Schwarting GA. P blood group regulation of glycosphingolipid levels in human erythrocytes. J Biol Chem 1979;254:11196.

312. Tomisawa S, Kogure T, Kuroume T, et al. P blood group and proneness to urine tract infection in Japanese children. Scand J Infect Dis 1989;21:403.

313. Clausen H, Hakomori SI. ABO and related histo-blood group antigens: immunochemical differences in carrier isotypes and their distribution. Vox Sang 1989;56:1.

314. Stapleton A, Nudelman E, Clausen H, Hakomori S, Stamm WE. Binding of uropathogenic *Escherichia coli* R45 to glycolipids extracted from vaginal epithelial cells is dependent on histo-blood group secretor status. J Clin Invest 1992;90:965.

315. Kinane E, Blackwell C, Brettle R, Weir D, Winstanley F, Elton R. ABO blood group secretor state and susceptibility to urinary tract infection. Br Med J 1982;285:7.

316. Jantausch BA, Criss VR, O'Donnell R, et al. Association of the Lewis blood group phenotypes with urinary tract infection in children. J Pediatr 1994;124:863.

317. Stapleton A, Hooton TM, Fennell C, Roberts PL, Stamm WE. Effect of secretor status on vaginal and rectal colonization with fimbriated *Escherichia coli* in women with and without recurrent urinary tract infection. J Infect Dis 1995;171:717.

318. Lomberg H, Jodal U, Leffler H, de Man P, Svanborg C. Blood group non-secretors have an increased inflammatory response to urinary tract infection. Scan J Infect Dis 1992;24:77.

319. Smellie JM, Poulton A, Prescod NP. Retrospective study of children with renal scarring associated with reflux and urinary infection. Br Med J 1994;308:1193.

320. Lidefelt KJ, Bollgren JI, Nord CE. Changes in periurethral microflora after antimicrobial drugs. Arch Dis Child 1991;66:683.

321. Donabedian H, O'Donnell E, Drill C, Lipton LM, Khuder SA, Burnham JC. Prevention of subsequent urinary tract infection in women by the use of anti-adherence antimicrobial agents: a double-blind comparison of enoxacin with co-trimoxazole. J Antimicrobial Chemother 1995;35:409.

322. Herthelius BM, Hedstrom KG, Möllby R, Nord CE, Pettersson L, Winberg J. Pathogenesis of urinary tract infection-amoxicillin induces genital *Escherichia coli* colonization. Infection 1988; 16:263.

323. Uehling D, Hopkins W, Dahmer L, Balish E. Phase I clinical trial of vaginal mucosal immunization for recurrent urinary tract infections. J Urol 1994;152:2308.

324. Ruttgers H, Grischke E. Elevation of secretory IgA antibodies in the urinary tract by immunostimulation for the pre-operative treatment and post-operative prevention of urinary tract infections. Urol Int 1987;42:424.

325. Schulman S, Corbusier A, Michiels M, Taenzer H. Oral immunotherapy of recurrent urinary tract infections: a double-blind placebo-controlled multicenter study. J Urol 1993;150:917.

326. Brooks S, Lyons J, Braude A. Immunization against retrograde pyelonephritis. Am J Pathol 1974;74:345.

327. Kaijser B, Larsson P, Olling S. Protection against ascending *Escherichia coli* pyelonephritis in rats and significance of local immunity. Infect Immunol 1978;20:78.

328. Kaijser B, Larsson P, Nimmich W, Soderstrom T. Antibodies of *Escherichia coli* K and O antigens in protection against acute pyelonephritis. Prog Allergy 1983;33:275.

329. Moayeri N, Collins CM, O'Hanley P. Efficacy of a *Proteus mirabilis* outer membrane protein vaccine in preventing experimental *Proteus* pyelonephritis in a BALB/c mouse model. Infect Immunol 1991;59:3778.

330. Pecha B, Low D, O'Hanley P. Gal-Gal pili vaccines prevent pyelonephritis by piliated *Escherichia coli* in a murine model. Single-component Gal-Gal pili vaccines prevent pyelonephritis by homologous and heterologous piliated *E. coli* strains. J Clin Invest 1989;83:2102.

331. Roberts JA, Hardaway B, Kaack MB, Fussell EF, Baskin G. Prevention of pyelonephritis by immunization with P-fimbriae. J Urol 1984;131:602.

332. Denich K, Blyn LB, Craiu A, et al. DNA sequences of three *papA* genes from uropathogenic *Escherichia coli* strains: evidence of structural and serological conservation. Infect Immunol 1991;59:3849.

333. Schmidt M, O'Hanley P, Lark D, Schoolnik GK. Synthetic peptides corresponding to protective epitopes of *Escherichia coli* digalactoside-binding pilin prevent infection in a murine pyelonephritis model. Proc Natl Acad Sci USA 1988;85:1247.

334. Langermann S, Palaszynski S, Barnhart M, et al. Prevention of mucosal *Escherichia coli* infection by FimH-adhesin-based systemic vaccination. Science 1997;276:607.

CHAPTER 27

Vesicoureteral Reflux

Martin Kaefer and David Diamond

HISTORY

The role of the ureter in unidirectional flow of urine from the kidney to the bladder was first noted by Galen in the first century AD.[1] In 1903 Sampson proposed a "ureterovesical lock mechanism" to describe the physiologic principle that served to prevent reflux.[2] Although vesicoureteral reflux (VUR) has long been recognized in humans and other species, the understanding that pathologic changes of the upper urinary tract could result from VUR was not appreciated until the pioneering work of Hutch in 1952.[3] He recognized a correlation between reflux and chronic renal damage from pyelonephritis and concluded that bacterial access to the upper urinary tract was significantly increased because of the retrograde flow of infected urine. Hutch's work in adult paraplegics was then applied to the pediatric population by Hodson, who recognized a similarly high correlation between reflux and chronic renal damage in children.[4] Tauffer is credited with performing the first ureteroneocystotomy in 1877.[5] Landmark advances in the surgical management of VUR by Vermooten, Hutch, Politano, Leadbetter, Paquin, Lich, Stephens, Glenn, Cohen, and others have provided a safe and effective means of managing this anatomic problem.[3, 6–11] The introduction of expectant therapy involving prophylactic antibiotics, first championed by Smellie, has dramatically increased our understanding of the natural history of reflux. Stephens, in identifying VUR in twins, suggested a genetic propensity for developing VUR.[12] Current work focuses on further defining the indications for surgical versus medical management and defining the genetic elements responsible for this disorder.[13, 14]

INCIDENCE (TABLE 27.1)

The true incidence of vesicoureteral reflux in normal infants is unknown. Many early studies point to a low incidence of reflux in asymptomatic children who have not had issuing indicated (approximately 1%).[14–17] Poor definition of the populations being studied, lack of standardized methods for testing for VUR, and the nonphysiologic means of assessing for reflux used in many of these early studies prevent us from drawing any absolute conclusions from this early work. A recent study by Zerin et al demonstrating a high incidence of VUR in children with prenatal hydronephrosis tends to question earlier conclusions regarding the low prevalence of reflux.[18, 19]

The incidence of VUR in a given population depends on many factors, including family history, race, gender, and age. Vesicoureteral reflux is the most commonly inherited anomaly of the genitourinary tract. Beginning with Stephens' initial observation of reflux in twins, many authors have sought to define the incidence of sibling reflux.[12, 20–24] In the largest cohort of siblings studied to date, Wan et al identified 144 cases of vesicoureteral reflux in 622 children for an overall prevalence of 27%.[25] This incidence of roughly 25% of siblings being affected is in agreement with most other historical series. As would be expected from the natural history of this disease, reflux is less frequently detected in siblings older than the index case relative to those that are younger (19% and 31%, respectively).[25, 26] Although having a sibling with VUR increases the incidence of developing reflux, few characteristics of the index case can predict the characteristics of the reflux in the sibling. Neither the grade of reflex nor presence of established scars in the index patient appears to correlate with reflux grade in the sibling.[26] This unpredictable variability in grade of reflux between family members initially lead many authors to propose a polygenic or multifactorial mode of inheritance.[27] A slightly higher rate of transmission from female to female (than from female to male) suggested an X-linked component to the model.[26] However, the inability to confirm a statistically significant correlation between sex of the index patient and incidence of sibling reflux does not support this contention. While a polygenic model is attractive, the 50% incidence of sibling reflux within the first 2 years of life, coupled with the higher incidence of VUR transmission from

TABLE 27.1. *Demographics of VUR*

Incidence of VUR relative to demographic characteristics (all grades of reflux included)		
Population	%	Author
General	0.5–1.0	Politano (1960)
Mode of presentation		
Prenatal sonography	38	Zerin (1993)
Assymptomatic bacteriuria	5–17	NOT (1975)
Symptomatic UTI	30–50	Smellie (1972)
Familial		
Sibling of index	8–33	Wan (1996), Noe (1992)
Twin sibling	66	Wan (1996)
Child of index	66	Noe (1992)
Age		
UTI (children/adults)	26.4/5.2	Baker (1966)
Sibling (<2/>2 years)	46/28	Noe (1992)
Gender (F/M)[1]	30–50/14	Smellie (1972)
Race[1]		
Black	12	Skoog (1991)
White	41	Skoog (1991)

[1]Percentage of individuals presenting with urinary tract infection.
NOT, Cooperative study of asymptomatic bacteriuria in school children in Newcastle upon type.

parent to child (66%) and for twin siblings (66%) suggests the possibility of an autosomal dominant mode of inheritance with variable penetrance.[25, 26]

An autosomal dominant mode of transmission is further suggested from experimental work involving the PAX family of transcriptional regulatory factors.[13] PAX genes are responsible in most species for body segmentation and cell specification.[28] One member of these highly conserved genes, PAX-2 is specifically expressed in the kidney by cells destined to become the ureter, renal pelvis, and collecting duct system.[29] Experimental ablation ("knock out") of one of the alleles (paired genes encoding for a molecule) can result in metanephric arrest and megaureter in mice, suggesting that it may play a role in ureteral development and VUR.[30] PAX-2 mutations occurring in humans are inherited in an autosomal dominant manner.[31] These mutations have been linked to specific syndromes that include vesicoureteral reflux.[30]

That the incidence of VUR varies among national groups and races further suggests a heritable nature to reflux.[32] Kunin et al were the first to draw attention to this racial difference.[33–35] In evaluating school children with asymptomatic bacteriuria, they found nearly one third the incidence of VUR in the black patients (9% black versus 21% white). Blacks also had nearly one third the incidence of asymptomatic bacteriuria (0.5% and 1.2%, respectively) resulting overall in a rate of identification of VUR in the black population that is 10-fold lower than in whites. Askari and Belman in evaluating children with symptomatic UTI noted an incidence of reflux in black children relative to white children of 1:3.4 (12% in blacks versus 41% in whites).[36]

Despite the lower incidence of VUR, Skoog and Belman found no significant differences in the mode of presentation, age at presentation, or age at resolution between these two groups.[37] Among whites, red hair appears to confer a slightly higher probability of reflux.[37]

The frequency with which VUR is identified is inversely proportional to age.[7] Baker et al, in their study of VUR in children with bacteriuria, found 70% of children younger than 1 year of age to have VUR as compared to 25% of children who had reached the age of 4.[38] Nearly every other study of VUR, regardless of mode of presentation, has confirmed this phenomenon.

Significant gender differences in the prevalence of reflux have also been appreciated. These gender-associated differences likewise depend on the age at presentation. Most VUR identified in children screened as a result of a febrile UTI or asymptomatic bacteriuria was seen in females.[39] In contrast, when patients presented for radiologic workup as a result of prenatal sonographic findings, the gender distribution was markedly different. Zerin found that reflux was as likely to be identified in males as in females, whereas most other neonatal studies found that up to 80% of neonates diagnosed prenatally with hydronephrosis were male.[19, 40–44] The higher incidence found in boys in these earlier studies may, in part, be a result of the increased frequency of hydronephrosis in male fetuses and a more consistent performance of cystography in male subjects caused by the need for excluding urethral pathology (i.e., posterior urethral valves). Regardless of age, when VUR is diagnosed it is more frequently of greater severity in boys than in girls.[22, 24, 39] Higher voiding detrusor pressures in boys may help explain this association.[9, 45]

ETIOLOGY

Under normal physiologic conditions the function of the ureterovesical junction (UVJ) is to facilitate the unidirectional flow of urine from the upper urinary tract to the bladder. Failure to perform this function can be manifested in obstruction or vesicoureteral reflux. When left untreated, the severity and pathologic consequences of VUR can range from uncomplicated, spontaneous resolution to severe, irreversible damage to the upper urinary tract.

Normal Physiology of the UVJ

The role of the ureter in propelling urine unidirectionally from the kidney was first noted by Galen in the first century.[1] He came to the conclusion that "liquid can enter the bladder through the ureters, but is unable to go back again the same way" by observing that when the urethra was ligated, urine could find no egress from the bladder.[46] The valvular role that the UVJ plays depends on the anatomic relationship between the ureter and the bladder.[2] The ureter, composed of three muscle layers (inner longitudinal, middle circular, outer longitudinal), travels in a retroperitoneal course from the kidney to the bladder. After penetrating the bladder wall, the ureter takes a medial course as it travels from the external aspect of the detrusor into the bladder lumen. Under normal conditions, the ureter is securely anchored to the bladder wall throughout its entire transmural course. The inner longitudinal layer of the ureter continues into the bladder where the fibers then fan out, travelling medially to merge with similar fibers from the contralateral ureter, and inferiorly to end in the bladder neck. The extension of this inner longitudinal layer of muscle thereby makes up the superficial trigone. In a similar fashion, the adventitial layer of the ureter (also known as Waldeyer's Sheath) continues inferomedially from the ureteral orifice and is in continuity with the deep trigone.[47] This anatomic arrangement serves to maintain a competent one-way valve at the UVJ. This valve mechanism is best described by the flap valve principle (Fig. 27.1).[48] Pressure elevation within the reservoir is effectively transmitted to a supple, thin-walled, small diameter conduit (ureter) in a submucosal location, thereby compressing its lumen against the firmer wall of the storage reservoir.[8]

The variables that influence the effectiveness of the flap valve include adequate tunnel length, appropriate muscular backing, intact trigonal muscular tone, and an adequate storage reservoir. Adequate tunnel length to lumen ratio is perhaps the most important variable determining the success of the flap valve mechanism.[8] Paquin identified a 5:1 ratio of ureteral tunnel length to orifice diameter in nonrefluxing children and a 1.4:1 ratio in children with VUR. Suppleness of the conduit

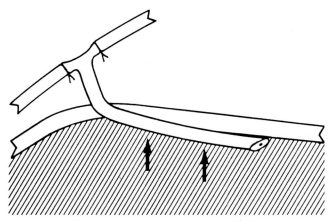

FIG. 27.1. The flap valve principle maintains that pressure elevation within the reservoir is effectively transmitted to a supple, thin-walled, small-diameter conduit (ureter; *arrows*) in a submucosal location, thereby compressing its lumen against the firmer wall of the storage reservoir. Reprinted with permission from Hinman F Jr. Functional classification of conduits for continent urinary diversion. J Urol 1990; 144:27–30.

and firmness of the reservoir wall (i.e., muscle backing) play important roles in providing a successful continence mechanism according to this principle. Integrity of the flap valve also depends on the presence of a low pressure, highly compliant reservoir with an adequate storage capacity.[29] As with any valvular mechanism, pressure above a certain threshold will serve to compromise its efficiency for providing unidirectional flow across the tubular lumen. A recent study of patients undergoing unilateral ureteroneocystotomy to determine the mechanism of contralateral new onset reflux supports this concept.[49] Diamond et al demonstrated a significant positive correlation between the grade of unilateral reflux that was surgically corrected and the onset of new contralateral VUR. This correlation supports the concept that reflux may result from elimination of a pop-off mechanism, thereby effectively reducing the favorable storage characteristics (i.e., capacity) of the reservoir.

Although the function of this valve is largely passive, there is reason to believe that an active component may also be operative. Tone of the trigonal musculature may be important for maintaining a competent ureterovesical junction, particularly during voiding.[50, 51] Early experimental work by Tanagho demonstrated that interruption of the trigone would lead to upward and lateral migration of the ureteral orifice and subsequently to reflux.[52] The same effect was achieved when paralysis of the ipsilateral trigone was created through unilateral lumbar sympathectomy. Electrical stimulation of the trigone had the opposite effect, leading to an inferomedial migration of the ureteral orifice and resistance to flow at the ureterovesical junction. Stephens emphasized the importance of the ureteral musculature itself. He thought that contraction of the longitudinal smooth muscle of the intramural ureter resulted in apposition of the floor and roof of the ureteral orifice.[30] Finally, Ekman et al have shown that diuresis may act to prevent reflux.[48, 53]

Pathophysiology of Vesicoureteral Reflux

Integrity of the flap valve mechanism depends on several intact anatomic relationships and physiologic parameters.[8] Any condition that alters these relationships can lead to compromise of the ureterovesical junction and VUR.

Sampson was the first to recognize the importance of the normal obliquity of the ureter during its intramural course in maintaining a competent valve mechanism. By reimplanting a ureter in an end-to-side fashion he noted that reflux recurred.[2] The minimal length-to-width ratio of ureter that must reside in the bladder to prevent reflux likely varies between patients. In general, once this ratio decreases to less than 3 : 1, reflux is more likely to occur.[54]

Conditions that weaken the muscular support that the bladder provides for the ureter can also lead to reflux. For a flap valve to function properly, the supple tube must be attached to and compressed against a stiff surface. Waldeyer's fascia serves to seal the potential space between the intramural tunnel wall and the ureter and thereby prevent herniation of the periureteral muscular support.[55] Attenuation of the muscle backing caused by a periureteral (Hutch) diverticulum (Fig. 27.2) or an everting ureterocoele can contribute to

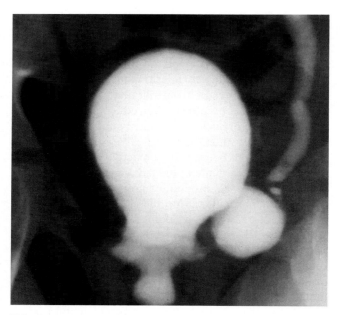

FIG. 27.2. In a periureteral diverticulum, attenuation of the muscle backing within the storage reservoir (bladder) results in the absence of a strong support against which the ureter can be compressed.

reflux.[47, 56–59] An increased prevalence of bladder diverticuli in Menkes' syndrome and Ehler-Danlos syndrome may result in VUR in these conditions.[60, 61] Finally, the likelihood of spontaneous resolution within completely duplicated systems appears not to be as high and may, in part, be the result of anatomic variables that attenuate or distort ureteral backing (i.e., ureterocoeles).[43]

Children with hyperreflexic bladders (i.e., uninhibited contractions) or bladder sphincter dyssynergia have higher than normal intravesical pressure that may contribute to the development of reflux.[62, 63] This viewpoint is supported by the work of Homsy et al who treated 37 cases of VUR and associated bladder hyperreflexia with anticholinergic medication. After an average follow-up of 30 months, 51% of their patients had resolution of the reflux and 11% had significant improvement in the degree of reflux.[64] Although this represents a higher rate of improvement than would be expected in the population as a whole, no proper control arm was included in this study. Further support for persistence of an infantile response to bladder filling (the uninhibited bladder of childhood) as a factor that may cause VUR comes from the work of Koff and Murtagh.[64, 65] They identified 62 neurologically normal children with VUR, 34 of whom had uninhibited bladder contractions associated with voluntary urethral sphincteric contractions, resulting in intermittent periods higher than normal intravesical pressure. Twenty six of the 34 with unbalanced bladder dynamics were treated with anticholinergic medication, whereas eight were not. After an average follow-up of 3.9 years the rates of resolution were revealing. Patients with uninhibited contractions treated with anticholinergic medications had a higher resolution rate than similar individuals who were not treated with anticholinergic medications (44% versus 33%).[66] Only 17% of ureters in bladders with normal urodynamics ceased refluxing during this time period. This demonstrates that not addressing dysfunctional voiding patterns as a factor contributing to VUR may lead to reduced success of medical and surgical management.

Bladder inflammation can contribute to vesicoureteral reflux.[67–70] Bumpus and later Auer and Seager observed that inflammation or periureteral induration could cause an otherwise normally functioning ureterovesical valve to permit reflux.[71, 72] They contended that inflammation led to a more rigid intramural ureter that was more resistant to collapse. Bacterial endotoxins that result in ureteral paralysis may also serve to lower the threshold of the ureter to reflux.[73, 74] Furthermore, inflammation can alter bladder dynamics, potentially causing uninhibited contractions, increasing intravesical pressure, and stressing the valve-like properties of the ureterovesical junction.

The term secondary reflux is used to describe reflux that results, at least in part, from other well-defined abnormalities of the lower urinary tract. Etiologies in-

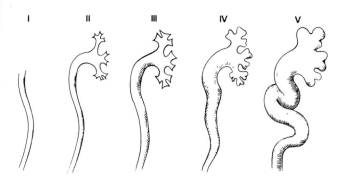

FIG. 27.3. IRS classification system for grading vesicoureteral reflux. Reprinted with permission from Report of the International Reflux Study Committee. Medical versus surgical treatment of primary vesicoureteral reflux: a prospective international reflux study in children. J Urol 1981;125: 277–283.

clude neurogenic bladder dysfunction, anatomic bladder outlet obstruction. (e.g., posterior urethral valves), or iatrogenic injury.[75] Unless these primary pathologies are addressed, the rate of reflux resolution will be substantially diminished relative to individuals with primary ureterovesical dysfunction. The etiologies responsible for secondary vesicoureteral reflux are described at length elsewhere in this text. The remainder of this chapter deals exclusively with the evaluation, natural history, and management of reflux related primarily to congenital anomalies of the ureterovesical junction.

CLASSIFICATION AND EVALUATION

Classification

The role of any grading or staging system is to classify a disease process with respect to its potential for responding to therapy and to the patient's ultimate prognosis. With VUR this should translate into the likelihood of spontaneous resolution and the probability of developing reflux-associated complications. The first grading systems included broad categories. As our imaging capabilities and understanding of the natural history of this disease improved, more refined classification systems have been devised. Nearly three decades ago,

more precise definitions of reflux led Heikel and Park-kulainen[76] and Dwoskin and Perlmutter[77] to propose better stratified classification systems. In 1981 these two systems were combined to create the well-recognized International Reflux Study (IRS) Classification of grades of vesicoureteral reflux (Fig. 27.3).[14] Table 27.2 indicates the likelihood of encountering each grade of reflux at presentation, a distribution that varies depending on the age at which the patient is first observed. The application of this system to many children has confirmed its utility in predicting the likelihood of spontaneous resolution for single system reflux.[78] The lower resolution provided by radionuclide cystography (RNC) has required the development of a separate grading system for this modality. The most widely accepted grading system used today for reflux identified on RNC is that proposed by Willi and Trevis.[79] This system is comprised of three grades that correspond to the following grades on VCUG: Grade I = IRS Grade I, Grade II = IRS Grade II or III, Grade III = IRS Grade IV or V.

While the cystographic findings emphasized in the IRS classification help predict outcome, additional factors may help to further enhance our ability to identify which individuals are more likely to show spontaneous resolution. As previously mentioned, the incidence of reflux highly depends on the age at which it is sought because reflux is known to resolve with time (see Natural History). Therefore, the age of the patient impacts significantly on the outcome of VUR. Possible explanations for reflux resolution over time include a lengthening of the intravesical ureter as axial growth occurs and developmental improvement in bladder dynamics.[39]

Three interdependent variables are potentially predictive of reflux resolution in that they provide anatomic assessment of the flap valve mechanism: ureteral tunnel length to diameter ratio, ureteral orifice morphology, and ureteral orifice position. The most frequently used classification of ureteral orifice position is that proposed by Mackie and Stephens in which orifice position is described relative to the normal position of the ureteral bud (Fig. 27.4).[80, 81] According to this theory, the more laterally displaced the ureteral orifice is the higher the incidence of reflux.[8] Although orifice position can be assessed using oblique films during a VCUG, a more

TABLE 27.2. *Distribution of reflux grades relative to mode of presentation*

Authors	No. of renal units	Age (average months)	Grade (%)				
			I	II	III	IV	V
Greenfield et al (1997)	835		22	45	21	9	3
Skoog et al (1991)							
White	493	39	4	50	37	6	3
Black	51	45	2	49	37	10	2
Peppas et al (1991)							
Duplicated system	70	30	6	40	27	16	11
Zerin et al (1993)	67	0	10	24	27	16	22

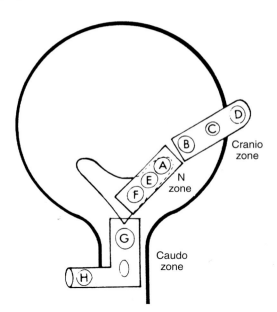

FIG. 27.4. The bladder and urethra showing three zones of ureteral orifices. *A, E,* and *F,* normal zone; *B, C,* and *D,* cranio zone (*D* in the diverticulum); *G* and *H,* caudo zone (*G* in the urethra and *H* in the sex duct). Reprinted with permission from Mackie, GG. Abnormalities of the ureteral bud. Urol Clin North Am 1978;5:161–174.

accurate assessment of lower ureteral anatomy requires that cystoscopy be performed under general anesthesia. Unfortunately all of these criteria are subjective. Ureteral orifice morphology, although sometimes helpful, can be described as abnormal in many children who do not have reflux.[65] In addition, these characteristics (i.e., ureteral orifice morphology) can change with varying degrees of bladder filling.[82] Thus, morphology is not an accurate prediction of reflux resolution.

Hinman introduced the concept of low-pressure and high-pressure reflux to describe VUR that occurred during the filling and emptying phases of the cystogram, respectively.[83] Mean bladder pressure at the time of reflux was higher in patients demonstrating reflux during the emptying phase as opposed to those demonstrating VUR during filling. Reflux occurring during the filling phase may represent an intrinsic defect that is less likely to undergo spontaneous resolution. Godley et al quantitated reflux with simultaneous RNC and urodynamic measurements and found several different patterns of VUR. Reflux during the low pressure filling phase occurred progressively throughout filling or incrementally with unstable bladder contractions. Maximal reflux during the voiding phase was typically seen as detrusor pressure fell.[84] Unfortunately, no prospective study with simultaneous pressure measurements has been performed to correlate the phase at which reflux occurs with the likelihood of spontaneous resolution.

EVALUATION

Mode of Presentation

The manner in which patients with vesicoureteral reflux present to the urologist is age dependent. Young infants with reflux and urinary tract infections most frequently have general signs and symptoms of fever, vomiting, and failure to thrive. Differentiating between pyelonephritis and other causes of sepsis may be difficult in this age group. Older children who have an active infection may have additional symptoms of flank pain and dysuria. Even in the absence of infection, reflux associated flank pain may be experienced during the act of voiding. In recent years, more infants and children are presenting before the onset of infection because of the widespread application of prenatal sonography and sibling screening.

Indications for Evaluation

Evaluation for vesicoureteral reflux should be performed after a single, well-documented urinary tract infection. Reflux is identified in 30 to 50% of children who undergo evaluation for significant bacteriuria, regardless of the presence or absence of symptoms.[85–87] Further support for an aggressive approach to evaluation comes from studies that have demonstrated a 5 to 17% incidence of scars on initial evaluation of children with VUR.[88–91] The lower incidence of reflux in black children prompted Askari and Belman to recommend that asymptomatic bacteriuria not be an indication for radiographic evaluation in black girls.[36] Findings by Kunin et al that none of the black children in their series with asymptomatic bacteriuria developed scars may support this position.[33, 92] However, most clinicians would agree that even in racial groups with a low incidence of VUR, frequent recurrences of asymptomatic bacteriuria or infections that do not respond to therapeutic measures should prompt a full evaluation.

When basing management decision on bacteriuria, it is important to clearly define what constitutes a significant urinary tract infection to reduce unnecessary evaluations. Specimens obtained by adhering a plastic bag to the perineum are useful only if no organisms grow. Any growth usually reflects the perineal flora. A bacterial count of >100,000 colony-forming unit (CFU) mL from a clean midstream collection or any significant growth from a catheterized specimen or suprapubic aspiration are considered positive.

The widespread availability of obstetric ultrasonography has increased the number of children that present with renal abnormalities before developing symptoms. It is generally felt that all neonates who have moderate to severe hydronephrosis or other renal abnormalities (e.g., ureterocoeles, cysts, etc.) should be started on prophylactic antibiotics and subject to full evaluation of the upper and lower urinary tracts after delivery. Differences of opinion remain, however, regarding the optimal management of the child with prenatally detected mild hydronephrosis or normal postnatal ultrasound. Zerin et al, in their review of 130 infants found to have renal abnormalities in utero, studied all patients with VCUG in the postnatal period.[19] Of those with normal postnatal ultrasound, 25% had vesicoureteral reflux. As a result, the authors recommend that all neonates with abnormal findings on prenatal ultrasound be studied with a VCUG regardless of postnatal ultrasonographic results. Findings by Najmaldin et al in which 14 of 46 (30%) refluxing units had no prenatal or postnatal hydronephrosis support this opinion that all children with abnormal renal findings on prenatal sonography should undergo full evaluation.[93] Others point out that most patients with a normal postnatal ultrasound who are found to have reflux have minor degrees of reflux and that they almost invariably will resolve spontaneously.[42, 43] They contend that a full radiologic workup is therefore not necessary in these individuals.

Siblings or children of a patient with vesicoureteral reflux require evaluation for vesicoureteral reflux. As emphasized earlier, siblings have a significantly increased chance of having VUR relative to the general population (Sibling of index, one-third; Child of index, two-thirds; Twin of sibling, two-thirds).[25, 26, 94] Although the incidence of reflux is lower in siblings who are older than the index patient (31% if younger than index versus 19% if older than index)[25] and the percent of positive studies drops off significantly with age (46% if <1.5 years old versus 28% if >1.5 years)[26,] the percentage is still significant enough to warrant screening of all siblings younger than 10 years of age. Support for this philosophy comes from Smellie et al, who found that new renal scars could develop up to age 10.[95]

Finally, various upper urinary tract abnormalities associated with an increased incidence of contralateral VUR should undergo evaluation. Limkakeng and Retik in evaluating children with unilateral renal agenesis were the first to note an increased incidence of reflux in the contralateral ureter (75%).[96] In addition, a high incidence of reflux into a hypoplastic blind ending ureter was noted. Song et al likewise found a high incidence of contralateral reflux (19 of 51 [37%]) in children with renal agenesis.[97] The incidence of VUR is also increased in children with a multicystic dysplastic kidney.[98, 99] Gough et al identified reflux in 20% (12 of 62) of contralateral kidneys, while Selzman and Elder identified this association in 15% (10 of 65). In the later series, males were more likely than females (22% and 7%, respectively) and whites were more likely than nonwhites (22% and 4%, respectively) to have associated contralateral reflux.[99]

History and Physical Examination

The importance of a complete history and physical examination cannot be overstated. Information obtained can significantly impact on management decisions and the likelihood of successful resolution. A thorough voiding history, including complaints of frequency, urgency, straining to void, enuresis, and encopresis may uncover an element of dysfunctional voiding. Van Gool et al identified an 18% prevalence of bladder and sphincter dysfunction in patients with primary VUR using a voiding pattern questionnaire.[100] A strong correlation between dysfunctional voiding, recurrent UTIs, and resolution of VUR (negative correlation with the latter) underscore the importance of this portion of the history. Examination of the underclothes for fecal soiling may serve as an additional clue to dysfunctional elimination habits. Physical examination must include palpation of the flanks and abdomen for any mass or tenderness. Careful inspection of the external genitalia for rashes suggestive of chronic wetting or anatomic abnormality is likewise important. Identification of cutaneous lesions on the back or an asymmetric gluteal cleft may be the first clue to the presence of an occult spinal dysraphism. Finally, because of the high incidence of associated hypertension in patients with VUR and associated renal scarring, blood pressure should be measured in all children suspected of having reflux.

Radiographic Evaluation

The specific radiographic tests to evaluate children for VUR will depend greatly on the mode of presentation, age of presentation, and availability of specific imaging modalities. In general, all patients who have significant bacteriuria should undergo lower urinary tract evaluation with a VCUG and upper urinary tract evaluation with an ultrasound. Children presenting for sibling screening should also undergo an evaluation. Because of the decreasing incidence of sibling reflux with age, Noe has suggested that a renal-bladder ultrasound will suffice in children older than 5 years who do not have a history of urinary tract infection.[26] Initial evaluation recommendations based on mode of presentation are shown in Table 27.3. The clinician may find it appropriate to modify these recommendations based on additional patient characteristics (i.e., compliance with follow-up, parental concern, etc.). A DMSA renal scan to further evaluate renal parenchymal anatomy and differential renal function may be warranted in any child noted to have an abnormality on these initial studies.

Radiographic evaluation for VUR begins with the voiding cystourethrogram (VCUG) (Fig. 27.5). Although this study can never be completely physiologic,

TABLE 27.3. *Indications for radiologic evaluation*

Indications for evaluation	Recommended radiographic tests
A single well-documented urinary tract infection (UTI)[1]	Age <10 years old: VCUG & US
Sibling	Male: Age <5 years old: RNC or low dose VCUG Age 5–10 years old: US Female: Age <10 years old: RNC or low dose VCUG
Unilateral renal agenesis Multicystic kidney	Age <10 years old: RNC or low dose VCUG
Prenatal hydronephrosis[2]	

US (age 1 month)
⊖ ↙   ↘ ⊕
Repeat US (3 months)
↙   ↓
⊖   ⊕ ⟶ VCUG

[1]Yield may be low in blacks.

[2]Recommendations for unilateral hydronephrosis. Bilateral and severe unilateral prenatal hydronephrosis deserves earlier evaluation.

using an instillation temperature of 37°C, with gravity flow at a height of no more than 80 cm H$_2$O will help to reduce artifact. A complete set of films including oblique views of the bladder and images during voiding should be obtained. The films are assessed for grade of reflux, presence of intrarenal reflux, location of ureteral insertion, presence of any associated periureteral pathology, and importantly, for adequacy of upper urinary tract drainage of the refluxed urine (to evaluate for the possibility of an associated UPJ or UVJ obstruction).

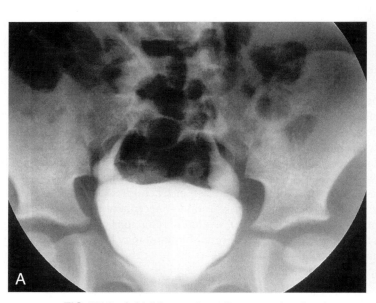
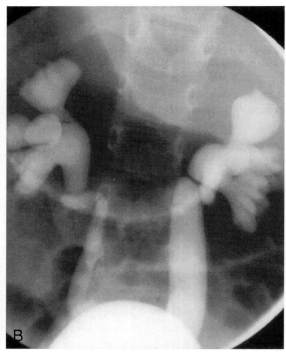

FIG. 27.5. A, Voiding cystourethrogram showing the contrast entering the distal ureters bilaterally during early filling. **B,** Bilateral grade IV reflux into the pelvicalyceal systems is demonstrated after the bladder is filled to capacity.

On occasion, reflux may be detected only intermittently by VCUG. The cyclic VCUG, as described by Paltiel et al, should be performed in all patients in whom one has a high suspicion of reflux.[101] This technique is especially appropriate for younger children who may spontaneously empty the bladder of contrast before it has been filled to an adequate capacity for a proper study. The proper time to perform a VCUG after a UTI remains controversial. Most clinicians think that the best time to perform a VCUG is after 2 to 3 weeks of antimicrobial therapy. They argue that bacterial endotoxins, which can result in ureteral stasis, may result in the false impression of a chronically dilated ureter if studies are performed too close to the time of infection.[73] Others feel that it is important to perform the study during or immediately after the UTI has been treated.[102] They contend that on rare occasions, reflux is present only during an active infection.

The most sensitive and accurate method of diagnosing VUR is the radionuclide cystogram (RNC) (Fig. 27.6). This study allows for continuous monitoring of bladder filling and emptying and permits detection of reflux at any time during the test. The primary advantage of this modality is a dramatic reduction in gonadal radiation dose (by as much as 200 fold).[79, 103] Disadvantages include failure to adequately image the urethra, false-negative results with grade I reflux, and an inability to differentiate between the various grades of reflux in the pelvicalyceal system.[79, 104] RNC is used primarily in the periodic evaluation of patients with reflux who have already had a VCUG for baseline anatomic definition. In addition, RNC is well-suited for the screening of a sibling for reflux and to check for reflux resolution after surgical reimplantation.

One further alternative that combines the advantages of standard VCUG (spatial resolution) and RNC (reduced radiation dose) is the tailored low-dose fluoroscopic voiding cystogram. As with the other two techniques, a catheter is placed and contrast material is instilled at body temperature using gravity. Once the bladder is full and voiding has begun, both kidneys are monitored fluoroscopically. Immediately after voiding is completed, the bladder is briefly imaged. Digital freeze-frame video images are stored and immediately refilmed. By eliminating preliminary and fluoroscopic spot films and using a low-dose fluoroscopic unit, the level of gonadal radiation is kept to less than 1.5 mrad. One obtains high resolution images of the bladder, UVJ, ureter, and kidney while exposing the gonadal structures to a radiation dose that is comparable to the lowest reported dosage with radionuclide techniques. This technique has proven efficacious in the longitudinal evaluation of patients with known reflux and in screening for familial reflux.[105, 106]

Ultrasound is also used in the evaluation of children suspected of having VUR. Valuable information pertaining to reflux that can be obtained from this modality includes renal size; presence of hydronephrosis or hydroureter, suggestion of ureteral duplication, and evidence for renal scarring. Doppler images may also indicate retrograde flow up the ureter.[107] In the presence of hydroureteronephrosis, temporal changes in ureteral or pelvic diameter and urothelial thickening may also increase one's suspicion that reflux is present. However, taken alone both of these findings lack specificity because obstructive etiologies of hydronephrosis (i.e., posterior urethral valves) may also improve with bladder emptying. Finally, it is important to note that while useful information can be obtained from this modality, a normal ultrasound does not exclude the possibility of vesicoureteral reflux. This is especially true in the immediate postnatal period when a state of relative dehydration exists.

Once reflux has been positively identified, a functional evaluation of the upper urinary tract is appropriate to obtain baseline assessment of renal function. Traditionally an intravenous pyelogram was used for this purpose. More objective measurements of differential renal function and renal scar distribution can be obtained with renal nuclear scintigraphy (i.e., DMSA).[108] Most recently, single photon computerized tomography (SPECT) using [99]m technetium-labeled DMSA has been used to provide three-dimensional imaging for calculation of individual kidney function. This information can be useful when contralateral pathology

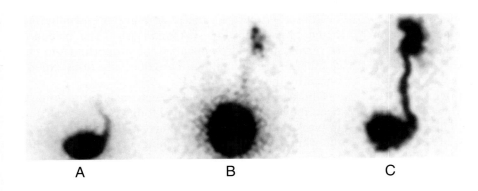

FIG. 27.6. Radionuclide cystograms showing grade I reflux into the ureter alone **(A)**, grade II reflux into the ureter and kidney without dilation of the renal pelvis **(B)** and grade III reflux with distortion of the ureter and pelvicalyceal system **(C)**.

exists (in contrast to the simple differential function obtained by standard DMSA).[109]

Cystoscopy, frequently advocated for evaluation of VUR, has in recent times been deemphasized because of the added risk and cost of an anesthetic. In addition, although information regarding orifice morphology and tunnel length may be obtained, there can be considerable variation of observed findings among different examiners. A review of the cystoscopic data obtained for the International Reflux Study found a poor correlation between cystoscopic findings and resolution of reflux. However, cystoscopy is appropriate at the time of definitive surgical treatment of VUR. Findings of acute inflammation will likely dissuade the clinician from proceeding with open repair until bacteriologic confirmation of sterile urine is obtained. Of equal importance is the identification of occult pathology (i.e., duplication, ureterocele, or posterior urethral valves) that could influence specific surgical decisions (i.e., ureterocele incision or valvular resection).

Uninhibited bladder contractions have been identified in many cases of reflux with recurrent breakthrough infections.[65] Urodynamic evaluation has therefore been advocated by some authors as a means of identifying this population with unstable bladders. However, the law yield of identifying abnormalities on urodynamic studies in the VUR population as a whole makes such an approach impractical.

Laboratory evaluation should include a baseline determination of serum creatinine. Urinary measurements of various tubular enzymes and cytokines, although predictive of renal injury, are not of sufficient sensitivity or specificity to warrant their routine use in the evaluation and management of children with VUR.[110, 111]

SEQUELAE OF REFLUX

Renal Scarring

Convincing evidence that renal scarring could be the result of VUR was first put forth by Hodson who demonstrated that 97% of children with scars showed evidence of reflux on voiding cystourethrography.[4] Hodson made the additional observation that scarring almost always occurred in the polar segments of the kidney. This latter phenomenon is best explained by the increased frequency of intrarenal reflux noted in the upper and lower poles of the kidney. Intrarenal reflux is identified almost exclusively in those regions in which calyces contain compound papillae (papillae fused with adjacent papillae) in which the papillary ducts open at right angles to the calyx rather than at oblique angles (Fig. 27.7).[112, 113] Papillary ducts that exit at an oblique angle share a common geometry with the intravesical ureter, which makes them more likely to close as a flap valve and thereby resist intrarenal reflux. Studies of papillary

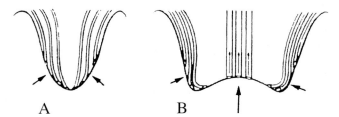

FIG. 27.7. A, Convex papillary ducts exit at an oblique angle and share a common geometry with the intravesical ureter, making them more likely to close as a flap valve and thereby resist intrarenal reflux (nonrefluxing papilla). **B,** Compound papillary ducts (papillae fused with adjacent papillae) open at right angles rather than at oblique angles and are thereby less resistant to the retrograde flow of urine (refluxing papilla). Reprinted with permission from Ransley PG, Risdon RA. Reflux and Renal Scarring, Br J Radiol 1978;14(suppl):1.

morphology in human cadaver kidneys indicate that at least two-thirds of kidneys possess papillae with this compound morphology.[75] Whitaker and Cuckow provided further experimental evidence to confirm the decreased resistance of polar papillae to intrarenal reflux. By injecting the pelvicalyceal systems of fresh pig kidneys with a dilute resin they were able to construct a high-resolution impression of the papillary morphology. Although the extent of the intrarenal reflux was variable, when it occurred it was usually polar.[114]

Irreversible renal damage in the form of parenchymal scarring is the most common pathologic sequel to reflux and associated urinary injection. From 5 to 30% of children presenting for initial evaluation of reflux will have a scar.[95, 115, 116] The incidence of scarring in children with asymptomatic bacteriuria is also significant (5–17%).[89, 90] Children without bacteriuria who undergo evaluation for sibling reflux have nearly a 14% incidence of scarring.[25] The specific incidence in any one study reflects the age and mode of presentation of the children being evaluated.

The likelihood of developing renal scarring depends on many factors. The grade of reflux has been demonstrated to be directly proportional to the incidence of scarring in most studies.[26, 62–65, 115] A higher incidence of scarring among males than females (20–22% versus 12%) has also been demonstrated, a difference that may be caused, in part, by the probability of encountering higher grade reflux in boys than in girls.[39] The incidence of renal scarring also appears to be proportional to the number of symptomatic urinary tract infections experienced by the patient.[117]

Differences in scarring between racial groups have been shown as well. Kunin et al found no renal scarring in blacks who were found to have VUR (versus 15.6% in whites) based on screening for asymptomatic bacteriuria.[33, 92] However, when children with VUR were identified based on a symptomatic infection, the racial distribution of associated renal scarring was different (23% black versus 13% white).[39] Other known risk factors for scarring include delay in treatment of VUR with infection and noncompliance with prophylactic antibiotics. These last two risk factors may help explain the differences in scarring between different epidemiologic groups.[95]

The age at which patients experiences their first episode of pyelonephritis is important. Patients who experience a febrile urinary tract infection before the age of 4 have a much greater likelihood of developing a scar than children who have their first episode of pyelonephritis at an older age.[95] Several factors may be responsible for this finding. Young children have more immature immune systems and therefore may have less resistance to combating developing infection when it occurs in the renal parenchyma. An intrinsically lower resistance of the papillary ducts to back pressure in younger children may likewise be important. Autopsy studies in children younger than 1 month of age demonstrate that intrarenal reflux may occur at pressures as low as 2 mm Hg. In contrast, the same degree of reflux in a 1-year-old child requires a back pressure of nearly 20 mm Hg.[118] Radiographically, intrarenal reflux is appreciated only in children younger than age 4.[119] This higher incidence of intrarenal reflux coupled with frequent uninhibited contractions that can occur in the neurologically immature bladder may translate into a greater susceptibility to renal damage. The nonspecfic presentation of neonates with pyelonephritis may also lead to delays in presentation and adequate treatment, thereby causing a more frequent occurrence of renal scarring.

Whether sterile reflux results in renal damage remains controversial. Early experimental work by Hodson, in which reflux and partial bladder outlet obstruction were surgically created (i.e., creating a secondary reflux scenario), produced renal damage that resembled radiologic scarring seen in children with reflux.[120] Other experimental work in which sterile reflux was created in the absence of secondary bladder pathology (i.e., creating a primary reflux scenario) did not produce renal scarring.[121, 122] Clinically, Smellie et al found that most kidneys with primary VUR grew at a normal rate and did not develop scarring if infection was controlled with prophylactic antibiotics.[123] In a meta-analysis of the world's reflux literature, Smellie and Normand identified 1,720 children with reflux who were observed serially with upper urinary tract studies.[124] Of the 83 who developed new scars, reflux was present in 80 and infection in 79. From these data it was concluded that in most cases, infection is needed for the development of acquired renal scarring.[124]

Dysplastic changes that resemble reflux nephropathy radiographically have been identified in neonates before any infection.[93] This supports the hypothesis of Mackie and Stephens that renal impairment associated with VUR can be caused by congenital abnormalities of the ureteral bud.[81] Others have concluded similarly that renal impairment associated with high-grade primary VUR is frequently present at birth and not secondary to subsequent infection.[43, 125] It remains unclear as to whether these changes associated with fetal VUR are primary or secondary to the reflux itself.

Hypertension

Reflux nephropathy is the most common cause of severe hypertension (HTN) in children[25, 26,] with HTN reported in up to 20% of children with established scars.[124] In one large study of reflux-associated hypertension, Wallace evaluated 166 originally normotensive patients who underwent successful ureteral reimplantation.[126] Overall, 12.8% of patients developed hypertension over the ensuing 10 years. Patients with bilateral scars had a statistically significant higher chance of developing HTN than did individuals with unilateral scarring (18.5% versus 11.3%). HTN did not develop in the absence of scarring. Although HTN only occurs in combination with renal scarring, it has been impossible to correlate the likelihood of developing hypertension with the grade of reflux or the extent of scarring,[127, 128] perhaps because of the limitations of IVP as a quantitative measure of the extent of renal damage. Quantitation of scarring with DMSA scanning may allow us to draw more refined conclusions regarding reflux, scar formation, and hypertension (Fig. 27.8). It remains imperative that all individuals with a history of VUR be observed long-term for the development of HTN.

Most individuals who develop HTN have nearly normal renal function. It appears unlikely that the onset of hypertension is related to renal failure in most cases. Rather, the mechanism for developing hypertension is likely renin dependent.[127, 129] The identification of specific cases of renin-mediated HTN supports such a mechanism.[130] Nevertheless, a large study of reflux associated hypertension by Savage et al did not find any direct correlation between plasma renin levels and blood pressure.[127]

Renal Function

The early effects of vesicoureteral reflux on renal function appear to be related to renal tubular dysfunction. Walker et al demonstrated concentrating defects in the kidneys of children with reflux and sterile urine.[131, 132] This defect in concentrating ability was inversely proportional to the grade of reflux and was most significant in kidneys with renal scarring. Correction of reflux served to improve this concentrating defect.[133–135] With continued damage and scarring, global renal function may deteriorate resulting in decreased glomerular function and chronic renal failure.[136] Patients with bilateral

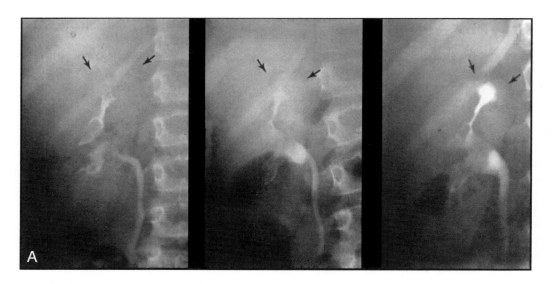

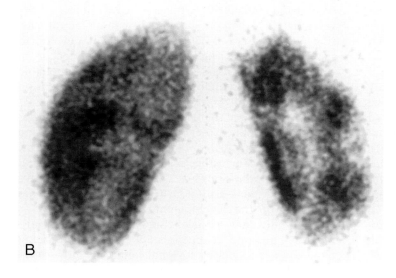

FIG. 27.8. A, IVP excretory urogram of the right kidney demonstrating progressive development of renal scarring in the upper pole (*arrows*). **B,** Posterior ^{99m}Tc-DMSA images (obtained with a pinhole collimator) of the right kidney showing an absence of tracer uptake in the extreme portion of the upper pole and areas of decreased tracer uptake in the lower pole and midpolar regions, indicative of diffuse scarring. Note that the left kidney has slightly decreased uptake at its upper and lower poles.

renal scarring, hypertension, or proteinuria appear to be at the highest risk for developing end stage renal disease.[137]

Secondary UPJ Obstruction

Vesicoureteral reflux and ureteropelvic junction obstruction can occur in the same renal unit.[138, 139] In a 10-year review of all patients undergoing evaluation for vesicoureteral reflux (N = 2800) or ureteropelvic junction obstruction (N = 200), Lebowitz and Blickman identified this association 21 times.[140] In as many as a third of these individuals high-grade reflux may play an etiologic role in development of the upper urinary tract obstruction.[138] Secondary UPJ obstruction is believed to result from the chronic effects of high-grade reflux on the upper urinary tract. Williams and later Whitaker proposed that atonicity of an overstretched renal pelvis prevented adequate formation and propagation of a

bolus of urine through the ureteropelvic junction.[141, 142] Johnston hypothesized that massive reflux could rapidly distend the upper urinary tract and result in angulation of the ureteropelvic junction.[143] Another contributing factor in the etiology of secondary UPJ obstruction may be inflammation (i.e., ureteritis and pyelonephritis) that can result in stenosis of the ureter.[144]

Proper cystographic evaluation of the child with reflux must include careful evaluation for signs of associated UPJ obstruction. Otherwise significant UPJ obstruction in association with mild reflux can be mistaken for severe vesicoureteral reflux alone.[140] Contrast that readily refluxes up the ureter but then abruptly stops before entering the renal pelvis is the first clue that UPJ obstruction may coexist (Fig. 27.9). Reflux into the pelvis on later films may also be suggestive of obstruction if the density of the contrast in the pelvis is diminished relative to the ureter. This is because of the dilutional effect of residual urine trapped in the renal pelvis. Postvoid films that reveal prompt drainage of contrast from the refluxing ureter with retention of contrast in the renal pelvis cinch the diagnosis. Hollowell et al have coined the term "pseudoobstruction" to describe simple overdilation of the renal pelvis by reflux.[138] Adequate drainage of contrast from the renal pelvis on postvoid films easily separates these individuals from those with significant obstructive pathology at the ureteropelvic junction. Once suspicion has been raised as to the presence of obstruction, the severity should be evaluated with intravenous pyelography or diuretic renography. Either functional study must be performed with a catheter draining the bladder to prevent reflux.

Determining whether a concomitant UPJ is secondary to reflux or simply coincidental may be difficult. Maizels et al described criteria to help differentiate between these two possibilities.[139] Their criteria included the appearance of the ureteropelvic junction on VCUG, orifice morphology, and the grade of reflux. An attempt was made to differentiate between simple tortuosity, mild kinks, and severe fixed kinks of the upper ureter. They further argued that high-grade reflux was strongly suggestive of reflux being the cause of the obstruction. Unfortunately, although UPJ and orifice morphology can be helpful, they remain subjective. Furthermore, proper classification of reflux with the IRS grading sys-

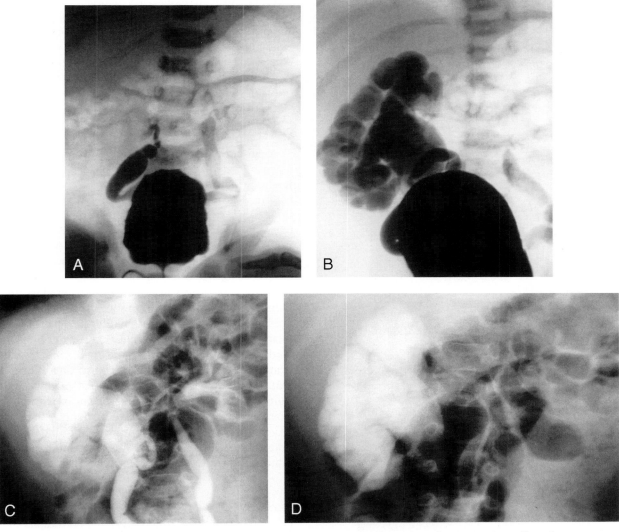

FIG. 27.9. A, In concomitant VUR and ureteral pelvic junction obstruction, the contrast readily refluxes up the ureter and then abruptly stops before entering the renal pelvis (right kidney). **B,** Reflux into the renal pelvis on later films. Note the reduced density of the contrast in the pelvis relative to the ureter. This is owing to the dilutional effect of residual urine trapped in the renal pelvis. **C and D,** Prevoid and postvoid films revealing prompt drainage of contrast from the refluxing ureter (and contralateral kidney) with retention of contrast in the right renal pelvis.

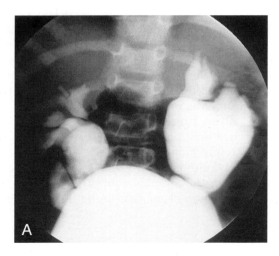

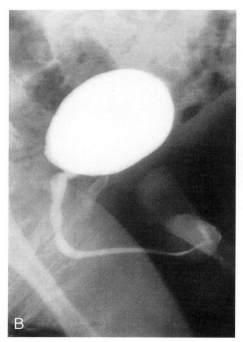

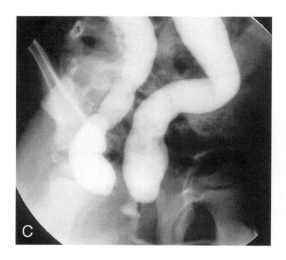

tem is impossible in the presence of obstruction. Because the renal pelvis is already dilated in cases of ureteropelvic obstruction, mild reflux and high-grade reflux can be expected to have a similar appearance.[140]

Megacystis-Megaureter Association

When massive bilateral reflux is present, the constant recycling of urine from the upper urinary tracts to the bladder can result in marked dilation of the ureters and bladder Fig. 27.10).[145] This constellation of findings, referred to as the Megacystis-Megaureter Association (MMA), is more frequently identified in males. The differentiation between MMA and infravesical obstruction (i.e., posterior urethral valves) is made with a VCUG. This makes the prenatal distinction difficult. Findings suggestive of MMA include a thin-walled bladder and variation in the degree of hydronephrosis during the ultrasound examination.[145] In addition, normal renal echogenicity on prenatal sonographic examination is consistent with the diagnosis of a nonobstructive etiology in the context of a dilated bladder and bilateral hydroureteronephrosis.[146]

NATURAL HISTORY

An understanding of the natural history of VUR plays a central role in determining appropriate management. Reflux grade remains the best predictive parameter of eventual resolution (Table 27.4).[147] When urinary tract infections are prevented, as many as 87% of grade 1, 63% of grade 2, 53% of grade 3, and 33% of grade 4 reflux will resolve within 3 years.[78] Although this trend is frequently noted, resolution rates between individual grades of reflux often do not reach statistical significance. A report by Tamminen-Mobius et al for the IRS identified no significant difference in resolution between grades III and IV.[148] This is likely the result of several factors, including the variability in reflux grade between studies and the inherent limitations of a stepwise classification system for a disease that exists on a continuum.[54] Data pertaining to the resolution of higher grades of reflux remain relatively sparse because of the surgical treatment bias in treating these patients.

VUR has a tendency to improve spontaneously with time, most likely because of the lengthening of the intramural and intravesical ureter commenserate with axial

---

FIG. 27.10. A, VCUG filling phase demonstrating massive bilateral reflux associated with MMA. **B,** VCUG Voiding phase showing normal urethral anatomy and no evidence of obstruction. **C,** VCUG after the voiding phase showing residual urine in the upper urinary tracts, which subsequently drained back into the bladder.

TABLE 27.4. *Frequency of resolution relative to reflux grade*

Authors	Length of follow-up (months)	Grade (% resolution)			
		I	II	III	IV
Bellinger (1984)	30	87	63	53	33
Arant (1992)	60	82	80	46	—
Greenfield (1997)	38	69	56	49	—

—Information not available.

somatic growth.[8, 71] Therefore, the more growth potential that remains, the more likely it is that VUR will resolve spontaneously. A change in voiding dynamics as the individual progresses from an infantile to a mature voiding pattern may also contribute to spontaneous improvement. Among children with VUR with a symptomatic UTI (average age, 3 years), 30 to 35% can be expected to have a reduction of reflux grade each year.[147] Of children with lower grades of reflux (grades I, II, or III) who show spontaneous resolution, greater than 90% will do so within 5 years.[23] Neonates diagnosed with reflux caused by prenatal hydronephrosis have a higher chance of resolution than older children.[19, 42, 149] This holds true even for the higher grades of reflux.[149]

Other patient characteristics have been shown to impact on the likelihood of reflux resolution. Cessation of VUR is observed significantly more often in children with unilateral (40 of 74, 54%) than with bilateral (18 of 154, 12%) reflux (p < 0.001).[148] Spontaneous resolution is less likely to happen when it occurs in the lower pole of duplex systems.[150–152] Blacks who resolve their reflux do so at a much faster rate than do whites (14.6 months versus 21.4 months).[39]

MANAGEMENT OF VESICO-URETERIC REFLUX

The management of primary vesico-ureteral reflux is based on the principles that reflux represents a mechanical problem at the uretero-vesical junction, which can resolve spontaneously with time and that sterile, low pressure reflux is harmless to the kidney. It was on these principles that Smellie based her landmark clinical study on the medical management of vesico-ureteral reflux.[153] During the same period, improved operative techniques to correct reflux were being developed such that the surgical option, if necessary, became a more attractive one.

Medical Management of Reflux

Smellie was the first to show that vesico-ureteral reflux could be effectively managed medically, while awaiting spontaneous reflux resolution.[154] Her approach entailed the use of continuous, low-dose antibi-

otics, interval urine cultures, instructions regarding proper perineal hygiene, and avoidance of constipation. Smellie demonstrated that this approach could effectively protect the kidney from pyelonephritic scarring until reflux resolved or the decision to operate was made.

Because the most grades I and II reflux resolve spontaneously, a medical approach has been favored and supported by the results of several well-done clinical studies.[155] Grade V reflux has an exceedingly low likelihood of spontaneous resolution and has been historically regarded as a surgical problem.[156] The greatest controversy has surrounded the optimal management of grades III and IV vesico-ureteral reflux. In an attempt to resolve this controversy, an International Reflux Study was undertaken in 1981 to prospectively compare results in patients with grades III and IV vesico-ureteral reflux randomized to medical versus surgical management.[157] This study, published in 1992, concluded that both approaches were equally effective in preventing further renal scarring (new scars developed in 19 of 155 children treated medically and 20 of 151 children treated surgically), but that patients assigned to the medical arm had a higher incidence of pyelonephritis than those treated surgically.[158, 159] These results were consistent with those from the Birmingham Reflux Study Group of 1987, which also demonstrated that new scar formation occurred infrequently but equally among medically and surgically treated patients.[160] An intriguing study by Arant in 1992 indicated that in a group of 59 patients observed with optimal medical management, new renal scars occurred in 10% of patients with grades I and II reflux and 28% with grade III reflux.[161] He suggested that, while prospective clinical trials comparing medical versus surgical treatment for low grade reflux were unlikely to be undertaken, they may be of interest. Nonetheless, based on the available data, it seemed reasonable to conclude that a medical or surgical approach should be equally effective in protecting the kidney from reflux nephropathy.

Based on Smellie's work, the importance of continuous low-dose antibiotic prophylaxis as opposed to intermittent short courses of an antibiotic to treat recurrent infection has become well accepted.[153] The preferred antibiotics are Trimethaprim-sulfamethoxazole (TMP-

SMX) and nitrofurantoin because they achieve high urinary concentrations, are active against a broad spectrum of urinary pathogens, have minimal effect on bowel bacterial flora, have few side effects, and are inexpensive. A low-dose (TMP-SMX 2 mg/kg/day [based on the TMP component], nitrofurantoin 2 mg/kg/day) is administered at bedtime. Urine cultures are obtained every 3 months and whenever the child has symptoms suggestive of urinary tract infection. The importance of vigorous hydration and frequent bladder emptying are emphasized, as is the importance of avoiding constipation. It has become well established that associated bladder instability may prolong the time before reflux resolution.[162] Thus one should elicit any relevant history suggestive of bladder instability, such as daytime wetting, and treat that patient accordingly with spasmolytic or anticholinergic medication. After an initial fluoroscopic VCUG, the child's reflux status may be reassessed at 1- or 2-year intervals with radionuclide cystogram or low-dose fluoroscopic VCUGs, depending on the severity of the reflux and age of the child. A baseline DMSA renal scan should be performed to rule out parenchymal scarring and assess relative renal function. This routine is followed until reflux resolution is documented on one well-performed study.

For the individual patient, the optimal approach for treatment depends on several factors and practical considerations. The grade of reflux and the determination that no coexistent uretero-vesical junction pathology exists, based on VCUG, are critical. The patient's age is an important factor. It has been demonstrated that after the first year of life, the likelihood of spontaneous reflux resolution is fairly constant, from 10 to 30% per year. However, the longer an individual patient's reflux remains unchanged, the less likely spontaneous resolution becomes.[147] Prolonged follow-up entails repeated radiographic studies requiring instrumentation, ongoing antibiotic prophylaxis, and repeat urine cultures; thus, compliance is a major issue. For certain children and families, the routine may become burdensome. In addition, as the child approaches puberty, the bladder descends from its abdominal location deeper into the pelvis, making the anatomy slightly less accessible to surgical reconstruction. Thus, as the child approaches age 10 or 11, it is desirable to have a strong sense as to that child's likelihood of spontaneous reflux resolution.

There are certain classic contraindications to the medical management of reflux. From an anatomic perspective, the ureter entering a Hutch diverticulum is best treated surgically. Similarly, an occult ureterocele associated with reflux should be treated. In these settings, spontaneous reflux resolution will not occur and prolonged antibiotic prophylaxis and repeat studies are inappropriate. Breakthrough febrile urinary tract infections indicate that antibiotic prophylaxis is ineffective

and surgical protection of the kidney should be undertaken. If the family or child are noncompliant with medical management, then antireflux surgery should be performed. A relative indication for surgical correction is the coexistence of significant renal scarring and reflux.

Surgical Management of Vesico-Ureteral Reflux

The surgical correction of vesico-ureteral reflux was pioneered by Leadbetter and Politano and Paquin in the 1950s and most clearly established the principles necessary for successful surgical outcome.[7, 8] These included adequate detrusor backing for the ureter, with the ratio of ureteral tunnel length to ureteral lumenal diameter of four or five to one. Paquin's criteria for success have enabled experienced pediatric urologists to achieve greater than a 95% success rate with standard transvesical antireflux procedures for ureters of normal caliber.[163] However, clinical experience has demonstrated that despite good tunnel length, a maximal ureteral lumenal diameter can be exceeded in the setting of a refluxing megaureter, allowing persistent reflux despite the 5:1 ratio unless tapering of the ureter is performed. Several modifications to Leadbetter and Politano's original approach have been made, all affording success rates of greater than 95%.[164]

A renewed interest has been demonstrated in extravesical ureteral reimplantation over the past decade.[165, 166] This has been associated with decreased morbidity and length of hospital stay as well as success rates that have approached the standard transvesical antireflux techniques.[167]

Also within the past decade, a new direction in antireflux surgery was taken in the transurethral correction of reflux, based on the work by Puri and O'Donnell.[168] While the success rates with the transurethral techniques have not approached those of open surgery, the markedly reduced morbidity have made this alternative appealing.[169]

Surgical Techniques

At the time of planned surgical correction for reflux, it is advisable to perform cystoscopy in many cases. This enables one to rule out an acute cystitis that would make reconstructive surgery inadvisable or occult pathology such as a duplication anomaly that may have been unrecognized radiographically.

Leadbetter-Politano Procedure (Fig. 27.11)

In the classic Leadbetter-Politano ureteral reimplantation, the ureters are freed up from their hiatus in the bladder and brought through a new hiatus superior and

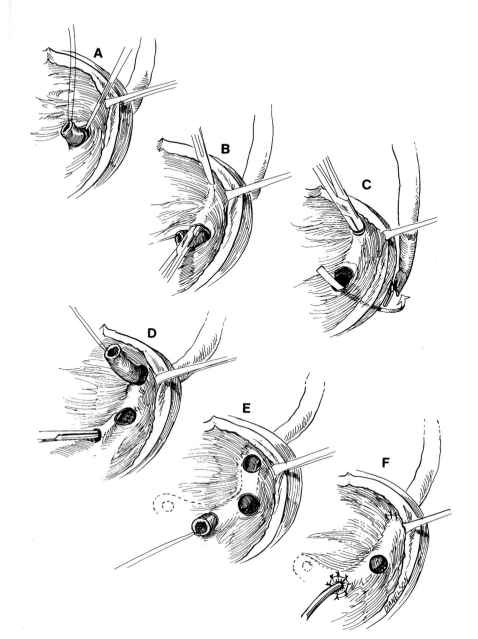

FIG. 27.11. A, For the Leadbetter–Politano technique, the ureter is freed up from its hiatus in the bladder. **B–D,** The ureter is brought through a new hiatus superior and lateral to the original one. **E and F,** A long submucosal tunnel is created as the ureter courses from its new hiatal opening toward the bladder neck. Reprinted with permission from Walsh PC, Retik AB, Stamey TA, Vaughan ED, eds., Campbell's Urology. 6th ed. Philadelphia: Saunders, 1992. King, Lowell R. Vesicoureteral Reflux, Megaureter and Ureteral Reimplantation. Chapter 44 pp. 1689–1742.

lateral to the original one. This allows a long submucosal tunnel to be created as the ureter courses from its new hiatal opening toward the bladder neck. The advantages of this approach have been its high success and low complication rates, and positioning of the ureteric orifice in an accessible location for transurethral catheterization, if necessary.[170] The disadvantages of the Leadbetter-Politano technique seem related to creation of the new hiatus.[171] Because this typically entails a blind maneuver, on rare occasions the ureter has been brought through bowel or vagina in the course of creating the new hiatus. Rarely, kinking of the ureter has also been

observed in the early postoperative period or even years later after a pubertal growth spurt.

Paquin Technique

The Paquin technique uses transvesical and extravesical exposure of the new superolaterally located hiatus.[8] While it is similar in principle to the Leadbetter-Politano operation, its enhanced exposure avoids the potential blind dissection of the new hiatus in the original operation. Its success rate (96%) is equivalent to the Leadbetter-Politano procedure.[163] The Paquin technique is particularly applicable to dilated ureters and may be effectively combined with a psoas hitch procedure.

Glenn-Anderson Technique (Fig. 27.12)

In 1967, Glenn and Anderson described their technique of ureteral advancement.[172] This entails freeing of the ureter from its intramural attachments and advancing it distally in a submucosal tunnel toward the bladder neck. A new hiatus is not created and therefore certain potential complications such as ureteral kinking can be avoided. The limitation of the Glenn-Anderson technique is its applicability to laterally displaced orifices, allowing adequate tunnel length to be created. A subsequent modification by Glenn in which the original hiatus was extended proximally thereby enhancing tunnel length, extends the indications for this technique.[173] High success rates (98%) have been reported.[174] The one disadvantage of this technique is the occasional technical difficulty of performing the distal anastomosis near the bladder neck, to achieve adequate tunnel length.

Cohen Technique (Fig. 27.13)

The most widely used surgical technique to correct reflux is that described by Cohen, in 1975.[175] Cohen overcame the limitations of the Glenn-Anderson technique by bringing the ureters transtrigonally to the opposite bladder wall to achieve adequate tunnel length. This allows one to perform the distal anastomosis with ease, while using the original hiatus. Success with the Cohen technique has been reported to be as high as 99%, and therefore it has become the gold standard against which all antireflux techniques are compared.[176, 177] The one disadvantage of the Cohen technique is that the reimplanted ureteric orifice becomes relatively inaccessible to transurethral instrumentation. However, in this era of percutaneous intervention, this limitation appears to be small.

Extravesical: Lich-Gregoir (Fig. 27.14)

The extravesical approach to ureteral reimplantation was described Lich and Gregoir in the early 1960s.[178, 179]

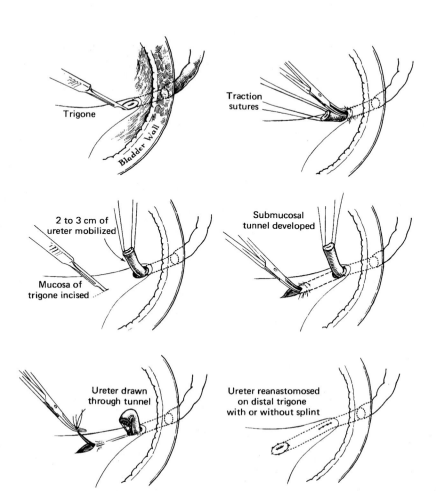

FIG. 27.12. For the Glenn–Anderson technique, the distal ureter is mobilized and the submucosal tunnel is developed distally toward the bladder neck. Reprinted with permission from Glenn JF, ed., Urologic Surgery. 2nd ed. New York: Harper & Row, 1975, p. 281. Politano VA. Vesicoureteral Reflux, 4th ed. 1991, pp. 272–293.

This technique entails freeing up of the distal ureter from outside the bladder without detaching the ureter from its hiatus. After exposing the hiatus, the bladder muscle is split to create a long trough, allowing mucosa to bulge out much as one would perform a pyloromyotomy. The ureter is laid into a submucosal trough and bladder muscle is carefully approximated over it, creating a long submucosal tunnel. In experienced hands, the success rates with the Lich-Gregoir approach have approximated those of the Leadbetter-Politano procedure (90–98%).[180, 181] The advantages of this technique include considerably less morbidity by avoiding a cystotomy and potentially fewer obstructive complications at the level of the ureteric orifice by not dismembering it. There appears to be two major disadvantages to this technique. When bilateral Lich-Gregoir reimplantations have been performed, transient urinary retention has been reported in up to 16% of patients.[182] No long-term areflexia has been reported, however. In addition, the extravesical approach may be less applicable to the ureter requiring a tapering procedure.

STING Transurethral Correction of Reflux

The technique of endoscopic correction of reflux was developed by Puri and O'Donnell in the early 1980s using polytetrafluorethylene (Teflon) paste.[168] In their approach, small quantities of Teflon paste (<0.2 mL) were injected transurethrally beneath the ureteric orifice, creating a volcano configuration. This technique, which is a 15-minute outpatient procedure, was successful in correcting reflux in 80% of cases treated once. If the initial injection failed, a second injection could be performed, which increased overall success rates to 89%.[183] The enthusiasm for this technique has been tempered by concerns regarding the long-term implications of injectable Teflon because the particles have been demonstrated to migrate to distant sites in the body (i.e., lung).[184] As a result, alternative injectable substances have been developed.

Frey and coworkers have used injectable collagen in the manner of Puri.[169] Because of collagen's different physical chemical properties, larger volumes have been injected (up to 4.8 mL/ureter). Over time, some volume loss has been noted with collagen, making reinjection necessary more often. Frey has reported success rates

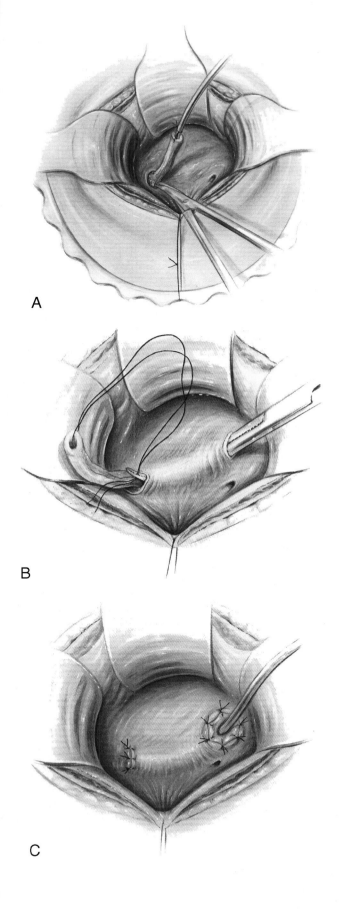

FIG. 27.13. A, For the Cohen technique, the ureter is mobilized from the detrusor attachments. **B,** It is then brought through a transtrigonal submucosal tunnel. **C,** The ureter is anastomosed to the bladder. Reprinted with permission from Eckstein HB, Hohenfellner R, Williams DI, eds., Surgical Pediatric Urology. Philadelphia: Saunders, 1977. The Cohen technique of ureteroneocystostomy. Cohen SJ. pp. 269–274.

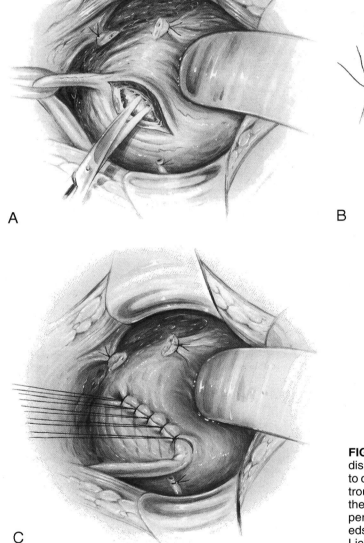

A

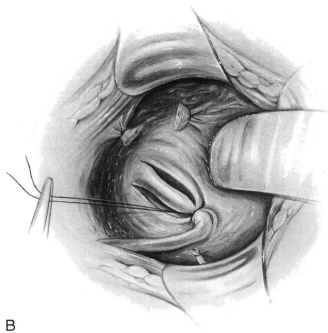

B

C

FIG. 27.14. A, For the Lich–Gregoir technique, the ureter is dissected to the hiatus, and then the bladder muscle is divided to create a long trough. **B,** The ureter is placed in a submucosal trough. **C,** The bladder muscle is carefully approximated over the ureter, creating a long submucosal tunnel. Reprinted with permission from Eckstein HB, Hohenfellner R, Williams DI, eds., Surgical Pediatric Urology. Philadelphia: Saunders, 1977. Lich-Gregori operation. Gregoir W. pp. 265–268.

of 63% with one injection, which can be increased to 79% with a second injection.[169] The primary disadvantage of collagen remains the uncertainty that successful correction of reflux will persist over time.

The search continues for an injectable substance that remains in its subureteric location, maintains its volume, and is nonreactive. One exciting area of investigation is the work of Atala et al, using autologous tissue (chondrocytes, smooth muscle) to serve as the injectable bulking agent to correct reflux.[185]

REFERENCES

1. Polk HC. Notes on Galenic Urology. Urol Surv 1965;15:2.
2. Sampson JA. Ascending renal infection: with special reference to the reflux of urine from the bladder into the ureters as an etiological factor in its causation and maintenance. Johns Hopkins Hosp Bull 1903;14:344–352.
3. Hutch JA. Vesico-ureteral reflux in the paraplegic: cause and correction. J Urol 1952;68:457–467.
4. Hodson CJ. The radiologic diagnosis of pyelonephritis. Proc R Soc Med 1959;52:669.
5. Bovee JW. A critical survey of ureteral implantation. Ann Surg 1900;31:165.

6. Vermooten V, Neuswanger OH. Effects on the upper urinary tract in dogs of an incompetent ureterovesical valve. J Urol 1934;32:330.

7. Politano VA, Leadbetter WF. An operative technique for the correction of vesicoureteral reflux. J Urol 1958;79:932.

8. Paquin AJ. Ureterovesical anastomosis: the description and evaluation of a technique. J Urol 1959;82:573.

9. Lich R, Howerton LW, Davis LA. Recurrent urosepsis in children. J Urol 1961;86:554.

10. Glenn JF, Anderson EE. Distal tunnel ureteral reimplantation. Trans Am Assoc Genitourin Surg 1966;58:37–41.

11. Cohen MH, Rotner MB. A new method to create a submucosal ureteral tunnel. J Urol 1969;102:567–568.

12. Stephens FD, Joske RA, Simmons RT. Megaureter with vesicoureteric reflux in twins. Aust N Z J Surg 1955;24:192.

13. Anonymous. Vesicoureteric reflux: all in the genes? Report of a meeting of physicians at the Hospital for Sick Children, Great Ormond Street, London [clinical conference]. Lancet 1996;348:725–728.

14. Anonymous. Medical versus surgical treatment of primary vesicoureteral reflux: a prospective international reflux study in children. J Urol 1981;125:277–283.

15. Politano VA. Vesicoureteral reflux in children. JAMA 1960;172:1252.

16. Ransley PG. Vesicoureteric reflux: continuing surgical dilemma. Urology 1978;12:246–255.

17. Iannacconne G. Ureteral reflux in normal infants. Acta Radio 1955;44:451.

18. Lebowitz RL. Neonatal vesicoureteral reflux: what do we know? [editorial; comment]. Radiology 1993;187:17.

19. Zerin JM, Ritchey ML, Chang AC. Incidental vesicoureteral reflux in neonates with antenatally detected hydronephrosis and other renal abnormalities. Radiology 1993;187:157–160.

20. Bredin HC, Winchester P, McGovern JH, Degnan M. Family study of vesicoureteral reflux. J Urol 1975;113:623–625.

21. Dwoskin JY. Sibling uropathology. J Urol 1976;115:726–727.

22. de Vargas A, Evans K, Ransley P, et al. A family study of vesicoureteric reflux. J Med Genet 1978;15:85–96.

23. Jerkins GR, Noe HN. Familial vesicoureteral reflux: a prospective study. J Urol 1982;128:774–778.

24. Van den Abbeele AD, Treves ST, Lebowitz RL, et al. Vesicoureteral reflux in asymptomatic siblings of patients with known reflux: Radionuclide cystography. Pediatrics 1987;79:147.

25. Wan J, Greenfield SP, Ng M, Zerin M, Ritchey ML, Bloom D. Sibling reflux: a dual center retrospective study. J Urol 1996;156:677–679.

26. Noe HN. The long-term results of prospective sibling reflux screening. J Urol 1992;148:1739–1742.

27. Burger RH, Burger SE. Genetic determinants of urologic disease. Urol Clin North Am 1974;1:419–440.

28. Gruss P, Walther C. Pax in development. Cell 1992;69:719–722.

29. Keller SA, Jones JM, Boyl A, et al. Kidney and retinal defects (Krd), a transgene-induced mutation with a deletion of mouse chromosome 19 that includes the Pax2 locus. Genomics 1994;23:309–320.

30. Torres M, Gomex-Pardo E, Dressler, GR, Gruss P. Pax-2 controls multiple steps of urogenital development. Development 1995;121:4057–4065.

31. Sanyanusin P, Schimmenti LA, McNoe LA, et al. Mutation of the PAX2 gene in a family with optic nerve colobomas, renal anomalies and vesicoureteral reflux. Nat Genet 1995;9:358–363.

32. West W, Venugopal S. The low frequency of reflux in Jamaican children. Pediatr Radiol 1993;23:91–593.

33. Kunin CM. The natural history of recurrent bacteriuria in schoolgirls. N Engl J Med 1970;282:1443–1448.

34. Kunin CM. Urinary tract infections in children. Hosp Pract 1976;11:91–98.

35. Kuntz DH. Does ureteric reflux protect against calculus formation? Br J Urol 1977;49:80.

36. Askari A, Belman AB. Vesicoureteral reflux in black girls. J Urol 1982;127:747–748.

37. Urrutia EJ, Lebowitz RL. Relationship between hair/eye color and primary vesicoureteral reflux in children. Urol Radiol 1985;7:23–24.

38. Baker R, Masted W, Maylath J, Shuman I. Relation of age, sex, and infection to reflux: Data indicating high spontaneous cure rate in pediatric patients. J Urol 1966;95:26.

39. Skoog SJ, Belman AB. Primary vesicoureteral reflux in the black child. Pediatrics 1991;87:538–543.

40. Scott JE. Fetal ureteric reflux. Br J Urol 1987;59:291–296.

41. Marra G, Barbieri G, Moioli C, Assael BM, Grumieri G, Caccamo ML. Mild fetal hydronephrosis indicating vesicoureteric reflux. Arch Dis Child Fetal Neonatal Ed 1994;70:F147–F149; discussion 149–150.

42. Gordon AC, Thomas DF, Arthur RJ, Irving HC, Smith SE. Prenatally diagnosed reflux: a follow-up study. Br J Urol 1990;65:407–412.

43. Anderson PA, Rickwood AM. Features of primary vesicoureteric reflux detected by prenatal sonography. Br J Urol 1991;67:267–271.

44. Paltiel HJ, Lebowitz RL. Neonatal hydronephrosis due to primary vesicoureteral reflux: trends in diagnosis and treatment. Radiology 1989;170:787–789.

45. Chandra M, Maddix H, McVicar M. Transient urodynamic dysfunction of infancy: relationship to urinary tract infections and vesicoureteral reflux. J Urol 1996;155:673–677.

46. Galen. De naturalibus facultatibus. (Galen on the natural faculties, with English translation by Arthur John Brock) In: Heinemann W, ed. The Loeb classical library. London: Appleton and Company, 1916:339.

47. Hutch JA. The mesodermal component: its embryology, anatomy, physiology and role in prevention of vesicoureteral reflux. J Urol 1972;108:406–410.

48. Hinman FJ. Functional classification of conduits for continent urinary diversion. J Urol 1990;144:27.

49. Diamond DA, Rabinowitz R, Hoenig D, Caldamone AA. The mechanism of new onset contralateral reflux following unilateral ureteroneocystostomy. J Urol 1996;156:665–667.

50. Hinman FJ, Miller EA, Hutch JA, et al. Low pressure reflux relation of vesicoureteral reflux to intravesical pressure. J Urol 1962;88:758.

51. Hutch JA, Bunge RG, Flocks RH. Vesicoureteral reflux in children. J Urol 1955;74:607.

52. Tanagho EA, Meyers FH, Smith DR. The trigone: anatomical and physiological considerations, I In relation to the ureterovesical junction. J Urol 1968;100:623–632.

53. Ekman H, Jacobsson B, Kock NG, Sundin T. High diuresis, a factor in preventing vesicoureteral reflux. J Urol 1966;95:511–515.

54. Walker RD. Vesicoureteral reflux. In: Gillenwater JY, Grayhack JT, Howards SS, Duckett JW, eds. Adult and Pediatric Urology. Philadelphia: Mosby Year Book, 1991.

55. Stephens FD. The vesicoureteral hiatus and paraureteral diverticula. Trans Am Assoc Genitourin Surg 1978;70:47–51.

56. Hutch JA. Saccule formation at the ureterovesical junction in smooth walled bladders. J Urol 1961;86:390.

57. Uehling DT, Broskewitz, RC. Initiation of vesicoureteral reflux after heminephrectomy for ureterocele. Urology 1989;33:302–304.

58. Bellah RD, Long FR, Canning DA. Ureterocele eversion with vesicoureteral reflux in duplex kidneys: findings at voiding cystourethrography. AJR Am J Roentgenol 1995;165:409–413.

59. Chapman S, Bolton R. Intraureteric eversion and reflux into a simple ureterocele. Br J Radiol 1984;57:333–334.

60. Levard G, Aigrain Y, Ferkadji L et al. Urinary bladder diverticula and the Ehlers-Danlos syndrome in children. J Pediatr Surg 1989;24:1184.

61. Harcke HT, Capitanio MA, Grover WD, Valdes-Dopena M. Bladder diverticuli and Menke's syndrome. Radiology 1977;124:459–461.

62. Sillen U, Hjalmas K, Aili M, Bjure J, Hanson E, Hansson S. Pronounced detrusor hypercontractility in infants with gross bilateral reflux. J Urol 1992;148:598–599.

63. Sillen U, Bachelard M, Hermanson G, Hjalmas K. Gross bilateral reflux in infants: gradual decrease of initial detrusor hypercontractility. J Urol 1996;155:668–672.

64. Homsy YL, Nsouli I, Hamburger B, Laberge I, Schick E. Effects of oxybutynin on vesicoureteral reflux in children. J Urol 1985;134:1168–1171.

65. Koff SA, Lapides J, Piazza DH. Association of urinary tract infection and reflux with uninhibited bladder contractions and voluntary sphincteric obstruction. J Urol 1979;122:373–376.
66. Koff SA, Murtagh DS. The uninhibited bladder in children: effect of treatment on recurrence of urinary infection and on vesicoureteral reflux resolution. J Urol 1983;130:1138–1141.
67. Jerkins GR, Noe HN, Hill D. Treatment of complications of cyclophosphamide cystitis. J Urol 1988;139:923–925.
68. Roberts JA. Reflux nephropathy follows obstruction or infection. Semin Urol 1986;4:70–73.
69. Roberts JA, Kaack MB, Morvant AB. Vesicoureteral reflux in the primate, IV: Infection as cause of prolonged high-grade reflux. Pediatrics 1988;82:91–95.
70. Roberts JA. Effect of urinary tract infection on maturation of the ureterovesical junction. Surg Forum 1975;26:596–598.
71. Bumpus HC. Urinary reflux. J Urol 1924;12:341.
72. Auer J, Seager LD. Experimental local bladder edema causing urine reflux into ureter. J Exp Med 1937;66:741.
73. Teague N, Boyarsky S. Further effects of coliform bacteria on ureteral peristalsis. J Urol 1968;99:720.
74. Lennon GM, Ryan PC, Fitzpatrick JM. The ureter in vitro: normal motility and response to urinary pathogens. Br J Urol 1993;72:284.
75. Tamminen TE, Kaprio EA. The relation of the shape of renal papillae and of collecting duct openings to intrarenal reflux. Br J Urol 1977;49:345.
76. Heikel PE, Parkkulainen KV. Vesico-ureteric reflux in children: a classification and results of conservative treatment. Ann Radiol 1966;9:37.
77. Dwoskin JY, Perlmutter AD. Vesicoureteral reflux in children: a computerized review. J Urol 1973;109:888–890.
78. Bellinger MF, Duckett JW. Vesicoureteral reflux: a comparison of non-surgical and surgical management. Contrib Nephrol 1984;39:81–93.
79. Willi U, Treves S. Radionuclide voiding cystography. Urol Radiol 1983;5:161–173, 175.
80. Mackie GG, Awang H, Stephens FD. The ureteric orifice: the embryologic key to radiologic status of duplex kidneys. J Pediatr Surg 1975;10:473–481.
81. Mackie GG. Abnormalities of the ureteral bud. Urol Clin North Am 1978;5:161–174.
82. King LR. Vesicoureteral reflux, megaureter and ureteral reimplantation. In Walsh PC, Retik AB, Stamey TA, Vaughan ED, eds. Campbell's Urology, 6th ed. Philadelphia: W.B. Saunders, 1992.
83. Hinman F Jr, Miller ER, Hutch JA, Gainey MD, Cox CE, Goodfriend FB, Marshall S. Low pressure reflux: relation of vesicoureteral reflux in intravesical pressure. J Urol 1962;88:758.
84. Godley ML, Ransley PG, Parkhouse HF, Gordon I, Evans K, Peters AM. Quantitation of vesico-ureteral reflux by radionuclide cystography and urodynamics. Pediatr Nephrol 1990;4:485–490.
85. Smellie J. Do urinary tract infections really matter in children? Proc R Soc Med 1972;65:513–514.
86. Govan DE, Fair WR, Friedland GW, Filly RA. Management of children with urinary tract infections: the Stanford experience. Urology 1975;6:273–286.
87. Belman AB. Urinary tract infection and reflux [editorial]. JAM 1981;246:74.
88. Asscher AW, McLachlan MS, Jones RV, et al. Screening for asymptomatic urinary-tract infection in schoolgirls. A two-centre feasibility study. Lancet 1973;2:1–4.
89. Anonymous. Asymptomatic bacteriuria in schoolchildren in Newcastle upon Tyne. Arch Dis Child 1975;50:90–102.
90. Anonymous. Sequelae of covert bacteriuria in schoolgirls. A four-year follow-up study. Lancet 1978;1:889–893.
91. Savage DC, Wilson MI, McHardy M, Dewar DA, Fee WM. Covert bacteriuria of childhood. A clinical and epidemiological study. Arch Dis Child 1973;48:8–20.
92. Kunin CM. A ten-year study of bacteriuria in schoolgirls: final report of bacteriologic, urologic, and epidemiologic findings. J Infect Dis 1970;122:382–393.
93. Najmaldin A, Burge DM, Atwell JD. Fetal vesicoureteric reflux. Br J Urol 1990;65:403–406.
94. Noe HN, Wyatt RJ, Peeden JN Jr, Rivas ML. The transmission of vesicoureteral reflux from parent to child. J Urol 1992;148:1869–1871.
95. Smellie JM, Ransley PG, Normand IC, Prescod N, Edwards D. Development of new renal scars: a collaborative study. Br Med J (Clin Res Ed) 1985;290:1957–1960.
96. Limkakeng, AD, Retik AB. Unilateral renal agenesis with hypoplastic ureter: observations on the contralateral urinary tract and report of 4 cases. J Urol 1972;108:149–152.
97. Song JT, Ritchey ML, Zerin JM, Bloom DA. Incidence of vesicoureteral reflux in children with unilateral renal agenesis. J Urol 1995;153:1249–1251.
98. Gough DC, Postlethwaite RJ, Lewis MA, Bruce J. Multicystic renal dysplasia diagnosed in the antenatal period: a note of caution. Br J Urol 1995;76:244–248.
99. Selzman AA, Elder JS. Contralateral vesicoureteral reflux in children with a multicystic kidney. J Urol 1995;153:1252–1254.
100. van Gool JD, Hjalmas K, Tamminen-Mobius T, Olbing H. Historical clues to the complex of dysfunctional voiding, urinary tract infection and vesicoureteral reflux. The International Reflux Study in Children. J Urol 1992;148:1699–1702.
101. Paltiel HJ, Rupich RC, Kiruluta HG. Enhanced detection of vesicoureteral reflux in infants and children with use of cyclic voiding cystourethrography. Radiology 1992;184:753–755.
102. Kaplan GW. Postinfection reflux. Soc Pediatr Urology Newsletter, 1980:April 9.
103. Peeden JN Jr, Noe HN. Is it practical to screen for familial vesicoureteral reflux within a private pediatric practice? Pediatrics 1992;89:758–760.
104. Conway JJ, King LR, Belman AB, Thorson T. Jr. Detection of vesicoureteral reflux with radionuclide cystography. A comparison study with roentgenographic cystography. Am J Roentgenol Radium Ther Nucl Med 1972;115:720–727.
105. Kleinman PK, Diamond DA, Karellas A, Spevak MR, Nimkin K, Belanger P. Tailored low-dose fluoroscopic voiding cystourethrography for the reevaluation of vesicoureteral reflux in girls. AJR Am J Roentgenol 1994;1156;162:1151–1154; discussion 1155–1156.
106. Diamond DA, Kleinman PK, Spevak M, Nimkin K, Belanger P, Karellas A. The tailored low dose fluoroscopic voiding cystogram for familial reflux screening. J Urol 1996;155:681–682.
107. Nishizawa O, Ishida H, Sugaya K, Kohama T, Harada T, Tsuchida S. Application of Doppler color flow imaging method on the detection of vesicoureteral reflux. Tohoku J Exp Med 1989;159:163–164.
108. Andrich MP, Majd M. Diagnostic imaging in the evaluation of the first urinary tract infection in infants and young children. Pediatrics 1992;90:436–441.
109. Groshar D, Ember OM, Frenkel A, Front D. Renal function and technetium-99m dimercaptosuccinic acid uptake in single kidneys: the value of in vivo SPECT quantitation. J Nucl Med 1991;32:766.
110. Carr MC, Peters CA, Retik AB, Mandell J. Urinary levels of renal tubular enzyme N-acetyl-beta-D-glucosaminidase in relation to grade of vesicoureteral reflux. J Urol 1991;146:654–656.
111. Haraoka M, Senoh K, Ogata N, Furukawa M, Matsumoto T, Kumazawa J. Elevated interleukin-8 levels in the urine of children with renal scarring and/or vesicoureteral reflux. J Urol 1996;155:678–680.
112. Ransley PG, Risdon RA. Renal papillae and intrarenal reflux in the pig. Lancet 1974;2:1114.
113. Ransley PG, Risdon RA. Renal papillary morphology in infants and young children. Urol Res 1975;3:111–113.
114. Whitaker RH, Cuckow PM. A method of demonstrating intrarenal reflux. Br J Urol 1994;73:572–574.
115. Winter AL, Hardy BE, Alton DJ, Arbus GS, Churchill BM. Acquired renal scars in children. J Urol 1983;129:1190–1194.
116. Filly RA, Friedland GW, Govan DE, Fair WR. Urinary tract infections in children. Part II, Roentgenologic aspects. West J Med 1974;121:374–381.
117. Winberg J, Bergstrom T, Jacobsson B. Morbidity, age and sex distribution, recurrences and renal scarring in symptomatic urinary tract infection in childhood. Kidney Int 1975;8:s101.
118. Funston MR, Cremin BJ. Intrarenal reflux-papillary morphology

and pressure relationships in children's necropsy kidneys. Br J Urol 1978;51:665–670.

119. Rolleston GL, Maling TM, Hodson CJ. Intrarenal reflux and the scarred kidney. Arch Dis Child 1974;49:531–539.

120. Hodson CJ, Maling TM, McManamon PJ, Lewis MG. The pathogenesis of reflux nephropathy (chronic atrophic pyelonephritis). Br J Radiol 1975;suppl:1–26.

121. Ransley PG, Risdon RA. Reflux nephropathy: effects of antimicrobial therapy on the evolution of the early pyelonephritic scar. Kidney Int 1981;20:733–742.

122. Roberts JA, Fischman NH, Thomas R. Vesicoureteral reflux in the primate IV: does reflux harm the kidney? J Urol 1982; 128:650–652.

123. Smellie JM, Edwards D, Normand IC, Prescod N. Effect of vesicoureteric reflux on renal growth in children with urinary tract infection. Arch Dis Child 1981;56:593–600.

124. Smellie J, Normand C. Reflux nephropathy in childhood. In: Hodson J, Kincaid-Smith P, eds. Reflux Nephropath, NY: Masson Publishing, USA, 1979;14–20.

125. Crabbe DC, Thomas DF, Gordon AC, Irving HC, Arthur RJ, Smith SE. Use of 99mtechnetium-dimercaptosuccinic acid to study patterns of renal damage associated with prenatally detected vesicoureteral reflux. J Urol 1992;148:1229–1231.

126. Wallace DM, Rothwell DL, Williams DI. The long-term follow-up of surgically treated vesicoureteric reflux. Br J Urol 1978; 50:479–484.

127. Savage JM, Koh CT, Shah V, Barratt TM, Dillon MJ. Five year prospective study of plasma renin activity and blood pressure in patients with longstanding reflux nephropathy. Arch Dis Child 1987;62:678–682.

128. Braren V, West JC Jr, Boerth RC, Harmon CM. Management of children with hypertension from reflux or obstructive nephropathy. Urology 1988;32:228–234.

129. Savage JM, Dillon MJ, Shah V, Barratt TM, Williams DI. Renin and blood-pressure in children with renal scarring and vesicoureteric reflux. Lancet 1978;2:441–444.

130. Siegler RL. Renin-dependent hypertension in children with reflux nephropathy. Urology 1976;7:474–478.

131. Walker D, Richard GA. A critical evaluation of urethral obstruction in female children. Pediatrics 1973;51:272–277.

132. Uehling DT. Effect of vesicoureteral reflux on concentrating ability. J Urol 1971;106:947–950.

133. Uehling DT, Wear JB Jr. Concentrating ability after antireflux operation. J Urol 1976;116:83–84.

134. Walker RD. Renal functional changes associated with vesicoureteral reflux. Urol Clin North Am 1990;17:307–316.

135. Walker RD, Garin EH. Urinary prostaglandin E2 in patients with vesicoureteral reflux. Child Nephrol Urol 1990;10:18–21.

136. Kincaid-Smith P. Glomerular and vascular lesions in chronic atrophic pyelonephritis and reflux nephropathy. Adv Nephrol 1975;5:3.

137. Torres VE, Malek RS, Svensson JP. Vesicoureteral reflux in the adult, II: Nephropathy, hypertension and stones. J Urol 1983; 130:41–44.

138. Hollowell JG, Altman HG, Snyder HMD, Duckett JW. Coexisting ureteropelvic junction obstruction and vesicoureteral reflux: diagnostic and therapeutic implications. J Urol 1989;142:490–493; discussion 501.

139. Maizels M, Smith CK, Firlit CF. The management of children with vesicoureteral reflux and ureteropelvic junction obstruction. J Urol 1984;131:722–727.

140. Lebowitz RL, Blickman JG. The coexistence of ureteropelvic junction obstruction and reflux. AJR Am J Roentgenol 1983; 140:231–238.

141. Williams DI. Vesico-ureteric reflux. In: Aiken CE, Williams DI, Barnes RW, Ljunggren EJC, Boshamer K, eds. Encyclopedia of Urologogy. Berlin: Springer-Verlag 1974;119–125.

142. Whitaker RH. Reflux induced pelvi-ureteric obstruction. Br J Urol 1976;48:555–560.

143. Johnston JH. Upper urinary tract obstruction. In: Williams, DI, Johnston JH, eds. Paediatric Urology, 2nd ed. London: Butterworth Scientific, 1982;195.

144. Shopfner CE. Ureteropelvic junction obstruction. Am J Roentgen 1966;98:148.

145. Mandell J, Lebowitz RL, Peters CA, Estroff JA, Retik AB, Benacerraf BR. Prenatal diagnosis of the megacystis-megaureter association. J Urol 1992;148:1487–1489.

146. Kaefer M, Peters C, Retik A, Benacerraf B. Criteria for differentiating between obstructive and nonobstructive etiologies of bladder distension using prenatal sonography. Pediatrics 1996;Abstract.

147. Skoog SJ, Belman AB, Majd M. A nonsurgical approach to the management of primary vesicoureteral reflux. J Urol 1987;138: 941–946.

148. Tamminen-Mobius T, Brunier E, Ebel KD, et al. Cessation of vesicoureteral reflux for 5 years in infants and children allocated to medical treatment. The International Reflux Study in Children. J Urol 1992;148:1662–1666.

149. Steele BT, Robitaille P, DeMaria J, Grignon A. Follow-up evaluation of prenatally recognized vesicoureteric reflux. J Pediatr 1989;115:95–96.

150. Kaplan WE, Nasrallah P, King LR. Reflux in complete duplication in children. J Urol 1978;120:220–222.

151. Peppas DS, Skoog SJ, Canning DA, Belman AB. Nonsurgical management of primary vesicoureteral reflux in complete ureteral duplication: is it justified? J Urol 1991;146:1594–1595.

152. Fehrenbaker LG, Kelalis PP, Stickler GB. Vesicoureteral reflux and ureteral duplication in children. J Urol 1972;107:862–864.

153. Smellie JM, Gruneberg RN, Leakey A, Atkin WS. Long-term low-dose cotrimoxazole in prophylaxis of childhood urinary tract infection: clinical aspects. Br Med J 1976;2:203–206.

154. Smellie JM, Poulton A, Prescod NP. Retrospective study of children with renal scarring associated with reflux and urinary infection. BMJ 1994;308:1193–1196.

155. Scholtmeijer RJ. Treatment of vesicoureteric reflux. Results of a prospective study. Br J Urol 1993;71:346–349.

156. Belman AB, Skoog SJ. Nonsurgical approach to the management of vesicoureteral reflux in children. Pediatr Infect Dis J 1989;8: 556–559.

157. Anonymous. Medical versus surgical treatment of primary vesicoureteral reflux: report of the International Reflux Study Committee. Pediatrics 1981;67:392–400.

158. Weiss R, Duckett J, Spitzer A. Results of a randomized clinical trial of medical versus surgical management of infants and children with grades III and IV primary vesicoureteral reflux (United States). The International Reflux Study in Children. J Urol 1992;148:1667–1673.

159. Jodal U, Koskimies O, Hanson E, et al. Infection pattern in children with vesicoureteral reflux randomly allocated to operation or long-term antibacterial prophylaxis. The International Reflux Study in Children. J Urol 1992;148:1650–1652.

160. Group, B.R.S. Prospective trial of operative versus non-operative treatment of severe vesicoureteric reflux in children: five years observation. Br Med J (Clinical Research Edition) 1987; 295:237.

161. Arant BS Jr. Medical management of mild and moderate vesicoureteral reflux: followup studies of infants and young children. A preliminary report of the Southwest Pediatric Nephrology Study Group. J Urol 1992;148:1683–1687.

162. Koff SA. Relationship between dysfunctional voiding and reflux. J Urol 1992;148:1703–1705.

163. Woodard JR, Keats G. Ureteral reimplantation: Paquin's procedure after 12 years. J Urol 1973;109:891–894.

164. Hendren W. Ureteral reimplantation in children. J Pediatr Surg 1968;3:649–664.

165. Houle AM, McLorie GA, Heritz DM, McKenna PH, Churchill BM, Khoury, AE. Extravesical nondismembered ureteroplasty with detrusorrhaphy: a renewed technique to correct vesicoureteral reflux in children. J Urol 1992;148:704–707.

166. Burbige KA, Miller M, Connor JP. Extravesical ureteral reimplantation: results in 128 patients. J Urol 1996;155:1721–1722.

167. Zaontz MR, Maizels M, Sugar EC, Firlit CF. Detrusorrhaphy: extravesical ureteral advancement to correct vesicoureteral reflux in children. J Urol 1987;138:947–949.

168. O'Donnell B, Puri P. Treatment of vesicoureteric reflux by endoscopic injection of Teflon. Br Med J (Clin Res Ed) 1984;289:7–9.

169. Frey P, Lutz N, Jenny P, Herzog B. Endoscopic subureteral

collagen injection for the treatment of vesicoureteral reflux in infants and children. J Urol 1995;154:804–807.

170. Politano V. One hundred reimplantations and five years. J Urol 1963;90:696–701.

171. Burbige KA. Ureteral reimplantation: a comparison of results with the cross-trigonal and Politano-Leadbetter techniques in 120 patients. J Urol 1991;146:1352–1353.

172. Glenn JF, Anderson EE. Distal tunnel ureteral reimplantation. J Urol 1967;97:623–626.

173. Glenn JF, Anderson EE. Technical considerations in distal tunnel ureteral reimplantation. J Urol 1978;119:194–198.

174. Gonzales ET, Glenn JF, Anderson EE. Results of distal tunnel ureteral reimplantation. J Urol 1972;107:572–575.

175. Cohen S. Ureterozystoneostomie. Eine neue antirefluxtechnik. Akt Urol 1975;6:1–8.

176. Ehrlich RM. Success of the transvesical advancement technique for vesicoureteral reflux. J Urol 1982;128:554–557.

177. Ahmed S. Ureteral reimplantation by the transverse advancement technique. J Urol 1978;119:547–550.

178. Lich R, Howerton L, Goode L, et al. The uretero-vesical junction of the newborn. J Urol 1964;92:436.

179. Gregoir W, Van Regermorter G. Le reflux vesico-ureteral congenital. Urology International 1964;18:122.

180. Heimbach D, Bruhl P, Mallmann R. Lich-Gregoir anti-reflux procedure: indications and results with 283 vesicoureteral units. Scand J Urol Nephrol 1995;29:311–316.

181. Marberger M, Altwein JE, Straub E, Wulff SH, Hohenfellner R. The Lich-Gregoir antireflux plasty: experiences with 371 children. J Urol 1978;120:216–219.

182. Linn R, Ginesin Y, Bolkier M, Levin DR. Lich-Gregoir antireflux operation: a surgical experience and 5-20 years of follow-up in 149 ureters. Eur Urol 1989;16:200–203.

183. Puri P. Ten year experience with subureteric Teflon (polytetra-fluoroethylene) injection (STING) in the treatment of vesico-ureteric reflux. Br J Urol 1995;75:126–131.

184. Malizia A, Reiman H, Myers R, et al. Migration and granulomatous reaction after periurethral injection of polytef (Teflon). JAMA 1984;251:3277.

185. Atala A, Kim W, Paige KT, Vacanti CA, Retik AB. Endoscopic treatment of vesicoureteral reflux with a chondrocyte-alginate suspension. J Urol 1994;152:641–643; discussion 644.

CHAPTER 28

Hypospadias

David R. Roth

Hypospadias is the most common congenital anomaly of the penis and occurs in approximately 0.32% of males in the United States.[1] The term "hypospadias" is used to describe an abnormal configuration of the penis in which the urethral meatus is located on the ventrum of the penis proximal to the distalmost part of the glans. (If the meatus is located on the dorsal surface of the penis, the condition is termed "epispadias" rather than hypospadias.) Hypospadias varies in degree—from the more common glandular defect to a relatively rare, severe scrotal and perineal abnormality. The most common defects are the more distal abnormalities, but proximal hypospadias is seen regularly in busy pediatric urology referral centers.

Although hypospadias may be an isolated abnormality, it is generally, although not always, associated with an incomplete prepuce (dorsal hood) and chordee (ventral bending of the penile shaft). Often hypospadias is described by degrees with a first degree having the meatus between the glans and the distal shaft, second degree having the meatus between the midshaft and the proximal shaft, and the third degree with the meatus being penoscrotal, scrotal, or perineal. The severity of the chordee is not considered in this system, although it is very important in planning any surgical correction. Therefore, a more informative grading system was introduced by Barcat in 1973[2] that described the location of the meatus after the chordee, if any, has been released (Table 28.1).

Additionally, the following factors should be considered: the size of the meatus; the presence, degree, and location of chordee; and whether the chordee appears to be secondary to skin tethering; the thickness and dysplasia (if any) of the ventral skin; and the amount of dorsal skin (hood) present. All of these factors are important in planning a surgical correction and may influence the choice of surgical procedure to be utilized. Additionally, a description of the penis, rather than a grading of the defect, will provide more meaningful information for any physician consulted in the future.

In the past, evaluation of children with hypospadias sometimes included an intravenous pyelogram and/or voiding cystourethrogram. However, studies have shown that the incidence of associated upper urinary tract abnormalities is quite low and screening of the kidneys is not necessary.[3] Two studies[4, 5] have demonstrated that reflux is present in 10 to 17% of boys with hypospadias. The reflux is generally low grade and not of clinical importance. Therefore, most pediatric urologists restrict radiographic evaluation to those patients who would otherwise undergo x-rays for other indications, most commonly a history of urinary tract infection. Cystoscopy has no place in the routine evaluation of a child with hypospadias. A prominent utricle may be identified on voiding cystography, especially if the child has bilateral undescended testes as well. In that condition it may be associated with abnormal chromosomal analysis, but in all other circumstances it has no significance other than its potential to complicate catheterization of the urethra. Surgical treatment of a large utricle is unnecessary and may actually be detrimental given the intimate anatomic association of the external urethral sphincter and the verumontanum.

EMBRYOLOGY AND ETIOLOGY

The embryologic origin of the hypospadias defect lies in the development of the external genitalia. Penile development occurs early in the first trimester of pregnancy. The penis is formed by elongation of the genital tubercle, which can be identified within the first several weeks of gestation. The urethra is formed by three separate processes. The proximalmost part is the extension of the Wolffian duct system and includes the urethra from the bladder neck to the verumontanum. Hypospadias is not seen in this area. From the verumontanum to the glans, the urethra is formed by the infolding of the margins of the urethral groove, which is an elongation of the urethral folds and extension of the urogenital sinus. The labial scrotal folds close over the urethra to form the skin of the scrotum and penile shaft. The glandular

TABLE 28.1. *Classification of hypospadias according to meatal location after release of curvature*

Anterior hypospadias
    Glandular (meatus situated on the inferior surface of the glans)
    Coronal (meatus situated in the balanopenile furrow)
    Anterior penile (meatus situated in the distal third of the shaft)
Middle hypospadias
    Middle penile (meatus situated in the distal third of the shaft)
Posterior hypospadias
    Posterior penile (meatus situated in the posterior third of the shaft)
    Penoscrotal (meatus situated at the base of the shaft in front of the scrotum)
    Scrotal (meatus situated on the scrotum or between the genital swellings)
    Perineal (meatus situated behind the scrotum or behind the genital swellings)

Modified from Gillenwater J, Grayhack J, Howards SS, Duckett JW, eds. Adult and pediatric urology. 2nd ed. Chicago: Mosby–Year Book, 1991:2104.

urethra develops by the ingrowth of ectoderm from the tip of the penis. These cells canalize, forming the glandular urethra. The penile and glandular urethras meet at the corona, a common site of hypospadias. The prepuce is formed toward the end of the first trimester by the continued rolling of the genital folds. In hypospadias this process is incomplete because full closure of the glans does not occur. This failure gives rise both to an incomplete prepuce with a prominent dorsal hood and to a flattened appearance of the glans commonly observed in boys with hypospadias. Chordee may be a result of dystrophic ventral penile skin that tethers the penis. Sometimes, however, the bending persists because of a disproportion in the development of the corporal bodies or dense fibrous tissue along the corpus spongiosum. Often it is impossible to determine preoperatively the exact etiology of the chordee and the techniques that will be required to release it.

Although a definite cause for hypospadias has been identified in only a few cases, the presence of a genetic component is implied by the increased incidence of hypospadias in relatives of a boy with hypospadias.[1] Urethral development occurs under the influence of dihydrotestosterone, which is converted in peripheral tissues from testosterone by 5-α reductase. Therefore, the development of hypospadias can be related either to a reduction in 5-α reductase activity, to a lack of testosterone production, or to failure of the local receptors to recognize the hormone once it has been produced. A genetic abnormality has been identified in at least one child with hypospadias, but a cohesive definitive theory to explain most instances of hypospadias in children has yet to be proposed.[6]

SURGICAL GOALS AND PRINCIPLES

For decades surgical correction of hypospadias has been undertaken in an attempt to provide function and appearance of the penis that are as nearly normal as possible. Until recently, the goals of the procedure were limited to bringing the meatus "close" to the glans to allow the child to void standing, removing the chordee to allow for normal intercourse, and giving the phallus an appearance of a normally circumcised penis when observed from a distance. The surgery often was performed in stages with the expectation of completing all surgery by the time the child was 2 years old. Currently, our goals, although similar, are more exacting. The surgical outcome ideally should be a penis that appears normal to more than a causal observation. The meatus should be well placed on the tip of the glans and have a slitlike appearance. There should be glandular tissue proximal to the meatus and a mucosal collar of prepucial skin[7] distal to a smooth penile shaft. The child should be able to stand to void and the penis must be straight when erect. Because of advances in surgical techniques and anesthesia, these objectives can be achieved in most cases.

At pediatric referral centers throughout the country, urologists have had the opportunity to treat many cases of hypospadias and other unusual penile anomalies. Optical magnification by either surgical loupes (2X to 4X) or the operating microscope has become the standard throughout the country for all hypospadias surgery and offers significant benefits in performance of these procedures involving small sutures and delicate tissues. Fine (7-0 and 8-0), absorbable (catgut, chromic, Vicryl, Dexon, or PDS) sutures and delicate ophthalmic instruments are used throughout the procedure. Penile dressings, once bulky and cumbersome, have become simple—often a single piece of Op-Site, (a semipermeable, bio-occlusive dressing) that, in some cases, can be removed at home by the parents. Pediatric anesthesia has become widespread and safe. Regional, caudal anesthesia allows the child to remain comfortable for hours and to go home shortly after the surgical procedure.[8] Soft silastic tubes are used for urinary drainage and are often drained directly into a diaper to allow easy postoperative care. Although many physicians no longer use urinary diversion tubes, I continue to use them in almost all patients. We now operate on these youngsters when they are 6 months of age or younger and perform almost all procedures on an outpatient basis. With rare exceptions, a single-stage operation accomplishes the stated goals with limited complications.

Although there are more than 200 named surgical procedures to correct hypospadias, there are a few general concepts that are common to all. Close, preoperative inspection of the penis and groin are imperative to eliminate the possibility of operating in an area of diaper rash. The procedure is elective and can easily be delayed if the patient is not in the best of health. Perioperative antibiotics (a broad-spectrum cephalosporin) should be considered for any repeat operation or a procedure utilizing a free graft or a prepucial flap. Simple, meatal-based flaps or less-involved procedures can be performed safely without antibiotics.

Complete correction of any ventral penile chordee is imperative prior to completion of the operation and must be accomplished before the urethroplasty because the urethral meatus may move proximally as the penis is straightened and the ventrum extended. The use of an artificial erection[9] achieved by the injection of normal saline directly into the corpora cavernosum has become a mainstay of all hypospadias techniques to identify any residual chordee. In many cases, the chordee can be released by the sharp excision of fibrous tissue on the ventral corpora cavernosum along the corpus spongiosum. If any chordee remains after this dissection, it must be corrected. Nesbit described a plication procedure in which the dorsal lateral Buck's fascia is elevated off the corpora cavernosum and a wedge of tunica albuginea is removed. Closure of this defect by plication will often straighten the penis. If the chordee persists, the urethral plate must be elevated and a wedge of tunica albuginea from the ventrum removed. To close this defect and allow the penis to become straight, the ventrum is grafted with either tunica vaginalis from around the testis[10] or a dermal graft from the groin.[11] A second artificial erection must be performed to confirm that the penis is straight before the urethroplasty is begun.

A meatus that is normal in appearance and well placed on the glans should be possible in almost all cases. In the past, because of reluctance to operate on or even incise the glans penis, a subcoronal meatus was an acceptable final result. That is no longer the case, and the glans can be safely divided to bring the neourethra to its tip. Hypospadias surgery has advanced to the point that the glans is completely split to allow placement of a neourethra well into the glans. Anticipated problems of meatal stenosis and glans stricture do not occur, and the glans heals nicely, rarely leaving a significant scar. Injection of 0.5% lidocaine with 1:200,000 epinephrine directly into the glans penis or a tourniquet applied to the base of the penis during the operation will control the typically brisk glandular bleeding and allow completion of operative procedures in a relatively blood-free operative field. Closure of the glans with fine, absorb-

able suture gives an excellent cosmetic result with the scar often being almost invisible.

Most complicated hypospadias surgery use a technique for bringing in "new" skin to form a neourethra. This skin can either be vascularized, as in a meatal-based or prepucial flap, or non-vascularized, as with a graft from the prepucial skin, distant split-thickness skin, or buccal mucosal tissue. Both methods can provide excellent results, but most surgeons have a preference (based on training, personal experience, or bias) of one over the other. Because operative plans are often modified during the operative procedure to correct hypospadias, it is important for the surgeon to be familiar with several approaches.

The use of barrier tissue, either local or distant, has been found to be very beneficial in hypospadias surgery. A time-honored principle of reconstructive surgery has been that suture lines should be separated, since overlying suture lines are thought to increase the likelihood of breakdown of repairs and subsequent fistula formation. When it is not possible to offset the suture lines, vascularized flaps with blood supply based on the inner surface of the prepuce, parameatal region, scrotum, or even the tunica vaginalis can be used to provide separation between suture line and vascular support for underlying tissues. This approach should decrease the incidence of fistulae and improve ingrowth of blood vessels for free grafts.

Skin closure of the penile shaft, especially the dorsum, is very important, and because that area is most visible to parents and others, the skin there should be as flat as possible. At the same time, although the ventral skin is less visible, redundant skin should not remain at the conclusion of the procedure. The goal is to have the penis look as normal as possible before the child leaves the operating room. Subcutaneous skin closure with fine, absorbable suture will give an excellent appearance to subsequent scars and avoid unsightly skin tracks. The technique resulting in overlapping Byars flaps, which were once popular, has been replaced in many centers by techniques giving a single ventral midline scar that mimics the normal median raphe.[12] Construction of a glanular meatus with an apparent slit well placed at the tip should be possible in almost all cases.

Currently, patient immobilization and hospitalization are no longer needed for the repair of any but the most severe cases of hypospadias. Almost all patients are discharged on the day of surgery. The use of short, small-caliber, silastic urethral catheters that drain directly into the diaper has eliminated the turmoil associated with closed drainage systems and has not increased the incidence of urinary tract infections[13] or wound breakdown. These tubes are readily accepted by parents, easy to manage, and, while in place, negate the possibility of postoperative urinary retention. They are easily removed in the office, or in some cases even at home, 3 to 5 days after distal penile repairs and 10 to 14 days after grafts and prepucial flaps. For patient comfort, anticholinergic medication is prescribed as long as the catheter remains indwelling. The use of caudal anesthesia has significantly improved the postoperative course of these boys and has greatly decreased the need for both parenteral and home analgesics. The placement of a caudal anesthetic is rapid and safe, and its effects will last for several hours.[8] A simple dressing of Op-site or Tegaderm, both of which are semipermeable, is generally sufficient to decrease edema and keep the wound clean for all repairs. Occasionally, a pressure dressing with 1-inch cling may be considered when there appears to be slightly more than usual bleeding.

HYPOSPADIAS REPAIR

Hypospadias surgery can be classified by the type of procedure performed, and that generally is determined by the location of the original meatus (Table 28.2). The distal repairs usually can be performed without the use of either skin flaps or grafts. Advancement procedures such as the MAGPI,[14] urethral advancement,[15] or the Glans Approximation Procedure (GAP)[16] are often performed for distal lesions. If the meatus is more proximal, an attempt to preserve the urethral plate is appropriate, and techniques such as meatal-based flaps,[17] Barcat,[18] Horton Devine,[19] modified Tiersch-Duplay,[20] prepucial flaps,[21] or free grafts (onlay) are used for the repair. The midshaft or proximal meatus with significant chordee may require division of the urethral plate, which in turn would require construction with a tubularized graft[22] or a flap from the prepuce.[23] For the most severe cases, an approach combining both local tubularization of the proximal skin and a flap for a distal neourethra may be

TABLE 28.2. *Surgical procedures and degree of hypospadias*

Distal hypospadias
  MAGPI[a]
  Advancement[a]
  GAP[a]
Midshaft hypospadias
  Mathieu[a]
  Horton Devine
  Mastarde
  Barcat
  Modified GAP or Tiersch-Duplay[a]
Proximal repairs
  Duckett Ti[a]
  Onlay[a]
  Hodgson
  ASOPA
  Prepucial free graft[a]
  Two-stage[a]
  Combined
  Buccal mucosal

[a]Described in text.

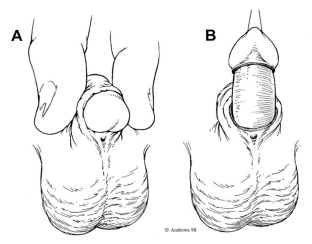

FIG. 28.1. As the chordee is released (**A**), the location of the meatus can slip proximally (**B**).

required.[24] A two-stage repair, although often derided in national meetings, still has a place in the treatment of very severe hypospadias associated with significant chordee.[25] In all cases, it is necessary to complete correction of any chordee before undertaking the urethroplasty, and this correction often modifies the location of the urethral meatus because it may slip proximally when the penis straightens (Fig. 28.1).

Because there are more than 200 reported techniques for the repair of hypospadias, it would be impossible to describe each procedure in detail. Therefore, discussion will be limited to those procedures that I commonly employ to repair each level of hypospadias.

Release of Chordee

The initial goal of any hypospadias repair is the confirmation of a straight penis. Before the urethroplasty is begun, an artificial erection is created by injecting either normal or heparinized saline into the corporal bodies after compression has been applied to the base of the penis. If the penis is curved after repair of the urethra, the subsequent release of chordee could jeopardize the neourethra. Therefore, once the penis has been degloved, the surgeon should artificially induce an erection by injecting saline into one of the corpora while compressing the base of the penis. If the penis is straight, the repair of the urethra can proceed. On the other hand, if there is ventral bending of the penis, a formal release of chordee is required. The straightening is begun by removing all the ventral fibrous tissue that overlies the corpus spongiosum and corpora cavernosa. Particular attention should be directed to the junction between the spongiosum and cavernosa because of the layer of tissue that often resides there. Once the glistening tunica albuginea of the corpora is seen, further removal of tissue will not be helpful and may cause troublesome bleeding. An artificial erection is obtained at that time. If chordee remains, the penis must be straightened by either shortening the dorsum or lengthening the ventrum. In most cases, penile length is adequate, and dorsal plications will accomplish the straightening without adversely affecting penile length. The technique was initially described by Nesbit.[26] However, it has been modified subsequently.[27,28] The dorsal neurovascular tissue should be elevated off the corpora cavernosa at the point of maximal curvature. At the dorsolateral angle, bilateral longitudinal incisions in the tunica albuginea are made. These are closed horizontally with 4-0 braided permanent suture and the curvature thus corrected. Artificial induction of an erection is repeated to confirm the absence of persistent bending. A second set of plications rarely is required.

In those instances of extreme chordee, consideration of ventral grafting of the tunica albuginea is appropriate. The urethral plate is elevated, and an incision of the tunica is made at the point of maximal curvature. A graft is harvested from the tunica vaginalis around the testis and used to close the defect in the corpora. This is sewn in place with fine, absorbable suture. A repeat artificial erection should confirm the absence of any residual chordee.

MAGPI

The meatal advancement and glans plasty (MAGPI)[14] for the treatment of a penis with a glandular or coronal meatus without chordee enjoyed widespread support and enthusiasm when first introduced. The procedure is relatively simple, and, because it does not involve a urethroplasty, has a minimal complication rate. Subsequent criticisms concerning the final cosmetic result, especially the blunting of the glans, have led to the limitation of this procedure to correction of only the most distal defects. The MAGPI essentially consists of incising the urethral groove from the meatus to the tip of the penis, suturing the meatus to the tip (with 7-0 Vicryl) and bringing glandular wings proximal to the neomeatus (Fig. 28.2). Penile shaft skin is reapproximated in a standard fashion. The procedure does not so much move the urethra as modify its appearance and its relationship to the remainder of the glans. If the indications have been extended so that more proximal defects are being treated, tension may develop on the advancement, giving the penis a bull-nosed appearance. Therefore, other techniques have, to a great extent, supplanted the MAGPI.

Urethral Advancement

Urethral advancement is used to correct many distal defects, especially those with the meatus at the coronal margin or just distal to it on the glans. The procedure

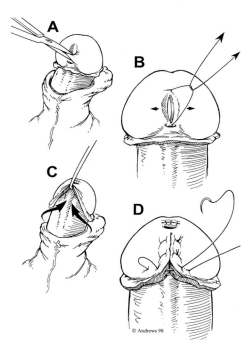

FIG. 28.2. **A,** For MAGPI, the penis has been degloved, and the chordee released. The incision is made between the meatus and the tip of the penis. **B,** Interrupted sutures are used to close this gap. **C,** Glandular tissue is drawn distally. **D,** Glandular sutures are placed to reapproximate the glans proximal to the neomeatus. Reprinted with permission from Kalais, King, and Belman, eds., Clinical pediatric urology, 3rd ed. Philadelphia: Lippincott-Raven, 1992:635.

is begun by degloving the penis to the penoscrotal angle. A mucosal collar is incorporated into the skin incision as described by Firlit.[7] An artificial erection is obtained to confirm that the penis is straight, and if it is not, release of the chordee is undertaken. Then the urethral meatus is circumscribed and the dissection continued proximally until the urethra is sufficiently free so that the meatus can easily and without tension be brought into the distal glans. The glans is injected with 1 mL of 0.5% lidocaine with 1:200,000 epinephrine and split in its midline with a circular segment excised at the midline location of the proposed neomeatus. The glans may be debulked, especially distally, to allow placement of the urethra into it. Glandular wings are developed by elevating the glans off the tips of the corpora cavernosa. The urethra is placed in the glans with the meatus easily reaching the tip. The meatus is tacked into place with interrupted sutures of 6-0 or 7-0 chromic or Vicryl. The glans is brought over the urethra and closed in two layers—the deep layer with 6-0 Vicryl in horizontal mattress sutures and the skin layer with simple 6-0 chromic running sutures—without excessive compression on the urethra. The penile shaft skin is then rotated and trimmed as necessary to cover the shaft. A stent can be placed and left for 3 to 5 days, although there are

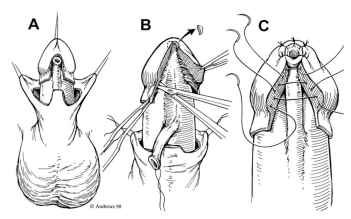

FIG. 28.3. **A,** For sleeve advancement urethroplasty, holding sutures are placed and a perimeatal M incision is made. **B,** Urethral mobilization is completed, the glans is bivalved, and the glans wings are created. Triangles of glanular epithelium are removed. **C,** Meatal sutures are placed, and the glans-plasty is performed. Modified from Spencer JR, Perlmutter, AD. Sleeve advancement distal hypospadias repair. J Urol 1990;144:523.

urologists who would not divert this repair (Fig. 28.3). As a neourethra is not constructed, complications are unusual and are generally restricted to meatal stenosis.

GAP and Modified Tiersch-Duplay Urethroplasty

The glans approximation procedure (GAP) was introduced by Zaontz in 1989.[16] With modifications, it can be used to deal with many forms of hypospadias.[20] Indeed, it has become the procedure I use most frequently. I like it particularly for boys with limited chordee and a meatus distal to the midshaft if the glans is of good size with a well-formed urethral plate. I begin by marking the penile skin and incorporating both a mucosal collar and a meatal-based skin flap on the ventrum if sufficient skin is present. If a flap cannot be used, the incision comes just proximal to the meatus. The flap can be used for a vascularized barrier layer over the neourethra after being de-epithelialized or for the neourethra itself if a GAP is abandoned and a flip-flap procedure performed. Skin incisions are then made and the penile shaft skin dropped back to the penoscrotal junction. The chordee is released and an artificial erection established to confirm the absence of any bending. Once it is determined that the penis is straight, the glans is injected with 1 mL of 0.5% lidocaine with 1:200,000 epinephrine. Lateral incisions, wide enough to allow closure over an 8F urethral catheter, are made along the urethral plate and extend onto the glans to the location of the proposed neomeatus. The glans incisions are deepened and brought laterally so that the glans ultimately will cover the neourethra without tension. In those instances in which closure is tight over an 8F catheter, the urethral

plate should be incised in its midline as described by Snodgrass.[29] This will allow the edges of the skin to cover the stent and will give the neourethra an adequate diameter. The resultant defect in the urethral plate re-epithelializes and has not been reported to cause any problems. Closure of the urethra is begun distally with 7-0 Vicryl and continued in a subcuticular manner toward the original meatus. Just before final closure, the excess skin of the meatal-based flap is excised, leaving only the vascular tissue that is brought distally and tacked in place with 7-0 Vicryl over the neourethra. If that tissue either is not available or is tethered tightly to the corpus spongiosum, vascularized tissue can be harvested from the inner layer of the prepuce or the tunica vaginalis to provide a barrier layer. The glans is closed and the penis recovered as in the previously described procedure (Fig. 28.4). The penis is dressed with Op-site, and a urethral catheter is left in place for 3 to 5 days.

Meatal-Based Flaps

The modified Mathieu or flip-flap hypospadias repair[17] is used for a penis with limited chordee or no chordee and a meatus that is generally between the midshaft and corona. The first part of the procedure is the same as that for the GAP. A circumferential incision is made about the dorsum of the penis with a flap based at the meatus on the ventrum. The length of the flap is the same as the distance that the urethra must be extended to reach the tip of the penis. The skin is dissected to the penoscrotal junction, and any chordee present is

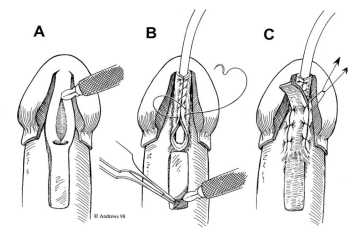

FIG. 28.4. **A,** For tubularized, incised plate urethroplasty, the penis is degloved and the chordee is released. Next, longitudinal incisions are made to separate urethral plate from the glans. Then a deep midline incision of urethral plate from the meatus to the glanular tip is performed. **B,** The urethral plate is tubularized over the catheter. **C,** Dorsal subcutaneous tissue is mobilized to cover the suture line before glans closure.

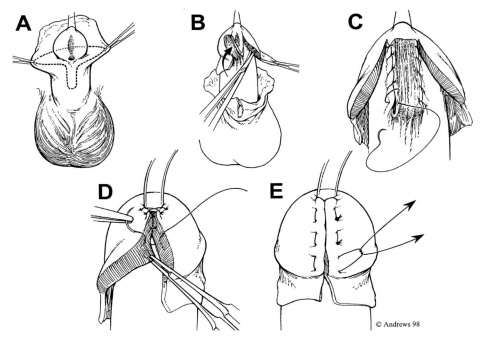

FIG. 28.5. **A,** For meatal-based flaps, skin incisions are made, incorporating a flap based on the meatus. **B,** Incisions are made to the distal glans, and the flap is flipped to the distal glans. **C,** The flap is sewn to the edges of the urethral plate. **D and E,** Glans closure is completed in two layers.

released in the same manner as with the GAP hypospadias repair. Once the chordee has been released, lateral incisions are marked on the glans that are parallel and in line with the lateral margins of the meatal-based flap. The technique of urethral plate incision described by Snodgrass[29] can be incorporated at this point if additional tissue is needed to close the neourethra over the catheter. The flap is then flipped (thus flip-flap) so that its original proximal border becomes the neomeatus (Fig. 28.5). The neourethra is then closed over an 8F catheter. Each lateral border is reapproximated with 7-0 Vicryl in a subcuticular manner. A barrier layer of vascular tissue from the flap, from the inner aspect of the prepuce, or from the tunica vaginalis should be used to provide additional coverage over the closure and thereby decrease the occurrence of fistulae. The closure of glans and skin is the same as for the GAP. The dressing and urethral catheter are left for 3 to 5 days.

Onlay

An onlay urethroplasty is more complicated than repairs that use local tissue and is thought to have a higher complication rate. This procedure generally is used when the quality or quantity of the local skin suggests that more limited surgery is inappropriate. As with both the flip-flap and GAP repairs, only limited chordee can be present because an intact urethral plate is essential for this procedure. Conceptually, the onlay repair is similar to the Mathieu repair. In this case, however, the tissue used to form the ventrum of the neourethra is a flap taken from the inner aspect of the prepuce or a graft from either the inner prepuce or a distant area (Fig. 28.6). The procedure begins with a circumferential incision just proximal to the corona. Once more, Firlit mucosal collars are incorporated into the incision lines. The ventral incision should come just proximal to the meatus. The penile shaft skin is dissected off Buck's fascia to the penoscrotal junction, and any existing chordee is released. An artificial erection is obtained to confirm complete straightening of the penis. The techniques for removing the chordee have been described earlier in this chapter. Once the penis is straight, a flap or graft is marked on the prepucial skin or other donor site. Often the graft is preferred to avoid bringing the bulk of a blood supply around the side of the penile shaft and into the distal glans. If a flap is elected, the blood supply is dissected from the inner prepuce, allowing the epithelium to rotate to the ventrum to form the ventral neourethra. When a graft is elected, the tissue is harvested from the inner prepuce, the thigh, or the buccal mucosa. The graft is defatted and transferred to the ventral neourethra. In both instances, an anastomosis between the urethral plate and flap or graft is completed with 7-0 Vicryl suture. A barrier layer of subcutaneous tissue should be brought over the neourethra to decrease the possibility of fistulae formation. The anastomosis is performed over an 8F silastic catheter that is left in place for 10 to 14 days. The glans is closed as it is in the other procedures. Skin coverage may be

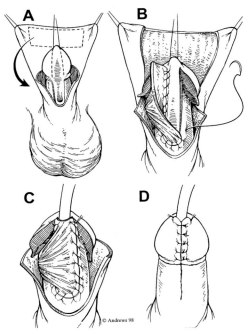

FIG. 28.6. A, For an onlay pedicle flap repair, the skin is freed up, leaving the distal urethral plate intact. **B,** Incisions are carried distally into the glans to Buck's fascia, and a segment of the hooded prepuce is freed on its pedicle and swung ventral. The lateral anastomosis to the urethral plate is made. **C,** The second lateral anastomosis is completed, the pedicle covers the flap. **D,** Glans closure is completed.

somewhat more challenging because of the blood supply to the flap, but it is achieved in the manner already described. The child is sent home on the day of surgery with a bio-occlusive dressing that is left in place for 4 to 7 days.

Tubularized Urethroplasties

Occasionally, the degree of chordee is such that the urethral plate must be divided to allow complete straightening of the penile shaft. In those cases, none of the previously described procedures are possible because they all require an intact plate. When the urethral plate is separated, a circumferential neourethra must be constructed. The introduction of a circular anastomosis increases the possibility of strictures, an additional cause of significant postoperative morbidity. Furthermore, the incidence of urethrocutaneous fistulae is increased, probably because of a more tenuous blood supply.

Both vascularized flaps and free grafts have been used to provide tissue for the neourethra. The transverse island hypospadias repair, which uses a flap from the inner prepuce, is often used for proximal shaft hypospadias repair.[23] The operation is begun by marking incision lines proximal to the corona on the dorsum and just proximal to the meatus. The shaft skin is incised and dissected to the penoscrotal junction. The chordee re-

lease is completed as in the other procedures. If, after release of all ventral fibrous tissue and Nesbit plications, there is residual chordee or tethering of the urethral plate, the plate must be incised to allow straightening of the shaft. Then a tubularized neourethra must be created.

In the transverse island repair, the tissue for the neourethra is harvested as a flap from the inner prepuce; this is the same tissue that is used for a vascularized onlay urethroplasty. It is brought to the ventrum with the vascular pedicle (which is based on the split blood supply of the prepuce) around the lateral edge of the penis. The flap is tubularized with fine, absorbable suture and anastomosed to the original urethral meatus. Spatulation of both the neourethra and original meatus should decrease the occurrence of anastomotic strictures. The distal flap is sewn to the distal glans after it has been prepared by incision and development of lateral wings to cover the neourethra. Glandular tissue is excised to allow for a perfect fit of the neourethra into the penile glans without traction on the subsequent glans closure. A vascularized barrier layer should be brought over the neourethra to minimize fistula development. Coverage of the glans and skin is performed as in the previously described procedures (Fig. 28.7).

A variation of the transverse island urethroplasty avoids the development of a separate vascular pedicle to the neourethra by bringing the overlying outer prepuce to the ventrum in continuity with the urethral flap. This prepucial skin is used as part of the skin coverage for the shaft. This technique removes the necessity for a barrier layer since the pedicle brings additional tissue with it. The main drawback of this technique is that the ventral skin closure has rectangular suture lines. On the other hand, there should be a lower incidence of fistulae (Fig. 28.8).

Some surgeons prefer a free graft[22] to the vascularized prepucial flap. The operation begins in the same manner as a transverse island repair. Once all of the chordee has been released, a rectangle of inner prepuce is harvested. The length of the graft is the length needed to bridge the defect, and the width is between 12 and 15 mm. The graft is defatted as with the onlay graft repair. A neourethra is built by tubularizing the graft over an 8F catheter using 7-0 and 8-0 Vicryl. The graft is then placed on the ventral penis as it is in the transverse island repair. The anastomosis to the original meatus is done with interrupted suture, and the edges are spatulated to decrease the occurrence of an anastomotic stricture. A vascularized barrier layer is brought over the neourethra as with the other procedures. Glans and skin closure are completed.

The dressing for both the tubularized flaps and grafts should be left in place for 3 to 5 days and the stent for 10 to 14 days. The child usually can be sent home on the day of the surgery.

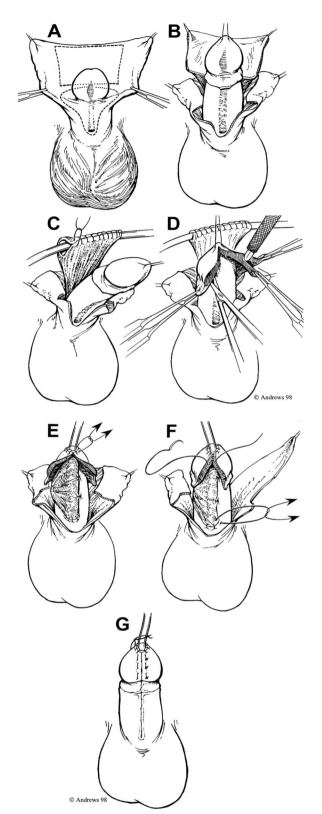

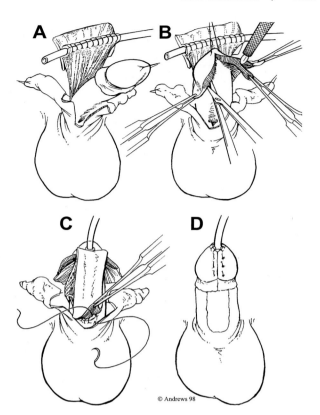

FIG. 28.8. A, In the modified transverse island repair, the flap is completed in continuity with the outer prepuce. B, The glans mobilization is the same. C, The proximal and distal anastomoses are completed. D, The completed repair includes the rectangular preputian skin in its ventral midline.

Two-Staged Repairs

Although most hypospadias repairs can be achieved with a single surgical procedure, some patients are best treated with a staged approach. These are the boys with proximal hypospadias, severe chordee, and minimal preputial skin. Although a decision concerning staging of hypospadias surgery often is not made until the initial procedure is under way, the possibility of staging usually is apparent at the preoperative evaluation and should be discussed with the parents.

A two-stage hypospadias repair (Fig. 28.9) is begun in a manner identical to that of a transverse island repair. After the chordee has been corrected, the presence of adequate preputial skin for a single-stage repair is established. If the length of the inner prepuce is less than

FIG. 28.7. A, For the transverse island repair, skin incisions are visualized. B, The incisions are made so the meatus falls to the midshaft or penoscrotal junction after release of the chordee. C, A tubularized flap with the blood supply, based on the inner aspect of the prepuce, is fashioned. D, The glans

is mobilized to allow the flap to be placed into the distal glans. E, Anastomoses between the original meatus and the flap and between the distal glans and the flap are performed. F, Additional vascular tissue is used to cover the lateral anastomosis, and glans closure is performed. G, Final appearance. The completed repair. Reprinted with permission from Glenn. Urologic surgery. 4th ed. Philadelphia: Lippincott, 1991.

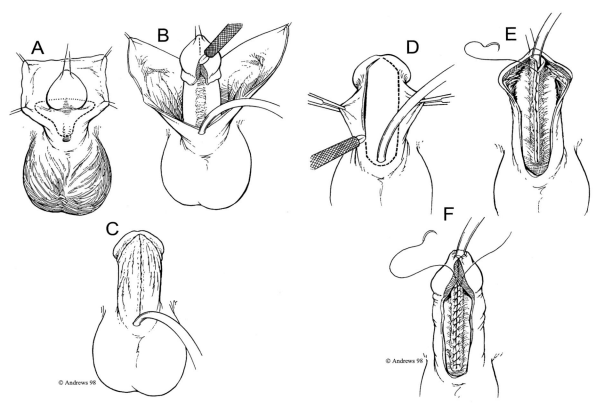

FIG. 28.9. A, The two-stage procedure is begun in a similar fashion to the transverse island repair. **B,** After completion of the chordee release, insufficient dorsal hood skin is available for a transverse island flap, and the dorsal hood is split in the dorsal midline. **C,** The dorsal shaft skin is then swept ventrally to cover the shaft with redundant skin in preparation for the second stage. **D,** In the second stage, the ventral skin is mobilized. **E,** The ventral skin is closed over a urethral stent. **F,** After the neourethra is covered with vascular tissue, glans closure is performed.

the defect from the urethral meatus to the tip of the glans, it is my preference to stage the repair. The dorsal prepuce is split in its midline to allow its transfer to the ventral penile shaft. The prepuce is spread along the ventral shaft so that a second procedure 6 months later will allow rolling in of a neourethra. The glans should be split to allow distal placement of preputial skin so there will be enough tissue for subsequent formation of a glanular urethra. A Foley catheter is inserted and is removed on the first postoperative day. A dressing is left for several days as there may be substantial edema associated with this procedure.

Six months later a neourethra is completed by the rolling together of the ventral skin that was transferred from the dorsal prepuce. This procedure is begun by confirming the absence of recurrent chordee when an artificial erection is elicited. If there is chordee, it must be corrected at this time. Once it is established that the penis is straight, the surgery is begun by marking a ventral channel 12 mm in width with its proximal edge incorporating the urethral meatus. Care is taken not to injure the urethral plate or to devascularize the skin coverage. Subcutaneous tissue should be mobilized to provide at least one and preferably two layers of tissue to cover the neoure-

thra. The urethra is rolled over an 8F stent and sutured with 7-0 Vicryl. The glanular urethra is rolled in a similar manner using the skin that was placed there during the first stage. The edges of the glans are brought together and the glans closed as in the other procedures. The skin closure is similar to that of other repairs. Throughout the procedure 7-0 Vicryl suture is used. A Zaontz catheter is left indwelling for 10 to 14 days, and a standard dressing remains in place for 3 to 5 days.

COMPLICATIONS

The complications most commonly seen with hypospadias are strictures, fistulae, and recurrent chordee. It is my belief that these are related for the most part to limited blood supply and subsequent infection, either overt or subclinical. Corrections of these complications require repeat operations, which can be challenging and may require completely taking down the earlier reconstruction. Indeed, preserving the initial repair may jeopardize the results of the second procedure. On the other hand, simple repairs can be done without involvement of the remainder of the urethroplasty. Complication rates vary depending on the degree of hypospadias and chordee. Generally speaking, the longer the urethroplasty and the worse the chordee, the greater the complication rate. For distal repairs, the complication rate should be less than 5%.[30] These complications generally are fistulae. However, for the more proximal hypospadias, complication rates of 25 to 40% are not unusual.[31, 32] These complications include strictures, fistulae, and recurrent chordee.

Repair of fistulae can be straightforward. A small fistula can be circumscribed, the tract removed and closure performed. Excellent results can be expected in these cases. More significant fistulae require more involved surgery. The tissue around the fistulae must be incised and layers developed. The fistula tract is closed with 7-0 Vicryl suture. Subcutaneous tissue is brought over the urethral closure as a second layer. If possible, a third layer of subcutaneous tissue is brought into the field. The last layer is the skin, which is closed with either subcuticular or simple Vicryl suture. Catheter drainage usually is not required. A standard dressing is used for the more involved cases.

Strictures are generally more troublesome than fistulae because they may cause urinary retention that can require immediate intervention. Most commonly, symptoms consist of straining to void and dysuria. Placement of a urethral catheter will temporize the matter, but usually signals the need for a repeat procedure. At times an optical urethrotomy may suffice, but often an open repeat urethroplasty is required. In those instances, complete exposure of the neourethra is often the only way to assess and repair the problem adequately. Rarely, dividing the stricture is sufficient; more often, additional tissue must be brought to the strictured area to increase the diameter of the urethra. On occasion, a complete reconstruction of the neourethra is necessary.

Recurrent chordee is repaired by once more degloving the penile shaft and identifying the point of maximal curvature. In the process of exposing the corpora cavernosa, it is important to preserve the neourethra if possible so that a further urethroplasty is not needed. Once the point of maximum curvature is found, a repeat plication should be performed. This usually will resolve the problem.

Unfortunately, when one complication is found, there may be others. It is important to be prepared to perform a major hypospadias revision whenever addressing a hypospadias complication. In many instances, a complete revision of the urethroplasty will be necessary, since an attempt to preserve a neourethra may jeopardize a subsequent revision. The family must therefore be prepared to accept major penile surgery whenever these problems are encountered.

REFERENCES

1. Bauer SB, Retik AB, Colodny AH. Genetic aspects of hypospadias. Urol Clin North Am 1981;8:559–564.
2. Barcat J. Current concepts of treatment. In: Horton CE, ed. Plastic and reconstructive surgery of the genital area. Boston: Little, Brown & Co, 1973.
3. Davenport, MacKinnon. The value of ultrasound screening of the upper urinary tract in hypospadias. Br J Urol 1988;62:595.
4. Shelton TB, Noe HN. The role of excretory urography in patients with hypospadias. J Urol 1985;134:97.
5. Shafir R, Hertz M, Boichis H, et al. Vesicoureteral reflux in boys with hypospadias. Urology 1982;20:29–32.
6. Sutherland RW, Wiener JS, Hicks JP, et al. Androgen receptor gene mutations are rarely associated with isolated penile hypospadias. J Urol 1996;156:828–831.
7. Firlit CF. The mucosal collar in hypospadias surgery. J Urol 1987;137:80–82.
8. Hannallah RS. Pediatric outpatient anesthesia. Urol Clin North Am 1987;14:51–62.
9. Gittes RF, McLaughlin AP III. Injection technique to induce penile erection. Urology 1974;4:473.
10. Perlmutter AD, Montgomery BT, Steinhardt GF. Tunica vaginalis free graft for the correction of chordee. J Urol 1985;134:311–313.
11. Horton CE Jr, Gearhart JP, Jeffs RD. Dermal grafts for correction of severe chordee associated with hypospadias. J Urol 1993;150:452–455.
12. Snodgrass W, Decter RM, Roth DR, Gonzales ET Jr. Management of the penile shaft skin in hypospadias repair: alternatives to Byars' flaps. J Pediatr Surg 1988;23:181–2.
13. Montagnino BA, Gonzales ET Jr, Roth DR. Open catheter drainage after urethral surgery. J Urol 1988;140:1250–1252.
14. Duckett JW. MAGPI (meatoplasty and glanuloplasty). Urol Clin North Am 1981;8:513–519.
15. Spencer JR, Perlmutter AD. Sleeve advancement distal hypospadias repair. J Urol 1990;144:523–525, discussion 530.
16. Zaontz MR. The GAP (glans approximation procedure) for glandular/coronal hypospadias. J Urol 1989;141:359–361.
17. Wacksman J. Modification of the one-stage flip-flap procedure to repair distal penile hypospadias. Urol Clin North Am 1981;8:527–530.
18. Barthold JS, Teer TL, Redman JF. Modified Barcat balanic groove technique for hypospadias repair: experience with 295 cases. J Urol 1996;155:1735–1737.
19. Devine JC, Horton CE. A one-stage hypospadias repair. J Urol 1961;85:166–172.
20. Snodgrass W. Tubularized, incised plate urethroplasty for distal hypospadias. J Urol 1994;151:464–465.
21. Elder JS, Duckett JW, Snyder HM. Onlay island flap in the repair of mid and distal penile hypospadias without chordee. J Urol 1987;138:376–379.
22. Stock JA, Cortez J, Scherz HC, Kaplan GW. The management of proximal hypospadias using a 1-stage hypospadias repair with a preputial free graft for neourethral construction and preputial pedicle flap for ventral skin coverage. J Urol 1994;152:2335–2337.
23. Duckett JW Jr. Transverse preputial island flap technique for repair of severe hypospadias. Urol Clin North Am 1980;7:423–430.
24. Flack CE, Walker RD III. Onlay-tube-onlay urethroplasty technique in primary perineal hypospadias surgery. J Urol 1995;154:837–839.
25. Retik AB, Bauer SB, Mandell J, et al. Management of severe hypospadias with a 2-stage repair. J Urol 1994;152:749–751.
26. Nesbit RM. Congenital curvature of the phallus. Report of three cases with description of corrective operation. J Urol 1965;93:230.
27. Yachia D. Modified corporoplasty for the treatment of penile curvature. J Urol 1990;143:80–82.
28. Baskin LS, Duckett JW, Ueoka K, et al. Changing concepts of hypospadias curvature lead to more onlay island flap procedures. J Urol 1994;151:191–196.
29. Snodgrass W, Koyle M, Manzoni G, et al. J Urol 1996;156:839–841.
30. Hakim S, Merguerian PA, Rabinowitz R, et al. J Urol 1996;156:836–838.
31. Barraza MA, Roth DR, Terry WJ, et al. One-stage reconstruction of moderately severe hypospadias. J Urol 1987;137:714–715.
32. Vyas PR, Roth DR, Perlmutter AD. Experience with free grafts in urethral reconstruction. J Urol 1987;137:471–474.

CHAPTER 29

Cryptorchidism

Richard I. Silver and Steven G. Docimo

The term cryptorchidism is derived from the Greek words *kryptos* and *orchis,* meaning "hidden" and "testis," respectively, and refers to absence of a testis from the scrotum. Although the adjectives "cryptorchid" and "undescended" in referring to a testis are often used interchangeably, they are not synonymous since cryptorchid testes may also be ectopic or absent. Cryptorchidism has been recognized for centuries, since the time of Galen and Vesalius,[1] but it was John Hunter in the eighteenth century who is credited with characterizing the features of the cryptorchid testis accurately. More than 200 years later, the cause of this condition remains poorly understood and the management is, in some instances, controversial. The clinical issues related to the etiology, diagnosis, and management of cryptorchidism are the focus of this chapter.

TESTICULAR DEVELOPMENT

Testicular development is determined at the time of conception by the presence of the *SRY* (*s*ex-determining *region Y* linked) gene on the short arm of the Y chromosome.[2] Embryogenesis begins in week 5 of gestation, when proliferation of coelomic epithelium and the underlying mesenchyme medial to the mesonephros produces the gonadal ridge. Epithelial primary sex cords then grow into the underlying mesenchyme,[3] resulting in the development of a cortex and medulla; the cortex regresses and the medulla develops. Primordial germ cells, present in the wall of the yolk sac from the fourth week of gestation, migrate by chemotaxis[4] along the dorsal mesentery of the hindgut to reach the gonadal ridge by week 6 of gestation. By week 7, the SRY gene protein induces the bipotential gonad to differentiate into a testis. Sertoli cells appear by week 8 and Leydig cells appear by week 10 to produce Müllerian-inhibiting substance and testosterone, respectively. These hormones cause involution of the Müllerian duct and differentiation of the Wolffian duct to provide normal male internal genitalia by week 13 of gestation. Development of the male external genitalia, including the scrotum, occurs between weeks 10 and 15 of gestation and results from the conversion of testosterone to dihydrotestosterone by the enzyme 5 α-reductase type 2[5] in the primordia of these tissues. This process is important because development of the scrotum allows for the ultimate descent of the testis out of the abdomen and pelvis to an extracorporeal position.

TESTICULAR DESCENT

Testicular descent into the cooler environment of the scrotum is necessary to allow for normal spermatogenesis and on an anatomical basis occurs in three separate stages: *(a)* transabdominal migration of the testis to the internal inguinal ring; *(b)* development of the processus vaginalis and the inguinal canal; and *(c)* transinguinal descent of the testis to the scrotum. Transabdominal migration of the testis begins during the fifth week of gestation. At this time, a band of mesenchyme called the gubernaculum attaches the caudal end of the gonad and Wolffian duct to the genital swellings, the precursors of the scrotum. As the embryo elongates and the kidney ascends, the testis remains anchored at the internal inguinal ring by the gubernaculum. In the third month of gestation, the processus vaginalis forms from the peritoneum as a potential space through the weakness in the abdominal wall adjacent to the gubernaculum and gradually extends into the inguinal canal and scrotum. The process of testicular descent remains dormant until the seventh month of gestation, when the gubernaculum swells as a result of an increased content of hyaluronic acid, distending the inguinal canal and scrotum. Transinguinal descent of the testis occurs very rapidly, usually between weeks 24 and 28 of gestation,[6] and is usually completed in the third trimester.[7] The epididymis appears to precede the testis into the scrotum.[8] Normally, the processus vaginalis completely obliterates prior to birth,[9] and the gubernaculum atrophies but persists as the gubernacular ligament. When the testis does not descend, the processus vaginalis remains patent more than 90% of the time.

Of neonates born with an undescended testis, the majority show spontaneous testicular descent. During the first trimester of pregnancy, testosterone production by the fetal testis is stimulated by maternal gonadotropins. If the testis is undescended at birth, descent during the first year of life is presumably caused by the burst of testosterone during the first 3 months, secondary to the hypothalamic-pituitary axis activation by loss of negative feedback from the maternal endocrine environment. Serum testosterone peaks at age 2 months and diminishes rapidly to trace levels by 6 months of age.[10] This hormonal surge may also be important for central nervous system (CNS) imprinting, spermatogenesis, and ultimate male behavioral patterns. Serum MIS also peaks during the first year of life in normal males[11] and has been thought by some to play a role in testicular descent, possibly the intraabdominal phase.[12] Functional insufficiency of the hypothalamic-pituitary system may result in cryptorchidism at birth and failed descent later in life.[10, 13, 14] However, hormonal evaluation of boys born with undescended testes during the first year of life has also shown no significant hormonal differences between those that exhibit testicular descent and those who do not.[15]

FACTORS IN TESTICULAR DESCENT

Knowledge regarding the factors responsible for descent of the testis has come from observations and experiments in nature and the laboratory. The observation by John Hunter that the testis may fail to descend because it is intrinsically abnormal, rather than being abnormal because it fails to descend, remains a focus of investigation and debate. Although animal models may not exactly represent testicular descent in man, current evidence indicates that testicular descent requires the interaction of hormonal and mechanical factors. Hormonal factors include the androgens testosterone and dihydrotestosterone, Müllerian inhibiting substance, descendin, epidermal growth factor, and estrogens. Specific mechanical factors implicated in the descent of the testis include the abdominal wall, the gubernaculum, the epididymis, and the genitofemoral nerve.

Hormonal Factors

Androgens

As early as 1931, it was suggested that an intact hypothalamic-pituitary-gonadal axis is essential for normal testicular descent.[16] Clinical evidence to support this includes syndromes with hypogonadism that are associated with bilateral cryptorchidism. Experimentally, descent of the testis is initiated by dihydrotestoster-

one, converted from gonadal testosterone by 5α-reductase.[17, 18] The theory that androgens are exclusive in promoting testicular descent has been weakened by the finding that anti-androgens prevent testicular descent in only 50% of animals,[19, 20] suggesting that other factors are also involved. The condition of unilateral cryptorchidism further suggests a local or partial role for androgens in this process. This partial role may be to effect only the transinguinal phase of descent.[18]

Normally, during the immediate postnatal period in male infants, there is a surge in testosterone that gradually subsides over a period of 6 months.[21] The postnatal rise in serum testosterone is lower in boys with cryptorchidism than in those with normal testicular descent.[22, 23] This appears to be caused by a primary deficiency in pituitary LH secretion, with FSH secretion being normal.[23]

Tissue-target sensitivity to androgens, requiring a normal androgen receptor (AR), is necessary for testicular descent.[24] Androgen receptor is present in the spinal cord near the cremaster nucleus before maximal androgen stimulation occurs.[25] However, a study of boys with isolated bilateral cryptorchidism, normal response to gonadotropins, and no other abnormalities of sexual differentiation revealed normal androgen receptor function.[26] Therefore, an AR mutation is a rare cause of cryptorchidism and is almost always associated with other genital anomalies.

Müllerian Inhibiting Substance

Some evidence suggests that Müllerian inhibiting substance (MIS) may play a role in testicular descent. Patients with MIS deficiency often have intraabdominal testicles. Mean serum MIS levels in boys with cryptorchidism are lower than in age-matched controls with scrotal testes, and boys with bilateral cryptorchidism have lower MIS levels than boys with unilateral cryptorchidism.[11, 27] MIS may initiate transabdominal migration, while androgens stimulate the inguinoscrotal descent.[28, 29]

Since cryptorchid testes may have histologic abnormalities that include Sertoli cells, whether or not a low MIS level is the cause or consequence of the cryptorchid condition has been unclear. In addition, significant evidence indicates that MIS plays no role in testicular descent. MIS is usually sufficient to cause regression of Müllerian structures in cryptorchid boys.[30–32] Experiments have shown that antibodies to MIS prevent regression of the Müllerian system, but do not prevent testicular descent,[33] and that genetic MIS deficiency created in laboratory mice does not impair testicular descent.[34] MIS deficiency probably prevents testicular descent indirectly by the obstruction produced by the persistent Müllerian structures, rather than by a direct lack of hormone.

Descendin

Recent evidence indicates that an androgen-independent factor produced by the testis, called descendin, has a specific local effect on gubernacular cell growth.[35, 36] Initial knowledge of this factor was deduced by the partial effect of androgen blockade on testicular descent and the lack of gubernacular growth in animals subjected to fetal orchidectomy.[36, 37] Since gubernacular growth is essential to testicular descent, lack of descendin may impair this process. The genetic and physical characteristics of this factor remain unknown.

Epidermal Growth Factor

Epidermal growth factor (EGF) can cause persistence of the Wolffian ducts even in the absence of androgens.[38] EGF has also been shown to act on the placenta and secondarily increase testosterone production. In mice, maternal EGF appears to precede the testosterone secretion by the fetal testis and may therefore play some role in testicular descent.[39] However, human correlation is lacking.

Estrogens

During gestation, the fetus is exposed to maternal estrogens via the placenta. Estrogens are thought to act independently of androgens to prevent gubernacular growth and cause persistence of the Müllerian ducts.[12, 40] Bernstein et al.[41] noted that male infants born to mothers with high free-estradiol levels had a higher frequency of cryptorchidism. Although increased maternal estrogens during gestation may prevent testicular descent, the exact mechanism has not been elucidated.

Mechanical Factors

Abdominal Wall and Intraabdominal Pressure

The idea that the abdominal wall and intraabdominal pressure are responsible for testicular descent was first proposed in 1969.[42] Intraabdominal pressure may work in conjunction with the patent processus vaginalis to place traction on the gubernaculum. Clinically, cryptorchidism is a consistent finding in males with prune belly syndrome and occurs with increased incidence in patients with other abdominal wall defects such as gastroschisis, omphalocele, and umbilical hernia.[43] Experimentally, an inert, free-floating testicular prosthesis placed in the abdomen of a rat will descend into the scrotum, a process that can be facilitated by androgens.[44, 45] However, experimental evidence also suggests that intact abdominal wall musculature is not necessary for testicular descent.[46, 47] Moreover, this factor does not easily explain unilateral cryptorchidism, since the abdominal wall and intraabdominal pressure should affect both testes equally.

Gubernaculum

First described and named by John Hunter in 1762, the gubernaculum is a fibrous band of mesenchyme that originates on the lower pole of the testis and cauda epididymis and fans out to insert in the scrotum. The term "gubernaculum" means helm or rudder, since the function of this structure was thought to guide the testis into the scrotum. Later, separate extrascrotal bands or "tails" were described by Lockwood, perhaps explaining the occurrence of testicular ectopia.[48] Although generally considered to be a key mechanical factor in testicular descent, the role of the gubernaculum has undergone intense study and debate, and its exact function remains unclear. It has been thought to cause testicular descent by traction,[49] muscular contraction,[50] or differential growth around a fixed point.[51] Evidence suggests that the gubernaculum is androgen sensitive and that the combination of hormonal and mechanical factors related to the gubernaculum result in testicular decent.[18, 52] Interestingly, although the presence of a gubernaculum appears to be necessary for normal testicular descent, an intact gubernaculum is not required.[45] Most likely, the gubernaculum, in conjunction with the processus vaginalis, serves to dilate the inguinal canal and thereby facilitate descent of the testis into the scrotum.

Epididymis

The epididymis precedes the testis into the scrotum and undergoes maturational changes coincident with testicular descent.[8, 53] The thought that the epididymis is a factor in testicular descent is also based on the fact that it is androgen dependent, adjacent to the gubernaculum, and often abnormal in boys with cryptorchidism. Proponents of this theory argue that cryptorchidism results from incomplete epididymal differentiation caused by androgen deficiency.[8] However, removal of the epididymis does not prevent testicular descent,[54] and epididymal anomalies are five times more common in patients with inguinal hernia than cryptorchidism.[55] It is most likely that cryptorchidism and epididymal anomalies coexist because of a local deficiency of androgens.

Genitofemoral Nerve

The genitofemoral nerve eminates from the cremaster nucleus at the L1 level of the spinal cord, innervates the cremaster muscle, and releases calcitonin gene-related peptide (CGRP). Androgen receptor has been found in the lumbar spinal cord of the rat near the cremaster nucleus prior to testicular descent, and the administration of gestational antiandrogens can decrease the number of motoneurons in this nucleus and increase the incidence of cryptorchidism.[25, 56] Transection of the genitofemoral nerve prevents gubernacular migration,[57] the cremaster muscle in the rat gubernaculum has CGRP receptors,[58] and CGRP enhances contraction of the rat gubernaculum in vitro.[59, 60] Evidence that the cremaster nucleus is sexually dimorphic and androgen dependent and that its efferent neuron secretes a neuropeptide that can cause contraction of the gubernaculum has implicated the genitofemoral nerve as a factor in testicular descent. However, evidence that masculinization of the cremasteric nucleus may not be androgen dependent[61-63] and that the gubernaculum of primates contains almost no muscle[6] suggest that, at least in humans, the genitofemoral nerve may not be critically involved.

DEFINITIONS AND CLASSIFICATION

A variety of definitions and classification systems have been developed in an attempt to communicate the physical findings related to cryptorchidism.[64, 65] The most important physical feature is whether the testis is palpable, since this directly influences clinical management. Palpable cryptorchid testes, approximately 80% of the total, include true undescended and ectopic testes. Retractile testes are often misdiagnosed as palpable undescended testes and will be discussed in this section. Nonpalpable testes comprise the remaining 20% and include intraabdominal, canalicular, and absent testes.

Palpable Testes

Undescended Testis

A true *undescended testis* is found along the normal path of descent. Therefore, these testes are found in the abdomen, inguinal canal, and upper scrotum. Diminished spermatic cord length and fixation of the spermatic vessels in the retroperitoneum are common features. Some testes may move in and out of the internal inguinal ring and are then called "peeping" (Fig. 29.1A & B). The terms "emergent" or "gliding" have been used to describe the undescended testis that moves in and out of the external inguinal ring, with a patent processus vaginalis and gubernaculum,[64] but since these terms have also been used for testes at the internal ring, they are best avoided. Higher testes are associated with more ductal anomalies[69] and a greater incidence of inguinal hernia.[67]

Ectopic Testis

An *ectopic testis* is one that has deviated from the path of normal descent to a site outside the ipsilateral hemiscrotum. The most common site of ectopia is the

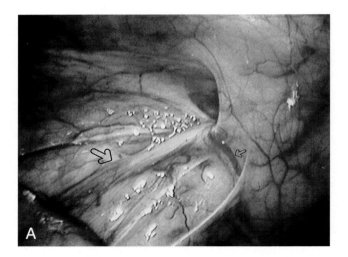

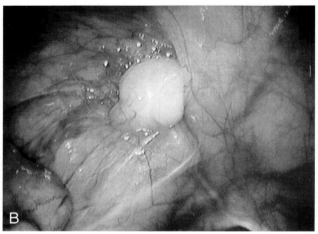

FIG. 29.1. **A,** Laparoscopic exploration of a patient with a nonpalpable testis reveals left gonadal vessels (*large arrow*) and vas deferens (*small arrow*) joining to exit the pelvis via the ipsilateral internal inguinal ring. **B,** Manual pressure on the left groin of the same patient causes the previously nonvisible and nonpalpable left testis to appear in the internal inguinal ring.

superficial inguinal pouch of Denis-Browne[68] the space between Scarpa's fascia and the external oblique fascia above the external inguinal ring. Less common sites of ectopia include femoral, pubic, penopubic, penile, and perineal positions. In rare cases, a testis will cross the scrotal septum or descend into the opposite inguinal canal or hemiscrotum, a condition known as transverse testicular ectopia.[69] Testicular ectopia can also occur in the anterior abdominal wall,[70] behind the bladder,[71] and other intraabdominal positions. Ectopic descent is thought to result from overdevelopment of one segment of the gubernaculum, that is, a tail of Lockwood, or from scrotal inlet obstruction. The accurate diagnosis of an ectopic testis, in contrast to an undescended or retractile testis, is important because the ectopic testis is fixed in position by fibrous attachments. Therefore, since it will not descend either spontaneously or with medical therapy, surgery will be necessary to place it in the scrotum.

Retractile Testis

A *retractile testis* is one that has completed the process of descent, but may be found in the groin because of an overactive cremasteric reflex, a function of the genitofemoral nerve that is present in all boys over 2 years of age.[72] When the reflex is elicited by tactile stimulation of the thigh, the cremaster muscle contracts and draws the testis out of the scrotum. A retractile testis can be manipulated into the scrotum, remains in the scrotum (at least temporarily) after its release, and is of normal size.[73] Retractile testes should be monitored during childhood since they can, on rare occasions, become truly undescended.[73] Examination of an "undescended" testis under anesthesia prior to orchidopexy may reveal that it is in the scrotum, indicating that it is retractile and obviating the need for surgery.

Nonpalpable Testes

Nonpalpable testes, approximately 20% of all cryptorchid testes, are usually intraabdominal, but can also be found in the inguinal canal or just inside the internal inguinal ring.[74] On rare occasions, a testis can be found at or above the level of the kidney. Approximately 20% of nonpalpable testes, or 4% of all cryptorchid testes, are absent[74–77] and another 30% of nonpalpable testes, or 6% of the total, are atrophic or rudimentary.

Intraabdominal Testes

Two variants of intraabdominal testis have been described, the closed-ring and open-ring variants. In the closed-ring variant, most commonly associated with the prune belly syndrome, the processus vaginalis does not develop, the gubernaculum is absent, and the internal inguinal ring is closed. With the open-ring variant, a patent processus vaginalis exists and the gubernaculum passes through it; the testis may be "peeping" into the canal, depending on the size of the processus vaginalis and the length of the testicular vessels.[64]

Absent Testes

Although unilateral absence, or monorchidism, occurs in 4% of patients with cryptorchidism, bilateral absence, or anorchidism, occurs in less than 1%.[75] Absence of the testis may result from atrophy following intrauterine torsion,[67] or testicular agenesis.

Vanishing Testis

The term vanishing testis was coined by Scott[78] to describe the condition in which testicular vessels and a vas deferens are found on surgical exploration, but not a testis. The etiology of a vanishing testis is presumed to be torsion of the gonadal vessels in utero after the development of the external genitalia.[79] Supporting evidence includes the common finding of hemosiderin and calcium deposits in testicular remnants found on exploration.[79–81] The majority of cases of in utero testicular torsion occur during transinguinal migration of the testis in the third trimester.[82] The presence of Wolffian duct structures, and the absence of Müllerian structures, indicate that an ipsilateral testis was present during gestation. In cases of a unilateral nonpalpable testis, both nonpalpable and vanishing testes are more common on the left. However, the relative likelihood of vanishing testis when the testis is nonpalpable is approximately the same on each side.[83]

Testicular Agenesis

A testis may fail to develop because of failure of the gonadal ridge to form or its blood supply to develop. Embryonic testicular regression can be seen in 46, XY agonadal individuals with either male or female phenotypes.[84, 85] The variable phenotypic appearance, including the presence and form of the internal genitalia, relates to the time during gestation when the testis is lost. The key clinical sign indicating testicular agenesis, rather than a vanished testis, is the presence of ipsilateral Müllerian structures.[86] This entity is much less common than the vanishing testis syndrome. True congenital absence of one testis is extremely rare,[87] and absence of both would result in a female phenotype.

BILATERAL UNDESCENDED TESTES

Between 10 and 25% of patients with cryptorchidism have bilateral undescended testes, representing approximately 1/600 male births,[1, 88] and this can be a normal physical finding in premature male neonates. It is estimated that at least 6% of patients with bilateral undescended testes have an endocrine disorder as the etiology.[89] Others have suggested that it is a manifestation of hypogonadotropic hypogonadism.[90]

Bilateral Nonpalpable Testes

The condition of bilateral nonpalpable testes represents a special situation that may have life-threatening implications, especially in association with severe hypospadias. The differential diagnosis includes anorchidism and ambiguous genitalia caused by female pseudohermaphroditism or another intersex condition. Congenital adrenal hyperplasia must be excluded. A karyotype, endocrine testing, and radiographic contrast studies provide the necessary information to make the diagnosis.

TABLE 29.1. *Evaluation of bilateral cryptorchidism*

	Cryptorchidism	Anorchidism	Female pseudohermaphroditism
Karyotype	46 XY	46 XY	46 XX
Serum testosterone			
Baseline	Normal	Low	Variable
HCG stimulation test	Positive	Negative	Negative
Gonadotropins	Normal	Increased	Normal
MIS	Positive	Negative	Negative
Adrenal steroid precursors	Normal	Normal	Increased
Ultrasound			
Gonads	Testes or negative	Negative	Ovaries or negative
Internal ducts	Negative	Negative	Uterus/Müllerian system
Genitogram	Male urethra	Male urethra	Urogenital sinus and/or Müllerian structures
Laparoscopy			
Gonads	Testes	Blind ending vessels	Ovaries
Internal ducts	Wolffian	Wolffian	Müllerian

When a male genotype is identified, endocrine studies may be useful to differentiate bilateral cryptorchidism from anorchia.[91, 92] Human chorionic gonadotropin (HCG) administration can be used to stimulate testosterone production by testicular tissue to detect its presence biochemically and may also cause the gonads to become palpable by physical examination. However, false-negative HCG stimulation testing can occur because of an unresponsive population of Leydig cells.[93] Therefore, HCG stimulation testing is combined with the measurement of gonadotropins to diagnose anorchia. Markedly elevated gonadotropins before puberty are indicative of anorchidism,[91] but all boys with normal serum gonadotropin levels must undergo exploration regardless of the outcome of the HCG stimulation test. Measurement of serum MIS can provide additional evidence that testicular tissue is present.[94] Thus, with a male genotype, the diagnosis of anorchia can be made with a low serum testosterone, a negative HCG stimulation test, increased serum gonadotropins, a negative serum MIS, normal levels of adrenal steroid precursors, and radiographic studies demonstrating the absence of Müllerian structures. In equivocal cases, laparoscopy or open surgical exploration may be required to confirm the diagnosis of anorchia (Table 29.1).

TESTICULAR ASCENT

An *ascended testis* refers to a cryptorchid testis, usually palpable, that had been previously identified as descended in the scrotum. This diagnosis has been controversial and is considered by some to be a misdiagnosis because of an error in physical examination.[95] However, the collective experience of qualified examiners suggests that this is a real phenomenon.[96–102] Since reported cases are rare, a specific incidence has not been determined, but approximately 2% of retractile testes are thought to become ascended. Affected individuals usually present as young children of grade-school age. The etiology is unclear, but is thought to be the relative shortening, or lack of elongation, of spermatic cord structures as the affected child grows.[103] This theory is supported by the finding of a fibrous remnant within the spermatic cord, thought to represent the obliterated processus vaginalis.[104] This structure may limit growth of the spermatic cord and cause the attached testis to appear to ascend. Ascent of the testis may also be iatrogenic and may occur after an inguinal hernia repair when the testis is not properly relocated in the scrotum.[105]

INCIDENCE AND NATURAL HISTORY

Since testicular descent is completed during the third trimester of gestation, the incidence of cryptorchidism depends to some extent on the age of the child examined. Boys born prematurely have an incidence of cryptorchidism of approximately 33%, which decreases to 3 to 5% for the full-term infant. By 1 year of age, the incidence is approximately 0.8 to 1.0%.[67, 106] Most undescended testes that descend spontaneously do so during the first 3 months after term, and few will descend after that.[107] Unilateral cryptorchidism (68%) is more than twice as common as bilateral cryptorchidism (32%), and the right side (70%) is affected more often than the left (30%).[108, 109] Reports on the incidence of cryptorchidism may overestimate the true incidence if retractile or ascended testes are included in the data.

RISK FACTORS

Gestational Factors

An increased risk of cryptorchidism has been associated with maternal estrogen use during gestation.[110–113] Male infants of mothers who have taken DES have an 8 to 17% incidence of cryptorchidism,[112, 114–116] although not all studies report the same findings.[117–119] Maternal obesity, Cesarean section, low birth weight and prematurity are also associated with cryptorchidism, increasing the relative risk to twice that of the general population.[120] There is also evidence to suggest that mothers of cryptorchid boys have shorter menses and later menarche than that of controls[121] and an increased tendency toward threatened abortions, prior miscarriage, and decreased fertility.[119] These findings may reflect altered hormonal physiology or placental function in the mother with consequences affecting the fetus. Interestingly, maternal blood group type B[122] and breech labor[110] have been suggested as additional risk factors. Race does not appear to be a significant risk factor.

Genetic Factors

Multiple reports have cited the strong familial clustering of cryptorchidism.[123–126] Approximately 14% of boys with cryptorchidism come from families in which other males are also affected.[67] Evidence suggests that cryptorchidism within a family is transmitted in a multifactorial pattern. Fathers are affected with an incidence of approximately 4% and siblings with an incidence of 6 to 10%.[121, 127] Although autosomal dominant inheritance with incomplete penetrance has been suggested,[128] studies of Mendelian chromosomal transmission in cryptorchidism have been unrevealing.[129, 130] Karyotype analysis of testicular biopsies indicates that cryptorchidism is not related to abnormal testicular cytogenetics.[130] The increased incidence of cryptorchidism in first-degree and second-degree relatives warrants counseling and monitoring families with cryptorchidism for its appearance in subsequent male children, including nephews and cousins.

Environmental Factors

Although geographic location does not appear to influence the development of cryptorchidism, some studies have identified a seasonal variation in the incidence of cryptorchidism. This finding may be related to a concomitant variation in the production of maternal pituitary gonadotropins. However, the season of greatest incidence has varied between studies.[120, 131]

ASSOCIATED ANOMALIES

Associated anomalies increase the relative risk of cryptorchidism to 13 times the incidence in the general population.[120] Because of the multiple factors involved in normal testicular descent, a wide variety of clinical syndromes that affect genetic integrity, as well as the endocrine, musculoskeletal, and nervous systems, can be associated with this condition (Table 29.2). For exam-

ple, abnormalities in chromosome number such as autosomal trisomy, triploidy, and Klinefelters syndrome (XXY) are commonly associated with cryptorchidism. Deficiencies in pituitary function, testosterone production, 5α-reductase activity, and androgen receptor sensitivity effectively interrupt androgen activity, and cryptorchidism is common in affected individuals. Infants with defects in the abdominal wall such as omphalocele, gastroschisis, and umbilical hernia,[43] as well as prune belly syndrome and bladder and cloacal exstrophy, often have undescended testes. Anatomic intraabdominal abnormalities also appear to predispose to this condition, since 19% of boys born with imperforate anus have undescended testes.[132] Cryptorchidism is commonly present with abnormal structure or function of the central nervous system, including myelomeningocele, with a 15% incidence of cryptorchidism overall[133] and a 50% incidence in those affected above L4; CNS dysfunction;[111] mental retardation and cerebral palsy;[134, 135] and spina bifida and spinal cord transection.[136]

Urinary Tract

Although some studies have shown an association of upper urinary tract anomalies with cryptorchidism,[137, 138] others demonstrate that the yield of unselected screening is no greater than that in the general population. Therefore, routine screening with an intravenous pyelogram (IVP) or renal ultrasound is not recommended.[139–141] Patients who should be screened include those with genital tract or skeletal anomalies or those with signs or symptoms of urinary tract malformation.[142] Interestingly, cryptorchidism occurs twelve times more commonly in boys with posterior urethral valves[143] and more than three times more frequently in boys with Wilms' tumor.[144]

Genital Tract

External Genitalia

The presence of hypospadias in association with cryptorchidism suggests an intersex condition, including mixed gonadal dysgenesis and male pseudohermaphroditism.[145–147] Appropriate investigation is warranted to exclude this possibility.

The Epididymis and Vas Deferens

Wolffian duct abnormalities have been reported in 30 to 79% of undescended testes, including agenesis of the epididymis and vas deferens, atresia or discontinuity between the testis and epididymis, and elongation of the epididymis.[53, 55, 148–151] Patients with bilateral[152] or nonpalpable undescended testes have a higher incidence of such anomalies,[150] and the more proximal the location

TABLE 29.2. *Syndromes associated with cryptorchidism*

Cryptorchidism: Common		Cryptorchidism: Less Common	
Syndrome	Classification	Syndrome	Classification
Aarskog (Facia-digital-genital)	X	Basal-cell nevus	AD
Androgen insensitivity	E	Beckwith-Wiedemann	S
Anencephaly	E	Coffin-Siris	S
Cleft lip/palate (holoprosencephalis)	E	Diastrophic dwarfism	AR
Cockayne	AR	Ellis-van Creveld	AR
Cornelia de Lange	S	Exstrophy of bladder, cloaca	AN
Cryptophthalmos	AR	Fanconi pancytopenia	AR
Dubowitz	AR	Femoral hypoplasia-unusual facies	S
Hypopituitarism	E	Fetal hydantoin	AQ
Kallman's	E	Fraser	AR
Laurence-Moon-Biedl	AR	Gorlin frontometaphyseal hypoplasia	S
Lowe (oculocerebrorenal)	X	Hallermann-Streiff	S
Meckel-Gruber	AR	Klinefelter, and variants	S
Noonan	S	Popliteal web	AD
Opitz	AD	Robinow	AR
Pituitary aplasia-hypoplasia	E	Rubella	AQ
Prader-Willi	S	Saethre-Chotzen	AD
Prune-belly	AN	Seckel	AR
Roberts	AR	Steinert myotonic dystrophy	AD
Rubinstein-Taybi	S	Treacher-Collins	AD
Septic-optic dysplasia	E	Trisomy 8	A
Smith-Lemli-Opitz	AR	Trisomy 21 (Down)	A
Testicular enzymatic defects	E	XYY	S
Triploidy	A	Zellweger (Cerebrohepatorenal)	AR
Trisomy 13	A	5p- (Cri-du-chat)	A
Trisomy 18 (Edwards)	A	21 q	A
4p- (Wolf-Hirschhorn)	A		
5α-reductase deficiency	E		
13 q	A		
18 q	A		

Reprinted with permission from Kogan S. Cryptorchidism. In: Kelalis PP, King LR, Belman AB, eds. Clinical pediatric urology. Vol. 2. Philadelphia: Saunders, 1992:1058.

A, autosomal; *AD*, autosomal dominant; *AR*, autosomal recessive; *X*, X-linked; *S*, sporadic; *AN*, anomalads; *AQ*, acquired; *E*, endocrine.

of the testis, the more severe the epididymal malformation.[66] An elongated, or "long-looping," vas deferens is usually associated with an intraabdominal testis, but may be seen with an inguinal testis. Epididymal abnormalities are clinically important for three reasons. First, an abnormal vas deferens and epididymis may preclude the option of orchidopexy based on collateral blood supply through these organs. Second, in cases of disjunction between the testis and epididymis, epididymal tissue may be present in the scrotum and mistaken for an atrophic testis if surgical exploration is not performed.[153,154] Third, epididymal anomalies may be the cause of future infertility despite a technically successful orchidopexy.[151]

DIAGNOSIS

History

Evaluation of the boy with cryptorchidism includes a thorough history from his mother regarding the use of drugs such as sex steroids during her pregnancy that might impair testicular descent or cause ambiguous genitalia. Family history of cryptorchidism, genetic or hormonal disorders, and anosmia is sought. Caretakers are asked whether the testis has ever been seen in the scrotum. A history of an inguinal mass or low abdominal pain may suggest an associated hernia or testicular torsion. If the child has had previous groin surgery, testicular ascent or secondary cryptorchidism must be considered. Individuals who present as adults and are sexually active may be questioned regarding evidence of fertility, including documentation of paternity and/or semen quality.

Physical Examination

Physical examination should be performed in a warm, comfortable room to minimize patient anxiety. A complete examination is performed for signs of clinical syndromes associated with cryptorchidism and for signs of virilization in older children and adults. Examination of the abdomen and flank is performed to identify any masses, scars, or hernias. The penis is examined to exclude micropenis and hypospadias, and the scrotum is examined for hypoplasia. If one normal testis is present and descended in the scrotum, its size, shape, volume, consistency, and position are determined. Compensatory hypertrophy of a solitary scrotal testis may suggest absence of its mate,[155-157] but this finding is variable and not reliable enough for diagnosis.[158] The groin and spermatic cord on each side are palpated to feel for evidence of an inguinal hernia and a vas deferens.

Physical search for a cryptorchid testis is best performed with warm hands to try to prevent a cremasteric reflex. Examining fingers are swept from the hip above the internal inguinal ring and along the inguinal canal toward the scrotum. Lubricant on the fingertips may allow the fingers to slide easily over the skin and improve the ability to feel a testis. All sites known for ectopic testicular migration are carefully examined. In contrast to lymph nodes, which are generally small, firm, and relatively fixed, palpable inguinal and ectopic testes are usually larger, softer, and somewhat mobile. The child may be examined in several positions, including supine, sitting, squatting, and standing, if the testis is difficult to identify. This is especially helpful for the older or obese child. If a testis is found, the size, shape, volume, consistency, and position are noted and compared with the descended mate. If the testis is retractile, it should easily reach the scrotum and remain there, at least temporarily, on release. Difficulty differentiating the retractile from the truly undescended testis may explain the varying success of hormonal therapy, as well as the fact that the incidence of orchidopexy in some studies exceeds the expected incidence of cryptorchidism.[159]

Localization Studies

Historically, radiographic localization studies have been used to attempt to identify the nonpalpable testis. The rationale for these studies has been that those with absent testes could be spared unnecessary surgery and those with inguinal or abdominal testes could receive a properly tailored operation. Studies such as pneumoperitoneography,[160] contrast herniography,[161, 162] arteriography,[163, 164] and spermatic venography[165-171] have been used. However, these localization techniques have fallen into disfavor for many reasons. Not only are these techniques invasive, expensive, and difficult to perform, they also require radiation exposure and often an anesthetic. Most importantly, these techniques are unreliable. Modern imaging techniques such as ultrasound,[172, 173] computerized tomography (CT),[174-177] and magnetic resonance imaging (MRI)[178-182] are noninvasive, easier to perform, and more accurate in identifying an intraabdominal testis, but even these studies are associated with a false-negative rate of approximately 20%.

Localization studies are of value only when they are accurate enough to rely on for clinical management. Unfortunately, all radiographic localization studies suffer from deficiencies in sensitivity and specificity, none can prove that a testis is absent, and radiographic imaging for a cryptorchid testis is only 44% accurate overall.[183] For these reasons, and because of the potentially serious consequences of a falsely negative study, radiologic imaging is not recommended for routine localization of a unilateral, nonpalpable testis. Since such imaging will be followed by surgical intervention in almost all cases, regardless of the results, it is also unnecessary. At this time laparoscopy is the diagnostic procedure of choice for the nonpalpable testis because of its superior accuracy.[184, 185]

Radiographic imaging studies may be useful in certain circumstances, as judged by the individual health care provider. The judicious use of scrotal-inguinal ultrasound may help to identify nonpalpable inguinal and abdominal testes and to select patients who are likely to derive maximal benefit from laparoscopy,[186] although examination under anesthesia at the time of orchidopexy is likely to be equally helpful. Imaging is also reserved for very unusual cases such as ultrasonography of an overweight boy to identify a nonpalpable, inguinal testis and the follow-up of adolescents who, because of comorbid conditions, are not surgical candidates.

TREATMENT OF CRYPTORCHIDISM

Indications for Treatment

The primary goal in the treatment of cryptorchidism is to salvage healthy testes and position them in the scrotum. Factors that influence the decision and type of treatment include patient age, testis position, and the presence of a clinical syndrome or an intersex state. Therefore, treatment is individualized based on the clinical situation. In otherwise uncomplicated cases, the risks of untreated cryptorchidism include infertility, malignancy, inguinal hernia, torsion, and physical and psychologic trauma.

Histologic Changes and Fertility

Histologic Changes

At birth and into the first year of life, undescended testes have normal histology, including a normal population of germ cells (Fig. 29.2).[187-189] After 18 months, light microscopy shows a reduced number of germ cells and Leydig cells, retarded maturation of gonocytes into Ad spermatogonia, decreased seminiferous tubule diameter, and increased peritubular and perivascular collagen (Fig. 29.3).[190, 191] Electron microscopy at 1 to 2 years of age demonstrates a reduced germ-cell population, degeneration of Sertoli cells and mitochondria, loss of

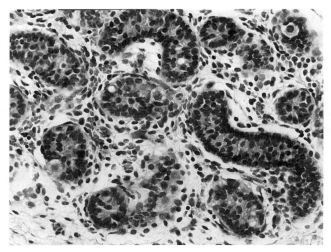

FIG. 29.2. Photomicrograph of a cryptorchid testis removed from a 1-year-old boy. Seminiferous tubules are present but contain only Sertoli cells, without germinal elements.

ribosomes from the cytoplasm and smooth endoplasmic reticulum, and peritubular hyalinization and fibrosis.[192–194] Such histologic changes can also be seen in a contralateral, descended testis after 2 years,[195] supporting Hunter's contention that in unilateral cryptorchidism both the undescended and scrotal testes are intrinsically abnormal.[196] Others believe that these findings result from deficient hormonal stimulation,[187, 190, 197] as opposed to an intrinsic testicular abnormality or abnormal testicular position.[198] However, histology correlates with testicular position, with worse features seen in

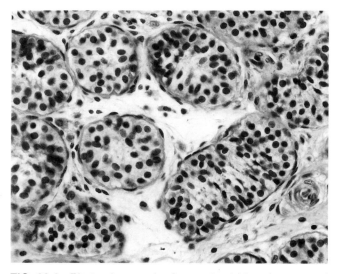

FIG. 29.3. Photomicrograph of a cryptorchid testis removed from the abdomen of an 11-year-old boy. Seminiferous tubules are of normal size, but contain only Sertoli cells. The absence of germ cells is abnormal and is characteristic of this condition. Leydig cells are scattered in the interstitium of the testis.

higher testes.[67, 199] Histologic changes in ascended testes are less severe and tend to occur later, but ultimately become evident.[200] Although it is felt that testicular maturation and fertility are normal in retractile testes,[201] changes in histology and semen analysis have been reported.[202–204] Grossly, histologic deterioration results in decreased testicular size and a softer consistency,[205] with higher testes demonstrating smaller testicular volume.[206]

Fertility

Clinically, the degenerative histologic changes seen in undescended testes result in decreased fertility, a well-recognized consequence of cryptorchidism.[207] The histologic changes of cryptorchidism can be graded by a fertility index,[208] initially devised by Mack,[209] and indirect evidence suggests that early surgical correction of the undescended testis improves its fertility potential.[208, 210–212] Even after orchidopexy, fertility is impaired in approximately 50 to 70% of men born with one undescended testis and up to 75% of those born with two undescended testes.[207, 213] Orchidopexy within the first year of life might improve these results. Without treatment, bilateral cryptorchidism results in infertility.[214]

Antisperm antibodies,[215–217] abnormalities of the epididymis and vas deferens, and surgical injury to the vas deferens during orchidopexy may contribute to infertility in patients with cryptorchidism. Assisted reproductive technology, including in vitro fertilization and intracytoplasmic sperm injection, may allow subfertile males with a history of cryptorchidism to achieve paternity.

Malignancy

Incidence

Individuals born with an undescended testis have an increased incidence of testicular malignancy over those born with scrotal testes. Since the incidence of testicular cancer in the general population is approximately one in 100,000 and that in the cryptorchid population is one in 2500, the relative risk is increased approximately 40-fold. Approximately 10% of all testis tumors develop in individuals with a history of an undescended testis. The incidence of malignant degeneration increases with the higher location of the undescended testis,[218–221] with a tumor four times more likely to occur in an abdominal than an inguinal testis.[1] Intraabdominal testes comprise 14% of undescended testes, but develop nearly 50% of associated testicular tumors.[218]

The reason for the increased risk of testicular cancer in cryptorchid patients is unclear. One theory implicates exposure to the increased temperature and pressure of the abdomen, while another theory (Hunter) implicates an intrinsic histologic abnormality within the testes. The observation that 10 to 20% of testicular tumors in cryptorchid patients occur in the normally descended testis[221,222] suggests that an intrinsic abnormality is present.

Although there has been some hope that early orchidopexy would lead to a decreased incidence of testicular cancer in boys born with cryptorchidism,[223,224] evidence that this occurs is lacking.[225] It is important for the patient's family to realize that malignancy can develop in undescended testes even after orchidopexy.[226]

Despite the increased incidence of testicular malignancy in boys born with cryptorchidism, the very low incidence of this disease in the general population makes the risk of cancer in these patients low enough that the removal of all undescended testes is unwarranted. Although orchidopexy does not yet appear to prevent development of a testicular tumor, it does allow for easy examination and detection of this process.

Pathology

The most common testicular tumor in untreated undescended testes is seminoma (Fig. 29.4), while that in successfully treated testes is embryonal carcinoma.[222] The lymphatic drainage of the testis is altered after orchidopexy, such that the inguinal lymph nodes may be the first involved if a testis tumor develops.[227] However, the number of cases in which inguinal metastases occur is small.[228] The approach to suspicious inguinal lymph nodes would be dictated by the tumor histology and stage.

Carcinoma in Situ

Testicular biopsy at the time of orchidopexy may reveal carcinoma in situ in both the undescended and the contralateral descended testis.[229,230] Ectopic testes may also harbor carcinoma in situ.[231] Carcinoma in situ is far more common in abdominal testes than in ones that are more descended.[232] However, such premalignant histologic changes may not be seen in cryptorchid testes treated before adulthood.[233] In addition, although some cases of carcinoma in situ may progress to testicular tumors, the fact that not all do makes the clinical significance and management of this finding controversial. Therefore, the routine use of testicular biopsy at orchidopexy cannot be recommended at this time.

Inguinal Hernia

Since closure of the processus vaginalis is a final step in testicular descent, a patent processus vaginalis, or indirect inguinal hernia, is commonly associated with undescended testes.[55] About 90% of undescended testes are associated with an occult inguinal hernia, especially those with more severe degrees of undescent and epididymal abnormalities,[9,67,234] while ectopic testes have this association in about 50% of cases.[234] Conversely, up to 6% of inguinal hernias are associated with an undescended testis.[235] The presence of a hernia sac may not be clinically evident by history or physical examination.[236,237]

Risk of Torsion

Testicular torsion may occur more frequently in undescended testes because normal scrotal attachments are absent.[238] Torsion of the testis in the inguinal canal is unusual, despite the fact that most undescended testes are found there, and may be related to the short cord and the presence of an associated hernia. When torsion does occur in an undescended testis, it often indicates the presence of testicular tumor.[239] Torsion in an undescended testis may be difficult to diagnose, but should be suspected in any male with groin or abdominal pain and an empty hemiscrotum.[240,241]

Risk of Trauma

A testis in the scrotum is mobile and one in the abdomen is surrounded by the abdominal wall. In both cases, the testis is protected from blunt trauma. However, a testis in the inguinal canal is subject to injury by compression against the pubic bone, which is obviated by orchidopexy or orchidectomy.

Psychologic Factors

The psychologic impact of an empty hemiscrotum is difficult to assess. Preoccupation with a solitary scrotal testis, wonder regarding the presence and location of a cryptorchid testis, embarrassment with peers and sexual partners, a tarnished body image, fear of sterility, and

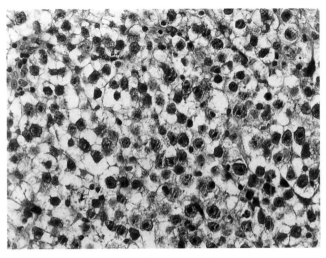

FIG. 29.4. Testicular seminoma.

other adverse personality changes may result as a consequence of cryptorchidism.[242] Theoretically, orchidopexy or placement of a testicular prosthesis could prevent such psychologic decompensation. In our experience, this has not seemed a particularly important issue, although formal psychologic testing has not been performed.

Patient Age

Therapy is usually carried out at about 1 year of age and should be completed before age 2. Since testes rarely descend after 3 months, surgery before the first birthday is reasonable and can be safely performed.[188] In cases of high intraabdominal testes such as in the prune belly syndrome, there may be anatomic and technical advantages to orchidopexy within the first 6 months of life.[243] Decisions regarding orchidopexy after age 2 are based on the benefit of the testis to the individual. Although an undescended testis may function poorly for fertility, the usefulness in terms of androgen production must be considered, especially in cases of a solitary testis. The anesthetic and surgical risk of orchidectomy become greater than the risk of testicular cancer after the age of 32 and removal is not indicated.[244] For some patients with comorbid conditions, the risks of surgery may be significant even before this age is reached.

NONSURGICAL THERAPY

Medical treatment for cryptorchidism is based on clinical and experimental evidence that a defect in the androgen hormone axis is related to testicular maldescent.[17, 22, 23] Human chorionic gonadotropin (HCG) and gonadotropin or luteinizing hormone releasing hormone (GnRH or LHRH) have been used to promote testicular descent. Human menopausal gonadotropin, synthetic analogs of LHRH, and combined hormonal therapy have also been used. Testosterone therapy is less successful because high, *local* levels of androgens are the key factor in testicular descent.[17, 245]

A recent meta-analysis of the hormonal treatment of cryptorchidism indicates that the success of LHRH (21%) is better than HCG (19%) to promote testicular descent, and both are better than placebo (4%), with non-randomized trials reporting better results than randomized trials.[246] This analysis confirms the findings of an earlier independent, randomized, double-blind study.[247] In addition to the choice of agent, patient selection is the key factor in attaining good results with medical therapy. Success of therapy is better for lower testes and is especially good for those high in the scrotum or at the external inguinal ring.[246] Retractile testes uniformly respond to therapy and the inclusion of retractile testes in some studies may overestimate the success of medical therapy.[247] The response rate is better for bilateral undescended testes, presumably because of a systemic defect in the androgen axis since gestation. After successful therapy, the patient should be reexamined periodically since 10 to 25% of successfully treated testes may reascend.[99, 248] If unsuccessful, there is no evidence that repeat courses are likely to be beneficial.

Hormonal therapy is contraindicated in newborns since spontaneous descent may occur. Hormonal therapy is usually ineffective for patients with prune belly syndrome because of the high intraabdominal testes with absent gubernacula. Hormonal therapy is also ineffective for ectopic testes or testes that are otherwise fixed in position because of scarring after prior inguinal surgery, although some favor such therapy to increase vascularity prior to reoperation.[249, 250] A clinically evident inguinal hernia associated with cryptorchidism will not close with hormonal therapy, and surgery should be performed to correct both conditions simultaneously. After puberty, there is no indication for hormonal therapy in the absence of an endocrinopathy.

Temporary side effects of hormonal therapy are related to the increase in circulating androgens and include penile enlargement, frequent erections, increased appetite, weight gain, and aggressive behavior. A potential complication of excessive hormonal therapy is premature closure of the epiphyseal plate, limiting long-bone growth. Possible effects on the CNS and behavior are not well documented.

Agents

HCG

Human chorionic gonadotropin (HCG) has been used since 1931 to treat undescended testes.[251] It is structurally similar to luteinizing hormone (LH) and stimulates endogenous testosterone production by the testis. A typical course of therapy is 1500 units intramuscularly for each square meter of body surface area twice a week for 4 weeks. To avoid complications, the total dose should not exceed 15,000 units. It is currently available for use in the United States.

LHRH

Since 1974, luteinizing hormone releasing hormone (LHRH) has been used to treat cryptorchidism[252] by stimulating gonadotropin secretion from the pituitary. It was initially administered intramuscularly, but has been used as a nasal spray since 1975.[253] A typical course of therapy consists of 1.2 mg/day, in divided doses, for 4 weeks. Results from European studies show that it is more effective than HCG. This form of therapy is not approved for use in the United States.

Combination Therapy

Combination therpy with HCG and LHRH has been used to treat cryptorchidism with the premise that the combining of agents will compensate for gonadotropin insufficiency that may have contributed to failed descent. Results have been variable, but appear to be better than that achieved with either HCG or LHRH as a single agent.[246, 254–256]

Buserelin

Buserelin is a synthetic superanalog of endogenous LHRH and is typically administered in very small doses, for example, 20 μg per day for 1 month. Buserelin therapy can induce testicular descent and improve germ-cell histology and spermiograms obtained after spontaneous descent or orchidopexy.[257–259] It is not approved for use in the United States.

SURGICAL THERAPY

History of Surgical Therapy

The term orchidopexy refers to the surgical transfer and fixation of an undescended testis to the scrotum. John Hunter in the 1700s provided the first descriptions of testicular anatomy and descent that set the stage for the surgical treatment of cryptorchidism. The first orchidopexy was attempted by Rosenmerkel in 1820,[260] but results were poor and the procedure was not accepted. In 1899 Bevan described the principles for successful orchidopexy (isolation and mobilization of the testis and spermatic cord, repair of an associated hernia, and scrotal fixation)[261] and in 1903 suggested that testicular vessels could be safely sacrificed in cases limited by their length.[262] In 1931 LaRoque modified Bevan's description to propose an antegrade approach from above the internal inguinal ring, with dissection proceeding distally.[263] In 1959 Fowler and Stephens described the collateral circulation of the testis,[264] providing scientific evidence that division of the spermatic vessels to achieve length was theoretically sound. In 1960 Prentiss described the triangular arrangement of the testicular vessels in the retroperitoneum and methods to lengthen the testicular vessels by releasing the lateral bands and dividing the inferior epigastric vessels and the floor of the inguinal canal.[265] Techniques of fixation have evolved from attaching the testis to the thigh with suture (Torek)[266] or a rubber band (Cabot and Nesbit)[267] or passing it through a hole in the scrotal septum (Ombredanne).[268] In 1931 Petrivalsky first described the creation of a scrotal subdartos pouch for placement of the testis,[269] which was later popularized by Lattimer[270] and Koop.[271] The current approaches to orchidopexy have all been derived from these foundations.

Surgical Anatomy

The testis is supplied by the structures of the spermatic cord within the inguinal canal. The spermatic cord contains the ilioinguinal (L1) and genital branch of the genitofemoral nerve (L1-L2), the cremaster muscle, the testicular vessels, the vas deferens, sympathetic and parasympathetic nerves, and the remnants of the processus vaginalis. The fascial coverings of the spermatic cord are the extensions of the abdominal counterparts: the external spermatic (external oblique), cremasteric or middle spermatic (internal oblique), and internal spermatic (transversalis) fascia.

The primary arterial blood supply of the testis is the testicular artery, also termed the gonadal or internal spermatic artery, a branch of the abdominal aorta. Additional collateral blood supply comes from the cremasteric or external spermatic artery and the artery of the vas deferens, which are branches of the inferior epigastric and inferior vesical arteries, respectively. Minor collateral contributions come from the anterior and posterior scrotal arteries, which are branches of the pudendal artery.[272] Venous drainage of the testis is through the pampiniform (L. pampinus, meaning tendril, the spirally coiling organ of a climbing plant) plexus of veins, which drains through the gonadal vein into the renal vein on the left and the inferior vena cava on the right. The gonadal vessels course in the retroperitoneum ventral to the ureter before entering the internal inguinal ring just lateral to the inferior epigastric vessels. Venous drainage of collateral vessels follows their arterial counterparts. It is important to recognize the indirect course of the testicular vessels to take advantage of additional vascular length available during orchidopexy.[265] Lymphatic drainage of the testis is to the retroperitoneal lymph nodes, but may be altered after orchidopexy to include the superficial inguinal lymph nodes.

Surgery for the Palpable Testis

The principles of orchidopexy include isolation of the testis, repair of an associated hernia, mobilization of the spermatic cord, and fixation of the testis in the scrotum. Although variations have been introduced in the last century, and the initial approach to palpable and nonpalpable testes may differ, these same basic principles are valid for all forms of orchidopexy.

Inguinal Orchidopexy

After the induction of anesthesia, the cremasteric reflex is blocked, and the patient is reexamined to exclude the diagnosis of a retractile testis. A transverse inguinal incision is made in a skin crease midway between the pubic tubercle and the anterior superior iliac spine. Scarpa's fascia, which is well developed in infants, is divided. Careful dissection is performed in this area to avoid inadvertent surgical injury to the testis, which may be in the superficial pouch.[68] The external oblique fascia is then incised in the direction of its fibers just medial to the inguinal ligament. The ilioinguinal nerve is identified and preserved. The testis may be located behind a hernia sac at this point. The anterior wall of the hernia can be opened to expose the testis, which is supported by a carefully placed stay suture. The gubernacular attachments are carefully divided to avoid injuring a "long-loop" vas deferens that may be present in the canal distal to the testis. The spermatic cord is freed proximally to the internal inguinal ring, and all cremaster muscle fibers are divided. The opened hernia sac is dissected from the anteromedial aspect of the cord to the level of the internal inguinal ring. The hernia sac is suture ligated at the internal inguinal ring with absorbable suture, and the ligated sac is held to expose the retroperitoneal space if necessary.

Division of cremasteric attachments and the hernia sac will, in most instances, provide adequate length for tension-free placement of the testis in the scrotum. If not, the internal inguinal ring is opened laterally, and the peritoneum is bluntly elevated off the testicular vessels. The lateral spermatic fascia, sometimes called the tethering bands of Denis Browne, is sharply divided. The floor of the inguinal canal can be divided to the pubis to perform a Prentiss maneuver,[265] dividing the inferior epigastric vessels and transposing the testicular vessels medially to provide a straight course to the scrotum. Alternatively, the testis and vessels can be passed underneath the epigastric vessels to preserve them with the same results.

Once the testis has been adequately mobilized, it is fixed within the scrotum. A subdartos pouch is created in the anterior wall of the scrotum and the tip of a hemostat is passed through the scrotal incision into the inguinal canal to grasp the stay suture and deliver the testis into the pouch. To provide additional security, a suture may be passed through the fibrous tissue beneath the lower pole of the testis, then through the scrotal skin using a Keith needle, and tied over a button. The specific placement of this suture is based on intratesticular arterial anatomy[273] to avoid the risk of testicular atrophy. The vascular pedicle is then inspected to confirm the absence of tension and torsion. The wounds are then closed anatomically in layers using absorbable suture. The procedure is generally performed on an outpatient basis.

The scrotal button and suture are usually removed 1 week after surgery. Patients are seen 3 months and 1 year later to determine testicular position and size. Recommendations are made for evaluation at puberty to confirm testicular growth and to teach self-examination. For those with congenital or surgical monorchia, warnings are given regarding the benefits of protection during contact sports.

Incidental Findings

At the time of orchidopexy, ectopic tissue may rarely be identified adjacent to the testis. Examples include spleen and liver tissue resulting from splenogonadal[274] and hepatogonadal fusion[275] and adrenal tissue in the form of an adrenal rest. Intraabdominal structures may descend into a patent processus vaginalis and may be present in a hernia sac in the spermatic cord. Examples include abdominal viscera such as bowel and omentum, as well as pelvic viscera such as the bladder. Preoperative awareness and intraoperative recognition of these variations in anatomy should allow proper management and prevent complications.

Surgery for the Nonpalpable Testis

Surgery for the nonpalpable testis has two goals: *(a)* to identify the presence or absence of the testicle (diagnostic) and, *(b)* if present, to achieve orchidopexy or orchidectomy (therapeutic). The easiest and most accurate way to achieve the first goal is diagnostic laparoscopy; the goal of successful orchidopexy for the intraabdominal testis has been more elusive.[276] Several approaches to the high undescended testis have been devised, none of which has been proven to be superior in a prospective fashion.

Laparoscopy

At this time, the most common indication for laparoscopy in the pediatric age group is for the evaluation of the nonpalpable testicle. Originally, the anatomic findings at laparoscopy were used only to plan an open surgical approach or to avoid open surgery altogether in approximately 40% of patients.[277-279] In recent years, Bloom[280] and Jordan et al.[281] have demonstrated that the intraabdominal testis can be brought down to the scrotum using laparoscopic techniques in single or staged procedures. Contraindications to laparoscopy may include prior abdominal surgery with potential scarring or a body habitus that will not allow for proper placement of ports and laparoscopes.

Diagnostic Laparoscopy

Abdominal access and insufflation are obtained as described elsewhere.[282] With the patient in Trendelenburg position, the normal anatomy of the pelvis in the child is distinct. The internal inguinal rings are located just lateral to the medial umbilical ligaments on each side. The examination is begun by looking at the internal ring on the side of the normal testis, if there is one. The spermatic vessels join the vas deferens, coursing medial to lateral, just prior to entering the inguinal canal. The affected side is then examined, and one of three possible observations will be made.

has been noted, but no clear genetic determinant has been identified. History is often unhelpful, and physical diagnosis can be unreliable. With the increased use of laparoscopy, radiographic localization procedures are obsolete in all but the most unusual cases. Hormonal testing can be especially useful to diagnose anorchia.

Medical therapy has limited success, but may improve later fertility. Surgical therapy is usually effective, but success relates to the initial position of the testis. Laparoscopy is particularly helpful for diagnosis and management in cases of a nonpalpable testis. Reoperative orchidopexy can be challenging, but can be successful with proper surgical approach. Although use of the testicular prosthesis to replace an absent or removed testis has diminished in recent years, the development of safe biomaterials may make this option more attractive in the future.

Despite the perception that cryptorchidism is a simple and common problem with an easy surgical solution, our understanding of testicular descent is elementary, and the surgical techniques for correcting maldescent require reexamination and improvement.

REFERENCES

1. Marshall FF, Elder JS. Cryptorchidism and related anomalies. New York: Praeger, 1982:118.
2. Page DC, Mosher R, Simpson EM, et al. The sex-determining region of the human Y chromosome encodes a finger protein. Cell 1987;51:1091.
3. Moore KL. The developing human. 3rd ed. Philadelphia: Saunders, 1982:479.
4. Josso N. Development and descent of the fetal testis in maldescensus testis. In: Bierich JR, Rager K, Ranke, MB, eds. Development and descent of the fetal testis in maldescensus testis. Baltimore: Urban & Schwarzenberg, 1977:3.
5. Wilson JD, Griffin JE, Russell DW. Steroid 5 alpha-reductase 2 deficiency. Endocr Rev 1993;14:577.
6. Heyns CF. The gubernaculum during testicular descent in the human fetus. J Anat 1987;153:93.
7. Rajfer J; Walsh PC. Testicular descent. Birth Defects 1977; 13:107.
8. Hadziselimovic F, Kruslin E. The role of the epididymis in descensus testis and the topographical relaionship between the testis and epididymis from the sixth month of pregnancy until immediately after birth. Anat Embryol (Berl) 1979;155:191.
9. Elder JS. Cryptorchidism: isolated and associated with other genitourinary defects. Pediatric Clin North Am 1987;34:1033.
10. Job JC, Toublanc JE, Chaussain JL, et al. The pituitary-gonadal axis in cryptorchid infants and children. Eur J Pediatr 1987;146(Suppl 2):S2.
11. Yamanaka J, Baker M, Metcalfe S, Hutson JM. Serum levels of Müllerian inhibiting substance in boys with cryptorchidism. J Pediatr Surg 1991;26:621.
12. Heyns CF, Hutson JM. Historical review of theories on testicular descent. J Urol 1995;153:754.
13. Job JC, Gendrel D, Safar A, Roger M, et al. Pituitary LH and FSH and testosterone secretion in infants with undescended testes. Acta Endocrinol 1977;85:644.
14. Job JC, Gendrel D. Endocrine aspects of cryptorchidism. Urol Clin North Am 1982;9:353.
15. De Muinck Keizer-Schrama SMPF, Hazebroek FWJ, Drop SLS, et al. Hormonal evaluation of boys born with undescended testes during their first year of life. J Clin Endocrinol Metab 1988; 66:159.
16. Engle ET. Experimentally induced descent of the testis in the Macacus monkey by hormones from the anterior pituitary and pregnancy urine. Endocrinology 1932;16:513.
17. Rajfer J, Walsh PC. Hormonal regulation of testicular descent: experimental and clinical observations. J Urol 1977;118:985.
18. Hutson JM, Donahoe PK. The hormonal control of testicular descent. Endocr Rev 1986;7:270.
19. Spencer JR, Torrado T, Sanchez RS, et al. Effects of flutamide and finasteride on rat testicular descent. Endocrinology 1991; 129:741.
20. Husmann DA, McPhaul MJ. Time-specific androgen blockade with flutamide inhibits testicular descent in the rat. Endocrinology 1991;129:1409.
21. Forest MG, Sizonenko PC, Cathiard AM, Bertrand J. Hypophyso-gonadal function in humans during the first year of life: evidence for testicular activity in early infancy. J Clin Invest 1974;53:819.
22. Gendrel D, Job JC, Roger M. Reduced post-natal rise of testosterone in plasma of cryptorchid infants. Acta Endocrinol 1978;89:372.
23. Gendrel D, Roger M, Job JC. Plasma gonadotropin and testosterone values in infants with cryptorchildism. J Pediatr 1980;97:217.
24. Hutson JM. Testicular feminization: a model for testicular descent in mice and men. J Pediatr Surg 1986;3:195.
25. Cain MP, Kramer SA, Tindall DJ, Husmann DA. Expression of androgen receptor protein within the lumbar spinal cord during ontologic development and following antiandrogen induced cryptorchidism. J Urol 1994;152:766.
26. Brown TR, Berkovitz GD, Gearhart JP. Androgen receptors in boys with isolated bilateral cryptorchidism. Am J Dis Child 1988;142:933.
27. Donahoe PK, Ito Y, Morikawa Y, Hendren WH. Müllerian inhibiting substance in human testes after birth. J Pediatr Surg 1977;12:323.
28. Habenicht UF, Neumann F. Hormonal regulation of testicular descent. Adv Anat Embryol Cell Biol 1983;81:1.
29. Hutson JM, Donahoe PK, Budzik GP. Müllerian inhibiting substance: a fetal hormone with surgical implications. Aust N Z J Surg 1985;55:599.
30. Brook CGD, Wagner H, Zachman M, et al. Familial occurrence of persistent mullerian structures in otherwise normal males. Br Med J 1973;1:771.
31. Sloan WR, Walsh PC. Familial persistent Müllerian duct syndrome. J Urol 1976;115:459.
32. Josso N, Fekete C, Cachin O, et al. Persistence of Müllerian ducts in male pseudohermaphroditism, and its relationship to cryptorchidism. Clin Endocrinol 1983;19:247.
33. Tran D, Picard J, Vigier B, et al. Persistence of Müllerian ducts in male rabbits passively immunized against bovine anti-Müllerian hormone during fetal life. Dev Biol 1986;116:160.
34. Behringer RR, Finegold MJ, Cate RL. Müllerian-inhibiting substance function during mammalian sexual development. Cell 1994;79:415.
35. Wensing CJ. The embryology of testicular descent. Horm Res 1988;30:144.
36. Husmann DA, Levy JB. Current concepts in the pathophysiology of testicular undescent. Urology 1995;46:267.
37. Fentener van Vlissingen JM, van Zoelen EJ, Ursem PJ, Wensing CJ. In vitro model of the first phase of testicular descent: identification of a low molecular weight factor from fetal testis involved in proliferation of gubernaculum testis cells and distinct from specified polypeptide growth factors in fetal gonadal hormones. Endocrinology 1988;123:2868.
38. Cain MP, Kramer SA, Tindall DJ, Husmann DA. Epidermal growth factor reverses antiandrogen induced cryptorchidism and epididymal development. J Urol 1994;152:770.
39. Cain MP, Kramer SA, Tindall DJ, Husmann DA. Alterations in maternal epidermal growth factor (EGF) effect testicular descent and epididymal development. Urology 1994;43:375.
40. Newbold RR, Suzuki Y, MacLachlan JA. Müllerian duct maintenance in heterotypic organ culture after in vivo exposure to diethylstilbesterol. Endocrinology 1984;115:1863.
41. Bernstein L, Pike MC, Depue RH, et al. Maternal hormone levels in early gestation of cryptorchid males: a case-control study. Br J Cancer 1988;58:379.

42. Gier HT, Marion GB. Development of mammalian testes and genital ducts. Biol Reprod 1969;1(Suppl 1):1.

43. Kaplan LM, Koyle MA, Kaplan GW, et al. Association between abdominal wall defects and cryptorchidism. J Urol 1986;136:645.

44. Frey HL, Peng S, Rajfer J. Synergy of abdominal pressure and androgens in testicular descent. Biol Reprod 1983;23:1233.

45. Frey HL, Rajfer J. Role of the gubernaculum and intraabdominal pressure in the process of testicular descent. J Urol 1984;131:574.

46. Quinlan DM, Gearhart JP, Jeffs RD. Abdominal wall defects and cryptorchidism: an animal model. J Urol 1988;140:1141.

47. Attah AA, Hutson JM. The role of intra-abdominal pressure in cryptorchidism. J Urol 1993;150:994.

48. Lockwood CB. The development and transition of the testicles: normal and abnormal. Br Med J 1987;1:444.

49. Sonneland SG. Undescended testicle. Surg Gynecol Obstet 1925;401:535.

50. Curling JB. Observations on the structure of the gubernaculum and on the descent of the testis in the fetus. Lancet 1840;2:70.

51. Wyndham NR. A morphological study of testicular descent. J Anat 1943;77:179.

52. Elder JS, Isaacs JT, Walsh PC. Androgen sensitivity of the gubernaculum testis: Evidence for hormonal/mechanical interactions in testicular descent. J Urol 1982;127:170.

53. Mininberg DT, Schlossberg S. The role of the epididymis in testicular descent. J Urol 1983;129:120.

54. Frey HL, Rajfer J. Epididymis does not play an important role in the process of testicular descent. Surg Forum 1982;33:617.

55. Elder JS. Epididymal anomalies associated with hydrocele/hernia and cryptorchidism: implications regarding testicular descent. J Urol 1992;148:624.

56. Husmann DA, Boone TB, McPhaul MJ. Flutamide-induced testicular undescent in the rat is associated with alterations in genitofemoral nerve morphology. J Urol 1994;151:509.

57. Fallat ME, Williams MPL, Farmer PJ, Hutson JM. Histologic evaluation of inguinoscrotal migration of the gubernaculum in rodents during testicular descent and its relationship to the genitofemoral nerve. Pediatr Surg Int 1992;7:265.

58. Yamanaka J, Metcalfe SA, Hutson JM, Mendelsohn FAO. Testicular descent. II. Ontogeny and response to denervation of calcitonin gene-related peptide receptors in neonatal rat gubernaculum. Endocrinology 1993;132:280.

59. Goh DW, Momose Y, Middlesworth W, Hutson JM. The relationship among calcitonin gene-related peptide, androgens and gubernacular development in 3 animal models of cryptorchidism. J Urol 1993;150:574.

60. Shono T, Goh DW, Momose Y, Hutson JM. Physiological effects in vitro of calcitonin gene-related peptide on gubernacular contractility with or without denervation. J Pediatr Surg 1995;30:591.

61. Barthold JS, Mahler HR, Newton BW. Lack of feminization of the cremaster nucleus in cryptorchid androgen insensitive rats. J Urol 1994;152:2280.

62. Barthold JS, Mahler HR, Sziszak TJ, Newton BW. Lack of feminization of the cremaster nucleus by prenatal flutamide administration in the rat and pig. J Urol 1994;156:767.

63. Goh DW, Farmer PJ, Hutson JM. Absence of normal sexual dimorphism of the genitofemoral nerve spinal nucleus in the mutant cryptorchid (TS) rat. J Reprod Fertil 1994;102:195.

64. Kaplan GW. Nomenclature of cryptorchidism. Eur J Pediatr 1993;152(Suppl 2):S17.

65. Beltran BF, Villegas AF. Clinical classification for undescended testes: experience in 1,010 orchidopexies. J Pediatr Surg 1988;23:444.

66. Canavese F, Lalla R, Linari A, et al. Surgical treatment of cryptorchidism. Eur J Pediatr 1993;152(Suppl 2):S43.

67. Scorer CG, Farrington GH. Congenital deformities of the testis and epididymis. New York: Appleton-Century-Crofts, 1972.

68. Browne D. The diagnosis of undescended testicle. Br Med J 1938;2:168.

69. Redman JF. Transverse testicular ectopia. Urology 1982;19:181.

70. Redman JF, Brizzolara JP. An unusual case of testicular ectopia. J Uro 1985;133:104.

71. Carmody E, Klotz L, Leonhardt C. Bilateral retrovesical testes: an unusual location for impalpable undescended testes. Abdominal Imaging 1993;18:301.

72. Caesar RE, Kaplan GW. The incidence of the cremasteric reflex in normal boys. J Urol 1994;152:779.

73. Wyllie GG. The retractile testis. Med J Aust 1984;140:403.

74. Redman JF. Impalpable testes: observations based on 208 consecutive operations for undescended testes. J Urol 1980;124:379.

75. Levitt SB, Kogan SJ, Engel RM, et al. The impalpable testis: a rational approach to management. J Urol 1978;120:515.

76. Smolko MJ, Kaplan GW, Brock WA. Location and fate of the nonpalpable testis in children J Urol 1983;129:1204.

77. Wright JE. Impalpable testis: a review of 100 boys. J Pediatr Surg 1986;21:151.

78. Abeyaratne MR, Aherne WA, Scott JES. The vanishing testis. Lancet 1969;2:822.

79. Kogan SJ, Gill B, Bennett B, et al. Human monorchism: a clinicopathological study of unilateral absent testes in 65 boys. J Urol 1986;135:758.

80. Huff DS, Wu HY, Snyder HM III, et al. Evidence in favor of the mechanical (intrauterine torsion) theory over the endocrinopathy (cryptorchidism) theory in the pathogenesis of testicular agenesis. J Urol 1991;146:630.

81. Turek PJ, Ewalt DH, Snyder HM III, et al. The absent cryptorchid testis: surgical findings and their implications for diagnosis and etiology. J Urol 1994;151:718.

82. Plotzker ED, Rushton HG, Belman AB, Skoog SJ. Laparoscopy for nonpalpable testes in childhood: is inguinal exploration also necessary when vas and vessels exit the inguinal ring? J Urol 1992;148:635.

83. Diamond DA, Caldamone AA, Elder JS. Prevalence of the vanishing testis in boys with a unilateral impalpable testis: is the side of presentation significant? J Urol 1994;152:502.

84. Edman CD, Winters AJ, Porter JC, et al. Embryonic testicular regression. A clinical spectrum of XY agonadal individuals. Obstet Gynecol 1977;49:208.

85. Josso N, Briard ML. Embryonic testicular regression syndrome: variable phenotypic expression in siblings. J Pediatr 1980;97:200.

86. Jost A. Problems of fetal endocrinology: the gonadal and hypophyseal hormones. Recent Prog Horm Res 1953;8:379.

87. Goldberg LM, Skaist LB, Morrow JW. Congenital absence of testes: anorchism and monorchism. J Urol 1974;111:840.

88. Brock WA. Bilateral cryptorchidism. In: Resnick MI, Kursh E, eds. Current therapy in genitourinary surgery. Toronto: Decker, 1987:302.

89. Hortling H, de la Chapelle A, Johansson C-J, et al. An endocrinologic follow-up study of operated cases of cryptorchidism. J Clin Endocrinol Metab 1967;27:120.

90. Snyder HM III. Bilatral undescended testes. Eur J Pediatr 1993;152(Suppl 2):S45.

91. Jarow JP, Berkovitz GD, Migeon CJ, et al. Elevation of serum gonadotropins establishes the diagnosis of anorchism in prepubertal boys with bilateral cryptorchidism. J Urol 1986;136:277.

92. Levitt, SB, Kogan SJ, Schneider KM, et al. Endocrine tests in phenotypic children with bilateral impalpable testes can reliably predict "congenital" anorchism. Urology 1978;11:11.

93. Bartone FF, Huseman CA, Maizels M, Firlit CF. Pitfalls in using human chorionic gonadotropin stimulation test to diagnose anorchia. J Urol 1984;132:563.

94. Lee MM, Donahoe PK, Silverman BL, et al. Measurements of serum mullerian inhibiting substance in the evaluation of children with nonpalpable gonads. N Engl J Med 1997;336:1480.

95. Rabinowitz R, Hulbert WC Jr. Late presentation of cryptorchidism: the etiology of testicular re-ascent. J Urol 1997;157:1892.

96. Docimo SG. Testicular descent and ascent in the first year of life. Urology 1996;48:458.

97. Schiffer KA, Kogan SJ, Reda EF, Levitt SB. Acquired undescended testes. Am J Dis Child 1987;141:106.

98. Robertson JF, Azmy AF, Cochran W. Assent to ascent of the testis. Br J Urol 1988;61:146.

99. Myers NA, Officer CB. Undescended testis: congenital or acquired? Austr Paediatr J 1975;11:76.

100. Villumsen AL, Zachau-Christiansen B. Spontaneous alterations in position of the testes. Arch Dis Child 1966;41:198.

101. Belman AB. Acquired undescended (ascended) testis: effects of human chorionic gonadotropin. J Urol 1988;140:1189.

102. Wright JE. Testes do ascend. Pediatr Surg Int 1989;4:269.

103. Atwell JD. Ascent of the testis: fact or fiction. Br J Urol 1985;57:474.
104. Clarnette TD, Rowe D, Hasthorpe S, Hutson JM. Incomplete disappearance of the processus vaginalis as a cause of ascending testis. J Urol 1997;157:1889.
105. Kaplan GW. Iatrogenic cryptorchidism resulting from hernia repair. Surg Gynecol Obst 1976;142:671.
106. Scorer CG. The descent of the testis. Arch Dis Child 1964;39:605.
107. Berkowitz GS, Lapinski RH, Dolgin SE, et al. Prevalence and natural history of cryptorchidism. Pediatrics 1993;92:44.
108. Gross RE, Jewett TC Jr. Surgical experiences from 1222 operations for undescended testis. J Am Med Assoc 1956;160:634.
109. Hadziselimovic F. Cryptorchidism. In: Gillenwater JY, Grayhack JT, Howards SS, Duckett JW, eds. Adult and pediatric urology. Chicago: Year Book Medical, 1987:2217.
110. Depue RH. Maternal and gestational factors affecting the risk of cryptorchidism and inguinal hernia. Int J Epidemiol 1984;13:311.
111. Depue RH. Cryptorchidism, an epidemiologic study with emphasis on the relationship to central nervous system dysfunction. Teratology 1988;37:301.
112. Gill WB, Schumacher GF, Bibbo M, et al. Association of diethylstilbestrol exposure in utero with cryptorchidism, testicular hypoplasia and semen abnormalities. J Urol 1979;122:36.
113. Panagiotopoulou K, Katsouyanni K, Petridou E, et al. Maternal age, parity, and pregnancy estrogens. Cancer Causes & Control 1990;1:119.
114. Whitehead ED, Leiter E. Genital abnormalities and abnormal semen analyses in male patients exposed to diethylstilbestrol in utero. J Urol 1981;125:47.
115. Niculescu AM. Effects of in utero exposure to DES on male progeny. J Obstet Gynecol Neonatal Nurs 1985;14:468.
116. Stillman RJ. In utero exposure to diethylstilbestrol: adverse effects on the reproductive tract and reproductive performance and male and female offspring. Am J Obstet Gynecol 1982;142:905.
117. McBride ML, Van den Steen N, Lamb CW, Gallagher RP. Maternal and gestational factors in cryptorchidism. Int J Epidemiol 1991;20:964.
118. Burton MH, Davies TW, Raggatt PR. Undescended testis and hormone levels in early pregnancy. J Epidemiol Commun Health 1987;41:127.
119. Davies TW, Williams DR, Whitaker RH. Risk factors for undescended testis. Int J Epidemiol 1986;15:197.
120. Berkowitz GS, Lapinski RH, Godbold JH, et al. Maternal and neonatal risk factors for cryptorchidism. Epidemiology 1995;6:127.
121. Czeizel A, Erodi E, Toth J. Genetics of undescended testis. J Urol 1981;126:528.
122. Swerdlow AJ, Wood KH, Smith PG. A case-control study of the aetiology of cryptorchidism. J Epidemiol Commun Health 1983;237:238.
123. Abrams HJ. Familial cryptorchidism (letter). Urology 1975;5:849.
124. Rezvani I, Rettig KR, DiGeorge AM. Inheritance of cryptorchidism. Pediatrics 1976;58:774.
125. Perrett L, O'Rourke DA. Hereditary cryptorchidism. Med J Aust 1969;1:1289.
126. Corbus BC, O'Conor VJ. The familial occurrence of undescended testes. Surg Gynecol Obstet 1922;34:237.
127. Jones IR, Young ID. Familial incidence of cryptorchidism. J Urol 1982;127:508.
128. Klein D, Ferrier P, Ammann F. La genetique de l'ectopic testiculaite. Pathol Biol (Paris) 1963;11:1214.
129. Dewald GW, Kelalis PP, Gordon H. Chromosomal studies in cryptorchidism. J Urol 1977;117:110.
130. Klugo R, Van DD, Weiss L. Cytogenic studies of cryptorchid testes. Urology 1978;11:255.
131. Czeizel A, Erodi E, Toth J. An epidemiological study on undescended testis. J Urol 1981;126:524.
132. Cortes D, Thorup JM, Nielsen OH, Beck BL. Cryptorchidism in boys with imperforate anus. J Pediatr Surg 1995;30:631.
133. Meyer S, Landau H. Precocious puberty in myelomeningocele patients. J. Pediatr Orthop 1984;4:28.
134. Cortada X, Kousseff BG. Cryptorchidism in mental retardation. J Urol 1984;131:674.
135. Rundle JSH, Primrose DA, Carachi R. Cryptorchidism in cerebral palsy. Br J Urol 1982;54:170.
136. Hutson JM, Beasley SW, Bryan AD. Cryptorchidism in spina bifida and spinal cord transection: a clue to the mechanism of transinguinal descent of the testis. J. Pediatr Surg 1988;23:275.
137. Grossman H, Ririe DG. The incidence of urinary tract anomalies in cryptorchid boys. Am J Roentgenol Rad Ther Nucl Med 1968;103:210.
138. Pappis CH, Argianas SA, Bousgas D, Athanasiades E. Unsuspected urological anomalies in asymptomatic cryptorchid boys. Pediatr Radiol 1988;18:51.
139. Kleinteich B, Popp W, Daniel P, Grahl KO. Excretory urography as a screening method for abnormalities of the upper urinary tract in asymptomatic boys with undescended testicles. Int Urol Nephrol 1981;13:77.
140. Waaler PE, Maurseth K. Letter: Cryptorchidism: is routine intravenous pyelography indicated? Arch Dis Child 1976;51:324.
141. Noe HN, Patterson TH. Screening urography in asymptomatic cryptorchid patients. J Urol 1978;119:669.
142. Noble MJ, Wacksman J. Screening excretory urography in patients with cryptorchidism or hypospadias: a survey and review of the literature. J Urol 1980;124:98.
143. Krueger RP, Hardy BE, Churchill BM. Cryptorchidism in boys with posterior urethral valves. J Urol 1980;124:101.
144. Breslow NE, Beckwith JB. Epidemiological features of Wilms' tumor: results of the National Wilms' Tumor Study. J Nat Cancer Inst 1982;68:429.
145. Rajfer J, Walsh PC. The incidence of intersexuality in patients with hypospadias and cryptorchidism. J Urol 1976;116:769.
146. Rohatgi M, Menon PS, Verma IC, Iyengar JK. The presence of intersexuality in patients with advanced hypospadias and undescended gonads. J Urol 1987;137:263.
147. Visser HK. Associated anomalies in undescended testes. Eur J Pediatr 1982;139:272.
148. Marshall FF, Shermeta DW. Epididymal abnormalities associated with undescended testis. J Urol 1979;121:341.
149. Heath AL, Man DW, Eckstein HB. Epididymal abnormalities associated with maldescent of the testis. J Pediatr Surg 1984;19:47.
150. Gill B, Kogan S, Starr S, et al. Significance of epididymal and ductal anomalies associated with testicular maldescent. J Urol 1989;142:556.
151. Koff W, Scaletscky R. Malformations of the epididymis in undescended testis. J Urol 1990;143:340.
152. Mininberg DT. The epididymis and testicular descent. Eur J Pediatr 1987;146(Suppl 2): S28.
153. Badenoch AW. Failure of the urogenital union. Surg Gynecol Obstet 1946;82:471.
154. Marshall FF, Weissman RM, Jeffs RD. Cryptorchidism: the surgical implications of non-union of the epididymis and testis. J Urol 1980;124:560.
155. Laron Z, Zilka E. Compensatory hypertrophy of testicle in unilateral cryptorchidism. J Clin Endocrinol Metab 1969;29:1409.
156. Tato L, Corgnati A, Boner A, et al. Unilateral cryptorchidism with compensatory hypertrophy of descended testicle in prepubertal boys. Horm Res 1978;9:185.
157. Koff SA. Does compensatory testicular enlargement predict monorchism? J Urol 1991;146:632.
158. Huff DS, Snyder HM III, Hadziselimovic F, et al. An absent testis is associated with contralateral testicular hypertrophy. J Urol 1992;148:627.
159. Olsen LH. Inter-observer variation in assessment of undescended testis. Analysis of kappa statistics as a coefficient of reliability. Br J Urol 1989;64:644.
160. Lunderquist A, Rafstedt S. Roentgenologic diagnosis of cryptorchidism. J Urol 1967;98:219.
161. White JJ, Shaker IJ, O KS, et al. Herniography: a diagnostic refinement in the management of cryptorchidism. Am Surg 1973;39:624.
162. Dwoskin JW, Kuhn JP. Herniagrams in undescended testes and hydroceles. J Urol 1973;109:520.
163. Khademi M, Seebode JJ, Falla A. Selective spermatic arteriography for localization of an impalpable undescended testis. Radiology 1980;136:627.

164. Ben-Menachem Y, deBerardinis MC, Salinas R. Localization of intra-abdominal testes by selective testicular arteriography: a case report. J Urol 1974;112:493.

165. Weiss RM, Glickman MG, Lytton B. Venographic localization of the non-palpable undescended testis in children. J Urol 1977;117:513.

166. Weiss RM, Glickman MG, Lytton B. Clinical implications of gonadal venography in the management of the non-palpable undescended testis. J Urol 1979;121:745.

167. Weiss RM, Glickman MG. Venography of the undescended testis. Urol Clin North Am 1982;9:387.

168. Pommerville P, Futter NG, McKay DE, Desmarais R. The role of gonadal venography in the management of the adult with non-palpable undescended testis. Br J Urol 1982;54:408.

169. Khan O, Williams G, Boley NB, Allison DJ. Testicular venography for the localization of the impalpable undescended testis. Br J Surg 1982;69:660.

170. Freeny PC, Cummings KB, Simmons JR. Selective testicular venography for localization of nonpalpable testis. Urology 1978;12:617.

171. Amin M, Wheeler CS. Selective testicular venography in abdominal cryptorchidism. J Urol 1976;115:760.

172. Kullendorff CM, Hederstrom E, Forsberg L. Preoperative ultrasonography of the undescended testis. Scand J Urol Nephrol 1985;19:13.

173. Wolverson MK, Houttuin E, Heiberg E, et al. Comparison of computed tomography with high-resolution realtime ultrasound in the localization of the impalpable undescended testis. Radiology 1983;146:133.

174. Wolverson MK, Jagannadharao B, Sundaram M, et al. CT in localization of impalpable cryptorchid testes. Am J Roentgenol 1980;134:725.

175. Rajfer J, Tauber A, Zinner N, et al. The use of computerized tomography scanning to localize the impalpable testis. J Urol 1983;129:972.

176. Lee JK, McClennan BL, Stanley RJ, Sagel SS. Utility of computed tomography in the localization of the undescended testis. Radiology 1980;135:121.

177. Green RJ. Computerized axial tomography vs spermatic venography in localization of cryptorchid testes. Urology 1985;26:513.

178. Kogan BA, Hricak H, Tanagho EA. Magnetic resonance imaging in genital anomalies. J Urol 1987;138:1028.

179. Beomonte ZB, Vicentini C, Masciocchi C, et al. Magnetic resonance imaging in the localization of undescended abdominal testes. Eur Urol 1990;17:145.

180. Troughton AH, Waring J, Longstaff A, Goddard PR. The role of magnetic resonance imaging in the investigation of undescended testes. Clin Radiol 1990; 41:178.

181. Miyano T, Kobayashi H, Shimomura H, et al. Magnetic resonance imaging for localizing the nonpalpable undescended testis. J Pediatr Surg 1991;26:607.

182. Maghnie M, Vanzulli A, Paesano P, et al. The accuracy of magnetic resonance imaging and ultrasonography compared with surgical findings in the localization of the undescended testis. Arch Pediatr Adolesc Med 1994;148:699.

183. Hrebinko RL, Bellinger MF. The limited role of imaging techniques in managing children with undescended testes. J Urol 1993;150:458.

184. Tennenbaum SY, Lerner SE, McAleer IM, et al. Preoperative laparoscopic localization of the nonpalpable testis: a critical analysis of a 10-year experience. J Urol 1994;151:732.

185. Moore RG, Peters CA, Bauer SB, et al. Laparoscopic evaluation of the nonpalpable testis: a prospective assessment of accuracy. J Urol 1994;151:728.

186. Cain MP, Garra B, Gibbons MD. Scrotal-inguinal ultrasonography: a technique for identifying the nonpalpable inguinal testis without laparoscopy. J Urol 1996;156:791.

187. Hadziselimovic F, Herzog B, Buser M. Development of cryptorchid testes. Eur J Pediatr 1987;146(Suppl 2):S8.

188. Kogan SJ, Tennenbaum S, Gill B, et al. Efficacy of orchiopexy by patient age 1 year for cryptorchidism. J Urol 1990;144:508.

189. Huff DS, Hadziselimovic F, Duckett JW, et al. Germ cell counts in semithin sections of biopsies of 115 unilaterally cryptorchid

testes. The experience from the Children's Hospital of Philadelphia. Eur J Pediatr 1987;146(Suppl 2):S225.

190. Huff DS, Hadziselimovic F, Snyder HM III, et al. Postnatal testicular maldevelopment in unilateral cryptorchidism. J Urol 1989;142:546.

191. Francavilla S, Santiemma, V, Francavilla F et al. Ultrastructural changes in the seminiferous tubule wall and intertubular blood vessels in human cryptorchidism. Arch Androl 1979;2:21.

192. Hadziselimovic F. Pathogenesis of cryptorchidism. In: Kogan SJ, Hafez ESE, eds. Pediatric andrology. The Hague: Martinus Nijhoff, 1981:147.

193. Mininberg DT, Rodger JC, Bedford JM. Ultrastructural evidence of the onset of testicular pathological conditions in the cryptorchid human testis within the first year of life. J Urol 1982;128:782.

194. Gaudio E, Paggiarino D, Carpino F. Structural and ultrastructural modifications of cryptorchid human testes. J Urol 1984; 131:292.

195. Mengel W, Hienz HA, Sippe WG II, Hecker WC. Studies on cryptorchidism: a comparison of histological findings in the germinative epithelium before and after the second year of life. J Pediatr Surg 1974;9:445.

196. Hecker, W, Hienz HA. Cryptorchidism and fertility. J Pediatr Surg 1967;2:513.

197. Huff DS, Hadziselimovic F, Snyder HM III, et al. Histologic maldevelopment of unilaterally cryptorchid testes and their descended partners. Eur J Pediatr 1993;152(Suppl 2):S10.

198. Cortes D, Thorup JM, Beck BL. Quantitative histology of germ cells in the undescended testes of human fetuses, neonates and infants. J Urol 1995;154:1188.

199. Hadziselimovic F. Cryptorchidism: management and implications. New York: Springer-Verlag, 1983.

200. Hadziselimovic F. Cryptorchidism. In: Gillenwater JY, Grayhack JT, Howards SS, Duckett JW, eds. Adult and pediatric urology. St. Louis: Mosby–Year Book, 1991:2217.

201. Puri P, Nixon HH. Bilateral retractile testes–subsequent effects on fertility. J Pediatr Surg 1977;12:563.

202. Nistal M, Paniagua R. Infertility in adult males with retractile testes. Fertil Steril 1984;41:395.

203. Ito H, Kataumi Z, Yanagi S, et al. Changes in the volume and histology of retractile testes in prepubertal boys. Int J Androl 1986;9:161.

204. Bremholm RT, Ingerslev HJ, Hostrup H. Bilateral spontaneous descent of the testis after the age of 10: subsequent effects on fertility. Br J Surg 1988;75:820.

205. Cendron M, Huff DS, Keating MA, et al. Anatomical, morphological and volumetric analysis: a review of 759 cases of testicular maldescent. J Urol 1993;149:570.

206. Puri P, Sparnon A. Relationship of primary site of testis to final testicular size in cryptorchid patients. Br J Urol 1990;66:208.

207. Kogan SJ. Fertility in cryptorchidism. An overview in 1987. Eur Pediatr 1987;146(Suppl 2):S21.

208. McAleer IM, Packer MG, Kaplan GW, et al. Fertility index analysis in cryptorchidism. J Urol 1995;153:1255.

209. Mack WS, Scott LS, Ferguson-Smith MA, Lenox B. Ectopic testis and true undescended testis: a histological comparison. J Pathol Bacteriol 1961;82:439.

210. Kiesewetter WB, Shull, WR, Fetterman, GH. Histologic changes in the testis following anatomically successful orchidopexy. J Pediatr Surg 1969;4:59.

211. Friedman RM, Lopez FJ, Tucker JA, et al. Fertility after cryptorchidism: a comparative analysis of early orchidopexy with and without concomitant hormonal therapy in the young male rat. J Urol 1994;151:227.

212. Ludwig G, Potempa J. [Fertility after orchidopexy]. [German]. Fortschritte der Andrologie 1974;3:160.

213. Cendron M, Keating MA, Huff DS, et al. Cryptorchidism, orchiopexy and infertility: a critical long-term retrospective analysis. J Urol 1989;142:559.

214. Lee PA. Fertility in cryptorchidism. Does treatment make a difference? Endocrinol Metab Clin North Am 1993;22:479.

215. Mininberg DT, Chen ME, Witkin SS. Antisperm antibodies in cryptorchid boys. Eur J Pediatr 1993;152(Suppl 2): S23.

216. Mengel W, Zimmermann FA. Immunologic aspects of cryptorchidism. Urol Clin North Am 1982;9:349.

217. Urry RL Carrell DT, Starr, NT, et al. The incidence of antisperm antibodies in infertility patients with a history of cryptorchidism. J Urol 1994;151:381.

218. Campbell HE. Incidence of malignant growth of the undescended testicle: A critical and statistical study. Arch Surg 1942;44:353.

219. Campbell HE. The incidence of malignant growth of the undescended testicle: a reply and re-evaluation. J Urol 1959;81:663.

220. Martin DC, Menck, HR. The undescended testis: management after puberty. J Urol 1975;114:77.

221. Martin DC. Malignancy in the cryptorchid testis. Urol Clin North Am 1982;9:371.

222. Batata, MA, Whitmore WJ, Chu FC, et al. Cryptorchidism and testicular cancer. J Urol 1980;124:382.

223. Whitaker RH. Management of the undescended testis. Br J Hosp Med 1970;4:25.

224. Martin DC. Malignancy and the undescended testis. In: Fonkalsrud EW, Mengel W, eds. The undescended testis. Chicago:Year Book Medical Publishers, 1981:144.

225. Pike MC, Chilvers C, Peckham MJ. Effect of age at orchidopexy on risk of testicular cancer. Lancet 1986;1:1246.

226. Altman BL, Malament M. Carcinoma of the testis following orchiopexy. J Urol 1967;97:498.

227. Witus WS, Sloss JH, Valk WL. Inguinal node metastases from testicular tumors developing after orchiopexy. J Urol 1959;81:669.

228. Lanteri VJ, Choudhury M, Pontes JE, et al. Treatment of testicular tumors arising in patients with previous inguinal and/or scrotal surgery. J Urol 1982;127:58.

229. Skakkebaek NE, Berthelsen JG, Muller J. Carcinoma-in-situ of the undescended testis. Urol Clin North Am 1982;9:377.

230. Skakkebaek NE. Carcinoma in situ of the testis: frequency and relationship to invasive germ cell tumours in infertile men. Histopathology 1978;2:157.

231. Williams TR, Brendler H. Carcinoma in situ of the ectopic testis. J Urol 1977;117:610.

232. Ford TF, Parkinson MC, Pryor JP. The undescended testis in adult life. Br J Urol 1985;57:181.

233. Muffly KE, McWhorter CA, Bartone FF, Gardner PJ. The absence of premalignant changes in the cryptorchid testis before adulthood. J Urol 1984;131:523.

234. Jones PG. Undescended testes. Aust Paediatr J. 1966;2:36.

235. Snyder WH Jr, Chaffin L. Inguinal hernia complicated by undescended testis. Am J Surg 1955;90:325.

236. Brereton RJ. Hernia and hydrocele in cryptorchidism. Lancet 1989;2:172.

237. Adamsen S, Borjesson B. Difficulty in detection of hernia and hydrocele in cryptorchidism. Lancet 1989;1:1259.

238. Schultz KE, Walker J. Testicular torsion in undescended testes. Ann Emerg Med 1984;13:567.

239. Riegler HC. Torsion of intra-abdominal testis: an unusual problem in diagnosis of the acute surgical abdomen. Surg Clin North Am 1972;52:371.

240. Mowad JJ, Konvolinka CW. Torsion of undescended testis. Urology 1978;12:567.

241. O'Riordan WD, Sherman NJ. Cryptorchidism and abdominal pain. J Am Coll Emerg Physi 1977;6:196.

242. Bell AI. Psychologic implications of scrotal sac and testes for the male child. Clin Pediatr 1974;13:838.

243. Woodard JR, Parrott TS. Reconstruction of the urinary tract in prune belly uropathy. J Urol 1978;119:824.

244. Farrer JH, Walker AH, Rajfer J. Management of the postpubertal cryptorchid testis: a statistical review. J Urol 1985;134:1071.

245. Rajfer J. Endocrinological study of testicular descent in the rabbit. J Surg Res 1982;33:158.

246. Pyorala S, Huttunen NP, Uhari M. A review and meta-analysis of hormonal treatment of cryptorchidism. J Clin Endocrinol Metab 1995;80:2795.

247. Rajfer J, Handelsman DJ, Swerdloff RS, et al. Hormonal therapy of cryptorchidism. A randomized, double-blind study comparing human chorionic gonadotropin and gonadotropin-releasing hormone. N Engl J Med 1986;314:466.

248. Colodny AH. Undescended testis-is surgery necessary? N Engl J Med 1986;314:510.

249. Urban MD, Lee PA, Lanes R, Migeon CJ. HCG stimulation in children with cryptorchidism. Clin Pediatr 1987;26:512.

250. Polascik TJ, Chan-Tack KM, Jeffs RD, Gearhart JP. Reappraisal of the role of human chorionic gonadotropin in the diagnosis and treatment of the nonpalpable testis: a 10-year experience. J Urol 1996;156:804.

251. Schapiro B. Ist der kryptorchismus chirurgisch oder hormonal zu behandeln? Deutsch Med Wochenschr 1931;57:718.

252. Bartsch G, Frick J. Therapeutic effects of luteinizing hormone releasing hormone (LH-RH) in cryptorchidism. Andrologia 1974;6:197.

253. Happ J, Kollman F, Krawehl C, et al. Intranasal GnRH therapy of maldescended testes. Horm Metab Res 1975;7:440.

254. Waldschmidt M Jr, Priefer A. Therapeutic results in cryptorchidism after combination therapy with LH-RH nasal spray and hCG. Eur J Pediatr 1987;146(Suppl 2):S31.

255. Lala R, Matarazzo P, Chiabotto P, et al. Combined therapy with LHRH and HCG in cryptorchid infants. Eur J Pediatr 1993;152(Suppl 2):S31.

256. Waldschmidt J, Doede T, Vygen I. The results of 9 years of experience with a combined treatment with LH-RH and HCG for cryptorchidism. Eur J Pediatr 1993;152(Suppl 2):S34.

257. Bica DT, Hadziselimovic F. Buserelin treatment of cryptorchidism: a randomized, double-blind, placebo-controlled study. J Urol 1992;148:617.

258. Hadziselimovic F, Huff D, Duckett J, et al. Treatment of cryptorchidism with low doses of buserelin over a 6-months period. Eur J Pediat 1987;146(Suppl 2):S56.

259. Hadziselimovic F, Herzog B. Treatment with a LH-RH analogue following successful orchiopexy markedly improves the chance of fertility later in life. Pediatrics 1996;98(Suppl):637.

260. Rosenmerkel JF. Veber die Radicalcur des in der Weiche liegenden Testikels bei nicht Descensus Desselben. Munich: J Lindauer, 1820.

261. Bevan AD. Operation for undescended testicle and congenital inguinal hernia. JAMA 1899;33:773.

262. Bevan AD. The surgical treatment of the undescended testicle. JAMA 1903;41:718.

263. LaRoque GP. A modification of Bevan's operation for undescended testicle. Ann Surg 1931;94:314.

264. Fowler R, Stephens FD. The role of testicular vascular anatomy in the salvage of high undescended testes. Aust N Z J Surg 1959;29:92.

265. Prentiss RJ, Weickgenant CJ, Moses JJ, Frazier DB. Undescended testis: surgical anatomy of spermatic vessels, spermatic surgical triangles, and lateral spermatic ligament. J Urol 1960;83:686.

266. Torek F. The technique of orchidopexy. NY Med J 1909;90:948.

267. Cabot H, Nesbit RM. Undescended testis: principles and methods of treatment. Arch Surg 1931;22:850.

268. Ombredanne L. Sur l'orchidopexie. Bull Soc Pediat Paris 1927;25:473.

269. Petrivalsky J. Zur Behandlung des Leistenhodens. Zentbl Chir 1931;58:1001.

270. Lattimer JK, Smith AM. Scrotal pouch techniques. Adjunct to orchiopexy. Urology 1975;5:137.

271. Koop CE. Technique of herniorraphy and orchidopexy. Birth Defects: Original Article Series 1977;13:293.

272. Skandalakis JE, Colborn GL, Pemberton LB, et al. The surgical anatomy of the inguinal area. II. Contemp Surg 1991;38:28.

273. Jarow JP. Clinical significance of intratesticular arterial anatomy. J Urol 1991;145:777.

274. Knorr PA, Borden TA. Splenogonadal fusion. Urology 1994;44:136.

275. Ferro F, Lais A, Boldrini R, et al. Hepatogonadal fusion. J Pediatr Surg 1996;31:435.

276. Docimo SG. The results of surgical therapy for cryptorchidism: a literature review and analysis. J Urol 1995;154:1148.

277. Castilho LN, Ferreira U, Netto NR, et al. Laparoscopic pediatric orchiectomy. J Endourol 1992;6:155.

278. Peters CA, Kavoussi LR. Pediatric endourology and laparoscopy. In: Walsh PC, Retik AB, Stamey TA, Vaughan ED, eds. Campbell's Urology. Philadelphia: Saunders, 1993:1.

279. Cortesi N, Ferrari P, Zambarda E, et al. Diagnosis of bilateral abdominal cryptorchidism by laparoscopy. Endoscopy 1976;8:33.
280. Bloom DA. Two-step orchiopexy with pelviscopic clip ligation of the spermatic vessels. J Urol 1991;145:1030.
281. Jordan GH, Winslow BH. Laparoscopic single stage and staged orchiopexy. J Urol 1994;152:1249.
282. Docimo SG, Jordan GH. Laparoscopic surgery in children. In: Marshall FF, ed. Textbook of operative urology. Philadelphia: Saunders, 1996:207.
283. Weiss RM, Seashore JH. Laparoscopy in the management of the nonpalpable testis. J Urol 1987;138:382.
284. Winfield HN, Donovan JF, See WA, et al. Urological laparoscopic surgery. J Urol 1991;146:941.
285. Guiney EJ, Corbally M, Malone PS. Laparoscopy and the management of the impalpable testis. Br J Urol 1989;63:313.
286. Jordan GH. Management of the abdominal nonpalpable undescended testicle. Altas Urologic Clin North Am 1993;1:49.
287. Naslund MJ, Gearhart JP, Jeffs RD. Laparoscopy: its selected use in patients with unilateral nonpalpable testis after human chorionic gonadotropin stimulation. J Urol 1989;142:108.
288. Boddy SA, Corkery JJ, Gornall P. The place of laparoscopy in the management of the impalpable testis. Br J Surg 1985;72:918.
289. Pan BS, Ooi LL, Mack PO. Laparoscopic assessment and orchidectomy for the undescended testis. Aust N. Z. J Surg 1994;64:118.
290. O'Donoghue J, Rogers E, Keeling P, Corcoran M. Laparoscopic removal of an intra-abdominal seminoma. Br J Urol 1993;71:109.
291. Beck RO, Nicholl P, Hickey NC, Black J. Laparoscopic excision of an intra-abdominal testis. Br J Urol 1992;70:105.
292. Stewart LH, Heasley RN, Loughridge WG. Laparoscopic removal of intra-abdominal testis. Br J Urol 1992;70:208.
293. Docimo SG, Moore RG, Adams J, Kavoussi LR. Laparoscopic orchiopexy for the high palpable undescended testis: preliminary experience. J Urol 1995;154:1513.
294. Moore RG, Kavoussi LR, Bloom DA, et al. Postoperative adhesion formation after urological laparoscopy in the pediatric population. J Urol 1995;153:792.
295. Rozanski TA, Wojno KJ, Bloom DA. The remnant orchiectomy. J Urol 1996;155:712.
296. Kogan SJ, Houman BZ, Reda EF, Levitt SB. Orchiopexy of the high undescended testis by division of the spermatic vessels: a critical review of 38 selected transections. J Urol 1989;141:1416.
297. Koff SA, Sethi PS. Treatment of high undescended testes by low spermatic vessel ligation: an alternative to the Fowler-Stephens technique. J Urol 1996;156:799.
298. Redman JF, Mooney, DK. Fowler-Stephens orchiopexy in a patient with prune belly syndrome and segmental atretic vas deferens. Urology 1993;41:130.
299. Stephens FD. Fowler-Stephens orchiopexy. Semin Urol 1988;6:103.
300. Ransley PC, Vordermark JS, Caldamone AA. Preliminary ligation of the gonadal vessels prior to orchiopexy for the intra-abdominal testicle: a staged Fowler-Stephens procedure. World J Urol 1984;2:266.
301. Elder JS. Two-stage Fowler-Stephens orchiopexy in the management of intra-abdominal testes. J Urol 1992;148:1239.
302. Elder JS. Laparoscopy and Fowler-Stephens orchiopexy in the management of the impalpable testis. Urol Clin North Am 1989;16:399.
303. Pascual JA, Villanueva MJ, Salido E, et al. Recovery of testicular blood flow following ligation of testicular vessels. J Urol 1989;142:549.
304. Ortolano V, Nasrallah PF. Spermatic vessel ligation (Fowler-Stephens maneuver): experimental results with regard to fertility. J Urol 1986;136:211.
305. Caldamone AA, Amaral JF. Laparoscopic stage 2 Fowler-Stephens orchiopexy. J Urol 1994;152:1253.
306. Bogaert GA, Kogan BA, Mevorach RA. Therapeutic laparoscopy for intra-abdominal testes. Urology 1993;42:182.
307. Joseph DB, Law S, Perez LM. Two-Stage Fowler-Stephens orchidopexy with laparoscopic clipping of the spermatic vessels. Pediatrics 1996;98:(Suppl 3):646.
308. King LR. Optimal treatment of children with undescended testes. J Urol 1984;131:734.
309. Levy DA, Abdul-Karim FW, Miraldi F, Elder JS. Effect of human chorionic gonadotropin before spermatic vessel ligation in the prepubertal rat testis. J Urol 1995;154:738.
310. Firor HV. Two-stage orchiopexy. Arch Surg 1971;102:598.
311. Corkery JJ. Staged orchiopexy-a new technique. J Pediatr Surg 1975;10:515.
312. Steinhardt GF, Kroovand RL, Perlmutter AD. Orchiopexy: planned 2-stage technique. J Urol 1985;133:434.
313. Kiesewetter WB, Mammen K, Kalyglou M. The rationale and results in two-stage orchidopexies. J Pediatr Surg 1981;16:631.
314. Persky L, Albert DJ. Staged orchiopexy. Surg Gynecol Obstet 1971;132:43.
315. Redman JF. The staged orchiopexy: a critical review of the literature. J Urol 1977;117:113.
316. Jones PF, Bagley FH. An abdominal extraperitoneal approach for the difficult orchidopexy. Br J Surg 1979;66:14.
317. Hodges CV, Behman AM, Attaran S. Transplantation of the internal spermatic artery: an experimental study. J Urol 1964;91:90.
318. Silber SJ, Kelly J. Successful autotransplantation of an intraabdominal testis to the scrotum by microvascular technique. J Urol 1976;115:452.
319. Wacksman J, Dinner M, Staffon RA. Technique of testicular autotransplantation using a microvascular anastomosis. Surg Gynecol Obstet 1980;150:399.
320. Martin DC, Salibian AH. Orchiopexy using microvascular surgical technique. J Urol 1980;123:435.
321. Harrison CB, Kaplan GW, Scherz HC, et al. Microvascular autotransplantation of the intra-abdominal testis. J Urol 1990;144:506.
322. Frey P, Bianchi A. Microvascular orchiopexy. Eur J Pediatr 1987;146(Suppl 2):S51.
323. Bukowski TP, Wacksman J, Billmire DA, Sheldon CA. Testicular autotransplantation for the intra-abdominal testis. Microsurgery 1995;16:290.
324. Bianchi A. Microvascular orchiopexy for high undescended testes. Br J Urol 1984;56:521.
325. Romas NA, Janecka I, Krisiloff M. Role of microsurgery in orchiopexy. Urology 1978;12:670.
326. Hinman F Jr. Alternatives to orchiopexy. J Urol 1980;123:548.
327. Smith AM, Lattimer JK. Psychosexual impact of undescended testes and implantation of prostheses. Med Aspects Human Sexuality 1975;9:62.
328. Elder JS, Keating MA, Duckett JW. Infant testicular prostheses. J Urol 1989;141:1413.
329. Girsdansky J, Newman HF. Use of a vitallium testicular implant. Am J Surg 1941;53:514.
330. Lakshmanan Y, Docimo SG. Testicular implants. J Long Term Effects Med Implants 1997;7:65.
331. Lattimer JK, Vakili BF, Smith AM, Morishima A. A natural-feeling testicular prosthesis. J Urol 1973;110:81.
332. Pidutti R, Morales A. Silicone gel-filled testicular prosthesis and systemic disease. Urology 1993;42:155.
333. Maizels M, Gomez F, Firlit CF. Surgical correction of the failed orchiopexy. J Urol 1983;130:955.
334. Livne PM, Savir A, Servadio C. Re-orchiopexy: advantages and disadvantages. Eur Urol 1990;18:137.
335. Cartwright PC, Velagapudi S, Snyder HM III, Keating MA. A surgical approach to reoperative orchiopexy. J Urol 1993;149:817.
336. Woodard JR, Trulock TS. Complications of orchiopexy. Urol Clin North Am 1983;10:537.
337. Beechey NN, Harriss D. Iatrogenic torsion of an undescended testis. Br J Urol 1990;66:552.
338. Hurren JS, Corder AP. Acute testicular torsion following orchidopexy for undescended testis. Br J Surg 1992;79:1292.
339. Colodny AH. Bladder injury during herniorrhaphy. Urology 1974;3:89.
340. Nguyen DH, Mitchell ME. Ureteral obstruction due to compression by the vas deferens following Fowler-Stephens orchiopexy. J Urol 1993;149:94.
341. Zeidan B, Brereton RJ. Unusual complication of the Fowler-Stephens orchidopexy. J Pediatr Surg 1988;23:381.

CHAPTER 30

Adolescent Varicocele

Evan J. Kass

A varicocele represents an abnormal dilation of the internal spermatic veins and the pampiniform plexus. This venous malformation has been recognized since the first century, when it was described by Celsus and termed a cirsocele. Curling in 1856 was one of the first to suggest a causal relationship between a varicocele and male infertility.[1] Barwell in 1885 devised a wire loop to entrap the dilated scrotal veins in an effort to cure the varicocele in 28 men,[2] but not until 1952 when Tulloch reported the return of spermatogenesis in an azospermic patient did widespread interest in the relationship between infertility and varicocele gain momentum.[3] Since that time, ligation of a varicocele has become the most common surgical procedure in males with infertility. Despite this experience in adults, the management of an adolescent with a varicocele is still controversial because of the extreme variability in both the severity of the varicocele-induced testicular injury and its time of onset. It is hoped that with an improved understanding of this unique problem, a protocol can be developed to identify those boys at risk for possible fertility problems and to allow physicians to intervene as early as possible.

ETIOLOGY

Several different etiologies have been offered to explain varicocele formation, the most common being incompetent or absent valves in the left internal spermatic vein, which allows retrograde blood flow into the pampiniform plexus.[4] The anatomic differences between the left and right internal spermatic veins are also thought to play an important role in varicocele formation. The right internal spermatic vein is approximately 10 cm shorter than the left and enters the inferior vena cava at an oblique angle in contrast with the longer, normally right-angled insertion of the left internal spermatic vein into the left renal vein. This anatomic difference may allow for the preferential transmission of higher hydrostatic venous pressures to the left pampiniform plexus and may explain the increased incidence of left sided varicocele formation.

Other investigators have suggested that a "nutcracker" effect in which the left renal vein is compressed as it passes between the aorta and the superior mesenteric artery contributes to varicocele formation. However, in a review of 659 varicoceles by Braedel et al.,[5] the nutcracker phenomenon was only demonstrated in three patients. They hypothesized that the embryogenic transformation of the primary venous system into the secondary system, with subsequent collateral venous development, resulted in varicocele formation. The subcardinal veins, the posterior cardinal veins, and the supracardinal veins eventually involute as the inferior vena cava is formed. Occasionally, as a result of disordered involution, there are persistent intercardinal anastomoses that could lead to development of an idiopathic left varicocele.

DIAGNOSIS

In the adolescent male, a varicocele is usually asymptomatic and therefore its detection is based on the routine physical examination of a healthy individual in the upright position. Varicoceles are rarely identified in boys younger than 10 years of age, and the incidence of varicocele detection gradually increases between 10 and 15 years of age,[6,7] ultimately involving 10 to 15% of males. Bilaterally palpable varicoceles are diagnosed in fewer than 2% of all males. Once present, the varicocele typically persists for the remainder of the individual's life; therefore, a varicocele detected in an adult male with infertility has been present since early adolescence. Because of this observation, it is important to examine all boys over the age of 10 years in both the standing and supine position to facilitate the early detection of a varicocele.[6]

A varicocele is classically graded by size during physical exam with the patient in the standing position. A grade I varicocele is small and can be palpated only with difficulty during a Valsava maneuver. A grade II varicocele is moderate in size, with the mass of veins being generally 1 to 2 cm in diameter and easily detected on physical exam. A grade III varicocele is large and easily visible through the scrotal skin and has a diameter of greater than 2 centimeters. Most adolescents with a varicocele have a grade I varicocele (9.4% of all adolescent males), 3.6% have a grade II varicocele, and 1.7% have a grade III varicocele.[6]

Since the majority of adolescents with a varicocele are asymptomatic and the varicocele is discovered during the routine physical examination performed by a primary care physician who is not specifically looking for or suspecting a varicocele, it is not surprising that in this circumstance a large varicocele is more likely to be identified than a small one. It is our observation that it is unusual for a teenager with a grade I varicocele to be referred for evaluation; yet the data from population surveys indicate that a grade I varicocele is in fact more common than a grade III varicocele.

Because no teenager generally presents for an evaluation of male infertility, it is important to consider whether the size of the varicocele is of any clinical relevance. Dubin and Amelar[8] suggested that the size of the varicocele is not critical, when they reported similar results with varicocele repair in men with grade I, II, or III varicocele. To confuse matters even further some investigators[9] have postulated that a nonpalpable subclinical varicocele detected through Doppler ultrasonography may have the same damaging effect as a higher-grade varicocele. Fariss and coworkers, in contrast, reported that men with a large varicocele had significantly lower sperm counts than did men with a small varicocele.[10]

At the present time, despite numerous publications concerning the adult male with a subclinical varicocele over the past 15 years, controversy still exists as to the need to diagnose and treat this adult population.[11, 12] Therefore, at the present time Doppler ultrasonography for the detection of a subclinical varicocele is not recommended for routine use in adolescents, and only a varicocele detected by physical examination should be considered potentially significant.

TESTICULAR HISTOLOGY

Testicular abnormalities can be demonstrated in both testes of an infertile adult male with a unilateral left varicocele.[13–15] The abnormalities described include incomplete maturation arrest at the spermatid and spermatocyte levels, decreased spermatogenesis, and tubular thickening with decreased tubular diameter. Typically, the pathologic lesions are more pronounced in the left testis, but the right is nearly always involved as well. Mcfadden and Mehan[16] suggested that the Leydig cell histology is more important than the tubular histology. They noted that when Leydig cell hyperplasia is present in infertile men with a varicocele, the pregnancy rate

after varicocele surgery is only 5%, but when Leydig cell atrophy is present, the pregnancy rate is 40%.

Hadziselimovic[17] also noted the importance of Leydig cell abnormalities in infertile adult men with a varicocele. He reported that Leydig cell hyperplasia indicated a very poor prognosis following varicocele correction whereas Leydig cell atrophy portended a better outcome irrespective of tubular pathology. These studies concluded that it is the grade of the pathologic changes in the Leydig-sertoli cell interrelationship and not the degree of the tubular pathology that ultimately decides whether varicocele surgery will be successful in restoring fertility.

Cameron et al.[18] evaluated testicular biopsies from men with a varicocele and described ultrastructural changes in the sertoli-cell cytoplasm. They believed that the sertoli cell was the primary site of injury and that the degree to which the cell was affected determined the extent to which the spermatogenic process was disrupted. Information about the potential reversibility of the histologic lesions in the testis after varicocele ligation is limited. Interestingly, Johnsonn and Agger[13] performed testis biopsies before and 1 year after varicocele ligation and noted that, although the operation for varicocele correction significantly improved the histologic appearance, few testes returned to a completely normal state.

The pathologic changes in the adolescent testis appear to be similar to those found in adults, but are generally less severe. Heinz and colleagues[19] performed testicular biopsies in 10 boys undergoing varicocele ligation and demonstrated histologic changes in the tubular epithelium, interstitium, and blood vessels. Kass and coworkers[20] demonstrated similar pathologic changes in the left testis in nine of 24 adolescents with grade II to III varicocele. The biopsy tissue from the contralateral testis demonstrated normal or near-normal histology in the majority of cases. Hadziselimovic[21] reported that there were proliferative endothelial lesions of the capillaries at the ultrastructural level, which preceded other histologic changes in the testes of boys with a varicocele. His group also noted that there is a progressive worsening of Leydig-cell damage between adolescence and adulthood, indicating that the degree of testicular injury may be related to the age of the patient. These studies suggest that abnormalities in the testicular histologic appearance may occur in association with a varicocele early in the natural history of the disease; however, the pathologic changes are generally less severe in adolescents than in adults and initially involve the testis that is ipsilateral to the varicocele.

The most widely publicized theory of testicular damage being caused by a varicocele is that it results from hyperthermia created in the testis. Normally, the temperature of arterial blood is cooled from the intraabdominal temperature of 37°C to the intratesticular temperature of 33 to 34°C.[22] Phillips and McKenzie were one of the first to demonstrate that increased scrotal temperatures associated with a varicocele had a significant adverse effect on testicular function and spermatogenesis.[23] Salisz and coworkers[24] reported that adolescents with a varicocele have a significant elevation of scrotal temperatures bilaterally when compared with controls and also noted that the temperature increase of the left testicle was greater than the right. They also noted that the higher the temperature of the left testis the greater the potential for volume loss on that side. Following successful varicocele surgery, scrotal temperatures decreased and were identical to controls.

In the experimental animal model, a surgically created unilateral varicocele induced testicular damage similar to that observed in humans in both the testis ipsilateral to the varicocele and the contralateral testis. Kay and coworkers[25] created a left-sided varicocele in rhesus monkeys and subsequently noted a bilateral increase in testicular temperature and a disorganization of the germinal epithelium in both testes. Subsequent surgical repair of the varicocele resulted in the return of testicular blood flow and temperature to normal levels. Other investigators[26, 27] reported similar histologic changes in their experimental model, with abnormalities first noted in the left testis, but ultimately affecting both testes. Leydig-cell hyperplasia was frequently demonstrated in the left testis, but was observed less commonly in the right. Fussell and colleagues[28] also demonstrated similar early ultrastructural changes in sertoli cells and spermatogonia in a varicocele model in a monkey.

These various experimental models correlate quite well with the histologic abnormalities in testis biopsies of humans with a varicocele. The varicocele-induced testicular injury initially appears to be mild and confined to the left testis. With time, the pathologic changes in the left testis progress and similar but milder lesions are eventually present in the supposedly uninvolved right testis. The literature clearly demonstrates that the earlier the varicocele is corrected, the better the prognosis; however, once Leydig-cell hyperplasia is present, the testicular damage may not be reversible.

TESTICULAR VOLUME

It is critical to measure the volume of both testes of an adolescent with a varicocele as it is a generally accepted concept that testicular volumes correlate well with semen quality and fertility, since 98% of the testicular mass is comprised of seminiferous tubules and germinal cells. Currently, the simplest way to facilitate the early detection of testicular growth failure is to measure testicular volume with a standard orchidometer. An alternative method for measuring testicular volume was developed by Nasu and colleagues and consists of a series of ellipsoid rings 1 to 30 mL in size that can be fitted over the testis.[29] Accurate testicular volume measurements are possible with either technique; however, some

experience is necessary before reproducible results can be achieved. Recently, it was suggested that ultrasonography may be a more accurate method for determining absolute testicular volume.[30] Other investigators have pointed out that the degree of correlation between ultrasonically determined testicular volumes and those measured with an orchidomiter depends primarily on the experience of the examiner, and the added expense of ultrasound volumetrics is not justified by any theoretic advantage in accuracy.[31]

Typically, there should be no more than a 2-mL difference in volume between the two testicles. In normal men, the average testicular volume is 24 ± 3 mL; however, because testicular volume varies with the stage of sexual maturity in adolescents, most investigators have used the right testis as the normal control in comparison of the volume of both testes.[32] Steeno et al. observed the loss of testicular volume and/or a change in the consistency of the testis ipsilateral to the varicocele in approximately one-third of boys with a grade II varicocele and in 80% of those with a grade III varicocele.[6] No such changes were noted in the left testis of individuals with a grade I varicocele.

Lipshultz and Corriere carefully measured testicular size in men with a varicocele and compared these measurements with an age-matched control group without a varicocele.[33] The left testis was significantly smaller in individuals with a varicocele, and often both testes were significantly smaller than those of the age-matched cohort. Lyons et al. reported volume loss in the left testis in 77% of 30 adolescent boys with a clearly palpable left varicocele.[34] These investigators suggested that the most damaging effect of a varicocele may occur in the rapidly growing testis of adolescence. Kass and Belman performed varicocele ligation on 20 adolescent males with a grade II to III left-sided varicocele and a loss of volume in the left testis.[35] The mean age was 13.8 years, and all had asymptomatic varicoceles discovered during routine physical examination. In no instance was infertility or testicular pain an indication for treatment. A significant increase in the volume of the left testis was noted in 16 of the 20 patients, with left testicular volume equaling the right side postoperatively in most cases. These results indicate that a moderate to large varicocele may be responsible for the retardation of testicular growth in adolescents and that early ligation of the varicocele may reverse this process. A small varicocele does not seem to have a significant effect on testicular growth. This observation may indicate that an individual with a large varicocele is at a greater risk for infertility than is an individual with a small varicocele, but longer-term studies are needed to confirm this data.

SEMEN ANALYSIS

Ethical considerations by both patients and physicians make it occasionally difficult to obtain a semen sample from adolescents, and even if it were always possible, the normal parameters have not yet been well defined prior to sexual maturity. It is important to know at what age semen parameters reach normal adult values and if a single normal semen analysis in an individual with a varicocele ensures normal potential for fertility in the future. Janczewski and Bablok evaluated semen specimens from 134 normal pubertal boys between 12 and 19 years of age.[36] Early in puberty, spermatozoa are absent from the ejaculate; however, semen quality gradually improves and achieves adult normal values 29 to 33 months after the onset of puberty.

There is a "classic stress pattern" attributed to varicoceles by the work of Macleod in which he noted subnormal motility, an increase in immature forms, and a shift in morphology from oval to tapered and amorphous sperm forms.[37] This pathognomonic semen pattern has been challenged for lacking specificity to varicoceles per se,[38] but there is indisputable evidence that sperm counts and motility are reduced and sperm morphology is affected in some form in patients with a varicocele. Baker and coworkers observed abnormal semen parameters in 92% of 651 varicocele patients being evaluated for infertility.[39]

It is important to note that the semen analysis in an individual with a varicocele may deteriorate over time. Cheval and Purcell evaluated 13 men aged 25 to 35 years with normal semen parameters and a palpable varicocele who were never treated.[40] Reevaluation at an average interval of 44.3 months later demonstrated a significant deterioration in sperm density (from mean baseline density of 90.4×10^6/mL to 14.9×10^6/mL at follow-up) and motility (mean baseline 63.1 to 36.1% at follow-up). The authors concluded that normal semen parameters in an individual with a varicocele should not be routinely expected to stay normal and that close follow-up is indicated even if the testis and semen analysis are normal initially. Gorelick and Goldstein also noted the potentially progressive nature of varicocele-induced testicular injury.[41] They reviewed 1099 consecutive patients with male-factor infertility and discovered a palpable varicocele in 35% of the men with primary infertility and 81% of the men with secondary infertility ($P < .001$). The age differences of the men and their partners between the two groups were too small to explain the decline in fertility. The period since the last known paternity in the men with secondary infertility averaged 8.8 years, leading the authors to conclude that a progressive detrimental effect of the varicocele was responsible for the observed loss of fertility in these patients. Witt and Lipshultz also noted that a varicocele occurred much more frequently in men with secondary infertility and also concluded that the detrimental effect of a varicocele in some men is an on-going, progressive process.[42]

GONADOTROPIN-RELEASING HORMONE STIMULATION

Ospina was the first to demonstrate a supranormal gonadotropin response to the intravenous administration of gonadotropin-releasing hormone (Gn-RH) in infertile men with a varicocele.[43] He postulated that the excessive release of gonadotropic hormones (primarily FSH) after Gn-RH stimulation is a result of an abnormality of the seminiferous tubules. Hudson and co-workers also demonstrated this excessive gonadotropin response to Gn-RH stimulation in infertile men with a varicocele.[44, 45] After varicocele ligation, those individuals whose sperm density improved also had normalization of their gonadotropin response. Men whose sperm density did not improve had identical hormonal responses before and after varicocele ligation. These studies suggest that in infertile men with a varicocele there is a significant abnormality in both testicular hormone synthesis and spermatogenesis which is potentially reversible by varicocele ligation.

Nagao and colleagues[46] measured the gonadotropin response to Gn-RH stimulation in three groups of men: first, those with normal fertility and no demonstrable varicocele; second, those men with normal fertility and a palpable varicocele; and third, those with documented infertility and a palpable varicocele. In comparison with normally fertile men, the infertile men with a varicocele demonstrated an exaggerated gonadotropin response to Gn-RH stimulation; however, some normally fertile men with a varicocele also had a supranormal response to Gn-RH stimulation. These studies indicate that hormonal abnormalities can be observed in both fertile and infertile men with a varicocele, suggesting that there is some degree of testicular dysfunction in many men with a varicocele, regardless of their fertility status. This varicocele-induced testicular injury may become clinically significant with increasing age.

Dickerman determined that measuring gonadotropin response to Gn-RH stimulation was useful for evaluation of testicular function in prepubertal boys.[47] Lipshultz reported that the FSH response to Gn-RH stimulation was twice as high as normal in men who had undergone orchiopexy in childhood and concluded that this FSH response indicated damage to the seminiferous tubules.[48] Okuyama et al. reported that there was a similarly exaggerated FSH response to Gn-RH stimulation in a small number of adolescent boys with a varicocele.[49]

Kass and colleagues measured the response to Gn-RH stimulation in 104 adolescent males 11 to 17 years of age with a palpable unilateral left-sided varicocele and compared it with that of a control group of aged-matched adolescents without evidence of testicular abnormalities.[50] Abnormal response was observed in approximately 30% of patients with a varicocele. They concluded that the Gn-RH stimulation test is helpful in identifying individuals with evidence of testicular dysfunction, and there is good reason to believe from similar studies in adults that the observed testicular dysfunction is directly related to the presence of a varicocele. Fujisawa and coworkers performed the Gn-RH stimulation test preoperatively and postoperatively on 30 infertile patients with a varicocele.[51] High ligation of the spermatic vein was performed in all patients and, in a group that became pregnant, the preoperative excessive response of luteinizing hormone to the Gn-RH test decreased significantly after surgery. This reduction in the luteinizing hormone response may be a valuable predictive parameter for responders after varicocele correction.

Su et al.[52] recently evaluated serum testosterone levels in 53 patients with varicoceles and found that varicocele ligation can result in a statistically significant increase in serum testosterone in infertile men with varicoceles, especially those with abnormally low values. Although this increase in testosterone does not directly improve semen quality, it further demonstrates the hormonal relationship involved with varicoceles.

TREATMENT

Before deciding on a procedure to correct a varicocele in an adolescent, consideration of the relative advantages and disadvantages of the various treatment modalities is critical. With regards to transvenous occlusion of the internal spermatic vein, there are variable methods of treatment. The percutaneous techniques include the use of stainless steel occluding spring coils, balloon occlusion and transcatheter antegrade or retrograde sclerotherapy of the internal spermatic vein with various sclerosing agents.[53, 54] Some of the advantages are lower cost, shorter recovery period and the requirement of only a local anesthetic. One disadvantage, even in centers with experienced interventional radiologists, is that this procedure may require 1 to 3 hours to complete. More importantly, transvenous occlusion cannot be accomplished in approximately 15% of individuals,[55] and the reported persistence rate of the varicocele with various radiographic techniques is at least as significant as that of surgical correction.[56] In addition, most medical centers do not have a radiologist with sufficient skill and experience with this procedure to justify its routine use. It may, however, have a role in patients who have previously undergone unsuccessful varicocele ligation. In this setting, the primary surgery may pose a potential serious risk to the collateral arterial blood flow, ultimately resulting in testicular atrophy. Under these circumstances, if an experienced radiologist is not available, referral to a specialized center is preferred.

Transperitoneal or retroperitoneal laparoscopic varicocele ligation is another alternative to open surgical correction. It was first introduced in 1990 by Donovan and Winfield in the correction of varicoceles in adults,[57] and the widespread use of this procedure in adolescents is still limited. Potential advantages of this procedure are the presumed shorter postoperative convalescence and the elimination of an abdominal incision. The disadvantages are numerous and include the requirement of a general anesthetic with endotracheal intubation; the potential complications of intraabdominal surgery such as bleeding, peritonitis, or bowel obstruction; and the increased cost of equipment.[58]

For most adolescents who undergo prophylactic varicocele correction, open surgical repair is the preferred treatment modality. Overall, there have been few significant surgical complications of varicocele ligation, except for postoperative persistence of the varicocele. Therefore, the preferred surgical technique should be that with the highest success rate. Coolsaet demonstrated that in adolescents with a large varicocele, there may be significant collateral flow through the external spermatic, ductus deferens, anterior and posterior scrotal, and saphenous veins.[59] He postulated if a suprainguinal ligation of the internal spermatic vein is performed, these collaterals would be missed, resulting in an operative failure. Despite these theoretical advantages, we had a failure rate of 16% with the Ivanissevich approach,[60] although optical magnification and other intraoperative techniques were utilized that had been purported to maximize success.[61] Because of this experience with the inguinal approach, we switched to the retroperitoneal approach, with preservation of the artery, on the premise there would be fewer venous collaterals at this higher level. Unfortunately, the varicocele persistence rate utilizing this method was 11%, which was not statistically different from the failure rate with the inguinal approach.

An attempt was then made to perform intraoperative, postligation spermatic venography in 30 patients undergoing artery-sparing varicocele ligation in an effort to reduce the rate of operative failure.[62] Unfortunately, this procedure did not significantly improve the surgical results. In addition, the procedure was frequently time consuming, frustrating to perform, subjected the patient to significant radiation exposure, and in many cases could not be completed because of technical reasons.

Significant frustration with this failure rate, despite the use of intraoperative venography, optical magnification, and Doppler probes, provided the incentive to use the technique originally described by Palomo.[63] Our results with this procedure have been substantially better than those with the artery-sparing surgical techniques. Additionally, the Palomo procedure is much simpler to perform, because it is no longer necessary to identify every venous collateral in an attempt to preserve the internal spermatic artery. So far, we have performed the Palomo procedure on more than 120 patients

TABLE 30.1. *Adolescent varicocele*

Group	No. pts.	Relative testicular volume % Preop.	Relative testicular volume % Postop.	Mean mos. follow-up
Artery sparing	36	73[a]	91	32
Palomo	36	72	92	18
Comparison	8	79	82	24

[a]Mean relative volume of Ivanissevich and modified Palomo groups.

and have noted a persistent varicocele in only two patients. Testicular atrophy has not been observed, and "rebound" growth of the left testis has been comparable with that after the artery-sparing procedures.[64] Indeed, we have noted that "catch-up" growth of the testis only occurs following successful surgery, and it does not matter whether the artery is preserved (Table 30.1).

Initially, there was concern that interruption of the internal spermatic artery could result in vascular compromise to the testis; however, to our knowledge, there has been no report of testicular atrophy after a Palomo procedure in any patient who has not had previous inguinal surgery. Hosli and Okuyama have reported excellent results with the Palomo technique in adolescents, without any testicular atrophy.[65, 66] Yamamoto and colleagues[67] conducted a randomized, prospective study in 66 infertile men with unilateral varicoceles comparing an artery-ligating with an artery-preserving-retroperitoneal (Palomo) procedure. They found a statistically significant improvement of sperm density and motility in the artery-ligated group, while the artery-preserved group showed only statistical improvement in sperm density. Postoperative loss of testicular volume was not observed in either group, and they concluded that artery-preserving surgery is neither advantageous nor warranted. Also of particular importance was the observation that preexisting testicular volume loss ipsilateral to the varicocele was reversed only after successful surgery; testicular growth failure was not reversed in any patient with a persistent varicocele.[64] Therefore, a failed operation to correct a varicocele appears to be more detrimental to the testis than is internal spermatic arterial disruption.

These data demonstrate that retroperitoneal ligation of the entire spermatic cord significantly decreases the risk of operative failure. It is hypothesized that there are collateral branches of the internal spermatic vein intimately associated with the internal spermatic artery that are not functionally significant unless the primary internal spermatic channels are ligated. These small venous channels are extremely difficult to identify and ligate and may not even be demonstrable on venography; however, after surgery the increased venous pressure associated with many of the large adolescent varicoceles facilitates blood flow through these collateral channels, thereby producing operative failure.[68] Inter-

estingly, Hirokowa et al.[69] surgically excised internal spermatic segments during Palomo varicocele repair and then had the specimens examined pathologically. In all specimens, intimately associated with the gonadal artery were the presence of two to five small internal spermatic venous channels. Additional significant collateral venous branches that are separate from the main retroperitoneal internal spermatic vessels must be rare, or the failure rate with the Palomo technique would be much higher. Certainly, these venous channels outside the main internal spermatic bundle may be seen radiographically, but they do not seem to be a significant cause of operative failure. Indeed, in our experience, venography in patients who have had a persistent varicocele after an artery-sparing procedure has uniformly shown a patent venous channel within the main internal spermatic vessel complex, which would have been ligated with the Palomo technique. We have not had a persistent varicocele result from a branch of the external spermatic, ductus deferens, or scrotal veins.

Postoperative hydrocele is a potential problem with any of the techniques used for varicocele ligation, but the risk may be greatest with the Palomo procedure because no attempt is made to preserve the lymphatics. We anticipate that with time, more patients will be identified with hydroceles; however, these hydroceles are usually asymptomatic and pose a less significant problem than does a persistent varicocele.

CURRENT APPROACH

The current data suggest that any individual with a palpable varicocele, even when there is previous fertility, is at risk of subsequent loss of testicular function and infertility. Because most varicoceles in adolescents are detected during routine physical examination and these patients' fertility status is untested, the accurate identification of all individuals at risk for future problems is probably beyond our capability at the present time. Certainly, many of these adolescents need to be treated, because there is convincing evidence a varicocele may have a progressively toxic effect on the testes that ultimately results in irreversible infertility if left untreated. Because of the fact that a varicocele can be detected in approximately 15% of adolescents and not everyone with a varicocele will be infertile if left untreated, routine varicocele ligation in all teenagers is not recommended. Virtually all investigators recommend selective surgical intervention for individuals with evidence of a varicocele-induced testicular injury who may be at increased risk for infertility.[70] For individuals without such abnormalities treatment is not currently recommended, because there is no evidence that prophylactic varicocele ligation in this setting is helpful.

At the current time, varicocele ligation is recommended for older teenagers or adults with a varicocele and abnormal semen parameters, because in this setting there is good evidence the varicocele is responsible for the impairment in testicular function and its associated infertility.

When it is not possible to obtain a semen sample in an adolescent with a varicocele, loss of testicular volume ipsilateral to the varicocele is considered to be the primary indication for surgical treatment. Okuyama and coworkers surgically corrected grade II and III varicoceles in 24 of 40 boys aged 11 to 17 years and followed all patients for a period of 15 to 64 months.[66] Testicular growth impairment was present in 16 of the 24 prior to surgery and in only 8 postoperatively. No new testicular atrophy developed in the treated group. Testicular growth impairment was present in 8 of the 16 unoperated patients at the initial visit; the growth impairment did not resolve spontaneously in any patient during follow-up, but 4 patients did develop new evidence of testicular atrophy. Most importantly, the surgically corrected group demonstrated significantly better semen quality in terms of sperm density, sperm motility, and percentage of morphologically normal spermatozoa.

Laven and associates randomly assigned 67 adolescent males between 17 and 20 years of age and with a palpable varicocele into treated and untreated groups.[71] A similar group of healthy volunteers served as controls. No statistically significant differences in the semen parameters were noted in the baseline samples, but one year later, the sperm concentration was significantly higher in the treated group compared to the untreated group. The initial mean testicular volume was significantly smaller in the varicocele group than the controls. The right testis was also smaller than normal in the varicocele patients, but statistical significance was not achieved. After one year of follow-up, the left testis of the treated and control groups were significantly larger than in the untreated group. The right testis volumes were also smaller than normal in the untreated group, but this again, was not statistically significant.

In the first study of its kind, Madgar and colleagues[72] concluded that varicoceles are associated with reduced fertility and seminal parameters and that varicocele correction significantly improves both abnormalities. They conducted a randomized, controlled, prospective study on 45 infertile couples whose male partner had a diagnosed varicocele and whose female partner had been evaluated and to be free of any obvious infertility factor. The first group of 20 men did not receive any treatment for 12 months after recruitment, while the second group of 25 men underwent high ligation of the spermatic vein. Within the first 12 months after surgery, group two had 15 pregnancies and the semen analysis statistically improved in sperm count, motility and morphology. Over the next two years there were 4 additional pregnancies for an overall pregnancy rate of 76%. In the first group at the end of 12 months, conception occurred in only two couples and the semen parameters had not changed; the rest of the men in group one then underwent high ligation of the spermatic vein. During the first year following surgery, eight pregnancies occurred and the semen analysis showed statistically significant improvement in the group. Four more pregnancies occurred in this group over the next two years for a pregnancy rate of 66.7%.

The Gn-RH stimulation test is an additional aid in the identification of individuals with early evidence of testicular injury. The initial hypothesis was that adolescents with a decrease in size of the left testis would be more likely to have an abnormal response; however, although there was a tendency for individuals with testicular volume loss to demonstrate an abnormal result and Gn-RH stimulation, there was no statistically significant relationship.[50] At the present time, the Gn-RH stimulation test may be helpful in evaluating adolescents who are too young or unable to provide a semen sample and who do not fulfill other criteria for varicocele correction surgery. An abnormal response to Gn-RH stimulation may identify a group that with increasing age may be at a higher risk for fertility problems. These individuals are probably best served by early varicocele ligation.

Additionally, it is reasonable to recommend surgical repair for the few individuals with a palpable bilateral varicocele or a large varicocele that is symptomatic. When none of the aforementioned criteria are present, surgery is not recommended, but the patients should be followed with annual visits until they have completed their families, because the detrimental effect of a varicocele on testicular function is a potentially progressive disorder with marked variation in time of onset and degree of injury. At the time of the annual re-evaluation, the volume of the testes is measured, and if possible, a semen analysis is obtained. When there is evidence of volume loss in either testis of deteriorating semen parameters, surgery is then recommended. Patients who are noncompliant or incapable of adhering to the follow-up protocol should be offered surgery, because without close follow-up, irreversible infertility may result.

CONCLUSION

Current recommendations for varicocele repair in adolescents are (a) the volume of the left testis is at least

3 mL less than the right, *(b)* the results of semen analysis are abnormal, *(c)* a large symptomatic varicocele is present, *(d)* bilaterally palpable varicoceles are present, or *(e)* the response of either luteinizing hormone or FSH to the Gn-RH stimulation test is supranormal. When surgery is necessary, the Palomo technique significantly decreases the risk of operative failure and has facilitated "rebound" growth of the left testis that is comparable to that after artery-sparing procedures.

It is important to note that there is potential for impaired fertility whenever a palpable varicocele is present. Unfortunately, no test or series of tests can predict with absolute certainty whether an adolescent with a varicocele will be fertile or infertile. Therefore, it is important to observe untreated patients yearly until they complete their families. Patients who are unwilling or unable to adhere to that protocol should be considered candidates for surgical correction.

REFERENCES

1. Curling JP. A practical treatise on the disease of the testis and spermatic cord and scrotum. Philadelphia: Blanchard & Lee, 1856.
2. Barwell R. One hundred cases of varicocele treated by the subcutaneous wire loop. Lancet 1985;1:978.
3. Tulloch WS. A consideration of sterility factors in the light of subsequent pregnancies. Trans Edinburgh Obstet Soc 1952;55:29.
4. Sigmund G, Gall H, Bahren W. Stop-type and short-type varicocele: venographic findings. Radiology 1987;163:105.
5. Braedel HU, Steffens J, Ziegler M. A possible ontogenic etiology for idiopathic left varicocele. J Urol 1994;151:62.
6. Steeno O, Knops J, Declerck L, et al. Prevention of fertility disorders by detection and treatment of varicocele at school and college age. Andrologia 1976;8(1):47.
7. Johnson DE, Pohl DR, Rivera-Corren H. Varicocele an innocuous condition? South Med J 1970;63:34.
8. Dubin L, Amelar RD. Varicocele size and results of varicocelectomy in selected subfertile men with varicocele. Fertil Steril 1970;21:606.
9. Greenberg SH, Lipshultz LI, Morganroth J. The use of the Doppler stethoscope in the evaluation of varicoceles. J Urol 1977;117:296.
10. Fariss BL, Fenner DK, Plymate SR, et al. Seminal characteristics in the presence of a varicocele as compared with those of expectant fathers and prevasectomy men. Fertil Steril 1981;35:325.
11. Marsman JWP, Schats R. The subclinical varicocele debate. Hum Reprod 1994;9:1.
12. Hirsh AV, Cameron KM, Tyler JP, et al. The doppler assessment of varicoceles and internal spermatic vein reflux in infertile men. Br J Urol 1980;52:50.
13. Agger P, Johnsen SG. Quantitative evaluation of testicular biopsies in varicocele. Fertil Steril 1978;29:52.
14. Charney CW. Effect of varicocele on fertility-Results of varicocelectomy. Fertil Steril 1962;13:47.
15. Ibrahim AA, Awad HA, El-Haggar S, Mitawi BA. Bilateral testicular biopsy in men with varicocele. Fertil Steril 1977;28:663.
16. McFadden MR, Mehan DJ. Testicular biopsies in 101 cases of varicocele. J Urol 1978;119:372.
17. Hadziselimovic F, Leibundgut B, DaRugna D. The value of testicular biopsy in patients with varicocele. J Urol 1986;135:707.
18. Cameron DF, Snydle FE, Ross MH, Drylie DM. Ultrastructural alterations in the adluminal testicular compartment in men with varicocele. Fertil Steril 1980;33:526.
19. Hienz HA, Voggenthaler J, Weissbach L. Histological findings in testes with varicocele during childhood and their therapeutic consequences. Eur J Pediatr 1980;133:139.
20. Kass EJ, Chandra RS, Belman AB. Testicular histology in the adolescent with a varicocele. Pediatrics 1987;79:996.
21. Hadziselimovic F, Herzog B, Liebundgut B, et al. Testicular and vascular changes in children and adults with varicocele. J Urol 1989;142:583.
22. Kass EJ, Salisz JA. The significance of scrotal temperature elevation in an adolescent with a varicocele. J Urol 1990;143(4):263A.
23. Philips RW, McKenzie FF. Thermoregulatory function and mechanism of the scrotum. Res Bull Univ Miss Agric Stat 1934;217.
24. Salisz JA, Kass EJ, Steinert BW. The significance of elevated scrotal temperature in an adolescent with a varicocele. In Zorgniotti AW, ed. Temperature and environmental effects on the testis. New York: Plenum Press, 1991:245–251.
25. Kay R, Alexander N, Baugham WL. Induced varicoceles in rhesus monkeys. Fertil Steril 1979;31:195.
26. Saypol DC, Howards SS, Turner TT, Miller ED Jr. Influence of surgically induced varicocele on testicular blood flow, temperature, and histoloty in adult rats and dogs. J Clin Invest 1981;68:39.
27. Green KF, Turner TT, Howards SS. Varicocele: reversal of the testicular blood flow and temperature effects by varicocele repair. J Urol 1984;131:1208.
28. Fussell EN, Lewis RW, Roberts JA, Harrison RM. Early ultrastructural findings in experimentally produced varicocele in the monkey testis. J Androl 1981;2:111.
29. Nasu T, Takihara H, Hirayama A. A new apparatus for the measurement of testicular volume. Jpn J Fertil Steril 1979;24:12.
30. Constabile RA, Skoog S, Randowich M. Testicular volume assessment in the adolescent with a varicocele. J Urol 1992;147:1348.
31. Behre HM, Nashan D, Nieschlag E. Objective measurement of testicular volume by ultrasonography: evaluation of the technique and comparison with orchidometer estimates. Int J Androl 1991;12:395.
32. Cockett ATK, Takihara H, Cosentino MJ. The varicocele. Fertil Steril 1984;41:5.
33. Lipshultz LI, Corriere JN Jr. Progressive testicular atrophy in the varicocele patient. J Urol 1977;117:175.
34. Lyons RP, Marshall S, Scott MP. Varicocele in childhood and adolescence: implication in adulthood infertility? Urology 1982;19:641.
35. Kass EJ, Belman AB. Reversal of testicular growth failure by varicocele ligation. J Urol 1987;137:475.
36. Janczewski Z, Bablok L. Semen characteristics in pubertal boys. I. Semen quality after first ejaculation. Arch Androl 1985;15:199.
37. MacLeod J. Seminal cytology in the presence of varicocele. Fertil Steril 1965;16:735.
38. Ayodeji O, Baker WG. Is there a specific abnormality of sperm morphology in men with varicoceles? Fertil Steril 1986;45:839.
39. Baker HW, Buger HG, DeKretser DM. Testicular vein ligation and fertility in men with varicoceles. Br Med J 1985;291:1678.
40. Cheval MJ, Purcell MH. Deterioration of semen parameters over time in men with untreated varicocele: Evidence of progressive testicular damage. Fertil Steril 1992;57:174.
41. Gorelick JI, Goldstein M. Loss of fertility in men with a varicocele. Fertil Steril 1992;57:174.
42. Witt MA, Lipshultz LI. Varicocele: A progressive or static lesion? Urology 1993;42:541.
43. Ospina LF. Augmented gonadotropin response to luteinizing hormone-releasing hormone (LH-RH) in infertile men with varicocele. Clin Res 1977;25:106a.
44. Hudson RW, Marrero RA, Trawford VA, McKay DE. Hormonal parameters in incidental varicoceles and those causing infertility. Fertil Steril 1986;45:692.
45. Hudson RW, Perez-Marrero RA, Crawford VA, McKay DE. Hormonal parameters of men with varicoceles before and after varicocelectomy. Fertil Steril 1985;43:905.
46. Nagao RR, Plymate SR, Berger RE, et al. Comparison of gonadal function between fertile and infertile men with varicoceles. Fertil Steril 1986;46:930.
47. Dickerman Z, Landman J, Prager-Lewin R, Laron Z. Evaluation of testicular function in prepubertal boys by means of the luteinizing hormone-releasing hormone test. Fertil Steril 1978;29:655.
48. Lipshultz LI, Caminos-Torres R, Greenspan CS, Snyder PJ. Testicular function after orchiopexy for unilaterally undescended testis. N Engl J Med 1976;295:15.

49. Okuyama A, Koide T, Itatani H, et al. Pituitary-gonadal function in schoolboys with varicocele and indications of varicocelectomy. Eur Urol 1981;7:92.

50. Kass EJ, Freitas JE, Salisz JA, Steinert BW. Pituitary gonadal dysfunction in adolescents with varicocele. Urology 1993;42:179.

51. Fujisawa M, Hayashi A, Imanishi O, et al. The significance of gonadotropin-releasing hormone test for predicting fertility after varicocelectomy. Fertil Steril 1994;61:779.

52. Su L, Goldstein M, Schlegel PN. The effect of varicocelectomy on serum testosterone levels in infertile men with varicoceles. J Urol 1995;154:1752.

53. Ferguson JM, Gillespie N, Chalmers N, et al. Percutaneous varicocele embolization in the treatment of infertility. Br J Radiol 1995;68:700.

54. Tauber R, Johnsen N. Antegrade scrotal sclerotherapy for the treatment of varicocele: technique and late results. J Urol 1994;151:386.

55. Porst H, Bahren W, Lenz M, Altwein JE. Percutaneous sclerotherapy of varicoceles-an alternative to conventional surgical methods. Br J Urol 1984;56:73.

56. Kaufman SL, Kadir S, Barth KH, et al. Mechanisms of recurrent varicocele after balloon occlusion or surgical ligation of the internal spermatic vein. Radiology 1983;147:435.

57. Donovan JF, Winfield HN. Laparoscopic varix ligation. J Urol 1992;47:77.

58. See WA, Mong TG, Weldon BC. Laparoscopic urology. St. Louis: Quality Medical Publishing 1993:183.

59. Coolsaet BLRA. The varicocele syndrome: venography determining the optimal level for surgical management. J Urol 1980;124:833.

60. Ivanissevich O. Left varicocele due to reflux. J Int Coll Surg 1960;34:742.

61. Kass EJ, Marcol B. Results of varicocele surgery in adolescents: A comparison of techniques. J Urol 1992;148:694.

62. Levitt S, Gill B, Katlowitz N, et al. Routine intraoperative post-ligation venography in the treatment of the pediatric varicocele. J Urol 1987;137:716.

63. Palomo A. Radical cure of varicocele by a new technique: preliminary report. J Urol 1949;61:604.

64. Atassi O, Kass EJ, Steinert BW. Testicular growth after successful varicocele correction in adolescents: Comparison of artery sparing techniques with the Palomo procedure. J Urol 1995;153:482.

65. Hosli PO. Varicocele-results after early treatment in children and adolescents. Z Kinderchir 1988;43:213.

66. Okuyama A, Nakamura M, Namiki M, et al. Surgical repair of varicocele at puberty: preventive treatment for fertility improvement. J Urol 1988;139:562.

67. Yamamoto M, Tsuji Y, Ohmura M, et al. Comparison of artery-ligating and artery-preserving varicocelectomy: Effect on postoperative spermatogenesis. Andrologia 1995;27:37.

68. Gorenstein A, Katz S, Schiller M. Varicocele in children: "to treat or not to treat"-venographic and manometric studies. J Pediatr Surg 1986;21:1046.

69. Hirokawa M, Matsushita K, Iwamoto T, et al. Assessment of Palomo's operative method for infertile varicocele. Andrologia 1993;25:47.

70. Kass EJ, Freitas JE, Bour JB. Adolescent varicocele: objective indications for treatment. J Urol 1989;142:579.

71. Laven JSE, Haans LCF, Mali WPTM, et al. Effects of varicocele treatment in adolescents: a randomized study. Fertil Steril 1992;58:756.

72. Madgar I, Weissenberg R, Lunenfeld B, et al. Controlled trial of high spermatic vein ligation for varicocele in infertile men. Fertil Steril 1995;63:120.

CHAPTER 31

Other Disorders of the Penis and Scrotum

Thomas H. Bartholomew and Bradley McIver

When a woman gives birth to an infant
That has no well marked sex,
Calamity and affliction will seize upon the land;
The master of the house will have no happiness.
—Babylonian Stone Tablet
1700 BC

A most pivotal and resolute decree in human experience involves the declaration of gender at the time of birth. Disorders of the genitalia in babies are especially troubling for parents. This is perhaps because of the profound and subconscious emotional significance of these reproductive structures or the consequent impact of deformities on future generations. Whether instinctive or socially acquired, concern over genital disorder seems at times exaggerated. Early consideration, thoughtful reassurance or treatment benefits parents in these times and ideally eliminates fears of discovery and embarrassment later for the child.

It is beyond the scope of this chapter to touch on every genital disorder. Specific reference is available elsewhere in this text regarding hypospadias, cryptorchidism, and intersex states.

THE PREPUCE

The skin of the penis folds on itself to cover the glans for a variable distance. In the 10th fetal week a small epithelial tag forms at the penile tip (Fig. 31.1).[1] This tag becomes a pronounced fold by 12 weeks, which grows inward and ventrally surrounding the glans at birth. The inner epithelial layer of this fold is fused with the glans epithelium and thus will not retract in most newborns. The complete development of the prepuce occurs after closure of the urethra. In cases of incomplete urethral closure (e.g., hypospadias) ventral development of the prepuce is incomplete. Thus the typical hypospadic penis will have an absence of the ventral prepuce.

PHYSIOLOGIC PREPUCE RETRACTION

Oster[2] recorded more than 9,000 observations in Danish boys in the 1960s, considerably advancing our understanding of the natural history of the prepuce. He demonstrated that foreskin separation is a progression that results in 99% of males achieving retraction by age 17. Limited experience leads some well-intentioned care givers to believe that this physiologic inability to retract the prepuce in youngsters is pathologic and to encourage abruption of this plane in infants. The progressive separation that will occur is, in part, caused by enlarging accumulations of trapped, desquamated cells that painlessly and bloodlessly separate the epithelial surfaces. These whitish masses of infant smegma are typically sterile and emerge from the edge of the prepuce as it retracts. They are often visible through the thin translucent prepuce and may arouse concern in parents.

PHIMOSIS

Phimosis is the inability to retract the foreskin. It could be further defined as physiologic, as in infancy and childhood, or pathologic. Pathologic phimosis results from inflammatory or traumatic injury to the prepuce resulting in an acquired inelastic scar that prevents retraction. Forceful disruption of physiologic adhesions in infants no doubt encourages pathologic phimosis. Recurrent posthitis (inflammation of the prepuce) may also result in such dense scarring that circumcision becomes necessary. Urine trapping inside the small preputial aperture is an unusual result of phimosis that will be best treated by circumcision.

PARAPHIMOSIS

Paraphimosis (Fig. 31.2) develops when the preputial aperture is retracted proximal to the corona of the glans. The loose inner preputial epithelium is so elastic that in a short time edema prevents replacement of the aper-

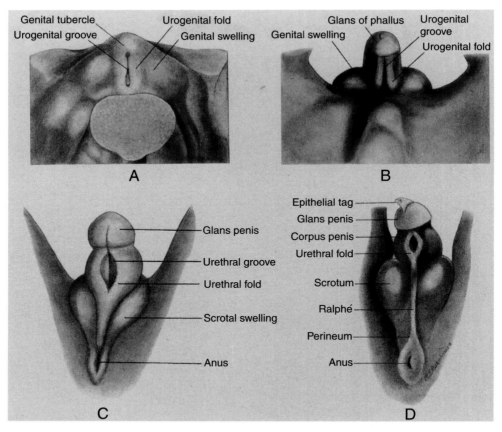

FIG. 31.1. A, A 3-mm embryo of indifferent sex with paired genital tubercles. **B,** A 21-mm embryo of indifferent sex with fused tubercles. **C,** At 10 weeks, the scrotal anlage approach the midline. **D,** At 12 weeks, the genitalia are recognizably male Reprinted with permission from Arey LB. Developmental anatomy: a textbook and laboratory manual of embryology. 7th ed. Philadelphia: Saunders, 1974.

ture distal to the glans and edema; pain and venous congestion progress.

Emergency room reduction of the paraphimosis is almost always successful. Compressing the area with an elastic bandage for 10 minutes or with a pediatric blood pressure cuff inflated to diastolic blood pressure level makes the reduction easier. If neglected for several days, the tight preputial aperture may need surgical division.

NEWBORN CIRCUMCISION

The true origins of circumcision have been lost in the mists of earliest history. Depicted as a ceremonial act in man's oldest writings, circumcision practices of the 33rd Century BC are shown in religious settings in hieroglyphic records of that era. Today, circumcision is performed on nearly half of this country's newborn males but, despite our medical advances, still remains a ritualistic and culturally driven procedure.

Medical reasons to perform newborn circumcision are established fact. Certainly infant circumcision offers nearly absolute protection against carcinoma of the penis. No specific component of penile secretions has been shown to produce cancer, but adequate hygiene will decrease the risk of penile carcinoma if carried out conscientiously. Newborn circumcision significantly reduces the risk of urinary tract infection in the first 12 months of life[3] and should be encouraged in infants with vesicoureteral reflux.

Specific medical reasons not to circumcise newborns should be recognized. Abnormal penile development may require surgical correction and this often involves use of the foreskin. In this regard, hypospadias, chordee, epispadias, or a penis that is small or unusual in appearance is a contraindication to circumcision. Bleeding disorders, prematurity, and systemic illness are other medical contraindications to circumcision. Less distinct arguments with broader application against circumcision regard the relative risk of complication after the operation.

Complications of Newborn Circumcision

Gee and Ansell[4] reviewed the complications of 5,521 neonatal circumcisions involving the Plastibell and Gomco techniques. The cumulative complication rate was 0.2%. There was no significant difference between the two techniques for the various complications except for infection (Fig. 31.2). Wound infection occurred in 0.14% of the patients circumcised with the Gomco technique and 0.72% with the Plastibell, a fivefold difference.

Depending on how it is defined, meatal stenosis is probably the most common delayed complication of circumcision. Although often overdiagnosed, it is of significance only if it interferes with bladder emptying by causing obstructive changes in the stream. It seems to

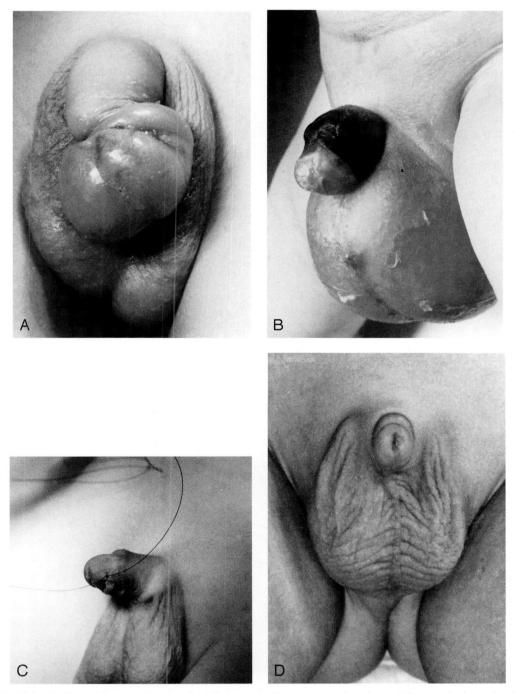

FIG. 31.2. A, Paraphimosis showing that the constricting prepuce has been left retracted proximal to the glans. **B,** Infection after circumcision that has advanced enough to require surgical debridement. **C,** Skin bridges can usually be ligated as an office procedure. **D,** Penis concealed by the scar caused by circumcision.

be nearly exclusively found in circumcised boys and is probably related to irritation of the unprotected edges of the meatus. The clinically significant stenotic meatus is best evaluated by observation of the stream. Upward deflection, a fine, unusually forceful stream, and a consistent prolongation on emptying of more that 20 seconds indicates a significant stenosis. When these features are present, the problem is solved with a urethral meatotomy using EMLA anesthetic in the office or as a day surgery procedure.

Surplus foreskin remaining after circumcision is of consequence only if it interferes with penile hygiene. If the prepuce remnant covers the glans at rest, adhesions are likely to persist or reform, making hygiene less than fool-proof. Doctor visits for "penis problems" are six times more common in uncircumcised boys as opposed to circumcised boys mostly because of the difficulty with hygiene.[5] This persistent adherence may require revisions of circumcision later in infancy.

Separation of the circumcision line is probably a result of removing too much skin. The shaft appears denuded and at first the appearance may be alarming. Conservative management with wet to dry dressings or antibiotic ointment leads to healing by secondary intention and a normal appearance. Temptations to skin graft or resuture should be resisted.

Dense skin bridges covering the coronal sulcus can be prevented by separation of the skin edges in the first weeks after a circumcision. This is the main benefit of a follow-up evaluation. When these skin bridges persist they can be safely eliminated by circumligation with strong suture as an office procedure (Fig. 31.2). Concealed penis (Fig. 31.2) has a most serious appearance wherein the circumcision scar forms over the glans. In most cases the patient voids without difficulty through the scar's aperture and a conservative approach may be followed. By 12 months the dense scar is soft and more elastic and often allows the glans to emerge. If surgical revision is needed, a Heineke-Mikulicz maneuver at the 3 o'clock and 9 o'clock positions will release the trapped glans. Parental exposure of the penis is essential in the first postoperative weeks to prevent reconcealment of the glans with healing.

THE PENIS

The penis develops from the paired genital tubercles visible as swellings ventral to the cloacal membrane in the three millimeter embryo (Fig. 31.1). With elongation these tubercles fuse superiorly leaving a urogenital groove inferiorly. The genital swellings, lateral to the tubercles, develop further, inferiorly fusing to form the

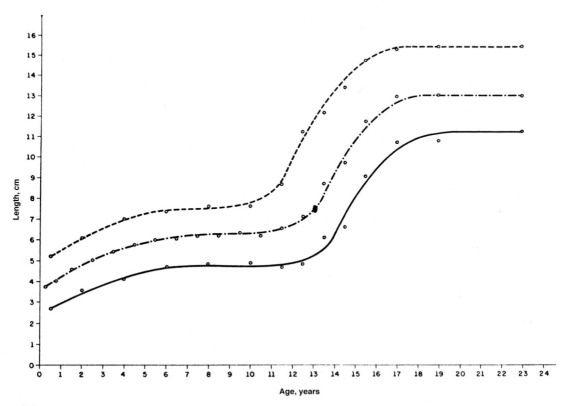

FIG. 31.3. Penile length growth curve from birth to maturity. *Dashed line,* 9th decide; *dotted and dashed line,* median; *solid line, 1st decile.* Reprinted with permission from Schonfeld WA. Primary and secondary sexual characteristics. Am J Dis Child 1943;65:535–549.

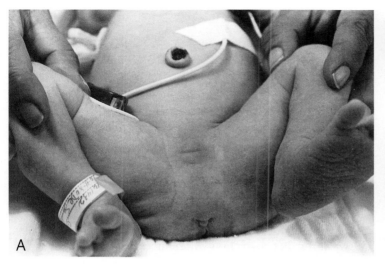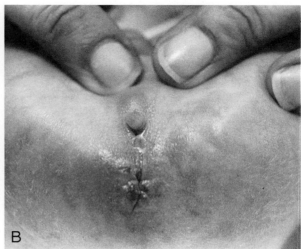

FIG. 31.4. A, In aphallia, the scrotum is hypoplastic and the testes are undescended. **B,** A midline appendage anterior to the anus is typical.

scrotum. By the 12th week, the genitalia can be identified as male. The urogenital folds close over from proximal to distal enclosing the urogenital groove to form the urethra. At term the stretched penile length is 3.5 cm on average with a standard deviation of 0.4 centimeters (Fig. 31.3).[6]

ABSENCE OF THE PENIS-APHALLIA

This rare anomaly (Fig. 31.4) results from absence of the genital tubercles and has been reported in fewer than 100 cases worldwide. Three varieties have been described based on the relationship of the urethra to the anal sphincter: postsphincteric, presphincteric, and urethral atresia.[7] The more proximal the bladder outlet the more severe are the associated anomalies and the higher the mortality. If present, the scrotum and testes are usually normal. A consistent feature in aphallia is a midline skin tag anterior to the anus containing a urethral opening. More than half of these patients will have associated anomalies, especially of the genitourinary system, including undescended testes and renal aplasia or dysplasia. Imperforate anus is common as is rectal atresia or rectovesical fistula. Prompt evaluation should be initiated at birth with female gender assignment being the rule. Orchiectomy and feminizing genioplasty will lead to suitable gender identity.

DIPHALLIA

Diphallia (Fig. 31.5) is also a rare condition and varies from a small accessory penis to complete or true diphallia. In this latter variety each penis contains a urethra, which join to drain a single bladder or drain separate duplicated bladders. Varieties of hypospadias or epi-

spadias are not unusual. Imperforate anus is particularly common with diphallia. Prompt evaluation would include retrograde imaging studies, evaluation of other associated life-threatening conditions, and individualized functional considerations.

PENILE TORSION

This usually counter-clockwise[6] rotation of the penis on its long axis (Fig. 31.6) is common in hypospadias.

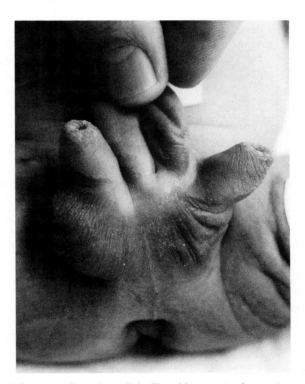

FIG. 31.5. Complete diphallia with an ectopic scrotum.

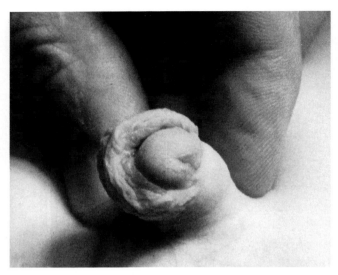

FIG. 31.6. A counterclockwise rotation is common in hypospadias.

Isolated examples of torsion are prevalent without hypospadias. An incidence of 1 in 80 males has been reported. Most cases involve less than 90° rotation and rarely cause a functional problem. Complete degloving of the shaft skin down to Bucks' fascia, starting from the circumcision line, followed by slight overcorrected reapplication of the skin will correct most cases, although rarely taking Bucks' fascia at the base of the penis is necessary to fully correct the abnormality.

Subtle degrees of chordee should be anticipated in such cases and evaluated with an artificial erection during this dissection. Keep in mind that otherwise insignificant distal urethral hypoplasia may accompany torsion, encouraging caution in separating the thin ventral skin over such underdeveloped or absent corpora spongiosa.

CHORDEE

This condition usually implies ventral bending of the penis. Kaplan and Lamm[8] demonstrated this as a normal stage in fetal penile development that may be a transient finding in a third of premature males.

Though usually associated with hypospadias, chordee can be present as an isolated finding. Lateral or dorsal "chordee" is also possible. The penis is characteristically normal in appearance while flaccid with no visible or palpable anomaly. With erection the deformity becomes obvious. Fortunately, mild cases are the rule, but with severe angulation, correction is needed. The argument for postponing this intervention until after puberty is compelling. There should be little risk in infancy or childhood of discovery or embarrassment because the deformity is only seen with erection. The surgical correction may involve elimination of corporal disproportion

and if carried out in infancy may worsen or improve with penile growth.

Documentation of the degree of angulation is awkward in the teenager in the office setting. Home Polaroid photography can be used to see the erect penis and document the defect accurately. Minor bending that will not lead to buckling with intercourse should not cause dysfunction. Bends of 45° or more will cause difficulty.

Surgical correction centers on the Nesbit[9] principle of shortening the longer or convex side, removing ellipses of tunica albuginea. An artificial erection is created after the penis is degloved by injecting intravenous saline solution into the corpus cavernosum while a rubberband tourniquet is constricting the base of the penis. The degloving alone can correct the angulation and thus no further dissection will be necessary, but this has not been our experience. If the chordee persists, the neurovascular bundle is elevated away from the site of the tunical ellipses. Small elliptical segments of the tunica are excised and the defect closed with inverted fine prolene suture (Fig. 31.7).[10]

The artificial erection is repeated to assess the adequacy of the repair. It is better to take several smaller wedges than one large wedge to avoid postoperative angulation at the surgical site.

PRIAPISM

Priapism for the pediatric patient is most commonly secondary to sickle cell disease. It is the persistent unwanted painful erection of the penis. It results from an accumulation and sludging of rigid sickle cells in the corpora cavernosa. The incidence has been reported in 6 to 76% of boys younger than 21 years[11] with homozygous sickle cell disease. Transient <2 hours) priapism is more common than prolonged priapism involving a single episode. These requires no specific intervention but may respond to simple measures at home (Table 31.1).[11] It may be useful to treat boys with recurrent transient episodes with pseudoephedrine 30 to 60 mg at bedtime to promote contraction of muscle fibers in the erectile tissue.

Prolonged priapism is treated with hydration and transfusion to increase Hgb A to 12 gm %. Pain control and alkalinization are also provided.

Aspiration and irrigation of the corpora with 1:1,000,000 solution of epinephrine has been successfully used by Ewalt et al to relieve pain and prevent corporal fibrosis.[11] They encourage this treatment for cases lasting more than 2 hours.

THE SCROTUM

Genital swellings form by the sixth week of fetal development lateral to the urogenital folds. With caudal migration and fusion during the fourth fetal month these hemiscrota fuse at the scrotal raphé to form the scrotum.

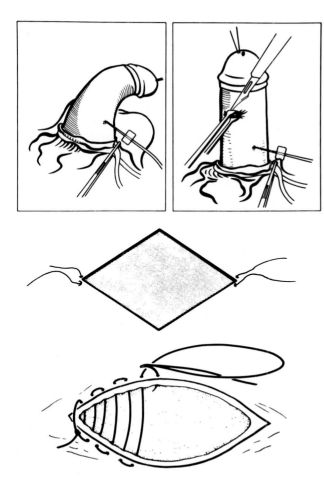

FIG. 31.7. An artificial erection demonstrating the point of angulation. Small elliptical segments are removed, followed by transverse closure. Reprinted with permission from Kelami A. Congenital penile deviation and its treatment with the Nesbit-Kelami technique. Br J Urol 1987;60:261–263.

Most anomalies of the scrotum occur in association with other urogenital anomalies. Because of the coincident nature of urethral, phallic, and scrotal embryologic development, severe cases of hypospadias can often be seen with scrotal anomalies. Bifid scrotum, ectopic scrotum and penoscrotal transposition are the common scrotal malformations.

TABLE 31.1. *Interventions reported as successful in terminating priapism*

Intervention	No. of patients (%)
Urination	15 (55)
Acetaminophen with codeine	13 (48)
Gentle exercise	9 (33)
Warm bath	8 (29)
Nothing	6 (22)
Total patients	27*

*More than one intervention was successful in some patients.

The inadequate fusion of hemiscrota leads to bifid scrotum. This is rarely an isolated event but is commonly found in severe hypospadias. Various degrees of penoscrotal transposition are possible from complete to partial. This is caused by failure or delay in urethral formation and incomplete fusion of the urethral folds. This prevents caudal migration and fusion of the genital swellings.

Successful correction of penoscrotal transposition or bifid scrotum can be safely combined with chordee release and hypospadias repair. The smooth hairless skin of the ventral penis will transfer upward in a Z plasty procedure, which is reproduced in a mirror image fashion on either side (Fig. 31.8). The rugate scrotal skin is thus rotated inferiorly to establish a normal fused appearance in the midline. Our results with this approach in combination with freegraft techniques for urethroplasty have been gratifying (Fig. 31.9).

Scrotal anlage may migrate to ectopic locations.[12] This could include perineal, inguinal, or medial thigh. In most cases the testis of the associated hemiscrotum retains its normal gubernacular relation and is found in the abnormally positioned scrotum.

ACQUIRED SCROTAL CONDITIONS

One of the most challenging arenas for the pediatric urologist to enter is the emergency room for evaluation of the boy with an acutely inflamed scrotum. Time is most important in successful elimination of testicular torsion and, unfortunately, numerous other scrotal conditions often make the distinction difficult.

There is a general reluctance on the part of primary care physicians to make a disposition on boys with scrotal swelling primarily because of the fear of missed torsion. A characteristic reaction to any cause of inflammation of the scrotum or testis involves scrotal swelling and the appearance of a hydrocele. Insect bites (Fig. 31.10), diaper rash, idiopathic scrotal edema, Henoch-Schonlein purpura, and epididymitis may convincingly mimic testis torsion. In some of these cases the testis can be pushed up into the inguinal area away from the region of redness confirming that the disease is in the scrotal wall and not arising from the testicle (Fig. 31.11).

Insect bites are common to the genitalia. Because of the closed conditions of underclothing multiple bites can occur before being noticed. There will often be itching and a central point of envenomation.

Diaper rash peaks in frequency in children around 9 to 12 months of age and is characterized by classical erythematous changes in the scrotal skin with satellite lesions. There is no involvement of the scrotal contents.

Mumps orchitis is a rarely seen inflammation of the testicle in boys. Orchitis is much more common in postpubertal males, and more commonly develops a few days after the onset of the parotitis. There is no treat-

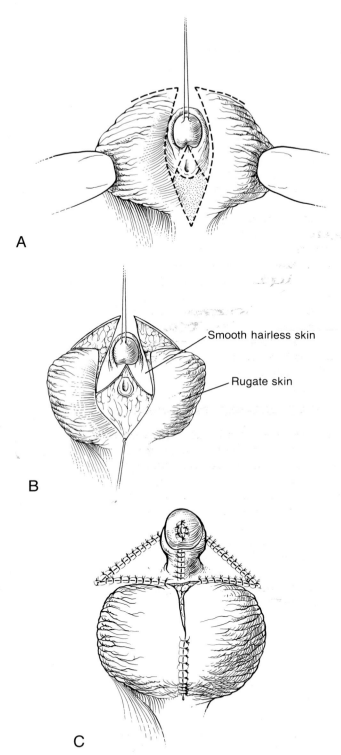

Smooth hairless skin

Rugate skin

FIG. 31.8. A, Incisions for the Z-plasty technique for correcting penoscrotal transposition. **B,** Transposition of the flaps moves the rugate scrotal halves inferiorly to the midline. **C,** Completion of the skin closure after urethroplasty.

ment of proven value, and the long-term effect is usually unilateral atrophy of the affected testicle.

Acute bacterial epididymitis in children is not a common occurrence, and it is often difficult to discern from torsion. The diagnosis frequently is made at scrotal exploration. Its presence should prompt a search for anatomic abnormalities that would allow entry of infection into the lumen of the vas deferens. Epididymitis is often the presenting sign of an ectopic ureter. It may also follow indwelling foley catheterization, especially after transurethral treatment of urethral valves. It can also be seen in infants with imperforate anus and a rectourethral fistula.

Henoch-Schonlein (H-S) purpura (Fig. 31.10) is a disorder of unknown etiology that is probably related to an autoimmune phenomenon. The syndrome is characterized by a purpuric rash, abdominal pain that is often associated with gastrointestinal bleeding, arthralgia, microscopic hematuria, proteinuria, and nephritis.

In a large series of 110 cases of children with H-S purpura, scrotal involvement was present in five (4.5%). However, the incidence of scrotal involvement with H-S purpura has been reported in up to 36%. It can present with symptoms similar to testicular torsion, and testicular scintography has been used to rule out torsion.[13]

The diagnosis can be made when the characteristic symptoms and skin lesions are present, but occasionally the scrotal pain can precede the purpura.[14] Torsion has been reported concurrently with H-S purpura. Therefore, careful physical examination is imperative, and exploration may be necessary in equivocal cases.[15]

Acute Idiopathic Scrotal Edema (AISE) is one of the more common nontorsion etiologies of the acute scrotum. AISE primarily occurs in prepubertal boys but has been reported in adults.[16] Patients with AISE typically have an acute onset of painless scrotal erythema. However, pain can be present mimicking torsion. The affected hemiscrotum becomes swollen, firm, and bright pink. The testicle itself is not involved in the inflammatory process. Typically, vital signs, urinalysis, and white blood cell count are normal. A normal testicular arterial flow on a Doppler sonogram can further confirm the diagnosis in equivocal cases. AISE can be difficult to distinguish from torsion, and when no diagnosis is clear, surgical exploration is mandatory. The swelling resolves spontaneously, without sequelae, in 1 to 3 days.[17]

The etiology of AISE is unclear, although there is a hypothesis that it is similar to angioneurotic edema, and, therefore, an allergic phenomenon. Najmaldin and Burge[18] found that 60% of boys in their series of patients with AISE had a history of allergy or had allergic manifestations, compared with 28% of controls (p<0.05). The incidence of AISE has been reported to be from 7 to 8% of cases of acute scrotum.[19]

AISE can spread from the scrotum to the penis, abdomen, or perineum. Up to 52% of cases can be bilateral,

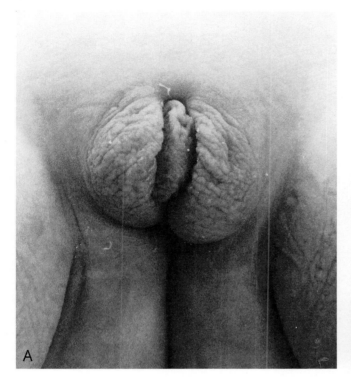
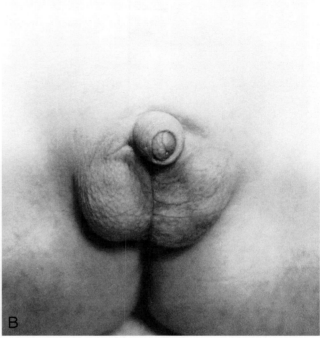

FIG. 31.9. A, In a bifid scrotum, the scrotal halves are separated in the midline by the hypospadic penis. **B,** Appearance after the correction of penoscrotal transposition.

and recurrence has been reported in up to 21%. Some have advocated treatment of AISE with antihistamines, given its proposed allergic etiology. Once the diagnosis is made, the most commonly recommended therapy is rest and reassurance.

SCROTAL GANGRENE

Fortunately, acute scrotal (Fournier's) gangrene is a rare entity in the pediatric population. However, its high mortality makes early diagnosis and treatment mandatory. Most pediatric cases involve infants 12 weeks old or younger, although the syndrome is possible at any age, and is much more common in immunocompromised adults. Lesions generally involve the scrotum, penis, or perineum and present as a gangrenous ulceration or erythematous patch of skin that is exquisitely tender to touch and may be tense or fluctuant. Systemic illness with fever, dehydration, or sepsis is commonly present; however, patients with scrotal gangrene can occasionally look remarkably well.

In infants, scrotal gangrene may follow systemic disease with cutaneous manifestations such as measles or varicella.[20] Also, recent circumcision (Fig. 31.2), diaper rash, and perineal skin infections can precede its onset. These minor skin abrasions serve as a route of entry of the infecting organisms, and the spread of infection within the subcutis invokes an obliterating endarteritis.[21]

The bacterial spread through the subcutaneous tissue along with the endarteritis invariably lead to ischemic necrosis of the scrotum. The infectious etiology is usually polymicrobrial, with organisms such as *E. coli, beta-hemolytic Streptococcus, Staphylococcus aureus, Bacteroides, Pseudomonas, Proteus,* and *Clostridium welchii.*[22] The testicle and spermatic cord usually are spared because the testicular artery is unaffected.

Early recognition of the syndrome is imperative as mortality rates range up to 45%. Prompt and aggressive debridement of all devitalized tissue along with broad spectrum antibiotic coverage is recommended, and can be life-saving. Severe cases may require extensive scrotal resection and placement of the testicles within a subcutaneous pouch in the medial thighs. While skin grafting may be necessary, healing by secondary intent in most cases is satisfactory once the necrotic tissue is removed.

THE TESTIS

Primordial undifferentiated germ cells begin a migration to the genital ridge in the third fetal week. By the eighth week the testis has distinctive features lying high in the retroperitoneum. Two stages of testicular descent have been described. In the first stage, mediated by Müllerian Inhibiting Substance, the testis migrates toward the internal inguinal ring by the seventh month.

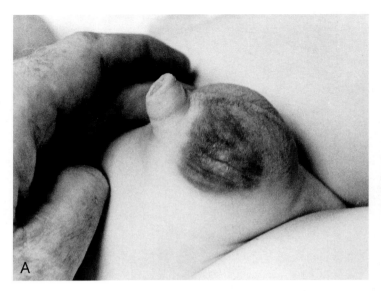

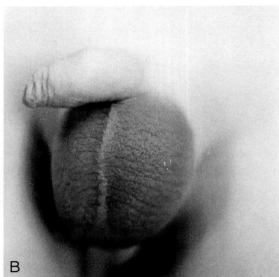

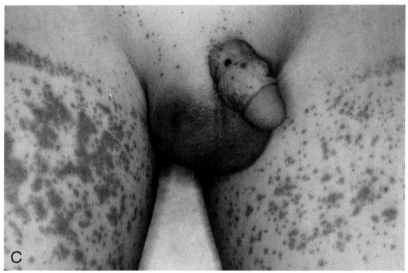

FIG. 31.10. A, Scrotal insect bite. **B,** Idiopathic scrotal edema, in which the scrotal wall has thickened. **C,** Henoch–Schonlein purpura involving the genitalia.

The descent into the scrotum may be mediated by testosterone and involves passage along the inguinal canal and requires the helmsman (the gubernaculum) and an intact genitofemoral nerve.

ABSENT TESTIS

When the testis is nonpalpable, the testis will be absent in up to 40% of patients.[23] Fortunately, this absence rarely is bilateral because unilateral occurrences are 30 times more common. Bloom[23] argues convincingly that this is the loss of a formed fetal testis rather than agenesis. The fetal testis produces MIS and causes regression of the ipsilateral Müllerian duct in the fetus if present at 16 weeks. Because Müllerian structures are uncommon in the monorchid patient, the strong implication is that the fetal testis was formed and present, precluding

fallopian tube or uterine development. The left side predominates in 67 to 81% of reports.[24] Blind-ending spermatic vessels, usually ending at the internal ring, are present in most patients.

Laparoscopy or thorough intraabdominal exploration is accepted as a means to establish the absence of a testis. The goal is accurate definition of the anatomy to prevent a misconception of an absent testes that unfortunately later becomes malignant.[25] If findings of late fetal loss are present, prophylactic fixation of the solitary contralateral testis is indicated. Participation in collision sports may be prohibited in such boys at the high school or college level. This may be an excessively restrictive approach and the significance of possible injury should be made clear to the family.

Bilateral testicular absence caused by late fetal loss results in a phenotypically normal male. The levels of gonadotropins are elevated and there is no response to

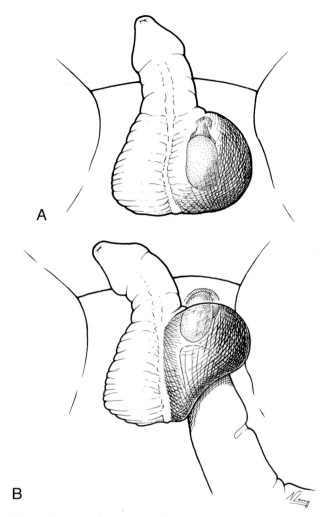

FIG. 31.11. In scrotal wall inflammation, the testicle can be displaced upward into the inguinal area away from the region of redness.

stimulation by hCG.[26] This rare abnormality is reported in 1 in 20,000 males.[27] Laparoscopic confirmation is advocated to eliminate the possibility of an occult dysplastic gonadal remnant (Bartone et al).[28] Scrotal appearance will be flat and hypoplastic in these patients, and placement of testicular protheses is indicated. Exogenous testosterone is required to properly virilize these patients at puberty.

HYPOPLASTIC TESTES

Testis size is approximately 1 mL in volume at birth and reaches a peak infant volume of approximately 2 mL at 2 months of age.[29] This correlates with elevated serum testosterone levels and erectile activity. Testicular volume decreases by 6 months to remain constant until puberty. Testicular growth is the first sign of pubertal development. Reduced unilateral testicular volume

may be related to maldescent, trauma, torsion, hernia repair, orchidopexy, or varicocele.

Bilateral small testes also can result from any of the above. Other signs of deficient secondary sexual features should be sought in such patients as well as abnormal FSH, LH, or testosterone levels.

TORSION OF THE TESTICLE

The sudden vascular insult of torsion arises in conjuction with the twisting of an unusually long artery that provides the dominant portion of blood supply to an organ. The internal spermatic artery is the longest end artery in the body and thus stands an increased chance of vascular "accident." The vessels to the testis are most often injured through rotation with warm ischemic injury destroying the testis within hours.

Five percent of torsions occur before birth or soon after (Fig. 31.12).[30] This perinatal rotation of the cord is proximal to the attachment of the tunica vaginalis that encloses the testis and is termed extravaginal torsion. These tissues have little attachment to the scrotal wall around the time of descent and so are free to rotate. Such patients seem to have little pain but only a firm solid mass in the scrotum. The scrotal skin is characteristically fixed to the necrotic gonad.

Inguinal exploration is suggested in the newborn with these findings to confirm the diagnosis and perhaps more importantly to fix the contralateral testis in place and prevent subsequent torsion (Fig. 31.13). Das and Singer[31] reported in their studies that this extravaginal type of torsion occurred prenatally in 72% and postnatally in 28%. Twenty-one percent were bilateral, 3% were asynchronous bilateral. Early surgery of the postnatal variety can result in testicular salvage.[32] The more prevalent prenatal variety has little salvage potential and surgery need not be considered an emergency nor necessarily justified.[33]

Intravaginal torsion takes place at levels distal to the investment of the tunica vaginalis and accounts for 95% of torsion of the spermatic cord. This can occur at any age but has an unexplained peak incidence at 13 years. (Fig. 31.12).[30] The risk of suffering a twist of the cord or an appendage of the testis, i.e., having an acute scrotum by age 25 is 1:160.[34] More cases involve the left testis than the right and bilateral cases account for 2%.

If the tunica vaginalis surrounds the gonad normally the posterior aspect of the testicle is fixed to the adjacent scrotal wall, and rotation within this space is unlikely. Anomalous suspension or a "bell clapper" deformity, however, is suggested as a prerequisite to torsion. The contraction of the cremasteric muscle has also been suggested as initiating the rotation that leads to torsion. It would seem plausible that this anomalous suspension is congenital but only at the time of pubertal growth

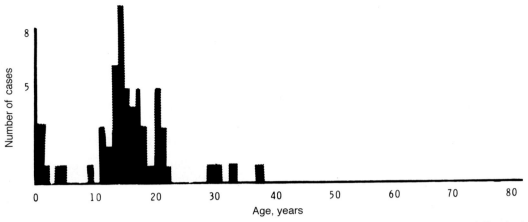

FIG. 31.12. Age distribution of testis torsion. Reprinted with permission from Bartsch G, et al. Testicular torsion: late results with special regard to fertility and endocrine function. J Urol 1980;124:375.

does the more massive testicle have the momentum to rotate into 360° or 720° of torsion.

Sudden and severe pain is the dominant feature of torsion. Approximately 25% of patients will also be nauseated. The nature of adolescent boys is such that they are loath to describe problems of this type to their parents and thus they experience even greater delay in obtaining medical evaluation. Barada et al[35] found a median time of 20 hours between onset of pain and medical evaluation of patients younger than 18 years of age compared with a 4 hour interval in patients older than 18 years.

Early examination demonstrates a high riding testis without a cremasteric reflex.[36] Initially there will be minimal erythema or edema of the overlying skin. In time

a reactive hydrocele, erythema and ecchymosis become more striking. Pain may lessen as the necrosis becomes more complete.

The problem most likely to mimic testicular torsion is epididymitis. There may be helpful findings supporting the diagnosis of epididymitis such as fever, leucocytosis, vasal, and prostatic tenderness, physical and laboratory findings expected to be normal in testes torsion. Epididymitis is uncommon prepubertally and should be a diagnosis of exclusion. Urinary tract infection supports the clinical impression of acute epididymitis. Also, 27% of patients with acute epididymitis will have a renal anomaly ipsilaterally. Finding such an anomaly on renal ultrasound might favor the diagnosis of epididymitis over testicular torsion in equivocal cases.

Doppler ultrasound can be helpful in verifying arterial flow in difficult cases although this technique is very operator dependent. The nuclear scan would seem ideal in the early stage of torsion in demonstrating diminished blood flow. The problem with either of these adjuncts is the time required with resulting delay in surgical exploration, which is definitive and halts progress of ischemia.

Attempts at manual detorsion in the emergency room can do no harm and may result in a dramatic cessation of pain. The spermatic cord can be infiltrated with 0.5% Xylocaine and the testes rotated outward. More than one rotation is usual. Immediate surgical exploration is still mandatory to ensure that complete detorsion has been achieved and to fix the contralateral testis in place. Placing ice around the scrotum before surgery will improve salvage by reducing warm ischemia time.

Salvage of ischemic testes is inversely related to duration of time the testis has been torsed. Krarup[37] evaluated patients who had treatment for testicular torsion

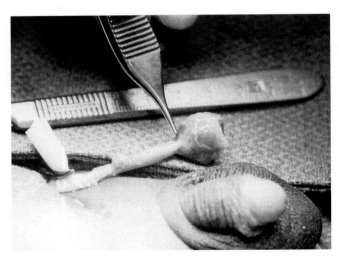

FIG. 31.13. Inguinal exposure of the necrotic extravaginal prenatal torsion.

with follow-up interviews, testicular sonography, and semen analysis. The fertility as judged by semen analysis was normal in only 1 of the 19 men investigated. The degree of atrophy of the twisted testicle was a function of the time elapsed between onset of symptoms and detorsion. Nine of 28 testes were of normal size and all had been explored in the first 10 hours of symptoms. Operations within 4 hours of torsion did not guarantee the survival of a full-sized testis but less atrophy was seen in that group. If 24 hours or more elapsed, total atrophy was found in most men at follow-up.

The cause for reduced sperm counts in patients with previous torsion is not yet clear. Theories of a sympathetic orchiopathy are supported by some animal studies.[38, 39] It is suggested that a testis that has undergone torsion may damage its fellow by producing some detrimental substance. Efforts to demonstrate this in long-term studies yield evidence to the contrary.[40] Evidence for sympathetic orchiopathy in man is even more fragmentary. Fraser[41] sought abnormalities in gonadal function in 47 patients 2 to 10 years after torsion and found no evidence of testicular autoimmunization using standard assays.

Other investigations suggested that infertility in patients with unilateral torsion may be a consequence of a preexisting testicular pathologic condition.[42] These studies show bilateral testicular disease in biopsies from patients at the time of unilateral testicular torsion. Significant preexisting abnormalities were found in most of the patients so evaluated.

APPENDICEAL TORSION

The appendages of the testis and epididymis represent Müllerian and Wolffian vestigial polyps. Due to their pedunculated nature, they are prone to torsion and infarction. The clinical feature in such cases can be typical. The age at appendiceal torsion is younger than that of true testicular torsion. Pain is often mild and gradual in onset. Although there is commonly a history of minor trauma, a causal relationship is difficult to establish. Symptoms are so vague and patients of this age are typically so unlikely to report genital symptoms that several days pass before they seek attention. In some cases the inflammatory reaction is so mild that the dark pea-sized appendix can be seen through the thin overlying skin, the blue dot sign[43] confirming the diagnosis. In other cases the inflammation is so pronounced that erythema and a reactive hydrocele obscure the findings and surgical exploration is needed to rule out torsion of the testicle. The signs and symptoms of an appendicial torsion are self-limiting and generally last from 2 to 4 days. Prolonged symptoms may warrant exploration and removal of a partially torsed, but ischemic appendage.

REFERENCES

1. Arey LB. Developmental Anatomy: A Textbook and Laboratory Manual of Embryology. Revised 7th ed. Philadelphia: W.B. Saunders, 1974.
2. Oster, J. Further fate of the foreskin. Arch Dis Child 1968;43:200.
3. Wiswell TE, Smith FR, Buss JW. Decreased incidence of urinary tract infections in circumcised male infants. Pediatrics 1985;75:901.
4. Gee WF, Ansell JS. Neonatal circumcision: a ten year overview. Pediatrics 1976;58:824.
5. Fergusson DM, Hons BA, et al. Neonatal circumcision and penile problems: an eight year longitudinal study. Pediatrics 1988;81:537.
6. Schonfeld WA. Primary and secondary sexual characteristics. Am J Dis Child 1943;65:539.
7. Skoog SJ, Belman AB. Aphallia, its classification and management. J Urol 1989;141:589.
8. Kaplan GW, Lamm DL. Embryogenesis of chordee. J Urol 1975;114:769.
9. Nesbit RM. Congenital curvature of the phallus: report of three cases with description of corrective operation. J Urol 1965;93:230.
10. Kelami, A. Congenital penile deviation and its treatment with the Nesbit-Kelami Technique. Br J Urol 1987;60:261.
11. Ewalt DH, Cavender JD, Buchanan GR. Characterization and incidence of priapism in boys with Sickle Cell Anemia. Presented at the American Academy Pediatric Urologic Section 1995, Accepted for publication in J Pediatr Hematol Oncol.
12. Lamm DL, Kaplan GW. Accessory and etopic strota. Urology 1977;9:149.
13. Katz S, et al. Surgical evaluation of Henoch-Schonlein Purpura. Arch Surg 1991;126:849–52.
14. Eadie DGA, Higgins PM. Apparent torsion of the testicle in a case of Henoch-Schonlein purpura. Br J Urol 1964;51:634.
15. Loh HS, Jalan OM. Testicular torsion in the Henoch-Schonlein syndrome. Br Med J 1974;ii:96.
16. Brandes SB, Chelsky MJ, Hanno PM. Adult acute idiopathic scrotal edema. Urology 1994;44(4):602–605.
17. Johnston JH. Abnormalities of the scrotum and testes. In: Williams DI, ed. Pediatric Urology. NY: Appleton-Century-Crofts 1970;470.
18. Najmaldin A, Burge DM. Acute idiopathic scrotal oedema: incidence, manifestations, and aetiology. Br J Urol 1987;74:634–635.
19. Nour S, MacKinnon AE. Acute scrotal swelling in children. J R Coll Surg Edinb 1991;36(6):392.
20. Werner H, Falk M. Acute gangrene of the scrotum in an 8 year old. J Pediatr 1964;65:133.
21. Adeyokunnu AA. Fourniers syndrome in infants. Clin Pediatr 1983;22(2):101–103.
22. Bloom DA, Wan J, Key D. Disorders of the male external genitalia and inguinal canal. In: Kelalis PP, King LR, Belman AB, eds. Clinical Pediatric Urology 3rd ed., Philadelphia. W. B. Saunders 1992;1028.
23. Bloom DA, Ayers JW, McGuire EJ. The role of laparscopy in the management of the nonpalpable testes. J Urol 1988;94:465.
24. Kogan SJ, Gill B, Bennett B. Human monorchism: a clinicopathologic study of unilateral absent testis in 65 boys. J Urol 1986;135:758.
25. Brothers LR III, Weber CH Jr, Ball TP Jr. Anorchism vs. cryptorchism: the importance of a diligent search for intra-abdominal testis. J Urol 1978;119:707.
26. Levitt SB, Kogan SJ, Schneider KM, et al. Endocrine test in phenotypic children with bilateral impalpable testes can reliably predict 'congenital' anorchism. Urology 1978;11:11.
27. Barrow M, Gough MH. Bilateral absence of testis. Lancet 1970;1:366.
28. Bartone FF, Huseman CA, Maizels M, Firlit CF. Pitfalls in Using Human Chorionic Gonadotropin Stimulation Test to Diagnose Anorchia. J Urol 1987;131:563.
29. Cassarola FG, Golden SM, Johnsonbaugh RE, et al. Testicular volume during early infancy. J Pediatr 1981;99:742.
30. Bartsch G, Frank St. Marberger H, Mikuz G. Testicular torsion: late results with special regard to fertility and endocrine function. J Urol 1980;124:375.
31. Das SE, Singer A. Controversies of perinatal torsion of the

spermatic cord: a review survey and recommendations. J Urol 1990;143:231.

32. Jerkins GR, Noe HN, et al. Spermatic cord torsion in the neonate. J Urol 1983;129:121.

33. Cumming DC, Hyndmon CM, Deacon JSR. Intrauterine testicular torsion: not an emergency. Urology 1979;14:603.

34. Williamson RCN. Torsion of the testis and allied conditions. Br J Surg 1976;63:465.

35. Barada JH, Weingarten JL, Cromie WJ. Testicular salvage and age related delay in the presentation of testicular torsion. J Urol 1989;142:746.

36. Rabinowitz R. The importance of the cremasteric reflex in acute scrotal swelling in children. J Urol 1984;132:89.

37. Krarup T. The testis after torsion. Br J Urol 1978;50:43.

38. Harrison RG, Lewis Jones DI, et al. Mechanism of damage to the contralateral testis in rats with an ischaemic testis. Lancet 1981;II:723.

39. Nagler HM, de Vere White R. The effect of testicular torsion on the contralateral testis. J Urol 1990;65:225.

40. Anderson JD, Williamson RCN. Fertility after torsion of the spermatic cord. Br J Surg 1985;72:237.

41. Fraser I, Slater N, et al. Testicular torsion does not cause autoimmunization in man. Br J Surg 1985;72:237.

42. Hadžiselimović F, Snyder A, Duckett J, Howards S. Testicular histology in children with unilateral testicular torsion. J Urol 1986;136:208.

43. Dresner ML. Torsed appendage: diagnosis and management, blue dot sign. Urology 1973;1:63.

CHAPTER 32

Intersex States

Julia Spencer Barthold and Ricardo González

Intersexuality, particularly when associated with genital ambiguity, has been a subject of fascination and controversy throughout recorded history. As reviewed by van Niekerk,[1] the Greeks romanticized intersexuality and applied the concept to many of their gods, but by the Middle Ages intersexuals were subject to persecution. New and Kitzinger resurrected the enduring legend of Pope Joan, an alleged female pope with apparent genital ambiguity.[2] Official records of such a papacy do not exist, but subsequent voluminous writings describe a probable genetic female with congenital adrenal hyperplasia who was condemned for her sex and removed from office after delivering a child. One piece of evidence that appears to support her existence is the "porphyry chair," a red marble chair with a perforated seat allegedly used after 1099 AD to palpate the genitalia of the prospective pope during installation ceremonies to confirm his male gender. That intersex disorders can be diagnosed neonatally and sometimes prenatally, and definitively treated early in life has ushered in a new era of controversy. Some affected individuals and others interested in the field urge that strict categorization of intersex newborns as male or female and early surgical intervention be avoided, and that individuals with intersex be allowed to choose to live as male, female, or "intersexual" when old enough to decide for themselves.[3,4,5]

Intersexuality is classically defined as the expression of male and female physical and sexual characteristics within the same individual. For practical purposes, any instance of abnormal sexual determination or differentiation is considered an intersex state. In the past, these disorders were classified based primarily on phenotype and, when available, karyotypic, histologic, radiologic, and endocrine data. More precise classification is possible based on molecular data. The most significant recent discovery is identification of the SRY (*sex determining region of the Y* chromosome) gene and confirmation that it is a prerequisite for testicular determination. However, genetic analysis of intersex subjects has shown that testis determination can occur in the absence of SRY or fail in the presence of SRY, confirming that sex chromosome complement alone does not determine the fate of the bipotential gonad. Furthermore, recent data suggest that syndromes once thought to be distinct may represent a spectrum of diseases of similar etiology. Moreover, a range of phenotypes may be present in individuals with the same genetic mutation. Although phenotypic classifications help diagnose individual patients, intersex states are best characterized primarily as abnormalities of gonadal determination (differentiation and maintenance of the bipotential gonad as ovary or testis) or of genital differentiation (development of the internal and external genitalia along masculine or feminine lines). This classification scheme is used throughout this review.

OVERVIEW OF NORMAL SEXUAL DIFFERENTIATION

Development of sexual phenotype depends on the degree of testicular determination and by subsequent testicular function (see Chapters 9, 10, and 38 for details of gonadal and genital development). Evidence suggests that multiple genes are required for formation of the bipotential gonad and for subsequent development of testis and ovary. However, whereas the female phenotype develops by default in the absence of a functional testis, normal male development requires timely and complete testicular determination, differentiation, and function.

Gonadal Determination

At least two genes, WT-1 (the Wilms' tumor gene) and Ftz-F1, a gene encoding steroidogenic factor-1 (SF-1) are known to be reqired for development of the bipotential gonad (Fig. 32.1) because gonads of any type do not develop in transgenic mice homozygous for a deletion of either gene.[6,7] However, once the gonad is formed, the pivotal event in sexual differentiation is

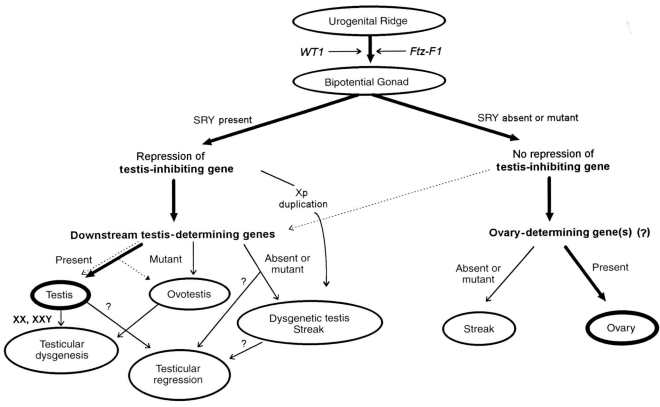

FIG. 32.1. Proposed scheme for gonadal determination.[36, 37] The normal pathways for testis and ovary determination are indicated by bold arrows. The genes for Wilms' tumor (WT1) and steroidogenic factor 1 (Ftz-F1) are required for formation of the bipotential gonad. If SRY (sex-determining region, Y chromosome) is present, a putative testis inhibiting gene is repressed, allowing activation of downstream testis-determining genes. Absence or mutation of one of these genes leads to complete or partial gonadal dysgenesis (streak, dysgenetic testis, or testicular regression) or true hermaphroditism (ovotestis). In the absence of SRY, the ovarian pathway is activated; however, if the putative testis-inhibiting gene is absent or mutant (dotted lines) or an activating mutation of a downstream testis-determining gene is present testis determination will proceed.

presence or absence of testis determination. The testicular determination pathway is activated by SRY, a gene located on the short arm of the Y chromosome that encodes a transcription factor containing a conserved HMG (high mobility group) DNA-binding domain.[8, 9] To explain testicular development in 46,XX, SRY-negative subjects and lack thereof in 46,XY, SRY-positive males, it has recently been hypothesized that the SRY protein negatively regulates a downstream inhibitory gene in the testicular determination pathway (Fig. 32.1).[10] This putative gene, thought to act as a link between the testis and ovary determining pathways, may be located on the short arm of the X chromosome (Xp) at a locus variously termed TDF-X (*testis determining factor-X* chromosome),[11, 12] SRVX (*sex reversal X*)[13] or, most commonly, DSS (*dosage-sensitive sex reversal*).[14] Observations that support the theory that DSS inhibits testicular development include the finding of testicular differentiation in 46,XX subject with an Xp deletion[15]

and Xp duplication associated with XY sex reversal caused presumably by double dosage of the inhibitory gene that cannot be repressed by SRY.[16, 17] Furthermore, deletion of Xp in 46,XY individuals is compatible with normal male development.[15]

Other downstream, X-linked, or autosomal genes appear to be required for testis determination, based on studies of familial transmission of gonadal dysgenesis syndromes and XX sex reversal. Mutations in these genes may result in failure of normal testicular development (gonadal dysgenesis) or escape from regulation by SRY (testis development in the absence of a Y chromosome or SRY; demonstrated by the dotted lines in Fig. 32.1). Those downstream testis determining genes that have been identified include SOX9 (an *SRY*-like HMG b*ox* gene located on chromosome 17),[18] and genes located on 10q[19] and 9p.[20] Mutations in testis determining genes downstream of SRY appear to produce a spectrum of phenotypes (Fig. 32.1), including complete gonadal dysgenesis (streak gonads), dysgenetic testes, and possibly absence of testes in intersex individuals (testicular regression syndrome); these entities are discussed in detail later.

In the absence of SRY, the "default" pathway is ovarian development. However, evidence suggests that specific genes are required for ovarian determination because gonadal dysgenesis occurs in 45,X females (Turner's syndrome) and in some 46,XX females through autosomal recessive inheritance.

Genital Differentiation

Once the testis determination pathway is initiated, male sexual development depends on complete development and maintenance of a functional testis. The critical events for each sex are shown in Figure 32.2.[21-25] The earliest event in the gonad destined to be a testis is

appearance of Sertoli cells and almost simultaneous expression of Müllerian inhibiting substance (MIS), which is secreted from these cells.[26] Subsequently, Leydig cell secretion of testosterone (T) begins, a process that may initially be independent of gonadotropins,[27] but which is subsequently stimulated by placental human chorionic gonadotropin (hCG) and then fetal luteinizing hormone (LH). MIS and T appear to control all phases of male genital differentiation, except for testicular descent, which may require another testicular hormone or factor in addition to T.[28] Ipsilateral Wolffian duct development requires local production of T, which may diffuse down the duct to produce its effect.[29] If T production is delayed or insufficient, or androgen insensitivity is present, irreversible regression of the Wolffian duct occurs by the 9th week of gestation. Similarly, Müllerian duct stabilization occurs after the 7th week in the absence of MIS secretion or function. Masculinization of the external genitalia

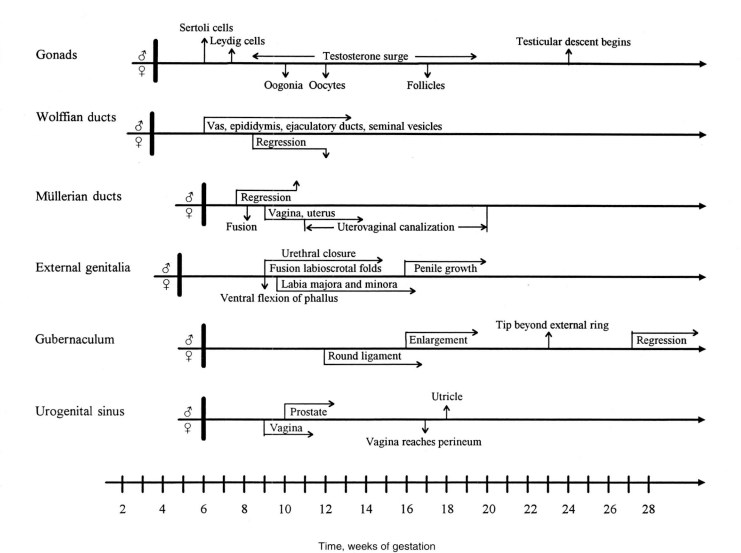

FIG. 32.2. Timeline of genital differentiation in male and female human fetuses.[21-25]

largely depends on the enzyme steroid 5α-reductase type 2, which converts T to dihydrotestosterone (DHT).

Animal and clinical studies suggest interplay between MIS and sex steroidal function in fetal and postnatal life.[26, 30] For example, MIS overproduction in transgenic mice causes ovarian germ cell loss and Sertoli cell differentiation in females (gonadal sex reversal) and impaired T synthesis with hypospadias and cryptorchidism in males. Conversely, mice lacking the MIS or MIS receptor gene have normal gonadal development and testicular descent but persistence of Müllerian-derived structures. Fetal Müllerian ducts exposed to exogenous estrogen become resistant to MIS, and MIS levels are abnormally high in androgen insensitivity syndrome. The significance of these observations vis à vis normal sexual differentiation remains poorly understood.

The mechanism by which SRY triggers production of testicular hormones also remains largely unknown. Several gene products appear to be upregulated by SRY, at least indirectly.[31, 32] One of the most important of these proteins is SF-1, which is expressed in multiple sites within the embryonic reproductive tract including the bipotential gonad, Sertoli and Leydig cells, and the hypothalamus and pituitary.[33] SF-1 appears to play a role in gonadal determination (see earlier) and in regulation of genes for MIS, the steroid hydroxylases (which encode enzymes required for testosterone biosynthesis), aromatase, gonadotropins, and the gonadotropin-releasing hormone receptor. SF-1 may also regulate the DAX-1 gene,[34] located on Xp and a possible candidate for the DSS testis inhibitory gene.[35] A link between SRY and expression of the MIS gene has also been identified, but the effect is indirect.[8, 31]

In summary, the master switch for testis determination is SRY, which interrupts the programmed differentiation of the gonad into an ovary, triggered by a putative testis-inhibiting gene. SRY probably represses gene(s) in the ovary determining pathway and upregulates a spectrum of genes required for differentiation of the testis and for the timely secretion of hormones required for successful male genital differentiation.

ABNORMALITIES OF GONADAL DETERMINATION

Gonadal determination disorders comprise a spectrum of diseases ranging from complete absence of gonadal development to delayed gonadal failure caused by intrinsic developmental anomalies (Table 32.1). The former group includes failed gonadal development in genetic males and females with complete gonadal dysgenesis caused by genetic abnormalities of sex or autosomal chromosomes. The term partial gonadal dysgenesis is used to refer to a group of related disorders in which partial testicular determination occurred at some point during development, and includes the syndromes of mixed gonadal dysgenesis, dysgenetic male pseudo-hermaphroditism, and some cases of testicular regression.[36, 37] Available clinical and genetic data suggest that these syndromes are different phenotypic manifestations of a common disease process. Rare cases of true hermaphroditism and 46,XX sex reversal may also represent forms of partial gonadal dysgenesis. Finally, diseases associated with normal testicular determination in utero but subsequent testicular failure include true hermaphroditism, classical 46,XX sex reversal, and Klinefelter's syndrome.

Complete Gonadal Dysgenesis

If there is no testicular determination, the bipotential gonad continues along the ovarian determination pathway. If a single X chromosome is present, as in individuals with a 45,X karyotype (Turner's syndrome) the gonad differentiates as an ovary but subsequently degenerates into a streak gonad comprised of ovarian-like stroma and few or no germ cells.[38] Indirect evidence suggests that the streak gonads found in patients with "pure" (XX or XY) gonadal dysgenesis are also degenerated ovaries.[36, 39, 40] XX and XY gonadal dysgenesis are distinguished from Turner's syndrome because they usually lack the associated stigmata observed in patients with a 45,X chromosomal complement. However, sexual differentiation is similar in the three groups.

XY Gonadal Dysgenesis

Etiology

Also called XY sex reversal or Swyer's syndrome, XY complete gonadal dysgenesis is caused by absence of testicular determination despite presence of a Y chromosome. Familial incidence in some cases suggests X-linked recessive or male-limited autosomal dominant inheritance.[39, 40] In approximately 15% of cases, mutations in SRY can be detected, and in most of these the mutation affects the DNA binding domain of the protein.[41, 42] In some instances the mutation was present in other phenotypically normal male family members, demonstrating variable expression of the abnormal genotype. In some cases more extensive Y chromosomal deletion or translocation is present. Other causes of isolated XY gonadal dysgenesis in otherwise normal individuals have not been well characterized but are presumably caused by mutations in regulatory regions adjacent to the SRY gene or in other X-chromosomal or autosomal testis determining genes.

Clinical Features

Presentation is typically that of a phenotypic female with normal or hypoplastic external genitalia and de-

TABLE 32.1. *Characteristics of intersex disorders classified by genital phenotype*

Syndrome	Typical genital phenotype	Karyotype	Type of gonad	WD	MD	Testicular position	Puberty*	Gonadal tumor/fertility	Other clinical features	Genetic mutations identified	Diagnosis
21-hydroxylase deficiency (CAH)	Ambiguous	XX	Ovary	−	+	–	Virilization	No/Yes	Salt wasting	CYP21	↑17α-hydroxyprogesterone
11-hydroxylase deficiency (CAH)	Ambiguous	XX	Ovary	−	+	–	Virilization	No/Yes	HTN, ↓K+	CYP11β1	↑11-deoxycortisol, ↑DOC
3β-hydroxysteroid dehydrogenase deficiency (CAH)	Ambiguous	XY	Testis	+	−	Labioscrotal inguinal	Virilization or gynecomastia	No/No	Salt wasting	3β-HSD type II	↑DHEA, ↑17α-hydroxy-pregnenolone
17β-hydroxysteroid dehydrogenase deficiency	Ambiguous	XY	Testis	+	−	Usually inguinal, variable	Virilization or gynecomastia	No/No	↑LH, FSH (adult)	17β-HSD type 3	↑Androstenedione/T ratio (±hCG stimulation)
5α-reductase 2 deficiency	Ambiguous	XY	Testis	+	−	Inguinal, labioscrotal	Virilization	No/No	↑LH (adult)	SRD5A2	↑T/DHT ratio (±hCG stimulation)
Partial androgen insensitivity (PAIS)	Ambiguous	XY	Testis	±	±	Inguinal, labioscrotal	Partial virilization	Yes/No	↑or N LH and T	AR	AR analysis, ↓SHBG suppression by stanazol
True hermaphroditism	Ambiguous	XX, XX/XY or XY	Ovotestis, Ovary, Testis	±	+	Palpable in 60% of patients	Virilization or feminization	Rare/Rare (females)		Y translocation or SRY− (rare)	Gonadal histology
Partial gonadal dysgenesis	Ambiguous	X0/XY, XY	Testis, streak, regression	±	+	Inguinal, scrotal, abdominal	Virilization	Yes/No	±Turner stigmata	Majority unknown	Gonadal histology
XX sex reversal	Male (classic) Ambiguous	XX	Testis	+	−	Usually scrotal	Virilization, gynecomastia	No/No	Short stature	Y translocation	Gonadal histology
Klinefelter's syndrome	Male	XXY or mosaics	Testis	+	−	Scrotal	Virilization, gynecomastia	No/No	Tall stature	Karyotype	Karyotype
Persistent Müllerian duct syndrome	Male	XY	Testis	+	+	Scrotal, transverse ectopy, abdominal	Normal virilization	Yes/No	↓serum MIS (~50%)	MIS, MIS receptor	Surgical exploration
Complete androgen insensitivity (CAIS)	Female	XY	Testis	Rare	±	Inguinal, abdominal, labioscrotal	Gynecomastia	Yes/No	Taller than normal ♀	AR	↑or normal T, ↑LH, AR analysis
17α-hydroxylase/17,20 lyase deficiency (CAH)	Female	XY	Testis	+	−	Abdominal, inguinal	Absent	No/No	HTN, ↓K+	P450c17	↑corticosterone, DOC, pregnenolone, progesterone
Leydig cell agenesis	Female	XY	Testis	+	−	Usually inguinal	Absent	No/No		LH receptor, abnormal Y	No T response to hCG, nl androgen precursors, ↑LH
Turner's syndrome	Female	X0/XX, X0	Streak	−	+	–	Absent	No/No	Stigmata		Karyotype
XY gonadal dysgenesis	Female	XY	Streak	Very rare	+	–	Absent	Yes/No	±Turner stigmata	SRY, WT1, SOX9, Xp duplication	Gonadal histology, ↑LH, ↑FSH, no T response to hCG stimulation
XX gonadal dysgenesis	Female	XX	Streak	−	+	–	Absent	No/No		FSH receptor	Gonadal histology, ↑LH, ↑FSH

*Possible changes at puberty in untreated individuals.

WD, Wolffian duct structures; MD, Müllerian duct structures; DOC, deoxycorticosterone; DHEA, dihydroepiandrosterone; LH, luteinizing hormone; FSH, follicle stimulating hormone; T, testosterone; AR, androgen receptor; SHBG, sex hormone binding globulin; MIS, Müllerian inhibiting substance.

layed pubertal development.[36, 39] In rare cases, minimal virilization may be present. Müllerian ductal structures are present and Wolffian duct derivatives usually absent except for occasional microscopic remnants. Adult height tends to be greater than normal females, presumably because of the presence of Y-linked growth gene(s), but shorter than normal males because of the absence of androgens.[43, 44] Endocrine studies show normal female levels of T and elevated, castrate range serum LH and FSH. Streak gonads are present bilaterally and are comprised of ovarian-type stroma with primitive or absent germ cells. Ovarian follicles have been observed in fetuses and young children, suggesting that streak gonads are degenerated ovaries. Cases may be familial or sporadic; however, expression of the disorder within families may show phenotypic variability with regard to the degree of gonadal dysgenesis. Occasional patients with the stigmata of Turner's syndrome have been reported; most of these have deletions of the short arm of the Y chromosome (Yp) that encompass SRY and a putative "anti-Turner" gene on Yp.[36, 45]

The risk of gonadal malignancy is significantly increased in streak gonads when Y chromosomal material is present. Although there are reports of gonadoblastoma in the absence of Y genetic material in the older literature, newer molecular data suggest that this rarely occurs.[46–48] Recent data suggest that a gonadoblastoma locus (GBY) is present on the proximal long arm of the Y chromosome, which predisposes dysgenetic gonads to malignant degeneration.[49, 50] Gonadoblastoma is comprised of primitive germ cells, immature Sertoli or granulosa cells with or without Leydig or lutein-type cells and is considered an in situ germ cell tumor.[46, 51] It occurs in 25 to 60% of individuals with XY gonadal dysgenesis, is more common in familial cases, and is frequently bilateral. More aggressive secondary malignancies such as dysgerminoma/seminoma and nonseminomatous germ cell tumors may arise in up to 50% and 10% of cases, respectively. Gonadoblastoma or dysgerminoma may be present in streak or dysgenetic gonads in early infancy or childhood, whereas the more malignant germ cell tumors are usually diagnosed at puberty or later.

Associated Syndromes

Several known genetic mutations produce syndromes that are associated with XY complete gonadal dysgenesis, which include duplication of the short arm of chromosome X (Xp), mutations in the autosomal genes WT-1 (Denys-Drash syndrome) and SOX9 (campomelic dysplasia), and deletions of 10q and 9p.

The specific gene on Xp that is responsible for sex reversal has not been identified but is most frequently referred to as DSS (dosage sensitive sex reversal).[16, 17] It is hypothesized that the duplicated gene escapes X inactivation, and is therefore expressed in double dos-

age, which disrupts testis formation despite expression of SRY. The possibility that DSS may be the testis inhibitory gene that is theoretically repressed by SRY in the testis determining pathway (Fig. 32.1) awaits confirmation. Patients with Xp duplication encompassing the DSS critical region (Xp 21.3) have complete or partial gonadal dysgenesis and frequently have associated somatic anomalies including facial dysmorphism, cleft palate, cardiac anomalies, and mental retardation.

Denys-Drash syndrome occurs in patients with mutations in WT1 and is characterized by female or ambiguous genitalia in 46,XY individuals, progressive nephropathy and Wilms' tumor.[52, 53] The gonadal phenotype is markedly variable; of cases in which it was documented, 73% had complete or partial gonadal dysgenesis; the coexistence of ovarian and testicular tissue (true hermaphroditism) was also reported. Müllerian ductal differentiation was observed adjacent to testes, suggesting that abnormal testicular differentiation had occurred. Nephropathy and Wilms' tumor are usually identified within the first and second years of life, respectively. Denys-Drash syndrome should be distinguished from other syndromes associated with renal disease and abnormal sexual differentiation. In the Frasier syndrome, nephropathy and complete gonadal dysgenesis occur in the absence of mutations in the WT1 gene.[54] WT1 mutations have been identified in the WAGR syndrome (Wilms' tumor, aniridia, genitourinary abnormalities, and mental retardation), but nephropathy and gonadal dysgenesis do not occur.[52] In addition, WT1 mutations have not been linked to isolated cases of XY gonadal dysgenesis or genital malformation.[55, 56] In summary, a spectrum of gonadal and genital anomalies is seen in patients with mutations of WT1, but associated renal anomalies are always present.

Mutations in the SOX9 gene, located on chromosome 17, are associated with campomelic dysplasia (dwarfism) with or without XY sex reversal.[57] Affected individuals have multiple skeletal malformations and the disease is usually lethal. Most commonly, 46,XY-affected individuals have complete gonadal dysgenesis, although partial gonadal dysgenesis is also seen, and markedly different phenotypes have been seen in unrelated patients with the same mutation. Similarly, terminal deletions of the short arm of chromosome 9 (9p)[20] and the long arm of chromosome 10 (10q)[19] may cause complete gonadal dysgenesis and multiple somatic anomalies including microcephaly, facial anomalies, and widely spaced nipples. Both 9p and 10q deletions are also associated with ambiguous genitalia and partial gonadal dysgenesis.

Management

The diagnosis is confirmed by karyotypic analysis and identification of streak gonads, uterus, and Fallopian tubes. Gonadectomy is indicated at the time of diagnosis because of the risk of malignancy. Estrogen replacement therapy is indicated at the time of expected puberty (see management of Turner's syndrome, later).

XX Gonadal Dysgenesis

Etiology

"Pure" gonadal dysgenesis in females with a normal 46,XX chromosomal complement is likely a heterogeneous disorder that is sporadic or inherited as an autosomal recessive trait.[39, 58] Two known causes include mutations of WT1 (Denys-Drash syndrome) in 46,XX individuals[52] and a point mutation of the FSH receptor gene.[59]

Clinical Features and Management

As with the XY form of "pure" gonadal dysgenesis, affected individuals have primary or, less commonly, early secondary ovarian failure. Streak gonads, normal female genitalia, and Müllerian ductal structures are present, although primordial follicles may be seen in the group with an FSH receptor mutation.[59] Unlike patients with XY gonadal dysgenesis, stature is in the normal female range and there is no increased risk of gonadal tumor.

Turner's Syndrome

Individuals with complete or mosaic X monosomy (45,X or 45,X/46,XX) or with significant deletions of an X chromosome may have gonadal dysgenesis and somatic features characteristic of Turner's syndrome.[38, 60]

Etiology

Recently, sensitive detection techniques have shown that 45,X/46,XX mosaicism is present in as many as 74% of cases of Turner's syndrome. Considering that approximately 99% of 45,X embryos abort spontaneously, a mosaic karyotype may improve the likelihood of fetal survival. The incidence of classic Turner's syndrome is approximately 1 in 2,000 live female births. Turner stigmata are also observed in patients with specific deletions of the short or long arms of the X or Y chromosomes.[36, 45, 61] Therefore, it is theorized that homologous genes that are not subject to X-inactivation are present on both sex chromosomes, and normally prevent Turner-type stigmata in males and females; haploinsufficiency of one of these "anti-Turner" genes results in characteristics of Turner's syndrome.[61]

Clinical Features

Patients may be diagnosed prenatally by karyotype analysis or by findings of nuchal fold thickening, cystic hygroma, horseshoe kidney, or cardiac anomalies. However, it is important to note that most 45,X/46,XX individuals identified by prenatal screening have a normal phenotype.[62] Postnatal features leading to the diagnosis include webbed neck, low hairline and swelling of extremities caused by congenital lymphedema, shield chest, and widely spaced nipples. Other anomalies include aortic valvular defect, coarctation of the aorta, horseshoe kidney, or other renal anomalies. Later manifestations include impaired somatic growth and absent puberty. Although some degree of pubertal development is possible in up to 25% of girls, menstruation is rare. Pathologic study of 45,X fetuses shows that ovaries differentiate but subsequently degenerate to form streak gonads. Gonadoblastoma does not occur in the absence of Y chromosomal material.

Management

Growth hormone treatment is recommended beginning early in childhood. Graded estrogen therapy is recommended, and when begun at 14 to 15 years of age rather than earlier, final height is optimized.[60] Pregnancy is possible using donor eggs and assisted reproductive techniques, and has also occurred spontaneously in rare instances.

Partial Gonadal Dysgenesis

In the presence of SRY, impaired testicular determination or differentiation results in partial gonadal dysgenesis. Although the phenotypic manifestations are variable, the pathophysiology of each syndrome is thought to be similar. Patients usually have a 46,XY, 45,X/46,XY, or other mosaic karyotype and streak, absent or dysgenetic gonads. Combinations may include a streak gonad and dysgenetic testis (mixed gonadal dysgenesis) (Fig. 32.3), bilateral dysgenetic testes (dysgenetic male pseudohermaphroditism) or absence of one or both testes (embryonic testicular regression sequence).[36, 37, 63–65]

Etiology

Karyotype may be 45,X/46,XY or 46,XY, although the former is more common in patients who have the clinical picture of mixed gonadal dysgenesis. Nevertheless, prenatal diagnosis has shown that most individuals (95%) with 45,X/46,XY or related mosaicisms have a normal male phenotype.[66] The difference between the prenatally diagnosed cases and those with abnormal genital development and 45,X/46,XY mosaicism postnatally is unknown. One explanation may be related to the type of cell line differentiation within the gonads. For example, Sugarman et al reported a patient with peripheral mosaicism whose streak

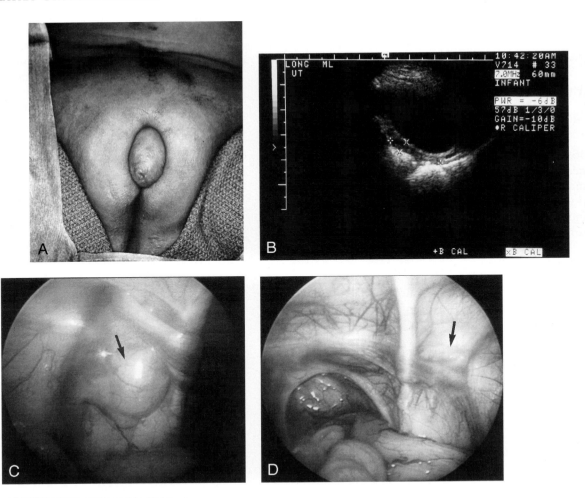

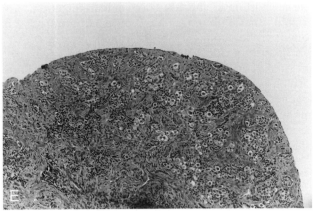

FIG. 32.3. Case of partial gonadal dysgenesis in a 3-month-old 46,XY infant without palpable gonads assigned a female sex of rearing. After hCG, serum T and T:DHT ratio were normal. A macroscopically normal left testis and a right streak gonad and fallopian tube were removed and clitoroplasty and vaginoplasty performed. **A,** Photograph of ambiguous genitalia with a 1.5 cm phallus, urogenital sinus (not shown) and feminine labioscrotal folds. **B,** Pelvic ultrasound showing a uterus identified by cursors. **C,** Laparoscopic view of right testis (*arrow*) proximal to internal ring. **D,** Laparoscopic view of left streak gonad and fallopian tube (*arrow*). **E,** Photomicrograph of the streak gonad with disorganized ovarian-type stroma and many primitive follicles (reduced from ×125).

gonad was comprised of 45,X cells while the contralateral normal testis contained Y chromosome-bearing cells.[67]

Mutations within the SRY gene itself result in complete gonadal dysgenesis, although the partial form is reported in a patient with a mutation upstream of SRY.[68] By contrast, many of the mutations reported for other putative sex determining regions, which result in com-

plete XY gonadal dysgenesis (such as Xp duplication, 10q deletion, WT1 mutations [Denys-Drash syndrome] or mutations in X-linked genes), are also reported in cases of partial gonadal dysgenesis. However, the etiology of gonadal dysgenesis remains unknown in most cases. Some cases of embryonic testicular regression appear to be inherited through an X-linked or autosomal mechanism.[37, 69]

Clinical Features

Deficient virilization, i.e., ambiguous genitalia or hypospadias with cryptorchidism, is seen in most patients with partial gonadal dysgenesis (Fig. 32.3). If severe feminization is present, the diagnosis may be delayed until virilization occurs at puberty; conversely, feminization of a phenotypic male may be caused by an estrogen-secreting gonadoblastoma. Rarely, fully masculinized external genitalia are present. However, all patients have a uterus and at least one fallopian tube, and variable degrees of Wolffian duct differentiation. Up to a third of patients with 46,XY or mosaic karyotype have Turner stigmata or isolated short stature, likely because of deletion of critical region(s) on the X or Y chromosome.

Gonadal development consists of a dysgenetic or apparently normal testis and a contralateral dysgenetic testis, streak, or absent gonad. The available data suggest that a spectrum of gonadal development may occur within the same individual or in familial cases,[36, 37] possibly because of intrinsic asymmetry in embryologic development of the gonad or to mosaicism within the gonads. Impaired Müllerian inhibition and virilization in these individuals, irrespective of the histology of the gonads, suggests inadequate or delayed fetal testicular function. It was recently reported that dysgenetic testes express MIS,[70] so that persistence of Müllerian ducts is likely caused by insufficient or delayed production of the hormone. Embryonic testicular regression (absence of one or both gonads in 46,XY feminized individuals) was originally hypothesized to be caused by sudden loss of testicular tissue at a critical point in gestation.[71, 72] However, incongruity between the degree of masculinization and Müllerian duct regression in many individuals suggests that the testis is abnormal before regressing and that this syndrome is another manifestation of gonadal dysgenesis[37] (see Fig. 32.1). These patients are differentiated from cases of testicular absence in phenotypically normal males, which is likely because of testicular loss late in gestation after sexual differentiation is complete. Referred to as "testicular regression" by some authors,[73] this is more commonly called "vanishing testis syndrome."

Streak gonads contain ovarian type stroma and rare poorly developed tubules.[74, 75] Occasional primordial follicles may be present in infants and young children (Fig. 32.3), but should not lead to the misdiagnosis of true hermaphroditism. As many as a third of these streak gonads have adjacent epididymal structures. Dysgenetic testes may appear normal grossly, but microscopic abnormalities include disorganization of the hilar region, hypoplastic tubules surrounded by ovarian or fibrotic stroma, and discontinuity of the tunica albuginea. The risk of gonadoblastoma in patients with the partial (as

in the complete) form of gonadal dysgenesis is reportedly 15 to 30%.[46, 63, 64] As stated earlier, gonadoblastoma is frequently associated with malignant germ cell tumors; typical CIS may also be seen in patients with partial gonadal dysgenesis.[76, 77] The incidence of gonadoblastoma appears to be higher in more undervirilized patients and the most common associated karyotype is 46,XY.[51, 63] Although the degree of impairment of testicular descent correlates with risk of malignancy, tumors have also been reported in scrotal testes.[51] In half of the cases in which the original gonadal histology is evident, the tumor was shown to arise within a dysgenetic testis.

Management

Female sex of rearing is preferred in patients with severe undervirilization, particularly because the gonads are at risk for malignancy and chance for fertility is essentially nil, even when mature spermatozoa are present in a descended testis. Streak gonads and undescended testes should be removed at the time of diagnosis. If male gender is chosen before or at the time of diagnosis, management of a scrotal testis remains controversial. Testicular biopsy has been advocated, but prepubertal histologic findings may not reflect the risk of malignancy.[75] All testes that are not removed should be observed closely, possibly with serial biopsy.

True Hermaphroditism

Ovarian and testicular determination in the same individual is called true hermaphroditism (TH). The diagnosis is reserved for cases in which the coexistence of seminiferous tubules and normal ovarian tissue is proven by histology, and should not be used in cases of dysgenetic gonads in young infants in whom scattered primordial follicles may be present. As with other disorders of gonadal determination besides Turner's syndrome, the disease is rare and is familial in a subset of patients.[78]

Etiology

The cause of TH is multifactorial and varies geographically.[1, 78] Overall, the most common karyotype, recorded in 70% of cases, is 46,XX and is almost exclusively seen in African blacks. 46,XX/46,XY or other mosaicism (such as 45,X/46,XY) is present in 20%, 46,XY in 7%, and other karyotypes in the remainder of cases. Mutations in the SRY gene in individuals with a 46,XY cell line and translocation of Y chromosomal material, including SRY, to an X chromosome are reported rarely (10% or less of cases).[79–82] When SRY is present, possible explanations for the coexistence of ovarian and testicular determination include gonadal mosaicism, X-inactivation of a proportion of Y-bearing X chromosomes within gonadal cells, or mutation of downstream testis determining genes with only partial expression of SRY. In individuals identified as SRY-negative, possible causes include mosaicism limited to the gonad[83] or mutation of a testis-inhibiting gene, which may be X-linked and undergo X-inactivation in some gonadal cells but not others.[80, 81] A case of TH that supports the latter mechanism is that of a 46,XX, SRY-negative individual with a deletion of distal Xp, including the putative testis-inhibitory DSS region.[15] Recent data also suggest that TH may exist in a spectrum of related gonadal differentiation disorders. For example, TH and XX sex reversal have occurred within the same family, suggesting that they represent alternative phenotypes of the same genetic defect.[84, 85] Similarly, it is theorized that dysgenetic testes may be degenerated ovotestes and that partial gonadal dysgenesis and TH may also represent a spectrum of related diseases.[36]

Clinical Features

Patients most commonly have ambiguous genitalia, although near-normal female or male genitalia may be present. Although a correlation between karyotype (presence of a Y chromosome) and phenotype has been suggested,[1] this has been unconfirmed by more recent data.[78] Rarely, well-masculinized patients may present after puberty with gynecomastia, cyclical hematuria, or scrotal pain secondary to ruptured ovarian follicles.[86] One or both gonads are palpable in at least 60% of patients,[1] most commonly on the right side[87] and may be irregularly shaped in some cases. A vagina and uterus are each reported in 80 to 100% of cases. Typically, the urogenital sinus is short and the uterus is abnormal (lacking a cervix, unicornuate or bicornuate, or hypoplastic).[1]

Data from two large reviews suggest that the most common gonad found is the ovotestis (50%), followed by ovary (30%) and testis (20%).[1, 83] Combinations, in order of frequency, are ovotestis/ovary (34%), bilateral ovotestis or ovary and testis (both 27%), and ovotestis/testis (12%). Testes occur more commonly on the right side and ovaries on the left, and the degree of descent of a testis or ovotestis is proportional to the percentage of testicular tissue present. Ovaries are usually in normal position; occasionally one is found prolapsed into an inguinal hernia or accompanying the contralateral testis into the scrotum. The ovarian and testicular tissue is situated end-to-end in most ovotestes; however, one cell type may be confined to the hilum in up to 20% of cases. The internal ducts are usually appropriate for the gonad if it is an ovary or testis; ovotestes are associated with a Fallopian tube more commonly than a vas or epididymis, and rarely both types of ducts may be present.

While ovarian histology and function is potentially normal, seminiferous tubular development and endocrine function of testicular tissue, irrespective of position or coexistence of ovarian tissue, is typically abnormal.[87-89] Spermatogonia may be present in infancy but usually disappear by early childhood. Interstitial fibrosis, tubular hyalinization, and infrequent spermatogenesis are reported in individuals raised as males, with fertility almost unheard of. Similarly, testosterone secretion is subnormal in most patients raised as males. By contrast, 21 pregnancies have been reported in patients raised as females; almost all have one ovary and a normal uterus.[83] Gonadal malignancy is rare, with an incidence of gonadoblastoma, dysgerminoma, and other germ cell tumors each occurring in approximately 1% of reported patients.[83]

Management

The diagnosis of TH is suspected in 46,XX patients with ambiguous genitalia, a combination of Müllerian and Wolffian derivatives and testosterone secretion, and requires biopsy-proven presence of ovarian and testicular tissue. Ovotestes usually have a grossly visible and palpable demarcation between the ovarian and testicular portions; the former is hard, and the latter soft. If no demarcation is apparent, ultrasound and testicular bivalving and biopsy are necessary. Gonadectomy is necessary if the inappropriate gonadal tissue cannot be completely removed. Adequate excision of testicular tissue can be confirmed postoperatively by measurement of stimulated androgen levels or serum MIS, which is undetectable when no testicular tissue is present.[90] Unfortunately, ovarian function cannot be evaluated prepubertally, but if significant ovarian tissue is left in situ, it may manifest as gynecomastia at puberty. In patients raised as males, all remaining testicular tissue should be left or placed in a scrotal location.[88] Despite biopsy, an erroneous diagnosis of partial XY gonadal dysgenesis or XX sex reversal with genital ambiguity may be made in certain cases if isolated islands of ovarian tissue are missed.

In an older series reported by van Niekerk, 75% of cases of TH were raised as males, possibly because most of them were evaluated medically during later childhood and adolescence.[1] van Niekerk stressed that sex reassignment should be performed in older individuals only when the gender identity is discordant with the sex of rearing. A female sex of rearing has been advocated more recently for most patients because of the potential for childbearing and the impaired exocrine and endocrine testicular function.[88] In a recent series, most patients were first evaluated in infancy, and only 8 of 22 (36%) were assigned a male sex of rearing because of significant virilization, normal hCG stimulation studies, an abnormal or absent uterus, or family concerns.[83]

These patients responded to hormonal stimulation with growth of the penis to appropriate size for age. However, testosterone supplementation may be required to initiate or sustain puberty if the quality or quantity of remaining testicular tissue is inadequate.

XX Sex Reversal

Testicular development alone in 46,XX individuals is considered XX sex reversal or XX maleness, and is estimated to be present in 1 in 20,000 to 30,000 males.[91] As with other abnormalities of gonadal determination, the etiology is multifactorial and a spectrum of phenotypes is seen.

Etiology

Translocation of part of the short arm of the Y chromosome, including SRY, to an X chromosome is demonstrable in approximately a third of the cases.[92, 93] Most commonly, SRY is present in fully masculinized patients and absent in undervirilized patients, although exceptions are reported.[94, 95] The etiology of testis determination in the absence of SRY is unknown, but may be related to loss of function of a testis-inhibiting gene (either autosomal or X-linked) or gain of function of a downstream testis-determining gene despite absence of SRY (see Fig. 32.1). Abbas et al noted phenotypic similarities between cases of SRY-negative TH and XX sex reversal, and postulate that the same genetic defect may produce either disease.[96] This is supported by the finding of both syndromes within the same family.[84, 85]

Clinical Features

"Classical" XX sex reversal (80–90% of cases) is typically diagnosed when normal males are evaluated for infertility, gynecomastia, or after karyotyping.[91, 94] Gynecomastia occurs in association with hyperestrogenism at puberty. XX males are also shorter than normal males presumably because of absence of a Y-linked growth gene.[43, 44] The earliest manifestation of testicular failure is absence of spermatogonia in early childhood.[91] Testosterone response to hCG stimulation and serum gonadotropins may be normal before puberty, but subsequent hypergonadotropic hypogonadism is the rule. Small, firm testes with impaired spermatogenesis and infertility are features shared with Klinefelter's syndrome (see later). The recent finding of Y-linked genes responsible for spermatogenesis on the long arm of the Y chromosome may explain the progressive testicular dysgenesis seen in XX males who may be missing these sequences.[97] Some patients (10%) have hypospadias, micropenis or cryptorchidism, or overt genital ambiguity;[92, 94–96] some have dysgenetic testes and persistent Müllerian structures.[98] These cases may represent a link in the testis

determination pathway between XX TH and XX sex reversal. There is no reported increased risk of gonadal malignancy in XX sex reversal.[46]

Management

The severity of genital ambiguity, when present, is not usually sufficient to warrant female sex of rearing. However, as in Klinefelter's syndrome, androgen production is often impaired at puberty in classic and nonclassic XX males and replacement therapy is required.[98]

Klinefelter's Syndrome

In males with at least one additional X chromosome, testicular determination occurs normally but is followed by testicular failure, which is well established by puberty. This disorder is called Klinefelter's syndrome and is present in approximately 0.1% of live male births.[99]

Etiology

Subjects most frequently have a 47,XXY karyotype that, in most cases, is caused by nondisjunction in the developing zygote, which results in 24,XX ova or 24,XY sperm. Other karyotypes that produce the syndrome include 46,XY/47,XXY mosaics, those with additional X or Y chromosomes (e.g., 48,XXXY, 48,XXYY, etc.) and 46,XX males with translocated Y chromosomal sequences.

Clinical Features

Patients most frequently present in the peripubertal period with infertility and gynecomastia. Occasional cases are identified during childhood because of genital anomalies (hypospadias, cryptorchidism, micropenis) or behavioral or learning disabilities. Although testes may be small and firm throughout childhood, the diagnosis is typically not made based on this finding because prepubertal testicular size is variable. Loss of germ cells appears to occur in infancy, followed by tubular fibrosis and hyalinization at puberty.[100] Also at puberty, gonadotropin values become elevated, serum estradiol may be high, and serum T is low normal.[101] The resultant elevated estradiol/testosterone ratio may produce gynecomastia. Adult height is greater than in normal males and is associated with excessive growth of the lower extremities (eunichoid habitus). Although gonadal germ cell tumors may occur, cases of Klinefelter's syndrome appear to be disproportionally represented in the group of individuals who have extragonadal germ cell tumors.[102, 103]

Because serum T plateaus in early adolescence and progressively decreases during adulthood in men with Klinefelter's syndrome, early treatment with androgen replacement therapy is advised beginning at age 12.[101] The objectives of therapy are gradual pubertal onset, treatment of hypergonadotropism with prevention of gynecomastia, and beneficial effects on behavior, libido, and strength.

DISORDERS OF GENITAL DIFFERENTIATION

If gonadal determination proceeds normally based on karyotypic sex, intersex states may still occur because of excess or insufficient production of androgens, insufficient MIS, or end organ responsiveness to these hormones. The generic terminology used in cases of genital ambiguity with normal testicular or ovarian development is male pseudohermaphroditism and female pseudohermaphroditism, respectively; however, categorization based on the underlying disease process is preferable (Table 32.1). Virilization of females is caused by congenital adrenal hyperplasia (CAH) or fetal exposure to other endogenous or exogenous sources of excess androgen. In genetic males, undervirilization is caused by defects in androgen biosynthesis with or without CAH or by androgen insensitivity. Persistent Müllerian duct syndrome in males is secondary to MIS deficiency or insensitivity. Finally, abnormal genital differentiation may occur in the presence of normal gonadal development and function, but may present clinical features that mimic those of the classic intersex states.

Congenital Adrenal Hyperplasia

Any defect in adrenal steroidogenesis that results in impaired production of cortisol and ACTH-induced adrenal hyperplasia is considered a form of congenital adrenal hyperplasia or CAH[104, 105] (Fig. 32.4). Biosynthetic defects that produce CAH and virilization of female fetuses include 21-hydroxylase, 11β-hydroxylase, and 3β-hydroxysteroid dehydrogenase (3β-HSD) deficiency. In contrast, the steroidogenic defects in males that produce undervirilization with associated CAH include side chain cleavage (SCC) enzyme (or 20,22 desmolase), 3β-HSD, and 17α-hydroxylase/17,20-lyase deficiency. Of all cases of CAH, 90 to 95% are caused by 21-hydroxylase deficiency and the remainder most commonly by deficiency of 11β-hydroxylase; deficiencies of 3β-HSD, 17α-hydroxylase/17,20-lyase, and particularly SCC are rare.

21-Hydroxylase Deficiency

21-hydroxylase, also known as P450c21, catalyzes the conversion of progesterone and 17α-hydroxyprogesterone to deoxycorticosterone (DOC) and 11-deoxycortisol, respectively (Fig. 32.4). The classical form of steroid 21-hydroxylase deficiency is the most common cause of ambiguous genitalia in the neonatal period.[104] Screening studies indicate an incidence of approximately 1 in 15,000 live births although there is marked geographical variability.[106] Underproduction of cortisol and aldosterone leads to salt wasting in many cases and accumulation of androgenic steroids with masculinization of the female fetus.

Etiology

Mode of inheritance is autosomal recessive, as with all disorders of adrenal steroidogenesis. Several mutations in the CYP21 gene, which is located on the short arm of chromosome 6 and encodes the 21-hydroxylase enzyme, have been identified.[105] In general, absence of enzyme activity is associated with classic salt wasting disease, while severely and moderately reduced activity results in simple virilizing and nonclassical forms, respectively. However, different phenotypes may be seen in patients with the same mutation.[107]

Clinical Features

Three phenotypes of the disease are described: classical forms including the salt wasting and simple virilizing types and the nonclassical phenotype. The latter occurs in up to 1% of the population and does not produce intersexuality. In the classic forms, the genitalia are typically ambiguous, but the degree of masculinization may range from mild clitoral hypertrophy to formation of a complete phallic urethra (Fig. 32.5). Similarly, variable degrees of labial fusion, rugation of the fused labia minora, and urogenital sinus formation are seen. In general, salt wasting is associated with more severe virilization of the external genitalia and urogenital sinus.[108] Virilization of internal genitalia and gonadal descent do not occur, presumably because early local testosterone production is required for these processes. Salt wasting occurs in 75% of patients with classical disease and is evident within the first 2 weeks of life. Features include hyponatremia, hypokalemia, and inappropriate natriuresis with low serum aldosterone and elevated plasma renin activity (PRA). Individuals with the simple virilizing form also have reduced aldosterone production, but levels are sufficient to prevent clinical salt wasting.

The diagnosis of 21-hydroxylase deficiency is suspected in a masculinized infant without palpable gonads and with Müllerian derivatives evident on pelvic ultrasound or rectal examination, and is confirmed by the presence of a 46,XX karyotype and a 50- to 100-fold increase in serum 17α-hydroxyprogesterone. Increased levels of serum dihydroepiandrosterone (DHEA), androstenedione, and T are also present.

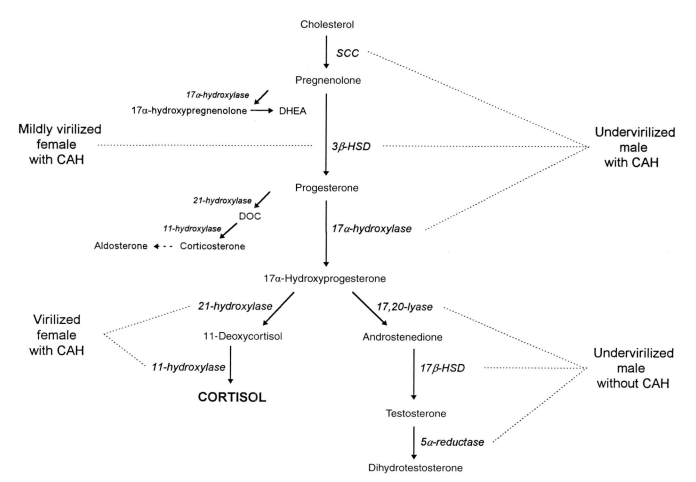

FIG. 32.4. Defects in steroid biosynthesis associated with abnormal genital differentiation. SCC, side chain cleavage; CAH, congenital adrenal hyperplasia; DHEA, dihydroepiandrosterone; HSD, hydroxysteroid dehydrogenase; DOC, deoxycorticosterone.

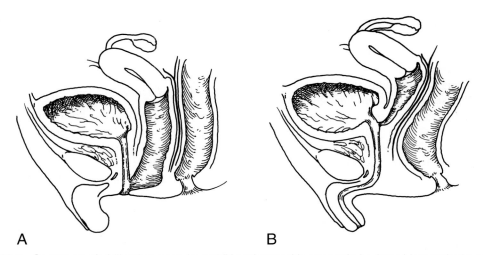

A   B

FIG. 32.5. Spectrum of virilization seen in 46,XX patients with congenital adrenal hyperplasia caused by 21-hydroxylase deficiency. **A,** Clitoromegaly with distal urethrovaginal confluence and short urogenital sinus. **B,** Complete phallic urethra with high urethrovaginal confluence and long urogenital sinus.

Pubertal development is delayed, menses irregular, and fertility uncommon in girls who are noncompliant with medical therapy.[109] In addition, fertility rates are markedly reduced in patients with the salt wasting form of the disease. Psychosocial evaluation suggests that affected females may exhibit "tomboyish" behavior and delayed or reduced heterosexual activity. Some investigators report an increased incidence of homosexuality.[109, 110] Most patients appear to be satisfied with their female gender identity, and limited data suggest an inferior outcome if the diagnosis is delayed and male sex assignment made.[111]

Treatment

Medical therapy involves treatment with hydrocortisone to inhibit overproduction of ACTH and androgenic steroids, and with 9α-fluorohydrocortisone (Fluorinef) to prevent salt wasting. Patients with simple virilizing disease may also benefit from mineralocorticoid therapy if PRA is elevated. Serial measurements of PRA, 17α-hydroxyprogesterone, and serum androgens are used to monitor therapy. Gender assignment should always be female because of the potential for fertility, and early feminizing surgery is advocated by most surgeons. Surgical therapy includes clitoroplasty, feminizing genitoplasty, and vaginoplasty (see Surgical Treatment of Ambiguous Genitalia).

Prenatal Diagnosis and Treatment

The risk of abnormal genital differentiation can be markedly reduced in fetuses with a known family history of CAH caused by 21-hydroxylase deficiency.[112] After confirmation of pregnancy, maternal dexamethasone (20 μg/kg/day given twice daily) is started at 5 weeks of gestation. Karyotyping and analysis of the CYP21 gene using allele-specific polymerase chain reaction are performed on samples retrieved by chorionic villus sampling at 9 to 11 weeks' gestation or amniocentesis at 15 to 18 weeks' gestation. In addition, amniotic fluid 17α-hydroxyprogesterone may be diagnostic. If the fetus is male or CYP21 analysis is normal, treatment is stopped, although occasional false-negative and false-positive results are reported. Virilization was absent or minimal in most of the affected fetuses when treatment was started at or before 10 weeks' gestation, without apparent significant fetal side effects. However, there are concerns regarding the potential long-term negative effects of this therapy, particularly because many fetuses are treated needlessly before genetic analysis is complete.[113]

11β-Hydroxylase Deficiency

11β-hydroxylase, also known as P45011β, catalyzes the conversion of 11-deoxycortisol to cortisol and DOC to corticosterone (Fig. 32.4). Deficiency results in impaired production of cortisol and overproduction of androgens and other steroids with mineralocorticoid activity.[104, 105, 114]

Etiology

Two genes on the long arm of chromosome 8 encode 11β-hydroxylase (CYP11B) isoenzymes; defects in CYP11B1 result in virilizing CAH. At least 10 mutations of the CYP11B1 gene have been identified, all resulting in complete absence of the 11β-hydroxylase enzyme. Nevertheless, significant variability in phenotype is seen between affected individuals.

Clinical Features

Genital ambiguity manifest as variable degrees of masculinization ranging from mild clitoromegaly to a phallic urethra and a variably long urogenital sinus is seen. Hypertension is usually present but may be mild or absent in the first few years of life. Hypokalemic alkalosis caused by mineralocorticoid excess is present in some patients. Salt wasting occurs occasionally in infancy when DOC levels are relatively low or may be precipitated by glucocorticoid therapy. Untreated females undergo further virilization at puberty, whereas males exhibit precocious puberty. There is poor correlation between the degree of virilization, hypertension, and hypokalemia. Diagnosis rests on the finding of elevated levels of 11-deoxycortisol and DOC.

Treatment

Female sex assignment with appropriate feminizing surgery, as for 21-hydroxylase deficiency, is indicated. Medical management includes glucocorticoids and, if indicated, antihypertensives. Although prenatal diagnosis and therapy is theoretically possible, reported experience with its use is lacking.

3β-Hydroxysteroid Dehydrogenase (3β-HSD) Deficiency

3β-HSD catalyzes the conversion of Δ⁴ to Δ⁵ steroids: pregnenolone to progesterone, 17α-hydroxypregnenolone to 17α-hydroxyprogesterone, and the androgenic precursors DHEA and androstenediol to androstenedione and testosterone, respectively (Fig. 32.4). Reduced enzyme activity results in impaired production of cortisol, aldosterone, and sex steroids.[104, 105, 115]

Etiology

The 3β-HSD gene maps to the short arm of chromosome 1 and exists in two forms, types I and II, the latter form expressed predominantly in the adrenals and gonads. Mutations of the type II gene have been linked to 3β-HSD deficiency, with complete loss of enzymatic activity associated with the salt-wasting form of the disease and low levels of activity usually associated with the non–salt-wasting form.[116] As with 21-hydroxylase deficiency, a nonclassic form associated with normal genital differentiation but postpubertal virilization in females occurs at a much higher frequency than the classic form of the disease, but its genetic basis is unknown.[104]

Clinical Features

The severity of the defect in cortisol production may result in poor survival and consequently the apparent rarity of the disease.[104] Salt wasting with hyperkalemic acidosis is usually present. Overproduction of DHEA is sufficient to cause slight virilization in some females characterized by mild clitoromegaly and, rarely, labial fusion. In males, a range of phenotypes from normal female to normal male is seen; however, the most common is moderate to severe hypospadias with or without cryptorchidism, suggesting that the steroidogenic defect is less severe in the testis than the adrenal.[117] An increased incidence of testicular neoplasia has not been reported in this or other testosterone biosynthesis disorders despite the presence of cryptorchidism.[46, 47] As with other forms of CAH, the severity of the enzymatic defect does not correlate directly with the degree of abnormal genital differentiation. Diagnosis is based on increased levels of serum 17α-hydroxypregnenolone and DHEA.

Treatment

Gender assignment in males is based on adequacy of virilization, as for other causes of ambiguous genitalia (see later). However, adoption of a male gender role at puberty after female sex of rearing has been reported.[118] In addition to glucocorticoid therapy, mineralocorticoid replacement is necessary in patients with salt wasting. Sex steroid replacement is necessary at puberty in both sexes.

17α-Hydroxylase/17,20-Lyase Deficiency

Initially thought to be separate enzymatic steps in steroidogenesis, the 17α-hydroxylase and 17,20-lyase (desmolase) reactions (Fig. 32.4) are now known to be catalyzed by the same cytochrome P450 enzyme, P450c17. 17α-Hydroxylation of progesterone and pregnenolone produces 17α-progesterone and 17α-pregnenolone, which are converted by 17,20-lyase to androstenedione and DHEA, respectively. Deficiency of both enzymatic activities is usually present, resulting

in impaired production of glucocorticoids and sex steroids and overproduction of mineralocorticoids.[119, 120] Rarely, isolated 17α-hydroxylase or 17,20-lyase deficiency occurs.

Etiology

The gene encoding the common enzyme, P450c17, is located on chromosome 10 and several mutations associated with the syndrome have been identified. The molecular basis for incomplete forms of the enzyme deficiency is incompletely understood.

Clinical Features

Affected males usually have complete absence of virilization similar to that seen in androgen insensitivity, with female external genitalia, a blind-ending vagina, absence of Müllerian derivatives, and abdominal or inguinal testes. Occasional patients with partial enzyme defects have ambiguous genitalia. Hypertension and hypokalemia are present in 85 to 90% of cases, although salt wasting may be present in infancy. Clinical glucocorticoid insufficiency is rare, possibly because of overproduction of corticosterone. Serum pregnenolone, progesterone, corticosterone, and DOC are elevated. The genital phenotype of males with isolated 17,20-lyase deficiency is similar to that observed in cases of 17α-hydroxylase/17,20-lyase deficiency. Diagnosis is based on normal serum levels of cortisol and aldosterone and increased ratios of 17α-hydroxypregnenolone to DHEA and 17α-progesterone to androstenedione.

Treatment

Bilateral orchiectomy is performed in phenotypic females at the time of hernia repair or after workup for delayed puberty, and at the time of diagnosis in patients with abnormal genitalia assigned a female gender. Medical therapy is as for patients with 11β-hydroxylase deficiency.

SCC Deficiency

Deficient function of the side chain cleavage (SCC) enzyme (also known as P450SCC, 20,22 desmolase or cholesterol desmolase) that catalyzes conversion of cholesterol to pregnenolone results in profound deficiencies in all adrenal and gonadal steroids.[104] The syndrome is also called congenital lipoid adrenal hyperplasia because of accumulation of cholesterol in adrenal cortical cells. Possibly in part because of a high risk of early lethality, SCC deficiency is diagnosed rarely. Findings include absent or minimal virilization of males, severe salt loss and lethal Addisonian crisis. Laboratory data show decreased levels of all adrenal and gonadal steroids, hyponatremia, hypokalemia, and metabolic acidosis. The molecular basis for the disease remains unknown. Survivors require glucocorticoid, mineralocorticoid, and sex steroid replacement.

Other Causes of Virilization of Genetic Females

Exposure of the female fetus to external sources of sex steroids such as the maternal ovary or adrenal or maternal ingestion may produce masculinization. In addition, placental aromatase deficiency has been reported in a virilized female.[121]

Deficient Testosterone Biosynthesis Without CAH

Impaired testicular testosterone production in patients with normal adrenal steroidogenesis may also produce impaired genital differentiation in males. Such disorders include isolated 17,20-lyase deficiency (see earlier), 17β-hydroxysteroid dehydrogenase deficiency, and Leydig cell agenesis.

17β-Hydroxysteroid Dehydrogenase (17β-HSD) Deficiency

17β-HSD (17-ketosteroid reductase) catalyzes the conversion of several androgenic and estrogenic precursors to their more active metabolites, including androstenedione to T (Fig. 32.4). As with the androgen biosynthesis defects associated with CAH, inheritance is autosomal recessive and incidence is rare.[122] A group of affected males has been identified among the Arabs of Gaza.

Etiology

Four isozymes of 17β-HSD have been identified; the type 3 enzyme is limited to the testis and its deficiency is responsible for the clinical syndrome.[123] The gene encoding 17β-HSD type 3 is located on the long arm of chromosome 9. A variety of mutations has been identified resulting in absent or markedly reduced enzyme activity.

Clinical Features

Males have feminine external genitalia with mild to moderate degrees of clitoral hypertrophy but with a separate urethra and blind-ending vaginal pouch.[117, 122] Wolffian derivatives develop normally, suggesting that their masculinization is possible in response to androstenedione or low levels of T. Testes are usually inguinal but may be intra-abdominal or labioscrotal in location. The diagnosis is often made at puberty, when progressive virilization associated with penile growth, attainment of male secondary sex characteristics, testicular descent, and a change of gender identity may occur.

Although the gender conversion has been attributed to favorable cultural conditions in Gaza, successful gender conversion was also described in an American patient,[124] suggesting that prenatal and postnatal hormonal factors may overcome sex of rearing with regard to gender identity in some individuals. Gynecomastia occurs at puberty in approximately 50% of patients.[124] Diagnosis is based on an increased serum androstendione:T ratio in unstimulated pubertal or adult patients and after hCG stimulation in infants and children; serum T may be within the normal range. Postpubertal serum LH and FSH are increased. The surge in androgen production at puberty with accompanying virilization may be caused by conversion of androgen precursors, primarily androstenedione, to T by nonmutant 17β-HSD isozymes in extragonadal sites and to increased 5α-reductase activity.[123] Spermatogenesis is incomplete, even after early orchidopexy and timely T replacement therapy.[122] Although the risk of testicular malignancy in testosterone biosynthesis disorders is reportedly not increased,[46, 47] a nonseminomatous germ cell tumor was reported in a case of 17β-HSD deficiency occurring in a previously inguinal testis 15 years after orchidopexy at age 14.[124]

Treatment

When identified in infancy, male gender assignment has been advocated if a significant penile growth response to T therapy is seen.[122] Normal penile size was reported in a few of these patients after puberty, but it is unclear if adult penile size and function will be adequate in all patients treated early in life. In addition, recommendations for male gender assignment are based on characteristics of Gaza males that may not pertain to other cases: affected subjects may be more readily identified early in life, there is cultural bias toward male sex of rearing, and significant residual enzyme activity is present. Female gender assignment is more prevalent in other parts of the world, and may be advantageous because of the markedly feminized genitalia. Subjects raised as females should undergo early clitoroplasty and gonadectomy.

Leydig Cell Agenesis

This rare disorder, comprising less than 20 published cases reviewed in 1991, is referred to in the literature as Leydig cell agenesis, hypoplasia, hypofunction, or abnormal differentiation.[125]

Etiology

The absence of histologically identifiable Leydig cells and of testosterone production in response to hCG, without evidence of a specific enzyme deficiency, supports abnormal functioning of gonadotropin receptors in reported patients.[125] In some cases, reduced binding to LH receptors was documented, and more recently, specific mutations in the LH receptor in two families have been identified.[126, 127] In another case, an abnormal Y chromosome with loss of a portion of the long arm was identified, suggesting that a gene in this region is required for Leydig cell development.[128]

Clinical Features

Patients typically present at or after puberty with a phenotype similar to that seen in 17β-HSD deficiency.[129] The external genitalia are feminine or slightly masculinized with mild clitoromegaly, posterior labial fusion, a blind ending vagina, or a distal urogenital sinus. Overt genital ambiguity[125] and micropenis[126] have also been reported. Testes are usually inguinal but may be abdominal or labioscrotal. Wolffian ductal structures are present and Müllerian derivatives absent. Laboratory studies confirm female levels of T with no response to hCG. Postpubertal serum LH is elevated but FSH is normal. Histology of the testes reveals undifferentiated cells in the interstitium but few or no Leydig cells, and no germ cell differentiation beyond spermatogonia or spermatocytes.

Treatment

Female sex of rearing with orchiectomy, feminizing surgery, if necessary, and estrogen replacement is indicated.

Steroid 5α-Reductase 2 Deficiency

A defect in the enzyme that catalyzes the conversion of T to DHT, an androgen with much higher affinity for its receptor that is responsible for masculinization of the external genitalia and prostate, results in a syndrome originally called pseudovaginal perineoscrotal hypospadias or familial incomplete male pseudohermaphroditism, type 2.[130, 131] This rare syndrome has been reported in more than 50 families worldwide.[132]

Etiology

5α-Reductase deficiency is an autosomal recessive disorder, with a rate of documented consanguinity in affected families of almost 40%.[133] Recently, two separate 5α-reductase isoenzymes were identified; type 1, which is present in skin and other nongenital tissues, and type 2, which is expressed in genital tissues and is deficient in affected males.[132] The gene encoding 5α-reductase 2, SRD5A2, has been localized to chromosome 2; more than 35 homozygous or compound heterozygous mutations in the gene have been identified.[132] There appears to be a positive correlation between the percentage of residual activity of the mutant enzyme and the degree of fetal virilization.[134]

Clinical Features

Affected individuals are typically 46,XY males with moderate to severe genital ambiguity at birth. Most patients have an abnormally small penis with severe hypospadias, variable degrees of scrotal development, and a urogenital sinus or separate urethral and vaginal openings. Testes are inguinal or labioscrotal and Wolffian duct development is normal. Occasional patients may be completely feminized or have a normally developed small penis, and different phenotypes may be seen within a single family despite documentation of identical genotype.[135] In untreated patients, marked virilization occurs at puberty characterized by moderate penile growth (although ultimate penile size remains significantly smaller than normal), testicular descent, acquisition of a male habitus, absence of gynecomastia, and/or change of gender identity from female to male.[132] Postnatal virilization may be mediated by increasing serum T or by DHT synthesized by the intact type 1 or mutant type 2 isoenzyme.[132, 133] Masculinization of the brain may occur in the fetal or postnatal period because male gender identity may be evident before puberty in some subjects raised as girls. Testicular histology may be normal in infants and adults with descended testes.[74] In some individuals, sperm production has been documented, but fertility has not been reported. There are no published reports of testicular malignancy.[46, 47]

Diagnosis is based on an elevated T:DHT ratio (normal = 14 ± 5), which is obtained after hCG stimulation in prepubertal patients.[136] Serum LH and FSH may be normal or slightly elevated. Differentiation between 5α-reductase deficiency and partial androgen insensitivity may be difficult in some cases because secondary 5α-reductase deficiency may be present in patients with androgen receptor defects.[137] Differential diagnosis may be based on the presence or absence of gynecomastia, the ratio of urinary 5β- to 5α-glucocorticoid metabolites or molecular genetic analysis.

Treatment

In patients diagnosed in infancy, appropriate treatment remains unclear. Male gender assignment has been recommended because replacement therapy may facilitate genital reconstruction and further virilization occurs at puberty. However, even after long-term treatment of adults with androgens mean penile size was only 5.8 cm (normal adult median = approximately 13 cm).[132] It has not been determined if prepubertal therapy will increase postpubertal penile size. Although some patients function well as males by choice after puberty despite small penile size, cultural factors may contribute to this success in some cases; others retain a female social sex or have inadequate male sexual function. In patients assigned or acquiring a male gender, androgen replacement therapy with high-dose T or with parenteral or transcutaneous DHT, if available, should be considered in addition to orchidopexy and hypospadias repair, although the long-term effects of such therapy are unknown.[132] In patients raised as girls, gonadectomy should be performed as early as possible, followed by appropriate feminizing surgery.

Androgen Insensitivity Syndrome (AIS)

Morris reviewed a large series of patients with a female phenotype, male karyotype, and bilateral testes, and gave the first comprehensive description of a disorder that he termed "testicular feminization."[138] Other groups of patients with "testicular feminization" but with varying degrees of virilization were originally classified as Reifenstein's, Gilbert-Dreyfus, or Lubs' syndromes or as incomplete male pseudohermaphroditism, type 1; these cases are recognized as variable manifestations of the same disease.[139] All these patients have insensitivity or resistance of the androgen receptor (AR) to androgen action, and therefore the more accurate and appropriate terminology used is complete or partial androgen insensitivity syndrome (CAIS, PAIS). CAIS is the most common cause of feminization of 46,XY males with testicular determination (male pseudohermaphroditism) and is estimated to occur in at least 1 of 20,000 male births. The prevalence of PAIS is unknown but in its various forms may be as common as CAIS.

Etiology

AIS is caused by familial (X-linked recessive) or de novo mutations in the AR gene. More than 200 different mutations have been identified, several that far surpass the incidence of mutation in other steroid receptor genes despite that the AR gene was the last of these genes to be cloned.[139, 140] The AR gene is located on the long arm of the X chromosome and encodes a protein transcription factor that has DNA- and steroid-binding domains. The AR has highest affinity for DHT, less for T and low affinity for adrenal androgens and other sex steroids. Mutations in the AR gene in AIS are typically single base mutations although a few deletions and insertions have been reported. Complete deletions or mutations that result in absent androgen binding result in CAIS, whereas single base mutations produce a wide range of phenotypes that includes complete and partial AIS. In some cases, no mutations within the coding region of the AR have been found. The effect of each mutation on phenotype is difficult to predict because the degree of virilization is variable in patients with different mutations at the same site and even between and within families with the same mutation and degree of AR binding activity. Phenotypic variability may be caused by variable fetal androgen production and the observation that as little as 10% of normal AR function may result in significant masculinization of the fetus.[139]

Clinical Features

Patients with CAIS are normal phenotypic females who present during childhood with one or both testes palpable in an inguinal hernia (comprising an estimated 1–2% of all girls presenting with hernia) or with amenorrhea at puberty.[139] A few are diagnosed based on discrepancy between prenatal karyotype and phenotype at birth. These girls have normal or small clitoral and labial size, a blind-ending, usually short vagina, and hypoplastic or vestigial Müllerian or Wolffian ductal derivatives in up to a third of the cases. Possible explanations for incomplete Müllerian regression include participation by androgen in MIS action or unopposed estrogen effect in AIS causing stabilization of Müllerian ducts.[141] Testes are usually intraabdominal or inguinal but may be labial in location. At puberty, development of breasts and a female habitus occurs normally but pubic and axillary hair is sparse or absent. Adult height is greater than average for females, presumably because of the presence of Y-linked gene(s). Patients with PAIS have a wide spectrum of genital development that varies from normal females with development of sexual hair at puberty, mild virilization (clitoromegaly, separate urethral and vaginal openings, or partial labial fusion), moderate virilization (perineal hypospadias with micropenis or ambiguous phallus, urogenital sinus, variable degrees of scrotal development, and cryptorchidism) to rare cases of isolated hypospadias or normal male genital differentiation with infertility. Wolffian duct differentiation varies from rudimentary to complete, and Müllerian duct remnants may also be present. At puberty, further virilization or variable degrees of gynecomastia may occur.

In CAIS and PAIS, testicular histology is characterized by immature tubules, loss of germ cells with increasing age, Leydig cell hyperplasia, hamartomatous nodules, or Sertoli cell adenomas.[142] In PAIS, testicular histology may be normal before puberty, but tubules subsequently become atrophic and hyalinized; spermatozoa are rarely seen. The incidence of malignant tumors of the testis is estimated to be 5 to 10%, with seminoma most common, but nonseminomatous germ cell tumors and other malignancies also reported.[74] There have been no well-documented prepubertal cases, and the tumor risk appears greater in older patients and in those with CAIS. By contrast, intratubular germ cell neoplasia has been identified in prepubertal subjects with partial but not complete AIS, with a similar incidence in inguinal and labioscrotal testes.[143]

Diagnosis of AIS is based on clinical and family history, endocrine studies and, if indicated, androgen binding analysis in genital skin fibroblasts or molecular genetic studies.[139] Prepubertal serum T, LH, FSH, and androgen precursors are normal, although T, LH, and MIS levels may be abnormally high in patients with PAIS during early infancy.[30, 144] Postpubertally, serum LH is high, and T, estrogen, and FSH are normal or elevated. The T:DHT ratio (after hCG stimulation in childhood) is usually normal but may be elevated, indicative of secondary 5α-reductase deficiency. Androgens suppress serum sex hormone binding globulin (SHBG) in normal males but not in cases of AIS; therefore, measurement of SHBG inhibition by the anabolic steroid stanozolol has been recommended as an additional diagnostic test for AIS.[145]

Treatment

In cases of CAIS, gonadectomy is indicated, but vaginal augmentation may or may not be required. In patients who have inguinal hernia(e) before puberty, orchiectomy is indicated at the time of hernia repair to confirm the diagnosis and because of the risk of neoplasia and psychologic concerns associated with the procedure in the postpubertal patient. In PAIS, orchiectomy is indicated as soon as the diagnosis is made to avoid further virilization in patients raised as females. In patients with a predominantly male phenotype (i.e., perineal hypospadias and micropenis, or Reifenstein's syndrome), male gender assignment is usual but not always successful. Unfortunately, in patients diagnosed prepubertally, predicting the adequacy of virilization in adulthood may not be possible based on family history or characterization of the genetic defect. Unlike adults,[132] some children respond well to high dose androgen therapy,[146] but data supporting the durability of this response are unavailable. Similarly, although molecular genetic diagnosis is available for identification of carriers and fetuses at risk for a specific mutation, prenatal counseling is complicated because the phenotype of affected offspring is unpredictable.[147–149]

Persistent Müllerian Duct Syndrome

Isolated failure of Müllerian duct regression in otherwise normal males, originally termed hernia uteri inguinalis, is called persistent Müllerian duct syndrome (PMDS). This is a rare disorder with fewer than 200 cases reported in the literature.[150]

Etiology

PMDS is caused by absent or impaired synthesis of MIS or insensitivity of the MIS receptor.[151] The disease is transmitted through autosomal recessive inheritance.

A variety of mutations in the MIS gene, located on chromosome 19, have been identified,[151] as has a mutation in the recently cloned MIS receptor gene located on chromosome 12.[152] MIS gene defects may result in impaired quantity or function of the MIS protein, and phenotypic variability has been reported within families.

Clinical Features

Patients are normally virilized, 46,XY males who have cryptorchidism with or without a clinical hernia and normal penile development.[153] Most patients have one scrotal or one inguinal testis prolapsing into a hernia sac and approximately a third of these have transverse testicular ectopia. Approximately 10% have bilateral abdominal testes. Several cases of monorchia suggestive of vanishing testis syndrome have been reported.[150, 154] It is theorized that these testes are more prone to torsion because of absence of a gubernacular remnant. Vasa, epididymides, fallopian tubes (located in the mesosalpinx), and a uterus are present.[153] However, some reports suggest that an abnormal epididymis or vas may result in impaired communication with the testis or urethra.[155, 156] Serum MIS in normal males remains elevated during the first 2 years of life and declines significantly after midpuberty.[30] Levels were unmeasurable or low in approximately two thirds of prepubertal patients with PMDS reported by Imbeaud et al; in these cases, significant mutations in the MIS gene were found.[151] Serum T, LH, and FSH, when measured, are typically normal, even in adults.[154, 157, 158]

Histologically, the testes are normal before puberty. However, generalized or focal impairment of spermatogenesis has often been observed postpubertally, even in scrotal testes that did not require orchidopexy.[155, 157–159] In addition, limited semen analysis data have shown azoospermia, oligospermia, or impaired motility, and paternity has not been well-documented in men with PMDS. Martin et al[158] suggest that partial ductal obstruction may explain the abnormal semen quality; transgenic mice that lack MIS production or receptors are usually infertile despite normal testicular spermatogenesis, suggesting that there is a sperm transport problem.[26] Patency of the distal vas, which is embedded in the uterus, has not been systematically studied in patients with PMDS.

The risk of testicular tumor in patients with PMDS may be as high as 10% based on 14 cases in more than 150 reports of the syndrome published as of 1994.[160, 161] Seminoma is the most common risk but nonseminomatous germ cell tumors and intratubular germ cell neoplasia have also been reported. In one case, embryonal carcinoma was diagnosed in a scrotal testis of a 16-year-old boy subsequent to bilateral orchidopexy for abdominal testes in infancy.[162]

Treatment

Orchidopexy and herniorrhaphy are recommended at the time of diagnosis, but controversy surrounds the need for concomitant removal of the Müllerian remnants. No complications associated with their persistence have been reported. However, excision may be necessary to facilitate orchidopexy in some cases. Although fertility is unlikely, some authors recommend removal of the uterine corpus and proximal fallopian tubes with preservation of the cervical and vaginal remnants to avoid injury to the vas.[153, 163]

Other Abnormalities of Genital Differentiation

The presence of an underlying intersex condition should be considered in certain patients who have isolated genital abnormalities such as micropenis, penile agenesis, hypospadias with cryptorchidism, prostatic utricular enlargement, and Müllerian dysgenesis.

Micropenis

Penile size of more than 2 or 2.5 standard deviations (SD) below the mean for age (see Table 32.2) in the presence of otherwise normal anatomic development of the penis is called micropenis or microphallus, although the latter term is also used when hypospadias is additionally present.[164, 165] Cryptorchidism may also be present. The etiology may be any process resulting in impaired androgen production during the second or third trimesters of gestation, after urethral closure is complete. Most commonly, micropenis is caused by fetal hypogonadotropic hypogonadism, but it may be secondary to isolated growth hormone deficiency, associated with a known syndrome, or idiopathic. As discussed earlier, micropenis occasionally occurs in patients with Kleinfelter's syndrome, XX sex reversal, partial gonadal dysgenesis, testicular regression, androgen biosynthesis defects, PAIS, or 5α-reductase deficiency. These disorders may be excluded by karyotypic, endocrine, and molecular genetic analysis. Testicular function and penile response may be assessed in infancy by hCG stimulation: 500 to 1500 International Units (IU) intramuscularly every other day for 5 to 7 days[166] or every day for 3 days[167] with measurement of serum T before and 24 to 48 hours after the last injection. Parenteral T therapy, 25 to 50 mg testosterone enanthate or cypionate every 3 to 4 weeks for three to four doses,[164, 165] may be more effective in assessing penile growth potential, particularly in patients with a poor hormonal or clinical response to hCG. Recently, Choi et al reported that transdermal DHT produced durable normalization of penile length in patients with micropenis for up to 1 year after treatment, even in cases previously unresponsive to T.[168] Better results were obtained in peripubertal boys than in younger boys, the reverse of the results obtained with T.[169] Unfortunately, there are a paucity of data documenting ultimate penile size and adequacy of sexual function in adults who responded well to therapy for micropenis in infancy or childhood. Some evidence suggests that a good prepubertal response does not ensure adequate penile size in adulthood, particularly in patients with inadequate gonadal function and that psychosexual function is widely variable in adults with micropenis.[170-172]

Penile Agenesis

Complete absence of the penis in 46,XY males with testes should not be confused with true intersex states,

TABLE 32.2. *Penile and clitoral dimensions according to age*

Age	Stretched penile length (cm)		Clitoral length (cm)		Clitoral width (cm)		Clitoral index (mm²)
	Mean	*−2.5 SD*	*Mean*	*+2.5 SD*	*Mean*	*+2.5 SD*	*Length × width*
Newborn							
28 weeks	2.2	1.1					
30 weeks	2.5	1.4					
32 weeks	2.8	1.7	0.7	1.0	0.6	0.8	
34 weeks	3.0	1.9					
36 weeks	3.2	2.1	0.5	0.8	0.5	0.7	
38 weeks	3.5	2.4					
40 weeks	3.5–3.7	2.0–2.5	0.4	0.7	0.3–0.4	0.5–0.7	
Birth to 5 months	3.9	1.9	0.5	0.8	0.4	0.7	15 (1–8 years)
6–12 months	4.3	2.3					
1–2 years	4.7	2.6					
2–3 years	5.1	2.9					
3–4 years	5.5	3.3					
4–5 years	5.7	3.5					
5–11 years	6.0–6.4	<4.0					17 (8–13 years)
Adult	13.3	9.3	1.6	2.7	0.3	0.6	19–21 (+2.5 SD = 39)

SD, standard deviation.

but also requires prompt consideration of gender assignment. The anomaly is rare and is typically associated with a urethral opening in the anus or perineum and descended testes in a normal scrotum. Early female gender assignment with orchiectomy is advocated because of historical evidence of poor outcome in subjects raised as males.[173, 174]

Hypospadias and Cryptorchidism

While isolated hypospadias or cryptorchidism is rarely the presenting feature of intersex, a combination of both anomalies is reported to be associated with an underlying intersex state in 25 to 100% of cases.[175–177] However, analysis of these data shows that intersex is much more common in patients with a hypospadiac microphallus or proximal hypospadias in association with cryptorchidism than in patients with normal penile size and midshaft or distal hypospadias. For example, in the series of Rajfer and Walsh,[176] of 22 patients with normal penile length, 3 had gonadal dysgenesis, 1 had TH, and 2 had "male pseudohermaphroditism" of undetermined etiology, whereas of 23 patients with microphallus, 18 had a diagnosis of intersex or unspecified male pseudohermaphroditism. Therefore, although it is clear that patients with intersex caused by abnormal gonadal determination or defined abnormalities of hormonal synthesis and function may have an otherwise normal hypospadiac penis with cryptorchidism, most have ambiguous genitalia. To identify intersex in otherwise normal-appearing males with hypospadias and cryptorchidism, it seems prudent to obtain at least a karyotype if the hypospadias is severe or neither gonad is palpable and to perform a biopsy on any testis that is macroscopically abnormal or associated with Müllerian remnants at the time of planned orchidopexy.

In patients with isolated hypospadias, a search for defects in androgen biosynthesis or action has been largely unfruitful. Androgen receptor concentration or binding in genital tissue from patients with hypospadias did not differ significantly from control values[178, 179] and mutations of the AR gene have been identified in only 2 of 50 subjects with isolated hypospadias; one had a perineal and the other a distal penile meatus.[180, 181]

Enlarged Prostatic Utricle

The origin of the prostatic utricle, a small sac-like structure located within the verumontanum, is controversial but, as postulated for the distal vagina in the female, is likely comprised of epithelium of Müllerian, urogenital sinus, and possibly Wolffian origin.[182] An enlarged utricle is also referred to in the literature as a vagina masculinus or Müllerian duct remnant, and is observed in 56% of patients with proximal hypospadias.[183, 184] Approximately half of these patients also have cryptorchidism. Utricular enlargement in association with hypospadias and cryptorchidism has been des-

ignated "male pseudohermaphroditism" by some authors, even when no specific intersex condition has been identified.[176] However, not all of these patients have intersex.[183, 185] Furthermore, isolated utricular enlargement in the absence of a cervix, uterus, or tubes is more likely caused by insufficient masculinization of the urogenital sinus than to MIS deficiency, making the term "Müllerian remnant" misnomer.[183, 184, 186] Surgical treatment is usually unnecessary, although the symptomatic utricle may be removed by a transtrigonal or posterior sagittal approach, with care to avoid injury to the associated vasa.[185]

Müllerian Dysgenesis

Partial or complete vaginal agenesis with uterine and sometimes renal malformations in phenotypic, endocrinologically normal XX females is called Mayer-Rokitansky or Mayer-Rokitansky-Küster-Hauser syndrome and occurs in fewer than 1 in 5,000 female births.[187, 188] Patients typically present at puberty with amenorrhea or abdominal pain caused by hematometrocolpos. On examination, the vagina may be short and blind-ending (Fig. 32.6), as also seen in patients with CAIS. Defects range from uterine or vaginal duplication to increasing degrees of vaginal, uterine, tubal, and even ovarian agenesis. Urinary tract anomalies are present in 30 to 40% of cases; renal agenesis is associated with a greater severity of ipsilateral Müllerian dysgenesis. The preferred method of vaginal reconstruction in cases of agenesis differs between urologists and gynecologists, but in experienced hands progressive vaginal dilatation, skin graft, and bowel vaginoplasty have all been successful.[189]

EVALUATION OF AMBIGUOUS GENITALIA

Identification of ambiguous genitalia at birth necessitates complete evaluation of the patient on an urgent

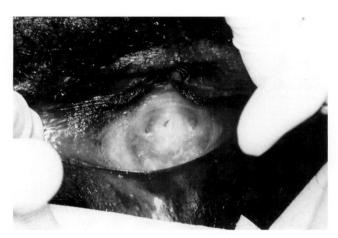

FIG. 32.6. Perineum of a postpubertal female with 46,XX phenotype, hypoplastic uterus, and blind-ending vagina (Müllerian dysgenesis).

basis to determine the underlying etiology (if possible), assign the appropriate gender, and prevent any associated complications. In one large series of patients with ambiguous genitalia during a 25-year period, a definitive diagnosis was made in 80% of cases.[190] CAH in girls was most common (53%), followed by partial gonadal dysgenesis, malformation syndromes, AIS, testosterone biosynthesis defect, and PMDS. Patient management is based less on chromosomal sex than on status of internal and external genitalia, potential for fertility or malignancy and parental bias. Optimally, interdisciplinary management of patients and family counseling should be available routinely.

History and Physical Examination

History of systemic symptoms such as failure to thrive or vomiting should be elicited. Family history of significance includes other individuals with genital or somatic malformations or unexplained reproductive disorders and maternal exposures during pregnancy.

Abnormal phallic size should be documented based on established norms, taking gestational age into account (Table 32.2).[164, 191–196] Specifically, a penis smaller than 2.0 cm or a clitoris larger than 7 mm (>2.5 SDs below or above the mean, respectively) is present in a newborn with ambiguous genitalia, thereby excluding boys with a normally sized hypospadiac penis with cryptorchidism from this diagnosis. Patients with isolated micropenis and normal urethral and scrotal development may also have intersex disorders, as discussed earlier but are not considered to have ambiguous genitalia. Documentation of the presence or absence of palpable gonad(s), hernia, urethral and vaginal openings, labial fusion, scrotal development, and a palpable cervix on transrectal examination is important. The presence of Turner stigmata or other congenital anomalies should also be noted. These initial observations will dictate which additional studies are indicated (Fig. 32.7).

Additional Studies

Karyotypic analysis of peripheral blood leukocytes is necessary in all patients and has replaced the buccal smear as a method of sex chromosome analysis. By far the most likely diagnosis in patients with a 46,XX chromosomal complement and no palpable gonads is CAH, most commonly 21-hydroxylase deficiency. Measurement of serum adrenal steroids and electrolytes will determine the appropriate diagnosis, although hormone levels may be inconclusive or inaccurate in the early postnatal period and serial studies may be neces-

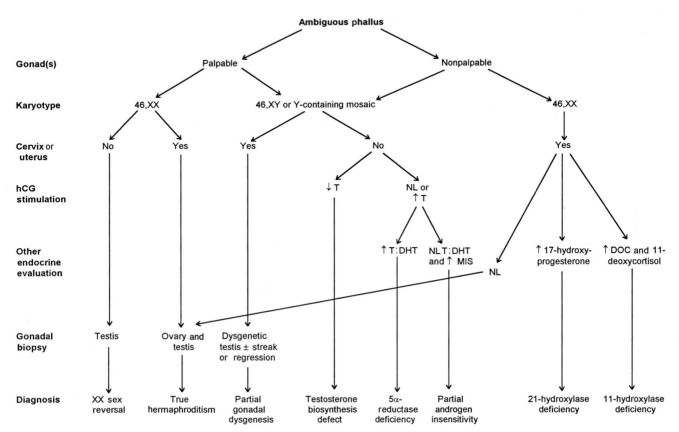

FIG. 32.7. Evaluation of patients with ambiguous genitalia. T, testosterone; DHT, dihydrotesterone; DOC, deoxycorticosterone; MIS; Müllerian inhibiting substance; NL, normal.

sary.[197, 198] Ultrasound can be used to accurately identify a normal uterus and ovaries in most newborns to support the diagnosis of CAH before the onset of salt wasting.[199, 200] However, adrenal enlargement is not necessarily present.[201] Retrograde genitography and cystoscopy are also important to confirm presence of a cervix and identify the level of urethrovaginal confluence as an aid in planning surgery.

CAH can be excluded in patients with other forms of intersex associated with a 46,XX karyotype and ambiguous genitalia when uterine or cervical hypoplasia or absence, palpable gonads, and normal adrenal steroids are present (Fig. 32.7). Gonadal exploration is required for confirmation of true hermaphroditism by biopsy, removal of inappropriate gonadal tissue and orchidopexy as indicated. In the rare cases of XX sex reversal with genital ambiguity, testes only are present but may be dysgenetic and require biopsy or removal.

In patients with a 46,XY or Y-containing karyotype, differentiation between an abnormality of gonadal determination (partial gonadal dysgenesis or true hermaphroditism) and of androgen production or action must be made. Persistence of Müllerian duct derivatives can usually be demonstrated in the former group by examination pelvic ultrasound, genitography, or laparoscopy. A definitive diagnosis is made in this group by gonadal biopsy, and studies of hypothalamic-pituitary-gonadal axis function are useful only to identify the presence or degree of functioning testicular tissue, preoperatively or postoperatively. Measurement of serum MIS can also be used to confirm the presence of testicular tissue in prepubertal patients without the need for hCG stimulation.[90] Dysgenetic testes, if placed or retained in the scrotum, require close follow-up to monitor for malignancy.

Measurement of T, DHT, DHEA, and androstenedione before and after administration of hCG is required in prepubertal patients to differentiate between abnormal testosterone biosynthesis with or without CAH, 5α-reductase deficiency, and PAIS. Standard dosage is 500 to 2000 IU of hCG given intramuscularly for 3 days with endocrine studies repeated on day 4.[166, 202] Because the response to hCG is normal in PAIS, abnormal elevation of serum T or MIS in early infancy,[30, 144] poor penile growth in response to androgen stimulation (as described earlier for cases of micropenis) or molecular genetic studies may be used to confirm the diagnosis. Patients with little or no penile growth response to hCG or depot testosterone are expected to have poor pubertal virilization. Serum LH and FSH may be useful in older patients (see Table 32.1) or to help diagnose anorchia.

Gender Assignment

It has been known for many years that sex of rearing should be decided as early as possible to avoid psychologic trauma to family and child.[203, 204] The most com-

monly used criteria for choice of gender include phallic size and potential for growth, and fertility potential. Fertility and normal sexual function are feasible in females with CAH, and a female sex of rearing is routine in these cases. In other conditions presenting with ambiguous genitalia, sex of rearing is usually based on the adequacy of virilization of the genitalia, i.e., it is recommended that patients with a phallus that is very small or poorly responsive to androgen stimulation be assigned as females.[190, 198]

Recently, this standard use of penile size as a major criterion for gender assignment has been challenged by some former patients and their advocates.[4, 5, 205] Longitudinal studies suggest that some adults happily retain or adopt a male gender identity despite a small penis that is inadequate for intercourse and, in some cases, absence of functioning testes.[172, 206] For example, a recent report describes reversion to a male gender role in a patient who underwent sex reassignment in infancy after penile loss from a circumcision injury.[207] Similarly, some patients with 5α-RD,[208, 209] 17β-hydroxysteroid dehydrogenase deficiency,[118, 122, 124] and PAIS[210] exhibit a male gender identity, sometimes evident prepubertally, despite deficient virilization and female sex of rearing. These examples suggest that virilization of the brain occurs in the prenatal and perhaps early postnatal periods, and may not be supplanted by female sex of rearing. In other patients, female sex reassignment is successful.[211] Unfortunately, it is impossible to predict ultimate penile size, gender identity, and adequacy of sexual functioning based solely on penile size and response to hormonal stimulation in infancy.

Because of the difficulty in predicting outcome in individual patients, it has been suggested that an intersex individual chose his or her own gender when old enough and that "cosmetic" surgical intervention, i.e., clitoral recession, vaginoplasty, or hypospadias repair, be avoided early in life.[205] This recommendation seems unrealistic because of the resultant parental ambivalence, the unpredictability of pubertal changes in untreated patients (Table 32.1), and the likelihood of stigmatization and its ill effects during childhood.[206, 211] Rather than adopt absolute criteria for gender assignment, it seems reasonable to assess each case individually and decide on appropriate gender based on degree of virilization, gonadal function, the predicted efficacy of hormonal therapy during and after puberty, and the natural history of the disease. The patient's family should be aware of the potential issues and their preferences given serious consideration. Before gender determination, all caregivers should refer to a newborn as "your baby," not "he" or "she," and avoid inconsistency of information in discussions with the patient's family.[204] Early and long-term counseling of patient and family are important. When raised as girls, patients with testicular tissue should undergo early postnatal gonadectomy as soon as is feasible to reduce the risk of further viriliza-

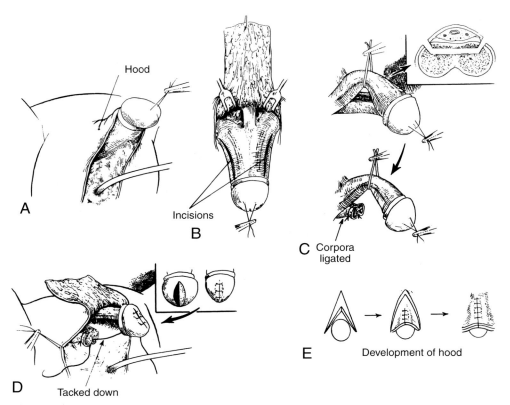

FIG. 32.8. Reduction clitoroplasty. **A,** Degloving of clitoris after circumcising incision. **B,** Incisions in lateral tunica albuginea to allow isolation of ventral corporal bodies. **C,** Resection of corporal bodies. **D,** Reduction of glans and suture of glans to corporal stump. **E,** Recreation of clitoral hood in patients without residual dorsal preputial skin.

tion. The feasibility of penile construction should be considered in association with male sex of rearing because it reportedly yields satisfactory results in children and adolescents.[212] However, follow-up is limited and the expertise required for the procedure is available at few centers. Ultimately, the acquisition of more long-term psychosexual data from patients with a history of ambiguous genitalia will be crucial for their improved management.

SURGICAL MANAGEMENT OF INTERSEX

Surgical procedures may be indicated for diagnosis and management of intersex disorders. In patients with palpable gonads or a Y chromosome-containing karyotype, gonadal biopsy is required to establish the diagnosis when partial gonadal dysgenesis, XX sex reversal with genital ambiguity or true hermaphroditism is suspected. Surgical reconstruction of the genitalia and removal of inappropriate gonadal tissue is then performed based on gender assignment.

Laparoscopy/Laparotomy

Evaluation of abdominal gonads and internal genitalia may be indicated in patients with abnormalities of gonadal determination. These cases include those with

sex chromosomal mosaicism, palpable gonads despite 46,XX karyotype, and discordant Müllerian development in 46,XY and 46,XX individuals (see Fig. 32.7). Diagnostic laparoscopy may be used in the initial evaluation of these cases or of patients with complete gonadal dysgenesis or Müllerian dysgenesis syndromes. Laparoscopic surgery is advocated for biopsy of gonads and removal of those that are dysgenetic or inappropriate to the sex of rearing and for excision of Müllerian structures in males.[213] However, laparotomy facilitates deep longitudinal gonadal biopsies, if necessary, and removal of gonadal tissue discordant with the sex of rearing in cases of true hermaphroditism. Therefore, we prefer laparotomy with a Pfannensteil incision when gonadal biopsy, partial gonadectomy, orchidopexy, or bowel vaginoplasty may be indicated. Removal of Müllerian structures may facilitate orchidopexy in patients with PMDS, but is not performed routinely. However, it should be noted that rare cases of uterine adenocarcinoma have been reported in patients with gonadal dysgenesis after long-term unopposed estrogen therapy.[75]

Clitoroplasty

Phallic reduction in individuals raised as girls is usually performed early in the neonatal period or soon after

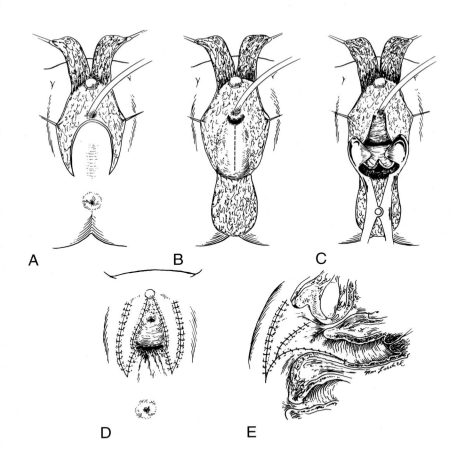

FIG. 32.9. Flap vaginoplasty after Fortunoff[229] in cases with low urethrovaginal confluence. **A,** Mobilization of U-shaped flap with preservation of subcutaneous tissue. **B,** Longitudinal incision of urogenital sinus. **C,** Visualization of apex of incision in vagina aided by placement of a nasal speculum. **D,** Advancement of perineal flap with anastomosis to posterior vagina and creation of labia minora using bivalved preputial skin. **E,** Lateral view of completed repair.

diagnosis. Early feminizing surgery is optimal to achieve a genital appearance consistent with the sex of rearing as soon as possible, and because concomitant vaginoplasty and perineoplasty is feasible in many cases.

Some patients report normal sexual function after clitorectomy,[203, 214] but this procedure has been abandoned in favor of more anatomically conservative techniques. Recession of the intact clitoris has produced unsatisfactory results in some cases because of persistent enlargement or painful erection of the clitoris postoperatively.[215–217] Most surgeons now perform clitoral reduction, using techniques that involve corporal resection with sparing of the neurovascular bundle[218] or subtunical removal of erectile tissue.[219] Little data regarding the functional results of clitoroplasty in infancy are available because these procedures are rarely performed and data regarding sexual function may be difficult to collect. Normal "erotic sensation" or orgasmic function has been reported in most patients available for long-term follow-up after clitoral recession[215, 217] or reduction,[216] including those who underwent the recession procedure in infancy.[220] Unfortunately, no long-term results of infant reduction clitoroplasty are available. Recently, Gearhart et al reported preservation of pudendal evoked potentials after reduction clitoroplasty,[221] but this finding may not correlate with ultimate sexual function.[222]

We use a technique of corporal resection that maximizes preservation of the neurovascular bundle. The tunica albuginea is incised lateral to the bundle on each side and a median strip left with it (Fig. 32.8). A dorsal wedge of glans is removed, if necessary, to achieve normal glanular diameter. In addition, when inadequate phallic skin remains for recreation of the clitoral hood, this can be achieved by a technique based on the Heineke-Mikulicz principle (Fig. 32.8E).

Vaginoplasty

Creation of a functional vagina is required in two distinct groups of patients assigned a female sex of rearing: (a) those with urethrovaginal confluence, most commonly genetic females with CAH and (b) cases of vaginal absence or inadequacy in females with Müllerian dysgenesis or in genetic males with impaired testicular function, AIS, micropenis, or penile agenesis. Vaginoplasty is performed using perineal flaps in the former group, but vaginal replacement, usually with bowel, may be required in the latter group. The optimal timing of surgery has been controversial. Because postpubertal revision is frequently required when vaginoplasty is performed in childhood,[223] some surgeons have recommended deferring primary surgery until adolescence or

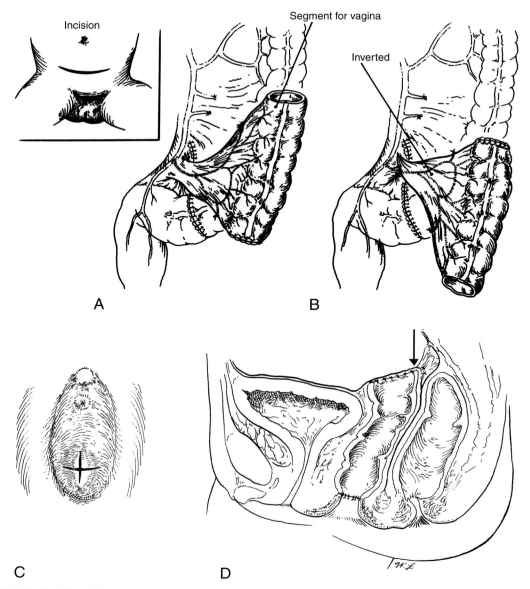

FIG. 32.10. Sigmoid vaginoplasty. **A,** Isolation of 10 to 15 cm segment of the lower sigmoid colon with preservation of the marginal artery. **B,** Closure of the distal sigmoid and inversion of the segment by 180°, which does not compromise its blood supply and allows it to reach the perineum more easily. **C,** Cruciate incision in vestible into blind-ending vagina. **D,** After completion of anastomosis of sigmoid segment to introital skin. Proximal neovagina is secured to the parietal peritoneum and presacral fascia to prevent prolapse.

postponing exteriorization of the high vagina until 2 to 3 years of age.[224, 225] More recently, one stage total genital reconstruction in young infants by an experienced surgeon is recommended in all cases, based on the premise that the potential for psychological trauma is reduced if a vagina is in place before puberty, even if the need for surgical revision is likely at that time.[226–228] The benefit of estrogenization during the first month of life has also been cited in support of early reconstructive surgery.[228] In addition, it is advantageous to use phallic skin mobi-

lized at the time of clitoroplasty, which is usually performed early to normalize the baby's external appearance, for creation of the labia minora or anterior vaginal wall.

Flap vaginoplasty as originally described by Fortunoff et al[229] is the standard procedure used when the vagina enters the mid or distal urethra (Fig. 32.9). Clitoroplasty is performed simultaneously and preputial skin is used to create a clitoral hood and labia minora. For severe masculinization of the urogenital sinus (see Fig. 32.5B), options include a pull-through procedure,[230] or use of local preputial[226, 231] or buttock[227] flaps for vaginal reconstruction. We use preputial skin to construct the vestibule and anterior vaginal wall and avoid cutback of the urogenital sinus.[226] In some cases, a long urogenital sinus can be used to augment the anterior vagina or remucosalize the perineal surface (Chapter 38, Figure 38.9). We do not use routine vaginal dilation postoperatively.

In the second group of patients in whom only a distal vagina is present, options include gradual vaginal amplification through dilation, skin graft urethroplasty (McIndoe technique), or bowel vaginoplasty.[189] The first two techniques, applicable only to adult females, have variable success rates and require continued vaginal dilation or intercourse to maintain capacity.[189, 214] By contrast, bowel can be used for vaginoplasty at any age, does not undergo shrinkage, and its mucus secretion provides a source of vaginal lubrication.[232] The sigmoid colon may be preferable because of its location. A reversed loop is used (Fig. 32.10) and anastomosed to

a cruciate opening in the blind-ending distal vaginal remnant. If the vestibule is absent and the perineum is flat, a tissue expander can be placed initially to generate flaps for anastomosis to the bowel[233] (Fig. 32.11), thereby avoiding the functional and cosmetic problems associated with direct anastomosis of bowel to the perineum.

As with clitoroplasty, minimal data are available to assess long-term sexual function after flap or bowel vaginoplasty performed in young children. The available data suggest that most patients undergoing vaginoplasty early in life will need later revision for introital stenosis and that secondary procedures are best performed after puberty.[223, 230, 234] However, surgery in infancy does not necessarily increase the risk of complications. Success after reoperation is likely, although routine vaginal dilation is necessary postoperatively. After bowel vaginoplasty, introital stenosis, vaginal prolapse, and excessive mucus production may occur but appear to be uncommon.[232] The risk of these complications may be minimized by using generous perineal flaps, securing

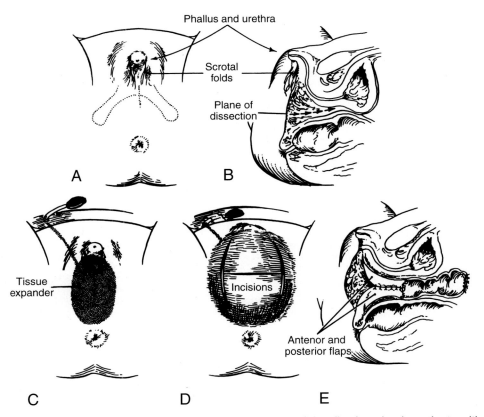

FIG. 32.11. Method of generating skin flaps for construction of the distal vagina in patients with a flat perineum using tissue expansion. **A,** Preoperative appearance. **B,** Lateral view showing plane of dissection in male-type pelvis between urethra and rectum. **C,** Placement of tissue expander in midline perineum. The injection port is placed externally with a suprapubic stab incision and gradual inflation of the reservoir accomplished with weekly injections to tolerance of sterile saline to a total volume of 100 to 150 mL. **D,** Incisions into expanded skin flaps at time of vaginoplasty. **E,** Lateral view showing suture of perineal flaps laterally and proximally to previously prepared sigmoid neovaginal segment.

the isolated loop of bowel to the sacrum, and avoiding use of an excessively long bowel segment.

REFERENCES

1. van Niekerk WA. True Hermaphroditism: Clinical, Morphologic and Cytogenetic Aspects. Hagerstown: Harper and Row, 1974; 1–5.
2. New MI, Kitzinger ES. President's address: Pope Joan: A recognizable syndrome. J Clin Endocrinol Metab 1993;76:3.
3. Diamond M. Prenatal predisposition and the clinical management of some pediatric conditions. J Sex Marital Ther 1996; 22:139.
4. Fausto-Sterling A. The five sexes: why male and female are not enough. Sciences 1993;Mar/Apr:20.
5. Chase C. Intersexual rights. Sciences 1993;July/Aug:3.
6. Kreidberg JA, Sariola H, Loring JM, et al. WT-1 is required for early kidney development. Cell 1993;74:679.
7. Luo X, Ikeda Y, Parker KL. A cell-specific nuclear receptor is essential for adrenal and gonadal development and sexual differentiation. Cell 1994;77:481.
8. Lovell-Badge R, Hacker A. The molecular genetics of sry and its role in mammalian sex determination. Phil Trans R Soc Lond B 1995;350:205.
9. Capel B. The role of sry in cellular events underlying mammalian sex determination. Curr Topics Devel Biol 1996;32:1.
10. McElreavey K, Vilain E, Abbas N, Herskowitz I, Fellous M. A regulatory cascade hypothesis for mammalian sex determination: SRY represses a negative regulator of male development. Proc Natl Acad Sci USA 1993;90:3368.
11. Ogata T, Hawkins JR, Taylor A, Matsuo N, Hata J, Goodfellow PN. Sex reversal in a child with a 46,X,Yp+ karyotype: support for the existence of a gene(s), located in distal Xp, involved in testis formation. J Med Genet 1992;29:226.
12. Ogata T, Matsuo N. Testis determining gene(s) on the X chromosome short arm: chromosomal localization and possible role in testis determination. J Med Genet 1994;31:349.
13. Arn P, Chen H, Tuck-Muller CM, et al. SRVX, a sex reversing locus in Xp21.2→p22.11. Hum Genet 1994;93:389.
14. Bardoni B, Zanaria E, Guioli S, et al. A dosage sensitive locus at chromosome Xp21 is involved in male to female sex reversal. Nature Genet 1994;7:487.
15. Tar A, Sólyom J, Györvári B, et al. Testicular development in an SRY-negative 46,XX individual harboring a distal Xp deletion. Hum Genet 1995;96:464.
16. Zanaria E, Bardoni B, Dabovic B, et al. Xp duplications and sex reversal. Phil Trans R Soc Lond B 1995;350:291.
17. Baumstark A, Barbi G, Djalali M, et al. Xp-duplications with and without sex reversal. Hum Genet 1996;97:79.
18. Da Silva SM, Hacker A, Harley V, Goodfellow P, Swain A, Lovell-Badge R. sox9 expression during gonadal development implies a conserved role for the gene in testis differentiation in mammals and birds. Nature Genet 1996;14:62.
19. Wilkie AOM, Campbell, FM, Daubeney P, et al. Complete and partial XY sex reversal associated with terminal deletion of 10q: report of 2 cases and literature review. Am J Med Genet 1993;46:597.
20. Bennett CP, Docherty Z, Robb SA, Ramani P, Hawkins JR, Grant D. Deletion 9p and sex reversal. J Med Genet 1993;30:518.
21. Jirasek JE. Development of the Genital System and Male Pseudohermaphroditism. Baltimore: Johns Hopkins Press 1971;3–41.
22. Arey LB. Developmental Anatomy. Philadelphia: W.B. Saunders 1974;315–341.
23. Josso N. Anatomy and endocrinology of fetal sex differentiation. In: DeGroot LJ, ed. Endocrinology. Philadelphia: W.B. Saunders 1995;1888–1900.
24. Heyns CF. The gubernaculum during testicular descent in the human fetus. J Anat 1987;153:93.
25. Winter JSD, Faiman C, Reyes FI. Sex steroid production by the human fetus: its role in morphogenesis and control by gonadotropins. Birth Defects 1977;13:41.
26. Mishina Y, Rey R, Finegold MJ, et al. Genetic analysis of the Müllerian-inhibiting substance signal transduction pathway in mammalian sexual differentiation. Genes Dev 1996;10:2577.
27. Word RA, George FW, Wilson JD, Carr BR. Testosterone synthesis and adenylate cyclase activity in the early human fetal testis appear to be independent of human chorionic gonadotropin control. J Clin Endocrinol Metab 1989;69:204
28. Husmann DA, Levy JB. Current concepts in the pathophysiology of testicular undescent. Urology 1995;46:267.
29. Tong SY, Hutson JM, Watts LM. Does testosterone diffuse down the wolffian duct during sexual differentiation? J Urol 1996;155: 2057.
30. Rey R, Josso N. Regulation of testicular anti-Müllerian hormone secretion. Eur J Endocrinol 1996;135:144.
31. Haqq CM, King C-Y, Ukiyama E, et al. Molecular basis of mammalian sexual determination: activation of Müllerian inhibiting substance gene expression by SRY. Science 1994;266:1494.
32. Shen W-H, Moore CCD, Ikeda Y, Parker KL, Ingraham HA. Nuclear receptor steroidogenic factor 1 regulates the Müllerian inhibiting substance gene: a link to the sex determination cascade. Cell 1994;77:651.
33. Ingraham HA, Lala DS, Ikeda Y, et al. The nuclear receptor steroidogenic factor 1 acts at multiple levels of the reproductive axis. Genes Devel 1994;8:2302.
34. Burris TP, Guo W, Le T, McCabe ERB. Identification of a putative steroidogenic factor-1 response element in the DAX-1 promoter. Biochem Biophys Res Commun 1995;214:576.
35. Swain A, Zanaria E, Hacker A, Lovell-Badge R, Camerino G. Mouse Dax1 expression is consistent with a role in sex determination as well as in adrenal and hypothalamus function. Nature Genet 1996;12:404.
36. Berkovitz GD, Fechner PY, Zacur HW, et al. Clinical and pathologic spectrum of 46,XY gonadal dysgenesis: its relevance to the understanding of sex differentiation. Medicine 1991;70:375.
37. Marcantonio SM, Fechner PY, Migeon CJ, Perlman EJ, Berkovitz GD. Embryonic testicular regression sequence: a part of the clinical spectrum of 46,XY gonadal dysgenesis. Am J Med Genet 1994;49:1.
38. Lippe B. Turner syndrome. Endocrinol Metab Clin North Am 1991;20:121.
39. Simpson JL, Christakos AC, Horwith M, Silverman FS. Gonadal dysgenesis in individuals with apparently normal chromosomal complements: tabulation of cases and compilation of genetic data. Birth Defects 1971;7:215.
40. German J, Simpson JL, Chaganti RSK, Summitt RL, Reid LB, Merkatz IR. Genetically determined sex-reversal in 46,XY humans. Science 1978;202:53.
41. Hawkins JR. Genetics of XY sex reversal. J Endocrinol 1995; 147:183.
42. Pivnick EK, Wachtel S, Woods D, Simpson JL, Bishop CE. Mutations in the conserved domain of SRY are uncommon in XY gonadal dysgenesis. Hum Genet 1992;90:308.
43. Ogata T, Tomita K, Hida A, Matsuo N, Nakhori Y, Nakagome Y. Chromosomal localisation of a Y specific growth gene(s). J Med Genet 1995;32:572.
44. Salo P, Kääriäinen H, Page DC, de la Chapelle A. Deletion mapping of stature determinants on the long arm of the Y chromosome. Hum Genet 1995;95:283.
45. Ogata T, Tyler-Smith C, Purvis-Smith S, Turner G. Chromosomal localisation of a gene(s) for Turner stigmata on Yp. J Med Genet 1993;30:918.
46. Verp MS, Simpson JL. Abnormal sexual differentiation and neoplasia. Cancer Genet Cytogenet 1987;25:191.
47. Savage MO, Lowe DG. Gonadal neoplasia and abnormal sexual differentiation. Clin Endocrinol 1990;32:519.
48. Page DC. Hypothesis: a Y-chromosomal gene causes gonadoblastoma in dysgenetic gonads. Development 1987;101(S):151.
49. Tsuchiya K, Reijo R, Page DC, Disteche CM. Gonadoblastoma: molecular definition of the susceptibility region on the Y chromosome. Am J Hum Genet 1995;57:1400.
50. Salo P, Kääriäinen H, Petrovic V, Peltomäki P, Page DC, de al Chapelle A. Molecular mapping of the putative gonadoblastoma locus on the Y chromosome. Genes Chromosomes Cancer 1995;14:210.
51. Scully RE. Neoplasia associated with anomalous sexual develop-

ment and abnormal sex chromosomes. Pediatr Adolesc Endocrinol 1981;8:203.

52. Mueller RF. The Denys-Drash syndrome. J Med Genet 1994; 31:471.

53. Pelletier J, Bruening W, Kashtan CE, et al. Germline mutations in the Wilms' tumor suppressor gene are associated with abnormal urogenital development in Denys-Drash syndrome. Cell 1991;67:437.

54. Poulat F, Amorin D, König A, et al. Distinct molecular origins for Denys-Drash and Frasier syndromes. Hum Genet 1993;91:285.

55. Nordenskjöld A, Fricke G, Anvret M. Absence of mutations in the WT1 gene in patients with XY gonadal dysgenesis. Hum Genet 1995;96:102.

56. Clarkson PA, Davies HR, Williams DM, Chaudhary R, Hughes IA, Patterson MN. Mutational screening of the Wilms's tumour gene, WT1, in males with genital abnormalities. J Med Genet 1993;30:767.

57. Schafer AJ, Foster JW, Kwok C, Weller PA, Guioli S, Goodfellow PN. Campomelic dysplasia with XY sex reversal: diverse phenotypes resulting from mutations in a single gene. Ann N Y Acad Sci 1996;785:137.

58. Aittomäki K. The genetics of XX gonadal dysgenesis. Am J Hum Genet 1994;54:844.

59. Aittomäki K, Herva R, Stenman U-H, et al. Clinical features of primary ovarian failure caused by a point mutation in the follicle-stimulating hormone receptor gene. J Clin Endocrinol Metab 1996;81:3722.

60. Saenger P. Turner's syndrome. N Engl J Med 1996;335:1749.

61. Barbaux S, Vilain E, Raoul O, et al. Proximal deletions of the long arm of the Y chromosome suggest a critical region associated with a specific subset of characteristic Turner stigmata. Hum Molec Genet 1995;4:1565.

62. Koeberl DD, McGillivray B, Sybert VP. Prenatal diagnosis of 45,X/46,XX mosaicism and 45,X: implications for postnatal outcome. Am J Hum Genet 1995;57:661.

63. Davidoff F, Federman DD. Mixed gonadal dysgenesis. Pediatrics 1973;52:725.

64. Rajfer J, Walsh PC. Mixed gonadal dysgenesis - dysgenetic male pseudohermaphroditism. Pediatr Adolesc Endocrinol 1981;8:105.

65. Borer JG, Nitti VW, Glassberg KI. Mixed gonadal dysgenesis and dysgenetic male pseudohermaphroditism. J Urol 1995;153:1267.

66. Chang HJ, Clark RD, Bachman H. The phenotype of 45,X/46,XY mosaicism: an analysis of 92 prenatally diagnosed cases. Am J Hum Genet 1990;46:156.

67. Sugarman ID, Crolla JA, Malone PS. Mixed gonadal dysgenesis and cell line differentiation. Case presentation and literature review. Clin Genet 1994;46:313.

68. McElreavey K, Vilain E, Barbaux S, et al. Loss of sequences 3' to the testis-determining gene, SRY, including the Y pseudoautosomal boundary associated with partial testicular determination. Proc Natl Acad Sci USA 1996;93:8590.

69. Mendonça BB, Barbosa AS, Arnhold IJP, McElreavey K, Fellous M, Moreira-Filho CA. Gonadal agenesis in XX and XY sisters: evidence for the involvement of an autosomal gene. Am J Med Genet 1994;52:39.

70. Rey R, Al-Attar L, Louis F, et al. Testicular dysgenesis does not affect expression of anti-Müllerian hormone by Sertoli cells in premeiotic seminiferous tubules. Am J Pathol 1996;148:1689.

71. Edman CD, Winters AJ, Porter JC, Wilson J, MacDonald PC. Embryonic testicular regression: a clinical spectrum of XY agonadal individuals. Obstet Gynecol 1977;49:208.

72. Coulam CB. Testicular regression syndrome. Obstet Gynecol 1979;53:44.

73. Smith NM, Byard RW, Bourne AJ. Testicular regression syndrome—a pathological study of 77 cases. Histopathology 1991; 19:269.

74. Rutgers JL, Scully RE. Pathology of the testis in intersex syndromes. Semin Diagn Pathol 1987;4:275.

75. Robboy SJ, Miller T, Donahoe PK, et al. Dysgenesis of testicular and streak gonads in the syndrome of mixed gonadal dysgenesis: perspective derived from a clinicopathologic analysis of twenty-one cases. Hum Pathol 1982;13:700.

76. Müller J, Skakkebaek NE, Ritzén M, Plöen L, Petersen KE.

77. Ramani P, Yeung CK, Habeebu SSM. Testicular intratubular germ cell neoplasia in children and adolescents with intersex. Am J Surg Pathol 1993;17:1124.

78. Krob G, Braun A, Kuhnle U. True hermaphroditism: geographical distribution, clinical findings, chromosomes and gonadal histology. Eur J Pediatr 1994;153:2.

79. Braun A, Kammerer S, Cleve H, Löhrs U, Schwarz H-P, Kuhnle U. True hermaphrodism in a 46,XY individual, caused by a postzygotic somatic point mutation in the male gonadal sex-determining locus (SRY): molecular genetics and histological findings in a sporadic case. Am J Hum Genet 1993;52:578.

80. Fechner PY, Rosenberg C, Stetten G, et al. Nonrandom inactivation of the Y-bearing X chromosome in a 46,XX individual: evidence for the etiology of 46,XX true hermaphroditism. Cytogenet. Cell Genet 1994;66:22.

81. McElreavey K, Rappaport R, Vilain E, et al. The minority of 46,XX true hermaphrodites are positive for the Y-DNA sequence including SRY. Hum Genet 1992;90:121.

82. Berkovitz GD, Fechner PY, Marcantonio SM, et al. The role of the sex-determining region of the Y chromosome (SRY) in the etiology of 46,XX true hermaphroditism. Hum Genet 1992;88: 411.

83. Hadjiathanasiou CG, Brauner R, Lortat-Jacob S, et al. True hermaphroditism: genetic variants and clinical management. J Pediatr 1994;125:738.

84. Kuhnle U, Schwarz HP, Löhrs U, Stengel-Ruthkowski S, Cleve H, Braun A. Familial true hermaphroditism: paternal and maternal transmission of true hermaphroditism (46,XX) and XX maleness in the absence of Y-chromosomal sequences. Hum Genet 1993;92:571.

85. Ramos ES, Moreira-Filho CA, Vicente YAMVA, et al. SRY-negative true hermaphrodites and an XX male in two generations of the same family. Hum Genet 1996;97:596.

86. Kropp BP, Keating MA, Moshang T, Duckett JW. True hermaphroditism and normal male genitalia: an unusual presentation. Urology 1995;46:736.

87. Aaronson IA. True hermaphroditism. A review of 41 cases with observations on testicular histology and function. Br J Urol 1985;57:775.

88. Nihoul-Fékété C, Lortat-Jacob S, Cachin O, Josso N. Preservation of gonadal function in true hermaphroditism. J Pediatr Surg 1984;19:50.

89. Van Niekerk WA, Retief AE. The gonads of human true hermaphrodites. Hum Genet 1981;58:117.

90. Gustafson ML, Lee MM, Asmundson L, MacLaughlin DT, Donahoe PK. Müllerian inhibiting substance in the diagnosis and management of intersex and gonadal abnormalities. J Pediatr Surg 1993;28:439.

91. de la Chapelle A. Nature and origin of males with XX sex chromosomes. Am J Hum Genet 1972;24:71.

92. de la Chapelle A. The Y-chromosomal and autosomal testis-determining genes. Development 1987;101(suppl):33.

93. Fechner PY, Marcantonio SM, Jaswaney V, et al. The role of the sex-determining region Y gene in the etiology of 46,XX maleness. J Clin Endocrinol Metab 1993;76:690.

94. Boucekkine C, Toublanc JE, Abbas N, et al. Clinical and anatomical spectrum in XX sex reversed patients. Relationship to the presence of Y specific DNA-sequences. Clin Endocrinol 1994; 40:733.

95. Boucekkine C, Toublanc JE, Abbas N, et al. The sole presence of the testis-determining region of the Y chromosome (SRY) in 46,XX patients is associated with phenotypic variability. Horm Res 1992;37:236.

96. Abbas NE, Toublanc JE, Boucekkine C, et al. A possible common origin of "Y-negative" human XX males and XX true hermaphrodites. Hum Genet 1990;84:356.

97. Reijo R, Lee T-Y, Salo P, et al. Diverse spermatogenic defects in humans caused by Y chromosome deletions encompassing a novel RNA-binding protein gene. Nature Genet 1995;10:383.

98. Turner B, Fechner PY, Fuqua JS, et al. Combined Leydig cell and Sertoli cell dysfunction in 46,XX males lacking the sex determining region Y gene. Am J Med Genet 1995;57:440.

Carcinoma in situ of the testis in children with 45X/46,XY gonadal dysgenesis. J Pediatr 1985;106:431.

99. Schwartz ID, Root AW. The Klinefelter syndrome of testicular dysgenesis. Endocrinol Metab Clin North Am 1991;20:153.

100. Müller J, Skakkebaek NE, Ratcliffe SG. Quantified testicular histology in boys with sex chromosome abnormalities. Int J Androl 1995;18:57.

101. Winter JSD. Androgen therapy in Klinefelter syndrome during adolescence. Birth Defects 1991;26:235.

102. Sogge MR, McDonald SD, Cofold PB. The malignant potential of the dysgenetic germ cell in Klinefelter's syndrome. Am J Med 1979;66:515.

103. Tay HP, Bidair M, Shabaik A, Gilbaugh JH III, Schmidt JD. Primary yolk sac tumor of the prostate in a patient with Klinefelter's syndrome. J Urol 1995;153:1066.

104. New MI. Congenital adrenal hyperplasia. In: DeGroot LJ, ed. Endocrinology. Philadelphia: WB Saunders 1995;1813–1835.

105. Laue L, Rennert OM. Congenital adrenal hyperplasia: molecular genetics and alternative approaches to treatment. Adv Pediatr 1995;42:113.

106. Pang S, Wallace MA, Hofman L, et al. Worldwide experience in newborn screening for classical congenital adrenal hyperplasia due to 21-hydroxylase deficiency. Pediatrics 1988;81:866.

107. Wilson RC, Mercado AB, Cheng KC, New MI. Steroid 21-hydroxylase deficiency: genotype may not predict phenotype. J Clin Endocrinol Metab 1995;80:2322.

108. Qazi QH, Thompson MW. Genital changes in congenital virilizing adrenal hyperplasia. J Pediatr 1972;80:653.

109. Mulaikal RM, Migeon CJ, Rock JA. Fertility rates in female patients with congenital adrenal hyperplasia due to 21-hydroxylase deficiency. N Engl J Med 1987;316:178.

110. Kuhnle U, Bullinger M, Schwarz HP. The quality of life in adult female patients with congenital adrenal hyperplasia: a comprehensive study of the impact of genital malformations and chronic disease on female patients life. Eur J Pediatr 1995;154:708.

111. Hochberg Z, Gardos M, Benderly A. Psychosexual outcome of assigned females and males with 46,XX virilizing congenital adrenal hyperplasia. Eur J Pediatr 1987;146:497.

112. Mercado AB, Wilson RC, Cheng KC, Wei J-Q, New MI. Prenatal treatment and diagnosis of congenital adrenal hyperplasia owing to steroid 21-hydroxylase deficiency. J Clin Endocrinol Metab 1995;80:2014.

113. Seckl JR, Miller WL. How safe is long-term prenatal glucocorticoid treatment? JAMA 1997;277:1077.

114. White PC, Curnow KM, Pascoe L. Disorders of steroid 11β-hydroxylase isoenzymes. Endocrine Rev 1994;14:421.

115. Bongiovanni AM. The adrenogenital syndrome with deficiency of 3β-hydroxysteroid dehydrogenase. J Clin Invest 1962;41:2086.

116. Simard J, Rheaume E, Mebarki F, et al. Molecular basis of human 3β-hydroxysteroid dehydrogenase deficiency. J Steroid Biochem Molec Biol 1995;53:127.

117. Peterson RE, Imperato-McGinley J. Male pseudohermaphroditism due to inherited deficiencies of testosterone biosynthesis. In: Serio M, et al, ed. Sexual Differentiation, Basic and Clinical Aspects. New York: Raven Press 1984;301–319.

118. Mendonca BB, Bloise W, Arnhold IJP et al. Male pseudohermaphroditism due to nonsalt-losing 3β-hydroxysteroid dehydrogenase deficiency: gender role change and absence of gynecomastia at puberty. J Steroid Biochem 1987;28:669.

119. Yanase T, Simpson ER, Waterman MR. 17α-hydroxylase/17,20-lyase deficiency: from clinical investigation to molecular definition. Endocrine Rev 1991;12:91.

120. Kater CE, Biglieri EG. Disorders of steroid 17α-hydroxylase deficiency. Endocrinol Metab Clin North Am 1994;23:341.

121. Shozu M, Akasofu K, Karada T, Kubota Y. A new cause of female pseudohermaphroditism: placental aromatase deficiency. J Clin Endocrinol Metab 1991;72:560.

122. Rösler A. Steroid 17β-hydroxysteroid dehydrogenase deficiency in man: an inherited form of male pseudohermaphroditism. J Steroid Biochem Molec Biol 1992;43:989.

123. Geissler WM, Davis DL, Wu L, et al. Male pseudohermaphroditism caused by mutations of testicular 17β-hydroxysteroid dehydrogenase 3. Nature Genet 1994;7:34.

124. Imperato-McGinley J, Peterson RE, Stoller R, Goodwin WE. Male pseudohermaphroditism secondary to 17β-hydroxysteroid dehydrogenase deficiency: gender role change with puberty. J Clin Endocrinol Metab 1979;49:391.

125. Martinez-Mora J, Sáez JM, Torán N, et al. Male pseudohermaphroditism due to Leydig cell agenesia and absence of testicular LH receptors. Clin Endocrinol 1991;34:485.

126. Latronico AC, Anasti J, Arnhold IJP, et al. Brief report: testicular and ovarian resistance to luteinizing hormone caused by inactivating mutations of the luteinizing hormone-receptor gene. N Engl J Med 1996;334:507.

127. Laue L, Wu S-M, Kudo M, et al. A nonsense mutation of the human luteinizing hormone receptor gene in Leydig cell hypoplasia. Hum Molec Genet 1995;4:1429.

128. Genuardi M, Bardoni B, Floridia G, et al. Dicentric chromosome Y associated with Leydig cell agenesis and sex reversal. Clin Genet 1995;47:38.

129. Berthezène F, Forest MG, Grimaud JA, Claustrat B, Mornex R. Leydig-cell agenesis: a cause of male pseudohermaphroditism. N Engl J Med 1976;295:969.

130. Imperato-McGinley J, Guerrero L, Gautier T, Peterson RE. Steroid 5α-reductase deficiency in man: an inherited form of male pseudohermaphroditism. Science 1974;186:1213.

131. Walsh PC, Madden JD, Harrod MJ, Goldstein JL, MacDonald PC, Wilson JD. Familial incomplete male pseudohermaphroditism, type 2: decreased dihydrotestosterone formation in pseudovaginal perineoscrotal hypospadias. N Engl J Med 1974;291:944.

132. Mendonca BB, Inacio M, Costa EMF, et al. Male pseudohermaphroditism due to steroid 5α-reductase 2 deficiency. Diagnosis, psychological evaluation, and management. Medicine 1996;75:64.

133. Forti G, Falchetti A, Santoro S, Davis DL, Wilson JD, Russell DW. Steroid 5α-reductase 2 deficiency: virilization in early infancy may be due to partial function of mutant enzyme. Clin Endocrinol 1996;44:477.

134. Thigpen AE, Davis DL, Milatovich A, et al. Molecular genetics of steroid 5α-reductase 2 deficiency. J Clin Invest 1992;90:799.

135. Sinnecker GHG, Hiort O, Dibbelt L, et al. Phenotypic classification of male pseudohermaphroditism due to steroid 5α-reductase deficiency. Am J Med Genet 1996;63:223.

136. Imperato-McGinley J, Gautier T, Pichardo M, Shackleton C. The diagnosis of 5α-reductase deficiency in infancy. J Clin Endocrinol Metab 1986;63:1313.

137. Imperato-McGinley J, Peterson RE, Gautier T, et al. Hormonal evaluation of a large kindred with complete androgen insensitivity: evidence for secondary 5α-reductase deficiency. J Clin Endocrinol Metab 1982;54:931.

138. Morris JM. The syndrome of testicular feminization in male pseudohermaphrodites. Am J Obstet Gynecol 1953;65:1193.

139. Quigley CA, DeBellis A, Marschke KB, El-Awady MK, Wilson EM, French FM. Androgen receptor defects: historical, clinical, and molecular perspectives. Endocrine Rev 1995;16:271.

140. Hiort O, Sinnecker GHG, Holterhus P-M, Nitsche EM, Kruse K. The clinical and molecular spectrum of androgen insensitivity syndromes. Am J Med Genet 1996;63:218.

141. Ulloa-Aguirre A, Méndez JP, Angeles A, del Castillo CF, Chávez B, Pérez-Palacios G. The presence of Müllerian remnants in the complete androgen insensitivity syndrome: a steroid hormone-mediated defect? Fertil Steril 1986;45:302.

142. Rutgers JL, Scully RE. The androgen insensitivity syndrome (testicular feminization): a clinicopathologic study of 43 cases. Int J Gynecol Pathol 1991;10:126.

143. Cassio A, Cacciari EM, D'Errico A, et al. Incidence of intratubular germ cell neoplasia in androgen insensitivity syndrome. Acta Endocrinologica 1990;123:416.

144. Lee PA, Brown TR, LaTorre HA. Diagnosis of the partial androgen insensitivity syndrome during infancy. JAMA 1986;255:2207.

145. Sinnecker G, Kohler S. Sex hormone-binding globulin response to the anabolic steroid stanozolol: evidence for its suitability as a biological androgen sensitivity test. J Clin Endocrinol Metab 1989;68:1195.

146. Grino PB, Isidro-Gutierrez RF, Griffin JE, Wilson JD. Androgen resistance associated with a qualitative abnormality of the androgen receptor and responsive to high dose androgen therapy. J Clin Endocrinol Metab 1989;68:578.

147. Batch JA, Davies HR, Evans BAJ, Hughes IA, Patterson MN. Phenotypic variation and detection of carrier status in the partial androgen insensitivity syndrome. Arch Dis Child 1993;68:453.

148. Lumbroso S, Lobaccaro J-M, Belon C, et al. Molecular prenatal exclusion of familial partial androgen insensitivity (Reifenstein syndrome). Eur J Endocrinol 1994;130:327.

149. Morel Y, Mebarki F, Forest MG. What are the indications for prenatal diagnosis in the androgen insensitivity syndrome? Facing clinical heterogeneity of phenotypes for the same genotype. Eur J Endocrinol 1994;130:325.

150. Souto CAV, da Costa Oliveira M, Telöken C, Paskulin G, Hoffmann K. Persistence of Müllerian duct derivative syndrome in 2 male patients with bilateral cryptorchidism. J Urol 1995;153:1637.

151. Imbeaud S, Carrè-Eusébe D, Rey R, Belville C, Josso N, Picard J-Y. Molecular genetics of the persistent Müllerian duct syndrome: a study of 19 families. Hum Molec Genet 1994;3:125.

152. Imbeaud S, Faure E, Lamarre I, et al. Insensitivity to anti-Müllerian hormone due to a mutation in the human anti-Müllerian hormone receptor. Nature Genet 1995;11:382.

153. Guerrier D, Tran D, Vanderwinden JM, et al. The persistent Müllerian duct syndrome: a molecular approach. J Clin Endocrinol Metab 1989;68:46.

154. Imbeaud S, Tey R, Berta P, et al. Testicular degeneration in three patients with the persistent Müllerian duct syndrome. Eur J Pediatr 1995;154:187.

155. Sloan WR, Walsh PC. Familial persistent Müllerian duct syndrome. J Urol 1976;115:459.

156. Mouli K, McCarthy P, Ray P, Ray V, Rosenthal IM. Persistent Müllerian duct syndrome in a man with transverse testicular ectopia. J Urol 1988;139:373.

157. Potashnik G, Sober I, Inbar I, Ben-Aderet N. Male Müllerian hermaphroditism: a case report of a rare cause of male infertility. Fertil Steril 1977;28:273.

158. Martin EL, Bennett AH, Cromie WJ. Persistent Müllerian duct syndrome with transverse testicular extopia and spermatogenesis. J Urol 1992;147:1615.

159. Brook CGD, Wagner H, Zachmann M, et al. Familial occurrence of persistent Müllerian structures in otherwise normal males. B Med J 1973;1:771.

160. Eastham JA, McEvoy K, Sullivan R, Chandrasoma P. A case of simultaneous bilateral nonseminomatous testicular tumors in persistent Müllerian duct syndrome. J Urol 1992;148:407.

161. Williams JC, Merguerian PA, Schned AR, Amdur RJ. Bilateral testicular carcinoma in situ in persistent Müllerian duct syndrome: a case report and literature review. Urology 1994;44:595.

162. Melman A, Leiter E, Perez JM, Driscoll D, Palmer C. The influence of neonatal orchiopexy upon the testis in persistent Müllerian duct syndrome. J Urol 1981;125:856.

163. Loeff DS, Imbeaud S, Reyes HM, Meller JL, Rosenthal IM. Surgical and genetic aspects of persistent Müllerian duct syndrome. J Pediatr Surg 1994;29:61.

164. Lee PA, Mazur T, Danish R, et al. Micropenis, I. Criteria, etiologies and classification. Johns Hopkins Med J 1980;146:156.

165. Aaronson IA. Micropenis: medical and surgical implications. J Urol 1994;152:4.

166. Forest MG. Pattern of the response of testosterone and its precursors to human chorionic gonadotropin stimulation in relation to age in infants and children. J Clin Endocrinol Metab 1979;49:132.

167. Almaguer MC, Saenger P, Linder BL. Phallic growth after hCG: a clinical index of androgen responsiveness. Clin Pediatr 1993;32:329.

168. Choi SK, Han SW, Kim DH, de Lignieres B. Transdermal dihydrotestosterone therapy and its effects on patients with microphallus. J Urol 1993;150:657.

169. Burstein S, Grumbach MM, Kaplan SL. Early determination of androgen-responsiveness is important in the management of microphallus. Lancet 1979;2:938.

170. Lee PA, Danish RK, Mazur T, Migeon CJ. Micropenis, III: Primary hypogonadism, partial androgen insensitivity syndrome, and idiopathic disorders. Johns Hopkins Med J 1980;147:175.

171. Money J, Lehne GK, Pierre-Jerome F. Micropenis: gender, erotosexual coping strategy, and behavioral health in nine pediatric cases followed to adulthood. Comp Psych 1985;26:29.

172. Reilly JM, Woodhouse CRJ. Small penis and the male sexual role. J Urol 1989;142:569.

173. Johnston WG, Yeatman GW, Weigel JW. Congenital absence of the penis. J Urol 1977;117:508.

174. Ciftci AO, Senocak ME, Büyükpamukçu N. Male gender assignment in penile agenesis: a case report and review of the literature. J Pediatr Surg 1995;30:1358.

175. Aarskog D. Intersex conditions masquerading as simple hypospadias. Birth Defects 1971;7:122.

176. Rajfer J, Walsh PC. The incidence of intersexuality in patients with hypospadias and cryptorchidism. J Urol 1976;116:769.

177. Rohatgi M, Menon PSN, Verma IC, Iyengar J. The presence of intersexuality in patients with advanced hypospadias and undescended gonads. J Urol 1987;137:263.

178. Gearhart JP, Linhard HR, Berkovitz GD, Jeffs RD, Brown TR. Androgen receptor levels and 5α-reductase activities in preputial skin and chordee tissue of boys with isolated hypospadias. J Urol 1988;140:1243.

179. Bentvelsen FM, Brinkmann AO, van der Linden JETM, Schröder FH, Nijman JM. Decreased immunoreactive androgen receptor levels are not the cause of isolated hypospadias. Brit J Urol 1995;76:384.

180. Alléra A, Herbst MA, Griffin JE, Wilson JD, Schweikert H-U, McPhaul MJ. Mutations of the androgen receptor coding sequence are infrequent in patients with isolated hypospadias. J Clin Endocrinol Metab 1995;80:2697.

181. Sutherland RW, Wiener JS, Hicks JP, et al. Androgen receptor gene mutations are rarely associated with isolated penile hypospadias. J Urol 1996;156:828.

182. Glenister TW. The development of the utricle and of the so-called 'middle' or 'median' lobe of the human prostate. J Anat 1962;96:443.

183. Devine CJ, Gonzalez-Serva L, Stecker JF, Devine PC, Horton CE. Utricular configuration in hypospadias and intersex. J Urol 1980;123:407.

184. Shima H, Yabumoto H, Okamoto E, Orestano L, Ikoma F. Testicular function in patients with hypospadias associated with enlarged prostatic utricle. Brit J Urol 1992;69:192.

185. Ritchey ML, Benson RC, Kramer SA, Kelalis PP. Management of Müllerian duct remnants in the male patient. J Urol 1988;140:795.

186. Wells LJ, Cavanagh MW, Maxwell EL. Genital abnormalities in castrated fetal rats and their prevention by means of testosterone propionate. Anat Rec 1954;118:109.

187. Vamer RE, Younger JB, Blackwell RE. Müllerian dysgenesis. J Reprod Med 1985;30:443.

188. Tarry WR, Duckett JW, Stephens FD. The Mayer-Rokitansky syndrome: pathogenesis, classification and management. J Urol 1986;136:648.

189. Seaman EK, Dean GE, Hensle TW. Vaginal agenesis, from diagnosis through reconstruction. Contemp Urol 1993;July:13.

190. Forest MG. Diagnosis and treatment of disorders of sexual development. In: DeGroot LJ, ed. Endocrinology Philadelphia: WB Saunders. 1995;1901–1937;

191. Feldman KW, Smith DW. Fetal phallic growth and penile standards for newborn male infants. J Pediatr 1975;86:395.

192. Yokoya S. Measurement of penile and clitoral size in pre-term and term newborns, infants, and children: toward earlier recognition of congenital endocrine disorders. Horumon to Rinsho 1983;31:1215.

193. Oberfield SE, Mondok A, Shahrivar F, Klein JF, Levine LS. Clitoral size in full-term infants. Am J Perinatol 1989;6:453.

194. Verkauf BS, von Thron J, O'Brien WF. Clitoral size in normal women. Obstet Gynecol 1992;80:41.

195. Sane K, Pescovitz OH. The clitoral index: a determination of clitoral size in normal girls and in girls with abnormal sexual development. J Pediatr 1992;120:264.

196. Tagatz GE, Kopher RA, Nagel TC, Okagaki T. The clitoral index: a bioassay of androgenic stimulation. Obstet Gynecol 1979;54:562.

197. De Peretti E, Forest MG. Pitfalls in the etiological diagnosis of congenital adrenal hyperplasia in the early postnatal period. Horm Res 1982;16:10.

198. Griffin JE, Wilson JD. Disorders of sexual differentiation. In:

Edited by Walsh PC, Retik AB, Stamey TA, Vaughan ED Jr, eds. *Campbell's Urology*. Philadelphia: WB Saunders 1992;1509–1542.

199. Kutteh WH, Santos-Ramos R, Ermel LD. Accuracy of ultrasonic detection of the uterus in normal newborn infants: implications for infants with ambiguous genitalia. Ultrasound Obstet Gynecol 1995;5:109.

200. Cohen HL, Shapiro MA, Mandel FS, Shapiro ML. Normal ovaries in neonates and infants: a sonographic study of 77 patients 1 day to 24 months old. AJR 1993;160:583.

201. Bryan PJ, Caldamone AA, Morrison SC, Yulish BS, Owens R. Ultrasound findings in the adrenogenital syndrome (congenital adrenal hyperplasia). J Ultrasound Med 1988;7:675.

202. Winter JSD, Taraska S, Faiman C. The hormonal response to HCG stimulation in male children and adolescents. J Clin Endocrinol 1972;34:348.

203. Money J, Hampson JG, Hampson JL. Hermaphroditism: recommendations concerning assignment of sex, change of sex and psychologic management. Bull Johns Hopkins Hosp 1955;97:284.

204. McCauley E. Disorders of sexual differentiation and development: psychological aspects. Pediatr Clin North Am 1990;37:1405.

205. Diamond M. Prenatal predisposition and the clinical management of some pediatric conditions. J Sex Marital Ther 1996;22:139.

206. Money J, Norman BF. Gender identity and gender transposition: longitudinal outcome study of 24 male hermaphrodites assigned as boys. J Sex Marital Ther 1987;13:75.

207. Diamond M, Sigmundson HK. Sex reassignment at birth: long-term review and clinical implications. Arch Pediatr Adolesc Med 1997;151:298.

208. Imperato-McGinley J, Peterson RE, Gautier T, Sturla E. Androgens and the evolution of male-gender identity among male pseudohermaphrodites with 5α-reductase deficiency. N Engl J Med 1979;300:1233.

209. Méndez JP, Ulloa-Aguirre A, Imperato-McGinley J, et al. Male pseudohermaphroditism due to primary 5α-reductase deficiency: variation in gender identity reversal in seven Mexican patients from five different pedigrees. J Endocrinol Invest 1995;18:205.

210. Gooren L, Cohen-Kettenis PT. Development of male gender identity/role and a sexual orientation towards women in a 46, XY subject with an incomplete form of the androgen insensitivity syndrome. Arch Sex Behav 1991;20:459.

211. Money J, Devore H, Norman BF. Gender identity and gender transposition: longitudinal outcome study of 32 male hermaprodites raised as girls. J Sex Marital Ther 1986;12:165.

212. Gilbert DA, Jordan GH, Devine CJ, Winslow BH, Schlossberg SM. Phallic construction in prepubertal and adolescent boys. J Urol 1993;149:1521.

213. Yu TJ, Shu K, Kung FT, Eng HL, Chen HY. Use of laparoscopy in intersex patients. J Urol 1995;154:1193.

214. Costa EMF, Mendonca BB, Inácio M, Arnhold IJP, Silva FAQ, Lodovici O. Management of ambiguous genitalia in pseudohermaphrodites: new perspectives on vaginal dilatation. Fertil Steril 1997;67:229.

215. Sotiropoulos A, Morishima A, Homsy Y, Lattimer JK. Long-term assessment of genital reconstruction in female pseudohermaphrodites. J Urol 1976;115:599.

216. Allen LE, Hardy BE, Churchill BM. The surgical management of the enlarged clitoris. J Urol 1982;128:351.

217. Randolph J, Hung W, Rathlev MC. Clitoroplasty for females born with ambiguous genitalia: a long-term study of 37 patients. J Pediatr Surg 1981;16:882.

218. Rajfer J, Ehrlich RM, Goodwin WE. Reduction clitoroplasty via ventral approach. J Urol 1982;128:341.

219. Kogan SJ, Smey P, Levitt SB. Subtunical total reduction clitoroplasty: a safe modification of existing techniques. J Urol 1983;130:746.

220. Newman K, Randolph J, Parson S. Functional results in young women having clitoral reconstruction as infants. J Pediatr Surg 1992;27:180.

221. Gearhart JP, Burnett A, Owen JH. Measurement of pudendal evoked potentials during feminizing genitoplasty: technique and applications. J Urol 1995;153:486.

222. Chase C. Letter to the editor. J Urol 1995;153:1139.

223. Bailez MM, Gearhart JP, Migeon C, Rock J. Vaginal reconstruction after initial construction of the external genitalia in girls with salt-wasting adrenal hyperplasia. J Urol 1992;148:680.

224. Snyder HMcC III, Retik AB, Bauer ST, Colodny AH. Feminizing genitoplasty: a synthesis. J Urol 1983;129:1024.

225. Oesterling JE, Gearhart JP, Jeffs RD. A unified approach to early reconstructive surgery of the child with ambiguous genitalia. J Urol 1987;138:1079.

226. Gonzalez R, Fernandes ET. Single-stage feminization genitoplasty. J Urol 1990;143:776.

227. Donahoe PK, Gustafson ML. Early one-stage surgical reconstruction of the extremely high vagina in patients with congenital adrenal hyperplasia. J Pediatr Surg 1994;29:352.

228. de Jong TPVM, Boemers TML. Neonatal management of female intersex by clitorovaginoplasty. J Urol 1995;154:830.

229. Fortunoff S, Lattimer JK, Edson M. Vaginoplasty technique for female pseudohermaphrodites. Surg Gynecol Obstet 1964;118:545.

230. Hendren WH, Atala A. Repair of the high vagina in girls with severely masculinized anatomy from the adrenogenital syndrome. J Pediatr Surg 1995;30:91.

231. Passerini-Glazel G. A new 1-stage procedure for clitorovaginoplasty in severely masculinized female pseudohermaphrodites. J Urol 1989;142:565.

232. Hendren WH, Atala A. Use of bowel for vaginal reconstruction. J Urol 1994;152:752.

233. Patil U, Hixson FP. The role of tissue expanders in vaginoplasty for congenital malformations of the vagina. Brit J Urol 1992;70:554.

234. Azziz R, Mulaikal RM, Migeon CJ, Jones HW Jr, Rock JA. Congenital adrenal hyperplasia: long-term results following vaginal reconstruction. Fertil Steril 1986;46:1011.

CHAPTER 33

Menstrual Problems in the Adolescent

Lydia A. Shrier and S. Jean Emans

PUBERTAL MATURATION

Puberty is the biologic transition from childhood to adulthood. In young women, hormonal changes result in the development of secondary sex characteristics, changes in muscle mass and fat distribution, skeletal growth, and the onset of menses. Understanding normal pubertal progression and development is essential to identifying when abnormalities of puberty occur.

Hormonal Changes of Puberty

Activation of the hypothalamic-pituitary-ovarian (HPO) axis heralds the onset of puberty and precedes the development of physical changes. Production of adrenal sex steroids, including dehydroepiandrosterone (DHEA), androstenedione, and estrone, increases approximately 2 years before the HPO axis matures. Probably in response to a decreased sensitivity to the negative feedback system between the central nervous system and the gonads, the HPO axis is activated. The hypothalamus synthesizes and releases gonadotropin releasing hormone (GnRH) (Fig. 33.1). GnRH is released in a pulsatile fashion into the portal plexus of the pituitary and binds to receptors in the anterior pituitary. GnRH simulates the synthesis and release of two glycoproteins: follicle stimulating hormone (FSH) and luteinizing hormone (LH). In early puberty, the increased amounts of FSH and LH are only nocturnal, but by midpuberty increases are also apparent during the day.

The pulsatile release of gonadotropins stimulates the ovary, resulting in maturation of the germinal epithelium and synthesis of gonadal steroid hormones. In addition, the ovary produces insulin-like growth factor (IGF), inhibin, activin, and cytokines. The gonadal hormones feedback on gonadotropin secretion at the level of the hypothalamus (modulating the frequency and amplitude of GnRH) and at the level of the pituitary (affecting the amount of FSH and LH released in response to GnRH pulses). Negative feedback occurs with small amounts of estrogen, suppressing GnRH secre-

tion. In late puberty, estrogen secretion increases during midcycle and triggers a surge of LH and FSH, resulting in ovulation.

The development of the hypothalamic-pituitary-ovarian system is mostly complete at birth. By 14 weeks of gestation, the hypothalamic portal system is intact. By mid-gestation, the negative feedback system of gonadal steroids on the hypothalamus and pituitary is apparent. At 5 to 6 months gestation, 6 to 7 million oocytes are present. Through atresia, 1 to 2 million oocytes are present at birth and by puberty only 0.3 to 0.5 million remain.[1] Gonadotropin levels increase sharply by 5 days after birth to levels higher than found in prepuberty, probably in response to the decrease in placental estrogen. A transient increase in estradiol may be seen in female infants, especially in the first 3 months of life. Gonadotropin levels then gradually decrease to childhood levels, although FSH may not be maximally suppressed for 1 to 4 years. Females have an elevated FSH:LH ratio compared to males.[2]

During the years before puberty, there is down regulation of the hypothalamic pituitary system, with a decrease in the amplitude and frequency of GnRH pulses and a decrease in pituitary responsiveness to a single dose of GnRH.[3] This inactivity appears to be in response to a central nervous system signal because it occurs even in agonadal patients.[4] In prepubertal girls, GnRH pulses continue to persist at low levels with amplification during sleep, and the FSH:LH ratio is higher than in earlier or later stages. Prepubertal girls often show little LH response to a single dose of GnRH but have a considerable increase in FSH. However, if GnRH is given in a physiologic manner over time, the pituitary becomes responsive.

The ovary increases in size during the prepubertal years and shows active follicular growth and atresia. The vagina, approximately 4 cm in length at birth, grows only 0.5 to 1.0 cm during early childhood, but increases to 7.0 to 8.5 cm in late childhood. The uterus is approximately 2.5 cm in length in infancy, with the corpus-to-

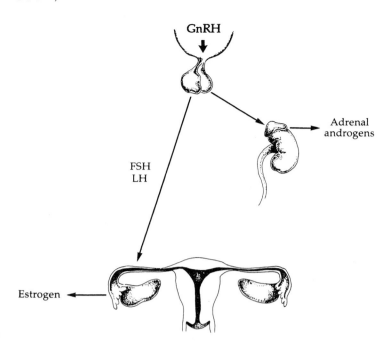

GnRH

FSH
LH

Adrenal
androgens

Estrogen

FIG. 33.1. Hormones responsible for the onset of puberty. The stimulus for the rise in adrenal androgens is unclear. *GnRH*, gonatropin releasing hormone; *FSH*, follicle-stimulating hormone; *LH*, luteinizing hormone.

cervix ratio slightly less than 1:1. This ratio reaches 1:1 at menarche and 3:1 in postmenarcheal adults.

The earliest change associated with pubertal maturation is adrenarche, the secretion of adrenal androgens (DHEA and its sulfate [DHEAS]) and androstenedione, which normally occurs between the ages of 6 and 8 years. This process involves the regrowth of the zona reticularis of the adrenal cortex, which regressed after birth, and increases in the activity of the microsomal enzyme p450c17. Adrenal androgens continue to increase through the ages of 13 to 15 years and are primarily responsible for the appearance of pubic and axillary hair (pubarche) in girls and the development of acne vulgaris.[5-7]

Around the age of 8 years, GnRH secretion is enhanced, first during sleep.[8] Pituitary responsiveness increases with increased secretion of LH and FSH (gonadarche).[9] LH responsiveness to exogenous GnRH testing also increases at this time, allowing for differentiation between pubertal and prepubertal patterns. Adrenarche and the age-related increase in gonadotropins occurs in patients with Turner syndrome, which suggests that ovarian sex steroids are not critical to the onset of puberty. Patients who have the onset of Addison's disease before puberty and patients with the onset of precocious puberty before age 6 can experience normal gonadarche without signs of adrenarche. Patients with constitutional delay of puberty frequently have delays in gonadarche and adrenarche.

During late prepuberty and early puberty, the episodic peaks of LH and FSH during sleep are gradually augmented. There is a greater increase in LH pulse amplitude than frequency.[10] Daytime pulsatility gradually increases. LH stimulates the theca interna cells of the ovary to synthesize precursors and FSH increases the enzyme aromatase, which is responsible for the conversion of androgen precursors to estrogen. Estrogen peaks 10 to 12 hours after the gonadotropin secretion.[9] The ovaries show increased follicular growth and may appear enlarged and "multicystic" on ultrasonography.

The onset of breast development (thelarche), estrogenization of the vaginal mucosa, and lengthening of the uterus occur with exposure to estrogen. The physiologic vaginal discharge of puberty (leukorrhea) results from the desquamation of epithelial cells and mucus from the estrogenized vaginal mucosa. As estrogen levels increase, growth hormone and IGF-1 levels increase and contribute to the growth spurt, which usually begins gradually at approximately the age of 9 years and reaches a peak by age 12 years.[11-14] The effect of estrogen is dose-related—low levels of estrogen stimulate growth hormone, IGF-1, and growth, whereas high levels of estrogen are associated with decreased growth hormone, IGF-1, and growth. Because bone age, as determined by Greulich and Pyle standards,[15] correlates best with pubertal age, a radiograph of the nondominant wrist and hand for bone age interpretation is useful when evaluating an individual with delayed or precocious puberty.

As puberty continues, nocturnal levels of FSH and LH are carried over into the daytime until the augmentation during sleep disappears. Before menarche, circulating estrogen levels in pubertal girls are somewhat cyclic, eventually enough to cause uterine bleeding. The

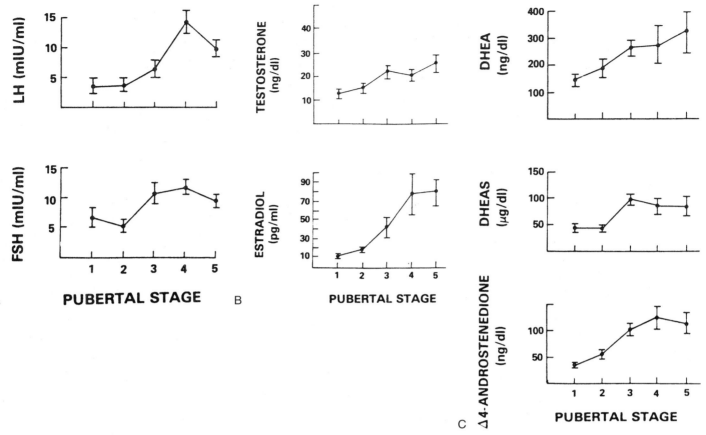

FIG. 33.2. Normal changes in luteinizing hormone (*LH*), follicle-stimulating hormone (*FSH*), testosterone, estradiol, dehydroepiandrostrone (*DHEA*), dehydroepiandrostrone sulfate (*DHEAS*), and Δ^9-androstenedione during puberty in girls. Reprinted with permission from Nottlemann ED, Susan EJ, Dorn LD, et al. Developmental processes in early adolescence: relations among chronologic age, pubertal stage, height, weight, and serum levels, of gonadotropins, sex steroids and adrenal androgens. J Adolesc Health Care 1987;8:246–260.

first 1 to 2 years after menarche are often characterized by anovulatory menses.[16–21] This time period coincides with the rapid growth of the uterus, vagina, fallopian tubes, and ovaries. With maturation, the biphasic positive feedback system develops, in which an increase in estrogen in the latter part of the follicular phase of the menstrual cycle triggers the surge of LH and FSH, which results in ovulation.

The normal changes of LH, FSH, estradiol, testosterone, DHEA, DHEAS, and androstenedione with puberty are shown in Figure 33.2.

Breast and Pubic Hair Development

In 1969, Marshall and Tanner recorded the rates of progression of pubertal development of 192 English schoolgirls.[22] These stages can be useful in assessing whether normal pubertal development is occurring. The Tanner stages (also known as Sexual Maturity Rating [SMR]) are as follows:[22, 23]

Breast (Fig. 33.3)

Stage B1. Prepubertal, elevation of the nipple only

Stage B2. Breast bud, elevation of the breast and nipple as a small mound, enlargement of the areolar diameter

Stage B3. Further enlargement of the breast and areola with no separation of the contours

Stage B4. Further enlargement with projection of the areola and nipple to form a secondary mound above the level of the breast

Stage B5. Mature, recession of the areola to the general contour of the breast, resulting in projection of the nipple only

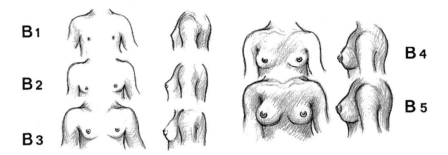

FIG. 33.3. The Tanner stages of female breast development. Modified from Grumbach MM, Styne DM. Puberty: ontogeny, neuroendocrinology, physiology, and disorders. In: Wilson JD, Foster DW, eds. Williams textbook of endocrinology, 8th ed. Philadelphia: Saunders, 1992; and from Marshall WA, Tanner JM. Variations in pattern of pubertal changes in girls. Arch Dis Child 1969;44:291–303.

Pubic Hair (Fig. 33.4)

Stage P_1. No pubic hair

Stage P_2. Sparse growth of long, downy, slightly pigmented, straight or only slightly curled hair along the labia

Stage P_3. Thicker, coarser, darker, and more curled hair extending sparsely over the junction of the pubis

Stage P_4. Hair is adult-type and spreads over the mons pubis but not to the medial surface of the thighs

Stage P_5. Hair is spread to the medial surface of the thighs (inverse triangle)

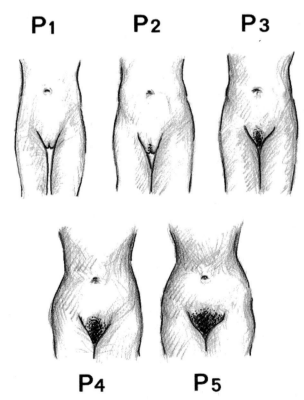

FIG. 33.4. The Tanner stages of female pubic hair development. Modified from Grumbach MM, Styne DM. Puberty: ontogeny, neuroendocrinology, physiology, and disorders. In: Wilson JD, Foster DW, eds.; Williams textbook of endocrinology, 8th ed. Philadelphia: Saunders, 1992; and from Marshall WA, Tanner JM. Variations in pattern of pubertal changes in girls. Arch Dis Child 1969;44:291–303.

The first sign of puberty in 85 to 92% of white girls is breast budding (stage B2), which usually begins around age 10.5 to 11 years and initially may be unilateral. The appearance of breast development usually corresponds to the onset of the growth spurt. In Tanner's series,[22] the mean interval from stage B2 to B5 was 4.2 years. Some girls pass from B3 directly to B5 and some remain in B4. Pubic hair development usually lags by approximately 6 months and appears at an average age of 11 to 12 years. Pubic hair may precede breast development as a normal variant, especially in black girls, but in some patients this may be a sign of an excess of androgens that later may cause hirsutism and menstrual irregularity. The mean interval from stage P_2 to P_5 is 2.7 years. In general, pubic hair will not advance beyond P_2 or P_3 without the presence of gonadal sex steroids. While the timing of the stages of pubertal development is variable, 98.8% of girls will have the first signs between ages 8 and 13 years. There is a high concordance between breast and pubic hair stage for black and white girls, with black girls being consistently more advanced than white girls for each chronologic age.[24]

Breast development before the age of 8 years is precocious and after 13 years is delayed, and requires further evaluation. It is also unlikely for a girl to reach B5 breast development without pubic hair development; if this occurs, androgen insensitivity (testicular feminization) syndrome or adrenal insufficiency should be considered. The development of pubic hair without breast maturation would suggest the presence of androgens alone, raising the possibility of estrogen deficiency, such as Kallmann's syndrome or Turner syndrome or, rarely, a virilized state, such as an intersex disorder.

Growth

The growth spurt depends on the onset of puberty. Growth charts are helpful in evaluating normal development. The growth charts commonly seen in the pediatrician's office use cross-sectional data from the National Health Statistics and do not clearly illustrate the pubertal growth spurt (Fig. 33.5).[25] Specialized growth charts using longitudinal data show normal, retarded, and ac-

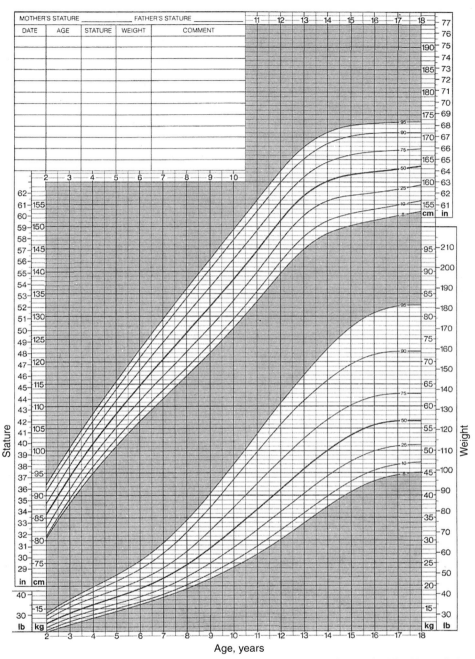

FIG. 33.5. Growth chart for girls aged 2 to 18 years showing National Center for Health statistics height and weight percentiles. Modified from Hamill PVV, Drizd TA, Johnson CL, et al. Physical growth: National Center for Health Statistics percentiles. Am J Clin Nutr 1979;32:607–629. Data from the National Center for Health Statistics (NCHS), Hyattsville, MD.

celerated patterns of growth (Fig. 33.6).[26] The inserts, the increment curves, represent the velocities of linear growth and weight gain. Peak height velocity (5.4 to 11.2 cm/year) is attained before Tanner stages B3 and PH2 in most adolescent girls. After menarche, growth slows to an average of 5 to 7.5 cm over the next 2 years.

The rate of pubertal development determines skeletal proportions. At puberty, the extremities rapidly lengthen, while the vertebral column elongates more gradually. As the epiphyses of the legs close, the vertebrae continue to add height for up to 2 years after menarche.

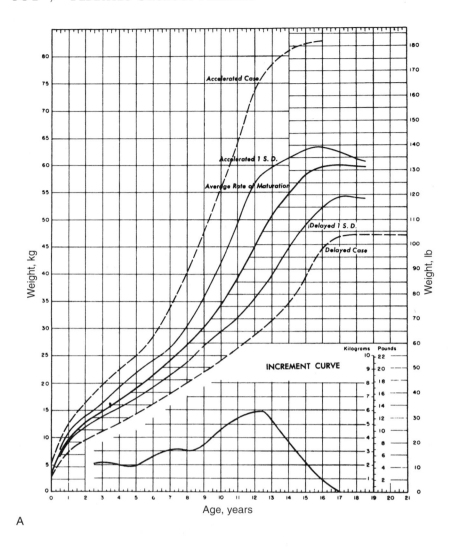

A

FIG. 33.6. Growth for girls by weight **(A)** and height **(B)**. Reprinted with permission from Bayley N. Growth curves of height and weight by age for boys and girls, scaled according to physical maturity. J Pediatr 1956;48:187.

Menarche

The mean age of menarche has been estimated to be 12.65 ± 1.2 years[16] to 13.46 ± 0.46 years,[22] and occurs slightly earlier in black girls than white girls. Most girls have reached stage 4 breast and pubic hair development by the time of menarche.[22]

In Tanner's series, the mean interval from breast development to menarche was 2.3 ± 0.1 years (range 0.5 to 5.8 years).[22] Awareness of this interval is useful in anticipatory counseling of the adolescent with breast buds regarding the onset of menses. During puberty, there is increased fat deposition, with a concurrent decrease in lean body mass from 80% to 75%. Pubertal weight gain accounts for 50% of adult ideal body weight. During the year of peak weight velocity, which follows peak height velocity by approximately 6 to 9 months, adolescent girls typically gain 4.6 to 10.6 kg.

In Frisch's studies,[27, 28] a minimum of 17% calculated body fat has been associated with menarche and a minimum of 22% for the maintenance of regular ovulatory cycles. Gymnasts, ballet dancers, and long-distance runners with reduced body weight and percentage body fat often have significant delays in pubertal development and onset of menses, especially if training began in the prepubertal years. Because aromatization of androgen precursors in fat produces estrogens, a low percentage of body fat may contribute to less estrogen, which is necessary for hypothalamic pituitary regulation and menarche. However, Frisch's hypothesis remains controversial because GnRH and gonadotropin secretion begins many years before menarche, percentage body fat was calculated, and weight at the time of menarche can vary tremendously in individual girls.

A retrospective study found that the interval between menarche and regular periods was approximately 14 months and the interval between menarche and painful, presumably ovulatory, cycles was approximately 24 months.[16–29] However, ovulatory cycles can begin in the first year postmenarche and may be associated with shortened luteal phases. Another study demonstrated that in the first 2 years after menarche, 55 to 82% of

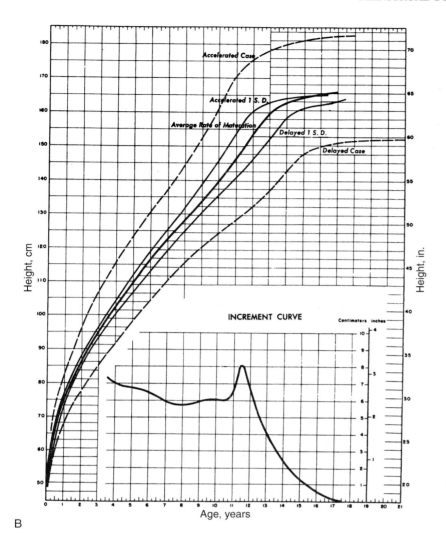

B

FIG. 33.6. *Continued.*

cycles were anovulatory.[30] By 3 years after menarche, the percentage of anovulatory cycles decreased to 50% and by 5 years to 10 to 20%.[5, 30] The later the age of menarche, the longer the interval before 50% of cycles are ovulatory. The interval was 1 year if menarche occurred at an age younger than 12 years, 3 years when menarche occurred at 12.0 to 12.9 years, and 4.5 years when menarche was after 13 years of age.[31]

Hormone Levels in Normal Ovulatory Cycles

Establishment of ovulatory cycles depends on the maturation of a positive feedback mechanism in which increasing estrogen levels trigger an LH surge at mid-cycle. The menstrual cycle is divided into follicular, ovulatory, and luteal phases (Fig. 33.7). In the early follicular phase, pulsatile GnRH released from the hypothalamus stimulates the secretion of FSH and LH from the pituitary. FSH increases the number of granulosa cells in the ovarian follicle and the number of FSH

receptors on the granulosa cells, and induces these cells to acquire an aromatizing enzyme for the conversion of androgen precursors to estradiol. Estradiol also increases the number of granulosa cells and the number of FSH receptors, leading to further amplification of the effect of FSH. The theca cells, stimulated by LH, secrete androstenedione, testosterone, and estradiol into the blood and into the follicle as substrate. By day 5 to 7 of the cycle, a single dominant follicle usually emerges. The rising estradiol level increases the number of glandular cells and stroma in the endometrium. By midfollicular phase, FSH is beginning to decline in part because of estrogen-mediated negative feedback. Inhibin, which is secreted by granulosa cells and blocks FSH synthesis and release, increases in the late follicular phase of the cycle parallel with estradiol. The highest levels of inhibin are found during the luteal phase and together with estradiol and progesterone appear to contribute to the regulation of FSH in this phase. FSH and inhibin levels are inversely related in the mid to late

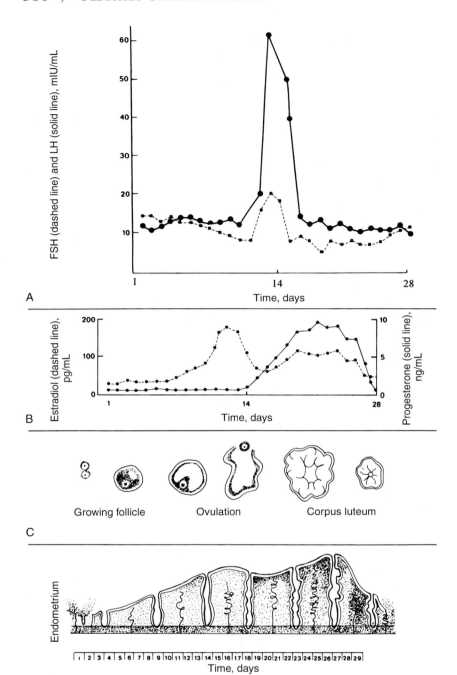

FIG. 33.7. Physiology of a normal ovulatory menstrual cycle: **A**, Gonadotropins; **B**, ovarian hormones; **C**, ovarian follicle; **D**, endometrium.

follicular phase and in the luteal phase.[32] Activins also secreted by the granulosa cells stimulate FSH secretion. The dominant follicle has the richest blood supply and produces the most estrogen and aromatase. The increased number of FSH receptors on the dominant follicle allows it to continue to respond even as increasing estrogen levels lower FSH. In the dominant follicle, estradiol levels are greater than androstenedione levels, whereas androstenedione levels are greater than estradiol levels in the atretic follicles.

In the periovulatory phase of the cycle, the dominant follicle is evident; it has increased receptors for LH and secretes increasing levels of estradiol. The rising estrogen levels produce a further proliferation of endometrium with mucosal thickening and glandular lengthening. The rising LH levels appear to induce a block in steroid pathways, which initiates secretion of 17-hydroxyprogesterone and progesterone and the gradual luteinization of the granulosa cells. The exact mechanism for the positive feedback effect of increasing estrogen and progesterone levels on the midcycle release of multiple pulses of LH is unknown. By midpuberty, the hypothalamic-pituitary system is capable of this positive feedback response. After the LH surge, the follicle ruptures and expels the oocyte.

The corpus luteum develops in response to LH levels and follicular rupture. As GnRH and LH are released in slower pulses, the corpus luteum is secreting progesterone and 17-hydroxyprogesterone. While plasma progesterone concentrations are stable during 24-hour studies in the early luteal phase and are unrelated to LH pulses, in the mid and late luteal phases the concentrations fluctuate significantly over 24 hours (from 2.3 to 40.1 ng/mL) and correlate with LH pulses.[33]

With increasing levels of progesterone and estrogen, the endometrium enters the secretory phase, which is characterized by coiling of the endometrial glands, increased vascularity of the stroma, and increased glycogen content of the epithelial cells. Maturation of the endometrium occurs by 8 or 9 days after ovulation and if fertilization of the ovum does not occur, regression begins. Evidence for ovulation and the occurrence of a luteal phase may be obtained by endometrial biopsy, basal body temperature charts, and measurement of serum progesterone levels of greater than 10 ng/mL.

Without pregnancy and its increasing placental human chorionic gonadotropin (HCG) levels, luteolysis begins and progesterone and estrogen levels fall. Unlike HCG, LH cannot sustain the corpus luteum for more than 14 days; thus, the luteal phase is usually of this duration. With the falling hormonal levels, the endometrium necroses and menstrual bleeding results. In the late luteal phase, FSH begins to increase to start new follicular development, and the next cycle begins.

DELAYED PUBERTY AND DISORDERS OF THE MENSTRUAL CYCLE

Disorders of the menstrual cycle include delayed menarche, primary and secondary amenorrhea, oligomenorrhea, and dysfunctional uterine bleeding. Menstrual irregularities may present with or without pubertal delay. It is helpful to consider the goal of the evaluation defining the source of the hypothalamic-pituitary-ovarian axis abnormality and to determine whether a genital anomaly is present. The differential diagnosis of delayed development can usually be divided based on the serum FSH levels into categories of hypergonadotropic hypogonadism (ovarian failure), hypogonadotropic hypogonadism (hypothalamic or pituitary dysfunction), and eugonadism (genital anomalies and polycystic ovary syndrome) (Table 33.1). These distinctions, along with a careful history and physical examination, will direct the laboratory evaluation and diagnostic testing.

TABLE 33.1 *Etiology of delayed puberty*

Hypergonadotropic hypogonadism (high FSH)
Gonadal dysgenesis
    Turner syndrome (45,X)
    Mosaic gonadal dysgenesis
    46,XY gonadal dysgenesis
Autoimmune oophoritis
46,XX premature ovarian failure
Ovarian failure secondary to radiation or chemotherapy
Resistant ovary syndrome
Postinfectious, posthemorrhagic, or postinfiltrative ovarian destruction
Galactosemia

Hypogonadotropic hypogonadism (low to normal FSH)
Physiologic delay
Chronic disease (cystic fibrosis, sickle cell disease, human immunodeficiency virus disease, renal disease, celiac disease, Crohn disease)
Anorexia nervosa
Female Athlete Triad
Lack of access to food (psychosocial)
Endocrinopathies
    Acquired hypothyroidism
    Diabetes mellitus
    Cushing syndrome
    Congenital adrenal hyperplasia
Hydrocephalus
Kallman syndrome (gonadotropin-releasing hormone deficiency)
Laurence-Moon-Biedl syndrome
Prader-Willi syndrome
Congenital and acquired central nervous system (CNS) defects
CNS tumors (prolactin-secreting and other pituitary adenomas, malignant pituitary tumors, craniopharyngiomas)
Brain abscess
Infiltrative lesions (tuberculosis, sarcoidosis, eosinophilic granuloma, Wegener granulomatosis, lymphocytic hypothysitis, CNS leukemia)
Postcranial radiation hypopituitarism
Other acquired hypopituitarism (head trauma, Sheehan's syndrome, pituitary infarction, autoimmune process)
"Empty sella" syndrome

Eugonadism
Obstructive genital anomalies
Androgen insensitivity
Polycystic ovary syndrome

Any girl who has not had any pubertal development by the age of 13 years is 2 standard deviations (SD) beyond the normal age of onset of puberty and should be evaluated. Absence of menarche by age 16 years is delayed menarche; primary amenorrhea is defined as no menarche by 18 years. The differential diagnosis for delayed menarche and primary amenorrhea depends as on the presence or absence of normal progression of pubertal development. Secondary amenorrhea should be evaluated at any time with a pregnancy test. Further workup of secondary amenorrhea is generally reserved for those patients in whom menses have been absent for 3 to 6 months without an obvious cause and for those with persistent oligomenorrhea, estrogen deficiency, or androgen excess.

The general approach to abnormalities in pubertal development involves a comprehensive, targeted history and physical examination. Key historical points may include:

- Family history, including heights of all family members, age of menarche and fertility of female relatives, history of ovarian tumors, and history of autoimmune endocrine disorders such as thyroiditis and Addison's disease.
- Neonatal history, including maternal ingestion of hormones, maternal history of miscarriages, birth weight, congenital anomalies, lymphedema (Turner syndrome), and neonatal problems suggestive of hypopituitarism such as hypoglycemia.
- Previous surgery, irradiation, or chemotherapy.
- Review of systems, emphasizing a history of chronic disease, abdominal pain, diarrhea, headaches, neurologic symptoms, ability to smell (Kallmann syndrome), weight changes, eating disorders, sexual activity, medications, substance abuse, emotional stresses, competitive athletics, and hirsutism.
- Age of initiation of pubertal development, if any, and rate of development.
- Longitudinal growth data plotted on appropriate charts.

The physical examination should include height and weight (plotted on growth charts), blood pressure, palpation of the thyroid gland, and Tanner staging of breast development and pubic hair. The breasts should be compressed to assess for galactorrhea. The examiner should look specifically for congenital anomalies, such as midline facial defects consistent with hypothalamic-pituitary dysfunction and somatic stigmata of Turner syndrome. A neurologic examination should include an assessment of the ability to smell, fundoscopic examination, and screening of visual fields by confrontation.

The gynecologic examination involves inspection of the external genitalia for clitoromegaly, estrogen effect, and hymenal appearance. In patients with no pubertal development, the etiology is likely an ovarian or hypothalamic-pituitary disorder, so visualization of the cervix is not essential. However, a rectoabdominal examination is useful for palpation of the cervix and the uterus in the nonobese prepubertal patient. If a congenital anomaly is suspected, the knee chest position may be used to visualize the vagina and the cervix in the unestrogenized patient.

The patient's pattern of growth can be useful in making a diagnosis. Failure of linear growth for several years may be seen with Crohn disease or an acquired endocrine disorder, or may indicate a bone age of 15 years or more and fusion of the epiphyses. In conditions with poor nutrition such as anorexia nervosa, inflammatory bowel disease, or celiac disease, the patient is usually underweight for height. In contrast, patients with acquired hypothyroidism, cortisol excess, and Turner syndrome are typically overweight for height. Obtaining a bone age can be useful in estimating final height in patients with delayed development. Menarche is more closely associated with bone age than with chronologic age. Assessment of percentage body fat may also be helpful in discussing potential etiologies for delayed puberty and amenorrhea with the patient. A clinical estimate of percentage body fat may be obtained by measuring triceps, biceps, subscapular, and suprailiac skinfold thickness.[34, 35]

Initial screening tests include a complete blood count (CBC), erythrocyte sedimentation rate (ESR), and serum thyroid stimulating hormone (TSH), FSH, and LH levels. A serum prolactin level may be included if the patient is suspected of having a central etiology for delayed puberty or amenorrhea; if a gonadal disorder is suspected because of short stature, measuring the prolactin can be delayed until the FSH level is known. A high ESR may indicate a chronic disease such as Crohn's disease. High LH and FSH levels are consistent with ovarian failure, whereas low to normal levels of LH and FSH suggest a central nervous system (CNS) etiology, such as a CNS tumor, hypopituitarism, or hypothalmic dysfunction, which may be primary or secondary to chronic disease, stress, or an eating disorder. A high FSH level should always be confirmed with a repeat level before conveying a definitive diagnosis of ovarian failure to the patient. Occasionally, the LH level is drawn during the midcycle surge and may be three times the baseline levels; the level should be redrawn if the patient has menses 2 weeks after the test was done. Constitutional delayed puberty is a possible diagnosis, although less common in girls than in boys. It tends to be familial and is associated with normal progression of puberty and fertility.

Hypergonadotropic Hypogonadism

Initial evaluation of the adolescent with elevated FSH levels in the absence of a history of radiation therapy or chemotherapy includes a karyotype. Patients may have an abnormal karyotype (such as 45,X Turner syndrome or, rarely, 46,XY gonadal dysgenesis) or a normal karyotype (such as autoimmune oophoritis, 46,XX premature ovarian failure, or ovarian failure associated with radiation or chemotherapy). In patients with 46,XX ovarian failure, evaluation should include a search for autoimmune etiology. In patients with hypertension, elevated FSH, and delayed puberty, serum levels of desoxycortisone and progesterone are obtained and may be elevated if 17-alpha hydroxylase deficiency is present.

Gonadal Dysgenesis

In gonadal dysgenesis the gonads consist of bilateral streaks of fibrous stroma without germ cells. Slightly more than half of the patients with gonadal dysgenesis have the classic 45,X karyotype (Turner syndrome), which occurs in approximately 1 in 2,000 live female births and 1 in 15 spontaneous abortions.[36] Stigmata of Turner syndrome include short stature, broad chest, webbed neck, low hairline, short fourth or fifth metacarpals, cubitus valgus, genu valgum, low-set ears, narrow higharched palate, micrognathia, lymphedema, and multiple pigmented nevi. The final height of patients with Turner syndrome ranges from 142 to 146.8 cm (56 to 57.8 inches) with a mean of 143 cm (56.3 inches).[37] Associated problems include cardiac anomalies in a third of the patients (bicuspid aortic valve, coarctation of the aorta, mitral valve prolapse, dissecting aneurysms), renal anomalies in 35 to 70% (horseshoe kidneys, unilateral pelvic kidney, rotational abnormalities, duplicated collecting systems, and rarely, ureteral pelvic obstruction and hydronephrosis), hearing impairment, otitis media and mastoiditis in a third, and an increased incidence of hypertension, achlorhydria, glucose intolerance, osteopenia, diabetes mellitus, Hashimoto thyroiditis, gastrointestinal vascular malformations, and possibly inflammatory bowel disease.[36-48] Intelligence is usually normal, although there have been reports of deficits in spatiotemporal processing, visual motor coordination, and specific learning skills.[36, 49]

A young adolescent with Turner syndrome has prepubertal female genitalia, bilateral streak gonads, and a normal uterus and vagina capable of responding to exogenous hormones. She may have sparse or absent pubic and axillary hair despite levels of DHEAS that correspond to Tanner PH2 or PH3. The adolescent with untreated Turner syndrome who has reached 15 or 16 years of age usually has pubic and axillary hair, but generally no breast development or estrogenization of the vaginal mucosa, representative of the lack of ovarian function. However, an estimated 5 to 15% of patients with Turner syndrome have spontaneous thelarche.

The other 40 to 50% of patients with gonadal dysgenesis have a mosaic karyotype (such as 46,XX/45,X) or a structural abnormality of the second X chromosome.[50, 51] Patients with mosaic karyotype are more likely to have pubertal maturation than patients with 45,X karyotype, but may have none, some, or all of the classic stigmata of Turner syndrome. Thus they may have (1) sexual infantilism, (2) some sexual development and primary amenorrhea, (3) secondary amenorrhea or irregular menses and short stature, or (4) regular menses and normal stature. Turner syndrome should be considered in patients with pubertal development and nonfamilial significant short stature because girls with mosaic karyotype who have some pubertal maturation may not have

elevated gonadotropin levels. Rarely spontaneous pregnancies have been reported in patients with 45,X and mosaic karyotypes, even in some with elevated FSH levels. These pregnancies have an increased risk of abortion, stillbirth, and chromosomally abnormal babies (Turner syndrome and Down syndrome).[52, 53] Genetic counseling and prenatal diagnosis is recommended for all patients with gonadal dysgenesis.

Patients with 45,X karyotype rarely may have undetected Y DNA (1 in 40 in one study of patients with Turner syndrome).[54] With polymerase chain reaction technology, the clinician can be aware of SRY sequences that correlate with the presence of Y-chromosomal DNA and anticipate virilization at puberty, the risk of a gonadal tumor, and the need to remove gonadal tissue. Older adolescent and adult patients without Y sequences should have annual pelvic examinations. If a pelvic examination is difficult, annual radiograph films for pelvic calcification or ultrasonography of the pelvis for gonadal tumors should be considered.

Patients with pure gonadal dysgenesis have normal or tall stature with the gonadal abnormality of Turner syndrome. They have little or no breast development and eunuchoid proportions. Gonadotropin levels are elevated and the karyotype is usually 46,XX or 46,XY. Patients with 46,XX ovarian failure may have a family history of premature menopause. Patients with 46,XY karyotype, streak gonads, a normal but infantile Müllerian system, and no sexual development have Swyer syndrome. Because of the presence of the Y chromosome, approximately 25% of these patients develop dysgerminomas or gonadoblastomas and thus require removal of the gonads. Patients with 47,XXX also may have ovarian failure and possibly neuropsychological impairment.[49]

Ovarian Failure Caused by Radiation or Chemotherapy

A history of a malignancy treated with radiation to the pelvis or abdomen or chemotherapy suggests a diagnosis of ovarian failure. The risk of ovarian failure increases with higher doses of radiation and older age at which the treatment was received. In addition, a patient who receives pelvic radiation therapy before puberty often has a small cervix and uterus despite estrogen therapy.

Children and adolescents are more resistant to the deleterious effects of chemotherapeutic agents than are adults. Adolescents may have amenorrhea and high gonadotropin levels while receiving chemotherapy and then sometimes have return of normal menstrual function and normal hormone levels months to years after completing therapy.

Autoimmune Oophoritis

Autoimmune oophoritis must be considered in any patient with normal karyotype and ovarian failure because of the risk of subsequent additional endocrinopathies. In adults with premature ovarian failure evaluated at medical centers, 18 to 50% have had evidence of autoimmune disease,[55–57] including thyroid disorders, Addison disease, hypoparathyroidism, myasthenia gravis, diabetes mellitus, pernicious anemia, and vitiligo. Women with premature ovarian failure often have antithyroglobulin and antithyroid microsomal antibodies. Antibodies against theca interna and corpus luteum cells, FSH receptors, and specific adrenal and ovarian enzymes, as well as antibodies to smooth muscle, gastric parietal cells, mitochondria, cell nucleus, pancreatic islet cells, and the adrenals have also been reported.[56–60]

Patients with autoimmune oophoritis may have a variable course; spontaneous remissions and the resumption of normal ovarian function is possible, but amenorrhea and infertility persist in most.[61, 62] For most patients, use of assisted reproductive technologies may be the best option for pregnancy.

Initial assessment of the patient with suspected autoimmune ovarian failure should include baseline TSH, morning cortisol, calcium, phosphorus, and CBC, as well as antibodies to thyroid, adrenals, ovaries, islet cells, and parietal cells. Patients may be screened for adrenal insufficiency with an adrenocorticotropin hormone (ACTH) test with measurement of cortisol levels at 0 and 30 or 60 minutes. The frequency of repeat testing has not been fully evaluated.

Other Causes of Ovarian Failure

In resistant ovary syndrome, a rare condition, the ovaries appear normal at laparoscopy with numerous primordial follicles on biopsy.[63] The defect may be a lack of an ovarian receptor for gonadotropin function or the presence of biologically inactive FSH and LH.

Deficiency of 17-alpha-hydroxylase, a rare disorder, is not true gonadal failure. Deficiency of this enzyme results in diminished synthesis of cortisol, androgens, and estrogens, and increased production of desoxycorticosterone, corticosterone, and progesterone. Patients have hypertension, hypokalemic alkalosis, infantile female external genitalia, absence of pubertal development, and primary amenorrhea with elevated gonadotropins. Patients with 46,XX karyotype have a female phenotype but no secondary sexual characteristics. Patients with 46,XY may have a female phenotype, vaginal agenesis, lack of müllerian structures, and (unlike patients with androgen insensitivity) lack of breast development.

Ovarian failure has been noted in patients with galactosemia,[64] myotonia dystrophica, trisomy 21,[65] sarcoidosis, and ataxia telangiectasia. Ovarian destruction also has occurred after mumps oophoritis, gonococcal salpingitis (rarely), ovarian hemorrhage, and ovarian infiltrative processes such as tuberculosis and mucopolysaccharidosis.

Hypogonadotropic Hypogonadism

Patients with delayed pubertal development and low to normal gonadotropin levels may have a central etiology such as chronic disease or malnutrition, a hypothalamic etiology such as Kallmann syndrome or a tumor, or a pituitary cause such as a microadenoma or infiltrative disease. A normal physiologic delay in puberty or menarche is a diagnosis of exclusion and warrants a complete medical evaluation before expectant management or hormonal therapy.

One of the most common causes of delayed puberty is poor nutrition, which frequently occurs with chronic diseases such as cystic fibrosis, sickle cell disease, human immunodeficiency virus disease, renal disease, celiac disease, and Crohn disease.[66–68] Some patients with Crohn disease have growth failure alone, but most will have a history of intermittent crampy abdominal pain, diarrhea, or constipation. The sedimentation rate is usually elevated, and mild anemia and hypoalbuminemia may be present. Renal problems associated with delayed growth include renal tubular acidosis, glomerular diseases treated with corticosteroids, and end-stage renal failure.

Adolescents with anorexia nervosa and other eating disorders may develop secondary amenorrhea, or less commonly, present with primary amenorrhea. Rarely, "fear of obesity" can cause growth failure even in prepubertal children.[69] Lack of access to food because of family psychosocial issues, alcoholism, drug abuse, poverty, or homelessness may also result in delayed development. Competitive athletes often experience delays in pubertal development and irregular menses.[70, 71] The concept of the Female Athlete Triad (disordered eating, amenorrhea, osteoporosis) has developed from the increasing recognition of the relationships among these conditions. The triad tends to occur in girls participating in activities to which body weight and composition is central, such as gymnastics, ballet, running, and figure skating. A highly structured life, social isolation, lack of supports, and a family history of disordered eating are associated with the condition. In contrast to the expected incidence of 2 to 5% of amenorrhea in adults, the incidence in athletes has been reported to be 3 to 66%.[72] One of the potential consequences of hypoestrogenic amenorrhea is decreased bone mass. Because most adult bone mass is acquired during the adolescent growth spurt,[73–82] studies have shown osteopenia in young adult women with exercise-related amenorrhea.[83–88]

Delayed puberty is also seen with endocrinopathies, such as acquired hypothyroidism, diabetes mellitus,[89] and Cushing syndrome. Like patients with malabsorptive disorders, patients with hypothyroidism may also present with slowed growth, but the latter tend to be overweight for height. Substance abuse and psychological problems also may be associated with delayed or interrupted puberty.

Hypothalamic dysfunction may be caused by a congenital defect such as Kallmann syndrome, a lack of pulsatile release of GnRH often associated with midline craniofacial defects or anosmia. Isolated GnRH deficiency may be difficult to distinguish from delayed puberty if the patient with delayed puberty has not begun to show a postpubertal response to GnRH or GnRH analogs. Gonadotropin deficiency may be more likely in a prepubertal patient with low or normal FSH if the bone age is older than 13 years, anosmia or panhypopituitarism is present, sleep-associated LH increase is lacking, and GnRH tests show a flat response.[90] Central lesions that cause delayed puberty include tumors, hydrocephalus, brain abscesses, and infiltrative lesions such as tuberculosis, sarcoidosis, eosinophilic granuloma, Wegener granulomatosis, lymphocytic hypophysitis, and CNS leukemia.[91]

Craniopharyngiomas usually present between the ages of 6 and 14 years with headaches, poor growth, delayed development, and diabetes insipidus. Patients who have had cranial radiation for leukemia therapy may have abnormal secretion of growth hormone or GnRH.[92, 93] Excess iron from hemochromatosis or transfusion therapy for thalassemia major can be associated with developmental delay. Hypogonadotropic hypogonadism is also seen in Laurence-Moon-Biedl and Prader-Willi syndromes.

Pituitary disorders associated with irregular menses include congenital or acquired hypopituitarism and tumors. Acquired hypopituitarism can follow head trauma,[94] postpartum shock and necrosis (Sheehan syndrome), pituitary infarction (such as in sickle cell disease), and rarely from an autoimmune process.[95] Prolactinomas are the most common pituitary tumors in adolescents and typically cause primary or secondary amenorrhea. A screening serum prolactin level should be obtained in patients with low or normal FSH and LH levels and delayed or interrupted puberty or menses. "Empty sella," a condition of multifactorial etiology, is also associated with hypothalamic pituitary dysfunction.[96] Nonfunctioning pituitary adenomas are generally not associated with amenorrhea and thus may not be diagnosed until imaging of the head occurs for other reasons.

Evaluation of hypogonadotropic hypogonadism thus focuses on determining the presence of systemic disease, malnutrition, CNS disorder, or endocrinopathy. Patients with low FSH levels should have a growth chart, neurologic examination, CBC, ESR, TSH, prolactin, bone age, and consideration of CNS imaging.

Hyperprolactinemia

Patients with prolactin-secreting pituitary adenomas may have galactorrhea, interrupted pubertal development, or primary or secondary amenorrhea. However, a third to a half of adolescents with secondary amenorrhea and hyperprolactinemia do not have galactorrhea, including most girls with primary amenorrhea and elevated prolactin levels. Thus, patients with amenorrhea and low to normal gonadotropin levels should have a serum prolactin measured. Other causes of hyperprolactinemia include physiologic stimuli (pregnancy, exercise, stress, breast stimulation, chest wall trauma, or surgery), medications or illicit drugs, hypothyroidism, and renal failure (decreased clearance of prolactin).

The evaluation of an adolescent with hyperprolactinemia should include a gynecologic history, menstrual history, medication and illicit drug use, hirsutism or acne, symptoms of hypothyroidism, visual changes, and headaches. The physical examination should include a neurologic assessment, including fundoscopic examination and a screen of visual fields by confrontation, thyroid palpation, vital signs, breast examination, and inspection for evidence of androgen excess and estrogenization by vaginal examination. Estrogen status should be assessed with a serum estradiol level, vaginal smear, or progestin challenge.

Treatment of a patient with a prolactin-secreting pituitary tumor depends on the size of the tumor, the patient's estrogen status, and her desire for fertility, and include observation, bromocriptine, surgery, and radiation.

Eugonadism

Eugonadism refers to normal estrogenization with a failure of a normal menstrual pattern. This category includes patients with genital anomalies and patients with polycystic ovary syndrome, who will often have normal to elevated estrogen levels with oligomenorrhea and hyperandrogenism. Patients with CNS disorders, systemic illnesses, stress, and weight loss may also be eugonadotropic if estrogen levels fall within the follicular range but normal cycles do not occur. Amenorrhea may occur after discontinuation of oral contraceptives, Depo-Provera, or Norplant. In the 1 to 2% of patients who develop amenorrhea after oral contraceptive pill use, approximately 95% revert to regular periods within 12 to 18 months.[97-99]

Secondary Amenorrhea

Secondary amenorrhea is defined as lack of menses for 3 to 6 months in a postmenarchal patient. Because one of the most common causes of secondary amenorrhea is pregnancy, a pregnancy test should be obtained whenever an adolescent is concerned about a period being late, even if only by 2 or 3 weeks. The pregnancy test should be performed even if the adolescent denies a history of sexual intercourse. Physical and emotional distress and environmental changes, such as going off to college, are stresses that most often explain missed periods. Adolescents involved in intensive athletic training may have menstrual irregularities, but each patient still must be considered individually for pregnancy or a significant medical disorder.

Adolescents may have irregular periods or amenorrhea for 3 to 6 months during the first 2 to 3 years after menarche. Patients who become amenorrheic for 4 months after regular cycles have been established or who have persistent oligomenorrhea (irregular, infrequent periods) or who have signs or symptoms of androgen excess such as hirsutism or acne should be evaluated. The medical history should include questions on stress, environmental changes, weight change, and involvement in competitive athletics. The review of systems should focus on evidence of hyperandrogenism (such as hirsutism and acne), CNS tumors (such as headaches, visual changes, and galactorrhea), and chronic disease, as well as any medication or illicit drug use. The physical examination should include fundoscopic examination and evaluation of visual fields by confrontation, palpa-

tion of the thyroid gland, measurement of blood pressure and pulse, and compression of the areolae for galactorrhea. Evidence of androgen excess, such as progressive hirsutism, clitoromegaly, or severe acne should be noted. Hirsutism may be quantified as the amount and distribution of long, coarse, pigmented hair (terminal hair), using the Ferriman-Gallwey scoring system.[100] Bimanual examination of the pelvis should be performed to assess for ovarian enlargement. After the medical history, physical examination, and pregnancy test, the estrogen status of patients with secondary amenorrhea should be assessed (Fig. 33.8). A vaginal smear, estradiol level, or progestin challenge test may be performed.

Most patients who withdraw from progesterone are normal; however, disorders such as polycystic ovary syndrome, ovarian tumors, Cushing disease, thyroid disease, and diabetes should be excluded by history, physical examination, and laboratory tests. Regardless of response to progesterone, patients with amenorrhea for more than 6 months or persistent oligomenorrhea without an explanation should be evaluated with measurement of serum FSH, LH, prolactin, and TSH. An elevated LH and a normal FSH is suggestive of polycystic ovary syndrome. In these patients and in any patient

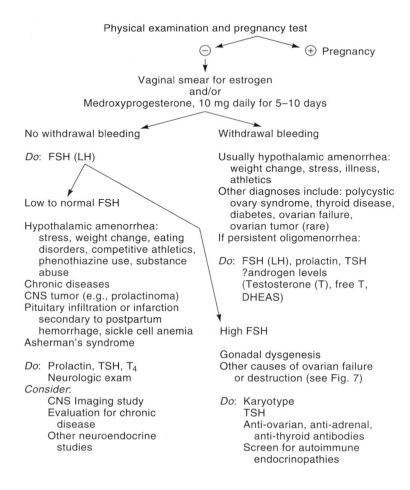

FIG. 33.8. Evaluation of secondary amenorrhea.

with signs of androgen excess, testosterone (free and total) and DHEAS should be measured. Patients who have withdrawal flow after a progesterone challenge often have hypothalamic amenorrhea from weight change, stress, illness, or athletics. In these patients, menses often return spontaneously without further intervention. If cyclic bleeding does not resume, medroxyprogesterone (Provera), given for 12 to 14 days, is usually given every 2 to 3 months. Patients who are underweight should be encouraged to gain weight. Birth control pills are generally used only in patients who require contraception or are hypoestrogenic over a prolonged period.

Polycystic Ovary Syndrome, Late Onset 21-Hydroxylase Deficiency, and Other Causes of Hirsutism

Polycystic ovary syndrome (PCOS) is a common cause of secondary amenorrhea and hirsutism among adolescent and young adult women. PCOS refers to a spectrum of disorders characterized by increased ovarian androgen production, often with abnormal gonadotropin secretion and insulin resistance.[101–107] LH levels are often elevated. The high LH levels stimulate excess androstenedione and testosterone secretion from the ovarian theca cells.[101, 102, 108] The action of testosterone is augmented because androgens decrease sex hormone binding globulin (SHBG) and result in increased circulating free testosterone. The low SHBG level also increases uptake of free androgens and peripheral conversion to estrogen. Thus patients with PCOS often have higher free estradiol levels than do normal women in the midfollicular phase of the menstrual cycle.[109, 110] FSH levels are generally slightly suppressed, resulting in an elevated LH:FSH ratio (usually >2). The low to normal FSH results in a deficiency of the aromatase required for the conversion of the androstenedione to estradiol in the ovarian follicle. The result is anovulation and androgen excess.

Clinical presentation is variable and may include hirsutism, obesity, oligomenorrhea, anovulation, and infertility. Ovaries may appear normal on ultrasound or they may be enlarged with a thickened capsule, multiple small peripheral cysts and increased stroma, or hyperthecosis. PCOS-like ovaries may also be seen in androgen excess from untreated congenital adrenocortical hyperplasia (CAH) and adrenal tumors or in any condition that causes chronic anovulation, such as Cushing disease, hypothyroidism, and hyperprolactinemia.

Patients with PCOS usually have a normal age of menarche, although occasionally they can have delayed menarche with hirsutism or virilization. Most adolescents with PCOS are overweight for height and may have an abnormal lipid profile.[111–113] Most patients will give a history of irregular menses from the time of menarche and often describe perimenarcheal onset of hirsutism or acne. Hyperinsulinemia is often present[101] and is associated with acanthosis nigricans (velvety, hyperpigmented skin over the nape of the neck, in the axillae, beneath the breasts, and in other intertriginous areas). HAIR-AN refers to the specific syndrome of hyperandrogenism (HA), insulin resistance (IR), and acanthosis nigricans (AN).

The differential diagnosis of irregular menses and hirsutism includes late onset 21-hydroxylase deficiency, 3 β-hydroxysteroid dehydrogenase deficiency, Cushing disease, and the rare ovarian or adrenal tumor. Late onset 21-hydroxylase deficiency, an autosomal recessive disorder, occurs in 1 to 10% of women with hirsutism[114–121] and is particularly prevalent among Ashkenzi Jews. The clinical presentation of late onset 21-hydroxylase deficiency may range from asymptomatic to hirsutism and irregular menses.

The initial laboratory evaluation of hirsutism and irregular menses usually elucidates the diagnosis and should include serum testosterone, free testosterone, DHEAS, LH, FSH, and prolactin. Thyroid function tests may also be obtained. If virilization is present or a tumor or late-onset CAH is under consideration, a first-morning serum 17-hydroxyprogesterone, DHEA, and androstenedione are also measured. If stigmata of Cushing disease are present, a 24-hour urine should be collected for free cortisol and a serum cortisol should be measured at 8 A.M. after an 11 P.M. dose of 1 mg of dexamethasone.

A testosterone level higher than 150 to 200 ng/dL, DHEAS higher than 700 μg/dL, or androstenedione higher than 500 ng/dL raises suspicion of a tumor or intersex disorder. ACTH testing is generally reserved for adolescents with clitoromegaly, elevated DHEAS, history of premature adrenarche, family history of CAH, ethnic history of a high prevalence of CAH, and a high baseline (7 to 8 A.M.) level of 17-hydroxyprogesterone (>200 ng/dL).

The treatment of PCOS depends on the degree of hirsutism and includes cyclic progestin, oral contraceptives, antiandrogens such as spironolactone, and GnRH agonists. Patients with hirsutism who are obese should be encouraged to lose weight to decrease peripheral conversion of androstenedione in fat cells and improve hyperinsulinism.[122–125] Facial bleach, depilatories, shaving, wax epilation, and electrolysis can help give the patient good cosmetic effects.

Hormone Replacement Therapy

For patients with significantly delayed development or irreversible estrogen deficiency, estrogen is recommended to normalize secondary sexual characteristics. Estrogen replacement can also reverse vaginal atrophy, decrease the risk of osteoporosis and fractures, and improve serum lipoprotein profiles.[126–131] To induce breast development, conjugated estrogens (Premarin) 0.3 mg or ethinyl estradiol 5 to 10 μg may be given daily for 6 to 12 months. To further enhance breast development and to initiate menses, the dose is increased and cyclic progestin is added. Oral contraceptives are recommended only for maintenance therapy and not to induce breast development. In patients with anorexia nervosa, the goal of therapy should be gradual weight gain and establishment of normal menstrual cycles. However, in the patient with amenorrhea who is not gaining weight, estrogen therapy should be instituted to attempt to preserve bone density, although results of prospective studies are few.

In patients with Turner syndrome, the initiation of estrogen replacement therapy must be considered carefully. The risks from bone demineralization must be weighed against the advancement of epiphyseal closure in these patients with short stature. Synthetic growth hormone can promote growth and is particularly beneficial when instituted early, but treatment is expensive. Because estrogen does not appear to advance growth when used with growth hormone,[132, 133] estrogen therapy can be delayed until around age 14 to 15 years (or after cessation of growth hormone therapy).

Patients with constitutional delay of puberty may desire hormone replacement therapy by the age of 14 to 15 years to promote normal breast development. Therapy can be stopped after the appearance of secondary sexual characteristics and menses. If no spontaneous development continues, then estrogen can be reinstituted for 6- to 12-month courses with periodic discontinuation of therapy to assess for hypothalamic functioning.

DYSFUNCTIONAL UTERINE BLEEDING

Irregular, heavy vaginal bleeding is common among adolescents. While dysfunctional uterine bleeding (DUB) can occur at menarche, more often a patient will have a history of 2 to 3 months of amenorrhea followed by frequent periods (metrorrhagia), which are prolonged (polymenorrhea) and heavy (hypermenorrhea).

The differential diagnosis for DUB is shown in Table 33.2. DUB may occur in the young adolescent secondary to anovulatory periods with incomplete shedding of a proliferative endometrium, or in the older adolescent with anovulatory cycles caused by stress or illness. Patients with other conditions that can cause an anovulatory state, such as eating disorders, weight changes, competitive athletics, drug abuse, endocrine disorders, and PCOS, may have DUB. Pregnancy and cervical or pelvic infections may also cause abnormal vaginal bleeding and must be excluded. Patients with bleeding disorders usually show other signs of bleeding, but patients with von Willebrand disease may have heavy menses since menarche.

TABLE 33.2 *Differential diagnosis of vaginal bleeding in the adolescent*

Dysfunctional uterine bleeding
Disorders of pregnancy: threatened, incomplete, or missed abortion; molar pregnancy; ectopic pregnancy
Pelvic inflammatory disease: salpingitis, endometritis
Blood dyscrasias: thrombocytopenia (e.g., idiopathic thrombocytopenic purpura, leukemia, aplastic anemia, hypersplenism), clotting disorders, von Willebrand's disase and other disorders of platelet function, iron deficiency
Endocrine disorders: hypothyroidism or hyperthyroidism, adrenal disease, diabetes mellitus, hyperprolactinemia, polycystic ovary syndrome, ovarian failure
Vaginal abnormalities: carcinoma, adenosis (secondary to maternal diethylstilbestrol)
Cervical problems: cervicitis, polyp, hemangioma, carcinoma
Uterine problems: congenital anomalies, submucous myoma, polyp, carcinoma, use of intrauterine contraceptive device, breakthrough bleeding associated with the use of oral contraceptives, ovulation bleeding
Ovarian cysts and tumors
Endometriosis
Systemic diseases
Trauma
Foreign body (e.g., retained tampon)
Medications: anticoagulants, platelet inhibitors, androgens

DUB may also be seen in patients with uterine abnormalities such as submucous myomas, congenital anomalies, IUD use, and breakthrough bleeding associated with oral contraceptive use. With congenital anomalies, the obstructed uterus or vagina will empty through a fistula slowly over the month. Carcinomas of the vagina and of the cervix are rare in adolescents. Cervical trauma, infections, and the rare cervical hemangioma may present with abnormal vaginal bleeding. Endometriosis and ovarian problems, such as tumors or cysts, also are associated with DUB.

Systemic illness may cause anovulation, interfere with coagulation, or cause local endometrial infection (e.g., tuberculosis). Trauma may occur from an acute fall, waterskiing, foreign objects introduced for masturbation or sexual play, or sexual assault. A retained tampon is usually associated with a foul-smelling discharge. Medications such as anticoagulants and platelet inhibitors can be associated with excessive bleeding. Athletes who use anabolic steroids may experience anovulatory cycles with DUB.

DUB that is cyclic is more commonly caused by a blood disorder or uterine problem, whereas acyclic bleeding infers anovulation. Normal cyclicity with superimposed abnormal bleeding is associated with foreign bodies, uterine polyps, vaginal malignancy, congenital uterine obstruction, infection, cervical abnormality, and endometriosis.

In addition to a careful history and general physical examination directed toward elucidating the differential diagnosis, initial evaluation should include a one-finger digital examination to check for foreign bodies and to palpate the cervix. A speculum examination should be performed if tolerated; if the hymenal opening is too small, a rectoabdominal examination in the lithotomy position is usually possible. Further evaluation with ultrasonography or examination under anesthesia may be considered if the patient does not respond to expectant management or hormonal therapy.

The patient with DUB who may be sexually active should have cultures for *Neisseria gonorrhoeae* and *Chlamydia trachomatis*. A wet prep and Papanicolaou smear can be obtained if there is no bleeding at the time of the examination. Laboratory tests should include a urine human chorionic gonadotropin (HCG) test and a CBC with differential and platelet count. Reticulocyte count is useful in patients with a history of particularly heavy bleeding who have a normal or mildly depressed hemoglobin. Other studies depend on the history of DUB and the physical examination.

Treatment

The assessment allows the clinician to determine if the patient with DUB can be observed for maturation of the HPO axis or if she requires medical treatment. The objectives of hormonal therapy are to administer estrogen to provide further endometrial proliferation and heal over the sites of bleeding and to administer progestins to induce endometrial stability. Treatment of mild DUB generally consists of observation, reassurance, and iron supplementation.

In moderate to severe DUB, oral contraceptives are usually prescribed, with doses ranging from one tablet a day up to one every 4 hours with severe menorrhagia for 21 days. One schedule uses 0.3 mg of norgestrel and 30 μg of ethinyl estradiol (Lo-Ovral) four times a day for 4 days, three times a day for 3 days, and twice a day for 14 days (a total of 21 days of therapy). Other monophasic oral contraceptives with 30 to 35 μg of estrogen have also been used in other schedules. Clinicians should be in contact with the patient to monitor for noncompliance with these increased doses of oral contraceptives, usually because of nausea, and to ensure the dose is sufficient to stop the bleeding. Pelvic pathology should be considered in patients for whom hormonal therapy does not control bleeding within 24 to 36 hours. Examination under anesthesia and dilation and curettage may rarely be required. In patients with significant anemia, noncyclic (continuous) oral contraceptives, should be given until the hemoglobin normalizes. Then the patient can be cycled for 3 to 4 months. Iron and folic acid supplementation should be instituted within 24 to 48 hours once the bleeding is controlled and the patient is stable.

Patients with a long history of anovulatory cycles and DUB have an increased risk of infertility and endometrial carcinoma.[134] These patients require long-term therapy with cyclic progestin for 14 days each month or oral contraceptives.

DYSMENORRHEA

Dysmenorrhea (pain with menses) is a common complaint among adolescent girls. The symptoms usually start 1 to 3 years postmenarche, and present as crampy lower abdominal pain a few hours to 2 days before each menstrual period. The cramps may be associated with nausea, vomiting, diarrhea, lower backache, thigh pain, headache, fatigue, anxiety, dizziness, or syncope. Evaluation of dysmenorrhea includes a menstrual history and a history of the timing of, treatment tried for, and degree of disability attributed to the dysmenorrhea. In the adolescent with mild cramps who has never been sexually active, examination may be limited to a general physical examination with inspection of the external genitalia. Patients with moderate or severe dysmenorrhea and those who are sexually active require a complete pelvic examination to exclude tenderness and masses, which may be associated with pelvic infection, endometriosis, or structural anomalies.

Treatment for patients with a normal examination may include nonsteroidal anti-inflammatory drugs (NSAIDs), such as naproxen sodium or ibuprofen taken with food. If NSAIDs are contraindicated in the patient, acetaminophen, with codeine if necessary, may be used. Generally, effective relief is obtained when the medication is given at the onset of menses, or 1 to 2 days before, and continued for the first 1 to 2 days of the cycle. A loading dose is helpful in patients who have sudden, severe symptoms. If a patient does not respond to NSAIDs or requires birth control, oral contraceptives should be prescribed. If severe cramps persist after 3 to 4 cycles on oral contraceptives or tenderness or nodularity is noted on examination, laparoscopy should be considered to exclude endometriosis and other organic disease.

ANOMALIES OF THE FEMALE GENITAL TRACT

Chapter 10 addresses the normal developmental embryology of the reproductive tract and Chapter 35 discusses the evaluation and treatment of ambiguous genitalia.

Anomalies of the female genital tract arise from abnormalities in development (agenesis or hypoplasia), vertical fusion (abnormal canalization of the junction between the Müllerian ducts and the urogenital sinus), or lateral fusion (duplications). The existence of varying diagnostic techniques and classification systems makes it difficult to determine the true incidence of Müllerian anomalies. Familial occurrence of Müllerian abnormalities has been reported.[135]

Obstructing genital anomalies usually present at birth with mucocolpos or at menarche with pain or a pelvic mass (hematocolpos). The pain may be cyclic or chronic. A noncommunicating rudimentary horn with a unicornuate uterus may result in an occult hematometra and dysmenorrhea. Nonobstructing lesions, such as complete duplication of the vagina, cervix, and uterus, may be asymptomatic. These lesions are most commonly diagnosed in women who have recurrent spontaneous abortions or are infertile. Genital examination may reveal an imperforate hymen, a vaginal dimple (vaginal agenesis), or a blind vaginal pouch.

Accurate diagnosis of Müllerian anomalies is important to determine whether surgical intervention is required. Transabdominal, transvaginal, or transperineal ultrasonography is useful in defining the anatomy.[136-139] MRI is preferred to define complicated obstructive anomalies[140-142] and also permits evaluation of the urinary system.[143] Hysterosalpingography has been traditionally used to identify an abnormal uterine cavity, but it cannot differentiate between a septate uterus and a true bicornuate uterus.[142]

Because the Müllerian ducts are closely associated with the mesonephric ducts during fetal development, there is a high association of coexisting anomalies. Genital malformations are often seen in cases of renal agenesis.[144, 145] Urinary tract abnormalities are associated with Müllerian anomalies in 20% of the cases.[146]

Other associated extragenital malformations include congenital scoliosis, limb bud deformity, lacrimal duct stenosis, external auditory canal stenosis, congenital heart disease, inguinal hernias, imperforate anus, and malposition of the ovary.[147-149] Obstructing Müllerian anomalies have been associated with endometriosis.[150]

Classification

The American Society for Reproductive Medicine (formerly the American Fertility Society [AFS]) classification includes six types of anomalies according to the degree of failure in the development of the Müllerian structures (Fig. 33.9),[151] and an additional class of anomalies related to diethylstilbestrol (DES) exposure in utero. To include abnormalities of the vagina, additional classifications have been described.[152, 153]

Class 1: *Segmental agenesis or hypoplasia.* The agenesis may involve the vagina, cervix, uterus, fallopian tubes, and ovaries. Mayer-Rokitansky-Kuster-Hauser syndrome is included in this class.

Class 2: *Unicornuate uterus.* The uterus may have a rudimentary uterine horn, which may communicate with the main uterine cavity. The rudimentary horn may contain endometrium. The kidney and ureter may be absent on the affected side.

Class 3: *Uterus didelphys.* Partial or complete failure of lateral Müllerian duct fusion is associated with partial or complete duplication of the vagina, cervix, and uterus.

Class 4: *Bicornate uterus.* The uterus may be complete or separate with two uterine bodies. There is a single-chamber vagina and cervix.

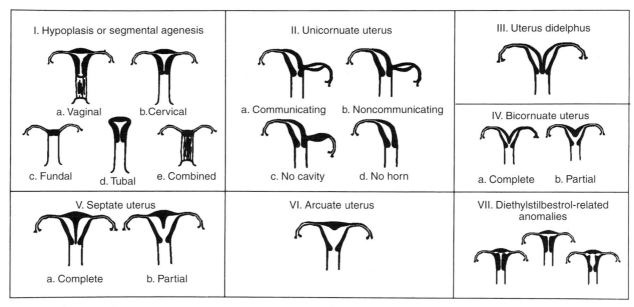

FIG. 33.9. Classification of Müllerian anomalies. Reprinted with permission from the American Fertility Society. The American Fertility Society Classification of adnexal adhesions, distal tubal occlusion secondary to tubal ligation, tubal pregnancies, Müllerian anomalies, and intrauterine adhesions. Fertil Steril 1988;49:944–955.

Class 5: *Septate uterus*. The uterus is a single organ with a partial or complete midline septum.

Class 6: *Arcuate uterus*. The uterus has a small septate indentation at the upper end of the fundus.

Class 7: *Diethylstilbestrol-related anomalies*.

Surgical intervention should be reserved for patients who have pain or reproductive difficulties. Asymptomatic patients with unobstructed anomalies may not need any treatment. Patients with a noncommunicating rudimentary horn associated with a unicornuate uterus may require surgical removal of the horn to relieve dysmenorrhea and prevent endometriosis from reflux. This procedure may be performed with operative laparoscopy or laparotomy.[153] Metroplasty may decrease the incidence of premature labor and adverse pregnancy outcomes. The uterus didelphys is usually asymptomatic and generally requires surgery only if the septum extends into the vagina and causes obstruction. Surgical repair of a septate or bicornuate uterus is indicated in a patient with a history of miscarriage. For a bicornuate uterus, a transabdominal approach is used to fuse the uterine horns. Operative hysteroscopy is used for resection of uterine septa.

Specific Anomalies of the Vagina

Disorders of Vertical Fusion of the Vagina

Disorders of vertical fusion result from incomplete canalization of the vagina and include imperforate hymen and transverse vaginal septum. The hymen, the junction of the sinovaginal bulbs and the urogenital sinus, is usually perforated during fetal development to establish a connection between the lumen of the vaginal canal and the vestibule. Imperforate hymen results when this perforation does not occur and is generally an isolated finding. Most cases are sporadic, although there are reports of familial clusters.[135] With routine examination of the genitalia, the diagnosis of imperforate hymen should be made early in a child's life. However, if a patient reaches menarcheal age before the diagnosis is made, she may have primary amenorrhea and a history of cyclic abdominal pain, often for years, or she may have no symptoms. On examination, the hymen is bluish and bulging and the vagina, distended with bloody, menstrual discharge may be noted on rectoabdominal palpation. In some cases the vagina may be large, resulting in nausea and vomiting, back pain, pain with defecation, or difficulty with urination. Hydronephrosis may result from mechanical obstruction of the ureters by the enlarged vagina.

Repair of the imperforate hymen can be accomplished on diagnosis, regardless of the age of the patient, but may be easier in the newborn period or in the postpubertal, premenarcheal state, when estrogen stimulation is present.[153] The gynecologic surgeon excises the hymen close to the hymenal ring. The fluid within the obstructed vagina, which may be under considerable pressure, is carefully evacuated. Puncture of a mucocolpos or hematocolpos should not be performed without definitive surgical repair because the fluid may not drain adequately and the small perforations will allow bacteria to ascend, possibly resulting in pelvic infection.

A transverse vaginal septum occurs when the junction between the Müllerian tubercle and sinovaginal bulb is incompletely canalized. The complete transverse vaginal septum is rare; most septa have a small central perforation but still may present with hematocolpos in the adolescent, mucocolpos in the child, or pyohematocolpos from ascending infection. Almost 50% of vaginal septi occur in the upper vagina, 40% in the middle vagina, and 14% in the lower vagina.[154] The external genitalia appear normal. The vagina is short and may be described as "blind pouch," but a mass is often palpable above the examining finger and on rectoabdominal palpation. Surgical treatment depends on septal thickness, which may be determined with ultrasonography or MRI. Incision of thin septi may be acceptable. For thicker septi, end-to-end anastomosis of the upper and lower vagina is necessary.[153] A Z-plasty technique may prevent scar formation perpendicular to the vaginal axis.[155]

Agenesis of the Vagina/Cervix/Uterus

Vaginal agenesis is second only to gonadal dysgenesis as a cause of primary amenorrhea, occurring with a frequency of 1 in 4,000 to 20,000 female births.[156] Vaginal agenesis is usually accompanied by uterine agenesis, but occasionally the uterus is normal but obstructed or rudimentary with a functional endometrium. Vaginal agenesis may also occur with cervical agenesis, which may present with pain and a distended uterus. In the Mayer-Rokitansky-Kuster-Hauser syndrome, in addition to the presentation of vaginal agenesis, patients often have skeletal, renal, and cardiac defects and, rarely, malposition of the ovary.[147–149] Patients are 46,XX and have normal ovaries and hormonal patterns, but have absent or rudimentary uteri. Complete vaginal agenesis is present in 75% of cases, while the remainder have a short vaginal pouch. Ultrasonography and MRI can help to define the anatomy preoperatively.

Patients with vaginal agenesis and obstruction require immediate surgery, whereas those with accompanying uterine agenesis can have elective reconstruction. Most patients prefer creation of a vagina in their mid-to-late teens, during the summer to avoid missing school and having to answer embarrassing questions from peers. The nonsurgical approach involves the use of graduated dilators (Frank method) and takes 3 to 9 months in the motivated patient.[157] In the lithotomy position, the patient presses the smallest dilator firmly against the vaginal dimple backward and inward to the point of mild discomfort, for at least 30 minutes three times a day for the first week. During the second week the patient inserts the dilator downward and inward in the line of the normal vaginal axis. The Ingram modification uses a bicycle seat to facilitate vaginal dilation.[158]

Surgical reconstruction is used when dilators are unsuccessful or if preferred by the patient. The McIndoe-Read vaginoplasty creates a vaginal canal with a split-thickness skin graft from the buttocks mounted on a mold.[159, 160] A transverse incision is made at the vaginal dimple and a cavity dissected through which the mold and skin graft are inserted. Dilators are used postoperatively for 6 months to prevent contraction of the graft. The Williams vulvoplasty uses a U-shaped incision and full-thickness skin flaps from the labia majora to create a pouch with a posterior axis.[161] The patient uses a dilator daily postoperatively for 3 to 4 weeks. This procedure is simpler and has fewer complications than the McIndoe-Read method, but results in a vagina with a markedly abnormal angle, and abnormally appearing external genitalia. The bowel may also be used for reconstruction and does not require postoperative dilation.[162–164] However, patients may be uncomfortable with the vaginal discharge and odor that results from the bowel mucosa.

Androgen Insensitivity

In androgen insensitivity (testicular feminization), a form of male pseudohermaphroditism, the patient has an XY genotype, testes in the abdomen or inguinal rings, and serum testosterone in the range of the normal male. However, because of androgen insensitivity and increased estrogen production, the patient has a female habitus and external genitalia, with good breast development. Therefore, patients with androgen insensitivity often have evaluation of delayed menarche. The end-organ failure to respond to adrenal and testicular androgens results in absent or sparse pubic and axillary hair. The vagina is short, with absent uterus and cervix.

The gonads in these patients have a high rate of malignancy, and should be removed after the patient has reached full height and breast development. Delaying gonadectomy until after adolescence is associated with better breast development; thus, prepubertal patients should be monitored for malignancy with rectoabdominal examination and pelvic imaging. After the gonads are removed, the patient should receive estrogen replacement therapy. The clinician must be sensitive to the issues of femininity and fertility that arise with these patients.

Female Genital Mutilation

Female genital multilation, also known by the misnomer "female circumcision," is practiced in approximately 26 African countries, the Middle East, and by Muslim peoples in Indonesia and Malaysia.[165, 166] The prevalence of the procedure in these regions ranges from 5 to 99%,[165] with an estimated 80 to 110 million women affected worldwide.[166] Female genital mutilation is associated with significant morbidity and even mortality, with short-and long-term physical, psychological, sexual, and reproductive effects in the survivors.

The procedure is usually performed in children from the ages of 4 to 10 years, most commonly at the age of 7 years.[165, 166] A classification scheme has been developed by Toubia[165] based on the degree of tissue removal and destruction:

Type I (clitoridectomy): Removal of a part of the clitoris or the whole organ.

Type II (clitoridectomy): Excision of the clitoris and part of the labia minora.

Type III (modified infibulation): Removal of the clitoris and the labia minora, with incision of the labia majora to create raw surfaces. The anterior two thirds of the labia majora are reapproximated to cover the urethra and introitus, leaving an opening of the lower third for the passage of urine and menstrual blood.

Type IV (total infibulation): Removal of the clitoris and the labia minora, with incision of the labia majora to create raw surfaces. The labia majora are reapproximated to cover the urethra and introitus, leaving a very small opening for the passage of urine and menstrual blood.

The procedure is usually performed without anesthesia by a midwife or village woman as a ritualistic right of passage into adult village society.[166] In types III and IV, the labial surfaces are reapproximated with sutures of silk or catgut or held together with thorns or twigs. The girl's legs are then bound from hips to ankles for up to 40 days so that scar tissue will form. Immediate risks from the procedure include pain, hemorrhage, damage to the urethra and anus, local infection, shock, sepsis, and death.[165, 166] Long-term risks include transmission of bloodborne pathogens from unsterilized instruments, pain, recurrent urinary tract infections, chronic vaginitis and endometritis, dysuria, dysmenorrhea, dyspareunia, and apareunia.[165, 166]

Women who have had female genital mutilation often require surgical revision before intercourse, with possible further revision before vaginal delivery. The surgeon must be aware of the cultural significance of this procedure and of the revision. One sensitive approach is to have the patient demonstrate with a hand-held mirror exactly what area of the genital region she wants revised. Figure 33.10 shows the prerevision and postrevision appearance of the genitals.

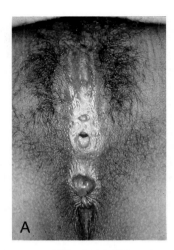

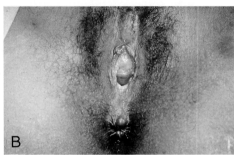

FIG. 33.10. Appearance of the genitals: prerevision **(A)** and postrevision **(B)**.

BREAST DEVELOPMENT AND ABNORMALITIES

Anatomy of the Normal Breast

The 6-week-old embryo develops the precursor to the breast as an ectodermal thickening along the "milk line" or "nipple line," which runs vertically from the axilla to the groin. The breast tissue that subsequently develops is made up of milk glands (alveoli) surrounded by myoepithelial strands and capillaries (Fig. 33.11). The alveoli connect through ducts that end in approximately 20 apertures on the areola. Adipose tissue surrounds glandular and duct tissue.

Examination of the Breast

The breast examination is an opportunity to educate the patient on breast anatomy and development, as well as in the older adolescent to teach her breast self-examination techniques.[167] The breast should be examined with the patient supine with her ipsilateral arm under her head to stretch the breast tissues on the chest wall. Tanner stage should be noted (see Fig. 33.3). If disorders of development are of concern, measurements of the areola, glandular breast tissue, and overall breast size (diameter of the fatty tissue of the breast mound) should be noted. The breast should be palpated in one of several ways: (1) in a pattern like spokes of a wheel, from the margin of the breast mound inward to the nipple,

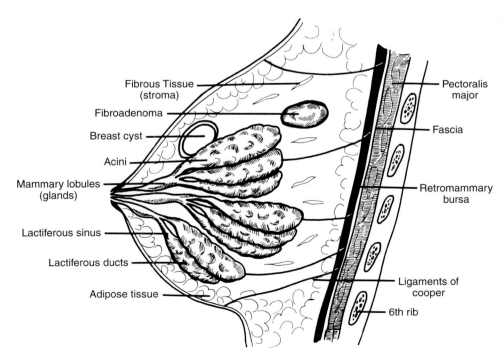

FIG. 33.11. Sagittal section showing the internal anatomy of the breast. Modified from Beach RK. Breast disorders. In: McAnarney ER, Kreipe RE, Orr DP, Comerci GD, eds., Textbook of adolescent medicine. Philadelphia: Saunders, 1992.

(2) in a pattern of concentric circles or a spiral inward, or (3) in a vertical or horizontal linear fashion. The examiner rotates the pads of his or her fingers to palpate for abnormalities. The areola should be compressed to express any discharge. The axillae should be palpated for breast tissue extending into this region and for lymphadenopathy.

Normal Variants of the Breast

Accessory breast tissue includes a supernumerary nipple (polythelia), breast tissue (polymastia), or both. Most accessory breast tissue occurs along the milk line. Rarely, accessory breast tissue can occur in the midline, in atypical locations. Excision may be appropriate to consider if the tissue changes during puberty or causes cosmetic problems. Supernumerary nipples may be associated with renal anomalies;[168, 169] renal ultrasonography is suggested in infants with supernumerary nipples and congenital anomalies.[170]

Diagnosis of accessory breast tissue should be considered whenever tissue exists, which changes in size with the menstrual cycle, regardless of its location. Normal breast tissue in the axilla is sometimes mistaken for accessory breast tissue. The patient may complain of premenstrual axillary discomfort or have axillary discomfort as the first sign of pregnancy.

Breast development often occurs asymmetrically and most adult women have one breast that is slightly larger than the other. Breast reduction or augmentation may be considered for those rare patients with marked asymmetry at Tanner stage B5 whose breasts have not grown during the previous 6 months, usually by age 15 to 18 years. Development must be completed before surgery, lest continued growth of one breast results again in asymmetry.

Rarely, breast asymmetry represents a mass from a juvenile fibroadenoma or cystosarcoma phylloides. These uncommon tumors usually present with a palpable mass on examination of the larger breast and are often associated with ipsilateral superficial venous engorgement. Ultrasonography is used to determine the presence of a mass in unclear cases.

Abnormalities of the Breast

Amastia, unilateral or bilateral absence of breast tissue, is rare. It is often associated with underdevelopment of the chest wall, as in Poland syndrome, or previous biopsy. Massive enlargement of the breast is called juvenile (formerly, virginal) hypertrophy and can occur unilaterally. This condition usually develops in Tanner stage B4 and may significantly regress by Tanner stage B5. The adolescent may have mechanical consequences of carrying large breasts, such as back pain and posture problems, or have cosmetic concerns. Fungal intertrigo can occur in the skin beneath the enlarged breast. Tumors must be excluded in patients with unilateral, rapidly progressive enlargement. Reduction mammoplasty is indicated in patients with significant symptoms.

Mastitis usually occurs in the peripartum period, but breast infections can occur in nonlactating adolescents. Many infections occur without known precipitating events and may be associated with ductal ectasia. Skin flora, such as staphylococci or streptococci, can gain entry to the breast tissue. Plucking or shaving periareolar hairs appears to predispose to infection. Mastitis is treated with antibiotics effective against penicillinase-resistant staphylococci and often requires incision and drainage. Disfigurement or scarring are potential consequences of the infection and its treatment.

Some adolescents may complain of irritation of the nipples from jogging or running. Nipple discomfort, abrasion, or a desquamating rash may result. This problem is most often caused by friction against clothing and may be alleviated by lubrication with petrolatum or protection with an adhesive bandage.[171]

Breast Discharge

Breast discharge can occur in adolescents and may be milky, serous, purulent, or bloody. Milky discharge has multiple fat droplets under magnification. Discharge from multiple duct openings is usally of hormonal etiology, whereas discharge from an isolated duct usually indicates local pathology. Occasionally, breast discharge emanates from the periareolar glands of Montgomery instead of a breast duct opening.[172] In adolescents, galactorrhea may represent breast manipulation from physical activity or sexual stimulation, trauma, pregnancy, medications that inhibit or suppress dopamine, hypothyroidism and other endocrinologic disorders, pituitary prolactinomas and other CNS tumors, hyperprolactinemia, and hypothalamic and pituitary disorders. The evaluation of hyperprolactinemia is discussed on page 591. Galactorrhea without hyperprolactinemia may resolve over several months if the adolescent is instructed not to stimulate secretion.

Serous or bloody discharge is often a symptom of intraductal papilloma. The discharge usually emanates from one isolated duct opening. Approximately half the time, a small mass can be palpated under the involved gland. The papilloma is treated with duct excision. Mammary duct ectasia may also be associated with nipple discharge. Duct ectasia is caused by metaplasia of the ductal epithelium, with occlusion of the duct by plugs of epithelial cells.

Breast Masses

Fibrocystic Changes

Most palpable breast masses in the adolescent are caused by fibrocystic changes or a fibroadenoma.[173] Fibrocystic changes involve nonpathologic physiologic response to cyclic hormonal stimulation. Clinically significant fibrocystic changes of the breast occur in approximately 10% of girls younger than 21 years of age. The most common symptom is bilateral breast pain or discomfort, generally in the upper and outer quadrants of the breast. The etiology of fibrocystic changes is unknown and does not appear to be related to caffeine intake.[174, 175] Pain is usually worse in the luteal phase of the menstrual cycle, suggesting progesterone involvement.[176]

On physical examination, the breasts are tender and the microcysts feel granular without discrete masses. The findings tend to vary during the patient's menstrual cycle and from month to month. Treatment may include a supportive bra and NSAIDs. Oral contraceptives are helpful in some cases. In women with fibrocystic changes, the risk for breast cancer is slightly increased if breast biopsy shows atypical hyperplasia.[177]

Fibroadenoma

Approximately 70% of breast masses surgically removed in adolescents are fibroadenomas.[178–181] Fibroadenomas are firm or rubbery, mobile masses with a clearly defined edge. They are palpable near the surface and tend to occur in the lateral quadrants of the breast. The mass may remain unchanged or increase in size with subsequent menstrual cycles. Recurrent or multiple fibroadenomas occur in 10 to 25% of patients.[172] Most patients elect excisional biopsy. A history of fibroadenoma in patients with a family history of breast cancer, complex histology, or proliferative disease is associated with an increased risk of breast cancer.[182]

Cystosarcoma Phylloides

Cystosarcoma phylloides is a rare tumor that is typically benign, but occasionally can be malignant.[183] These masses are usually large and circumscribed.[184] The nipple and the skin overlying the lesion may be affected. Biopsy is necessary for accurate diagnosis.[173]

Breast Cancer

Breast cancer is rare in adolescents.[180, 181, 185–188] Patients with previous radiation therapy to the chest have an increased risk of breast cancer at a young age and require monitoring with breast self-examination, regular check-ups, and mammography.[189–191] A family history of breast cancer in a first-degree relative and certain genetic syndromes are also associated with increased risk of breast cancer.[192–195]

Contusion

Trauma to the breast may produce a poorly defined, tender mass that resolves over several weeks. In severe trauma, the mass may take several months to resolve; palpable scar tissue occasionally may remain. Fat necrosis may present as a small, firm, immobile, superficial mass months after breast trauma.

REFERENCES

1. Speroff L, Glass RH, Kase NG. Clinical Gynecologic Endocrinology and Infertility, 5th ed. Philadelphia: Williams & Wilkins, 1994.
2. Lee PA. Neuroendocrinology of puberty. Semin Reprod Endocrinol 1988;6:13–20.
3. Besser GM, McNeilly AS, Anderson DC, et al. Hormonal responses to synthetic luteinizing hormone and follicle stimulating hormone in man. Br Med J 1972;3:267–271.
4. Ayerst Laboratories Inc. Factrel® (Gonadorelin Hydrochloride) Package Insert. New York, 1990.
5. Apter D, Pakarinen A, Hammond GL, et al. Adrenocortical function in puberty. Acta Paediatr Scand 1979;68:599.
6. Styne DM, Grumbach MM. Puberty in the male and female: its physiology and disorders. In: Yen SSC, Jaffe RB, eds. Reproductive Endocrinology. Philadelphia: WB Saunders, 1986.
7. Lucky AW, Biro FM, Huster GA, et al. Acne vulgaris in premenarchal girls. An early sign of puberty associated with rising levels of dehydroepiandrosterone. Arch Derm 1994;130:308–314.
8. Landy H, Boepple PA, Mansfield MJ, et al. Sleep modulation of neuroendocrine function: developmental changes in gonadotropin-releasing hormone during sexual maturation. Pediatr Res 1990;28:213–217.
9. Boyar RM, Wu RH, Roffwarg H, et al. Human puberty: 24-hour estradiol patterns in pubertal girls. J Clin Endocrinol Metab 1976;43:1418.
10. Yen SSC, Apter D, Bhtzow T, Laughlin GA. Gonadotropin releasing hormone pulse generator activity before and during sexual maturation in girls: new insights. Hum Reprod 1993; 8:66–71.
11. Rosenfield RL, Frulanetto R. Physiologic testosterone in estradiol induction of puberty increases plasma somatomedin-C. J Pediatr 1985;107:415.
12. Moll GW, Rosenfield RL, Fang VS. Administration of low-dose estrogen rapidly and directly stimulates growth hormone production. Am J Dis Child 1986;140:124.
13. Zachmann M, Prader A, Sobel EH, et al. Pubertal growth in patients with androgen insensitivity: indirect evidence for the importance of estrogens in pubertal growth of girls. J Pediatr 1986;108:694.
14. Rose SR, Municchi G, Barnes KM, et al. Spontaneous growth hormone secretion increases during puberty in normal girls and boys. J Clin Endocrinol Metab 1991;73:428 435.
15. Greulich WW, Pyle S. Radiographic Atlas of Skeletal Development of the Hand and Wrist. Standford, CA: Stanford University Press, 1959.
16. Zacharias L, Wurtman R. Age at menarche: genetic and environmental influences. N Engl J Med 1969;280:868.
17. MacMahon B. National health examination survey: age at menarche. DHEW Publication 74-1615, Series 11, No. 133, November 1973.
18. Apter D. Serum steroids and pituitary hormones in female puberty: a partly longitudinal study. Clin Endocrinol 1980;12:107.
19. Apter D, Viinikka L, Vihko R. Hormonal pattern of adolescent menstrual cycles. J Clin Endocrinol Metab 1978;47:944.
20. World Health Organization Task Force on Adolescent Reproductive Health. World Health Organization multicenter study on menstrual and ovulatory patterns in adolescent girls: I, A multicenter cross-sectional study of menarche. J Adol Health Care 1986;7:229–235.
21. World Health Organization Task Force on Adolescent Repro-

ductive Health. World Health Organization multicenter study on menstrual and ovulatory patterns in adolescent girls: II. Longitudinal study of menstrual patterns in the early postmenarcheal period, duration of bleeding episodes and menstrual cycles. J Adolesc Health Care 1986;7:236–244.

22. Marshall WA, Tanner JM. Variations in pattern of pubertal changes in girls. Arch Dis Child 1969;44:291.

23. Grumbach MM, Styne DM. Puberty: ontogeny, neuroendocrinology, physiology, and disorders. In: Wilson JD, Foster DW, eds. Williams Textbook of Endocrinology, 8th ed. Philadelphia: WB Saunders, 1992.

24. Harlan WR, Harlan EA, Grillo GP. Secondary sex characteristics of girls 12 to 17 years of age: the U.S. Health Examination Survey. J Pediatr 1980;96:1074.

25. Bayley N. Growth curves of height and weight by age for boys and girls, scaled according to physical maturity. J Pediatr 1956;48:187.

26. Hamill PVV, Drizd TA, Johnson CL, et al. Physical growth: National Center for Health Statistics percentiles. Am J Clin Nutr 1979;32:607.

27. Frisch RE. A method of prediction of age and menarche from height and weight at ages nine through thirteen years. Pediatrics 1974;53:384.

28. Frisch RE, McArthur JW. Menstrual cycles: fatness as a determinant of minimum weight necessary for their maintenance or onset. Science 1974;185:949.

29. Zacharias L, Wurtman RJ, Schatzoff M. Sexual maturation in contemporary American girls. Am J Obstet Gynecol 1970; 108:833.

30. Apter D, Bhtzow TL, Laughlin GA, Yen SCC. Gonadotropin releasing hormone pulse generator activity during pubertal transition in girls: pulsatile and diurnal patterns of circulating gonadotropins. J Clin Endocrinol Metab 1993;76:940–949.

31. Apter D, Vihko R. Serum pregnenolone, progesterone, 17-hydroxyprogesterone, testosterone, and 5 α-dihydrotestosterone during female puberty. J Clin Endocrinol Metab 1977;45:1039.

32. Tsonis CG, Messinis IE, Templeton AA, et al. Gonadotropic stimulation of inhibin secretion by the human ovary during the follicular and early luteal phase of the cycle. J Clin Endocrinol Metab 1988;66:915.

33. Filicori M, Butler JP, Crowley WF. Neuroendocrine regulation of the corpus luteum in the human: evidence for pulsatile progesterone secretion. J Clin Invest 1984;73:1638.

34. Duerenberg P, Pieters JJL, Hautvast JG. The assessment of the body fat percentage by skinfold thickness measurements in childhood and young adolescence. Br J Nutr 1990;63:293–303.

35. Pollock ML, Schmidt DH. Measurement of cardiorespiratory fitness and body composition in the clinical setting. Compr Ther 1980;6:12–27.

36. Stratakis CA, Rennert OM. Turner syndrome: molecular and cytogenetics, dysmorphology, endocrine, and other clinical manifestations and their management. Endocrinologist 1994; 4:442–453.

37. Rosenfeld RG. Turner syndrome: a guide for physicians. The Turner's Syndrome Society. Gardiner-Caldwell Synermed, 1992.

38. Ogata T, Matsuo N. Turner syndrome and female sex chromosome aberrations: deduction in the principal factors involved in the development of clinical features. Hum Genet 1995;95: 607–629.

39. Saenger P. Clinical review 48: the current status of diagnosis and therapeutic intervention in Turner's syndrome. J Clin Endocrinol Metab 1993;77:297–301.

40. Allen DB, Hendricks SA, Levy JM. Aortic dilation in Turner's syndrome. J Pediatr 1986;109:302.

41. AAP Committee on Genetics. Health supervision for children with Turner syndrome. Pediatrics 1995;16:1166.

42. Lippe B, Geffner ME, Dietrich RB, et al. Renal malformations in patients with Turner syndrome: imaging in 141 patients. Pediatrics 1988;82:852.

43. Neely EK, Marcus R, Rosenfeld RG, Bachrach LK. Turner syndrome adolescents receiving growth hormone are not osteopenic. J Clin Endocrinol Metab 1993;76:861–866.

44. Emans SJ, Grace E, Hoffer FA, Gundberg C, Ravnikar V, Woods ER. Estrogen deficiency in adolescents and young adults: impact on bone mineral content and effects of estrogen replacement therapy. Obstet Gynecol 1990;76:585–592.

45. Stepan JJ, Musilova J, Pacovsky V. Bone demineralization, biochemical indices of bone remodeling, and estrogen replacement therapy in adults with Turner's syndrome. J Bone Miner Res 1989;4:193–198.

46. Naeraa RW, Brixen K, Hansen RM, et al. Skeletal size and bone mineral content in Turner's syndrome: relation to karyotype, estrogen treatment, physical fitness, and bone turnover. Calcif Tissue Int 1991;49:77–83.

47. Rosenfield RG, Grumbach MM, eds. Turner Syndrome NY: Marcel Dekker, 1990.

48. Lippe B. Turner syndrome. Endocrinol Metab Clin North Am 1991;20:121–152.

49. Bender BG, Linden MG, Robinson A. Neuropsychological impairment in 42 adolescents with sex chromosome abnormalities. Am J Med Genet 1993;48:169–173.

50. Kleczkowska A, Dmoch E, Kubien E, Fryns JP, Van Den Berghe H. Cytogenetic findings in a consecutive series of 478 patients with Turner syndrome. The Leuven experience 1965–1989. Genet Counsel 1990;1:227 233. (Erratum) Genet Counsel 1991;2:130–131.

51. Temtamy SA, Ghali I, Salam MA, et al. Karyotype/phenotype correlation in females with short stature. Clin Genet 1992; 41:147–151.

52. Reyes FI, Koh KS, Faiman C. Fertility in women with gonadal dysgenesis. Am J Obstet Gynecol 1976;126:668.

53. Kaneko N, Kawagoe S, Hizoi M. 1990 Turner's syndrome—review of the literature with reference to a successful pregnancy outcome. Gynecol Obstet Invest 1990;29:81–87.

54. Krauss CM, Turksoy RN, Atkins L, et al. Familial premature ovarian failure due to an interstitial deletion of the long arm of the X-chromosome. N Engl J Med 1987;317:125.

55. Reindollar RH, Byrd JR, McDonough PG. Delayed sexual development: a study of 252 patients. Am J Obstet Gynecol 1981;140:371.

56. Alper MM, Garner PR. Premature ovarian failure: its relationship to autoimmune disease. Obstet Gynecol 1985;66:27.

57. Ahonen P, Miettinen A, Perheentupa J. Adrenal and steroidal cell antibodies in patients with autoimmune polyglandular disease type I and risk of adrenocortical and ovarian failure. J Clin Endocrinol Metab 1987;64:494.

58. Brelvisi L, Bombelli F, Sironi L, Doldi N. Organ-specific autoimmunity in patients with premature ovarian failure. J Endocrinol Invest 1993;16:889–892.

59. Smith BR, Furmaniak J. Editorial: adrenal and gonadal autoimmune diseases. J Clin Endocrinol Metab 1995;80:1502–1505.

60. Betterle C, Rossi A, Pria SD, et al. Premature ovarian failure: autoimmunity and natural history. J Clin Endocrinol 1993;39:35–43.

61. Alper MM, Garner MB, Seibel MM. Premature ovarian failure: current concepts. J Reprod Med 1986;31:699.

62. Rebar RW, Erickson GF, Yen SSC. Idiopathic premature ovarian failure: clinical and endocrine characteristics. Fertil Steril 1982;37:35.

63. Scully RE, ed. Case records of the Massachusetts General Hospital: case 46-1986. N Engl J Med 1986;315:1336.

64. Kaufman FR, Kogut MD, Donnell GN, et al. Hypergonadotrophic hypogonadism in female patients with galactosemia. N Engl J Med 1981;304:994.

65. Hsiang YH, Berkovitz GD, Bland GL, Midgeon CJ, Warren AC. Gonadal function in patients with down syndrome. Am J Med Genet 1987;27:449–458.

66. Finan AC, Elmer MA, Sasnow SR, et al. Nutritional factors and growth in children with sickle cell disease. Am J Dis Child 1988;142:237.

67. Platt OS, Rosenstock W, Espeland MA. Influence of sickle hemoglobinopathies on growth and development. N Engl J Med 1984;311:7.

68. Rosenbach Y, Dinari G, Zahavi I, et al. Short stature as the major manifestation of celiac disease in older children. Clin Pediatr 1986;25:13.

69. Pugliese MT, Lifshitz F, Grad G, et al. Fear of obesity: a cause of short stature and delayed puberty. N Engl J Med 1983;309:513.

70. Frisch RE, Gotz-Wolbergen AV, McArthur JW, et al. Delayed menarche and amenorrhea of college athletes in relation to age of onset of training. JAMA 1981;246:1559.
71. Warren MP. The effects of exercise on pubertal progression and reproductive function in girls. J Clin Endocrinol Metab 1980;51:1150.
72. Emans SJH, Goldstein DP. Pediatric and Adolescent Gynecology. Boston: Little, Brown and Company, 1990.
73. White CM, Hergenroeder AC, Klish WJ. Bone mineral density in 15- to 21-year-old eumenorrheic and amenorrheic subjects. AJDC 1992;146:31–35.
74. Theintz GE, Howald H, Weiss U, Sizonenko PC. Evidence for a reduction of growth potential in adolescent female gymnasts. J Pediatr 1993;122:306–313.
75. Mansfield MJ, Emans SJ. Growth in female gymnasts: should training decrease during puberty. J Pediatr 1993;122:237–239.
76. Bonjour JP, Theintz G, Buchs B, et al. Critical years and stages of puberty for spinal and femoral bone mass accumulation during adolescence. J Clin Endocrinol Metab 1991;73:555–563.
77. Theintz G, Buchs B, Rizzoli R, et al. Longitudinal monitoring of bone mass accumulation in healthy adolescent: evidence for a marked reduction after 16 years of age at the levels of lumbar spine and femoral neck in female subjects. J Clin Endocrinol Metab 1992;75:1060–1065.
78. Slemenda CW, Reister TK, Hui SL, et al. Influences on skeletal mineralization in children and adolescents: evidence for varying effects of sexual maturation and physical activity. J Pediatr 1994;125:210–217.
79. Gilsanz V, Roe TF, Mora S, et al. Changes in vertebral bone density in black girls and white girls during childhood and puberty. N Engl J Med 1991;325:1597–1600.
80. Lloyd T, Andon MB, Rollings N, et al. Calcium supplementation and bone mineral density in adolescent girls. JAMA 1993; 270:841–844.
81. Rubin K, Schirduan V, Gendreau P, et al. Predictors of axial and peripheral bone mineral density in healthy children and adolescents, with special attention to the role of puberty. J Pediatr 1993;123:863–870.
82. Recker RR, Davies KM, Hinders SM. Bone gain in young adult women. JAMA 1992;268:2403–2408.
83. Cann CE, Martin MC, Genant HK, et al. Decreased spinal mineral content in amenorrheic women. JAMA 1984;251:626.
84. Marcus R, Cann C, Madvig P, et al. Menstrual function and bone mass in elite women distance runners: endocrine and metabolic features. Ann Intern Med 1985;102:158.
85. Drinkwater BL, Nilson K, Chesnut CH, et al. Bone mineral content of amenorrheic and eumenorrheic athletes. N Engl J Med 1984;311:277.
86. Myerson M, Gutin B, Warren MP, et al. Total body bone density in amenorrheic runners. Obstet Gynecol 1992;79:973–978.
87. Louis O, Demeirleir K, Kalender W, et al. Low vertebral bone density values in young non-elite female runners. Int J Sports Med 1991;12:214–217.
88. Wolman RL, Clark P, McNally E, et al. Dietary calcium as a statistical determinant of spinal trabecular bone density in amenorrhoeic and oestrogen-replete athletes. Bone Mineral 1992;17:415–423.
89. Djursing H. Hypothalmic-pituitary-gonadal function in insulin-treated diabetic women with and without amenorrhea. Dan Med Bull 1987;34:139.
90. Rosenfield RL. Puberty and its disorders in girls. Endocrinol Metab Clin North Am 1991;20:15–42.
91. Vance ML. Hypopituitarism. N Engl J Med 1994;330:1651–1662.
92. Cicognani A, Cacciari E, Vecchi V, et al. Differential effects of 18- and 24-gy cranial irradiation on growth rate and growth hormone release in children with prolonged survival after acute lymphocytic leukemia. Am J Dis Child 1988;142:1199.
93. Costin G. Effect of low-dose cranial radiation on growth hormone secretory dynamics and hypothalamic-pituitary function. Am J Dis Child 1988;142:847.
94. Miller WL, Kaplan SL, Grumbach MM. Child abuse as a cause of posttraumatic hypopituitarism. N Engl J Med 1980;302:724.
95. Barkan AL, Kelch RP, Marshall JC. Isolated gonadotrope failure

in the polyglandular autoimmune syndrome. N Engl J Med 1985;312:1535.
96. Cacciari E, Zucchini S, Ambrosetto P, et al. Empty sella in children and adolescents with possible hypothalamic-pituitary disorders. J Clin Endocrinol Metab 1994;78:767–771.
97. Evrard J, Buxton BH, Erickson D. Amenorrhea following oral contraception. Am J Obstet Gynecol 1976;124:88.
98. Shearman RP. Prolonged secondary amenorrhea after oral contraceptive therapy: natural and unnatural history. Lancet 1971;2:64.
99. Shearman RP. Secondary amenorrhea after oral contraceptives: treatment and follow-up. Contraception 1975;2:123.
100. Ferriman D, Gallwey JD. Clinical assessment of body hair growth in women. J Clin Endocrinol Metab 1961;21:1440.
101. Barbieri RL, Smith S, Ryan KJ. The role of hyperinsulinemia in the pathogenesis of ovarian hyperandrogenism. Fertil Steril 1988;50:197.
102. McKenna TJ. Pathogenesis and treatment of polycystic ovary syndrome. N Engl J Med 1988;318:558.
103. Coney P. Polycystic ovarian disease: current concepts of pathophysiology and therapy. Fertil Steril 1984;42:667.
104. Lobo RA, Goebelsmann U. Effect of androgen excess on inappropriate gonadotropin secretion as found in the polycystic ovary syndrome. Am J Obstet Gynecol 1982;142:394.
105. Burghen GA, Givens JR, Kitabchi AE. Correlation of hyperandrogenism with hyperinsulinism in polycystic ovary disease. J Clin Endocrinol Metab 1980;50:113.
106. Shoupe D, Kumar DO, Lobo RA. Insulin resistance in polycystic ovary syndrome. Am J Obstet Gynecol 1983;147:588.
107. Loughlin T, Cunningham S, Moore A, et al. Adrenal abnormalities in polycystic ovary syndrome. J Clin Endocrinol Metab 1986;62:142.
108. Givens JR, Andersen RN, Wiser WL. The effectiveness of two oral contraceptives in suppressing plasma androstenedione, testosterone, LH, and FSH, and in stimulating plasma testosterone-binding capacity in hirsute women. Am J Obstet Gynecol 1976;124:333.
109. Waldstreicher J, Santoro NF, Hall JE, et al. Hyperfunction of the hypothalamic-pituitary axis in women with polycystic ovarian disease: indirect evidence for partial gonadotrophic desensitization. J Clin Endocrinol Metab 1988;66:165.
110. Lobo RA, Granger L, Goebelsmann U, et al. Elevations in unbound serum estradiol as a possible mechanism for inappropriate gonadotropin secretion in women with PCO. J Clin Endocrinol Metab 1981;52:156.
111. Mattsson L, Cullberg G, Hamgerber L, et al. Lipid metabolism in women with polycystic ovary syndrome: possible implications for an increased risk of coronary heart disease. Fertil Steril 1984;42:579.
112. Wild RA, Bartholomew MJ. The influence of body weight on lipoprotein lipids in patients with polycystic ovary syndrome. Am J Obstet Gynecol 1988;159:423.
113. Wild RA, Painter PC, Coulson PB, et al. Lipoprotein lipid concentrations and cardiovascular risk in women with polycystic ovary syndrome. J Clin Endocrinol Metab 1985;61:946.
114. Blankenstein J, Faiman C, Reyes F, et al. Adult onset familial adrenal hyperplasia due to incomplete 21-hydroxylase deficiency. Am J Med 1980;68:441.
115. Lobo RA, Goebelsmann U. Adult manifestation of congenital adrenal hyperplasia due to incomplete 21-hydroxylase deficiency mimicking polycystic ovary disease. Am J Obstet Gynecol 1980;138:720.
116. Migeon CJ, Rosewaks Z, Lee P, et al. The attenuated form of 21-hydroxylase deficiency as an allelic form of 21-hydroxylase deficiency. J Clin Endocrinol Metab 1980;51:647.
117. Kohn B, Levine LS, Pollack MS, et al. Late-onset steroid 21-hydroxylase deficiency: a variant of classical congenital adrenal hyperplasia. J Clin Endocrinol Metab 1982;55:817.
118. Pang S, Lerner A, Stoner E, et al. Late-onset adrenal steroid 3β-hydroxysteroid dehydrogenase deficiency: I, A cause of hirsutism in pubertal and postpubertal women. J Clin Endocrinol Metab 1985;60:428.
119. Emans SJ, Grace E, Fleischnick E, et al. Detection of late-onset

21-hydroxylase deficiency congenital adrenal hyperplasia in adolescents. Pediatrics 1983;72:690.

120. Chrousos GP, Loriaux DL, Mann DL, et al. Late-onset 21-hydroxylase deficiency mimicking idiopathic hirsutism or polycystic ovarian disease. Ann Intern Med 1982;96:143.

121. Benjamin F, Deutsch S, Saperstein H, et al. Prevalence of and markers for the attenuated form of congenital adrenal hyperplasia and hyperprolactinemia masquerading as polycystic ovarian disease. Fertil Steril 1986;46:215.

122. Reid RL, Van Vugt DA. Weight-related changes in reproductive function. Fertil Steril 1987;48:905.

123. Glass AR, Dahms WT, Abraham GE. Secondary amenorrhea in obesity: etiologic role of weight related androgen excess. Fertil Steril 1978;30:243.

124. Harlass FE, Playmate SR, Fariss BL. Weight loss is associated with correction of gonadotropin and sex steroid abnormalities in the obese anovulatory female. Fertil Steril 1984;42:649.

125. Hosseinian AH, Kim MH, Rosenfield C. Obesity and oligomenorrhea are associated with hyperandrogenism independent of hirsutism. J Clin Endocrinol Metab 1976;42:765.

126. Lindsay R. Estrogen therapy in the prevention and management of osteoporosis. Am J Obstet Gynecol 1987;156:1347.

127. Ettinger B, Genant HK, Cann CE. Long-term estrogen replacement therapy prevents bone loss and fractures. Ann Intern Med 1985;102:319.

128. Lobo RA, Pickar JH, Wild RA, Walsh B, Hirvonen E. Metabolic impact of adding medroxyprogesterone acetate to conjugated estrogen therapy in postmenopausal women. Obstet Gynecol 1994;84:987–995.

129. Grimes DA, Chaney EJ, Connell EB, et al, eds. Weighing the risks and benefits of hormone replacement therapy after menopause. The Contraception Report 1995;VI:1–15.

130. Davidson NE. Hormone-replacement therapy-breast versus heart versus bone. Editorial. N Engl J Med 1995;332:1638–1639.

131. Whitcroft SI, Crook D, Marsh MS, Ellerington MC, Whitehead MI, Stevenson JC. Long-term effects of oral and transdermal hormone replacement therapies on serum lipid and lipoprotein concentrations. Obstet Gynecol 1994;84:222–226.

132. Lodeweyckx MV, Massa AG, Maes M, et al. Growth-promoting effect of growth hormone and low dose ethinyl estradiol in girls with Turner's syndrome. J Clin Endocrinol Metab 1990; 70:122–126.

133. Massa G, Maes M, Heinrichs C, Vandeweghe M, Craen M, Lodeweyckx MV. Influence of spontaneous or induced puberty on the growth promoting effect of treatment with growth hormone in girls with Turner's syndrome. Clin Endocrinol 1993;38:253–260.

134. Southam AL, Richart RM. The prognosis for adolescents with menstrual abnormalities. Am J Obstet Gynecol 1966;94:637.

135. Usta IM, Awwad JT, Usta JA, et al. Imperforate hymen: report of an unusual familial occurrence. Obstet Gynecol 1993;82: 655–656.

136. Shatzkes DR, Haller JO, Velcek FT. Imaging of uterovaginal anomalies in the pediatric population. Urol Radiol 1991; 13:58–66.

137. Valdes C, Malini S, Malinak LR. Ultrasound evaluation of female genital tract anomalies: a review of 64 cases. Am J Obstet Gynecol 1984;149:285–290.

138. Scanlan KA, Pozniak MA, Fagerholm M, et al. Value of transperineal sonography in the assessment of vaginal atresia. AJR 1990;154:545–548.

139. Raga F, Bonilla-Musoles F, Blanes J, et al. Congenital müllerian anomalies: diagnostic accuracy of three-dimensional ultrasound. Fertil Steril 1996;65:523–528.

140. Markham SM, Parmley TH, Murphy AA, et al. Cervical agenesis combined with vaginal agenesis diagnosed by magnetic resonance imaging. Fertil Steril 1987;48:143–145.

141. Fedele L, Dorta M, Brioschi D, et al. Magnetic resonance imaging in Mayer-Rokitansky-Kuster-Hauser syndrome. Obstet Gynecol 1990;76:593–596.

142. Pellerito JS, McCarthy SM, Doyle MB, et al. Diagnosis of uterine anomalies: relative accuracy of MR imaging, endovaginal sonography, and hysterosalpingography. Radiology 1992;183:795–800.

143. Doyle MB. Magnetic resonance imaging in müllerian fusion defects. J Reprod Med 1992;37:33–38.

144. Erdogan E, Okan G, Daragenli O. Uterus didelphys with unilateral obstructed hemivagina and renal agenesis on the same side. Acta Obstet Gynecol Scand 1992;71:76–77.

145. Sheih CP, Li YW, Liao YJ, et al. Early detection of unilateral occlusion of duplicated müllerian ducts: the use of serial pelvic sonography for girls with renal agenesis. J Urol 1994; 151:708–710.

146. Sanfilippo JS. Strassman procedure for correction of a class II Müllerian anomaly in an adolescent. J Adolesc Health 1991; 12:63–66.

147. Pinsonneault O, Goldstein DP. Obstructing malformations of the uterus and vagina. Fertil Steril 1985;44:241.

148. Tran ATB, Arensman RM, Falterman KW. Diagnosis and management of hydrohematometrocolpos syndrome. Am J Dis Child 1987;141:632.

149. Golan A, Langer R, et al. Congenital anomalies of the Müllerian system. Fertil Steril 1989;51:747–755.

150. Olive DL, Henderson DY. Endometriosis and Müllerian anomalies. Obstet Gynecol 1987;69:412–415.

151. The American Fertility Society. The American Fertility Society classifications of adnexal adhesions, distal tubal occlusion, tubal occlusion secondary to tubal ligation, tubal pregnancies, Müllerian anomalies, and intrauterine adhesions. Fertil Steril 1988;49:944–955.

152. Goldstein DP, Laufer MR, Davis AJ. Gynecologic Surgery in Children and Adolescents: A Text Atlas. NY, Springer-Verlag, In press.

153. Laufer MR, Goldstein DP. Structural Anomalies of the Female Reproductive Tract. In: Emans SJ, Goldstein DP, Laufer MR, eds. Pediatric and Adolescent Gynecology, 4th ed. Philadelphia: Lippincott-Raven, 1998.

154. Lodi A. Contributo clinico statistico sulle malformazioni della vagina osservate nella clinica ostetrica e ginecologica di Milano dal 1906 al 1950. Ann Ostet Ginecol 1951;73:1246–1285.

155. Garcia RF. Z-plasty correction for congenital transverse vaginal septum. Am J Obstet Gynecol 1967;99:1164–1165.

156. Kim HH, Laufer MR. Developmental abnormalities of the female reproductive tract. Curr Opin Obstet Gynecol 1994; 6:518–525.

157. Frank RT. The formation of an artificial vagina without operation. Am J Obstet Gynecol 1938;35:1053–1055.

158. Ingram JM. The bicycle seat stool in the treatment of vaginal agenesis and stenosis: a preliminary report. Am J Obstet Gynecol 1981;140:867–873.

159. McIndoe AH, Banister JB. An operation for the cure of congenital absence of the vagina. J Obstet Gynaecol Br Commonw 1938;45:490.

160. McIndoe A. Treatment of congenital absence and obliterative conditions of the vagina. Br J Plast Surg 1950;2:254–267.

161. Williams EA. Congenital absence of the vagina—a simple operation for its relief. J Obstet Gynaecol Br Commonw 1964;71:511–512.

162. Wesley JR, Coran AG. Intestinal vaginoplasty for congenital absence of the vagina. J Pediatr Surg 1992;27:885–889.

163. Hensle T, Dean G. Vaginal replacement in children. J Urol 1992;148:677–679.

164. Hendren WH, Atala A. Use of bowel for vaginal reconstruction. J Urol 1994;152:752–755.

165. Toubia N. Female circumcision as a public health issue. N Engl J Med 1994;331:712–716.

166. Council on Scientific Affairs, American Medical Association. Female genital mutilation. JAMA 1995;274:1714–1716.

167. Hein K, Dell R, Cohen MI. Self–detection of a breast mass in adolescent females. J Adolesc Health Care 1982;3:15.

168. Kenney RD, Flippo JL, Black EB. Supernumerary nipples and renal anomalies in neonates. Am J Dis Child 1987;141:987.

169. Hersh JH, Bloom AS, Cromer AO, et al. Does a supernumerary nipple/renal field defect exist? Am J Dis Child 1987;141:989.

170. Goldstein DP, Emans SJ, Laufer MR. The Breast: examination and Lesions. In: Emans SJ, Goldstein DP, Laufer MR, eds. Pediatric and Adolescent Gynecology, 4th ed. Philadelphia: Lippincott-Raven, 1998.

171. Haycock CE. How I manage breast problems in athletes. Phys Sportsmed 1987;15:89.
172. Watkins F, Giacomantonio M, Salisbury S. Nipple discharge and breast lump related to Montgomery's tubercles in adolescent females. J Pediatr Surg 1988;23:718. Diehl T, Kaplan DW. Breast masses in adolescent females. J Adolesc Health Care 1985;6:353.
173. Neinstein LS. Review of breast masses in adolescents. Adolesc Pediatr Gynecol 1994;7:119–129.
174. Lubin F, Ron E, Wax Y, et al. A case-control study of caffeine and methylxanthines in benign breast disease. JAMA 1985;253:2388.
175. Shairer C, Brinton LA, Hoover RN. Methylxanthines and benign breast disease. Am J Epidemiol 1986;124:603.
176. Vorherr H. Fibrocystic breast disease: pathophysiology, patho-morphology, clinical picture, and management. Am J Obstet Gynecol 1986;154:161.
177. Dupont WD, Page DL. Risk factors for breast cancer in women with proliferative breast disease. N Engl J Med 1985;312:146–151.
178. Stone AM, Shanker IR, McCarthy K. Adolescent breast masses. Am J Surg 1977;134:275.
179. Goldstein DP, Miler V. Breast masses in adolescent females. Clin Pediatr 1982;21:17.
180. Simmons PS, Wold LE. Surgically treated breast disease in adolescent females: a retrospective review of 185 cases. Adolesc Pediatr Gynecol 1989;2:95–98.
181. Daniel W, Mathews M. Tumors of the breast in adolescent females. Pediatrics 1968;41:743.
182. Dupont WD, Page DL, Pari FF, et al. Long-term risk of breast cancer in women with fibroadenoma. N Engl J Med 1994;331:10–15.
183. Hart J, Layfield LJ, Trumbull WE, et al. Practical aspects in the diagnosis and management of cystosarcoma phylloides. Arch Surg 1988;123:1079.
184. Briggs RM, Walters M, Rosenthal D. Cystosarcoma phylloides in adolescent female patients. Am J Surg 1983;146:712–714.
185. Farrow J, Ashikari H. Breast lesions in young girls. Surg Clin North Am 1969;46:261.
186. Simpson L, Barson A. Breast tumors in infants and children: a 40-year review of cases at a children's hospital. Can Med Assoc J 1969;101:100.
187. Oberman H, Stephens P. Carcinoma of the breast in childhood. Cancer 1972;30:470.
188. Karl SR, Ballantine TV, Zaino R. Juvenile secretory carcinoma of the breast. Br J Surg 1987;74:214.
189. Bhatia S, Robinson LL, Oberlin O, et al. Breast cancer and other second neoplasms after childhood Hodgkin's disease. N Engl J Med 1996;334:745–751.
190. Tucker MA, Coleman CN, Cox RS, et al. Risk of second cancers after treatment for Hodgkin's disease. N Engl J Med 1988;318:76.
191. Squire R, Bianchi A, Jakate SM. Radiation-induced sarcoma of the breast in a female adolescent. Cancer 1988;61:2444.
192. Levine AJ. The p53 tumor-suppressor gene. N Engl J Med 1992;326:1350–1351.
193. Hall JM, Lee MK, Newman B, et al. Linkage of early-onset familial breast cancer to chromosome 17q21. Science 1990;250:1684–1689.
194. Narod SA, Feunteun J, Lynch HT, et al. Familial breast-ovarian cancer locus on chromosome 17q21-q23. Lancet 1991;338:82–83.
195. Ford D, Easton DF, Bishop DT, et al. Risks of cancer in BRCA1-mutation carriers. Lancet 1994;343:692–695.

CHAPTER 34

Urolithiasis in Children

Susan E. Thomas and F. Bruder Stapleton

Over the past 20 years, a better understanding of pediatric urolithiasis has evolved as a result of the evaluation and treatment of a growing number of pediatric patients. In 1975, Malek and Kelalis reported on their experience over a 20-year period (1950 to 1970) with 78 children with upper tract urinary calculi who were encountered among 145,000 new pediatric admissions.[1] More recently, Milliner and Murphy retrospectively analyzed 221 children with urolithiasis who were referred to the Mayo Clinic between 1965 and 1987 and were 16 years of age or younger at the time of diagnosis.[2] The prevalence of nephrolithiasis in American children varies from 1 in 1000 to 1 in 7600 hospital admissions depending on geographic region.[3] Children in the southeastern United States and in southern California appear to have the greatest risk for urinary calculi.[3] Although occasional studies report a slight male predominance, boys and girls appear to be affected equally. Urinary stones are found most often in Caucasian children and rarely affect African-American children. Urolithiasis is an important disease that has potentially lifelong implications in pediatric patients.

In this chapter, the metabolic causes of pediatric urolithiasis will be reviewed, as well as the current approach to the evaluation of urolithiasis in pediatric patients. When evaluating a pediatric patient, it is important to recognize that normal reference ranges vary depending on the stage of growth and development of the child. Also, therapeutic modalities effective in adults may not be suitable for a growing child. Current medical management and extracorporeal shock wave lithotripsy (ESWL) therapy will also be discussed.

CLINICAL MANIFESTATIONS

The diagnosis of urolithiasis in children may present a diagnostic challenge. The incapacitating flank, abdominal, or pelvic pain that typifies urinary stones in adults occurs in only 50% of children with urolithiasis.[3, 4, 5]

Symptoms of urolithiasis may vary with age.[2] Urinary tract infections are most commonly associated with stones in preschool children and are significant risk factors for stone formation in children with congenital urinary tract anomalies, with urinary diversion, or following urological surgery. Foreign material such as suture material or metallic clips may serve as a nidus for stone formation. For example, over 52% of children and young adults have been reported to develop urinary calculi following augmentation cystoplasty.[6] Hematuria, either microscopic or macroscopic, has been reported in 33% to 90% of children with stones[7] through all stages of childhood. Sterile pyuria is another common urinary abnormality in children with urolithiasis. Dysuria and urinary frequency should suggest bladder and/or urethral calculi.

In children, hematuria may be associated with hypercalciuria, hyperoxaluria or hyperuricosuria without overt urolithiasis.[7, 8] The hematuria may be microscopic or macroscopic and is seldom associated with abdominal or flank pain. Infants with hypercalciuria may exhibit irritability and have dysuria mimicking colic, in the absence of hematuria.[9] Some children complain of urinary frequency and/or dysuria with hypercalciuria. Often, children with hematuria associated with hypercalciuria have a strong family history of urolithiasis. Short-term follow-up studies indicate that 13 to 17% of children with this association develop urolithiasis within 5 years.

PATHOGENESIS OF STONE FORMATION

The formation of urinary calculi involves the disruption of a delicate balance of promoters and inhibitors of stone formation. Both physicochemical and anatomic factors are involved in this process (Table 34.1).[10]

Urine contains many solutes with differing concentrations and solubilities. The tendency for urine to form crystals is a function of the *free ion concentration* (per-

TABLE 34.1. *Factors affecting urinary stone formation*

Physicochemical factors
Degree of urinary supersaturation
    Solute excretion rate
    Urinary flow rate
    Urine pH
    Temperature
    Ionic strength of the urine
    Inhibitors of crystallization
        Ions: citrate, magnesium, pyrophosphate, sulfate,
            fluoride
        Trace elements: zinc, tin
        Glycosaminoglycans
        Glycoproteins: nephrocalcin, Tamm-Horsfall protein,
            B2-microglobulin, uropontin
Anatomic factors
Urinary stasis/recurrent infection
    Developmental anomalies
        Obstructive uropathy
        Vesicoureteral reflux
        Neurogenic bladder
    Foreign body

(Adapted from reference 10)

centage of the total ion concentration available to form a salt that can crystallize).[3] The product of the free ion concentrations is called the *activity product.* The *equilibrium solubility product* represents the activity product at equilibrium. The *activity product ratio* is the ratio of the activity to solubility products. When this value exceeds 1.0, there is a tendency for urinary crystals to form.[10] Urine normally exists in a supersaturated state called the *metastable zone.* This metastable zone exists because of the presence of inhibitors of crystal formation listed in Table 34.1. As the activity product rises, urinary crystals begin to form by a process called *nucleation.* The activity product at the point urinary crystals begin to form is called the *formation product.*[10] At this point the urine is considered oversaturated. When urinary crystals form in this manner, the process is called *homogenous nucleation.* Urinary crystals may precipitate at lower concentrations on foreign material, a process termed *heterogeneous nucleation.* This foreign material may also serve as a source of secondary infection. The formation of one crystal on a different crystal with a similar lattice structure is known as *epitaxy.*[3] Hyperuricosuria promotes the formation of calcium oxalate stones through this process.[11]

Urine pH influences crystal formation by affecting the solubility of stone-forming ions. Cystine and uric acid stones tend to form in acidic urine (pH <7.5, 6.0 respectively), while calcium phosphate stones tend to form in urine with a pH >6.5. Calcium oxalate solubility is not greatly affected by pH.[10] Citrate inhibits stone formation by forming complexes with calcium, thereby reducing the free ion available for crystal formation. Glycosaminoglycans inhibit the aggregation and growth of preformed crystals,[10] while glycoproteins inhibit all phases of crystallization.[11]

DISTRIBUTION OF CAUSATIVE FACTORS

Reports of causative factors for pediatric urolithiasis have varied widely in the literature. These differences largely depend on whether the authors were nephrologists or urologists, and on geographic location. As in adults, hypercalciuria represents the greatest factor in the development of urolithiasis (Table 34.2).

In our earlier review of pediatric patients in Memphis, Tennessee from 1979 to 1986,[12] we found that metabolic conditions accounted for 52% of the episodes of nephrolithiasis, while infection and idiopathic conditions represented 13.4% and 18.7%, respectively. These data are similar to the data for 221 children evaluated at the Mayo Clinic between 1965 and 1987.[2] In contrast, infec-

TABLE 34.2. *Causes of urolithiasis in children*

Underlying cause	USA[a] (%)	USA[b] (%)	USA[c] (%)	USA[d] (%)	Europe[e] (%)	Europe[f] (%)
Infection	13.4	18.6	2.0	4.3	43.5	30.1
Urinary tract anomalies			35.0	32.5	30.1	43.5
Hypercalciuria	42.0	22.6	27.4	7.9	7.4	8.9
Uric acid	3.6	3.6	1.6	4.5	0.4	0.5
Hyperoxaluria	2.7	11.3	0	2.4	1.0	1.0
Cystinuria	4.5	6.8	0	3.0	1.9	2.0
Idiopathic	18.7	24.9	26.0	28.3	14.1	14.0
Others	15.3	12.2	8.0	17.0	1.5	0

[a](Data taken from ref. 12.)
[b](Data taken from ref. 2.)
[c](Data taken from ref. 13.)
[d](Data taken from ref. 10.)
[e](Data taken from ref. 10.)
[f](Data taken from ref. 14.)

TABLE 34.3. *Metabolic disorders associated with nephrolithiasis*

CALCIUM LITHIASIS
Hypercalciuric states
Normocalcemic hypercalciuria
    Idiopathic hypercalciuria
        Absorptive (types I and II)
        Renal
    Distal renal tubular acidosis
    Generalized renal tubular dysfunction
    Hypertension
    Drug-induced (furosemide)
    Juvenile rheumatoid arthritis (15)
    Medullary sponge kidney
    Hyperprostaglandinuria
    Diabetes mellitus
    Hypothyroidism
    Hypophosphatemia
    Metabolic acidosis
    Expansion of extracellular fluid volume
Hypercalcemic hypercalciuria
    Associated with calcium resorption from bone
        Primary hyperparathyroidism
        Immobilization
        Hyperthyroidism
        Adrenocorticosteroid excess
            Endogenous (Cushing's syndrome)
            Exogenous corticosteroid therapy
        Adrenal insufficiency
        Osteolytic metastasis
    Associated with gastrointestinal hyperabsorption
        Hypervitaminosis D
        Idiopathic hypercalcemia of infancy
        Sarcoidosis
        Milk-alkali syndrome
    Malignancy
    Hyperalimentation
Hyperoxaluria
Hereditary hyperoxaluria types I and II
Enteric hyperoxaluria
Associated with pyridoxine deficiency
Hyperuricosuria
Hypocitraturia
Ketogenic diet
Associated with distal renal tubular acidosis
Due to gastrointestinal disease
Idiopathic

URIC ACID LITHIASIS
Familial/Idiopathic
Overproduction of Uric Acid
Inborn errors of metabolism
    HGPRT deficiency
        Partial
        Complete (Lesch-Nyhan syndrome)
    Glucose-6-phosphatase deficiency (type I
        glycogen storage disease)
    Increased phosphoribosyl pyrophosphate
        synthetase activity
Increased purine biosynthesis
    Lymphoproliferative/myeloproliferative disorders
    Polycythemia
Hyperuricosuria
High purine diet
    Excessive protein diet
    High dose pancreatic enzyme replacement
        therapy
Uricosuric drugs: sulfinpyrazone, high dose
    aspirin, ascorbic acid, phenylbutazone,
    probenecid
Defective tubular reabsorption
Chronic volume contraction
Gastrointestinal disease
Excessive cutaneous losses

STRUVITE LITHIASIS

CYSTINURIA

OTHER INBORN ERRORS OF METABOLISM
Hereditary Xanthinuria
Orotic Aciduria
Adenine Phosphoribosyltransferase deficiency

OTHER DRUG-ASSOCIATED LITHIASES
Allopurinol
Triamterene
Magnesium trisilicate containing antacids
Acetazolamide
Acyclovir
Theophylline
Vitamins C, D
Allopurinol (xanthine stones)

(Data taken from References 10, 15)

tion-related stones, often with genitourinary abnormalities, accounted for 37% of the episodes of urolithiasis at The Children's Hospital in Philadelphia.[13] Hypercalciuria is the most common metabolic abnormality in children with urolithiasis. Urinary tract infection remains a major cause of urolithiasis outside of North America. In Polinsky's review of the European literature, infection accounted for 43.5% of the episodes of nephrolithiasis.[10] According to Basaklar, nearly 75% of the pediatric stones in Europe were associated with infection or urinary anomalies.[14] (Table 34.3) shows the metabolic disorders associated with nephrolithiasis.

DIAGNOSTIC APPROACH TO PEDIATRIC UROLITHIASIS

At the initial evaluation of urolithiasis in a pediatric patient, a complete history and physical examination should be performed. The patient's age at presentation may provide clues to a particular metabolic cause for a urinary calculus. Particular attention to a family history of urolithiasis or hematuria is especially important. The physical examination should include an evaluation of growth and development, bone development, and blood pressure. A dietary history should be obtained with in-

TABLE 34.4. *Composition of urinary calculi in pediatric patients*

Component	%
Calcium oxalate	45–65
Calcium phosphate	14–29
Struvite	13
Cystine	5
Uric acid	4
Mixed/miscellaneous	4

quiries concerning any dietary excesses or deficiencies, vitamins, medications, and fluid intake. The urinary sediment should be examined for crystalluria. A step-by-step approach should include a thorough medical, metabolic, and radiographic evaluation for all children with a documented urinary calculus. If a stone is available, its analysis should be the first step in the evaluation (Table 34.4).

If stone analysis reveals a cystine, struvite, or uric acid calculus, the metabolic workup can be tailored to that cause. The finding of a calcium phosphate or calcium oxalate stone requires a broader metabolic evaluation, as outlined below. When a stone has not been recovered, or when the stone analysis reveals a calcium phosphate or calcium oxalate calculus, a 24-hour urine collection should be performed while the patient follows his or her customary diet. The urine should be analyzed for calcium, cystine, uric acid, oxalate, and citrate. It should be noted that citrate frequently is not included as part of the routine stone risk profile, and often must be ordered specifically. Normal values in school age children are listed in Table 34.5.[5] Normal values may differ significantly, depending on the age of the child.

Any abnormal values should be verified with a repeat collection. In children with repeated calculi and normal urinary values, a second urinary collection should be considered. Serum studies should also be performed, and should include calcium, magnesium, phosphorus, potassium, BUN, creatinine, bicarbonate, and uric acid. The possibility of a urinary tract infection should be ruled out in any child presenting with nephrolithiasis. Intact PTH levels should be determined in all children with hypercalciuria. A reduced urinary citrate level requires investigation of renal acidification ability, and may suggest distal renal tubular acidosis. Further

TABLE 34.5. *Normal urinary values for school age children*

Calcium	<4 mg/kg/day
Uric acid	<0.56 mg/dl GFR
Oxalate	<50 mg/1.73m2/day
Cystine	<60 mg/1.73m2/day
Citrate	>400 mg/g creatinine
Volume	>20 ml/kg/day

evaluation will be discussed in a problem oriented manner (as written).

CALCIUM LITHIASIS

Hypercalciuria

Increased urinary excretion of calcium is the most common metabolic cause for urolithiasis in children and in adults. Idiopathic hypercalciuria accounts for the largest percentage of children with this diagnosis. In a review of the cause of urolithiasis in 112 children, we reported that hypercalciuria was the most frequent cause of stone formation (42%).[12] No gender predilection was identified; however, a striking racial distribution was observed in this population in that few African-American children with idiopathic hypercalciuria and urolithiasis were identified. There are regional differences in the degree of hypercalciuria in children reported by various groups (Table 34.2).

Idiopathic hypercalciuria is defined as hypercalciuria that occurs in the absence of hypercalcemia, or when no other cause can be identified. Hypercalciuria may also occur secondary to a number of physiologic and hormonal influences associated with normal and elevated serum calcium levels (Table 34.3). Of the many conditions associated with hypercalciuria, furosemide therapy, prednisone or ACTH therapy, and distal renal tubular acidosis (RTA) are the most frequently associated with nephrolithiasis in children.[7, 16, 17]

Diagnosis of Hypercalciuria

Normal urinary excretion of calcium is less than 4 mg (0.1 mmol) per kg body weight per day.[7] In 24-hour and spot urine specimens, total calcium excretion is highly correlated with the ratio of urinary calcium to creatinine concentration (mg/mg). This ratio varies depending on the child's age, and normal values are listed in Table 34.6.

Urinary calcium excretion is significantly affected by the source of milk or type of formula: babies fed human milk have the highest urinary calcium excretion, whereas those fed soy-based formulas have the lowest

TABLE 34.6. *Normal urinary calcium/creatinine ratio values for fasting or 24 hour urinary calcium excretion**

Age	Calcium/creatinine ratio	
	mg/mg	mmol/mmol
0–6 mo	<0.8	<2.24
7–12 mo	<0.6	<1.68
>2 yr	<0.2	<0.56

*Measured by spot test in a fasting sample or in a 24 hour urine collection.
(Data taken from ref. 5)

calcium excretion.[18] Studies in preterm infants have confirmed the high neonatal calcium excretion, as well as the relationship between urinary calcium excretion and the type of milk source.[5, 18]

Idiopathic Hypercalciuria

Historically, idiopathic hypercalciuria has been divided into two distinct subtypes of hypercalciuria: renal and absorptive. Renal hypercalciuria was thought to result from a specific yet unidentified tubular defect leading to decreased reabsorption of calcium by the renal tubule. Absorptive hypercalciuria was defined by increased gastrointestinal absorption of calcium associated with a transient increase in serum calcium, following the ingestion of calcium-containing foods. When patients with absorptive hypercalciuria restricted their intake of dietary calcium, urinary calcium excretion returned to normal. Serum parathyroid hormone values were normal or low. The pathogenesis of absorptive hypercalciuria was incompletely understood. Some, patients with this disorder, but not the majority, had elevated serum 1,25 dihydroxyvitamin D_3 levels. Researchers believed that renal phosphate wasting may have been responsible for excessive serum $1,25(OH)_2D_3$ levels in some patients.[3]

Differentiating hypercalciuria into absorptive and renal categories was often difficult, and was further complicated by the finding that some children with renal (fasting) hypercalciuria demonstrated normal serum parathyroid concentrations. Further questions were raised with the finding that some patients with absorptive hypercalciuria continued to have hypercalciuria even during calcium restriction.[19] Coe et al. propose a "unifying hypothesis" that suggests that renal and absorptive hypercalciuria represent a continuum of the same disease process. Similar findings have recently been reported by Aladjem et al.[20] Presently, it appears that idiopathic hypercalciuria is the result of a uniform elevation of intestinal calcium absorption, and that a variable defect of renal calcium reabsorption exists.[19]

An interesting recent hypothesis proposes that idiopathic hypercalciuria is a disorder of monocytes, and that the proximal cause of hypercalciuria is bone resorption.[21] In this hypothesis, increased production of interleukin-1 (IL-1) from peripheral monocytes leads to increased prostaglandin-mediated bone resorption and increased $1,25(OH)_2D_3$-mediated gastrointestinal calcium absorption. While interesting, this hypothesis remains speculative. Langman,[22] however, has suggested in preliminary data that familial hypercalciuria is associated with bone demineralization.

Hypercalciuria may also result from an increased filtered calcium load as a result of increased bone resorption (hyperparathyroidism, hyperthyroidism, immobilization, acidosis, corticosteroid excess, or osteolytic metastasis), gastrointestinal hyperabsorption (hypervitaminosis D, sarcoid, or milk–alkali syndrome).

Diagnostic Evaluation

If at all possible, hypercalciuria should be diagnosed in a 24-hour urine collection. Urinary oxalate, citrate, and uric acid should also be examined. An abnormal result requires confirmation with a second sample in which urinary sodium is also measured. If spot urine specimens are used, a first morning fasting collection and a postprandial sample may be used. If only a single random sample is available, it is most helpful to obtain the sample 2 to 4 hours after a meal in which milk was given. In such a sample, if the ratio of urinary calcium to creatinine is <0.2 mg/mg, further evaluation for hypercalciuria is not necessary.[5] In the past, oral calcium loading tests were performed to differentiate between renal and absorptive hypercalciuria. This test is no longer routinely recommended in the evaluation of hypercalciuria in children.[23]

When hypercalciuria has been confirmed by two urine samples, the next step is to determine whether dietary manipulations can normalize urinary calcium excretion. If the second 24-hour urine collection reveals a high sodium intake, a third collection after 2 to 4 weeks of sodium restriction (2 to 3 gm of sodium per day) is indicated.[5] Important changes in urinary calcium have resulted from reduction in dietary sodium intake.[24] Serum should be obtained for electrolytes, BUN, creatinine, calcium, magnesium, phosphorus, and intact parathyroid hormone level.

Therapy

Therapy for hypercalciuria consists of promoting a high urinary flow rate, and restricting dietary sodium. Restriction of dietary calcium and the use of sodium cellulose phosphate can result in insufficient calcium for normal skeletal development, and should not be used. Recently, a reduced urinary potassium excretion has been noted in patients with urolithiasis.[25] In addition, increasing dietary potassium intake reduces urinary calcium excretion in adults.[26] Thus, children with hypercalciuria should be encouraged to eat a potassium-rich diet.

Hydrochlorothiazide (1 to 2 mg/kg/day) has been useful in children with hypercalciuria. The most common side effects include hypokalemia and hyperlipidemia. Plasma lipids should be monitored periodically in children receiving thiazide therapy. The long-term risks of thiazide therapy in children are not known. Citrate therapy is helpful if urinary citrate levels are low, or if hypercalciuria persists during thiazide therapy.

Distal Renal Tubular Acidosis

Nephrocalcinosis and nephrolithiasis are important complications of type I (distal) renal tubular acidosis. The pathogenesis is multifactorial and includes:

1. Constantly alkaline urinary pH, which promotes the precipitation of calcium phosphate salts,
2. Increased urinary calcium excretion from bone resorption,
3. Decreased urinary citrate.[7]

Interestingly, hypercalciuria has been implicated as a cause of urinary acidification defects.[27] Treatment with potassium citrate corrects the metabolic acidosis, hypokalemia, hypocitraturia, and hypercalciuria.[10]

OXALATE CALCULI

Oxalic acid is an end product of metabolism, and is excreted by the kidneys. Of the daily oxalate excretion, 10% to 15% derives from dietary sources and the remainder is the result of metabolism.[3] Dietary sources rich in oxalate are listed in Table 34.7.

Normal school children excrete <50mg/1.73m2/day of oxalate. Urinary oxalate excretion in infants may be fourfold or fivefold greater than in preschool children. Oxalate excretion is higher in formula-fed infants than in those fed human milk.[5] Increased oxalate excretion may result from increased dietary intake, an inborn error of metabolism, enteric hyperabsorption, or the excessive intake of oxalate precursors. As a result, calcium oxalate calculi may form in supersaturated urine. Calcium oxalate dihydrate crystals are pyramidal, while calcium oxalate monohydrate crystals are dumbbell-shaped (Figure 34.1).[11]

Primary Hyperoxaluria

Primary hyperoxaluria type I (PH-I) is inherited in an autosomal recessive fashion, and is a result of a deficiency of peroxisomal alanine:glyoxylate aminotransferase. Pyridoxine (B_6) is a cofactor for the AGT enzyme. The hyperoxaluria is associated with hyperglycollic aciduria. Primary hyperoxaluria type II is also inherited in an autosomal recessive manner, and is associated with a deficiency of cytosolic D-glycerate dehydrogenase (glyoxylate reductase). This disorder is associated with L-glyceric aciduria.[28] With a deficiency of the enzyme alanine: glyoxylate aminotransferase, there is increased synthesis and excretion of oxalate and glycolate. This is manifested clinically by the deposition of insoluble calcium oxalate, causing urolithiasis and nephrocalcinosis. If oxalate deposition in the kidneys is extensive, renal failure may ensue, with resultant oxalate deposition in tissues throughout the body causing systemic oxalosis. Both clinical and enzymic heterogeneity exist in PH I.[29] In most patients, the first symptoms of urolithiasis occur in childhood. However, initial presentation may be in the first few months of life or late in adulthood. Infantile oxalosis is the most severe form of primary hyperoxaluria type I.[30] Before the introduction of modern treatment modalities, an estimated 80% of PH I patients died from renal failure before they reached 20 years of age.[29] The normal AGT gene maps to chromosome 2q36-37 and consists of 11 exons spanning 10kb. The degree of enzyme activity does not seem to determine the onset or severity of PH I.[29]

Patients with primary hyperoxaluria most often present with symptoms referable to the genitourinary tract. Calcium oxalate calculi are radioopaque, and on renal biopsy birefringent crystals of calcium oxalate are seen throughout the parenchyma. Oxalate may be deposited in other tissues in the body as well. These tissues include bone marrow, retina, and cardiac tissue. Cardiac deposits may result in conduction defects, and cardiomyopathy and arterial lesions can result in limb gangrene. Crystalline retinopathy caused by deposition of calcium oxalate crystals has been noted in the fundi of patients with PH I.[30] If there is a clinical suspicion for hyperoxaluria, a urinary oxalate/creatinine ratio can be determined on a spot urine sample. Abnormal results should be qualified with a 24-hour urine collection for oxalate and creatinine. A low oxalate diet should be followed for 5 to 7 days prior to oxalate determinations. Normal urinary oxalate/creatinine ratios are listed in Table 34.8.

Definitive diagnosis requires a liver biopsy to assay the AGT activity. Prenatal diagnosis may be possible via chorionic villus sampling, and in the future may be possible with RFLP linkage analysis.[30]

Medical management includes measures to decrease urinary oxalate and calcium excretion.

Therapy includes promoting a high urinary flow 24 hours a day, and restricting dietary oxalate. In children with coexistent hypercalciuria, use of hydrochlorothiazide (1 to 2 mg/kg/day) may be beneficial. Restriction of dietary calcium could actually result in increased oxalate absorption via the gastrointestinal tract and should be avoided. Supplemental intake of vitamin C and D should also be avoided. Inhibitors of crystal growth including magnesium, citrate, and phosphate supplements

TABLE 34.7. *Selected dietary sources rich in oxalate*

Rhubarb	Beets
Nuts	Orange juice
Chocolate	Cranberry juice
Cocoa	Grape juice
Spinach	Gelatin
Tea	Black raspberries
Sweet potatoes	Okra
Pepper	Grits

(Data taken from ref. 3)

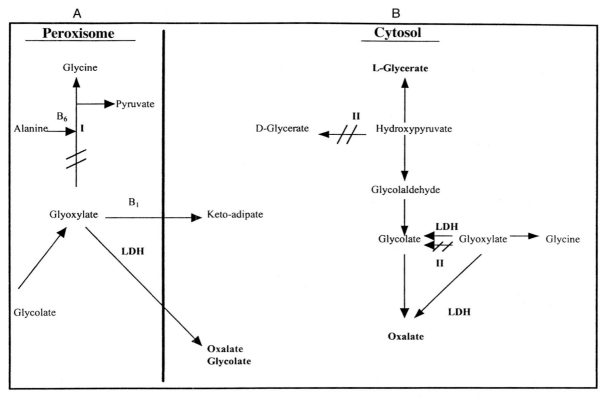

FIG. 34.1 Simplified pathway of oxalate metabolism.

A: Primary Hyperoxaluria Type I.
Defect of alanine: glyoxylate aminotransferase
Increased oxalate and glycolate
I = alanine:glyoxylate aminotransferase
B_1 = Thiamine pyrophosphate
B_6 = Pyridoxal phosphate

B: Primary Hyperoxaluria Type II.
Defect of D-Glycerate dehydrogenase
Increased Oxalate and L-Glycerate
II = D-Glycerate dehydrogenase
LDH = Lactate dehydrogenase

are routinely used. If renal insufficiency is present, the use of phosphate supplements is contraindicated. Some patients with PH I respond to pyridoxine. Occasionally there is complete restoration of the urinary oxalate level to the normal range, but more often the response is partial, with reduced, but still abnormal, oxalate excretion. Initial starting dose is 25 mg with a maximum of 250 mg/day. Urinary oxalate levels are followed as the dose is increased. Neurological toxicities have been attributed to high doses of pyridoxine (1000 mg).[30] The

ultimate therapy for primary hyperoxaluria is combined liver–kidney transplantation. The ultimate outcome depends on normalization of endogenous oxalate synthesis and maintenance of good renal function. Patients who are maintained on hemodialysis for long periods of time accumulate large oxalate loads that can destroy the transplanted kidney.

Enteric Hyperoxaluria

Increased urinary oxalate excretion may also accompany gastrointestinal disorders such as inflammatory bowel disease, pancreatitis, and small bowel resection. The increase appears to be caused by the both the increased bowel wall permeability to oxalate and by complexing of calcium by fatty acids that frees oxalate for absorption.[3]

Acquired Hyperoxaluria

Acquired hyperoxaluria has been recognized in association with several conditions: ethylene glycol poison-

TABLE 34.8. *Urine oxalate/urine creatinine in healthy children*

Age	UOX/UCr (mmol/mmol)* mean ± 2SD on logged data	
<1 year	0.061	*(0.015–0.26)*
1 to <5 years	0.036	*(0.011–0.12)*
5 to <12 years	0.030	*(0.0059–0.15)*
>12 years	0.013	*(0.0021–0.083)*

*UOX/UCr assumes normal renal function.
(Data taken from ref. 31)

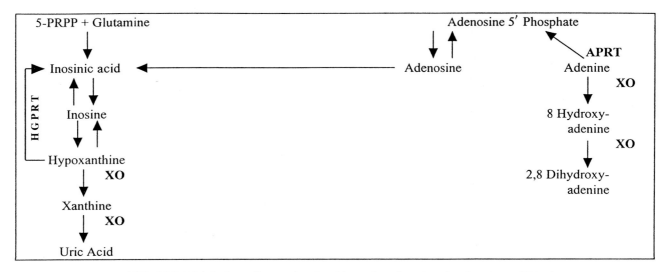

FIG. 34.2 Metabolic pathways involved in purine disorders leading to urolithiasis.
HGPRT = Hypoxanthine guanine phosphoribosyltransferase
APRT = Adenine phosphoribosyltransferase
XO = Xanthine oxidase

ing, hepatic cirrhosis, renal tubular acidosis, sarcoidosis, Shwachman's syndrome, cystic fibrosis, pyridoxine deficiency and following ingestion of large amounts of vitamin C.[3]

URIC ACID CALCULI

Uric acid calculi are responsible for 4% of urinary calculi in pediatric patients. Uric acid lithiasis can be associated with overproduction of uric acid, hyperuricosuria, or chronic volume contraction, or may be familial/idiopathic. Disorders associated with overproduction of uric acid include inborn errors of metabolism such as Lesch-Nyhan syndrome (Hypoxanthine-guanine phosphoribosyl transferase deficiency), and Type I glycogen storage disease (Glucose-6-phosphatase deficiency). Overproduction of uric acid is also associated with increased purine biosynthesis associated with lymphoproliferative and myeloproliferative disorders and polycythemia.[10] Hyperuricosuria may be the result of a high purine diet or uricosuric drugs, or from tubular defects such as an isolated defect in renal tubular urate reabsorption, or from generalized tubular dysfunction.[5] Patients with cystic fibrosis ingest a high purine load in the form of pancreatic enzyme supplementation, and may form uric acid stones.[32] Endemic uric acid stones are not uncommon in Southeast Asia and the Mediterranean. Such stones are not associated with hyperuricemia; however there is a familial tendency for urate stones in people from these regions.[7]

Uric acid, like oxalate, is an end product of metabolism. The kidney removes two thirds of the body's daily uric acid load, the remainder is removed by the gastrointestinal tract. Uric acid elimination by the kidney occurs through glomerular filtration, tubular reabsorption, tubular secretion, and postsecretory reabsorption. Children appear to have a greater capacity to increase uric acid excretion than do adults.[5] Therefore, increased production of uric acid cannot be excluded on the basis of a normal serum uric acid concentration. Uric acid excretion is increased in as many as 10% of patients with hypercalciuria and urolithiasis.[5] In adults, the fractional excretion of uric acid is 8% to 12%, with the total daily excretion being <700 mg (10 mg/kg) per day.[33] Uric acid excretion is extremely high in the neonatal period (fractional excretion $40 \pm 10\%$) and remains substantially higher than adult values throughout early childhood.[34] Uric acid crystals are a rhomboidal on microscopic analysis and radiolucent on radiographs.[11] In children, total urate excretion, excretion per unit of body weight, and fractional excretion of uric acid all vary with age. Therefore, age-related normal values must be used. In children older than 2 years of age, the amount of uric acid excreted per deciliter of glomerular filtrate does not vary with age. A normal value of less than 0.56 mg of uric acid/dl glomerular filtrate may be used in this population of children. The value may be calculated by the following formula:[5]

$$\frac{\text{Urine uric acid} \left(\frac{\text{mg}}{\text{dl}}\right) \times \text{Plasma creatinine} \left(\frac{\text{mg}}{\text{dl}}\right)}{\text{Urine creatinine (mg/dl)}}$$
$$= \text{mg/dl GFR}$$

Normal values for urinary uric acid excretion in children are listed in Table 34.9.[5]

TABLE 34.9. *Normal values for urinary uric acid excretion in children*

	Uric acid excretion*	
Age	mg/dl GRF	mmol/dl GFR
Preterm infant		
29–33 wk gestation	<8.8	<0.55
34–37 wk gestation	<4.6	<0.27
Term infant	<3.3	<0.20
>2 years	<0.56	<0.03

*Measured by spot test or 24-hour urine collection.
(Data taken from ref. 5)

Medical therapy for uric acid calculi includes efforts to maintain an alkaline urinary pH (>6.0), and a high urinary flow rate. Attempts should be made to identify a reversible cause of uric acid overproduction or excessive excretion. Urinary alkalinization may be achieved with sodium bicarbonate, sodium citrate, or potassium citrate. Therapy with allopurinol (5 to 10 mg/kg/day) should be considered prior to initiation of chemotherapy in children with myelo/lymphoproliferative disorders, or if the above measures fail to prevent further stone formation. Alkaline solutions have been effective in the chemolysis of uric acid stones. These stones can be dissolved with alkaline solutions, such as 0.1M sodium bicarbonate or tromethamine (THAM) via a nephrostomy tube.[35]

ADENINE PHOSPHORIBOSYL TRANSFERASE (APRT) DEFICIENCY

This is a rare disorder of purine metabolism, inherited in an autosomal recessive fashion and associated with a deficiency of the enzyme adenine phosphoribosyl transferase. This enzyme is active in the purine "salvage" pathway that reconverts adenosine to adenosine 5'-phosphate.[10] The APRT gene has been mapped to chromosome 16q24.[36] When this enzyme is absent, adenine accumulates and is metabolized by xanthine oxidase to 2,8-dihydroxyadenine. This compound is poorly soluble in urine, and may result in urinary calculi. These stones are radiolucent on plain radiographs. Special techniques, such as isotachophoresis or high-performance liquid chromatography, are required to distinguish these stones from uric acid.[3] Unlike uric acid calculi, alkalinization decreases the solubility of 2,8-dihydroxyadenine, but the condition responds to allopurinol therapy. A low purine diet is also recommended.

HEREDITARY XANTHINURIA

This is an inborn error of purine metabolism that is inherited in an autosomal recessive fashion. This disorder of purine metabolism is characterized by a complete deficiency of xanthine oxidase activity, which is responsible for the conversion of hypoxanthine and xanthine to uric acid.[10] Children with this disorder have low serum and urinary uric acid levels, while excretion of xanthine and hypoxanthine is elevated. Xanthine calculi are radiolucent. Xanthine urolithiasis has been seen in one third of affected patients; the majority remain completely asymptomatic, although myopathy and polyarteritis have also been described.[10] Xanthine calculi may also be a complication of allopurinol therapy.

OROTIC ACIDURIA

Orotic aciduria is a rare inborn error of pyrimidine metabolism that is recessively inherited and associated with urolithiasis. This disorder is characterized by onset during early infancy, growth failure, developmental delay, hypochromic anemia, and excessive urinary excretion of orotic acid (an intermediary in uridine synthesis.[10] Orotic acid calculi are radioopaque, and diagnosis is made by demonstrating increased urinary orotic acid levels. Beneficial results have followed treatment with uridine and glucocorticoids.[10]

CYSTINURIA

Cystine stones account for 5% of pediatric urinary calculi. Cystinuria is an inherited transport disorder characterized by excessive urinary excretion of cystine and the dibasic amino acids arginine, lysine, and ornithine. It results from the malfunction of a specific membrane transport system located in the brush-border membrane of the renal proximal straight tubule and the small intestine.[37] Children with this disorder present with urinary calculi as their sole manifestation owing to the limited solubility of cystine. Because of the nature of the metabolic defect, children with this disorder may suffer from recurrent urinary calculi in childhood and into adulthood. Cystinuria has been associated with hyperuricemia, uric acid urolithiasis, hemophilia, retinitis pigmentosa, muscular dystrophy, muscular hypotonia, trisomy 21, and hereditary pancreatitis.[5] Cystinuria has also been reported in patients with mental retardation or mental illness.[5] On a whole patients with cystinuria appear to have normal intelligence.

Children with this disorder often have renal colic in the second or third decade of life.[5] Cystine crystals are characteristically flat, hexagonal and colorless. Cystine crystals are diagnostic, but show up in only 19% to 26% of homozygous cystinuric patients.[37] Cystine stones are radioopaque on plain film. A sodium cyanide nitroprusside test may be used as a screening tool for cystinuria. A positive result should be followed by a 24-hour urine collection. Normal individuals excrete <60 mg of cystine/1.73m2/day, while patients who are homozygous for cystinuria may excrete >400 mg/1.73m2/day.[5]

Medical therapy consists of promoting a large fluid intake and achieves urinary alkalinization. When patients suffer from recurrent nephrolithiasis despite these measures, d-Penicillamine or Tiopronin may be used. Both compounds interact with cystine to form a thiol-disulfide exchange with cystine, which is more soluble in urine. Adverse effects associated with d-Penicillamine include gastrointestinal discomfort, loss of taste perception, bone marrow depression, proteinuria, membranous glomerulopathy, optic neuritis, myasthenia gravis, and trace metal deficiencies.[3] Similar side effects have been seen with Tiopronin. Captopril has been shown to form a thiol-cysteine mixed disulfide that is more soluble in urine than cystine. However, the hypocystinuric effect may be unrelated to and formation of the cysteine-captopril-disulfide compound. Little is known about side effects, owing to its limited use in cystinuric patients.[38] Rimatil is a newer chelating agent and is now in phase II clinical trials. Rimatil is a dithiol compound as opposed to a monothiol compound (d-Penicillamine, Tiopronin). Therefore, Rimatil is potentially more effective in forming a mixed disulfide complex with cysteine, thereby lowering cystine excretion in patients with cystinuria.[38]

Surgical intervention in patients with cystinuria is required when urinary calculi become infected or result in obstruction. Extracorporeal shock wave lithotripsy (ESWL) has been minimally successful. Percutaneous ultrasonic lithotripsy, which allows removal of large fragments, has been somewhat more successful.[37] Chemolysis is the process of kidney stone dissolution by chemical irrigation through nephrostomy tube systems.[35] Because of the pure content of cystine and uric acid calculi, these stones are more amenable to chemical dissolution. Cystine stones may be dissolved with sodium bicarbonate, but chemolysis of these stones usually requires stronger alkaline solutions, such as THAM-E (TRIS-hydroxymethyl aminomethane).[35] More commonly, cystine stones have been dissolved by using alkaline solutions in combination with thiol solutions.[35]

With aggressive medical and surgical management, the long-term outlook for patients with cystinuria is good. Renal function may eventually be compromised in up to a third of the patients; however, fewer than 5% progress to end-stage renal disease.[37]

STRUVITE CALCULI

The association between urolithiasis and urinary tract infection has long been recognized. Infections have been found to account for 13% to 40% of pediatric cases of urolithiasis.[5] Urinary infections produce calculi composed of struvite (magnesium-ammonium-phosphate) and carbonate apatite. On microscopic analysis, struvite crystals have a coffin-lid shape.[11] These stones form as a result of the bacterial enzyme urease, which hydrolyzes urinary urea to ammonia and carbon dioxide. This produces an alkaline urinary environment favors the formation of struvite calculi. Organisms known to produce ureas include Proteus, Klebsiella, Psuedomonas, Staphylococcus, Serratia, Candida, and Mycoplasma. Escherichia coli does not produce urease.[3] Struvite calculi may also be associated with congenital anomalies that cause stasis of urine. Urinary tract infections may be the primary cause of calculus formation, or may occur because of stones from other metabolic causes. In most children, stones related to infections are first discovered before the child is 5 years old. All races are affected, and boys account for 80% of the population.[3] These infection-related stones often form large radioopaque upper-tract stones called staghorn calculi. Infections may also produce a soft radiolucent mucoid substance called, "matrix concretion" that may calcify rapidly and account for the rapid formation of some infection-related calculi.[3] Because of their size, struvite calculi may be associated with obstruction, pyelonephritis, and urosepsis.

Despite recent advances in non-invasive technology, most struvite calculi in children are still removed surgically. Urease inhibitors have had limited use because of side effects, and are not yet approved for use in children.

It is advisable to delay detailed metabolic evaluation of children with infection-related calculi because urinary calcium excretion is markedly increased during acute pyelonephritis. Calcium excretion returns to normal after the stone is removed and the infection is cleared.[3]

X-LINKED RECESSIVE NEPHROLITHIASIS

X-linked recessive nephrolithiasis has been described in a large kindred from northern New York, with hereditary nephrolithiasis accompanied by urinary concentrating defects, nephrocalcinosis, renal insufficiency, and renal wasting of potassium, phosphate, calcium, and uric acid.[39] Within this family there were nine affected men belonging to a kindred consisting of 162 family members. The patients presented in childhood with calcium nephrolithiasis and proteinuria, with progression to nephrocalcinosis, urinary concentrating defects, and renal insufficiency.[39] Interpretation of renal biopsies revealed glomerulosclerosis, tubular atrophy, and interstitial fibrosis, and lacked evidence of other forms of hereditary nephritis. As the affected men reached adulthood, they developed abnormalities in the renal excretion of calcium, phosphate, potassium, and uric acid. One of the patients with X-linked nephrolithiasis underwent renal transplantation, and as of 1991 had retained his graft for 7 years without evidence of recurrence.[39] The primary defect causing the renal tubular disorder is unknown, however, the gene causing X-linked nephrolithiasis has been mapped to the pericentromeric region of the short arm of the X chromosome (Xp11.22).[40] Further investigation into the factors involved in the tubular dysfunction may provide information regarding treatment and prevention of renal insufficiency.

FACTITIOUS CALCULI

Urinary calculi have been reported as a manifestation of Munchausen's syndrome.[3] One example is a child whose mother claimed to have pass from the penile urethra. No metabolic or infectious cause for the stone was observed, and analysis of the stone determined it to be quartz.[3] When no metabolic or infectious cause can be found, and when there is a concern regarding the family dynamics, a factitious disorder should be considered.

ESWL THERAPY

A detailed review of the surgical management of childhood urolithiasis is beyond the scope of this chapter. The reader is referred to the following references: Cohen, et al.,[41] El-Damanhoury, et al.,[35] and Stapleton and Kroovand.[7] Extracorporeal shock wave lithotripsy was introduced for the treatment of urolithiasis by Chaussy et al. in 1980.[42, 43] Prior to this, urolithiasis was managed with medical therapy and open surgical techniques. Today, open surgical procedures are being replaced by less invasive techniques. Open surgery is still necessary, especially in children with malformations of the urinary tract, and those with cystine or staghorn calculi.

There has been an initial reluctance to use ESWL in children because the long-term consequences of shock wave therapy on renal and bone growth are unknown. Several animal studies have demonstrated the appearance of histologic changes when immature kidneys are subjected to shock waves. Parenchymal damage is thought to be proportional to the number of shocks received.[41] Thomas et al. found no evidence of retardation of linear growth (body height) in 12 children 2.2 to 15.3 years old (mean age 9.4) during follow-up periods ranging from 74 to 238 weeks. They evaluated renal function as measured by effective renal plasma flow via iodine hippurate I 131 scanning before and after ESWL and found no statistically significant difference between the treated and untreated kidneys.[42] Adams et al. reported no impairment of renal growth or permanent decline in renal function during a 3 year post-ESWL follow-up in children.[7] Corbally et al. reviewed the effects of ESWL on renal function in children aged 14 years or less who had undergone ESWL for renal tract calculi. They noted a 15% overall decrease in GFR after ESWL, a finding that was not statistically significant but nevertheless worrisome.[43] Concerns persist about potential renal damage and hypertension following

ESWL in the pediatric population. Its use in children should be carefully considered, and these children deserve long-term follow-up for potential complications.

The principles of this technique involve a shock wave generated within a water bath by an electrical discharge at the focus of a hemielliptical reflector. The shock wave is reflected to the kidney stone by biplanar fluoroscopy and is synchronized with the heart rate to avoid disturbing the cardiac induction system. The shock wave will deliver a pressure of 1 kilobar at the focal point (the stone). Because water has the same acoustic impedance as living tissue, the shock wave is able to traverse the soft tissues with minimal reflection. The wave impact against the stone results in dissolution of the stone. A typical treatment requires 1000 to 1500 shocks, after which the stone is pulverized to the consistency of sand.[3] First generation lithotripters provide shock wave energy over a small surface area, resulting in excellent stone fragmentation and a low retreatment rate. Because of pain and anxiety during treatment, general anesthesia is required for treatment of most pediatric patients. Second generation lithotripters deliver shock wave energy over a larger surface area for shock wave entry, cause less discomfort during treatment, and reduce requirements for anesthesia or analgesia.[7]

Contraindications for ESWL therapy include: lower ureteral calculi, bladder stones, distal ureteral obstruction, severe anatomical or functional abnormalities of the urinary tract, bleeding disorders, and uncontrolled hypertension. Patients unfit for anesthesia, and infants are poor candidates also. Staghorn calculi are a relative contraindication to ESWL. ESWL requires technical adaptation for use in children, including:

1. modification of the gantry,
2. careful shielding of the lung,
3. lowering of the water level to maintain the head in a position above the water level, and
4. protection of the exit sites of the shock wave with fluid bags.[4]

The surgical options for the treatment of pediatric stones are listed in Table 34.10.[44]

The overall results for treating children with renal calculi are similar to those for treating adults. Stone-free rates vary from 50% to 100% and depend primarily on the stone size, location, composition, and type of machine used.[41] Complications of ESWL therapy include entry site ecchymosis (common), pain, ureteral obstruction, subcapsular hematoma, branchial nerve palsy, cardiac arrhythmia, pancreatitis, and pulmonary contusion. The incidence of pulmonary contusion is reduced with appropriate shielding of the lung fields.

Long-term follow-up of children with urolithiasis is mandatory in order to preserve renal function, optimize growth, monitor for potentially deleterious side effects of medical and surgical therapies, apply new information

TABLE 34.10. *Surgical options for the treatment of pediatric stones*[44]

Location		Surgical options		
		First	Second	Third
Renal		ESWL	Percutaneous	Open surgery
Upper ureter		ESWL	Ureteroscopy	Open surgery
Lower ureter	Female	Ureteroscopy	Open surgery	
	Male	ESWL	Ureteroscopy	Open surgery

and technology as they become available, and prevent morbidity as the child enters into adulthood.

REFERENCES

1. Malek RS, Kelalis PP. Pediatric Nephrolithiasis. The Journal of Urology 1975;113:545–551.
2. Milliner DS, Murphy ME. Urolithiasis in Pediatric Patients. Mayo Clin Proc 1993;68:241–248.
3. Stapleton FB. Nephrolithiasis in Children. Pediatrics in Review 1989;11:21-21-30.
4. Gearhart JP, Herzberg GZ, Jeffs RD. Childhood Urolithiasis: Experiences and Advances. Pediatrics 1991;87:445–449.
5. Stapleton FB. Metabolic Stone Evaluation. In: Smith AD, Badlani GH, Bagley DH, Clayman RV, Jordan GH, Kavoussi LR, Lingeman JE, Preminger GM, Segura JW, eds. Smith's Textbook of Endourology, Quality Medical Publishing Inc., St. Louis, 1996; 1441–1452.
6. Palmer LS, Franco I, Kogan SJ, Reda E, Gill B, Levitt SB. Urolithiasis in Children Following Augmentation Cystoplasty. The Journal of Urology 1993;150:726–729.
7. Stapleton FB, Kroovand RL. Stones in Childhood. In: Coe FL, Favus MJ, Pak CYC, Parks JH, Preminger GM, eds. Kidney Stones: Medical and Surgical Management, Lippincott-Raven Publishers, Philadelphia, 1996;1065–1080.
8. Stapleton FB, Roy S, Noe HN, Jerkins G. Hypercalciuria in children with hematuria. N Engl J Med 1984;310:1345–1348.
9. Fivush B. Irrability and dysuria in infants with idiopathic hypercalciuria. Pediatr Nephrology 1990;4:262–263.
10. Polinsky MS, Kaiser BA, Baluarte HJ. Urolithiasis in Childhood. Pediatric Clinics of North America, 1987;34:683–710.
11. Coe FL, Parks, JH, Asplin JR. The Pathogenesis and Treatment of Kidney Stones. N Engl J Med 1992;327:1141–1151.
12. Stapleton FB, McKay CP, Noe HN. Urolithiasis in Children: The Role of Hypercalciuria. Pediatric Annals 1987;16:980–992.
13. Choi H, Snyder HM, Duckett JW. Urolithiasis in Childhood: Current Management. Journal of Pediatric Surgery 1987;22: 158–164.
14. Basaklar AC, Kale N. Experience with Childhood Urolithiasis—Report of 196 Cases. British Journal of Urology 1991;67:203–205.
15. Stapleton FB, Hanissian AS, Miller LA. Hypercalciuria in children with juvenile rheumatoid arthritis: Association with hematuria. Journal of Pediatrics 1985;107:235–239.
16. Brenner RJ, Spring DB, Sebastian A, McSherry EM, Genant HK, Palubinskas AJ, Morris RC. Incidence of radiographically evident bone disease, nephrocalcinosis, and nephrolithiasis in various types of renal tubular acidosis. N Engl J Med 1982;307:217–221.
17. Noe HN, Bryant JF, Roy S, Stapleton FB. Urolithiasis in Pre-Term Neonates Associated With Furosemide Therapy. The Journal of Urology 1984;132:93–94.
18. Hillman LS, Chow W, Salmons SS, Weaver E, Erickson M, Hansen J. Vitamin D metabolism, mineral homeostasis, and bone mineralization in term infants fed human milk, cow milk-based formula, or soy-based formula. Journal of Pediatrics 1988;112: 864–874.
19. Coe FL, Favus MJ, Crockett T, Strauss AL, Parks JH, Porat A, Gantt CL, Sherwood LM. Effects of Low-Calcium Diet on Urine Calcium Excretion, Parathyroid Function and Serum 1,25(OH)$_2$D$_3$ Levels in Patients with Idiopathic Hypercalciuria and in Normal Subjects. The American Journal of Medicine 1982;72:25–32.
20. Aladjem M, Barr J, Lahat E, Bistritzer T. Renal and Absorptive Hypercalciuria: A Metabolic Disturbance With Varying and Interchanging Modes of Expression. Pediatrics 1996;97:216–219.
21. Weisinger JR. New insights into the pathogenesis of idiopathic hypercalciuria: The role of bone. Kidney International 1996; 49:1507–1518.
22. Langman CB, Schmeissing KJ, Sailer DM. Children with genetic hypercalciuria exhibit thiazide response osteopenia (abst). Pediatr Res 1994;35:368A.
23. Stapleton FB. Idiopathic hypercalciuria: Association with isolated hematuria and risk for urolithiasis in children. The Southwest Pediatric Nephrology Study Group. Kidney International 1990; 37:807–811.
24. Muldowney FP, Freaney R, Moloney MF. Importance of dietary sodium in the hypercalciuria syndrome. Kidney International 1982;22:292–296.
25. Lawoyin S, Sismilich S, Browne R, Pak CYC. Bone Mineral Content in Patients With Calcium Urolithiasis. Metabolism 1979;28: 1250–1254.
26. Lemann H, Pleuss JA, Gray RW, Hoffman RC. Potassium administration increases and potassium deprivation reduces urinary calcium excretion in healthy adults. Kidney International 1991; 39:973–983.
27. Bonilia-Felix M, Villegas MO, Vehaskari VM. Renal Acidification in Children With Idiopathic Hypercalciuria. Journal of Pediatrics 1994;124:529–534.
28. Scheinman JI. Primary hyperoxaluria: Therapeutic strategies for the 90's. Kidney International 1991;40:389–399.
29. Danpure CJ, Jennings PR, Fryer P, Purdue PE, Allsop J. Primary Hyperoxaluria Type 1: Genotypic and Phenotypic Heterogeneity. J Inher Metab Dis 1994;17:487–499.
30. Leumann EP, Niederwieser A, Fanconi A. New aspects of infantile oxalosis. Pediatric Nephrology 1987;1:531–535.
31. Barratt TM, Danpure CJ. Hyperoxaluria. In: Holliday MA, Barratt TM, Avner ED, eds. Pediatric Nephrology 3rd ed. Williams & Wilkins Baltimore, 1994;557–571.
32. Langman CB, Moore ES. Pediatric Urolithiasis. In: Edelman CM, ed. Pediatric Kidney Disease 2nd ed. Little Brown & Co., Boston, 1992;2005–2012.
33. Baldree LA, Stapleton FB. Uric Acid Metabolism in Children. Pediatric Clinics of North America 1990;37:391–411.
34. Stapleton FB. Renal uric acid clearance in human neonates. Journal of Pediatrics 1983;103:290–294.
35. El-Damanhoury H, Burger R, Hohenfellner R. Surgical aspects of urolithiasis in children. Pediatric Nephrology 1991;5:339–347.
36. Fratini A, Simmers RN, Calleri DF, Hyland VJ, Tischfield JA, Stambrook PH, Sutherland GR. A new location for the human adenine phosphoribosyltransferase gene (APRT) distal the haptoglobin (HP) and fra (16) (q23) (FRA16D) loci. Cytogenet Cell Genet 1986;43:10–13.
37. Milliner DS. Cystinuria. Endocrinology and Metabolism Clinics of North America 1990;19:889–907.
38. Sakhaee K. Pathogenesis and Medical Management of Cystinuria. Seminars in Nephrology 1996;16:435–447.
39. Frymoyer PA, Scheinman SJ, Dunham PB, Jones DB, Hueber P, Schroeder ET. X-linked Recessive Nephrolithiasis With Renal Failure. N Engl J Med 1991;325:681–686.

40. Scheinman SJ, Pook MA, Wooding C, Pang JT, Frymoyer PA, Thakker RV. Mapping the Gene Causing X-Linked Recessive Nephrolithiasis to Xp11.22 by Linkage Studies. J Clin Invest 1993;91:2351–2357.

41. Cohen TD, Ehreth J, King LR, Preminger GM. Pediatric Urolithiasis: Medical and Surgical Management. Urology 1996; 47:292–303.

42. Chaussy CH, Brendel W, Schmiedt E. Extracorporeally Induced Destruction of Kidney Stones By Shock Waves. Lancet 1980; 2:1265–1268.

43. Schmiedt E, Chaussy CH. Extracorporeal Shock-Wave Lithotripsy (ESWL) of Kidney and Ureteric Stones. International Urology and Nephrology 1984;16:273–283.

44. Harmon EP, Neal DE, Thomas R. Pediatric urolithiasis: review of research and current management. Pediatric Nephrology 1994;8:508–512.

CHAPTER 35

Pediatric Oncology

Michael L. Ritchey

Treatment of solid tumors in children has evolved over the years. Before the availability of effective adjuvant treatment, surgery played the major role in treatment. When it was discovered that some solid tumors were responsive to radiation and chemotherapy, a multidisciplinary approach to treatment became important. These collaborative efforts have achieved significant improvements in the overall survival of children with cancer. However, we may have reached the limits in terms of survival that can be achieved with conventional therapy. Attention is now focused on the biologic features of solid tumors. This information can be used in several ways. Further stratification of children for treatment with conventional therapy may be possible if the biologic features are more predictive of risk for relapse than current surgical and pathologic staging. Novel treatment approaches based on our new understanding of tumor biology are also being tested and may provide answers for management of high-risk patients refractory to conventional treatment. Another goal of these therapies is to reduce therapy for children at low risk for relapse and thus minimize the morbidity secondary to late effects of treatment. This chapter reviews the progress in the treatment of urologic malignancies in children.

RENAL TUMORS

Wilms tumor is the most common primary malignant renal tumor of childhood. The most common benign solid tumor is congenital mesoblastic nephroma. There are many other less common malignancies; rhabdoid tumor of the kidney (RTK), clear cell sarcoma of the kidney (CCSK), and renal cell carcinoma (RCC). These latter tumors tend to be aggressive and less responsive to treatment. While survival for nephroblastoma has improved dramatically, the outcome for other renal malignancies encountered in children has remained relatively unchanged. New treatment modalities are being investigated to improve the survival of these high risk patients.

Wilms Tumor

Genetics and Epidemiology

The incidence rate of Wilms tumor is 8.1 cases per one million children or approximately 450 to 500 new cases annually in the United States.[1] Nephroblastoma is a disease of young children with a peak incidence in the fourth year of life for unilateral tumors. Bilateral tumors present earlier with a mean age at diagnosis of 29.5 months for boys and 32.6 months for girls.

Wilms tumors normally develop in otherwise healthy children, but 8% of cases occur in individuals with other recognized malformations.[2,3] The phenotypes associated with Wilms tumor can be classified as "overgrowth" or "nonovergrowth" syndromes. Overgrowth syndromes are the result of excessive prenatal and postnatal somatic growth such as macroglossia, nephromegaly, and hemihypertrophy.[3] The two most common overgrowth disorders associated with Wilms tumor are Beckwith-Wiedemann syndrome (BWS) and isolated hemihypertrophy, but others include Perlman, Sotos, and Simpson-Golabi-Behemel syndromes.[3-6] BWS is a familial disorder that is characterized by hemihypertrophy and excessive growth at the cellular and organ levels; there is also a 7.5% incidence of neoplasia including Wilms tumor, hepatoblastoma, and adrenocortical neoplasms.[3-5] Perlman syndrome shares some features with BWS but is associated with a distinctive facial appearance, an autosomal recessive pattern of inheritance, and a high risk for Wilms tumor.[6] Overall, children with these hemihypertrophy syndromes have a 3 to 5% risk of developing Wilms tumor.[3]

The list of nonovergrowth syndromes linked with Wilms tumor contains isolated (Congenital Nonsporatic) aniridia; genital malformations; trisomy 18; and the WAGR, Denys-Drash, and Bloom syndromes.[3,7] Genitourinary anomalies, such as hypospadias, cryptorchidism, and renal fusion anomalies, are found in 4.5% of patients with Wilms tumor. This represents more than a twofold increase over their occurrence in the general population but does not warrant screening for Wilms tumor in children with isolated genitourinary defects.[8–10] Denys and Drash independently described the syndrome that bears both of their names and includes male pseudohermaphroditism, nephropathy, and Wilms tumor. Since then more than 60 cases have been reported in the literature.[11] One should have a high index of suspicion for the development of these conditions in patients with male pseudohermaphroditism.[12] Aniridia is seen in 1.1% of patients with Wilms tumor. Aniridia and Wilms tumor occur in the WAGR syndrome characterized by the findings of Wilms tumor, aniridia, genitourinary malformations, and mental retardation.

The association of these syndromes and frequency of bilaterality has resulted in considerable interest in the pathogenesis of this embryonal neoplasm. Knudson and Strong proposed the two hit mutation theory for Wilms tumor formation similar to that proposed for retinoblastoma.[13] According to this hypothesis, both alleles of a tumor suppressor gene must be altered to permit neoplastic transformation. The first mutation is a constitutional lesion that is inherited from one parent or occurs as a denovo mutation. Because only one new event or second genetic hit is required, the likelihood of tumor formation is greater. The second event could be a gene mutation or gross loss of chromosomal material. With an initial germline mutation, the tumor would be heritable. Because only one additional mutation is required in familial cases, these patients would be expected to have an earlier age of onset and to have a greater incidence of multiple tumors. Familial Wilms tumors have been found to occur at an earlier age, but only 16% of familial cases are bilateral.[14] These tumors represent only 1 to 2% of all Wilms tumors, and their presence does not indicate as increased risk of tumors in the offspring of survivors of the disease.[15, 16] These observations suggest that Wilms tumor formation is more complex than initially thought and mechanisms other than inherited mutations may account for some of the bilateral and multicentric cases.[17]

The first recognized cytogenetically visible chromosomal abnormality in Wilms tumor was a constitutional deletion at the short arm of chromosome 11, 11p13, in patients with WAGR syndrome.[18] This provided the first clue to the location of the gene involved in Wilms tumor development. When sporadic Wilms tumors were analyzed, a third to a half of tumors were found to contain loss of heterozygosity (LOH) for DNA markers at 11p13.[19, 20] A gene named for Wilms tumor, *WT1*, was mapped to this locus, and alterations of this gene have been associated with Wilms tumor and genitourinary abnormalities.[9] An adjacent gene, *PAX6*, has been identified and linked with aniridia.[22]

WT1 appears to be a transcription factor that suppresses the expression of other genes. The genetic consequences of *WT1* inactivation appear to be restricted to organs that normally express this gene. *WT1* is expressed transiently in the developing kidney, and also in specific cells of the gonads. Mutations at the *WT1* locus, particularly males, may confer extensive genitourinary defects, most notably male pseudohermaphroditism.[11, 12] Mutations of the *WT1* gene were also detected in Wilms tumors associated with Denys-Drash syndrome, suggesting that *WT1* may be a tumor suppressor gene. The affected gonads and kidneys in patients with the Denys-Drash syndrome are heterozygous for germline mutations, implying that the *WT1* mutation acts dominantly with respect to genitourinary abnormalities.[23] However, only a few sporadic Wilms tumor cases have been shown to harbor *WT1* mutations.[23–25] There is variability in the penetrance of *WT1* mutations in terms of Wilms tumor development because tumors are found more frequently in *WT1* mutant individuals with Denys-Drash syndrome than in those with WAGR syndrome.[26]

A second Wilms tumor locus, 11p15.5 or WT2, on the short arm of chromosome 11 has been identified; it is distinct from *WT1*.[27] The BWS also maps to this location, but it is unknown if a single gene or adjacent genes are responsible for the syndrome and the tumor.[28] There is a fascinating dichotomy of parental alleles at *WT2*; the maternal allele is lost in cases of Wilms tumor, and the paternal allele seems to be duplicated in Beckwith-Wiedemann syndrome.[29] There are two candidates for WT2 located at 11p15, the insulin-like growth factor II gene (IGF II), and the H19 gene. The role of IGFII or H19 in Wilms tumorigenesis is still unknown.

Genetic linkage studies of families with an inherited susceptibility to development of Wilms tumor have suggested that other *WT* genes may exist.[30] LOH has been demonstrated at chromosome 16q in 20% of Wilms tumors and at 1p in 11%.[31] That this was not found to be a germline mutation suggests that this region may play a role in tumor progression rather than tumor initiation. Patients with tumor-specific LOH for chromosome 16q had a statistically significantly poorer 2-year relapse-free and overall survival than for those patients without LOH for chromosome 16q. This difference in outcome persisted after adjustment for histology and stage. Loss of 1p was associated with a worse outcome, although this difference did not reach statistical significance.[31] The most commonly altered tumor suppressor gene in human cancers, *p53*, was found to be mutated in only 4% of Wilms tumors in a large series, but all mutants had anaplastic histology.[32]

Pathology

In the typical Wilms tumor the adjacent normal renal parenchyma is compressed by the tumor and its pseudocapsule composed of compressed, atrophic renal tissues. Most tumors are soft and friable and hemorrhagic or necrotic areas are generally noted. Cysts occur and may be a dominant feature. Extrarenal locations are rare and are thought to arise from displaced metanephric elements or mesonephric remnants.

The microscopic features of nephroblastoma are variable.[33] The classic triphasic pattern includes varying proportions of three cell types: blastemal, stromal, and epithelial. Tumors that consist predominately of one or two of these elements are commonly encountered. The primitive blastemal cells usually show distinctive patterns that allow their recognition by experienced pathologists. It was once suggested that tumors with a predominant epithelial pattern were associated with a better outcome, but this has not been shown to be a significant predictor of survival with the excellent responses achieved by multimodal therapy.[34] It has been shown that tumors with a predominant differentiated pattern, epithelial or stromal, have a tendency for low stage at diagnosis suggesting that these tumors are less aggressive.[34] However, most diffusely blastemal tumors are stage III or IV at diagnosis. This suggests that these tumors are aggressive with a tendency to early dissemination.

Prognostic Factors

In initial National Wilms Tumor Study (NWTS) evaluations, patients were stratified for treatment by surgical and pathologic staging of the extent of the disease. In NWTS-1, it was noted that some tumors with "unfavorable" histologic features were associated with increased rates of relapse and death.[35] These included tumors of extreme nuclear atypia (anaplasia), and monomorphic sarcomatous appearing tumors. These latter tumors have been reclassified as CCSK and RTK and are no longer considered Wilms tumors (see later).

Anaplasia is defined by the presence of multipolar mitotic features and nuclei with increased chromatin and major diameters at least three times larger than adjacent cells. It is rare in the first 2 years of life, but the incidence increases to 13% in children age 5 years or older.[36] Anaplastic Wilms tumors are further stratified into focal and diffuse anaplasia.[37] The definition of focal anaplasia is based on a topographic principle. This requires that the anaplastic nuclear changes be confined to a specified region of the primary tumor and absent from the surrounding portions of the lesion. Diffuse anaplasia is diagnosed when anaplasia is present in more than one portion of the tumor or is found in any extrarenal or metastatic site. When the anaplastic component is completely removed, the stage I outcome is generally excellent.[38] However, if stage II to IV diffuse anaplasia is present with incomplete tumor removal, outcome is poor. This suggests that anaplasia is more a marker of chemoresistance than inherent aggressiveness of the tumor. Further evidence of this chemoresistance is the similar incidence of anaplasia in the national Wilms

tumor study (NWTSG) (5%) and in the International Society of Pediatric Oncology (SIOP) study (5.3%).[33] The latter group performs tumor removal after preoperative chemotherapy and the anaplastic cells appear to be unaffected, persisting after treatment.

Precursor lesions to Wilms tumor have been recognized for years. The preferred term is nephrogenic rest, defined as foci of abnormally persistent nephrogenic cells that can form a Wilms tumor.[39] They have been found in 1% of kidneys in infants on postmortem examination[40] and in 30 to 40% of kidneys removed for Wilms tumor.[41] Two distinct categories of nephrogenic rests have been identified, perilobar nephrogenic rest (PLNR) and intralobar nephrogenic rest (ILNR). This classification is based on the position of these lesions within the renal lobe.[42] PLNR are found in the periphery (Fig. 35.1) while ILNR can be found anywhere within the renal lobe. The presence of multiple or diffuse nephrogenic rests will lead to the diagnosis of nephroblastomatosis. A hyperplastic rest can be mistaken for a small Wilms tumor.

The presence of multiple rests in one kidney usually implies that nephrogenic rests are present in the other kidney,[42] and these patients are at risk for metachronous Wilms tumor. These patients need careful follow-up imaging to detect contralateral recurrence (Table 35.1) Because metachronous Wilms tumor occurs in patients previously treated with conventional chemotherapeutic regimens, nephrogenic rests cannot always be eradicated.

Biologic Parameters

Because of the excellent survival of most patients with favorable histology (FH) Wilms tumor, it has become increasingly difficult to find any particular histologic feature of a given tumor that will predict the risk of relapse. Several biologic factors are being investigated to further stratify patients with FH Wilms tumor for treatment. As noted earlier, chromosomal abnormalities of 16q and 1p are being evaluated prospectively in the NWTS study.

A relationship has been noted between tumor DNA content, measured by flow cytometry, and outcome in Wilms tumor. One study found that[43] those with small tetraploid patterns had a 69% 5-year survival, while those with stage III and IV tetraploid patterns in the tumor fared significantly worse with a 25% 5-year survival.[43] However, others have found that DNA ploidy was not a more accurate predictor of survival than histology and stage.[44]

Partin et al have used nuclear morphometric techniques to predict clinical outcome in patients with Wilms tumor.[45] An initial review of 27 Wilms tumor patients with favorable histology found a combination of three shape descriptors associated with a poor prognosis. A

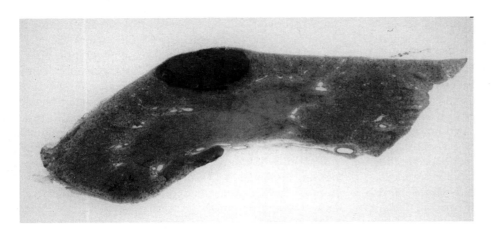

FIG. 35.1. A PLNR, composed of blastemal cells, is seen beneath the renal capsule (hematoxylin and eosin, ×40).

subsequent report identified two shape factors that could separate patients into groups with favorable and unfavorable outcome.[46] The 4-year relapse-free survival percentages for the two groups differed by more than 40%. Studies are underway to confirm these preliminary findings in a larger sample of patients.

Diagnosis and Preoperative Evaluation

The most common presentation is the incidental discovery of an abdominal mass. Gross hematuria, fever, and abdominal pain are other findings at diagnosis. The latter not infrequently results in exploration for presumed appendicitis. Rupture of the tumor with hemorrhage can result in the presentation of an acute abdomen. The propensity of Wilms tumor to grow into the renal vein and inferior vena cava can lead to atypical presentations. Varicocele, hepatomegaly caused by hepatic vein obstruction, ascites and congestive heart failure were found in less than 10% of patients with intracaval or atrial tumor extension in NWTS-3.[47] During the physical examination, it is important to note signs of associated Wilms tumor syndromes such as aniridia, hemihypertrophy, and genitourinary anomalies.

An emergent operation is unnecessary unless there is evidence of active bleeding or tumor rupture. Laboratory evaluation should include a complete peripheral blood count, platelet count, renal function tests, liver

TABLE 35.1. *Recommended follow-up imaging studies for children with renal neoplasms of proven histology and free of metastases at diagnosis*

Tumor type	Study	Schedule after therapy
Favorable histology Wilms tumor; Stage I anaplastic Wilms tumor	Chest films	6 wk and 3 mo postoperatively; then every 3 mo × 5, every 6 mo × 3, yearly × 2
Irradiated patients only	Irradiated bony structures[a]	Yearly to full growth, then every 5 y indefinitely[b]
Without NRs, Stages I and II	Abdominal ultrasound	Yearly × 3
Without NRs, Stage III	Abdominal ultrasound	As for chest films
With NRs, any stage[c]	Abdominal ultrasound	Every 3 mo × 10, every 6 mo × 5, yearly × 5
Stage II and III anaplastic	Chest films	As for favorable histology
	Abdominal ultrasound	Every 3 mo × 4; every 6 mo × 4
Renal cell carcinoma	Chest films	Like favorable histology
	Skeletal survey and bone scan	Like CCSK
Clear cell sarcoma (CCSK)	Brain MRI and/or opacified CT	When CCSK is established; then every 6 mo × 10
	Skeletal survey and bone scan	As for favorable histology
	Chest films	
Rhabdoid tumor	Brain MRI and/or opacified CT	As for CCSK
	Chest films	As for favorable histology
Mesoblastic nephroma[d]	Abdominal ultrasound	Every 3 mo × 6

[a]To include any irradiated osseous structures.

[b]To detect second neoplasms, benign (osteochondromas) or malignant.

[c]The panelists at the first International Conference on Molecular and Clinical Genetics of Childhood Renal Tumors, Albuquerque, New Mexico, May 1992 recommended a variation: every 3 months for 5 years or until age 7, whichever comes first.

[d]Data from the files of Dr. J.B. Beckwith reveal that 20 of 293 MN patients (7%) relapsed or had metastases at diagnosis; 4 of the 20 in the lungs, 1 of the 4 at diagnosis. All but 1 of the 19 relapses occurred within 1 year. Chest films for MN patients may be elected on a schedule such as every 3 months × 4, every 6 months × 2.

(Modified, with permission, from D'Angio GJ, Rosenberg H, Sharples K, Kelalis P, Breslow N, Green DM. Position paper: imaging methods for primary renal tumors of childhood: cost versus benefits. Med Pediatr Oncol 1993;21:205–212.)

function tests, serum calcium, and urinalysis. Elevation of the serum calcium can occur in children with congenital mesoblastic nephroma and rhabdoid tumor of the kidney. Children with nephroblastoma should be screened for acquired von Willebrand's disease, which has been found in 8% of newly diagnosed Wilms tumor patients.[48]

Elevated levels of hyaluronic acid and hyaluronic acid-stimulating activity have been reported in urine and serum of patients with Wilms tumor.[49, 50] After surgical removal of the tumor the levels returned to normal. Patients with persistent disease or relapse had significantly higher levels 1 to 6 months after surgery.[50] Elevated plasma renin levels have been reported in patietns with Wilms tumor, in addition to reduction in plasma levels after treatment.[51, 52] Recently, elevated plasma renin levels were noted in four children with relapse of Wilms tumor. In all cases, the renin level had decreased after initial tumor excision, but subsequently became elevated.

Imaging

Children with solid tumors undergo extensive imaging evaluation. The intent is to confirm the diagnosis and to define the extent of disease. However, all renal tumors share some similar features and cannot be readily distinguished preoperatively. Other important goals are to establish that there is contralateral functioning kidney before nephrectomy and to determine whether there is a solid renal tumor present. All of this information will help the surgeon plan for a major cancer operation. Even without a certain diagnosis, preoperative imaging should enable the surgeon to plan for a major cancer operation and avoid surgical complications.[53] Children entered on NWTS-3 who had an incorrect preoperative diagnosis were found to have an increased incidence of surgical complications.[54]

Ultrasonography is the initial study of choice for palpable abdominal masses.[55] In most cases, an experienced radiologist can determine if the mass is of renal origin and if cystic or solid. One important caveat is that some Wilms tumors are cystic and may mimic cystic nephroma. Another important role for ultrasound is to exclude intracaval tumor extension, which occurs in 4% of patients with Wilms tumor.[47]

Computerized tomography (CT) is performed in most children with renal masses and provides helpful anatomic and functional data. However, in today' cost conscious environment, it is important to assess whether these studies provide information that will alter medical management. There is some controversy regarding the utility of CT scans in the preoperative evaluation and their role in tumor staging.[56–58] Accurate staging of children with Wilms tumors is essential before initiating treatment as outcome is highly correlated with stage.[59]

CT with and without intravascular contrast can detect sharp demarcations between tumor and normal renal parenchyma and assess the relative function of the contralateral kidney. CT can suggest tumor extension into perirenal fat and adjacent organs, but only exploration can confirm it. In right-sided tumors, CT has a high false-positive rate for hepatic invasion, but it is 100% accurate when invasion is excluded.[60] Although CT can detect retroperitoneal adenopathy, benign nodal enlargement is commonly seen in children; therefore, adenopathy, even palpated at exploration, does not correlate well with metastatic disease.[61] CT is also of limited accuracy in excluding vascular invasion. However, the staging system used by the NWTSG relies on surgical findings and pathologic examination. Staging is divided into detection of distant metastases and defining the local extent of the tumor. The local tumor burden (regional lymph node involvement, residual disease, diffuse tumor spillage) determines whether the child receives abdominal irradiation and also the intensity of the chemotherapy regimen.

Magnetic resonance imaging (MRI) offers further advances over CT, including multiplanar views of the kidney and abdomen with superior soft-tissue contrast.[55] If extension of tumor into the IVC cannot be excluded by ultrasound, magnetic resonance imaging (MRI) is the next study ordered.[62] MRI is more effective in defining the extent of intravascular tumor extension including those with intracardiac extension. The drawbacks of MRI are its higher cost, lack of bowel contrast agent, and the susceptibility of motion artifact that makes sedation necessary in small children.

Controversy surrounds the use of CT to exclude contralateral renal involvement. Assessment of the contralateral kidney in pateints with Wilms tumor is essential because of increased incidence of bilaterality. The NWTSG protocol recommends formal exploration at the time of operation. Gerota's fascia is opened over the contralateral kidney to allow inspection and palpation of all surfaces. It has been proposed that contralateral renal exploration can be obviated with improved preoperative imaging.[63–65] Although several reports have found preoperative imaging including CT to be 100% accurate in confirming or excluding contralateral tumors, 7% of cases of synchronous bilateral Wilms tumor in NWTS-4 were missed by preoperative imaging and found only at surgery.[66] The NWTSG continues to recommend contralateral renal exploration to exclude synchronous contralateral Wilms tumor.

All patients with Wilms tumor should have a plain radiograph of the chest because the lungs are the most common site of metastasis.[55] If pulmonary metastases are seen, chest CT will not alter therapy, which includes the addition of doxorubicin to the chemotherapeutic regimen and the application of whole lung irradiation. The need for chest CT in patients with a negative plain

---

film is under debate, and it is unclear whether those with lesions detected by CT alone require more aggressive treatment.[67–69] A radionuclide bone scan and x-radiograph skeletal survey should be obtained postoperatively on all children with CCSK and RTK.[57] Brain imaging, using MRI or CT, should be obtained for all patients with CCSK and RTK. These tumors are associated with intracranial metastases.

Screening for Wilms Tumor

Routine screening by abdominal ultrasound is recommended for patients at high risk for developing Wilms tumor, including those with hemihypertrophy, BWS, and aniridia.[57] Sonography is recommended in high-risk children every 3 months until age 7 years, followed by physical examination every 6 months until somatic growth is complete.[3,57] Similar protocols have been proposed for observing multicystic dysplastic kidney for tumor development, although the risk of Wilms tumor is minimal.[70–72] Nephrogenic rests are found in 4.2% of multicystic dysplastic kidneys; in comparison, these rests are seen in only 0.2 to 0.95% of routine pediatric autopsies.[72] These lesions seem unlikely to undergo malignant transformation because only one case of Wilms tumor in a multicystic dysplastic kidney has been reported among the more than 7,000 cases registered with the NWTSG pathology center.[72]

There are conflicting data regarding whether screening for Wilms tumor in these high-risk groups detects tumors at an earlier stage. Green et al reported that patients with aniridia undergoing screening were more likely to have stage 1 tumors.[73] Another study of 13 high-risk children undergoing ultrasound screening did not report any significant difference in stage distribution between them and children not undergoing screening.[74] The authors suggested that abdominal palpation by the parents would be as effective as periodic imaging. It remains to be determined whether these screening efforts translate into improved survival.

Staging

The most important determinants of outcome in children with Wilms tumor are the histopathology and tumor stage. The staging system used by the NWTSG is summarized in Table 35.2. Stage I tumors are limited to the kidney and completely resected. The first signs of spread outside the kidney are in the renal sinus and lymphatic vessels. Penetration through the renal capsule is the next most common site of extrarenal spread. Tumors that penetrate the renal capsule are considered stage II lesions. Clear demonstration of tumor cells in the perirenal fat is required to document capsular penetration. Extensive involvement of the soft tissues of the renal sinus or the presence of tumor cells in blood or

TABLE 35.2. *Staging system of the national Wilms tumor study*

Stage	
I	Tumor is limited to the kidney and completely excised. The renal capsule is intact and the tumor did not rupture before removal. There is no residual tumor. The vessels of the renal sinus are not involved.
II	Tumor extends beyond the kidney, but is completely excised. There is regional extension of tumor (i.e., penetration of the renal capsule, extensive invasion of the renal sinus). The tumor may have been biopsied or there may be local spillage of tumor confined to the flank. Extrarenal vessels may contain tumor thrombus or be infiltrated by tumor.
III	Residual nonhematogenous tumor confined to the abdomen: lymph node involvement, diffuse peritoneal spillage before or during surgery, peritoneal implants, tumor beyond surgical margin grossly or microscopically, or tumor not completely removed.
IV	Hematogenous metastases (lung, liver, bone, brain, etc.) or lymph node metastases outside the abdominopelvic region are present.
V	Bilateral renal involvement at diagnosis.

lymphatic vessels of the sinus is considered a sign of stage II lesion.

The presence of lymph node metastases has an adverse outcome on survival, and therefore it is important that adequate lymph node sampling be performed during the course of removal of a nephroblastoma. Lymph node involvement confined to the abdomen is indicative of stage III. Local tumor extension is another important factor in identifying risk of tumor relapse. Patients with diffuse tumor spill are at increased risk of abdominal relapse and therefore are considered to have stage III disease and are given whole abdominal irradiation. For NWTS-3, the distribution of FH tumors was: stage I: 47%; stage II: 22%; stage III: 22%; and stage IV: 9%.[59]

Surgical Management

The surgeon has an important role in assessing local tumor extent. Accurate staging is essential for determining the appropriate chemotherapy regimen and the need for radiation therapy. In removing the tumor, the surgeon must be careful to avoid tumor rupture and spill that could increase the therapy needed. Likewise the completeness of the tumor resection can have an impact on patient survival. A transperitoneal approach is preferred. Once the peritoneal cavity is entered, the abdominal cavity is explored thoroughly. One should assess the liver, regional lymph nodes in the periaortic area, and look for other evidence of tumor spread. Exploration of the contralateral kidney should be performed before nephrectomy. The colon is reflected and Gerota's fascia opened so that the kidney can be inspected on all surfaces. A biopsy should be performed on any abnormalities of the kidney to exclude Wilms tumor or nephrogenic rests.

Radical nephrectomy is performed with sampling of regional lymph nodes, but formal lymph node dissection is not required.[61] Gentle handling of the tumor throughout the procedure is mandatory to avoid tumor spillage because these patients have a sixfold increase in local abdominal relapse.[59] Although early ligation of the renal vein does not appear to have an appreciable effect on survival, separate ligation is performed before mobilization of the tumor if, and only if, exposure is adequate. More importantly, the surgeon should be certain that the contralateral renal vessels, aorta, iliac, or superior mesenteric arteries have not been mistakenly ligated.[75] Palpation of the renal vein and IVC should be performed to exclude intravascular tumor extension before vessel ligation. For vena caval involvement below the level of the hepatic veins, the caval thrombus can be removed through cavotomy after proximal and distal vascular control is obtained. Generally the thrombus will be free-floating, but if there is adherence of the thrombus to the caval wall, the thrombus can often be delivered with the passage of a Fogarty or Foley balloon catheter. If the thrombus extends above the level of the hepatic veins, preoperative chemotherapy can shrink the tumor and thrombus,[76, 77] facilitating complete removal.

One should not overlook the morbidity of surgery, which can produce acute and late complications. A review of NWTS-3 patients undergoing primary nephrectomy found a 19% incidence of surgical complications.[54] The most common complications were hemorrhage and small bowel obstruction.[78] Several risk factors for increased surgical complications were identified, including higher local tumor stage, intravascular extension, en bloc resection of other visceral organs, and incorrect preoperative diagnosis. En bloc resection of all or parts of adjacent organs to which the tumor is adherent is generally not warranted. Wilms tumors often compress and adhere to adjacent structures without frank invasion.[54] If the tumor is found to be unresectable, biopsy of the tumor can be followed by chemotherapy or radiation therapy.[79, 80]

NWTS Trials

Important findings of the early NWTSG randomized clinical trials, NWTS-1, and NWTS-2, (1969–1978) included combination chemotherapy (which was more effective than single agents alone), identification of unfavorable histologic features of Wilms tumor, and identification of prognostic factors that allowed refinement of the staging system stratifying patients into high-risk and low-risk treatment groups.[81] It was recognized that the

presence of lymph node metastases had an adverse outcome on survival.[82, 83] This underscores the importance of adequate lymph node sampling during the course of removal of a nephroblastoma. Local tumor extension was another important factor identified that increased the risk of tumor relapse. Patients with diffuse tumor spill were therefore considered stage III and given whole abdominal irradiation.[59] This improved staging system was used in the design of subsequent trials in an attempt to further reduce the intensity of therapy for most patients while maintaining overall survival.

The findings of NWTS-3 (1979–1986) validated this approach. Patients with stage I, FH tumors can be treated successfully with an 11-week regimen of vincristine (VCR) and dactinomycin (AMD).[59] The 4-year relapse-free survival was 89%, and the overall survival was 95.6%. Patients with stage II FH tumors treated with AMD and VCR without postoperative radiation therapy (XRT) had a 4-year overall survival, equivalent to the 91.1% of patients who received doxorubicin (DOX) and XRT. The dosage of abdominal irradiation for patients with stage III FH tumors was reduced to 1,000 cGy. This was shown to be as effective as 2,000 cGy in preventing abdominal relapse if DOX is added to VCR and AMD. Four-year relapse-free survival for patients with stage III tumors was 82%, and the 4-year overall survival was 90.9%. Patients with stage IV FH tumors receive abdominal irradiation based on the local tumor stage and also receive 1,200 cGy to both lungs. The combination of VCR, AMD, and DOX produced a 4-year relapse-free survival of 79% and the overall survival was 80.9%.[83] There was no statistically significant improvement in survival when cyclophosphamide was added to the three-drug regimen.

The goals of the most recent intergroup study, NWTS-4 (1986–1994), were to further decrease treatment intensity for patients with favorable prognosis while trying to maintain their excellent survival. Another aim of the study was to decrease the cost of therapy through modification of the schedule of drug administration. Pulse-intensive regimens using single doses of AMD and DOX were compared to regimens using divided doses of the drugs. The pulse-intensive regimens were found to produce less hematologic toxicity than the standard regimens.[85] Patients treated with this regimen also achieve equivalent survival compared with the standard chemotherapy regimen.[86] The study was closed in September, 1994. Additional follow-up is required before outcome data will be reported.

Recommendations for treatment to be used in the recently opened intergroup study, NWTS-5, are outlined in Table 35.3. Patients will not be randomized for therapy, but instead biologic features of the tumors will be assessed. This study will attempt to verify the preliminary findings that LOH for chromosomes 16q and 1p are useful markers in identifying patients who will re-

TABLE 35.3. *Protocol for National Wilms Tumor Study-5*

	Radiotherapy	Chemotherapy
Stage I, II FH, and anaplasia	None	EE-4A—pulse-intensive AMD plus VCR (18 weeks)
Stage III, IV FH, and focal anaplasia II–IV	1,080cGy	DD-4A—pulse-intensive AMD, VCR, and DOX (24 weeks)
Stage II–IV diffuse anaplasia and CCSK	Yes[a]	Regimen I[b]
Stage I–IV Rhabdoid tumor of the kidney	Yes[a]	Regimen RTK[c]

[a]Radiation therapy is given to all patients with clear cell sarcoma. Patients with stage IV FH disease are given radiation based on the local tumor stage. Consult protocol for specific treatment.
[b]Regimen I: AMD, VCR, DOX, cyclophosphamide, and etopposide.
[c]Regimen RTK: Carboplatin, etoposide, and cyclophosphamide.
AMD, dactinomycin; VCR, vincristine; DOX, doxorubicin; FH, favorable histology; UH, unfavorable histology.

lapse.[31] If these variables are found to be predictive of clinical behavior, this information will then be used in subsequent clinical trials to stratify patients for therapy.

One aspect of the new protocol is the treatment of a select group of patients with stage 1 FH tumors by nephrectomy alone. The observation was made many years ago that children younger than age 2 years with tumors weighing less than 550 grams had an improved outcome even if adjuvant therapy was omitted.[87–89] Approximately 40% of patients with stage I tumors meet these criteria. A study of NWTS-4 patients with FH stage I tumors found that the 2-year relapse-free survival for patients younger than age 2 years with tumors weights less than 550 grams was 95.5%.[90] There was good correlation between age <2 years, tumor weight <550 grams, and negative microsubstaging variables that have been found to predict risk of relapse in stage 1 tumors.[91] Therefore, it was concluded that the variables of age and tumor weight could be more easily applied in clinical practice to stratify patients for treatment as they are easily determined.[90] Careful postoperative surveillance of this group of children will be necessary so that any relapses can be detected early.

The treatment for all other patients with stage I FH tumors and those with stage II FH and Stage I anaplastic Wilms tumor is the same. They will receive a pulse-intensive regimen of VCR and AMD for 18 weeks. Patients with stage III FH and Stage II–III focal anaplasia are treated with AMD, VCR, and DOX and 1,080 cGy abdominal irradiation. Patients with stage IV FH tumors receive abdominal irradiation based on the local tumor stage and 1,200 cGy to both lungs.

Children with stage II–IV diffuse anaplasia and stage I–IV clear cell sarcoma of the kidney will be treated with a new chemotherapeutic regimen combining VCR, ADR, cyclophosphamide, and etoposide in an attempt to further improve the survival of this high-risk group. All of these patients will receive irradiation to the tumor bed. Children with all stages of rhabdoid tumor of the kidney will be treated with carboplatin, cyclophosphamide, and etoposide. These patients will also receive abdominal irradiation.

Preoperative Chemotherapy

SIOP

The clinical protocols conducted by SIOP use preoperative therapy. The rationale is that the preoperative treatment decreases the risk of intraoperative rupture or spill.[92, 93] Preoperative treatment can produce dramatic reduction in the size of the primary tumor and facilitate surgical excision (Fig. 35.2). It is proposed that the neoadjuvant therapy will treat micrometastases and lead to a more favorable stage distribution at the time of surgery. More patients have "postchemotherapy stage I" tumors, and as a result, fewer patients receive postoperative radiation therapy. This was thought to be a significant advantage in terms of decreasing morbidity of treatment. When SIOP and NWTSG began their prospective studies, all children with Wilms tumor received postoperative radiation therapy. Over time, however, it became apparent to NWTSG investigators that radiation therapy was unnecessary for patients with stage I and II tumors.[59] Even children with stage IV disease who have organ confined tumors do not need abdominal irradiation. As a result, the number of children receiving abdominal irradiation has been decreasing steadily for NWTSG patients. For patients with nonmetastatic favorable histology, only 24% of children enrolled in NWTS were given XRT compared to 18% of SIOP patients.[94] The most recently completed and published studies by NWTSG and SIOP show similar survival for patients with nonmetastatic favorable histology Wilms tumor.[59, 95] There are differences in staging systems, but both groups have achieved excellent results.

One major concern regarding the routine use of preoperative chemotherapy is whether the "postchemotherapy" stage adequately defines the risk of relapse.[94] All tumor staging systems are designed to stratify patients into low- and high-risk groups. The goal is to select out high-risk patients for more intense therapy while minimizing treatment, and thus morbidity, for low-risk patients. The NWTSG relies on careful surgical and pathologic staging to determine treatment categories. The SIOP investigators use the postchemotherapy stage to determine the amount of postoperative therapy.

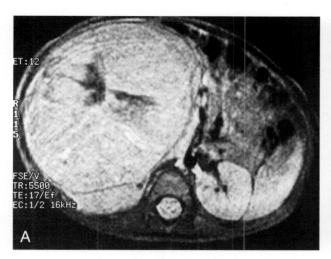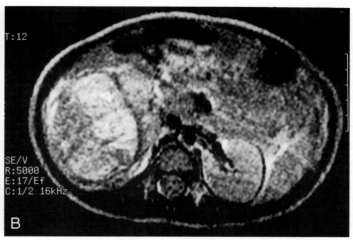

FIG. 35.2. **A,** MRI Scan showing a large, inoperable Wilms tumor. **B,** MRI scan of the same tumor after 6 weeks of chemotherapy. Reprinted with the permission of Mosby Year Book. Ritchey M, et al. Pediatric urologic oncology. In: Gillenwater J, ed. Adult and Pediatric Urology, 1996. Figure 58-11.

One important variable is the presence of lymph node involvement. NWTSG stage 3 patients with positive lymph nodes receive postoperative irradiation and the addition of doxorubicin to the chemotherapy regimen. In SIOP-6, "postchemotherapy stage II, node negative" patients were randomized to receive or not receive abdominal irradiation. The trial was stopped prematurely because of an excessive number of intraabdominal recurrences in nonirradiated patients.[95] Although the overall outcome between the two treatment arms was reported as no significant difference, subsequent SIOP trials added anthracycline to the chemotherapy regimen for "postchemotherapy stage II, node negative" patients.[94] Thus a larger percentage of SIOP patients than of NWTSG patients received this drug. This experience would suggest that staging the patient after chemotherapy may inadequately define the risk of relapse. Although preoperative therapy may destroy the evidence of extrarenal spread of disease, e.g., lymph node involvement or extracapsular extension, patients are still at an increased risk for relapse. This risk raises some concern regarding the utility of postchemotherapy stage, as opposed to staging at initial surgery used by the NWTSG, to predict tumor behavior.

The NWTSG recommends preoperative chemotherapy for some select groups of patients, including those with bilateral involvement,[96] tumors inoperable at surgical exploration,[80] and tumor extension into IVC above the hepatic veins (see earlier discussion).[77] For all other children, the NWTSG recommends primary nephrectomy.

Bilateral Disease

Synchronous bilateral nephroblastoma occurs in approximately 5% of children with metachronous lesions developing in only 1%.[96, 97] In the past, bilateral patients with Wilms tumor were managed with a primary surgical approach. In a review of 145 NWTS-2 and NWTS-3 patients, Blute et al found survival among patients treated with primary surgical resection was comparable to that of patients who had biopsy only, followed by preoperative chemotherapy, 83% at 2 years.[96] SIOP investigators have also reported good overall survival in patients treated with preoperative chemotherapy with a decrease in the incidence of residual disease.[98] One advantage of the latter approach is that more renal units will be spared if surgery is deferred until after the tumor burden is reduced.[97, 99] This is important because renal failure is a significant risk in patients with bilateral tumors.[100]

Therefore, the preferred approach for patients with bilateral Wilms tumor is initial biopsy followed by preoperative chemotherapy.[101] Radical excision of the tumor should not be performed at the initial operation. Bilateral biopsies should be obtained to confirm the presence of Wilms tumor in both kidneys and to define the histologic type, although sampling errors may occur. Suspicious lymph nodes should be biopsied, and a surgical stage assigned. After 6 weeks of chemotherapy the patient is reassessed with an abdominal CT to determine the feasibility of resection.

Bilateral nephrectomies and dialysis may rarely be required when the tumors do not respond to chemotherapy and radiation therapy. The recommended interval between successful completion of treatment of the Wilms tumor and renal transplantation varies. Some advocate a waiting period of 2 years to ensure that the patient does not develop metastatic disease; others have found that a 1-year interval is sufficient.[102]

Partial Nephrectomy in Unilateral Tumors

Concern about the late occurrence of renal dysfunction in children who have undergone unilateral nephrectomy has led some surgeons to recommend parenchymal sparing procedures for unilateral tumors to reduce the frequency of long-term complications of renal failure.[103, 104] There have been reports of patients with Wilms tumor who have developed renal failure, but they have been infrequent. A recent review of NWTSG patients with unilateral Wilms tumor found that the incidence of renal failure was 0.25% with a median follow-up of 6 years.[100] Most of those patients had the Denys-Drash syndrome. Such patients have intrinsic renal disease and generally have renal failure at diagnosis or inevitably progress to end stage renal disease. Another risk factor for the development of renal failure was irradiation of the remaining kidney.

Because most Wilms tumors are too large for a partial nephrectomy at initial presentation, pretreatment with chemotherapy is recommended to facilitate the surgery. However, staging of the patient after the chemotherapy could lead to inaccuracy as discussed earlier. Some authors rely on the preoperative imaging to select patients for partial nephrectomy and to stage the patient.[103, 104] There are no published studies prospectively correlating staging by imaging studies and surgical and pathologic staging.

After preoperative chemotherapy, 10% of patients may then be amenable to partial nephrectomy.[103] Some advocate enucleation of the tumor to allow parenchymal sparing procedures for even centrally located tumors where partial nephrectomy with a rim of renal tissue would be inadvisable.[104]

Inoperable Tumors

Approximately 5% of patients have large tumors found to be unresectable at surgery.[80, 95] Pretreatment with chemotherapy almost always reduces the bulk of the tumor and renders it resectable. However, this method does not result in improved survival rates but results in the loss of important staging information. Patients who are found to have unresectable tumor should be considered stage III and treated accordingly.[80] Once there is an adequate reduction in the size of the tumor to facilitate nephrectomy, then definitive resection should be completed. In general, the operative procedure can be performed within 6 weeks of initiating treatment. Serial imaging evaluation is helpful to assess response. Patients who do not respond can be considered for preoperative irradiation because this may produce enough shrinkage to facilitate nephrectomy. If the tumor remains inoperable, then biopsy of the primary tumor and accessible metastatic lesions should be performed. Patients with progressive disease have a poor prognosis and will require treatment with a different chemotherapeutic regimen.[80]

Treatment of Relapses

Results from NWTS-3 demonstrate that the risk of tumor relapse at 3 years is 9.6%, 11.8%, 22%, and 22%, respectively for stages I through IV. Relapses occurred in 36% and 45% of unfavorable histology patients stage I to III and IV.[59] Children with relapsed Wilms tumor have a variable prognosis, depending on the initial stage, site of relapse, time from initial diagnosis to relapse, and prior therapy. Adverse prognostic factors include previous treatment that included DOX, relapse less than 12 months after diagnosis, and intraabdominal relapse in previously abdominal irradiated patients.[105] In the past, treatment of these patients has been highly individualized. A prospective intergroup study with an uniform treatment for relapsed Wilms tumor is being conducted by the Children's Cancer Group and the Pediatric Oncology Group.[106] This protocol will evaluate a more aggressive approach, including the use of autologous bone marrow transplantation, particularly for those patients with adverse prognostic factors at the time of relapse.

Late Effects

As survival of patients with Wilms tumor has increased dramatically over the past 35 years, there has been an increasing cohort of long-term survivors of therapy. NWTSG patients who survive 5 years after completion of therapy are asked to participate in a late effects study. Numerous organ systems are subject to the late sequelae of anticancer therapy. Clinicians must become familiar with the spectrum of problems that face these children as they grow into adulthood.

Children treated for Wilms tumor are at increased risk for second malignant neoplasms (SMN). Investigators from the NWTSG have noted a 1.6% cumulative incidence of SMNs at 15 years after treatment.[107] Prior treatment for relapse, the amount of abdominal irradiation, and use of doxorubicin were associated with an increased incidence of SMNs.

Congestive heart failure is a well-known complication of treatment with anthracycline and the incidence is dose related.[108] In addition to the acute cardiotoxicity, reports are surfacing of cardiac failure up to 20 years after treatment.[109] In a preliminary review of patients entered on NWTS-1, -2, and -3, the frequency of congestive heart failure was 1.7% among patients treated with doxorubicin.[110] The risk was increased if the patient received whole lung irradiation. In light of these findings, all children who undergo treatment with these modalities should undergo periodic reevaluation.

Damage to reproductive systems can lead to problems with hormonal dysfunction and infertility. Gonadal radiation in males can result in temporary azoospermia and hypogonadism.[111] The severity of damage to the testis depends on the dose or radiation. Female patients with Wilms tumor who received abdominal radiation have a 12% incidence of ovarian failure.[112] In addition, women with prior abdominal radiation have the potential for adverse pregnancy outcomes. Perinatal mortality rates are higher, and infants are more likely to have low birth weights.[16]

Other Renal Tumors

Clear Cell Sarcoma of the Kidney (CCSK)

Not a Wilms tumor variant, this tumor is associated with a higher rate of relapse and death than favorable histology Wilms tumor. The tumor is also known as the 'bone-metastasizing renal tumor of childhood' because of its predilection for these sites.[113, 35] There are also more brain metastases with this entity.[114] CCSK accounts for 3% of renal tumors reported to the NWTS. Unlike tumors with anaplasia, stage I CCSK lesions are associated with increased rates of relapse. Studies have demonstrated that the use of doxorubicin is associated with a significant improvement in outcome for these children.[59]

Rhabdoid Tumor of the Kidney (RTK)

RTK was first identified by NWTSG pathologists in 1978.[35] This is a highly malignant tumor of the kidney that accounts for 2% of renal tumors registered to the NWTSG.[59] This tumor is typically seen in infants and very young children with a median age of 13 months. RTK metastasizes to the brain, which is exceedingly uncommon for Wilms tumor. There have been several cases of primary neuroectodermal tumors of the brain that have occurred separately in children with this neoplasm.[115] The prognosis of RTK remains dismal with conventional chemotherapeutic regimens and new treatment strategies are being developed for management of these children.

Solitary Multilocular Cyst

Solitary multilocular cyst, also known as multilocular cystic nephroma, is an uncommon, benign renal tumor with a bimodal incidence. Fifty percent of the multilocular cysts reported in the literature have been found in young children, usually boys. The second peak incidence occurs in adults, and unlike the pediatric cases is usually in women.[116] The most common feature of multilocular cyst of the kidney is an abdominal or renal mass found on routine physical examination. All cases of multilocular cystic renal disease have been unilateral. The gross appearance of the tumor is its most distinguishing feature. The cut surfaces reveal a well-circumscribed multilocular tumor composed of cysts ranging from several millimeters to several centimeters in greatest diameter. The tumor is well encapsulated and compresses the surrounding renal parenchyma.

Multilocular cyst is a benign lesion that is cured by nephrectomy; there have been no reports of tumor recurrence or metastases. Some of the smaller lesions can be managed by partial excision salvaging a portion of the kidney. If partial nephrectomy is considered, frozen section is indicated to exclude cystic, partially differentiated nephroblastoma.[117] This tumor has a similar gross appearance but has typical elements of Wilms tumor within the septa. These tumors are best managed by nephrectomy.

Renal Cell Carcinoma

Only 5% of renal cell carcinomas occur in children,[118, 119] generally presenting after age 5 years, and is the most common renal malignancy in the second decade of life. The signs and symptoms are similar to those of other solid renal tumors with an abdominal mass being the most common presentation in a child. Hematuria is more common in renal cell carcinoma than in Wilms tumor.[119]

Survival of children with renal cell carcinoma depends on complete resection of the tumor. Raney et al found that all children with stage I lesions survived, and others have reported 64 to 80% survival for stage I and II tumors.[120] Overall survival was approximately 50%. Age is also a prognostic factor with improved survival in children younger than 11 years.[120] These tumors do not appear responsive to chemotherapy or radiation therapy.

Congenital Mesoblastic Nephroma (CMN)

CMN is the most common renal tumor in infants with a mean age at diagnosis of 3.5 months.[121] The typical presentation is a newborn with an abdominal mass. In CMN, tumor induction is postulated to occur at a time when the multipotent blastema is predominately stromagenic.[122] There have been no cytogenetic or molecular markers discovered that are unique to CMN. The neoplasm is histologically distinct from Wilms tumor. The cell population is characterized by interlacing sheets of connective cells. Imaging studies cannot reliably distinguish CMN from other renal mass lesions.[123, 124]

Complete excision is curative for most patients with CMN. The growth pattern is one of local invasion and extension through the capsule.[121] Local recurrence has been reported in several patients with a cellular variant of CMN.[123, 124] This lesion is characterized by a high mitotic index and dense cellularity, but these features are present in 25% of CMN specimens.[125] Adequacy of surgical resection and age at diagnosis in these patients appear to be more important predictors of relapse than histology.[125] The risk of recurrence is thought to be lower in children younger than 3 months of age at diagnosis, but metastases have been reported in a few infants.[126] Neither chemotherapy nor radiation therapy is routinely recommended,[121] but adjuvant treatment should be considered for patients with cellular variants that are incompletely resected.[124]

GENITOURINARY RHABDOMYOSARCOMA

Rhabdomyosarcoma (RMS) is the most common soft tissue sarcoma in infants and children, accounting for approximately half of all pediatric soft tissue sarcomas and 15% of all pediatric solid tumors. Fifteen to twenty percent of all RMS arise from the genitourinary system.[127] The most common genitourinary sites are prostate, bladder, and vagina. Survival varies with site; special sites such as vagina and testes are associated with a better prognosis than bladder and prostate.[128, 129] There is a bimodal age distribution with a peak incidence in the first 2 years of life and again at adolescence.[130]

ETIOLOGY

Subgroups of children with a genetic predisposition to the development of RMS have been identified. The Li-Fraumeni syndrome associates childhood sarcomas with mothers who have an excess of premenopausal breast cancer and with siblings who have an increased risk of cancer.[131] A mutation of the p53 tumor suppressor gene was found in the tumors in all patients with this syndrome.[132] An increased incidence of RMS has been found in association with neurofibromatosis.[133]

Cytogenetic abnormalities have been noted in RMS. Embryonal RMS demonstrates LOH on chromosome 11p15, but at a different location than the WT2 implicated in the development of some Wilms tumors.[134, 135] Alveolar RMS is associated with a translocation between chromosomes 2 and 13 resulting in the formation of a chimeric protein.[136] PAX3, a DNA-binding protein on chromosome 2, is fused to the FKHR gene on chromosome 13. These genes may be involved in the pathogenesis of alveolar rhabdomyosarcoma. IGF-2 messenger RNA expression has been documented in alveolar and embryonal rhabdomyosarcoma.[137] Insulin-like growth factors (IGF) are known to stimulate myoblast proliferation and differentiation. Correlation of these molecular abnormalities with clinical behavior has not yet been performed.

Pathology and Patterns of Spread

There are several histologic variants of RMS. These recently have been reviewed by the pathology committee of the IRS.[138] The committee developed a new classification recognizing three major histology groups based on prognostic significance. Embryonal RMS is the most common subtype of RMS seen in children and accounts for must genitourinary tumors.[139-140] Embryonal RMS may occur in solid form arising in muscle groups, such as the trunk and extremities, or as the so-called sarcoma botryoides, a polypoid variety that occurs in hollow organs or body cavities such as the bladder or vagina. The botryoid and spindle variants of embryonal RMS are associated with an excellent survival rate. The second most common form is alveolar, which occurs more commonly in extremity lesions than at genitourinary sites and has a worse prognosis.[141, 140] Alveolar histology RMS also has a higher rate of spread to regional lymph nodes, local recurrence, bone marrow involvement and distant spread. The third category consists of undifferentiated tumors, which also fare poorly. Pleomorphic RMS is no longer considered to be a separate entity, but rather an anaplastic variant of the more common embryonal or alveolar RMS.[142]

The diagnosis of rhabdomyosarcoma can occasionally be difficult with conventional histologic techniques. In such cases, histology may be complemented by other studies, including electron microscopy, cytogenetics, immunohistochemistry, and DNA flow cytometry.[143] Advances in molecular biology have also helped in identification of difficult cases. Genes of the MyoD family are important in the differentiation of skeletal muscle.[136] MyoD gene expression is increased in rhabdomyosarcoma and is believed to represent failure of differentiation. MyoD expression is not thought to play a role in tumorigenesis, but may be a useful marker for identification of these tumors.[144]

Clinical Staging

Tumor stage at diagnosis is most predictive of clinical outcome.[145] Regional lymph node extension is fairly common and varies with site of the primary tumor. Metastatic spread of RMS is usually to the lungs. Clinical grouping was used in the early IRS studies (Table 35.4). One of the difficulties inherent in this system is that the stage depends to a large extent on the completeness of surgical excision. As the treatment of RMS has evolved, more patients have undergone biopsy only at the initial surgical procedure, leaving gross residual disease. This results in the shifting of more patients from group I to group III. Biologically equivalent tumors could end up in different categories depending on the aggressiveness of the initial surgical resection. A clinical staging system was devised for IRS-IV (Table 35.5).[146] This classifica-

TABLE 35.4. *IRS clinical grouping classification*

Group I	Localized disease completely resected
	Confined to organ of origin
	Contiguous involvement
Group II	Total gross resection with evidence of regional spread
	Microscopic residual
	Positive nodes but no microscopic residual
	Positive nodes but microscopic residual in nodes or margins
Group III	Complete resection with gross residual disease
	After biopsy only
	After gross or major resecton of the primary (>50%)
Group IV	Distant metastasis at diagnosis (lung, liver, bones, bone marrow, brain, and nonregional nodes)
	Positive cytology in CSF, pleural, or peritoneal fluid or implants on pleural or peritoneal surfaces are regarded as stage IV

tion relies on clinical findings from physical examination and laboratory and imaging studies. Tumor site, size, regional nodal involvement, and distant metastasis were most predictive of survival.

General Principles of Treatment

Radical surgical excision was the first effective treatment for RMS. For pelvic genitourinary tumors this consisted of total pelvic exenteration. It was later noted that RMS was radiosensitive, but high doses were required for local tumor control. In the 1960s, combination therapy was used with chemotherapy and radiation therapy after attempts at complete surgical excision.[147]

TABLE 35.5. *IRS pretreatment TGNM clinical staging based on clinical, radiographic, and laboratory examination and histology of biopsy*

Stage A:	Favorable site, nonmetastatic
Stage B:	Unfavorable, small, negative nodes, nonmetastatic
Stage C:	Unfavorable, bit or positive nodes, nonmetastatic
Stage D:	Any site, metastatic
Tumor:	$T_{site\ 1}$—Confined to site or origin
	$T_{site\ 2}$—Fixation to surrounding tissues
	<5 cm in size
	>5 cm in size
Histology:	G_1—Favorable histology (mixed, embryonal botryoid, other)
	G_2—Unfavorable histology (alveolar)
Regional lymph nodes:	N_0—regional lymph nodes not clinically involved
	N_1—regional lymph nodes clinically involved
Metastases:	M_0—No distant metastases
	M_{1site}—Metastases present

These efforts found that survival was significantly enhanced if chemotherapy was routinely administered after surgery.[148]

Because of the few patients encountered at any single institution, a cooperative effort was initiated to study the different therapeutic efforts for RMS.[139] During the early years of the IRS (1972–1978), radical surgical intervention before chemotherapy with or without radiation was standard. Once it was demonstrated that most patients would survive the disease, investigators explored the utilization of primary chemotherapy and radiation therapy to avoid exenterative surgery used for genitourinary RMS.[149, 150] A major aim of the protocols for patients with primary tumors in these sites in IRS-II (1978–1984) was preservation of a functional distal urinary tract, while maintaining the high survival rates achieved in IRS-I.[151] Unfortunately, primary chemotherapy with VAC (vincristine, dactinomycin, and cyclophosphamide) did not obviate the need for radiation therapy or radical surgery for patients with pelvic RMS. The percentage of patients alive at 3 years was the same for IRS-II as for IRS-I.[152] In IRS-III (1985–1991), intensification of therapy using a risk-based study design significantly improved overall treatment outcomes. This required more intensive chemotherapy for stage III tumors, but selected patients were able to receive decreased therapy.[153]

Several advances have been made during the IRS studies, including identification of histology, site, and extent of disease as prognostic factors;[146] reduced or eliminated radiation therapy for special groups or sites; and reduced need for radical surgery leading to increased bladder salvage from 25% to 60%[152, 154] and elimination of "routine" lymphadenectomy for localized paratesticular RMS.[155] These advances as they relate to genitourinary tumors are addressed in more detail later.

Specific Sites

Bladder and Prostate Tumors

Urinary obstruction is a frequent clinical presentation of RMS of the bladder or prostate. Signs and symptoms include urinary frequency, stranguria, acute urinary retention, and hematuria. On physical examination, an abdominal mass from a tumor or a distended bladder is often present. Tumors of the bladder usually occur as a botryoid form and grow intraluminally, usually at or near the trigone.[154] Prostatic RMS tends to present as a solid mass rather than in the botryoid form seen in the bladder. Determining the actual site of origin can be difficult. Imaging studies will reveal filling defects within the bladder or elevation of the bladder base in prostatic RMS. CT can delineate the extent of tumor and help evaluate the pelvic and retroperitoneal nodes. Cystoscopic evaluation establishes the diagnosis, and transurethral biopsies can be obtained.

In recent years, surgical treatment of RMS has become more conservative. Initial anterior pelvic exenteration is no longer considered to be the initial therapy in pelvic RMS.[156] Partial bladder resection of the bladder wall for primary tumors affecting the dome or sides of the bladder distant from the trigone is recommended as initial therapy or as a delayed procedure after chemotherapy. Although conservative surgical therapy for bladder tumors has not been as successful as for vaginal primaries, the bladder salvage rate has increased.[152, 157] With the intensification of treatment for pelvic RMS in IRS-III, 60% of patients retained a functional bladder at 4 years from diagnosis, and overall survival exceeds 85%.[158]

There are some concerns about this approach, particularly regarding the number of cases with residual disease after partial cystectomy. Among 22 patients undergoing conservative surgery as primary surgery, there were five instances of local relapse and one of distant relapse.[157] The estimated 3-year survival of 79% was similar to that noted for all patients with primary bladder tumors. However, others have noted that this is a select group of patients who should be expected to have a better prognosis than those with involvement of the bladder base and prostate.[159] In the most recent report from the IRS, partial cystectomy has been used in 40 patients, 33 before any other therapy.[152] Of the long-term survivors, 75% of the patients have no bladder-related symptoms. Bladder augmentation or substitution has been used in some of these patients to achieve good functional results.[160]

Unfortunately, most of these tumors arise from the trigonal area or prostate and are not amenable to local or partial resection. Prostatic involvement has been reported to be a significant predictor of a poor outcome.[128] Local recurrence is high if adequate resection is not accomplished. If chemotherapy does not result in adequate shrinkage to allow partial resection, then radical cystectomy may be necessary. Pelvic exenteration is also used for relapsed tumors.[152] Prostatectomy without cystectomy has been performed in selected patients with persistent disease or local relapse.[152, 161] However, local relapses have occurred in 40% of these patients. The difficulty of assuring complete surgical resection by frozen section can lead to local recurrence.[161]

Paratesticular RMS

Among primary genitourinary tumors, 7 to 10% are located in the paratesticular area.[162] The peak age of presentation ranges from 1 to 5 years of age.[155] Paratesticular RMS arises in the distal portion of the spermatic cord and may invade the testis or surrounding tissues. Paratesticular RMS is usually detected earlier than other genitourinary tumors. It often presents as a unilateral painless scrotal swelling or mass above the testis.

Physical examination reveals the presence a firm mass that usually is distinct from the testis. Ultrasound can confirm the solid nature of the lesion. At diagnosis, 60% of paratesticular tumors are stage I compared to 13% of RMS overall.[163] More than 90% of paratesticular RMS are embryonal in histology and are associated with a good prognosis.

Radical inguinal orchiectomy is recommended for initial treatment. If the tumor is removed with a transcrotal procedure, the risk of local recurrence and nonregional lymph node spread is increased. If cord elements remain after a transcrotal procedure, an inguinal exploration with removal of the remaining spermatic cord and a partial hemi scrotectomy including the earlier scrotal incision is performed.

Before effective chemotherapy, surgery alone produced a 50%, 2-year, relapse-free survival.[164] With current multimodal treatment, survival rates of 90% are expected.[155] An imaging evaluation is performed at diagnosis to exclude metastasis. Extension to retroperitoneal lymph nodes occurs in up to 30% of patients. CT is most frequently used to evaluate the retroperitoneum to identify nodal metastases,[145, 165] but even with advances in imaging there is a significant false-negative rate of CT, 14% for IRS-III patients with paratesticular RMS.[155]

The role of RPLND in paratesticular rhabdomyosarcoma is controversial.[155, 166-168] The initial use of RPLND was based on the management of non-RMS testicular malignancies. It was not thought that the node dissection itself was of therapeutic value but that it was indicated to stage the disease.[169] Patients found to have positive lymph nodes receive radiation therapy to the involved areas.

Arguments against the routine use of RPLND are that grossly involved retroperitoneal nodes can be detected by preoperative imaging studies and that there is significant morbidity associated with the surgery. Heyn et al reported a 10% incidence of intestinal obstruction, 8% ejaculatory dysfunction, and edema of the lower extremities in 5% of patients who had undergone RPLND for paratesticular RMS.[170] However, most of these patients underwent bilateral node dissection. A modified unilateral node dissection is appropriate for staging and, with the addition of nerve sparing techniques, may avoid some of the reported morbidity of node dissection.[171, 172] The capability of laparoscopy to identify retroperitoneal nodal disease in this setting remains to be evaluated, but it may offer a less morbid alternative to RPLND.

Another major argument against routine RPLND is that microscopic nodal disease can be treated effectively by chemotherapy. Olive et al reported on a group of 19 children with paratesticular RMS who had no clinical evidence of retroperitoneal nodal involvement.[166] Nodal recurrence developed in two patients (10.5%), one of whom did not receive any chemotherapy until relapse occurred. Both patients survived after salvage therapy. A subsequent study of the SIOP experience with 46 children with completely excised tumors and negative CT or lymphangiogram treated with intensive chemotherapy alone found that all children survived.[173] However, it should be noted that most of the children received doxorubicin or ifosfamide, both of which have potential for adverse late effects.

During IRS-III 121 children who had paratesticular RMS and had undergone RPLND were reported. Fourteen percent of patients with a negative clinical evaluation were found to have positive lymph nodes on pathologic evaluation.[155] Of the two patients who had nodal relapse, one had previously had a negative RPLND. This suggests a small risk of nodal relapse in these patients if regional radiation therapy and appropriate chemotherapy are received. The overall 5-year survival for the 98 patients with clinically negative nodes was 96%, but fewer than 10% of patients received doxorubicin or alkylating agents. Although the finding of positive retroperitoneal lymph nodes identified a group of patients with decreased survival, it is recommended that patients with clinically negative nodes undergo treatment with primary chemotherapy alone.[167] One exception may be children older than 10 years of age because these patients have a significantly worse prognosis.[155, 174]

Vaginal/Vulvar RMS

Vaginal and vulvar RMS generally present in the first few years of life with vaginal bleeding, discharge, or a vaginal mass. The clinical presentation can be striking if there is prolapse of the mass from the vaginal introitus. The diagnosis is made by vaginoscopy and biopsy of the lesion. The vaginal lesions usually arise from the anterior vaginal wall in the area of the embryonic vesicovaginal septum (urogenital sinus). Vaginal tumors may invade the vesicovaginal septum or bladder wall because of its proximity. Cystoscopy is warranted during initial evaluation and at intervals during follow-up.[175]

Vaginal lesions generally have embryonal or botryoid embryonal histology and have an excellent prognosis.[175] Vulvar lesions may have alveolar histology but, because most are localized, they also have a good prognosis. In addition to initial biopsy, clinical staging, including pelvic and chest CT, and a metastatic work-up are performed.

Anterior pelvic exenteration was frequently used to treat these patients. However, with the development of effective chemotherapy, attempts to preserve the vagina have become a priority. Definitive surgery is delayed until after an initial course of therapy.[176] Once an adequate response is demonstrated, repeat biopsies are obtained. If there is persistence of disease delayed tumor resection is performed, which may consist of partial vaginectomy or vaginectomy with hysterectomy.[175] In

IRS-III, 24 patients with vaginal primaries were treated with a primary chemotherapy protocol. At subsequent surgery, seven patients underwent partial or complete vaginectomy. Six of the latter patients had no viable tumor in the specimen. There was no local recurrence in any of the 24 patients.

Uterine RMS

Uterine RMS may present in two ways: as tumors originating from the cervix with vaginal bleeding or mass, or as tumors originating in the uterine body and presenting as an abdominal mass. Diagnosis is made by incisional or excisional biopsy (usually by dilation and curettage and transvaginal biopsy). More than 90% of uterine tumors are of embryonal histology.[177] In addition to biopsy, staging requires metastatic workup including pelvic examination and CT scans of the pelvis, abdomen and chest, examination of the bone marrow by biopsy or aspiration, cystoscopy, and vaginoscopy.

Older studies reported that patients with uterine RMS represent a distinct group of patients who present at a later age and have more limited response to treatment and thus poorer prognosis than those with vaginal RMS.[178, 179] However, more recent reports suggest that patients with uterine RMS were of the same age group (mean age 5.5 years) as the vaginal RMS patients. Patients treated by primary chemotherapy and delayed resection in IRS-III and pilot IRS-IV responded well to chemotherapy and conservative surgical intervention.[177] With this approach it may be possible to salvage the uterus, vagina, and bladder in many of these patients.[177]

TESTICULAR TUMORS

Testicular tumors are uncommon, representing 1 to 2% of all pediatric solid tumors. The peak incidence occurs in the first 2 years of life.[180, 181] The incidence of germ cell tumors is not as high as in adults, accounting for only 65% of prepubertal testicular tumors. A greater percentage of testicular lesions occurring in children are benign (Table 35.6).

Genetics and Etiology

There is a link between cryptorchidism and germ cell tumors of the testis, but these are rare in childhood.[182] In the German Society of Pediatric Oncology studies, 5% of patients had a history of cryptorchidism.[181] Germ cell tumors are thought to originate from pluripotent progenitor cells. Primordial germ cells migrate during embryogenesis to the gonads. This migratory pattern accounts for the variety of anatomic locations. Cytogenetic analysis of pediatric germ cell tumors reveals predominately diploid karyotypes. The tumor chromosomes are identical to those of the host cells, suggesting

TABLE 35.6. *Classification of prepubertal testicular tumors*

Germ cell tumors
    Yolk sac
    Teratoma
    Mixed germ cell
    Seminoma
Gonadal stromal tumors
    Leydig cell
    Sertoli cell
    Juvenile granulosa cell
    Mixed
Gonadoblastoma
Tumors of supporting tissues
    Fibroma
    Leiomyoma
    Hemangioma
Lymphomas and leukemias
Tumor-like lesions
    Epidermoid cyst
    Hyperplastic nodule secondary to congenital adrenal
       hyperplasia
Secondary tumors
Tumors of the adnexa

(Modified, with permission, from Kay R. Prepubertal testicular tumor registry. J Urol 1993;150:671.)

that they arise by meiotic division of the germ cell.[183] The most common cytogenetic abnormality occurs on the 12th chromosome. The short arm is duplicated, whereas the long arm is lost.[184]

Clinical Presentation and Diagnosis

The most common sign of a testicular tumor is a painless scrotal mass. There is often a delay between first recognition of the scrotal swelling by the parents and the initiation of treatment.[185] Some patients with hormonally active tumors may have nonpalpable intratesticular lesions.

The important feature of germ cell tumors is their production of biologic markers that can be detected in the serum. Alpha-fetoprotein (AFP) is a glycoprotein produced by the fetal yolk sac and found at highest levels in weeks 12 to 15 of gestation. Various benign and malignant conditions can produce elevations of AFP, including yolk sac tumors of the testis. AFP has a half-life of 5 days and degradation curves can be followed after orchiectomy to assess for residual disease. AFP levels are also monitored to detect tumor recurrence. The age of the child must be considered when monitoring serum levels of AFP.[186] AFP levels are high at birth and do not drop to adult levels (<10 ng/mL) until 8 months of age.[187] Recognition of this may eliminate unfounded concern regarding residual disease after orchiectomy for yolk sac tumor in a young infant.

The beta subunit of human chorionic gonadotropin (β-hCG) is a glycoprotein that is produced by em-

bryonal carcinoma and mixed teratomas. The half-life of β-hCG is approximately 24 hours. The normal value for β-hCG is less than 5 IU/L.

Ultrasound is useful in the evaluation of a scrotal mass. Hydrocele fluid around the testicle may prevent palpation of the testis. Ultrasound can detect small lesions not palpable on examination and identify cystic components of a teratoma of the testis or epidermoid cyst. If a benign lesion such as teratoma or epidermoid cyst is suspected preoperatively, a testicular sparing procedure can be considered.[188–190] Color Doppler ultrasound has been reported to be more effective than grayscale ultrasound in detecting intratesticular neoplasms in the pediatric population.[191] CT examination of the retroperitoneum is indicated in patients with malignant testis tumors. Chest radiograph or chest CT is mandatory to exclude pulmonary metastases.

Carcinoma in Situ

Carcinoma in situ (CIS) occurs in most patients with testicular tumors. It has been suggested that CIS is a precursor to the development of invasive germ cell tumor.[192] There is an increased incidence of CIS in subgroups of patients known to be at risk for the development of germ cell tumors including patients with cryptorchidism and intersex disorders.[193] CIS is diagnosed by histologic examination of the testis.

In the prepubertal patient, identification of CIS is more difficult. However a monoclonal antibody recently has been found that binds selectively to seminoma cells that may help detect this lesion.[194] Biopsies at the time of orchidopexy in prepubertal children have rarely demonstrated CIS. Hadziselimovic et al found a 0.4% (11 of 2,528) incidence of CIS in cryptorchid boys.[195] These patients have been observed a mean of 10.4 years. Only one child has reached puberty, but none has developed a testis tumor. The incidence of CIS in the prepubertal patient is significantly lower than that reported for adults. This may be accounted for by the difficulty in recognizing CIS in the prepubertal testis, but many cases may develop later in life. The prepubertal patient with CIS should be observed with a repeat biopsy after puberty because the natural history of the disease in younger patients is unknown.[195] An exception is the patient with androgen insensitivity or dysgenetic gonads.[196]

Germ Cell Tumors

Teratoma is a germ cell tumor with recognizable elements of more than one germ cell layer; endoderm, ectoderm, and mesoderm. The incidence of teratoma is lower than in adults, but it is the second most common testis tumor in children.[185] There may be underreporting of some of these benign tumors to the tumor registries, and reports from some single institutions have noted teratoma to be the most common prepubertal testicular tumor. These tumors generally appear well encapsulated on gross examination. There are multiple cysts present, but consistency on cross section varies with the amount of solid tissue present between the cysts. The microscopic appearance varies with the relative amounts of tissue derived from the different germ layers and the degree of maturation.[197]

Prepubertal teratomas have a benign clinical course that contrasts with the clinical behavior of teratomas in adults, where they have the propensity to metastasize.[197] Radical orchiectomy has been the mainstay of treatment of these tumors. However, ultrasound of the testis can demonstrate the cystic nature of this lesion suggesting the diagnosis of teratoma preoperatively. Other cystic lesions of the testis such as simple cysts of the tunica albuginea or epidermoid cyst must be considered in the differential diagnosis.[190] The latter lesions will generally have a hyperechoic center surrounded by an outer hypoechoic rim. If the preoperative evaluation suggests a benign intratesticular lesion, then a testicle-sparing procedure can be considered.[188, 190, 198] Theoretical concerns include incorrect diagnosis, the presence of multifocal microscopic disease within the testis, and tumor seeding. A detailed review of 21 cases of prepubertal teratoma at the Armed Forces Institute of Pathology did not reveal evidence of multifocal disease or carcinoma in situ of the adjacent testis.[188] Although only a limited number of patients have been treated with enucleation of the tumor, there have been no recurrences reported to date.

The most common prepubertal testicular tumor is yolk sac tumor or endodermal sinus tumor accounting for 60% of all tumors.[182] The peak incidence of childhood yolk sac tumors is in the first 2 years of life. The characteristic histologic finding in yolk sac tumors are Schiller-Duval bodies.[199] Eosinophilic cytoplasmic inclusions are common, and specialized staining techniques demonstrate the presence of AFP. Most tumors are confined to the testis at diagnosis. Radical inguinal orchiectomy is the standard initial therapy for all children with yolk sac tumors.

The lungs are the most common site of distant metastases. Spread to the retroperitoneal lymph nodes is uncommon, with an incidence of only 4 to 6%.[185, 200, 201] Retroperitoneal lymph node dissection (RPLND) has been performed for staging and treatment. Several reviews reported increased survival with the addition of RPLND.[202, 203] However, all of these patients were given adjuvant chemotherapy and radiation therapy if there were involved nodes.

Several factors have decreased the need for RPLND in children with yolk sac tumors. CT imaging of the retroperitoneum can identify most patients who have lymph node metastases, but there is a 15 to 20% false-negative rate.[204] The tumor marker, AFP, can detect residual or metastatic disease. If AFP levels are elevated at diagnosis, patients are observed prospectively. If they reach normal levels, the patient can be assumed to have localized disease. A subsequent increase in AFP is indicative of recurrence. Another justification for omitting RPLND is the ability to salvage relapsed patients with effective combination chemotherapy.[205, 206]

Several of the pediatric oncology cooperative groups in North America (Children's Cancer Group [CCG] and Pediatric Oncology Group [POG]), in Europe (German Society for Pediatric Oncology), and the United Kingdom (Children's Cancer Group) have recently completed studies of children with localized and advanced germ cell tumors.[181, 206, 207] The staging system used by the CCG/POG intergroup study is listed in Table 35.7.

Patients with clinical stage I tumors do not receive additional adjuvant treatment after radical orchiectomy. Chest radiograph and CT or MRI of the retroperitoneum are recommended once every 3 months and then every 6 months until 36 months after treatment. Tumor markers and physical examination are performed at more frequent intervals. Patients with normal or unknown tumor marker levels at diagnosis (marker negative) undergo ipsilateral retroperitoneal lymph node sampling because there is less reliable means of observing the patient for relapse than in marker positive patients.

Children who have previously undergone scrotal biopsy or transcrotal orchiectomy are classified stage II. The study protocol recommended ipsilateral hemiscrotectomy. This approach is no longer recommended in adult patients with gross contamination during removal of germ cell tumors.[208] Patients with persistent elevation of AFP undergo retroperitoneal lymph node sampling. All patients with stage II tumors receive chemotherapy (bleomycin, cisplatin, and etoposide). Children with stage III and IV germ cell tumors initially undergo retro-

TABLE 35.7. *Intergroup staging system for testicular germ cell tumors*

Stage	Extent of disease
I	Limited to testis (testes), completely resected by high inguinal orchiectomy; no clinical, radiographic, or histologic evidence of disease beyond the testes; tumor markers normal after appropriate half-life decline (AFP, 5 days; B-HCG, 16 hours). Patients with normal or unknown tumor markers at diagnosis must have a negative ipsilateral retroperitoneal node sampling to confirm stage I disease.
II	Transcrotal orchiectomy; microscopic disease in scrotum or high in spermatic cord (≤5 cm from proximal end); retroperitoneal lymph node involvement (≤2 cm) or persistently elevated increased tumor markers.
III	Retroperitoneal lymph node involvement (≤2 cm), but no visceral or extraabdominal involvement.
IV	Distant metastases, including liver.

peritoneal lymph node sampling followed by chemotherapy. At 12 weeks, patients with evidence of recurrent disease or elevation of tumor markers undergo surgery. Resection of residual retroperitoneal masses after chemotherapy is performed to establish a histologic diagnosis.[209] Patients with elevated tumor markers after chemotherapy also undergo biopsy or resection. Those patients with persistent viable tumor are then switched to another treatment regimen.

In the German study, 73 of 76 patients with yolk sac tumors had clinical stage I disease at diagnosis.[181] Of 56 patients who did not receive adjuvant chemotherapy, nine developed relapses requiring treatment. Fewer than 50% of the patients with malignant teratoma had stage I disease. Overall survival for all stages was 98.7% at a median of 60 months. Similar findings were reported by the United Kingdom Children's Cancer Study Group.[206]

Gonadal Stromal Tumors

Gonadal stromal tumors are the most common nongerminal testicular tumors in children. Leydig cell tumor is the most common gonadal stromal tumor, with a peak incidence at 4 to 5 years of age. The tumors can produce testosterone resulting in precocious puberty with accelerated skeletal and muscle development.[210] Precocious puberty secondary to pituitary lesions can be excluded by the finding of prepubertal LH and FSH levels with an increased serum testosterone. Other hormones produced by Leydig cell tumors include estrogens, progesterone, and corticosteroids, which can produce gynecomastia.

The differential diagnosis of Leydig cell tumors includes Leydig cell hyperplasia, tumors of adrenal rest tissue, and hyperplastic testicular nodules that develop in boys with poorly controlled congenital adrenal hyperplasia (CAH).[211] Testicular nodules in CAH tend to occur bilaterally, and a family history of CAH is helpful in making the diagnosis.[212] The hyperplastic nodules that develop in CAH resemble Leydig cells histologically but behave biochemically like adrenal cortical cells. Glucocorticoid replacement in CAH will generally produce regression of the hyperplastic nodules,[211] but the presence of fibrosis or calcification in the nodule may prevent this. Testicular sparing procedures can be considered for those patients with lesions unresponsive to steroids.[213] Leydig cell hyperplasia can be distinguished by normal levels of urinary 17-ketosteroids.

Leydig cell tumors appear well encapsulated with compression of the adjacent testicular tissue. They appear yellow to brown on cross-section reflecting the steroid production by the tumor. The pathognomonic histologic feature of Leydig cell tumor, Reinke's crystals, is present in approximately 40% of tumors.[197] Increased mitotic figures or other features suggestive of malignancy are absent in prepubertal Leydig cell tumors. Orchiectomy is adequate treatment in children.[185]

Sertoli cell tumor is the second most common gonadal stromal tumor in children. These tumors are not as actively metabolically as Leydig cell tumors, but gynecomastia has been reported.[214] The typical sign at diagnosis is a painless testicular mass, and orchiectomy generally is adequate treatment. These tumors present at an earlier age than Leydig cell tumors.

Gonadoblastomas are the most common tumors found in association with intersex disorders. Gonadoblastomas are small benign tumors that are bilateral in up to a third of cases. They occur in children with dysgenetic gonads and are associated with the presence of a Y chromosome in the karyotype.[215] The risk of tumor formation in patients with mixed gonadal dysgenesis is 25%,[216] and the incidence increases with age.[215] The germ cell component of gonadoblastoma is prone to malignant degeneration into seminoma and nonseminomatous tumors. Early gonadectomy is advocated as tumors have been reported in children younger than age 5 years.[217, 218] It has been recommended that all streak gonads in patients with gonadal dysgenesis be removed.[219] Patients with gonadal dysgenesis raised as females should have the gonads removed at diagnosis.[217, 218] In addition, all undescended testes should be removed, but scrotal testes can be preserved because they are less prone to develop a tumor. Carcinoma in situ has been demonstrated in gonadal biopsies of children with gonadal dysgenesis, and this has been suggested as a means of identifying those at risk for development of malignant germ cell tumors.[193, 196]

ADRENAL TUMORS

Neuroblastoma

Neuroblastoma is the most common extracranial solid tumor in children and is the most common malignant tumor of infancy. More than 60% of cases occur in children younger than age 2 years, and 97% are noted by the 10th year of life.[220] The overall incidence from birth to age 15 is 8.7 per million per year. Neuroblastoma is known to arise from cells of the neural crest that form the adrenal medulla and sympathetic ganglia. Tumors derived from the sympathetic nervous system are differentiated along two lines: the pheochromocytoma line (see later) and the sympathoblastoma line. The latter includes neuroblastoma, ganglioneuroblastoma, and ganglioneuroma. The variety of locations and degrees of differentiation of these tumors results in a wide range of clinical presentations and behavior.[221]

Genetics and Epidemiology

Familial cases of neuroblastoma have been reported.[222, 223] The median age at diagnosis for familial cases is 9 months, in control to a median age at diagnosis of 21 months for unselected patients with neuroblastoma. At least 20% of patients with familial neuroblastoma have bilateral adrenal or multifocal primary tumors. The risk of neuroblastoma developing in a sibling or offspring of patients with neuroblastoma is less than 6%.[222] These familial cases are thought to represent an autosomal dominant pattern of inheritance. Difficulties in detecting the incidence and penetrance of an inheritable susceptibility to neuroblastoma are caused by the high mortality rate, the complications of therapy that preclude reproduction of multigenerational pedigrees for evaluation, and frequent spontaneous regression and maturation of the tumor.

Karyotypic abnormalities found in neuroblastomas include chromosomal deletions, translocations, and cytogenetic evidence of gene amplification. Deletion of the short arm of chromosome 1 is found in 70 to 80% of neuroblastomas.[224] Deletions of chromosome 1 are found more frequently in children with advanced disease. There have been two reports of constitutional abnormalities involving the short arm of chromosome 1.[225, 226]

Embryology and Spontaneous Regression

In autopsy series of infants younger than 3 months of age, neuroblastoma in situ was found in 1 of 224 infants.[227] Neuroblastoma in situ has been described as small nodules of cells, found incidentally within the adrenal gland that are histologically indistinguishable from neuroblastoma. The incidence of in situ neuroblastoma is much greater than the incidence of clinical tumors, suggesting that spontaneous regression is common. It has been questioned whether these infant autopsy findings truly represent neuroblastoma in situ. Ikeda et al found that these neuroblastic nodules are present in all fetuses, and gradually regress.[228]

The concept of in situ neuroblastoma has been used to support the argument that many neuroblastomas arise and regress spontaneously. In several well-documented cases, infants with clinically evident neuroblastoma have had complete regression of their tumor.[229] Neuroblastoma and ganglioneuroblastoma are also remarkable for their ability to undergo maturation into benign ganglioneuroblastoma and ganglioneuroma. Most cases of spontaneous regression of childhood neuroblastoma occur in the first year of life, but account for only 1 to 2% of patients.[229]

Pathology

The three classic histopathologic patterns of neuroblastoma, ganglioneuroblastoma, and ganglioneuroma reflect a spectrum of maturation and differentiation. Neuroblastoma is characterized by a diffuse growth of small, round, blue cells. Ganglioneuroma is a histologically benign, fully differentiated counterpart of neuroblastoma. It consists of mature ganglion cells, Schwann cells, and nerve bundles. Ganglioneuroblastoma defines a heterogeneous group of tumors with histopathologic features spanning the extremes of maturation represented by neuroblastoma and ganglioneuroma. It is unclear whether ganglioneuroma arises de novo or by maturation of a preexisting neuroblastoma or ganglioneuroblastoma. Cases of metastatic lesions that have been observed to develop the histology of mature ganglioneuroma support the latter theory.[230] A histologic grading classification of neuroblastoma and ganglioneuroblastoma introduced by Shimada et al[231] has been shown to be predictive of outcome when combined with age.[232]

One of the important aspects of the *Shimada classification* is determining whether the tumor is stroma-poor or stroma-rich. Stroma-rich tumors can be separated into three subgroups: nodular, intermixed, or well-differentiated. Tumors in the latter two categories more closely resemble ganglioneuroblastoma or immature ganglioneuroma and are associated with better survival rates. The stroma-poor tumors can be divided into favorable and unfavorable subgroups based on the patient's age at diagnosis, degree of maturation, and the mitotic rate. Patients with stroma-poor tumors with unfavorable histopathologic features have a poor prognosis (<10% survival).[232] When compared with other clinical features, these histologic patterns were independently predictive of outcome.

Diagnosis and Preoperative Evaluation

The clinical manifestations of neuroblastoma depend on the location of the primary tumor, presence of metastases, and secretion of biochemical products. The most common site of origin is the abdomen, and physical examination will usually reveal a fixed, hard abdominal mass. Pelvic neuroblastomas arising from the organ of Zuckerkandl account for only 4% of tumors.[233] Extrinsic compression of the bowel and bladder can produce symptoms of urinary retention and constipation. Most ganglioneuromas are diagnosed in older children and are usually located in the posterior mediastinum and retroperitoneum with only a few arising in the adrenal glands.[234] Ganglioneuromas generally grow to a large size before they cause symptoms as a result of compression of adjacent structures.

Metastases are present in 70% of patients with neuroblastoma at diagnosis and can be responsible for a variety of the clinical signs and symptoms at presentation. Pain is the most frequent symptom. Several unique paraneoplastic syndromes have been associated with localized and disseminated neuroblastoma. Symptoms may mimic pheochromocytoma with paroxysmal hypertension, palpitation, flushing, and headache. Secretion of vasoactive intestinal peptide (VIP) by the tumor can produce severe watery diarrhea and hypokalemia.[235] Another unusual presentation of neuroblastoma is acute myoclonic encephalopathy.[236] Patients develop myoclonus, rapid multidirectional eye movements (opsoclonus), and ataxia. This syndrome may be related to antineural antibodies (e.g., anti-Hu) formed in response to the tumor.[237] These symptoms often disappear with successful therapy and may be associated with a more favorable outcome.[238]

Laboratory Evaluation and Screening

A complete blood count is essential. Anemia is noted in children with widespread bone marrow involvement. Studies suggest that marrow biopsies add substantially to the detection of marrow involvement by tumor compared to marrow aspirates alone.[239] It is recommended that two marrow aspirates and two biopsies be performed. The finding of unequivocal tumor in the marrow and elevated urinary catecholamines establishes the diagnosis of neuroblastoma. When sensitive techniques are used, increased levels of urinary metabolites of catecholamines vanillylmandelic acid (VMA) and homovanillic acid (HVA), are found in 90 to 95% of patients.[240] Therapy with various modalities has been shown to produce a reduction in catecholamine metabolite excretion in most patients.[241] These metabolites can also be studied to detect tumor relapse.

Measurement of urinary catecholamines also provides a noninvasive method for screening infants for neuroblastoma. The goal of screening programs is to detect disease at an earlier stage, which theoretically would lead to improved survival. Since the introduction of mass population screening in Japan, more patients have been diagnosed at younger than 1 year of age,[242] and most of these patients have had lower stage tumors.[243] Before mass screening started, 20% were diagnosed at younger than 1 year of age, whereas 55% were younger than 1 year of age after mass screening was instituted. There are biologic differences in tumors diagnosed by screening compared to tumors detected clinically.[244] These tumors are more likely to have a single copy of N-myc and a diploid chromosome pattern, both of which are associated with a favorable prognosis (see discussion later on prognostic factors).[245] In a large series of 357 patients with tumors diagnosed by mass screening, the overall survival was 97%.[243] This improved survival may not be caused by earlier detection, and these biologically favorable tumors may have a similar outcome detected clinically. It remains to be determined if screening will permit early detection of tumors with intermediate or unfavorable biologic features and thereby improve their prognosis.

Imaging

Calcification within the tumor is common and may be detected on plain radiographs. Ultrasound, which is obtained initially in most children with abdominal masses, will detect a solid tumor. CT and MRI provide more information about the extent of disease, including metastases. Invasion of the renal parenchyma is not uncommon and can be detected radiographically by CT.[246] MRI has advantages over CT in the evaluation of intraspinal tumor extension.[247] Bone scintigraphy and skeletal survey can be used to detect cortical bone metastases.[248] These lesions are found most commonly in the long bones and skull. A bone scan may detect metastases earlier than skeleton long bone films. The use of radiolabeled metaiodobenzylguanidine (MIBG) has become routine in the evaluation of patients with neuroblastoma.[249] This agent is taken up by the adrenergic secretory vesicles of the tumor cells in the primary and in metastatic sites. MIBG scintigraphy can be used to determine the extent of disease and also to detect recurrence of tumor after completion of therapy.[249] However, detection of additional disease by MIBG scans may have little impact on patient treatment.[250]

Staging

Several staging systems have been used in the treatment of neuroblastoma. They all have the common goal of stratifying patients for treatment. In general, the various staging systems give comparable results in distinguishing low-stage, good-prognosis patients from high-stage, poor-prognosis patients. The biggest differences arise when the staging systems are applied to the intermediate-stage patients. The recently proposed International Neuroblastoma Staging System (INSS) is based on clinical, radiographic, and surgical evaluation of children with neuroblastoma (Table 35.8).[251] In addition to the clinical features, there are many biologic studies that can be used to stratify patients for treatment.

Age is an important indicator of outcome,[252] with children aged 1 year or younger having a better survival rate than older children.[253] This difference may be attributable to more favorable biologic parameters in tumors diagnosed at this age. Stage of the disease is an independent prognostic indicator. The proportion of patients presenting with localized, regional, or metastatic disease is age dependent.[253] Virtually all patients with stage I tumors with complete resection of their primary tumor will survive. Patients with stage II tumors also have a more favorable survival, even though there may be incomplete excision.[254] Patients with advanced regional disease, stage III and stage IV, fare less well. The site of origin is of significance with a better survival noted for nonadrenal primary tumors.[233] Children with thoracic neuroblastoma have an improved survival even when this result is corrected for age and stage.[255]

TABLE 35.8. *International neuroblastoma staging system*

Stage	Description
I	Localized tumor confined to the area of origin; complete gross excision, with or without microscopic residual disease; identifiable ipsilateral and contralateral lymph nodes negative microscopically.
IIA	Unilateral tumor with incomplete gross excision; identifiable ipsilateral nonadherent lymph nodes negative microscopically.
IIB	Unilateral tumor with complete or incomplete gross excision; with positive ipsilateral nonadherent lymph nodes; identifiable contralateral lymph nodes negative microscopically.
III	Tumor infiltrating across the midline (vertebral column) with or without regional lymph node involvement; or unilateral tumor with contralateral regional lymph node involvement; or midline tumor with bilateral regional lymph node involvement or extension by infiltration.
IV	Dissemination of tumor to distant lymph nodes, bone, bone marrow, liver, or other organs (except as defined in stage IVS).
IVS	Localized primary tumor as defined for stage I or 2 with dissemination limited to liver, skin, or bone marrow (<10% tumor) in infants younger than 1 year.

A distinct group of infants with neuroblastoma present with distant liver, skin, and bone marrow metastases without radiologic evidence of bone metastases.[256] The median age of these infants is approximately 3 months. This group of patients, Stage IV-S (S, special) has an overall good prognosis ranging from 80 to 87% survival rate. Many of these tumors undergo spontaneous regression.[257, 258] Studies of children with stage IV-S neuroblastoma have not revealed adverse prognostic findings such as N-myc oncogene amplification (see later) typically seen in children with stage IV disease.[259]

Biologic Variables

The presence of homogenously staining regions (HSRs) and double minute chromosomes (DMs) has been noted in approximately a third of neuroblastoma tumors. These abnormalities are cytogenetic manifestations of gene amplification, and it has been found that the N-myc oncogene is mapped to these regions. The association of N-myc amplification with the pathogenesis of neuroblastoma is unclear,[221] but it has been shown that N-myc amplification is associated with an adverse prognosis.[260, 261] The poor prognosis associated with N-myc amplification is independent of patient age or stage of disease at presentation. Amplification is found in 5 to 10% of patients with low stages of disease and stage IV-S[259] but 30 to 40% of patients with advanced disease.[262, 263] However, not all patients with a poor outcome have N-myc amplification. Many advanced-stage

tumors lack N-myc amplification at diagnosis, and recurrence or progressive disease develops in most of these patients.

DNA content of tumor cells and ploidy number have been reported to have prognostic value in patients with neuroblastoma. Studies of DNA content measured by flow cytometry showed that a "hyperdiploid" karyotype (or increased DNA content) was associated with a favorable outcome.[264, 265] DNA diploidy and tetraploidy were associated with decreased survival. Deletions of the short arm of chromosome 1 are found in 70 to 80% of the near-diploid tumors that have been karyotyped.[262, 263] Preliminary studies suggest a correlation between lp deletion and poor survival.[262, 266] Because there is an association between N-myc amplification and lp deletion, it remains to be determined if this finding has independent prognostic significance.

Abnormalities of nerve growth receptors have been found in neuroblastoma. Increased expression of high-affinity nerve growth factor receptor correlates with an improved outcome.[267] Lack of expression of this growth factor receptor correlates with N-myc amplification and poor survival.[268]

Treatment

Multidisciplinary treatment is necessary for the management of most children with neuroblastoma. The extent to which surgery, chemotherapy, and radiotherapy are used in individual patients will vary depending on tumor stage, age, and other prognostic factors (Table 35.8).

Low-Risk Disease

Primary surgical excision plays a greater role in the management of children with low-stage disease. The goals of surgery are to establish the diagnosis, excise the tumor if localized, provide tissue for biologic studies, and to stage the tumor. Resectability of the primary tumor should take into consideration tumor location, mobility, relationship to major vessels, and overall prognosis of the patient. Surgical excision alone is adequate for Stage I neuroblastoma and for children with Stage II disease with favorable biologic characteristics.[253, 269] The Pediatric Oncology Group reviewed 101 children with localized neuroblastoma treated by surgical excision without routine postoperative adjuvant chemotherapy.[253] Nine patients developed relapses, but six were salvaged with chemotherapy. The overall survival for stage I and II exceeds 90%. Children older than 1 year of age with N-myc amplification, Shimada unfavorable histology, or significant amounts of occult bone marrow tumor by immunohistology may be at greater risk for relapse.[270]

Intermediate-Risk Disease

Included in this intermediate group are infants with stage 4 disease and all patients with stage 3 disease who have favorable biologic features—favorable Shimada classification, serum ferritin less than 143 ng/mL, and absence of N-myc amplification.[271] All patients with stage 3 disease younger than age 1 year regardless of biologic characteristics are in this group.[272] These patients should undergo surgical resection followed by postoperative chemotherapy. Radical resection probably is not justified in this group of patients. Radiation of the local tumor bed has been advocated for treatment of residual disease in patients with stage II disease. However, a report of 156 patients with stage II neuroblastoma found a 90% 6-year progression-free survival whether radiotherapy was used.[254]

The criteria for treatment of infants with stage IV-S tumors have yet to be standardized. Resection of the primary is not mandatory.[257, 273] Although excellent survival has been reported after surgery,[274] information regarding histologic prognostic factors was unavailable for all of these patients. Patients with extensive metastatic disease who are N-myc positive represent a high-risk group.[274] Infants younger than 6 weeks of age at diagnosis are also at increased risk.[273] These patients should be considered for a more aggressive treatment with chemotherapy or hepatic irradiation.

High-Risk Disease

Included in this category are all patients with stage 4 disease older than 1 year at diagnosis and patients with stage 3 disease older than 1 year with unfavorable biology—N-myc amplification, unfavorable Shimada classification, or serum ferritin greater than 143 ng/mL. Also at high risk are children with stage 2 disease and N-myc amplification and infants with stage 4 disease and N-myc amplification.

There is some debate about the aggresiveness of the surgical resection required for stage III lesions. With the efficacy of modern chemotherapy in reducing the size of primary tumors, sacrifice of vital structures to achieve resection at diagnosis should be avoided, particularly in young children in whom prognosis is excellent. A report of 58 patients with stage III disease found that 8 of 12 with initial complete excision and 12 of 14 with subsequent resection of the primary tumor were long-term survivors.[275] This contrasts with only 9 of 32 survivors among patients in whom complete tumor excision could not be accomplished. There was significant morbidity reported in association with the surgical procedures with 21 major complications. In a retrospective review, Kieley compared the results of radical tumor resection with those of more conventional surgery in patients with stage III and IV disease.[276] He found that survival in 46 patients treated with radical surgical procedures did not differ from that of 34 patients treated with more conventional surgery. Shorter et al also did not find any evidence that the extent of surgical resection had an impact on the survival of patients with stage IV disease.[277]

Usually the safest approach for advanced tumors is to defer tumor resection until after initial chemotherapy.[278] After chemotherapy the tumors are smaller and firmer with less risk of rupture and hemorrhage. Timing of surgery is generally 13 to 18 weeks after initiation of chemotherapy.[247] Some tumors will remain inoperable after chemotherapy. Other attempts at local tumor control for unresectable diseases have included the use of intraoperative radiation therapy. This technique has the advantage of delivering a higher dose of radiation to the operative field while sparing normal adjacent tissues.[247]

Several multiagent treatment regimens have been developed to treat high-risk patients with neuroblastoma. The goal of this treatment intensification is better disease control. Although initial response rates are improving with a prolonged time to progression of disease, relapse continues to be a major problem with 4-year overall survival of 10 to 20%.[279, 280] The dose intensification of chemotherapy needed for local tumor control results in significant myelosuppression, limiting the amount of therapy that can be given. This has prompted the use of autologous bone marrow transplantation after sublethal chemotherapy or total body irradiation.

The use of marrow-ablative chemoradiotherapy followed by autologous marrow reinfusion has resulted in complete remission in up to 40% of patients with recurrent stage IV disease.[281–283] However, a significant problem is the late risk of relapse. The presence of bulky disease results in increased failure. Tumor debulking with surgery or radiation therapy is warranted before autologous bone marrow transplantation. There are many questions yet to be resolved with this modality of treatment. Toxicity of bone marrow transplantation can be lethal, and the long-term complications that will occur in patients successfully transplanted are unknown. However, these risks are necessary given that long-term survival is difficult to achieve in these patients.

Another option in the treatment of metastatic neuroblastoma is the use of I[131] MIBG.[284] The finding that the primary tumor and metastatic areas take up this radiotracer suggested the possibility that therapeutic doses can be delivered to the tumor. The overall response rate is 30%. Other biologic targeted therapies being investigated are monoclonal antibodies to the GD2 ganglioside[285] and the use of cis-retinoic acid to induce maturation and growth arrest.[286]

REFERENCES

1. Breslow N, Olshan A, Beckwith JB, Green DM. Epidemiology of Wilms' tumor. Med Pediatr Oncol 1993;21:172.

2. Miller RW, Fraumeni JF, Mannnig MD. Association of Wilms tumor with aniridia, hemihypertrophy and other congenital malformations. N Engl J Med 1964;270:922.
3. Clericuzio CL, Johnson C. Screening for Wilms tumor in high-risk individuals. Hematol Oncol Clin North Am 1995;9:1253.
4. Beckwith JB. Macroglossia, omphalocele, adrenal cytomegaly, gigantism and hyperplastic visceromegaly. Birth Defects: Original Article Series 1969;5:188.
5. Sotelo-Avila C, Gonzalez-Crussi F, Fowler JW. Complete and incomplete forms of Beckwith-Wiedemann syndrome: Their oncogenic potential. J Pediatr 1980;96:47.
6. Perlman M, Levin M, Wittels B. Syndrome of fetal gigantism, renal hamartomas, and nephroblastomatosis with Wilms' tumor. Cancer 1975;35:1212.
7. Olson JM, Hamilton A, Breslow NE. Non-11p constitutional chromosome abnormalities in Wilms tumor patients. Med Pediatr Oncol 1995;24:305.
8. Breslow NE, Beckwith JB. Epidemiological features of Wilms' tumor: results of the National Wilms' Tumor Study. J Natl Cancer Inst 1982;68:429.
9. Drash A, Sherman F, Hartmann WH, Blizzard RM. A syndrome of pseudohermaphroditism, Wilms tumor, hypertension and degenerative renal disease. J Pediatr 1970;76:585.
10. Denys P, Malvaux P, Van Den Berghe H, Tanghe W, Proesmans W. Association d'un syndrome anatomo-pathologique de pseudohermaphrodisitism masculin, d'une tumeur de Wilms, d'une nephropathie parenchymateuse dt d'un mosaicism XX/XY. Arch Fr Pediatr 1967;24:729.
11. Coppes MJ, Huff V, Pelletier J. Denys-Drash syndrome: relating a clinical disorder to genetic alterations in the tumor suppressor gene WT1. J Pediatr 1993;123:673.
12. Tank ES, Melvin T. The association of Wilms' tumor with nephrologic disease. J Pediatr Surg 1990;25:724.
13. Knudson AG, Strong LC. Mutation and cancer: a model for Wilms' tumor of the kidney. J Natl Cancer Inst 1972;48:313.
14. Breslow N, Olson J, Moksness J, et al. Familial Wilms tumor: a descriptive study. Med Pediatr Oncol 1996;27:398.
15. Green DM, Fine NE, Li FP. Offspring of patients treated for unilateral Wilms' tumor in childhood. Cancer 1982;49:2285.
16. Li FP, Gimbrere K, Gelber RD, et al. Outcome of pregnancy in survivors of Wilms tumor. JAMA 1987;257:216.
17. Coppes MJ, Haber DA, Grundy P. Genetic events in the development of Wilms tumor: current concepts. N Engl J Med 1994;331:586.
18. Riccardi VM, Sujansky E, Smith AC, Francke U. Chromosomal imbalance in the aniridia-Wilms' tumor association: 11p interstitial deletion. Pediatrics 1978;61:604.
19. Koufos A, Hansen MF, Lampkin BC, et al. Loss of alleles at loci on human chromosome 11 during genesis of Wilms' tumor. Nature 1984;309:170–172.
20. Huff V. Inheritance and functionality of Wilms tumor genes. Cancer Bull 1994;46:255–259.
21. Call KM, Glaser T, Ito CY, et al. Isolation and characterization of a zinc finger polypeptide gene at the human chromosome 11. Cell 1990;55:827.
22. Ton CC, Hirvoven H, Miwa H, et al. Positional cloning and characterization of a paried box- and homeobox-containing gene from the aniridia region. Cell 1991;67:1059.
23. Huff V, Villalba F, Riccardi VM, et al. Alteration of the WT1 gene in patients with Wilms' tumor and genitourinary anomalies. Am J Hum Genet 1991;49:44 Abstract.
24. Pelletier J, Bruening W, Kashtan CE, et al. Germline mutations in the Wilms' tumor suppressor gene are associated with abnormal urogenital development in Denys-Drash syndrome. Cell 1991;67:437.
25. Varanasi R, Bardeesy N, Ghahremani M, et al. Fine structure analysis of the WT1 gene in sporadic Wilms tumor. Proc Natl Acad Sci USA 1994;91:3554.
26. Clericuzio CL. Screening for Wilms tumor in high-risk individuals. Dial Pediatr Urol 1996;19:2.
27. Reeve AE, Sih SA, Raizis AM, Feinberg AP. Loss of allelic heterozygosity at a second locus on chromosome 11 in sporadic Wilms' tumor cells. Molec Cell Biol 1989;44:711.
28. Koufos A, Grundy P, Morgan K, et al. Familial Wiedmann-

29. Beckwith syndrome and a second Wilms tumor locus both map to 11p15.5. Am J Hum Genet 1989;44:711–719.
30. Schroeder WT, Chao L, Dao DD, et al. Nonrandom loss of maternal chromosome 11 alleles in Wilms' tumors. Am J Hum Genet 1987;40:413.
30. Grundy P, Coppes MJ, Haber D. Molecular genetics of Wilms tumor. Hematol Oncol Clin North Am 1995;9:1201.
31. Grundy PE, Telzerow PE, Breslow N, et al. Loss of heterozygosity for chromosomes 16q and 1p in Wilms tumor predicts an adverse outcome. Cancer Res 1994;54:2331–2333.
32. Bardeesy N, Falkoff D, Petruzzi MJ, et al. Anaplastic Wilms tumour, a subtype displaying poor prognosis, harbours p53 gene mutations. Nat Genet 1994;7:91.
33. Schmidt D, Beckwith JB. Histopathology of childhood renal tumors. Hematol Oncol Clin North Am 1995;9:1179.
34. Beckwith JB, Zuppan CE, Browning NG, Moksness J, Breslow NE. Histological analysis of aggressiveness and responsiveness in Wilms tumor. Med Pediatr Oncol 1996;27:422.
35. Beckwith JB, Palmer NF. Histopathology and prognosis of Wilms tumor. Results from the National Wilms Tumor Study. Cancer 1978;41:1937–1948.
36. Bonadio JF, Storer B, Norkool P, et al. Anaplastic Wilms' tumor: clinical and pathological studies. J Clin Oncol 1985;3:513–520.
37. Faria P, Beckwith JB. A new definition of focal anaplasia (FA) in Wilms tumor identifies cases with good outcome. A report from the National Wilms Tumor Study. Mod Pathol 1993;6:3p. Abstract.
38. Zuppan CW, Beckwith JB, Luckey DW. Anaplasia in unilateral Wilms tumor: a report from the National Wilms Tumor Study Pathology Center. Hum Pathol 1988;19:1199.
39. Beckwith JB, Kiviat NB, Bonadio JF. Nephrogenic rests, nephroblastomatosis, and the pathogenesis of Wilms' tumor. Pediatr Pathol 1990;10:1–36.
40. Bennington JL, Beckwith JB. Tumors of the kidney, renal pelvis, ureter. In: Atlas of Tumor Pathology, Second Series, Fasicle 12. Bethesda: Armed Forces Institute of Pathology 1975.
41. Bove KE, McAdams AJ. The nephroblastomatosis complex and its relationship to Wilms' tumor: a clinicopathologic treatise. Perspect Pediatr Pathol 1976;3:185–223.
42. Beckwith JB. Precursor lesions of Wilms tumor: clinical and biological implications. Med Pediatr Oncol 1993;21:158–168.
43. Rainwater LM, Hosaka Y, Farrow GM, et al. Wilms tumors: relationship of nuclear deoxyribonucleic acid ploidy to patient survival. J Urol 1987;138:974.
44. Layfield LJ, Ritchie AWS, Ehrlich R. The relationship of deoxyribonucleic acid content to conventional prognostic factors in Wilms' tumor. J Urol 1989;142:1040–1043.
45. Partin AW, Walsh AC, Epstein JI, et al. Nuclear morphometry as a predictor of response to therapy in Wilms' tumor: A preliminary report. J Urol 1990;144:1222.
46. Partin AW, Yoo JK, Crooks D, et al. Prediction of disease-free survival after theray in Wilms' tumor using nuclear morphometric techniques. J Pediatr Surg 1994;29:456.
47. Ritchey ML, Kelalis PP, Breslow N, et al. Intracaval and atrial involvement with nephrobalastoma: review of National Wilms' Tumor Study-3. J Urol 1988;140:1113.
48. Coppes MJ, Zandvoort SWH, Sparling CR, et al. Acquired von Willebrand disease in Wilms tumor patients. J Clin Oncol 1993;10:1–7.
49. Stern M, Longaker MT, Adzick NS, et al. Hyaluronidase levels in urine from Wilms' tumor patients. J Natl Cancer Inst 1991;83:1569.
50. Lin RY, Argent PA, Sullivan KM, Stern R, Adzick NS. Urinary hyaluronic acid is a Wilms tumor marker. J Pediatr Surg 1995;30:304.
51. Voute PA, Van Der Meer J, Staugaard-Kloosterziel W. Plasma renin activity in Wilms' tumour. Acta Endocrinologica 1971;67:197.
52. Johnston MA, Carachi R, Lindop GBM, Leckie B. Inactive renin levels in recurrent nephroblastoma. J Pediatr Surg 1991;26:613–614.
53. Ritchey ML, Kelalis PP. Imaging of renal tumors. Curr Opin Urol 1992;2:428.
54. Ritchey ML, Kelalis PP, Breslow N, et al. Surgical complications

following nephrectomy for Wilms' tumor: A report of National Wilms' Tumor Study-3. Surg Gynecol Obstet 1992a;175:507.

55. Babyn P, Owens C, Gyepes M, D'Angio GJ. Imaging patients with Wilms tumor. Hematol Oncol Clin North Am 1995;9:1217.

56. Cohen MD. Staging of Wilms' tumor. Clin Radiol 1993;47:77.

57. D'Angio GJ, Rosenberg H, Sharples K, Kelalis P, Breslow N, Green DM. Position paper: imaging methods for primary renal tumors of childhood: cost versus benefits. Med Pediatr Oncol 1993;21:205–212.

58. Ditchfield MR, DeCampo JF, Waters KD, Nolan TM. Wilms' tumor: a rational use of preoperative imaging. Med Pediatr Oncol 1995;24:93–96.

59. D'Angio GJ, Breslow N, Beckwith JB, et al. Treatment of Wilms' tumor: results of the Third National Wilms' Tumor Study. Cancer 1989;64:349–360.

60. Ng YY, Hall-Craggs MA, Dicks-Mireaux C, Pritchard J. Wilms' tumour: Pre- and post-chemotherapy CT appearances. Clin Radiol 1991;43:255.

61. Othersen HB Jr, DeLorimer A, Hrabovsky E, et al. Surgical evaluation of lymph node metastases in Wilms' tumor. J Pediatr Surg 1990;25:3:1.

62. Weese DL, Applebaum H, Taber P. Mapping intravascular extension of Wilms' tumor with magnetic resonance imaging. J Pediatr Surg 1991;26:64.

63. Goleta-Dy A, Shaw PJ, Stevens MM. Re: the necessity of contralateral surgical exploration in Wilms' tumor with modern noninvasive imaging technique: a reassessment. (Letter). J Urol 1992;147:171.

64. Koo AS, Koyle MA, Hurwitz RS, et al. The necessity of contralateral surgical exploration in Wilms' tumor with modern noninvasive imaging technique: a reassessment. J Urol 1990;144:416–417.

65. Kessler O, Franco I, Jayabose S, Reda E, Levitt S, Brock W. Is contralateral exploration of the kidney necessary in patients with Wilms tumor? J Urol 1996;156:693.

66. Ritchey ML, Green DM, Breslow NE, Norkool P. Accuracy of current imaging modalities in the diagnosis of synchronous bilateral Wilms tumor. Cancer 1995;75:600.

67. Green DM, Fernbach DJ, Norkool P, Kollia G, D'Angio GJ. The treatment of Wilms' tumor patients with pulmonary metastases detected only with computed tomography: a report from the National Wilms' Tumor Study. J Clin Oncol 1991;9:1776–1781.

68. Wilimas J, Douglass EC, Magill HL, Fitch S, Hutsu HO. Significance of pulmonary computed tomography at diagnosis in Wilms' tumor. J Clin Oncol 1988;6:1144.

69. Cohen MD. Current controversey: is CT scan of the chest needed in patients with Wilms tumor? Am J Pediatr Hematol Oncol 1994;16:191–193.

70. Hartman GE, Smolik LM, Shochat S. The dilemma of the multicystic dysplastic kidney. Am J Dis Child 1986;140:925.

71. Oddone M, Marino C, Sergi C, et al. Wilms' tumor arising in a multicystic kidney. Pediatr Radiol 1994;24:236.

72. Beckwith JB. Wilms tumor in multicystic dysplastic kidneys: what is the risk? Dial Pediatr Urol 1996b;19:3–5.

73. Green DM, Breslow NE, Beckwith JB, Norkool P. Screening of children with hemihypertrophy, aniridia, and Beckwith-Wiedemann syndrome in patients in patients with Wilms' tumor: a report from the National Wilms Tumor Study. Med Pediatr Oncol 1993a;21:188–192.

74. Craft AW, Parker L, Stiller C, Cole M. Screening for Wilms tumour in patients with aniridia, Beckwith syndrome, or hemihypertrophy. Med Pediatr Oncol 1995;24:231–234.

75. Ritchey ML, Lally KP, Haase GM, Shochat SJ, Kelalis PP. Superior mesenteric artery injury during nephrectomy for Wilms' tumor. J Pediatr Surg 1992b;27:612.

76. Dykes EH, Marwaha RK, Dicks-Mireaux C, et al. Risks and benefits of percutaneous biopsy and primary chemotherapy in advanced Wilms' tumour. J Pediatr Surg 1991;26:610–2.

77. Ritchey ML, Kelalis PP, Haase GM, et al. Preoperative therapy for intracaval and atrial extension of Wilms' tumor. Cancer 1993a;71:41–4.

78. Ritchey ML, Kelalis P, Breslow N, Etzioni R, Haase G. Small bowel obstruction following nephrectomy for Wilms' tumor. Ann Surg 1993b;218:654.

79. Bracken RB, Sutow WW, Jaffe N, Ayala A, Guarda L. Preoperative chemotherapy for Wilms' tumor. Urology 1982;19:55–60.

80. Ritchey ML, Pringle K, Breslow N, et al. Management and outcome of inoperable Wilms tumor. A report of National Wilms' Tumor Study. Ann Surg 1994;220:683.

81. Farewell VT, D'Angio GJ, Breslow N, Norkool P. Retrospective validation of a new staging system for Wilms' tumor. Cancer Clin Trials 1981;4:167–171.

82. D'Angio GJ, Evans AE, Breslow N, et al. The treatment of Wilms' tumor: results of the National Wilms' Tumor Study. Cancer 1976;38:633–646.

83. D'Angio GJ, Evans A, Breslow N, et al. The treatment of Wilms' tumor: results of the Second National Wilms' Tumor Study. Cancer 1981;47:2302–2311.

84. Green DM, Breslow NE, Evans I, Moksness J, D'Angio GJ. Treatment of children with stage IV favorable histology Wilms tumor: a report from the National Wilms Tumor Study Group. Med Pediatr Oncol 1996;26:147.

85. Green DM, Breslow NE, Evans I, et al. Effect of dose intensity of chemotherapy on the hematological toxicity of the treatment of Wilms tumor. A report from the National Wilms Tumor Study. Am J Pediatr Hematol Oncol 1994c;16:207–212.

86. Green D, Breslow N, Beckwith J, et al. A comparison between single dose and divided dose administration of dactinomycin and doxorubicin. A report from the National Wilms Tumor Study Group. Proceedings of the American Society of Clinical Oncology, 1996.

87. Garcia M, Douglass C, Schlosser JV. Classification and prognosis in Wilms' tumor. Radiology 1963;80:574.

88. Green DM, Jaffee N. The role of chemotherapy in the treatment of Wilms' tumor. Cancer 1979;44:52.

89. Larsen E, Perez-Atayde A, Green DM, et al. Surgery only for the treatment of patients with stage I (Cassady) Wilms' tumor. Cancer 1990;66:264–266.

90. Green DM, Beckwith JB, Weeks DA, et al. The relationship between microsubstaging variables, tumor weight and age at diagnosis of children with stage I/favorable histology Wilms tumor. A report from the National Wilms Tumor Study. Cancer 1994b;74:1817–1820.

91. Weeks DA, Beckwith JB. Relapse-associated variables in stage I, favorable histology Wilms' tumor. Cancer 1987;60:1204.

92. Lemerle J, Voute PA, Tournade MF, et al. Preoperative versus postoperative radiotherapy, single versus multiple courses of actinomycin D, in the treatment of Wilms' tumor: preliminary results of a controlled clinical trial conducted by the International Society of Paediatric Oncology (SIOP). Cancer 1976;38:647.

93. Lemerle J, Voute PA, Tournade MF, et al. Effectiveness of preoperative chemotherapy in Wilms' tumor: results of an International Society of Paediatric Oncology (SIOP) clinical trial. J Clin Oncol 1983;1:604.

94. Green DM, Breslow NE, D'Angio GJ. The treatment of children with unilateral Wilms tumor. J Clin Oncol 1993c;11:1009–1010.

95. Tournade MF, Com-Nougue C, Voute PA, et al. Results of the sixth International Society of Pediatric Oncology Wilms' tumor trial and study: a risk-adapted therapeutic approach in Wilms' tumor. J Clin Oncol 1993;11:1014.

96. Blute ML, Kelalis PP, Offord KP, et al. Bilateral Wilms' tumor. J Urol 1987;138:968–973.

97. Montgomery BT, Kelalis PP, Blute ML, et al. Extended follow-up of bilateral Wilms' tumor: results of the National Wilms Tumor Study. J Urol 1991;146:514.

98. Coppes MJ, deKraker J, vanKijken PJ, et al. Bilateral Wilms' tumor: long-term survival and some epidemiological features. J Clin Oncol 1989;7:310–315.

99. Shaul DB, Srikanth MM, Ortega JA, Mahour GH. Treatment of bilateral Wilms' tumor: comparison of initial biopsy and chemotherapy to initial surgical resection in the preservation of renal mass and function. J Pediatr Surg 1992;27:1009.

100. Ritchey ML, Green DM, Thomas P, et al. Renal failure in Wilms tumor. Proceedings of SIOP, 25th Annual Meeting. Med Pediatr Oncol 1996;26:75–80.

101. Ritchey ML, Coppes M. The management of synchronous bilateral Wilms tumor. Hematol Oncol Clin North Am 1995;9:1303.

102. Penn I. Renal transplantation for Wilms' tumor: report of 20 cases. J Urol 1979;122:793.
103. McLorie GA, McKenna PH, Greenburg M, et al. Reduction in tumor burden allowing partial nephrectomy following preoperative chemotherapy in biopsy proved Wilms' tumor. J Urol 1991;146:509.
104. Cozzi F, Schiavetti A, Clerico A, et al. Tumor enucleation in unilateral Wilms' tumor: a pilot study. Med Pediatr Oncol 1995;25:313.
105. Grundy P, Breslow N, Green DM, et al. Prognostic factors for children with recurrent Wilms' tumor: results from the Second and Third National Wilms Tumor Study. J Clin Oncol 1989;7:638–647.
106. Tannous R, Coccia P, Sposto R, et al. Salvage intensive/sequential chemotherapy plus surgery for Wilms tumor: a Childrens Cancer Group study report. Proceedings of ASCO, 1995.
107. Breslow NE, Takashima JR, Whitton JA, et al. Second malignant neoplasms following treatment for Wilms' tumor: a report from the National Wilms' Tumor Study Group. J Clin Oncol 1995;13:1851–1859.
108. Gilladoga AC, Manuel C, Tan CT, et al. The cardiotoxicity of adriamycin and daunomycin in children. Cancer 1976;37:1070–1078.
109. Steinherz LJ, Steinherz PG, Tan CTC, et al. Cardiac toxicity 4 to 20 years after anthracycline therapy. JAMA 1991;266:1672.
110. Green DM, Breslow NE, Moksness J, D'Angio GJ. Congestive failure following initial therapy for Wilms tumor. A report from the National Wilms Tumor Study. Pediatr Res 1994d;35:161A. Abstract.
111. Kinsella TJ, Trivette G, Rowland J, et al. Long-term follow-up of testicular function following radiation for early-stage Hodgkin's disease. J Clin Oncol 1989;7:718–724.
112. Stillman RJ, Schinfeld JS, Schiff I, et al. Ovarian failure in long term survivors of childhood malignancy. Am J Obstet Gynecol 1987;139:62.
113. Marsden HB, Lawler W. Bone metastasizing renal tumour of childhood: histopathological and clinical review of 38 cases. Virchows Arch 1980;387:341.
114. Green DM, Breslow NE, Beckwith JB, et al. The treatment of children with clear cell sarcoma of the kidney. A report from the National Wilms Tumor Study Group. J Clin Oncol 1994a;12:2132–2137.
115. Bonnin JM, Rubenstein IJ, Palmer NF, Beckwith JB. The association of embryonal tumors originating in the kidney and the brain. Cancer 1984;54:2137–2146.
116. Banner MP, Pollack HM, Chatten J, Witzleben C. Multilocular renal cysts: radiologic-pathologic correlation. AJR 1981;136:239.
117. Joshi VV, Beckwith JB. Multilocular cyst of the kidney (cystic nephroma) and cystic, partially differentiated nephroblastoma. Terminology and criteria for diagnosis. Cancer 1989;64:466–479.
118. Hartman D, Davis C, Madewell J, Friedman A. Primary malignant tumors in the second decade of life: Wilms tumor versus renal cell carcinoma. J Urol 1982;127:888–891.
119. Broecker B. Renal cell carcinoma in children. Urology 1991;38:54–56.
120. Raney RB Jr, Palmer N, Sutow W, et al. Renal cell carcinoma in children. Med Pediatr Oncol 1983;11:91.
121. Howell CJ, Othersen HB, Kiviat NE, et al. Therapy and outcome in 51 children with mesoblastic nephroma: a report of the National Wilms' Tumor study. J Pediatr Surg 1982;17:826–830.
122. Tomlinson GE, Argyle JC, Velasco S, Nisen PD. Molecular characterization of congenital mesoblastic nephroma and its distinction from Wilms tumor. Cancer 1992;70:2358.
123. Joshi VJ, Kasznica J, Walters TR. Atypical mesoblastic nephroma: pathologic characterization of a potentially aggressive variant of conventional congenital mesoblatic nephroma. Arch Pathol Lab Med 1986;110:100–106.
124. Gormley TS, Skoog SJ, Jones RV, Maybee D. Cellular congenital mesoblastic nephroma: what are the options? J Urol 1989;142:479–483.
125. Beckwith JB. Congenital mesoblastic nephroma. When should we worry? Arch. Pathol Lab Med 1986;110:98–99.
126. Heidelberger KP, Ritchey ML, Dauser RC, McKeever PE, Beck-with JB. Congenital mesoblastic nephroma metastatic to the brain. Cancer 1993;72:2499–2502.
127. Maurer HM, Beltangady M, Gehan EA, et al. The Intergroup Rhabdomyosarcoma Study-I. A final report. Cancer 1988;61:209.
128. Crist WM, Garnsey L, Beltangady MS, et al. Prognostic factors in children with rhabdomyosarcoma: a report of the Intergroup Rhabdomyosarcoma Studies I and II. J Clin Oncol 1990;8:443.
129. Rodary C, Rey A, Olive D, et al. Prognostic factors in 281 children with non-metastatic rhabdomyosarcoma (RMS) at diagnosis. Med Pediatr Oncol 1988;16:71.
130. LaQualgia M, Heller G, Ghavami F, et al. The effect of age at diagnosis on outcome in rhabdomyosarcoma. Cancer 1994;73:109.
131. Li FP, Fraumeni JF Jr. Soft-tissue sarcomas, breast cancer, and other neoplasms. A familial syndrome? Ann Intern Med 1969;71:747.
132. Malkin D, Li FP, Strong LC, et al. Germ line p53 mutations in a familial syndrome of breast cancer, sarcomas, and other neoplasms. Science 1990;250:1233.
133. McKeen EA, Bodurtha J, Meadows AT, et al. Rhabdomyosarcoma complicating multiple neurofibromatosis. J Pediatr 1978;93:992.
134. Douglass EC, Valentine M, Etucabana E. A specific chromosomal abnormality in rhabdomyosarcoma. Cytogenet Cell Genet 1987;45:148.
135. Scrable HJ, Johnson DK, Rinchik EM, et al. Rhabdomyosarcoma associated locus and MyoD1 are synetic but separate loci on the short arm of chromosome 11. Proc Natl Acad Sci USA 1990;87:2182.
136. Parham DM. The molecular biology of childhood rhabdomyosarcoma. Semin Diagn Pathol 1994;11:39.
137. Leiroth D, Baserga R, Helman L, Roberts CT Jr. Insulin-like growth factors and cancer. Ann Intern Med 1995;12:54.
138. Asmar L, Gehan EA, Newton WA Jr, et al. Agreement among and within groups of pathologists in the classification of rhabdomyosarcoma and related childhood sarcomas: report of an international study of four pathology classifications. Cancer 1994;74:2579.
139. Maurer HM, Moon T, Donaldson M, et al. The Intergroup Rhabdomyosarcoma study. A preliminary report. Cancer 1977;40:2015.
140. Newton W, Soule EH, Hamoude A, et al. Histopathology of childhood sarcomas, Intergroup Rhabdomyosarcoma Studies I and II: Clinicopathologic classification. J Clin Oncol 1988;6:67.
141. Hays DM, Newton W Jr, Soule E, et al. Mortality among children with rhabdomyosarcoma of the alveolar histologic subtypes. J Pediatr Surg 1983;18:412.
142. Kodet R, Newton WA Jr, Hamoudi AB, et al. Childhood rhabdomyosarcoma with anaplastic (pleomorphic) features. Am J Surg Pathol 1993;17:443.
143. Shapiro DM, Parham DM, Douglas EC, et al. Relationship of tumor-cell ploidy to histologic subtype and treatment outcome in children and adolescents with unresectable rhabdomyosarcoma. J Clin Oncol 1991;9:159.
144. Dias P, Parham DM, Shapiro DN, et al. Monoclonal antibodies to the myogenic regulatory protein MyoD1: epitope mapping and diagnostic utility. Cancer Res 1992;52:6431.
145. Lawrence W Jr, Hays DM, Heyn R, et al. Lymphatic metastasis with childhood rhabdomyosarcoma. Cancer 1987a;60:910.
146. Lawrence W, Gehan EA, Hays DM, et al. Prognostic significance of staging factors of the UICC staging system in childhood rhabdomyosarcoma: a report from the Intergroup Rhabdomyosarcoma Study (IRS-II). J Clin Oncol 1987b;5:46.
147. Pinkel D, Pickren J. Rhabdomyosarcoma in children. JAMA 1961;175:293.
148. Heyn RM, Holland R, Newton WA Jr, et al. The role of combined chemotherapy in the treatment of rhabdomyosarcoma in children, Cancer 1974;34:2128.
149. Ortega JA. A therapeutic approach to childhood pelvic rhabdomyosarcoma without pelvic exenteration. J Pediatr 1979;94:205.
150. Voute PA, Vos A, deKraker J, Behrendt H. Rhabdomyosarcomas: chemotherapy and limited supplementary treatment to avoid mutilation. Natl Cancer Inst Monogr 1981;56:121.
151. Raney RB, Gehan EA, Hays DM, et al. Primary chemotherapy

with or without radiation therapy and or surgery for children with localized sarcoma of the bladder, prostate, vagina, uterus, and cervix. Cancer 1990;66:2072.

152. Hays DM. Bladder/prostate rhabdomyosarcoma: results of the multiinstitutional trials of the Intergroup rhabdomyosarcoma study. Semin Surg Oncol 1993;9:520.

153. Crist W, Gehan EA, Ragab AH, et al. The third intergroup rhabdomyosarcoma study. J Clin Oncol 1995;13:610.

154. Hays DM, Raney RB, Lawrence W, et al. Primary chemotherapy in the treatment of children with bladder-prostate tumors in the Intergroup Rhabdomyosarcoma Study (IRS-II). J Pediatr Surg 1982;17:812.

155. Weiner ES, Lawrence W, Hays D, et al. Retroperitoneal node biopsy in childhood paratesticular rhabdomyosarcoma. J Pediatr Surg 1994;29:171.

156. Raney B Jr, Heyn D, Hays DM, et al. Sequelae of treatment in 109 patients followed for 5 to 15 years after diagnosis of sarcoma of the bladder and prostate. Cancer 1993;71:2387.

157. Hays DM, Lawrence W, Crist W, et al. Partial cystectomy in the management of rhabdomyosarcoma of the bladder: a report from the Intergroup Rhabdomyosarcoma Study (IRS). J Pediatr Surg 1990a;25:719.

158. Hays DM, Raney RB, Wharam MD, et al. Children with vesical rhabdomyosarcoma (RMS) treated by partial cystectomy with neoadjuvant chemotherapy, with or without radiotherapy. A report from the Intergroup Rhabdomyosarcoma Study (IRS) Committee. J Pediatr Hematol Oncol 1995;17:46.

159. Fisch M, Burger R, Barthels U, et al. Surgery in rhabdomyosarcoma of the bladder, prostate and vagina. World J Urol 1995; 13:213.

160. Hicks BA, Hensle, TW, Burbige KA, Altman PR. Bladder management in children with genitourinary sarcoma. J Pediatr Surg 1993;28:1019.

161. McLorie GA, Abara OE, Churchill BM, et al. Rhabdomyosarcoma of the prostate in childhood: current challenges. J Pediatr Surg 1989;24:977.

162. Bruce J, Gough DCS. Long-term follow-up of children with testicular tumours: surgical issues. Br J Urol 1991;67:429.

163. deVries JD. Paratesticular rhabdomyosarcoma. World J Urol 1995;13:213.

164. Sutow WW, Sullivan MP, Ried HL, et al. Prognosis in childhood rhabdomyosarcoma. Cancer 1970;25:1385.

165. Raney RB Jr, Tefft M, Lawrence W Jr, et al. Paratesticular sarcoma in childhood and adolescence: a report from the Intergroup Rhabdomyosarcoma studies I and II, 1973-1983. Cancer 1987;60:2337.

166. Olive D, Flamant F, Zucker JM, et al. Paraaortic lymphadenectomy is not necessary in the treatment of localized paratesticular rhabdomyosarcoma. Cancer 1984;54:1283.

167. Rodary C, Flamant F, Maurer H, et al. Initial lymphadenectomy is not necessary in localized and completely resected paratesticular rhabdomyosarcoma. Med Pediatr Oncol 1992 20:430. Abstract.

168. Goldfarb B, Khoury AA, Greenberg M, et al. The role of retroperitoneal lymphadenectomy in localized paratesticular rhabdomyosarcoma. J Urol 1994;152:785.

169. Banowsky LH, Shultz GN. Sarcoma of the spermatic cord and tunics: review of the literature, case report and discussion of the role of retroperitoneal lymph node dissection. J Urol 1970; 103:628.

170. Heyn R, Raney B, Hays D, et al. Late effects of therapy in patients with paratesticular rhabdomyosarcoma. For the Intergroup Rhabdomyosarcoma Study Committee. J Clin Oncol 1992;10:614.

171. LaQuaglia M, Ghavimi F, Heller G, et al. Mortality in pediatric paratesticular rhabdomyosarcoma: a multivariate analysis. J Urol 1989;142:473.

172. Donohue JP, Foster, RS, Rowland RG, et al. Nerve-sparing retroperitoneal lymphadenectomy with preservation of ejaculation. J Urol 1990;144:287.

173. Olive-Sommelet D. Paratesticular rhabdomyosarcoma. International Society of Pediatric Oncology Protocol. Dial Pediatr Urol 1989;12(11):4.

174. Kattan J, Culine S, Terrier-Lacombe M, et al. Paratesticular rhabdomyosarcoma in adult patients: 16-year experience at Institut Gustav-Roussy. Ann Oncol 1993;4:871.

175. Andrassy RJ, Hays DM, Raney RB, et al. Conservative surgical management of vaginal and vulvar pediatric rhabdomyosarcoma: a report from the Intergroup Rhabdomyosarcoma Study III. J Pediatr Surg 1994;30:1034–1036.

176. Hays DM, Shimada H, Raney RB Jr, et al. Clinical staging and treatment results in 1985; rhabdomyosarcoma of the female genital tract among children and adolescents. Cancer 1988; 61:1893.

177. Corpron C, Andrassy RJ, Hays CM, et al. Conservative management of uterine rhabdomyosarcoma: a report from the Intergroup Rhabdomyosarcoma Studies III and IV Pilot. J Pediatr Surg 1994;30:942.

178. Hays DM, Raney RB, Lawrence W, et al. Rhabdomyosarcoma of the female urogenital tract. J Pediatr Surg 1981;16:828.

179. Hays DM, Shumada H, Raney RB, et al. Sarcomas of the vagina and uterus: The Intergroup Rhabdomyosarcoma Study. J Pediatr Surg 1985;20:718.

180. Li FP, Fraumeni JF Jr. Testicular cancers in children: epidemiologic characteristics. J Natl Cancer Inst 1972;48:1575.

181. Haas RJ, Schmidt P. Testicular germ-cell tumors in childhood and adolescence. World J Urol 1995;13:203.

182. Kay R. Prepubertal testicular tumor registry. J Urol 1993;150:671.

183. Hoffner L, Deka R, Chakravarti A, Urvashi S. Cytogenetics and origins of pediatric germ cell tumors. Cancer Genet Cytogenet 1994;74:54.

184. Murty VV, Dmitrovsky E, Bosl GJ, et al. Nonrandom chromosome abnormalities in testicular and ovarian germ cell tumor lines. Cancer Genet Cytogenet 1990;50:67.

185. Brosman SA. Testicular tumors in prepubertal children. Urology 1979;13:581.

186. Brewer JA, Tank ES. Yolk sac tumors and alpha-fetoprotein in first year of life. Urology 1993;42:79.

187. Wu JT, Book L, Sudar K. Serum alpha-fetoprotein (AFP) levels in normal infants. Pediatr Res 1981;15:50.

188. Rushton G, Belman AB, Sesterhenn I, et al. Testicular sparing surgery for prepubertal teratoma of the testis: a clinical and pathological study. J Urol 1990;144:726.

189. Grunert RT, Van Every MJ, Uehling DT. Bilateral epidermoid cysts of the testicle. J Urol 1992;147:1599.

190. Ross JH, Kay R, Elder J. Testis sparing surgery for pediatric epidermoid cysts of the testis. J Urol 1993;149:3553.

191. Luker GD, Siegel MJ. Pediatric testicular tumors: evaluation with gray-scale and color Doppler US. Radiology 1994;191:561.

192. Skakkebaek NE. Atypical germ cells in the adjacent "normal" tissue of testicular tumors. Acta Path Microbiol Scand 1975; 83:127-.

193. Muller J, Skakkebaek NE, Ritzen M, et al. Carcinoma in situ of the testis in children with 45,X/46,XY gonadal dysgenesis. J Pediatr 1985;106:431.

194. Hadziselimovic F, Herzog B, Emmons LR. The expression of CD44 adhesion molecules on seminoma cells: a new marker for early detection of tumor. Cancer 1996;77:429–430.

195. Hadziselimovic F. Increasing incidence of seminomas in cryptorchid boys and infertile males. Dialog Pediatr Urol 1996;19 (3):7.

196. Ramani P, Yeung C, Habeebu S. Testicula intratubular germ cell neoplasia in children and adolescents with intersex. Am J Surg Pathol 1993;17:124.

197. Mostofi FK, Price EB. Tumors of the male genital system. In: Atlas of Tumor Pathology. Washington, DC: Armed Forces Institute of Pathology, 2nd Series, Fasc 1973;8.

198. Altadonna V, Snyder HM, Rosenberg HK, Duckett JW. Simple cysts of the testis in children: preoperative diagnosis by ultrasound and excision with testicular preservation. J Urol 1988;140:1505.

199. Wold LE, Kramer SA, Farrow GM. Testicular yolk sac and embryonal carcinomas in pediatric patients: Comparative immunohistochemical and clinicopathologic study. Am J Clin Pathol 1984;81:427.

200. Exelby PR. Testicular cancer in children. Cancer 1980; 45(suppl):1803.

201. Bracken RB, Johnson DE, Cangir A, et al. Regional lymph

nodes in infants with embryonal carcinoma of testis. Urology 1978;11:376.

202. Staubitz WJ, Jewett TC Jr, Magoss IV, et al. Management of testicular tumors in children. J Urol 1965;94:683.

203. Hopkins TB, Jaffe N, Colodny A, et al. The management of testicular tumors in children. J Urol 1978;120:96.

204. Pizzocara G, Zanoni F, Salvioni R, et al. Difficulties of a surveillance study omitting retroperitoneal lymphadenectomy in clinical stage I nonseminomatous germ cell tumors of the testis. J Urol 1987;138:1393.

205. Kramer SA, Wold LE, Gilchrist GS, et al. Yolk sac carcinoma: an immunohistochemical and clinicopathological review. J Urol 1984;131:315.

206. Mann JR, Pearson D, Barrett A, et al. Results of the United Kingdom Children's Cancer Study Group's malignant germ cell tumor studies. Cancer 1989;63:1657.

207. Ablin A, Krailo M, Ramsay N, et al. Biologic characteristics and response to therapy in 89 patients with malignant germ cell tumours (MCGT): A Children's Cancer Study Group (CCG) Study. Med Pediatr Oncol 1987;15:294.

208. Giguere JK, Stablein DM, Spaulding JT, et al. The clinical significance of unconventional orchiectomy approaches in testicular cancer: a report from the testicular cancer intergroup study. J Urol 1988;139:1225.

209. Uehling DT, Phillips E. Residual retroperitoneal mass following chemotherapy for infantile yolk sac tumor. J Urol 1994;152:185.

210. Urban MD, Lee PA, Plotnick LP, et al. The diagnosis of Leydig cell tumors in childhood. Am J Dis Child 1978;132:494.

211. Srikath MS, West BR, Ishitani M, et al. Benign testicular tumors in children with congenital adrenal hyperplasia. J Pediatr Surg 1992;27:639.

212. Bokemeyer C, Kuczyk M, Schoffski P, Schmoll H. Familial occurrence of Leydig cell tumors: A report of a case in a father and his adult son. J Urol 1993;150:1509.

213. Skoog SJ, Walker BR, Winslow B, Canning DA. Testicular sparing surgery for steroid unresponsive testicular 'tumors' of the adrenogenital syndrome. J Urol 1996;155:319A.

214. Gabrilove JL, Freiberg EK, Leiter E, et al. Feminizing and non-feminizing Sertoli cell tumors. J Urol 1980;124:757.

215. Manuel M, Kayatama K, Jones HW Jr. The age of occurrence of gonadal tumors in intersex patients with a Y-chromosome. Am J Obstet Gynec 1976;124:293.

216. Schellas HF. Malignant potential of the dysgenetic gonad, I and II. Obstet Gynecol 1974;44:298.

217. Olsen MM, Caldamone AA, Jackson CL, Zinn A. Gonadoblastoma in infancy: Indications for early gonadectomy in 46XY gonadal dysgenesis. J Pediatr Surg 1988;23:270.

218. Gourlay WA, Johnson HW, Pantzar JT, et al. Gonadal tumors in disorders of sexual differentiation. Urology 1994;43:537.

219. Aarskog D. Clinical and cytogenetic studies in hypospadias. Acta Paediatr Scand 1970;203(suppl):1.

220. Matthay KK. Neuroblastoma: a clinical challenge and biologic puzzle. CA. Cancer J Clin 1995;45:179–192.

221. Brodeur GM. Neuroblastoma and other peripheral neuroectodermal tumors. In: Fernbach D.J, Vietti T.J, eds. Clinical Pediatric Oncology. St. Louis. Mosby Year Book 4th ed., 1991;337.

222. Kushner BH, Gilbert F, Helson L. Familial neuroblastoma: case reports, literature review and etiologic considerations. Cancer 1986;57:1887-1893.

223. Knudson AG Jr, Strong LC. Mutation and cancer: neuroblastoma and pheochromocytoma. Man J Hum Genet 1972;24:514–532.

224. Brodeur GM, Green AA, Hayes FA. Cytogenetic studies of primary human neuroblastomas. Prog Cancer Res Ther 1980;12:73–80.

225. Lampert F, Rudolph B, Christiansen H, Franke F. Identical chromosome 1p breakpoint abnormality in both the tumor and the constitutional karyotype of a patient with neuroblastoma. Cancer Genet Cytogenet 1988;34:235.

226. Laureys G, Speleman F, Opdenakker G, Leroy J. Constitutional translocation t(l;17)(p36;12-21) in a patient with neuroblastoma. Genes Lehman EP: Neuroblastoma. With report of a case. J Med Res 1981;36:309–326.

227. Beckwith JB, Perrin EV. In situ neuroblastomas: a contribution to the natural history of neural crest tumors. Am J Pathol 1963;43:1089–1104.

228. Ikeda Y, Lister J, Bouton JM, Buyukpamukcu M. Congenital neuroblastoma, neuroblastoma in situ, and the normal fetal development of the adrenal. J Pediatr Surg 1981;16:636.

229. Everson TC, Cole WH. Spontaneous Regression of Cancer. Philadelphia: WB Saunders. 1966;88–163.

230. Hayes FA, Green AA, Rao BN. Clinical manifestations of ganglioneuroma. Cancer 1989;63:1211–1214.

231. Shimada H, Chatten J, Newton WA Jr, et al. Histopathologic prognostic factors in neuroblastic tumors; Definition of subtypes of ganglioneuroblastoma and an age-linked classification of neuroblastomas. J Natl Cancer Inst 1984;73:405–416.

232. Chatten J, Shimada H, Sather HN, et al. Prognstic value of histopathology in advanced neuroblastoma: a report from the Childrens Cancer Study Group. Hum Pathol 1988;19:1187–1198.

233. Haase GM, O'Leary MC, Stram DO, et al. Pelvic neuroblastoma—implications for a new favorable subgroup: a Children's Cancer Group experience. Ann Surg Oncol 1995;2:516–523.

234. Enzinger FM, Weiss SW. Soft tissue tumors. St Louis: CV Mosby 1988;828–831.

235. Cooney DR, Voorhess ML, Fisher JE, et al. Vasoactive intestinal peptide producing neuroblastoma. J Pediatr Surg 1982;17:821–825.

236. Farrelly C, Daneman A, Chan HSL, Martin DJ. Occult neuroblastoma presenting with opsomyoclonus: utility of computed tomography. AJR 1984;142:807–810.

237. Fisher PG, Wechsler D, Singer HS. Anti-Hu antibody in a neuroblastoma-associated paraneoplastic syndrome. Pediatr Neurol 1994;10:309–312.

238. Altman AJ, Baehner RL. Favorable prognosis for survival in children with coincident opsomyoclonus and neuroblastoma. Cancer 1976;37:846.

239. Franklin IM, Pritchard J. Detection of bone marrow invasion by neuroblastoma is improved by sampling at two sites with both aspirates and trephine biopsies. J Clin Pathol 1983;36:1215.

240. Williams CM, Greer M. Homovanillic acid and vanillylmandelic acid in diagnosis of neuroblastoma. JAMA 1963;183:836–840.

241. Gerson JM, Koop CE. Neuroblastoma. Semin Oncol 1974;11:35.

242. Ishimoto K, Kiyokawa N, Fujita H, et al. Problems of mass screening for neuroblastoma: analysis of false-negative cases. J Pediatr Surg 1990;25:398–401.

243. Sawada T. Past and future of neuroblastoma screening in Japan. Am J Pediatr Hematol Oncol 1992;14:320–326.

244. Hayashi Y, Hanada R, Yamamoto K. Biology of neuroblastoma in Japan found by screening. Am J Pediatr Hematol Oncol 1992;14:342–347.

245. Ishimoto K, Kiyokawa N, Fujita H, et al. Biological analysis of neuroblastoma in mass screened negative cases. In: Evans AE, et al. eds. Advances in Neuroblastoma Research 3 1991;602–608.

246. Albregts AE, Cohen MD, Galliani CA. Neuroblastoma invading the kidney. J Pediatr Surg 1994;29:930–933.

247. Azizkhan RG, Haase GM. Current biologic and therapeutic implications in the surgery of neuroblastoma. Semin Surg Oncol 1993;9:493–501.

248. Heisel MA, Miller JH, Reid BS, Siegel SE. Radionuclide bone scan in neuroblastoma. Pediatrics 1983;71:206.

249. Geatti O, Shapiro B, Sisson J, Hutchison R, Mallette S, Eyre P, Beierwaltes WH. Iodine-131 metaiodobenzylguanidine scintigraphy for the location of neuroblastoma: preliminary experience in ten cases. J Nucl Med 1985;26:736–742.

250. Andrich MP, Shalaby-Rana E, Movassaghi N, Majd M. The role of Iodine-Metaiodobenzylguanidine scanning in the correlative imaging of patients with neuroblastoma. Pediatrics, 1996;97:246–250.

251. Haase GM, Atkinson JB, Stram DO, et al. Surgical management and outcome of locoregional neuroblastoma: comparison of the Childrens Cancer Group and the International Staging Systems. J Pediatr Surg 1995;30:289–295.

252. Breslow N, McCann B. Statistical estimation of prognosis for children with neuroblastoma. Cancer Res 1971;31:2098–2103.

253. Nitschke R, Smith EI, Shochat S, et al. Localized neuroblastoma

treated by surgery: a Pediatric Oncology Group Study. J Clin Oncol 1988;6:1271–1279.

254. Matthay KK, Sather HM, Seeger RC, et al. Excellent outcome of stage II neuroblastoma is independent of residual disease and radiation therapy. J Clin Oncol 1989;7:236–244.

255. Adams GA, Shochat SJ, Smith EI, et al. Thoracic neuroblastoma: a Pediatric Oncology Group study. J Pediatr Surg 1993;28: 372–377.

256. Evans AE, Chatten J, D'Angio GJ, et al. A review of 17 IV-S neuroblastoma patients at the Children's Hospital of Philadelphia. Cancer 1980;45:833–839.

257. Evans AE, D'Angio GJ, Propert K, et al. Prognostic factors in neuroblastoma. Cancer 1987;59:1853–1859.

258. Haas D, Ablin AR, Miller C, et al. Complete pathologic maturation and regression on stage IV-S neuroblastoma without treatment. Cancer 1990;62:2572–2575.

259. Hachitanda Y, Ishimoto K, Shimada H. Stage IVS neuroblastoma: Histopathology of 27 cases compared with conventional neuroblastomas. Lab Invest 1991;64:5P(26).

260. Seeger RC, Brodeur GM, Sather H, et al. Association of multiple copies of the N-myc oncogene with rapid progression of neuroblastomas. N Engl J Med 1985;313:1111–1116.

261. Seeger RC, Wada R, Brodeur GM, et al. Expression of N-*myc* by neuroblastomas with one or multiple copies of the oncogene. Prog Clin Biol Res 1988;271:41.

262. Brodeur GM, Fong, CT. Molecular biology and genetics of human neuroblastoma. Cancer Genet Cytogenet 1989;41:153–174.

263. Brodeur GM. Neuroblastoma—clinical applications of molecular parameters. Brain Pathol 1990;1:47.

264. Look AT, Hayes FA, Nitschke R, McWilliams NB, Green AA. Cellular DNA content as a predictor of response to chemotherapy in infants with unresectable neuroblastoma. N Engl J Med 1984;311:231–235.

265. Kusafuka T, Fukuzawa M, Oue T, Yoneda A, Okada A, Satani M. DNA flow cytometric analysis of neuroblastoma: distinction of tetraploidy subset. J Pediatr Surg 1994;29:543–547.

266. Hayashi Y, Kanda N, Inaba T, et al. Cytogenetic findings and prognosis in neuroblastoma with emphasis on marker chromosome 1. Cancer 1989;63:126.

267. Nakagawara A, Arima-Nakagawara M, Scavarda NJ, et al. Association between high levels of expression of the TRK gene and favorable outcome in human neuroblastoma. N Engl J Med 1993;328:847–854.

268. Suzuki T, Bogenmann E, Shimada H, et al. Lack of high-affinity nerve growth factor receptors in aggressive neuroblastomas. J Natl Cancer Inst 1993;85:377–384.

269. O'Neill JA, Littman P, Blitzer P, et al. The role of surgery in localized neuroblastoma. J Pediatr Surg 1985;20:708.

270. Moss TJ, Reynolds CP, Sather HN, et al. Prognostic value of immunocytologic detection of bone marrow metastases in neuroblastoma. N Engl J Med 1991;324:219–226.

271. Matthay KK, Seeger RC, Stram D, et al. Prognosis for stage IV neuroblastoma less than one year at diagnosis: a prospective

Childrens Cancer Group study. Proc Am Soc Clin Oncol 1995; 14:446.

272. Matthay KK, Seeger RC, Haase G, et al. Treatment and outcome for stage III neuroblastoma based on prospective biologic staging. Med Pediatr Oncol; 1994;23:173.

273. Nickerson HJ, Nesbit ME, Grosfeld JL, et al. Comparison of stage IV and IV-S neuroblastomas in the first year of life. Med Pediatr Oncol 1985;13:261–268.

274. Martinez DA, King DR, Ginn-Pease ME, et al. Resection of the primary tumor is appropriate for children with stage IV-S neuroblastoma: An analysis of 37 patients. J Pediatr Surg 1992;27:1016–1021.

275. Haase GM, Wong KY, de Lorimier AA, et al. Improvement in survival after excision of primary tumor in stage III neuroblastoma. J Pediatr Surg 1989;24:194–200.

276. Kiely EM. The surgical challenge of neuroblastoma. J Pediatr Surg 1994;29:128–133.

277. Shorter NA, Davidoff AM, Evans A, Ross A, Zeigler MM. O'Neill JA Jr. The role of surgery in the management of stage IV neuroblastoma: a single institution study. Med Pediatr Oncol 1995;24:287–291.

278. Shochat SJ. Update on solid tumor management. Surg Clin North Am 1992;72:1417–1428.

279. Campbell LA, Seeger RC, Harris RE, et al. Escalating dose of continous infusion combination chemotherapy for refractory neuroblastoma. J Clin Oncol 1993;11:623–629.

280. Haase GM, O'Leary MC, Ramsay N, et al. Aggressive surgery combined with intensive chemotherapy improves survival in poor risk neuroblastoma. J Pediatr Surg 1991;26:1141–1146.

281. Matthay KK, O'Leary MC, Ramsay NK, et al. Role of myeloablative therapy in improved outcome for high risk neuroblastoma: review of recent Children's Cancer Group results. Eur J Cancer 1995;31A:572–575.

282. Dinndorf P, Johnson L, Gaynon P, et al. Outcome of autologous (auto) vs. allogeneic (allo) bone marrow transplantation in 25 children with neuroblastoma (nb) and unfavorable features (UPF). J Cell Biochem 1992;16A(suppl):201.

283. Seeger RC, Villablanca JG, Matthay KK, et al. Intensive chemoradiotherapy and autologous bone marrow transplantation for poor prognosis neuroblastoma. Prog Clin Biol Res 1991;366: 527–534.

284. Hutchinson RJ, Sisson JC, Shapiro B, et al. I[131]-metaiodobenzylguanidine treatment in patients with refractory advanced neuroblastoma. Am J Clin Oncol 1992;15:226–232.

285. Murray JL, Cunningham JE, Brewer H, et al. Phase I trial of murine monoclonal antibody 14G2a administered by prolonged intravenous infusion in patients with neuroectodermal tumors. J Clin Oncol 1994;12:184–193.

286. Finklestein JZ, Krailo MD, Lenarsky C, et al. 13-Cis-retinoic acid in the treatment of children with metastatic neuroblastoma unresponsive to conventional chemotherapy: Report from the Childrens Cancer Study Group. Med Pediatr Oncol 1992;20: 307–311.

CHAPTER 36

Hydrocele/Hernia

Laurence S. Baskin and Barry A. Kogan

A hydrocele can be defined as an accumulation of fluid around the testicle. There are two types of hydroceles: 1) communicating and 2) noncommunicating (Fig. 36.1). A communicating hydrocele is caused by a persistence of a patent processus vaginalis with the same pathophysiology as an indirect hernia (see later), but with a smaller opening, preventing bowel from entering. The fluid around the testis is peritoneal fluid, which is a congenital defect. In contrast, a noncommunicating hydrocele has no connection to the peritoneum. Noncommunicating hydroceles are rare in children, occurring mostly in adolescents and adults. The fluid comes from the mesothelial lining of the tunica vaginalis and is often the result of inflammation of the testis or epididymis. This is an acquired lesion. Hydroceles recognized at birth will often resolve spontaneously by the first birthday. Whether this results from delayed closure of a patent processus vaginalis or represents fluid "trapped" at the time of testicular descent remains unknown. But it is clear that the majority of hydroceles in the neonate resolve spontaneously and do not recur.

A hernia is defined as a protrusion of an organ or tissue through an abnormal opening. In urology the most common type of hernia is an inguinal hernia. In pediatric urology two types of groin hernias exist: 1) indirect and 2) direct (Inguinal versus Femoral) (Fig. 36.2). Indirect inguinal hernias are caused by persistence of a patent processus vaginalis. This defect is congenital and allows protrusion of peritoneal contents (usually small intestine but also, on occasion, omentum, mesentery, appendix, ovary, etc.) through the internal inguinal ring, along the spermatic cord, for a variable distance, in some cases as far as the scrotum. This may become "incarcerated" if it cannot be reduced back into the peritoneum. If so, the pressure of the hernia may alter blood flow to the testis, which can be damaged from ischemia. In addition, the blood flow to the bowel may be affected, and in this circumstance is called a strangulated hernia. Direct inguinal hernias are a weakness in the floor of the inguinal canal. This is an acquired condition and is uncommon in children. Femoral hernias are caused by a weakness at the femoral canal and are rare in children.

EMBRYOLOGY

During the third month of gestation the peritoneal lining of the abdominal cavity protrudes out of the internal inguinal ring after the gubernaculum, as it courses down the inguinal canal past the external inguinal ring and into the scrotum (or in girls, to the labia majora) where it becomes attached. This is the processus vaginalis. Late in gestation the testis descends along the same path, from the retroperitoneal space, through the inguinal canal, just posterior to the processus vaginalis, and into the scrotum. At approximately the time of birth, the portion of the processus vaginalis between the peritoneum and the scrotum obliterates, separating the residual tunica vaginalis in the scrotum from the peritoneum. If the processus does not obliterate, it is said to remain patent.[1]

For obvious embryologic reasons, premature infants will have a much higher rate of patency of the processus vaginalis than will full-term infants.[2] If the patent processus is large enough to allow bowel to enter, there is an indirect inguinal hernia. If the processus is patent but the connection small, a communicating hydrocele is likely to result when peritoneal fluid enters the inguinal canal. If the processus obliterates, a noncommunicating hydrocele may result from and in association with secretion of fluid into the residual tunica vaginalis. This is usually associated with inflammation in the scrotum.

INCIDENCE

Approximately 1 to 3% of full-term children will have a hernia/hydrocele. In premature infants, the rate is approximately three times as high, depending on the degree of prematurity.[2-4] Approximately 10% of children with hernia/hydrocele will have a family history, although there is no known inheritance pattern or gene

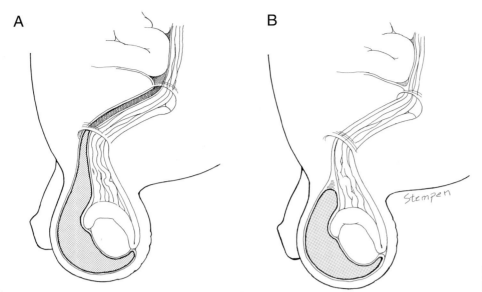

FIG. 36.1. Communicating **(A)** and noncommunicating **(B)** hydroceles.

identified. At least a third are diagnosed before 6 months of age. The male to female ratio is 8:1. The right to left ratio is 2:1, and approximately 16% are bilateral.[4] Several diseases have been associated with an increased incidence of hernia/hydrocele.[5–7] Patients with cystic fibrosis have an incidence of up to 15%. Infants with connective tissue abnormalities such as Ehlers-Danlos and Hunter-Hurler Syndromes have a higher risk for hernia/hydrocele and a higher recurrence rate after repair.[8] Some investigators have noted that recurrence of a repaired inguinal hernia may at times be the first sign of one of these connective tissue diseases.[8] Children with congenital dislocation of the hip or

chronic peritoneal dialysis, preterm infants with intraventricular hemorrhage, and children with myelomeningocele with a ventriculo-peritoneal shunt are also at increased risk for hernias/hydroceles.

DIAGNOSIS

The diagnosis is made in most cases by observation, often by the parents. A lump or bulge will be present in the groin, scrotum, or labium. The lesion is noted particularly at times of increased intra-abdominal pressure, e.g., when the child is crying or straining. Generally, the lump will disappear soon after the intra-

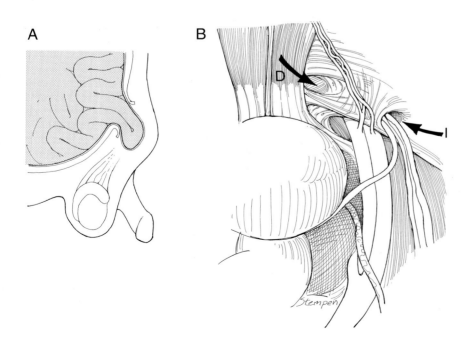

FIG. 36.2. A, Inguinal hernia. **B,** Direct (*D*) and indirect (*I*) hernias.

abdominal pressure returns to normal. In older children, the enlargement may be progressive during the day, and will recede during naps or at night. When present, the diagnosis is clear-cut. On occasion, the lesion is reported by the parents, but cannot be demonstrated in the office, even when the child is crying or straining. Sometimes, the examiner can elicit a "silk glove" sign, in which the layers of the processus vaginalis can be felt around the spermatic cord feeling like "silk rubbing on silk" in the absence of a lump. There may be a bluish discoloration underneath the skin because it filters out the yellow, giving a hint of blue. This has been mistaken at times for an incarcerated hernia. Sometimes the upper extent of the hydrocele will help differentiate it from a hernia. Alternatively, the parents can bring in a photograph to document the bulge, or if the parents are good historians, plans for repair can be based on history alone.

Because hydroceles in the first year of life do not require surgical intervention, it is important to differentiate them from hernias. Most often the physical examination is clear-cut with bowel clearly palpable as distinct from fluid. Sometimes, bowel sounds can be heard in the sac. Transillumination is of no value because hydrocele fluid and bowel fluid or air will transmit light. Needle aspiration is dangerous for fear that one could puncture or lacerate the bowel wall. In some circumstances, a plain abdominal radiograph or an ultrasound will be useful if air/fluid interfaces can be identified in the scrotum. Onset of an acute tense hydrocele in which the testis is not palpable at all may warrant a scrotal ultrasound to ensure the "normalness" of the testis and avoid misdiagnosing a hydrocele from ominous testicular pathology.

When the diagnosis of a hernia is unclear, some surgeons have recommended herniography. A 60% iothalamate solution is injected blindly into the peritoneum using a small needle. The child is placed upright for 10 minutes and a radiograph taken to determine if the contrast outlines the patent processus vaginalis. The diagnostic accuracy is high. Complications include the obvious potential for bowel injury, contrast reactions, and peritoneal irritation from the hyperosmolar contrast. In practice, this procedure is rarely useful.

An attempt should be made to reduce the hernia/hydrocele by keeping the child calm and applying gentle pressure on the lump.[3,5] Bowel will most often be reduced easily. Fluid in the sac may also reduce easily. An interesting circumstance occurs when there is a large hydrocele noted in the scrotum that does not reduce easily. Although there is some parental pressure to repair the hydrocele because of its obvious appearance, that it does not reduce easily suggests that the connection with the peritoneum is small. In infants, these may resolve spontaneously.

A special circumstance is the incarcerated hernia.[6]

Any child with symptoms of a bowel obstruction, i.e., vomiting and abdominal distention, should be examined carefully for a hernia. In these cases, the mass is usually tender, and sometimes there is skin erythema. The hernia may be palpable on rectal examination or confirmed by plain radiograph or ultrasound. An attempt to reduce the hernia should be made as described earlier. If it cannot be reduced, emergent operative intervention is needed. If it can be reduced, the child should be observed closely for signs of bowel injury. Operative repair should be performed soon after.

TREATMENT

There is no medical management for hernias/hydroceles, and the use of trusses is of historical interest only. Hernias will persist indefinitely and will almost always come to repair at some time. Hydroceles may resolve spontaneously during the first year of life. Consequently, in most circumstances, a period of observation is justified.

Hernias in premature infants should be repaired before hospital discharge, but most hernias and communicating hydroceles in children can be repaired as an outpatient surgical procedure with minimal discomfort and morbidity.[9] Surgical repair is performed by ligating the processus vaginalis at the internal inguinal ring, thereby separating the peritoneum from the distal tunica vaginalis. The success rate approaches 99% and the major risk is from the anesthetic. There is some danger of damage to spermatic cord structures because the processus vaginalis is intimately attached to them. In normal circumstances, the risk is approximately 1%. If surgery on an incarcerated hernia is necessary, the risk is significantly higher, as high as 6 to 10%, although it is unclear whether the damage is related to the repair or the prolonged incarceration, which can significantly reduce testicular blood flow because of swelling and increased pressure at the internal ring and compression of the spermatic vessels.

TECHNIQUE

Hernia and communicating hydrocele surgery can be performed in the outpatient setting using general anesthetic. To relieve postoperative pain it is standard practice to supplement the general anesthetic with an ilioinguinal nerve block or a caudal anesthetic.[3,11] After routine skin preparation an incision is made in the groin skin crease: crossing vessels are pushed aside with the use of small retractors. Scarpa's fascia is grasped and incised with blunt scissors, exposing the external oblique aponeurosis. The inguinal ligament is defined as a constant landmark of the groin, aiding in correct identification of the external ring and spermatic cord. Blunt dissection exposes the external inguinal ring where the bulging hernia sac frequently is visible. An incision is then made in the external oblique aponeurosis after separation of the cremasteric fibers and the ileoinguinal nerve, which are directly beneath the external oblique aponeurosis.

The hernia sac typically is found lying within the inguinal canal anterior and slightly medial to the spermatic cord. The anterior aspect is grasped with smooth forceps, delivering the sac and the spermatic cord into the wound. The cremasteric muscle is then bluntly dissected off the hernia sac with care taken to leave the spermatic cord and associated vessels undisturbed. Optical magnification is useful because of the small size of the structures, especially in young children. The vas deferens and spermatic vessels are never directly "held or picked-up" during the entire procedure.

The dissection is most easily performed close to the internal ring away from the testicle. After the sac is completely dissected from the vas deferens and spermatic cord, a hemostat is passed around the sac distally. The proximal sac is opened where it is exposed, releasing any hydrocele fluid. No attempt is made to remove the sac from the testicle. After the sac has been divided, the cord is separated from the sac to the internal ring. At this time, laparoscopic inspection of the contralateral internal ring can be performed through the patent hernia sac (Fig. 36.3). The sac is then twisted one to two full turns and ligated at the level of the internal inguinal ring. It is unnecessary to reconstruct the internal ring. The external oblique aponeurosis is closed, Scarpa's fascia reapproximated, and the skin approximated with a subcuticular skin closure. The testis is gently replaced into the scrotum by traction on the gubernaculum.

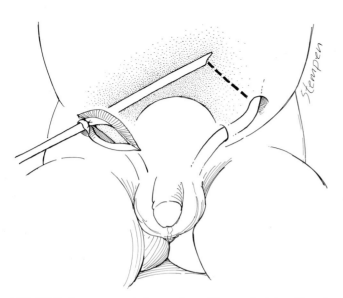

FIG. 36.3. Laparoscopic inspection of the contralateral inguinal ring at the time of hernia or hydrocele repair.

Contralateral Exploration

In infants, at the time of inguinal hernia repair, it is appropriate to explore the contralateral groin because approximately 60% will have a contralateral patent processus vaginalis.[6, 12–14] In older children the rate of positive exploration is much lower; thus, in most circumstances, contralateral surgery is not indicated. To be more certain, some authors have recommended intraoperative herniography, peritoneal carbon dioxide insufflation, and laparoscopy [is done infraumbilically or via the symptomatic hernia sac at the time of repair (Fig. 36.3)]. These techniques will likely determine the presence of a patent processus contralaterally. The unresolved issue is the meaning of an open processus vaginalis that has been clinically asymptomatic. Simply put, we do not know the true subsequent incidence of symptomatic hernia/hydroceles in patients who have an asymptomatic patent process vaginalis or open internal ring at laparoscopic inspection. The incidence of patent process vaginalis at autopsy in men without symptomatic hernia is 20%.[1]

Considering the incidence of inguinal hernias/hydroceles, it seems reasonable to explore the asymptomatic contralateral side in all males younger than 2 years of age and in infants and children with associated risk factors as described earlier. In healthy males older than 2 the incidence of a subsequent contralateral hernia seems low and bilateral exploration is not routinely warranted. Because females have a 50% incidence of bilateral hernia and the chance of injuring the reproductive organs during surgery is low, it is recommended that bilateral exploration and repair be performed at all ages in girls.

SPECIAL CIRCUMSTANCES

Testicular Feminization

Approximately 2 to 3% of girls with hernias will be found to have a testis within the hernia sac.[16] These girls have Testicular Feminization syndrome. They will have completely normal external genitalia, a shallow vaginal cavity, and should still be raised as females.

Depending on the philosophy of the local pediatric endocrine group, the testes may be left in place until after puberty (after which they should be removed because of the risk of gonadoblastoma), or removed at the time of hernia repair because of the risk of virilization if the syndrome is incomplete. These girls will be normal except for infertility and the need for hormone replacement. Although the likelihood of encountering a female child with unsuspected testicular feminization is remote, it is prudent for the surgeon performing herniorrhaphy on a female to be certain a normal ovary is observed through the open hernia sac at the internal ring or, alternatively to do vaginoscopy and document the presence of a normal uterine cervix.

Increased Intraabdominal Pressure

Communicating hydroceles are unlikely to resolve spontaneously in children with increased intraabdominal fluid. This is seen in children on peritoneal dialysis and those with ventriculoperitoneal shunts.[7] Early surgical repair is indicated. In these cases, there is a higher recurrence rate and repair should be performed with particular precision—in some cases, consider tightening of the internal ring beneath the spermatic cord.

Hernia Uterine Inguinale

Hernia Uteri Inguinale ia a rare disorder of intersexuality in males. Hernia Uteri Inguinale results when there is persistence of Müllerian structures secondary to the failure of paracrine secretion of Anti Müllerian Hormone (AMH) or to an AMH receptor defect.[15] Affected males are not ambiguous at birth and generally present later with undescended testes for orchiopexy or with inguinal hernias. At the time of the surgery Wolffian and Müllerian duct derivatives are present, with an epididymis and vas in proximity to an ipsilateral uterus, fallopian tube, and upper vagina. Care should be taken when excising the Müllerian remnants because these structures are intimately related to the vas deferens and injury to this structure can occur. No cases of uterine or vaginal malignancies have been reported in these patients when these structures are left in situ.

Connective Tissue Disorders

Hernias are more common in children with connective tissue disorders. In particular, children with Ehlers-Danlos and Hurler-Hunter syndromes are prone to hernias. As noted earlier, many children develop the hernias before the diagnosis of the disorder is made.[8]

REFERENCES

1. Rowe MI, Copelson LW, Clatworthy HW. The patent processus vaginalis and the inguinal hernia. J Pediatr Surg 1969;4:102.
2. Boocock GR, Todd PJ. Inguinal hernias are common in preterm infants. Arch Dis Child 1985;60:669.
3. Weber T, Tracy T. Groin hernia and hydroceles. In: Ashcraft K, Holder T, eds. Pediatric Surgery. Philadelphia: WB Saunders, 1993;562.
4. Rowe MI, Marchildon MV. Inguinal hernia and hydrocele in infants and children. Surg Clin North Am 1981;61:1137.
5. Nakayama DK, Rowe MI. Inguinal hernia and the acute scrotum in infants and children. Pediatr Rev 1989;11:87.
6. Rowe MI, Clatworthy HW. Incarcerated and strangulated hernias in children. A statistical study of high-risk factors. Arch Surg 1970;101:136.
7. Moazam F, Glenn JD, Kaplan BJ, Talbert JL, Mickle JP. Inguinal hernias after ventriculoperitoneal shunt procedures in pediatric patients. Surg Gynecol Obstet 1984;159:570.
8. Grosfeld JL, Minnick K, Shedd F, West KW, Rescorla FJ, Vane DW. Inguinal hernia in children: factors affecting recurrence in 62 cases. J Pediatr Surg 1991;26:283.
9. Stylianos S, Jacir NN, Harris BH. Incarceration of inguinal hernia in infants prior to elective repair. J Pediatr Surg 1993;28:582.
10. Puri P, Guiney EJ, O'Donnell B. Inguinal hernia in infants: the fate of the testis following incarceration. J Pediatr Surg 1984;19:44.
11. Moss RL, Hatch EI Jr. Inguinal hernia repair in early infancy. Am J Surg 1991;161:596.
12. Given JP, Rubin SZ. Occurrence of contralateral inguinal hernia following unilateral repair in a pediatric hospital. J Pediatr Surg 1989;24:963.
13. Rescorla FJ, Grosfeld JL. Inguinal hernia repair in the perinatal period and early infancy: clinical considerations. J Pediatr Surg 1984;19:832.
14. Rowe MI, Clatworthy HW Jr. The other side of the pediatric inguinal hernia. Surg Clin North Am 1971;51:1371.
15. Grossman PA, Wolf SA, Hopkins W, Paradise NF. The efficacy of laparoscopic examination of the internal inguinal ring in children. J Pediatr Surg 1995;30:214.
16. Blyth B, Churchill B. Intersex. In: Gillenwater J, Grayhack J, Howards S, Duckett J, eds. Adult and pediatric urology. St Louis: Mosby, 1996;2591.

CHAPTER 37

Imperforate Anus and Caudal Regression Syndrome

Jaffer H. Bashey and Steven J. Skoog

In 1960 Bernard Duhamel introduced the syndrome of caudal regression as a spectrum of anomalies from the "mermaid to imperforation."[1] This syndrome is the best example of coincidentally occurring congenital anomalies with their origin in a regional error in embryologic organization. At the fourth to fifth week of gestation an error in the simultaneous development of the terminal bowel, the kidney, the urinary bladder, and the lumbosacral spine from a common mesodermal origin put all these organs in harm's way.[2] Although the patient has an imperforate anus, this is only the tip of the iceberg, and a coordinated evaluation of all the potential components of the caudal regression syndrome must be performed.

Too often the genitourinary system is overlooked at birth in favor of the immediate concerns related to the imperforate anus. However, primary or secondary urologic abnormalities may represent the most significant source of acute and long-term morbidity for these patients.[3-6] Consequently, early involvement of the urologist in the clinical care team is imperative to provide the best care for these patients. This team should include the primary care provider, surgeon, urologist, gastroenterologist, and a nurse specialist. At times a neurosurgeon and orthopedic specialist are necessary.

This chapter reviews the embryology and embryopathology of anorectal malformations. A classification system is proposed that is anatomically and management based. The location of the terminal bowel in relation to the levator ani muscles is predictive of the presence of associated anomalies in other organ systems.[6,7] An in-depth review of the associated anomalies is presented because it acquaints the reader with the array of potential problems that can be present in patients with anorectal malformations. The VATER and VACTERL associations are explained and reviewed.

The numerous urologic anomalies associated with anorectal malformations requires the urologist to be aggressive and forthright in the evaluation and management of patients. Virtually any congenital anomaly of the upper and lower urinary tract can be present in these patients.[8] A high percentage of patients with anorectal malformations will have neurogenic bladders, which further complicates the picture.[9-11] This chapter reviews the management of the urologic manifestations of anorectal malformations with particular emphasis on diagnosis and treatment of the rectourinary fistula, obstructive uropathy, vesicoureteral reflux, neurogenic bladder, and urinary tract infections.

EMBRYOLOGY

The cloaca is an endoderm-lined cavity that first becomes apparent in the 12- to 15-day embryo.[12] The cloaca contacts the surface ectoderm forming the cloacal membrane.[13] Just before 4 weeks gestation, the cloaca receives the hindgut, allantois, and mesonephric (Wolffian) ducts.[13] Beginning at approximately 4 weeks gestation, the cloaca is partitioned in the coronal plane by the craniocaudal migration of the mesodermal urorectal septum (Fig. 37.1).[13] The urorectal septum is a composite structure of two integrated mesodermal septal systems.[14] The first of the septal systems is Tourneux's fold, which is a coronal plate that migrates caudally and is responsible for forming the urorectal septum down to Müller's tubercle, the site of the future verumontanum in males.[13] The second septal system is composed of Rathke's folds, which form as indentations in the lateral walls of the cloaca and migrate toward the midline. Rathke's folds predominate in forming the urorectal septum caudally near the cloacal membrane.[13] Partitioning of the cloaca is generally completed by week seven of gestation, creating a separate anterior urogenital sinus and a posterior anorectal system.[14]

Meanwhile, on the surface of the embryo, mesoderm has built up around the cloacal membrane creating the

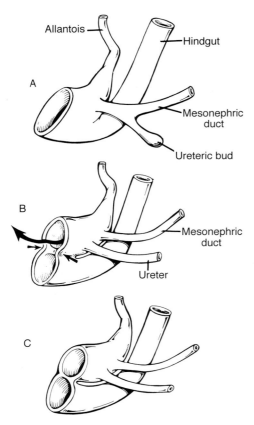

FIG. 37.1. Cloacal division and formation of the genitourinary tract. The developing urorectal septum and genitourinary structures are in close proximity. *Large arrow,* migration of Tourneux's fold; *small arrows,* migration of Rathke's folds. Reprinted with permission from Brock WA, Peña A: Cloacal abnormalities and imperforate anus. In: Kelalis PP, King LR, Belman AB, eds., Clinical pediatric urology, 3rd ed. Philadelphia: Saunders. 1992;921.

anal tubercles posteriorly and the genital folds and genital tubercle anteriorly. The depression formed by these structures is termed the external cloaca. The cloacal membrane atrophies and the external cloaca is divided by the caudal extension of the urorectal septum. The distal point of the urorectal septum forms the perineal body. More superficially the external cloaca is divided by medial migration of the mesoderm of the genital folds. The anal tubercles will contribute to the external sphincter complex of the anus. The genital folds and genital tubercle contribute to the formation of the urethra and genitalia.[13]

Simultaneous to division of the cloaca and creation of the definitive gastrointestinal tract, major developmental events are occurring in the genitourinary tract and the lumbosacral spine.[8] The mesonephric (Wolffian) ducts join the cloaca laterally and give rise to the ureteral buds. The close proximity of the ureteral bud, mesonephric duct and urorectal septum can be appreciated

in Figure 37.1. The ureteral bud contacts and induces the metanephric blastema to form the kidney and definitive urinary collecting system.[14] After cloacal partitioning, the mesonephric ducts open into the posterior wall of the urogenital sinus at Müller's Tubercle.[13] Eventually the mesonephric ducts and ureter will migrate, transpose, and possess different orifices within the urogenital system.[13] The epididymis, vas deferens, and seminal vesicle are derived from the distal portion of the mesonephric duct on each side.[14] In the female, the mesonephric (Wolffian) ducts atrophy and the paramesonephric (Müllerian) ducts fuse in the midline directly posterior to the urogenital sinus and develop into the uterus, Fallopian tubes, and most of the vagina.[14]

The vertebrae of the spine develop in a craniocaudal direction from condensation of the paraxial mesoderm that forms the somites.[15] The lower extremity limb buds are derived from somites 25 to 29.[2] The key events in caudal skeletal formation occur in the embryonic period between 4 and 8 weeks, concurrent with cloacal division.[15]

Improper division of the cloaca accounts for must anorectal malformations.[16] Anorectal malformations that result in imperforate anus are classified as high, intermediate, or low depending on the position of the terminal bowel in relation to the levator ani muscles.[17] Disturbances in Tourneux's and Rathke's folds, which form the urorectal septum, result in high anorectal malformations in males with a fistulous tract from the rectum to the urinary tract above the verumontanum.[16] In females urorectal septal defects lead to high or intermediate anorectal malformations with fistulous communication between the rectum and the genital structures above the vestibule.[16] In females, the Müllerian system is interposed between the rectum and urinary tract.[16] Rare fistulas to the bladder can occur in females when associated with a bifid or duplicated Müllerian system.[16] Disordered division of the external cloaca or improper dissolution of the anal membrane leads to malformations that are of an intermediate or low nature in the male and low malformations in the female.[16] In a few anorectal malformations there is no fistula from the bowel.[17]

The inciting event that adversely affects formation of the anorectum can also influence abnormal development of structures such as the mesonepric (Wolffian) ducts, ureteral bud, metanephric blastema, paramesonephric (Müllerian) ducts, lumbosacral spine, and the lower limbs, which share a close embryologic association.[2] Their common mesodermal origins are described in Figure 37.2. Defective partitioning of the cloaca can also cause malformations of the pelvic and perineal musculature that contribute anatomically to the continence mechanism.[13] The structures that form the caudal embryo are in close proximity during early development.

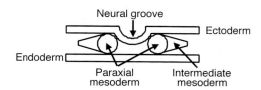

FIG. 37.2. Cross section of the trilaminar embryo showing the mesodermal precursors. The structures involved in caudal regression syndrome are derived from mesoderm: the spine and limb buds from the paraxial mesoderm and the kidneys and urorectal septum from the intermediate mesoderm.

The mesonephric duct enters the urogenital sinus at the level of the 28th somite. This corresponds to the position of the future first sacral vertebra.[7] The metanephric blastema is originally located at the level of the future second and third sacral vertebrae.[7] It is essential for the ureteral bud to contact the metanephric blastema to induce renal development, and the ureteral bud must enter the urogenital sinus in a precise manner or anomalies will occur.[8] An embryologic injury in the region of the 28th somite at 4 to 5 weeks gestation can account for the high association of genitourinary and spinal anomalies with imperforate anus.[7]

Clinically, high anorectal malformations occur at an earlier stage of development and are associated with more frequent and severe disturbances of the upper urinary tract because of faulty formation and migration of the ureteral bud. Also, lumbosacral spinal anomalies are more frequent and pronounced with high anorectal malformations.[7] Low anorectal malformations are thought to occur later in embryologic development and, as predicted embryologically, to carry with them a lower incidence of associated anomalies.[7]

An unmistakable embryopathogenic association between multiple caudal organ system anomalies is witnessed in terms of developmental timing, structural proximity, and derivation from a common mesodermal source. Disordered mesodermal migration from the primitive streak that forms the intraembryonic mesoderm, reduced cellular proliferation, and accelerated physiologic cell death in the caudal region are suggested mechanisms by which these anomalies may occur.[18-20] A recognized association between caudal regression syndrome and maternal diabetes exists.[21, 22] The exact mechanism of diabetic embryopathy is unknown; however, possible causes are hypoglycemia and hyperglycemia, somatomedin inhibitors, ketone production, altered archadonic acid metabolism, diminished turnover of phosphoinositide, or oxygen free radicals.[2, 21] Substances such as retinoids can cause caudal regression syndrome in animal models.[19] Mesodermal disturbances are not limited to the caudal region. Associations between imperforate anus and malformations of numerous vital structures in the more cranial portion of the embryo are recognized.[23, 24]

CLASSIFICATION, INCIDENCE, AND TYPES OF ANORECTAL MALFORMATIONS

Classification

Anorectal malformations span a wide and complex continuum of anomalies. Complete classification of these anomalies has been difficult, especially in the presence of numerous rare variants of the condition. Problems in conveying clinical information in the past occurred secondary to concurrent usage of several different classification systems.[25]

To remedy this problem, in 1970 a Pediatric Surgical Congress was held in Melbourne, Australia to establish a single system for classification of anorectal malformations.[17] The International Classification was designed to be anatomically descriptive in its nomenclature and to adhere to commonly held embryologic principles.[26] Major categories were designated as high, intermediate, or low based on the position of the terminal bowel in relation to the puborectalis sling of the levator ani muscles. The malformations were also listed in accordance with the sex of the patients.[17] The International Classification enjoyed wide scale acceptance and usage, supplanting the previously favored Ladd Gross classification system.[8, 17, 27]

Some critics, although in favor of the approach of the International Classification, found it to be too detailed and complex for practical usage and teaching purposes.[28] This was the motivation for convening a study group of pediatric surgeons in 1984 at the Wingspread Convention Center in Wisconsin. The Wingspread Classification of Anorectal Malformations retained many of the fundamental concepts of the International Classification but created a more manageable system by combining many of the rare anomalies into single categories.[17]

More recently, Peña proposed a classification system based on the terminal anatomic position of the fistula from the bowel and on the necessity of protective neonatal colostomy. This system is oriented toward the clinical management of anorectal malformations and is strongly predictive of associated genitourinary malformations in any given category.[29]

In Figure 37.3, a unified classification of anorectal malformations is presented. It combines the anatomically descriptive aspects of the anomalies with information pertaining to immediate and definitive surgical management. As indicated, intermediate malformations are clinically segregated with high malformations and require a protective colostomy in the neonatal period.[30] Low malformations are addressed in the neonatal period using a perineal approach, and colostomy is not

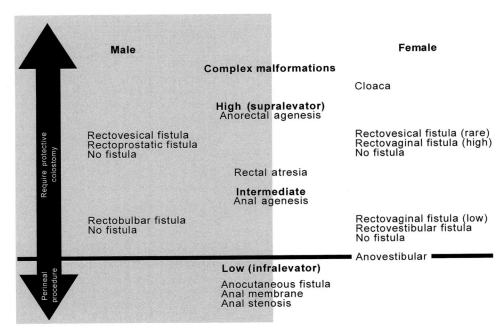

FIG. 37.3. Classification of anorectal malformations. High and intermediate anorectal malformations are grouped together and require protective colostomy in the neonatal period. Low anorectal malformations are treated with a perineal procedure in the neonatal period.

required.[30] The ability to classify anorectal malformations accurately has significant clinical relevance for predicting the potential presence of associated anomalies in other organ systems.[6,7]

Incidence

Anorectal malformations occur in approximately 1 in 5,000 births.[31] A slight male predominance is observed with males being affected in 53 to 64% of cases and females in 36 to 47% of cases.[5,31–34] Overall, low malformations are more common than high malformations, accounting for 53 to 60% of lesions;[31–34] however, high malformations involve males twice as often as females.[31,33] Examination of all high malformations reveals a fistulous communication to the urinary tract in 80% of males and to the genital tract in 87% of females.[31,32] Because males with high lesions have fistulas that enter the urinary tract and these are rare in females, the expected incidence of rectourinary fistulas in patients with imperforate anus is approximately 25%.[25]

Persistent cloacal malformations in females represent up to 10% of all anorectal anomalies in some series.[3,5] Anatomically, in cloacal anomalies the gastrointestinal, reproductive, and urinary tracts share a common channel of variable size that communicates with the exterior in the perineum.[36] Cloacal anomalies are discussed in Chapter 38.

Types of Anorectal Malformations

Anorectal Agenesis

In high (supralevator) anorectal malformations, the rectal pouch ends above the puborectalis muscle. Anorectal agenesis implies that the disal rectum and anus have not formed. In the most common variants of this malformation, fistulous communications to the genitourinary tract are present.[37]

Rectoprostatic Fistula

Rectoprostatic fistula is the most common high anorectal malformation in the male (Fig. 37.4). It accounts for approximately 80% of the cases in which there is a fistula to the urinary tract.[31] The fistula is usually fine and enters adjacent to the ejaculatory ducts and verumontanum. If the fistula opens cranial to the verumontanum, then the ejaculatory ducts and prostatic tissue are located cephalad to their normal positions. The fistula rarely can open between the verumontanum and the bulbous urethra. In this instance, the ejaculatory ducts and prostatic tissue retain their normal configuration.[37] Figure 37.5 shows a rectoprostatic fistula compared to other fistulas associated with anorectal malformations.

Rectovaginal Fistula

Rectovaginal fistulas (Fig. 37.5C) are described in the literature as being common, making up most high and

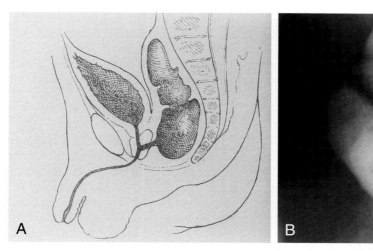

FIG. 37.4. A, A schematic representation of a rectoprostatic fistula. **B,** Contrast radiographic image. Note the catheter in the bladder.

intermediate lesions in females.[31, 38] This is disputed by Peña who discovered only eight true rectovaginal fistulas in a series of more then 632 patients with imperforate anus.[30] He ascribes this discrepancy to the misdiagnosis of persistent cloaca as rectovaginal fistulas and the mislabeling of vestibular fistulas as vaginal. Smith discovered many instances in the literature in which fistulas in a vestibular location were included under the heading of vaginal fistula.[31]

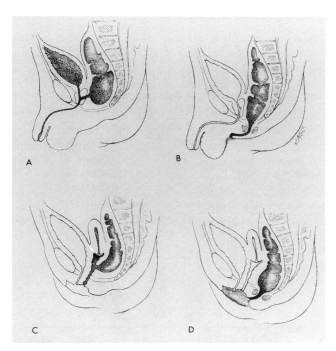

FIG. 37.5. Common fistulas found in anorectal malformations. **A,** Supralevator imperforate anus. **B,** Infralevator with cutaneous fistula at base of scrotum. **C,** Supralevator with upper vaginal fistula. **D,** Infralevator with posterior fourchette fistula.

Rectovesical Fistula

Rectovesical fistulas are uncommon in males, representing 6 to 13% of rectourinary fistulas.[31, 38] This malformation is rare in females because of the interposition of the Müllerian structures.[39] When rectovesical fistulas occur in females, which is in fewer than 1%, they are associated with varying degrees of duplication of the Müllerian structures.[31, 37, 38] In males and females the rectovesical fistula is likely to enter the bladder at the vesical neck or base.[37]

As with cloacal anomalies, rectovesical fistulas portend high risk of associated serious anomalies of the urinary tract, spine, and other organ systems.[37, 40]

Anorectal Agenesis Without a Fistula

Anorectal agenesis without a fistula accounts for approximately 15% of high anorectal malformations.[31, 38] The rectum ends blindly without any communication to the genitourinary tract.[37]

Rectal Atresia

Rectal atresia is a rare malformation accounting for lower than 2% of cases worldwide.[41] The terminal bowel ends blindly with the anus being normally formed without connection between the two. In rectal atresia, there is usually a fibrous cord connecting the proximal bowel to the anus, which has been shown microscopically to represent atretic bowel.[42] The atretic segment between the rectum and anus commonly spans a distance ranging from 0 to 2 cm.[41] The sphincteric mechanisms of the bowel are normal. This malformation is hypothesized to occur at a later stage of development than other anorectal malformations.[37] The lesion is thought to be secondary to an intrauterine vascular insult to the vessels supplying the lower rectum.[43] This is distinct from the process of disordered cloacal partitioning that causes other anorectal malformations.

Apart from the rare occurrence of other atretic bowel segments in association with rectal atresia, concomitant anomalies of other organ systems are infrequent. In a series of 67 patients with rectal atresia, no associated genitourinary anomalies were discovered.[41]

Anal Agenesis

Anal agenesis comprises the intermediate malformations. The most frequent intermediate male malformations is anal agenesis without a fistula. The close association of the rectal wall with the urethra makes dissection in this area difficult. Anal agenesis without a fistula is rarely seen in females.[37, 39]

Rectobulbar Fistula

This intermediate malformation is less common than anal agenesis without a fistula in males.[37] A fistulous communication is present between the rectum and bulbous urethra. The rectum ends superior to the bulbocavernosus muscle. The fistula, which at times is wide, enters the bulbous urethra below the membranous urethra. This fistula can often be accessed endoscopically. Rarely the fistula may end more distally along the anterior urethra and represent a narrow passage that has to travel for a portion of its course in the cavernous tissue.[37] Rectobulbar and anterior urethral fistulas can be associated with other deformities of the inner genital folds such as hypospadias, cleft scrotum, and bifid scrotum.[37, 44]

Vestibular Fistulas

Fistulous communication from the anorectum to the vestibule is the single most common anorectal malformation in females.[31, 35, 39] The outlet of the fistula is located at the posterior fourchette, which is distal to the hymenal ring. When a rectovestibular fistula is present, the terminal bowel lies within the pelvic muscular diaphragm and is connected to the vestibule by a long slender fistula that traverses the puborectalis muscle.[39] In rare circumstances the terminal bowel may be located well above the puborectalis muscle and still communicate with the vestibule, signifying a high-lying malformation.[39]

Anovestibular is the more frequent variety of vestibular fistula (Fig. 37.5D).[39] It emanates from the anterior aspect of the anus, which is in a low lying position, having passed through the pelvic muscular diaphragm. The fistula is often widely patent, allowing adequate passage of meconium without intestinal obstruction.[17, 39] Many think anovestibular fistulas should be classified and treated clinically as an intermediate type mal-

formation.[30, 39] The fundamental embryologic derangements of rectovestibular and anovestibular fistulas appear to be the same.[17] As shown in Figure 37.3, anovestibular fistula is classified between intermediate and low malformations for the reasons, given.

Low Malformations

Low malformations have a visible but abnormal termination of the bowel in most instances.[8] Fistulous communications from the distal bowel in low anorectal malformations exit onto the perineum. In males the fistula is commonly anterior to the expected anal site along the median raphe at the posterior base of the scrotum (Fig. 37.5B). However, it may open as far forward as the distal penile shaft adjacent to the glans. In females the fistula opens at a perineal or vulvar site. There are situations when low malformations have no external opening. In anal stenosis the anus is normally located but narrow. In the presence of an anal membrane, passage of meconium is impeded by persistence of this structure.[35]

The critical objective of recognizing and classifying the various anorectal malformations is to distinguish high and intermediate lesions from low lesions because their management strategies are different. The severity of the anorectal malformation also predicts the incidence of associated anomalies.

ASSOCIATED ANOMALIES

A complete understanding of the anomalies associated with imperforate anus is vital because these anomalies are often life-threatening and may be a cause of significant morbidity.[6] Associated anomalies occur in approximately 40 to 70% of patients with imperforate anus.[6] The frequency of associated anomalies for high anorectal malformations is twice that associated with low anorectal malformations (Fig. 37.6).[6] Anomalies in-

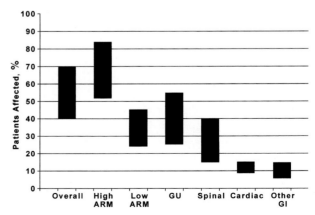

FIG. 37.6. Anomalies associated with anorectal malformations.

volving the genitourinary, vertebral, cardiac, gastrointestinal, musculoskeletal, and nervous systems are commonly encountered.[6] The association of anorectal malformations with multiple organ system anomalies occurs in a nonrandom nanner, prompting the assignment of a mutual embryopathogenic mechanism.[20]

Duhamel introduced the term "syndrome of caudal regression" to describe the observed association between multiple malformations affecting the caudal region.[1] In its most severe form, the syndrome of caudal regression comprises imperforate anus, agenesis of the genitourinary system except the gonads, lumbosacral spinal anomalies, and fusion of the lower extremities, which is termed sirenomelia.[1, 45] Duhamel cited experimental evidence that demonstrated that this striking anomaly resulted from destruction of the axial portion of the caudal region during early embryogenesis. More localized caudal injuries resulted in the creation of the individual anomalies that comprised the syndrome. He postulated that the formation of a "siren monster" and isolated imperforate anus represent two extremes of a continuum of malformations.[1] The embryologic theories and clinically acknowledged constellation of anomalies associated with imperforate anus lend support of Duhamel's insights.

Other anomalies distinct from the caudal malformations may also occur in individuals with imperforate anus. In 1972, Quan and Smith coined the acronym VATER association to describe the nonrandom occurrence of several concurrent anomalies.[23] VATER represented Vertebral defects, Anal atresia, Tracheoesophageal fistula with Esophageal atresia, and Radial dysplasia. Shortly thereafter renal dysplasia was included.[46] The association has been expanded further to VACTERL, which incorporates Cardiac and Limb defects.[47] The identification of three or more of the anomalies in given patient warrants the diagnosis of VACTERAL association.[23, 48, 49] Radial dysplasia is the most variable finding in the association.[50] In a series reported by Weaver et al, more than 60% of patients had five major concurrent anomalies including vertebral, anorectal, tracheoesophageal, renal, and cardiovascular.[50] Sixty to ninety percent of patients with VACTERL have upper urinary tract pathology.[48, 50] Genital anomalies are found frequently in this association.[50]

Anorectal malformations are part of an array of recognized syndromes. In many syndromes there is overlap in the constituent anomalies.[6] For example, anorectal malformations are a component of the axial mesodermal dysplasia spectrum in which features of caudal regression syndrome are found with the oculo-auriculovertebral and cardiac stigmata of Goldenhar's syndrome.[24] It should be appreciated that VACTERL and axial mesodermal dysplasia possess anomalies such as cardiac, upper gastrointestinal, and craniofacial anomalies that are

disparate from those found in the tail end in caudal regression syndrome. The postulated mechanism for these global malformations is a mesodermal disturbance during early organogenesis, which usually occurs in the absence of chromosomal abnormalities.[23, 24, 47–49]

Anorectal malformations can be associated with extensive abnormalities in other organ systems. Many times these patients are referred with syndromic designations. Knowledge of the potential anomalies helps to guide a thoughtful and thorough evaluation and treatment plan.

Genitourinary Anomalies

The genitourinary tract incurs the most anomalies of any organ system in association with anorectal malformations.[31] This is true even with the fistulous communications from the bowel to the lower genitourinary tract being considered part of the primary anomaly.[7, 8, 27] The overall incidence of associated genitourinary anomalies with anorectal malformations is 26 to 55%[3–5, 32, 33, 38, 51–54] Many of these urologic anomalies are occult but can progress to cause significant morbidity if unrecognized. The wide variance is attributable to the intensity of urologic investigation.[40] The underestimate of the true incidence of associated urologic anomalies was recognized by investigators in the late 1960s and early 1970s. At that time urologic evaluation was not carried out on a routine basis.[5, 44, 55] High anorectal malformations have an incidence of associated urologic abnormalities ranging from 38 to 70%.[3–5, 32, 38, 51] They tend to be more severe and have a greater likelihood of being multiple.[25] Patients with low anorectal malformations are affected by associated urologic anomalies at a lower yet still significant rate of 14 to 24% (Fig. 37.7).[4, 5, 32, 38, 51]

Urologic anomalies greatly influence morbidity and

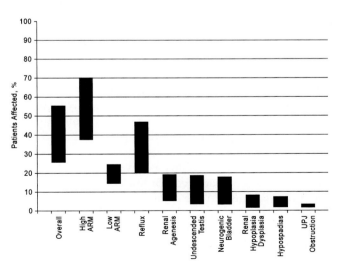

FIG. 37.7. Genitourinary anomalies in patients with anorectal malformations.

mortality of infants with anorectal malformations.[56] Hoekstra and coworkers in their series of 150 patients with anorectal malformations had a mortality rate of 16%. Three fourths of these deaths were related to genitourinary anomalies.[3] Wiener and Kiesewetter, in a series of 200 patients, found an overall mortality of 17%, and 5% of their patients had urinary tract lesions that were incompatible with life. In long-term follow-up, a third of their patients with genitourinary anomalies died.[4] Belman and King found 20 upper urinary tract anomalies in 65 patients with high imperforate anus; 80% of these anomalies posed a significant threat to renal function.[5]

The high frequency and severity of upper urinary tract involvement in patients with high anorectal malformations is explained by the close developmental timing and proximity of the genitourinary and gastrointestinal tracts. As the cloaca is being divided, the ureteric bud is interacting with the metanephric blastema and the urogenital sinus. An early simultaneous insult to gastrointestinal and genitourinary formation leads to the occurrence of the most commonly observed anomalies: vesicoureteral reflux and unilateral renal agenesis. Other common anomalies are renal hypoplasia, dysplasia, and ureteropelvic junction obstruction, which represent similar yet less pronounced aberrations.[8, 40]

Vesicoureteral Reflux

Vesicoureteral reflux was the most underdiagnosed urologic entity associated with imperforate anus. More recently, vesicoureteral reflux has been documented in 20 to 47% of patients with imperforate anus, making it the most frequently encountered associated genitourinary anomaly (Fig. 37.7)[3, 27, 31, 32, 57] The lower incidence of vesicoureteral reflux reported in earlier series stemmed from the lack of cystograms performed on a routine basis.[3–5, 27, 33] Those with high anorectal malformations more frequently exhibit vesicoureteral reflux than those with low malformations.[3, 32, 33, 54, 57] The potential impact of vesicoureteral reflux in the clinical course of patients with imperforate anus cannot be overemphasized. Early recognition is imperative. This is most readily facilitated by performance of a voiding cystourethrogram (VCUG) in the neonatal period. Intravenous urogram and ultrasound are inadequate to exclude vesicoureteral reflux.[58] Often vesicoureteral reflux is severe and bilateral or associated with a badly compromised or absent contralateral renal unit.[32, 58] The common occurrence of urinary tract infection and neurogenic bladder in patients with anorectal malformations accentuates the impact of vesicoureteral reflux on renal function, which underscores the importance of early diagnosis. Vesicoureteral reflux is an associated anomaly in which proper management can greatly influence outcome.

Renal Agenesis

Renal agenesis is the second most common genitourinary anomaly in patients with imperforate anus. Renal agenesis is often associated with multiple anomalies of other organ systems.[4] Bilateral agenesis occurs in 1 to 2.5% of cases of imperforate anus.[3, 4, 32, 53] In total, bilateral or unilateral renal agenesis occurs in 5 to 19% of patients (Fig. 37.7).[3, 4, 32, 33, 53, 54] Renal agenesis is more common in high anorectal malformations, occurring in 17 to 19% of patients.[32] It occurs in approximately 5% of patients with low lesions.[32] Failure of the ureteral bud to sprout from the mesonephric duct and induce the metanephric blastema is the cause of renal agenesis. This event takes place at approximately 4 weeks gestation, which explains the propensity of this anomaly to occur with high anorectal anomalies.[8]

When unilateral renal agenesis is identified, it is essential to uncover potential threats to the contralateral solitary kidney, which include vesicoureteral reflux, urinary tract infections, obstruction, and neurogenic bladder dysfunction.

Other Upper Urinary Tract Anomalies

Less severe embryologic disturbances of upper urinary tract formation than those resulting in renal agenesis occur in association with anorectal malformation. Renal hypoplasia and dysplasia occurs in 2 to 8% of patients.[3–5, 32, 53, 54] Other anatomic anomalies include renal ectopia, malrotation, and fusion abnormalities.[5] Rare fusion abnormalities can occur such as midline fusion in which both kidneys are drained by a common renal pelvis and ureter.[59] The ureter can be affected in isolation, producing duplication, ureteropelvic junction obstruction, or midureteral obstruction. Ureteropelvic junction obstruction occurs in 2 to 3% of patients with anorectal malformations.[3, 54, 55] Upper urinary tract anatomic arrangements can become bizarre, such as the reported bilateral ureteral triplication with crossed fused ectopia of the kidneys.[60]

Anomalies caused by ureteral incorporation into the urogenital sinus can result in ureterovesical junction obstruction, ureterocele, and ectopic ureter.[3–5, 54] A striking example of the pathology produced by improper separation of the ureteral bud from the Wolffian duct is ectopic communication between the vas deferens and ureter.[61–63] A strong association of this rare anomaly with imperforate anus exists.[62, 63] The communication between the vas deferens and the urinary collecting system can be as high as the renal calyceal system.[61] This type of anomaly can result clinically in a high incidence of epididymitis in patients with anorectal malformations.[61]

At times, a phenomenon of transient hydroureteronephrosis in newborns with imperforate anus has been described.[55, 64, 65] The etiology is thought to be ureteral compression by the dilated imperforate bowel and the condition resolves after decompressive colostomy. Knowledge of this situation is important during evaluation of the newborn, especially when entertaining the possibility of urologic intervention.[27]

Lower Urinary Tract Anomalies

With anorectal malformations, anomalies of the lower urinary tract can occur. When present, they are often not in isolation but are associated with globally pervasive disordered embryogenesis. These include absence of the bladder, duplication, of the bladder, exstrophy, urachal anomalies, and megacystis. Megacystis may be part of the triad or prune belly syndrome, with associated poor abdominal wall musculature and cryptorchidism, or secondary to urogenital sinus outlet obstruction.[4, 51, 55]

A lesion of great potential harm in a patient with imperforate anus is posterior urethral valves, which are seen in approximately 1 to 2% of patients.[3, 52, 54] Bladder outlet obstruction coupled with the presence of a rectourinary fistula, urinary tract infection, and vesicoureteral reflux into a solitary kidney with poor function can spell disaster. Although uncommon, posterior urethral valves and congenital urethral strictures are anomalies that can be diagnosed by voiding cystourethrography and require early attention.

Genital Anomalies

Genital anomalies occur frequently in patients with imperforate anus, resulting from abnormal external cloacal, genital fold, and genital tubercle formation. Hypospadias occurs in 2 to 7% of patients with imperforate anus but can occur with a frequency of 23% in males with high anorectal malformations.[3, 40, 53, 61, 66] The hypospadias lesion may be severe, especially when associated with an H-type rectourethral fistula.[64] Other male genital lesions include epispadias, urethral duplication or atresia, micropenis, bifid or duplicated penis, penile ectopia, or absence and scrotal anomalies.[3, 51, 52, 55]

Cryptorchidism has been recognized in 18% of males with imperforate anus.[55, 67] The positions of the undescended testes and their histologic characteristics are similar to patients with cryptorchidism without imperforate anus.[67] The correlation between cryptorchidism and anomalies of the genitourinary system and spine is strong. An 80% rate of undescended testes is present when both systems contained anomalies.[67] The gonads themselves are derived from outside the disordered developmental field responsible for imperforate anus and its associated anomalies. However, the Wolffian ducts and gubernaculum are mesodermally derived structures postulated to be important in testicular descent. Malformations in these structures in imperforate anus may adversely affect testicular migration.[67] In addition, the genitofemoral nerve, also important in animal models of testicular descent, may be adversely affected by associated spinal anomalies commonly seen in patients with anorectal malformations.[67]

Female genital anomalies can manifest as long-term obstetric and gynecologic problems. Primary vaginal and uterine anomalies have been encountered in 30 to 35% of females with anorectal malformations excluding the fistulous communications present to the genital structures.[68] The most common vaginal anomalies are the presence of a sagittal vaginal septum followed by vaginal agenesis.[68] Improper fusion of the Müllerian ducts can lead to various degrees of uterovaginal septation or duplication. These anomalies lead to problems with menses and conception, an increased spontaneous abortion rate, a decreased live birth rate, and the need for high risk obstetric care.[68, 69]

Spinal Anomalies

Bony spinal defects occur in 15 to 40% of patients with imperforate anus.[3, 32, 51, 55, 70, 71] As seen with other anomalies, the incidence is greater in high anorectal malformations.[38] These abnormalities typically affect the lumbosacral spine with the most common anomalies being complete or partial sacral agenesis and hemivertebral defects (Fig. 37.8).[6] Spinal anomalies tend to parallel the severity of gastrointestinal and genitourinary anomalies because these systems are developing concurrently and are susceptible to the same embryologic insult.[8] According to Brock, the presence of a sacral anomaly in his series coincided with the presence of a genitourinary anomaly in 72% of cases.[54] Sacral bony alterations can signal absence of the ventral sacral nerve roots or hypoplasia of the conus medullaris.[44] Nerve roots may be present in the absence of their corresponding vertebral segment.[72]

Previously, all spinal anomalies and neurologic lesions associated with imperforate anus and sacral dysplasia were thought to be static in nature.[44] However, it has been established that reversible, progressive dysraphic lesions of the spinal cord occur with alarming frequency in patients with anorectal malformations.[70, 71, 73–77] These lesions are amenable to neurosurgical intervention.[74, 78] Dysraphism results from the abnormal closure of the neural tube resulting in anomalous development of the midline neural, bony, and soft tissue structures. The spinal cord can become fixed to adjacent tissues at the site of the defect, resulting in tethering. The inability of the conus medullaris to ascend with growth, causes mechanical, metabolic, and vascular compromise of the spinal cord resulting in neurologic impairment.[70, 78] Spinal cord dysraphism is obvious in some instances such as myelomeningocele but in most patients with imperforate anus, it is occult. Occult spinal dysraphism is esti-

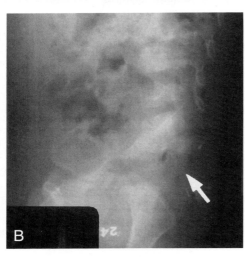

FIG. 37.8. A, Ap view demonstrating sacral agenesis. **B,** Lateral view of the same patient. Arrows, expected site of the sacrum.

mated to occur in 14 to 36% of patients with imperforate anus.[70, 71] Lesions consist of spinal cord tethering, thickened filum terminale, lipomyelomeningocele, anterior sacral meningocele, dermal sinus tracts, dural sac morphologic aberrations, split cord malformations, and syringomyelia. These can all lead to insidious progressive neurologic dysfunction.[70, 71, 73–78] It is important to realize that dysraphic lesions can be present even with a normal spinal radiograph of the sacrum.[9, 70] Magnetic resonance imaging (MRI) of patients with anorectal malformations and a normal spinal radiograph may demonstrate spinal cord dysraphism in 21% of these patients.[70] With a sacral anomaly present, approximately 46% of patients will

have an abnormal MRI suggestive of dysraphism.[70] A finding of spinal cord tethering may be found in 44% of high malformations and 27% of low malformations.[70] The concern for the clinician regarding these spinal anomalies is the resultant neurologic impairment that can affect the bladder, bowel, and musculoskeletal systems.

Cardiac Anomalies

Cardiac anomalies occur with a frequency of 9 to 15% in association with anorectal malformations. This group of anomalies can be life-threatening. The most common cardiac anomalies present are ventricular septal defects and Tetralogy of Fallot.[6]

Other Gastrointestinal Anomalies

Apart from genitourinary and spinal abnormalities, the next most common anomaly is esophageal atresia with or without a tracheoesophageal fistula.[8] It occurs in approximately 10% of cases of anorectal malformations.[6] Although more common in high anorectal malformations, its occurrence with low-lying lesions should not be overlooked. The next most common associated gastrointestinal anomaly is duodenal atresia.[6]

Overt Hirschsprung's disease has occasionally been associated with imperforate anus. A more important association is whether lower intestinal motility problems so often encountered in anorectal malformations may be related to incomplete ganglion cell migration to the affected terminal bowel segment.[6]

MANAGEMENT

The realization that anorectal malformations do not occur in isolation but rather are part of a multisystem anomaly has dictated the need for a multidisciplinary team approach to management. The anorectal anomaly is usually the presenting diagnosis, but clinical efforts cannot be solely concentrated on its management. A prompt comprehensive search for additional pathology must be initiated at birth especially in light of the potential life-threatening anomalies that often accompany anorectal malformations. This type of comprehensive care is best facilitated by early involvement of the urologist and other health care professionals. This policy fosters continuity of care to address the long-term issues that arise in these patients. Initial care of patients with anorectal malformations should be provided in a facility equipped to meet their complex needs.

A systematic approach to the initial management of patients born with an anorectal malformation is presented in Figure 37.8. The main objectives in the initial evaluation are determination of the level of the anorectal malformation and identification of life-threatening associated anomalies in other organ systems. The former allows a decision regarding appropriate initial surgical management and the latter allows intervention for urgent and life threatening anomalies. Early identification of associated anomalies provides a basis for further diagnostic and treatment strategies.

Prenatal Diagnosis

Management may begin before birth of the infant if prenatal ultrasound findings consistent with an anorectal malformation or caudal regression syndrome are discovered. The high-risk maternal group in which screening is advocated are mothers with diabetes, in whom all congenital anomalies that have their origin between 4 to 8 weeks of gestation are increased.[2] Prenatal sonographic findings indicative of anorectal malformations are dilated bowel, intraluminal calcification of meconium when a rectourinary fistula is present, and abnormal findings in the associated organ systems such as the genitourinary, musculoskeletal, and cardiac systems.[79, 80] It can be appreciated that many of these prenatal ultrasound findings are nonspecific and may not be present in many cases, reducing the sensitivity of ultrasound in this capacity. At 25 to 30 weeks gestation, ultrasound has been able to predict the presence of imperforate anus by demonstrating the absence of anal ultrasonographic characteristics in the perineum.[81] Potential urologic information from the prenatal ultrasound include the presence of hydronephrosis, absence of a renal unit, megacystis, or rare findings such as megalourethra.[82] Caudal malformations in the musculoskeletal system may also be discovered. Prenatal diagnosis allows the opportunity to offer the family prenatal counseling.[22] It alerts the clinician to the need for immediate postnatal diagnosis and treatment of these disorders.

Physical Assessment

In the newborn discovered to have imperforate anus, physical examination and urinalysis will allow determination of the level of the anorectal malformation in most patients.[30] Physical examination commences with a general inspection of the infant's well-being. A nasogastric tube should be passed to rule out esophageal atresia. If there is difficulty in passing the nasogastric tube, then water-soluble contrast studies should be obtained.[8] The nasogastric tube also facilitates bowel decompression. Signs and symptoms of cardiopulmonary status must be noted. Any evidence of abnormalities should prompt assessment with chest radiograph, electrocardiogram, and echocardiogram. The abdomen is palpated for masses representing hydronephrosis. The umbilicus should be assessed for urachal anomalies. The back is examined for spinal abnormalities and signs of dysraphism, such as cutaneous dimpling, a sacral sinus,

sacral pigmentation, hypertrichosis, or a sacral mass. Obvious myelomeningocele can be present. The male genitalia is assessed for undescended testis, urethral anomalies including hypospadias and epispadias, and scrotal development. Complete evaluation of the limbs and neurologic status is necessary, which includes motor and sensory evaluation and reflexes. The integrity of the sacral reflex arc should be determined by testing saddle sensation. Digital rectal examination is performed in cases of rectal atresia and anorectal stenosis that have a normal external appearance.[8]

Perineal inspection strives to identify a fistulous opening or an abnormal termination of the bowel. Usually one must allow 24 hours to elapse after birth for meconium to be observed through narrow fistulas.[12, 30] Perineal fistulas in the male are usually found anterior to the normal anal site along the median raphe posterior to the scrotum. However, the fistula at times can be as far forward as the glans penis. The fistula may appear as a black ribbon-like structure that is produced by meconium lying in a subepithelial position or the fistula may be signaled by a skin tag. Careful inspection is mandatory because the fistula may be marked by only a small drop of meconium.[30] Persistent anal membrane appears as a bulging epithelial veil with meconium visible behind it. Irregular epithelium at the expected anal site with a small opening is indicative of anal stenosis.[12]

Examination of the female with an anorectal malformation is facilitated by placement in the lithotomy position. Perineal fistulas are similar to those found in males. They often exit at the vulva. Vestibular fistulas are located outside the hymenal ring at the posterior fourchette. Vaginal fistulas are located inside the hymenal ring.[30] The urethral meatus must be identified. The presence of a single perineal opening in a female is evidence of a persistent cloaca, the management of which is discussed in Chapter 38.

The lack of any anal features and a flat bottom are findings consistent with a high anorectal malformation (Fig. 37.9). Additional clues to a high anorectal malformation are air or meconium emanating from the urethra. Also, the urine should be examined for meconium or squamous epithelial cells. These findings signify a high anorectal malformation with a rectourinary fistula.[40] Some anorectal malformations do not have fistulas or the clinical findings may be indeterminate in identifying the level of the bowel, in which case radiologic assessment is indicated.[30]

Radiologic Assessment

Level of the Anorectal Malformation

An invertogram or a prone cross table lateral radiograph can determine the distance of the gas shadow in the terminal bowel from the anal dimple that is marked

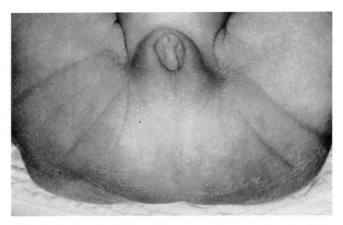

FIG. 37.9. Female infant with a cloacal anomaly and a flat, or rocker, bottom.

with a radiopaque object. A distance greater than 1 cm indicates a high malformation and less than 1 cm indicates a low malformation. Results obtained from the simpler cross table lateral radiograph are as reliable as the traditional invertogram without subjecting the patient to the potential complications of being placed in an upside down position. Sixteen to twenty-four hours must be allowed to elapse until gas can reliably be expected to reach the terminal bowel.[30] Passage of a nasogastric tube does not interfere with these tests as long as gas has entered the small bowel before placement.[8]

Other studies that may be used for anatomic definition are direct injection contrast fistulogram and imaging modalities such as ultrasound, CT scan, and MRI.[28]

Associated Anomalies

Radiologic diagnosis of associated anomalies begins in the newborn period (Fig. 37.10).

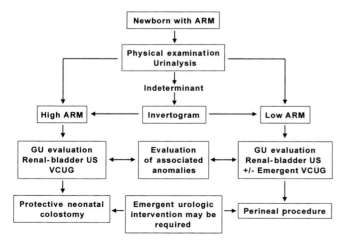

FIG. 37.10. Initial management of a newborn with an anorectal malformation. *ARM,* anorectal malformation; *GU,* genitourinary; *US,* ultrasound; *VCUG,* voiding cystourethrogram.

Urinary tract evaluation should begin before any surgical intervention for the anorectal malformation.[56] In all cases a renal bladder ultrasound is obtained to identify hydronephrosis and to check the number and appearance of the kidneys. Information regarding the bladder is also obtained. In patients with high anorectal malformations, a VCUG should also be performed before any surgical intervention. In low anorectal malformations, the VCUG may be performed on a less emergent basis if the urinary tract is sonographically normal. The VCUG is diagnostic of such conditions as reflux, neurogenic bladder, poor vesical emptying, posterior urethral valves, and ureterocele. The VCUG can potentially delineate a rectourinary fistula and give anatomic information regarding the level of the anorectal malformation.

Assessment of the lumbosacral spine should be performed in all patients with anorectal malformations.[44, 56] Plain radiographs should include a frontal view for the detection of hemivertebrae and a lateral view to determine the number of vertebral segments.[6] All patients with anorectal malformations should undergo further imaging of the lumbosacral spine regardless of the results of the plain film survey.

High-resolution ultrasound of the spine is an excellent screening modality for detection of spinal dysraphism.[83] Ultrasound is easy, inexpensive, does not require sedation, and can be accomplished for the spine concurrently with the urinary tract evaluation.[71] Ultrasound appears to be as accurate as MRI in detecting intraspinal pathology; however, the abnormalities are more anatomically defined with MRI.[83] Thus a normal plain film series and ultrasound of the spine makes MRI unnecessary. If abnormalities are found on spinal ultrasound then further delineation with MRI should be considered. Ultrasound is feasible early in life when the spine is poorly ossified. This period lasts until 3 months of age.[70, 74] Poor ossification may allow subtle lumbosacral bony abnormalities to go unnoticed on plain films. Children found to have evidence of spinal cord dysraphism are referred appropriately for neurosurgical evaluation.

Early Urologic Intervention

The impetus for early urologic evaluation is to uncover situations requiring emergent neonatal urologic intervention, which can be coordinated under the same anesthetic as surgical intervention for the anorectal anomaly (Fig. 37.10). Such instances include high-grade reflux, obstruction, and anomalies associated with diminished renal function.

High-grade reflux, especially when associated with neurogenic bladder dysfunction or urinary tract infection, is an indication for early urologic intervention. Vesicostomy is an effective means for decompressing the urinary tract in this situation.

Obstructive lesions can be treated by providing proximal drainage or by addressing the anomaly directly. Lower urinary tract anomalies that may be amenable to immediate endoscopic treatment are posterior urethral valves and ureteroceles causing ureteral or bladder neck obstruction, respectively. Congenital urethral strictures and urethral atresia may require vesicostomy.

Upper urinary tract obstruction, when bilateral or associated with a solitary kidney, demands immediate attention. Hydrocolpos requires early intervention when it results in lower urinary tract obstruction. Treatment includes intermittent catheterization, vesicostomy, or vaginostomy.[27, 40, 56]

Surgical Management of Anorectal Malformations

Surgical therapy is based on determination of the level of the anorectal malformation. Low anorectal malformations are managed by a perineal procedure in the neonatal period, which may represent a cutback procedure or an anoplasty that places the anus within the external sphincter. Anal membranes are incised and anal stenotic lesions are dilated.[30]

The remainder of anorectal malformations representing high and intermediate anomalies are managed in the neonatal period by creation of a temporary protective diverting colostomy.[30] This provides intestinal decompression and diverts the fecal stream away from the urinary tract and site of the future definitive anorectal repair. Individual preference largely dictates the colonic site from which the colostomy is fashioned. The type and site of the colostomy impact clinically. The colostomy should be fully divided because loop colostomies have a greater tendency to prolapse and there is spillover of stool into the distal limb posing a threat of urinary tract infection and compromised healing of the definitive anorectoplasty.[15] The colostomy should not be too distal, otherwise mobilization of the colon at the time of definitive repair may be impeded. A colostomy that is too proximal may act as a reservoir for urine accumulation if a rectourinary fistula is present. This can lead to severe metabolic consequences. It is prudent to evacuate the distal limb of the colostomy mechanically and with antibiotic irrigation at the time of surgery.[30]

After the patient has been stabilized, the timing of definitive repair of high and intermediate anorectal malformations is decided. This varies from 1 to 12 months, depending on the practice of the specific surgeon, the general condition of the patient including the presence of associated anomalies and adequate growth, and the type of anorectal malformation present.[12] A useful test for defining anorectal anatomy before definitive repair is a distal colostogram. This study shows the height of the rectum and the exact position and course of any fistulous communications. At times high pressures are required to overcome the resistance of a fistula to fully

display its position. This study helps guide planning of the definitive repair.[30]

The standard of care for definitive repair of high and intermediate anorectal malformations is through a posterior sagittal anorectoplasty, the most popular procedure for addressing these lesions.[12] The patient is placed in a prone position with the table jack-knifed to elevate the pelvis. The midline sagittal incision begins over the mid-sacrum and extends forward to the middle of the external sphincter (Fig. 37.11). This gives excellent exposure of the entire region. An electrical muscle stimulator is used throughout the procedure to identify the muscular continence complex that is divided exactly in the midline (Fig. 37.11). This avoids injury to the pelvic nerves that lie laterally and preserves the integrity of the continence muscles.[30] One must be certain that no paralytic agents are being used in the anesthetic.[84]

The bowel is identified and opened in the midline. The fistula is identified from within the bowel lumen, allowing precise division of the fistula under direct vision. In cases of rectourethral fistulae a catheter should be present in the urethra to mark its extent. The plane superior to the fistula between the bowel and the vagina in the female or the urethra in the male is indistinct and requires meticulous dissection. The distal bowel is mobilized to reach the skin without tension. The distal bowel is tapered to fit within the muscular continence mechanism. The muscular complex is approximated in the midline around the bowel. An abdominal approach must be combined with the posterior sagittal anorectoplasty in approximately 10% of cases to reach and mobilize a high distal bowel segment.[30] In addition to approaching high and intermediate anorectal malformations posterosagittally, strong consideration should be given to repairing female anovestibular fistulas with this approach after colostomy. This may reduce the rate of infection, dehiscence, and need for reoperation, when compared to a primary perineal procedure to correct this lesion in the neonatal period.[30, 54]

Anal dilation begins 2 weeks after definitive surgery and the colostomy is closed after progression of dilation to the desired size is reached. The frequency of dilation is then gradually tapered. The key factors in subsequent fecal continence are consistency of the stool, adequacy of sacral innervation, the severity of the initial anorectal malformation, the quality of the pelvic muscular complex, and the psychosocial constitution of the patient and family.[30, 54]

In the past, most surgical complications were secondary to improper division of rectourinary fistulas. Inherent to older pull-through procedures was the poorly visualized step of dividing the fistula.[30] Complications include urethral stricture and recurrent fistula.[27] The urethra can be completely transected if it is tented up at the time of division of the fistula. If the fistula is

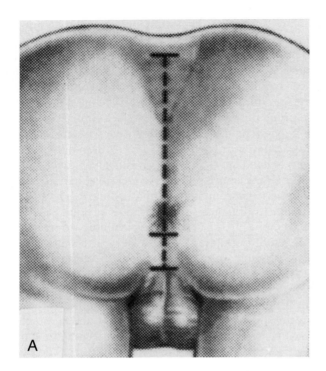

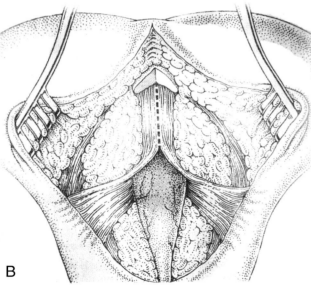

FIG. 37.11. A, Skin incision for the posterior sagittal approach for the repair of high and intermediate anorectal malformations. **B,** Division of the muscular continence complex in the midline.

divided too close to the bowel, a resultant urethral diverticulum or retained rectal pouch can develop.[51]

Urethral strictures resulting from fistula division are managed by proximal urinary diversion with vesicostomy in the very young patient. Older patients are treated with dilation, direct vision urethrotomy, or urethroplasty depending on the nature of the stricture. Stricture may also develop from injudicious use of indwelling catheters and instrumentation of the urethra.

Urethral diverticula or retained rectal pouches may lead to calculus formation, urinary infection, constipation, and incontinence. Urethral diverticula or retained rectal pouches are not always visualized by voiding cystourethrography, and other imaging modalities may be required.[85] Figure 37.12 demonstrates the VCUG and MRI appearance of a large retained rectal pouch that was excised by a combination posterior sagittal and abdominal approach.

Other complications of anorectal surgery with urologic implications can occur. Nerve injury from lateral dissection results in neurogenic bladder dysfunction. Direct injury to other genitourinary structures such as the pelvic reproductive organs, the bladder neck, and the ureters can occur.[27, 40]

The advantages of the posterior sagittal approach are multiple. It provides superb exposure to the anatomic area of interest. This allows clear access to the fistula, avoidance of injury to the lateral pelvic nerves, and it affords identification of other vital pelvic structures.[54] Criticism of the posterior sagittal anorectoplasty include the effect of deliberate division of the puborectalis muscle on fecal continence, and tapering of the bowel and direct anastomosis to the skin without flaps, which potentially may lead to anal stenosis.[28]

Urologic Management

Depending on the result of initial urinary tract screening, additional evaluation may be necessary, which may include laboratory evaluation, renal scintigraphy, intravenous urography, or endoscopic assessment. Many patients require urodynamic evaluation. Management issues are the control of urinary tract infection, treatment of vesicoureteral reflux, relief of obstruction, preservation of renal function, complications related to rectourinary fistulas, repairing genital anomalies, and addressing the sequelae of neurogenic bladder dysfunction. None of these issues are mutually exclusive and an integrated treatment approach is required to optimize outcomes.

Urinary Tract Infections

Urinary tract infection must be suspected in any child with an anorectal malformation. This is especially true if fevers or sepsis are present because the urinary tract is a common source.[40] The incidence of urinary tract infection reported in the literature ranges from 21 to 48%.[32] Factors that promote urinary tract infection in patients with anorectal malformations are the presence of a rectourinary fistula, stasis of urine caused by associated urinary tract anomalies, neurogenic bladder dysfunction, and iatrogenic abnormalities.[4, 51]

The risk a rectourinary fistula poses in urinary tract contamination is diminished by diversion of the fecal stream with a colostomy. When serious infection is

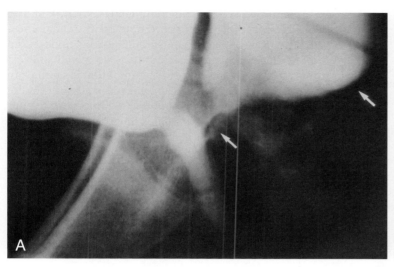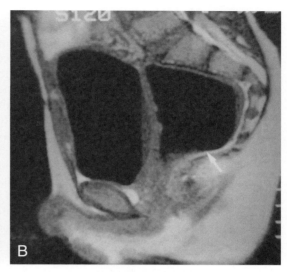

FIG. 37.12. VCUG (**A**) MRI Scan (**B**) of a large retained rectal pouch. *Arrows*, the extent of the pouch.

found, some other factor besides the fistula is usually operant.[4, 51] An otherwise normal urinary tract is frequently effective at clearing contamination from a fistula.[4, 51] Measures to reduce the chance of urinary tract infection when a fistula is present are prophylactic antibiotics, antibiotic wash-out of the distal limb of the colostomy, and adequate urinary tract drainage. If conservative management is unsuccessful in eradicating infection, then early anorectoplasty with fistula division may be required. An associated anomaly linked to persistent infection may need to be addressed before definitive anorectoplasty. The effects of urinary tract infection caused by obstruction or reflux can be devastating.[4, 51]

The phenomenon of recurrent epididymitis occurs with some frequency in males with imperforate anus and can persist even after closure of a rectourinary fistula.[40] Potential causes include the fistula, neurogenic bladder dysfunction, strictures, abnormal ejaculatory ducts, urethral diverticula, and ectopic insertion of the vas deferens, yet in some instances the cause is idiopathic.[25, 40, 44, 57] In persistent cases, vasectomy may be required.[44]

Vesicoureteral Reflux

Vesicoureteral reflux is managed similarly to otherwise healthy individuals keeping in mind confounding factors. These include infection, neurogenic bladder dysfunction, the need to definitively repair the anorectal malformation, and the presence of renal insufficiency. Treatment of primary vesicoureteral reflux is grade dependent. Lesser degrees of reflux (International Grade I–III) in patients with anorectal malformations are likely to resolve with conservative management.[57] Prophylactic antibiotic therapy is instituted to

prevent urinary tract infection. These patients must be followed closely to detect evidence of infection, renal scarring, and progression to higher grades of reflux. Vesicoureteral reflux is unlikely to resolve in the presence of high intravesical pressures. Treatment with timed voiding, intermittent catheterization, and anticholinergic medications may be necessary.

Severe degrees of vesicoureteral reflux (International Grade IV and V) may require early surgical intervention if urinary infection cannot be controlled with prophylactic antibiotics and bladder drainage. Vesicostomy, a less complicated procedure, is favored in the newborn period.[8, 27] Ureteral reimplantation should precede anorectoplasty especially if tapering of the ureters is required. If reimplantation is performed after anorectoplasty an intravesical and extravesical approach is necesssary due to scarring behind the bladder.[40] Reflux is the most common indication requiring a urologic operation in patients with anorectal malformations.[27]

Obstruction

Treatment of obstruction is cause specific. Often, temporary drainage with percutaneous nephrostomy is required. The most frequent cause of upper urinary tract obstruction in patients with anorectal malformations is ureteropelvic junction obstruction.[3, 54, 55] The diagnosis is made by ultrasound and a radioisotope renal scan with an agent such as mercaptoacetyltriglycine (MAG_3). The approach to management is similar to that in patients without anorectal malformation as long as infection or a solitary kidney are not issues. Repair can proceed when most prudent by a flank or dorsal lumbotomy incision. An advantage of a dorsal lumbotomy incision is the avoidance of the colostomy site.[32]

Renal Insufficiency

It is not surprising that many patients with imperforate anus progress to end-stage renal disease secondary to their congenital and acquired urinary tract abnormalities. Bilateral upper urinary tract anomalies occur in 14% of patients.[32] Mortality from renal failure can range from 6.4% for high anorectal malformations to 1.1% for low anorectal malformations. Males suffer a higher mortality in both categories.[32]

Preservation of renal function begins in the neonatal period with early diagnosis of urinary tract anomalies and concentrates on stabilization or correction of reversible pathology such as reflux, urinary tract infection, obstruction, and neurogenic bladder dysfunction. Surveillance must be long-term because there is a great propensity for renal deterioration in these patients. Modern techniques of pediatric renal replacement therapy, including peritoneal dialysis and renal transplantation, have been successful during infancy in patients with anorectal malformations.[86] Renal transplantation is performed after definitive repair of the anorectal malformation and closure of the colostomy because of the risk of infection and the necessity of immunosuppression.[86] Early renal transplantation provides potential for improved growth and development.[87]

Hyperchloremic Metabolic Acidosis

Before division of the fistula, passage of urine in a retrograde fashion through the fistula into the distal limb of the bowel can lead to stasis of urine with its resultant metabolic consequences. Chloride ions are absorbed and bicarbonate is excreted, leading to hyperchloremic hypokalemic metabolic acidosis.[44, 55, 88] This situation is analogous to the metabolic derangements witnessed when urinary diversion is undertaken to the sigmoid colon (ureterosigmoidostomy).[27, 44] Contributing factors include proximally placed colostomies, poor renal function, dehydration, and distal urinary tract obstruction, which may be found in up to 50% of cases.[88] Hall et al. reported a case of male infant with a high anorectal malformation who underwent transverse colostomy. His rectourethral fistula acted as a one-way valve filling the distal bowel, resulting initially in mild acidosis. Corrective measures were not initiated before discharge. The patient soon returned with fatal dehydration, pneumonitis, and electrolyte disturbances.[55] Management of hyperchloremic metabolic acidosis entails monitoring serum electrolytes, oral alkalinizing agents, and assurance of adequate vesical emptying with intermittent catheterization or vesicostomy.[27] Refractory acidosis may require early division of the fistula.

Genital Anomalies

Genital anomalies in patients with anorectal malformations are managed in the same time frames used for other children. Hypospadias repair is undertaken at 6 to 18 months of age and coordinated with other procedures. Hypospadias repair should not be undertaken before division of a rectourinary fistula and anorectoplasty because the risk of contamination is significant. Undescended testes are managed surgically in the first year of life when aspects related to the imperforate anus and other associated anomalies have been stabilized.

Vaginoplasty is best delayed until the child is older.[68] Early vaginoplasty has been identified as a risk factor for subsequent vaginal scarring.[68] In cloacal malformations the vaginal reconstruction is accomplished at the time of definitive repair with the posterior sagittal approach.[30, 36]

Neurogenic Bladder Dysfunction

The incidence of neurogenic bladder dysfunction in patients with anorectal malformations is high.[4, 9–11] All patterns of neurogenic bladder dysfunction can be encountered, including upper and lower motor neuron lesions.[9, 10, 72, 89] Goals in the management of neurogenic bladder dysfunction include preservation of renal function, minimization of urinary tract infection, and achievement of continence.[10]

The etiologies of neurogenic bladder dysfunction in patients with anorectal malformations are tethered spinal cord associated with dysraphism, hypoplasia of the conus medullaris, and pelvic nerve injury from repair of the anorectal malformation.[27, 40] Early in life the adequacy of vesical emptying must be determined.[56] This information is obtained from results of the bladder ultrasound and VCUG. The patient should be observed to void. Monitoring of serial catheterized bladder volumes is undertaken if failure to empty is suspected. Any indication of neurogenic bladder dysfunction should prompt evaluation with formal urodynamic studies. Often the only evidence of a subtle neurologic lesion is bladder dysfunction. The percentage of patients with detrusor hyperreflexia and detrusor sphincter dyssynergia is high.[10, 90]

Management of neurogenic bladder dysfunction is based on the urodynamic evaluation. Initially, failure to empty is managed with intermittent catheterization and elevated intravesical pressures are treated with a regimen of anticholinergic medications to decrease bladder wall tension and improve compliance.

Catheterization in a patient with imperforate anus may be problematic in the presence of a rectourinary fistula, a urethral diverticulum, urethral stricture, or urethral tortuosity.[11] This may be overcome by use of a coudé-tipped catheter, urethral reconstruction, or continent appendicovesicostomy.

More extensive problems of poor detrusor compliance with failure to empty are managed with augmentation cystoplasty. Augmentation cystoplasty is required to improve compliance if anticholinergics fail and upper urinary tract deterioration continues. Although numerous bowel segments can be used for augmentation cystoplasty, special considerations are necessary in patients with anorectal malformations. Previous colostomy and anorectoplasty can affect the blood supply of the colon.[56] Preservation of the ileocecal valve reduces the chance of changing stool consistency, which can result in fecal incontinence.[56] The appendix should be preserved at all times for potential use in urinary tract reconstruction.[91] Situations in which sphincteric incontinence is present are treated with bladder neck reconstructive techniques or procedures that use the Mitrofanoff principle.[56]

Close surveillance is required in all patients with neurogenic bladder dysfunction during periods of apparent stabilization. Deterioration can be sudden and cause irreversible damage if left uncorrected.

SUMMARY

The infant and child with an anorectal malformation presents a true challenge to all those who care for them. This challenge for the urologist is life-long because the associated abnormalities within the urinary tract pose significant long-term risks. A comprehensive understanding of the embryologic basis for the multiple anomalies associated with anorectal malformation provides the framework for treatment. The classification system proposed allows the clinician to predict the immediate need for colostomy and determines the probability of other organ system anomalies. An algorithm has been presented to help in the initial assessment and management of the infant with an anorectal malformation. The urologic management of the rectourinary fistula, obstruction, vesicoureteral reflux, neurogenic bladder dysfunction, urinary tract infection, and genital malformations has been reviewed with special emphasis on the team approach in the care of patients with caudal regression syndrome.

REFERENCES

1. Duhamel B. From the mermaid to anal imperforation: the syndrome of caudal regression. Arch Dis Child 1961;36:152.
2. Opitz JM. Blastogenesis and the "primary field" in human development. Birth Defects: Original Article Series. 1993;29(1):3.
3. Hoekstra WJ, Scholtmeijer RJ, Molenaar JC, Schreeve RH, Schroeder FH. Urogenital tract abnormalities associated with congenital anorectal anomalies. J Urol 1983;130:962.
4. Wiener ES, Kiesewetter WB. Urologic abnormalities associated with imperforate anus. J Pediatr Surg 1973;8:151.
5. Belman AB, King LR. Urinary tract abnormalities associated with imperforate anus. J Urol 1972;108:823.
6. Smith ED, Saeki M. Associated anomalies. Birth Defects: Original Article Series 1988;24(4):501.
7. Belman AB. Urinary problems associated with imperforate anus. In: Kelalis PP, King LR, Belman AB, eds. Clinical Pediatric Urology, 2nd ed. Philadelphia: W.B. Saunders Co, 1985;793–804.
8. Churchill BM, Hardy BE, Stephens CA. Urologic aspects of mal-

9. Kakizaki H, Nonomura K, Asano Y, Shinno Y, Ameda K, Koyanagi T. Pre-existing neurogenic voiding dysfunction in children with imperforate anus: problems in management. J Urol 1994;151:1041.
10. Ralph DJ, Woodhouse CRJ, Ransley PG. The management of the neuropathic bladder in adolescents with imperforate anus. J Urol 1992;148:366.
11. Sheldon C, Cormier M, Crone K, Wacksman J. Occult neurovesical dysfunction in children with imperforate anus and its variants. J Pediatr Surg 1991;26:49.
12. Grosfeld JL. Anorectal anomalies. In: Zuidema GD, Condon RE, eds. Shackeford's Surgery of the Alimentary Tract. 4th ed. Philadelphia: WB Saunders, 1996;450–464.
13. Stephens FD. Congenital Malformation of the Urinary Tract. New York: Praeger, 1983;2–14.
14. Larsen WJ. Human Embryology, 1st ed. New York: Churchill-Livingstone, 1993;220;235–256.
15. Moore KL. The Developing Human, 4th ed. Philadelphia: W.B. Saunders Co. 1988;337–339.
16. Stephens FD. Embryology of the cloaca and embryogenesis of anorectal malformations. Birth Defects: Original Article Series. 1988;24(4):177.
17. Smith ED. Classification. Birth Defects: Original Article Series. 1988;24(4):211.
18. Kallen B, Winberg J. Caudal mesoderm pattern anomalies: from renal agenesis to sirenomelia. Teratology 1974;9:99.
19. Mesrobian H-GJ, Sessions RP, Lloyd RA, Sulik KK. Cloacal and urogenital abnormalities induced by etretinate in mice. J Urol 1994;152:675.
20. Alles AJ, Sulik KK. A review of caudal dysgenesis and its pathogenesis as illustrated in an animal model. Birth Defects: Original Article Series, 1993;29:83.
21. Goto MP, Goldman AS. Diabetic embryopathy. Curr Opin Pediatr 1994;6:486.
22. Adra A, Cordero D, Mejides A, Yasin S, Salman F, O'Sullivan MJ. Caudal regression syndrome: etiopathogenesis, prenatal diagnosis, and perinatal management. Obstet Gynecol Surv 1994;49:508.
23. Quan L, Smith DW. The VATER association: vertebral defects, anal atresia, tracheoesophageal fistula with esophageal atresia, radial dysplasia. Birth Defects: Original Article Series 1972;8:75.
24. Russell LJ, Weaver DD, Bull MJ. The axial mesodermal dysplasia spectrum. Pediatrics 1981;67:176.
25. Parrot TS. Urologic implications of imperforate anus. Urology 1977;10:407.
26. Santulli TV, Kiesewetter WB, Bill AH Jr. Anorectal anomalies: a suggested international classification. J Pediatr Surg 1970;5:281.
27. Parrott TS. Urologic implications of anorectal malformations. Urol Clin North Am 1985;12:13.
28. Smith ED. The bathwater needs changing, but don't throw out the baby: an overview of anorectal anomalies. J Pediatr Surg 1987;22:335.
29. Brock WA, Peña A. Cloacal abnormalities and imperforate anus. In: Kelalis PP, King LR, Belman AB, eds. Clinical Pediatric Urology, 3rd ed. Philadelphia: W.B. Saunders, 1992;920–942.
30. Peña A. Current management of anorectal anomalies. Surg Clin North Am 1992;72:1393.
31. Smith ED. Incidence, frequency of types and etiology of anorectal malformation. Birth Defects: Original Article Series, 1988;24(4):231.
32. McLorie GA, Sheldon CA, Fleisher M, Churchill BM. The genitourinary system in patients with imperforate anus. J Pediatr Surg 1987;22:1100.
33. Wendelken JR, Sethney HT, Halverstadt DB. Urologic abnormalities associated with imperforate anus. Urology 1977;10:239.
34. Wiener ES, Kiesewetter WB. Urologic abnormalities associated with imperforate anus. J Pediatr Surg 1973;8:151.
35. Peña A. Imperforate anus and cloacal malformations. In: Ashcraft KW, Holden TM, eds. Pediatric Surgery, 2nd ed. Philadelphia, W.B. Saunders, 1993;372–392.
36. Hendren WH. Cloacal malformations: experience with 105 cases. J Pediatr Surg 1992;27:890.

formations and common abnormalities of the anus and rectum. Urol Clin North Am 1978;5(1):141.

37. Smith ED, Stephens FD. High, intermediate, and low anomalies in the male. Birth Defects: Original Article Series 1988;24(4):17.

38. Santulli TV, Schullinger JN, Kiesewetter WB, Bill AH Jr. Imperforate anus: a survey from the members of the surgical section of the American Academy of Pediatrics. J Pediatr Surg 1971;6:484.

39. DeVries PA. High, intermediate and low anomalies in the female. Birth Defects: Original Article Series 1988;24(4):73.

40. Brock WA, Peña A. Urologic implications of imperforate anus. AUA Update Series 1991;10(26):202.

41. Dorairazan T. Anorectal atresia. Birth Defects: Original Article Series 1988;24(4):105.

42. Magnus RV. Rectal atresia as distinguished from rectal agenesis. J Pediatr Surg 1968;3:593.

43. Partridge HD, Gough MH. Congenital abnormalities of the anus and rectum. Br J Surg 1961;49:37.

44. Williams DI, Grant J. Urological complications of imperforate anus. Br J Urol 1969;41:660.

45. Rossi R, Holzgreve W, Rehder H. Extreme hypotrophy of the lower body pole, extensive hypoplasia of the spinal column and multiple anomalies of abdominal organs: a maximal variant of the caudal regression sequence. Clin Dysmorph 1995;4:87.

46. Quan L, Smith DW. The VATER association. J Pediatr 1973;82:104.

47. Kimura K, Dietzek AM. VATER syndrome: significance in urology. Dial Pediatr Urol 1987;10(1):8.

48. Uehling DT, Gilbert E, Chesney R. Urologic implications of the VATER association. J Urol 1983;129:352.

49. Duncan PA, Shapiro LR, Klein RM. Sacrococcygeal dysgenesis association. Am J Med Gene 1991;4:153.

50. Weaver DD, Mapstone CL, Yu P. The VATER Association. Am J Dis Childhood 1986;140:225.

51. Smith ED. Urinary anomalies and complications in imperforate anus and rectum. J Pediatr Surg 1968;3:337.

52. Carlton CE Jr, Harberg FJ, Fry FM. Urologic complications of imperforate anus. J Urol 1973;109:737.

53. Parrot TS, Woodard JR. Importance of cystourethrography in neonates with imperforate anus. Urology 1979;13:607.

54. Brock WA. Anorectal malformations: urologic implications. Dial Pediatr Urol 1987;10(1):1.

55. Hall JW, Tank ES, Lapides J. Urogenital anomalies and complications associated with imperforate anus. J Urol 1970;103:810.

56. Sheldon CA, Gilbert A, Lewis AG, Aiken J, Ziegler MM. Surgical implications of genitourinary tract anomalies in patients with imperforate anus. J Urol 1994;152:196.

57. Narasimharoa KL, Prasad GR, Mukhopadhyay B, Katari YAS, Mitra SK, Pathak IC. Vesicoureteral reflux in neonates with anorectal anomalies. Br J Urol 1983;55:268.

58. Rickwood AMK, Spitz L. Primary vesicoureteric reflux in neonates with imperforate anus. Arch Dis Child 1980;55:149.

59. Currarino G, Weisbruch GJ. Transverse fusion of the renal pelvis and single ureter. Urol Radiol 1989;11:88.

60. Golomb J, Ehrlich RM. Bilateral ureteral triplication with crossed ectopic fused kidneys associated with the VACTERL syndrome. J Urol 1989;141:1398.

61. Hicks CM, Skoog SJ, Done S. Ectopic vas deferens, imperforate anus and hypospadias: a new triad. J Urol 1989;141:586.

62. Schwarz R, Stephens FD. The persisting mesonephric duct: high junction of vas deferens and ureter. J Urol 1978;120:592.

63. Gibbons MD, Cromie WJ, Duckett JW Jr. Ectopic vas deferens. J Urol 1978;120:597.

64. Munn R, Schillinger JF. Urologic abnormalities found with imperforate anus. Urol 1983;21:260.

65. Rickwood AMK. Transient ureteric dilation in neonates with imperforate anus: a report of four cases. Br J Urol 1978;50:16.

66. Metts JC III, Kotkin L, Adams MC, Brock JW III. Incidence of genital malformations in patients with imperforate anus: a review of 131 patients. Pediatrics 1996;98 (suppl 2):601.

67. Cortes D, Thorup JM, Nielsen OH, Beck BL. Cryptorchidism in boys with imperforate anus. J Pediatr Surg 1995;30:631.

68. Fleming SE, Hall R, Gysler M, McLorie GA. Imperforate anus in females: frequency of genital tract involvement, incidence of associated anomalies, and functional outcome. J Pediatr Surg 1986;21:146.

69. Hall R, Fleming S, Gysler M, McLorie G. The genital tract in female children with imperforate anus. Am J Obstet Gynecol 1985;151:169.

70. Long FR, Hunter JV, Mahboubi S, Kalmus A, Templeton JM. Tethered cord and associated vertebral anomalies in children and infants with imperforate anus: evaluation with magnetic resonance imaging and plain radiography. Radiology 1996;200:377.

71. Tsakayannis DE, Shamberger RC. Association of imperforate anus with occult spinal dysraphism. J Pediatr Surg 1995;30:1010.

72. Boemers TM, vanGool JD, deJong TPVM, Bax KMA. Urodynamic evaluation of children with the caudal regression syndrome. J Urol 1994;151:1038.

73. Carson JA, Barnes PD, Tunell WP, Smith EI, Jolley SG. Imperforate anus: the neurologic implications of sacral abnormalities. J Pediatr Surg 1984;19:838.

74. Karrer FM, Flannery AM, Nelson MD Jr, McLone DG, Raffensperger JG. Anorectal malformations: Evaluation of associated spinal dysraphic syndromes. J Pediatr Surg 1988;23:45.

75. Davidoff AM, Thompson CV, Grimm JK, Shorter NA, Filston HC, Oakes WJ. Occult spinal dysraphism in patients with anal agenesis. J Pediatr Surg 1991;26:1001.

76. Appignani BA, Jaramillo D, Barnes PD, Poussaint TY. Dysraphic myelodysplasias associated with urogenital and anorectal anomalies: prevalence and types seen with magnetic resonance imaging. Am J Radiol 1994;163:1200.

77. Rivosecchi M, Lucchetti MC, Zaccara A, DeGennaro M, Fariello G. Spinal dysraphism detected by magnetic resonance imaging in patients with anorectal anomalies: incidence and clinical significance. J Pediatr Surg 1995;30:488.

78. Melhem ER. Tethered cord and associated anomalies in children and infants with imperforate anus: evaluation with magnetic resonance imaging and plain radiography (editorial). Radiology 1996;200:318.

78. Foster LS, Kogan BA, Cogen PH, Edwards MSB. Bladder function in patients with lipomyelomeningocele. J Urol 1990;143:984.

79. Harris RD, Nyberg DA, Mack LA, Weinberger E. Anorectal atresia: prenatal sonographic diagnosis. Am J Radiol 1987;149:395.

80. Mandell J, Lillehei CW, Greene M, Benacerraf BR. The prenatal diagnosis of imperforate anus with rectourinary fistula: dilated fetal colon with enterolithiasis. J Pediatr Surg 1992;27:82.

81. Guzman ER, Ranzini A, Day-Salvatore D, Weinberger B, Spigland N, Vintzileos A. The prenatal ultrasonographic visualization of imperforate anus in monamniotic twins. J Ultrasound Med 1995;14:547.

82. Dillon E, Rose PG, Scott JE. Case report: the antenatal ultrasound diagnosis of megalourethra. Clin Radiol 1994;49:354.

83. Rohrschneider WK, Forsting M, Darge K, Tröger J. Diagnostic value of spinal ultrasound: comparative study with magnetic resonance imaging in pediatric patients. Radiology 1996;200:383.

84. Kuhn EJ, Skoog SJ, Nicely ER. The posterior saggital approach to posterior urethral anomalies. J Urol 1994;151:1365.

85. Vinnicombe SJ, Good CD, Hall CM. Posterior urethral diverticula: a complication of surgery for high anorectal malformation. Pediatr Radiol 1996;26:120.

86. Sharma AK, Kashtan CE, Nevins TE. The management of end stage renal disease in infants with imperforate anus. Pediatr Nephrol 1993;7:721.

87. Davis ID, Chang PN, Nevins TE. Successful renal transplantation accelerates development in young uremic children. Pediatrics 1990;86:594.

88. Caldamore AA, Emmens RW, Rabinowitz R. Hyperchloremic acidosis and imperforate anus. J Urol 1979;122:817.

90. Greenfield SP, Fera M. Urodynamic evaluation of the patient with an imperforate anus: a prospective study. J Urol 1991;146:539.

91. Sheldon CA, Gilbert A. Use of the appendix for urethral reconstruction in children with congenital anomalies of the bladder. Surgery 1992;112:805.

CHAPTER 38

Urogenital Sinus and Cloaca

Ricardo González and Julia Spencer Barthold

The development of the lower urinary tract, internal genitalia, and anorectum in females is intimately related, and abnormal development often involves all three systems. This chapter reviews the anomalies that result from persistence of the urogenital sinus and cloaca and their surgical correction. A thorough appreciation of the development of these organs is essential to understanding their malformations.

EMBRYOLOGY

Normal Development

The hindgut of the 4 week (4 mm stage) embryo ends in a dilated caudal portion, the cloaca (which also receives the allantois), the Wolffian ducts, and the post-anal gut. The cloacal membrane separates this endodermal cavity from the ectoderm. Shortly thereafter (5 mm stage) the cloaca is divided in the coronal plane by the urorectal septum, which grows caudally from the angle between the allantois and the hindgut and the separation of the primitive rectum from the urogenital sinus is complete by the 6th week (16 mm stage) (Fig. 38.1).[1] Others think that the caudal descent of the urorectal septum progresses only as far as the point where Müller's ducts join the cloaca (Müller's tubercle) and that caudal to this point the division progresses by ingrowth of the mesenchyme from both sides (Rathke's plicae) (Fig. 38.2). This dual origin of the cloacal septum has been emphasized by Stephens[2] and explains the common location of the urethrorectal fistula at the level of the verumontanum in males with high anal atresia.

Around this time (4th week), the developing mesonephric ducts migrating caudally join the cloaca anterolaterally above the cloacal membrane, and after the partition of the cloaca is completed they canalize and enter the cloaca near Müller's tubercle. Through a process of atrophy of the roof of the orifice the openings are moved cranially and give rise to the ureters and the trigone. In the absence of testes, vasa deferentia do not develop. It is beyond the scope of this chapter to discuss the development of the upper urinary tract.

The embryology of the female urethra and the vagina are related. Although the origin of the vagina remains somewhat controversial[3] the following explanation seems acceptable and useful. After the cloacal septum separates the hindgut from the urogenital sinus, the fused caudal end of the paired Müllerian ducts comes in contact with the posterior aspect of the sinus at the point where its wall has thickened to form the Müllerian tubercle.[4] This contact induces the formation of two paired structures composed of thickened urogenital sinus epithelium, the sinovaginal bulbs, which extend from the caudal end of the Müllerian ducts to the urogenital sinus. The sinovaginal bulbs soon become fused and form the vaginal plate, which eventually develops a lumen. The vagina thus developed remains separate from the sinus by the hymen, which becomes perforated later in fetal life.

One of the points of controversy is whether the Müllerian ducts contribute to the development of the vagina but most embryologists agree that the Müllerian ducts play a preponderant role in the development of the vagina above the hymen.[5] The distal part of the urogenital sinus exstrophies and everts to become the vestibule. The vagina and the urethra thus acquire separate openings in the vulva.

The origin of the sinovaginal bulbs has been studied in organ culture by Bok and Drews.[6] These authors have shown that the sinovaginal bulbs are the caudal segments of the mesonephric (Wolffian) ducts and that this fusion between the distal Wolffian and Müllerian ducts is prevented by testosterone, a view also supported by observations in the testicular feminization mutation mouse (Fig. 38.3).[7]

The vaginal epithelium is derived from the endoderm of the urogenital sinus and the fibromuscular wall of the vagina develops from the surrounding mesenchyme. A commonly held view is that the junction between the endodermal vaginal epithelium and the mesodermal epithelium derived from Müller's ducts (such as the

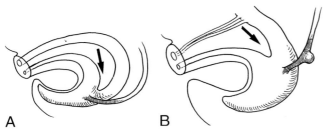

FIG. 38.1. Division of the cloaca by downgrowth of the cloacal septum (*arrows*) in a 4-mm **(A)** and 6-mm **(B)** embryo. Modified from Kelly HA, Burnam CF. Diseases of the kidneys, ureters and bladder. New York: Appleton, 1922.

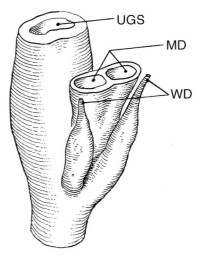

FIG. 38.3. Fusion of the distal Wolffian ducts (*WD*) with the Müllerian ducts (*MD*) to form the sinovaginal bulbs, which remain separated from the urogenital sinus (*UGS*) by the hymen. Modified from Bok G, Drews U. The role of the Wolffian ducts in the development of the vagina: an organ culture study. J Embryol Exper Morphol 1983;73:275–295.

endometrium) occurs at the level of the cervix but others think that the epithelium of the proximal vagina is also mesodermal. Ufelder and Robboy postulate that the entire vagina above the hymen is Müllerian but that the Müllerian epithelium is replaced by endodermal epithelium to the level of the cervical os.[8] Other evidence suggests that the caudal two fifths of the vaginal epithelium derives from the urogenital sinus and the cranial three fifths is of Müllerian origin.[9]

During the septation of the cloaca, the genital folds develop from the mesoderm around the cloacal membrane and the membrane becomes deep. The depression distal to the membrane is the external cloaca. The uro-anal septum, which will become the perineal body, develops deeply from the caudal extension of the urorectal septum and superficially from medial extensions of the genital folds.

Abnormal Development

Persistence of the urogenital sinus is seen with or without associated anorectal anomalies. Agenesis of Rathke's plicae and failure of migration of Müller's ducts to the vestibule results in a persistent cloaca with a septate or nonseptate vagina and uterus.[2] Persistence of the urogenital sinus after the urorectal septation has taken place may be caused by defective caudal migration of Müller's ducts or failure of the distal sinus to exstrophy and evert. Under the influence of male hormones, the urogenital sinus elongates and the Müllerian ducts remain connected to the sinus.

CLASSIFICATION

The persistence of the urogenital sinus in a female can be classified into three broad categories:[10] 1) simple, which includes patients with normal anus and rectum and without intersex conditions, 2) associated with intersexual states (see Chapter 32), 3) associated with anorectal anomalies (persistent cloaca) (Fig. 38.4).

PRESENTATION

Ultrasonographic suspicion of hydrometrocolpos in a fetus may represent indirect evidence of a persistent urogenital sinus or cloaca.[11] The persistence of a urogenital sinus associated with intersex states or anorectal anomalies is usually obvious at birth. Absence of the anus in cases of persistence of the cloaca or an enlarged clitoris and rugated labial folds in cases of intersex are characteristic and pathognomonic findings. Absence of the intergluteal crease suggests total or partial sacral agenesis. Palpation and imaging studies of the lower spine confirm sacral maldevelopment. When the junction of the vagina with the sinus is obstructed, uterine

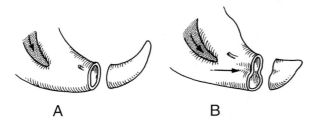

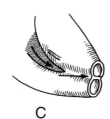

FIG. 38.2. Subdivision of the cloaca by downgrowth of the cloacal septum and lateral growth of Rathke's plicae (*arrows*). The cephalad migration of the Wolffian duct to the point at which the lateral and cephalad septa meet is also depicted. Modified from Stephens FD. Congenital malformations of the rectum and genitourinary tracts. London: Livingston, 1963.

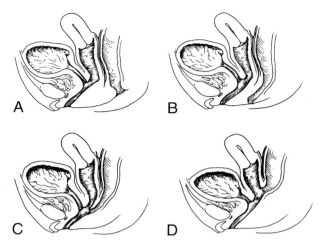

FIG. 38.4. Classification of persistent urogenital sinus not associated with intersex: **(A)** with normal anus and rectum; **(B)** with perineal anus; **(C)** low-confluence persistent cloaca; **(D)** high-confluence persistent cloaca.

and vaginal secretions produced under the influence of maternal estrogens accumulate and neonatal presentation with hydrometrocolpos is common. Hydrometrocolpos can also be the result of voiding through the urethra into the vagina when the sinus distal to their junction is stenotic. Meconium drainage into the vagina may also contibute to its dilation. In a series of 54 patients with cloaca, hydrometrocolpos was present in 14.[12]

The examination of the vulva of a newborn requires familiarity with the normal anatomy. Under the influence of maternal estrogens, the labia are turgid and vaginal secretions are often present. Identification of a separate introitus and urethral meatus is aided by gently pulling the labia majora downward and apart from each other with the patient supine and the legs abducted. It may be necessary to examine the infant more than once over the first 2 weeks of life if the normalcy of the anatomy is in question. The anus, the perineal body, and their relationship to the vulva should be noted (Fig. 38.5).

A midline abdominal mass in a newborn girl with only one or two perineal openings is most likely due to hydrometrocolpos and should be evaluated promptly. Associated hydronephrosis with or without bladder distention is common. Hydrometrocolpos may also result from imperforate hymen or vaginal septation, which are described elsewhere in this book.

Simple cases of persistent urogenital sinus may present at birth with hydrometrocolpos or later in life with urinary tract infections or urinary incontinence. The incontinence may be caused by an associated urethral or bladder neck malformation but more often is the result of vaginal voiding. The bladder empties into the vagina, which then drains in an incontinent fashion.

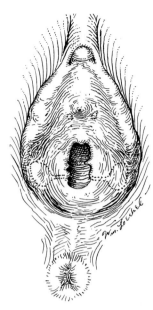

FIG. 38.5. Anatomy of the normal prepubertal vulva. From front to back the illustration depicts the clitoral hood and the glans clitoris. Behind are structures of the vestibule with the urethral meatus, the hymen and vaginal introitus and posterior fourchette. The *broken lines* depict Bartholin glands. The vestibule is flanked by the labia minora. Behind the fourchette is the perineal body which separates the vulva from the anus.

In other cases, the urethra is short (hypospadiac) and enters the proximal anterior vaginal wall. The channel distal to this point may be wide and serve as a vagina but is the urogenital sinus. Women with this anatomy may be asymptomatic or may have urinary tract infections or incontinence caused by urethral incompetence.

EVALUATION

Simple Urogenital Sinus

The goals in the evaluation in these cases are: 1) definition of the anatomy to plan surgical strategy, 2) detection of associated anomalies, predominantly in the urinary and genital tracts, and 3) definition of the mechanism of incontinence when appropriate. Retrograde contrast studies (genitogram),[13] voiding cystourethrography, endoscopy, and urodynamic evaluations when appropriate are essential. Renal ultrasonography helps define upper urinary tract anatomy, and pelvic ultrasonography allows definition of the internal genital anatomy. Laparoscopy and, at times, exploratory laparotomy at the time of the repair may be necessary to define the anatomy of the internal genitalia.

Intersex

In cases of intersex the general evaluation should follow the guidelines outlined in Chapter 32. In patients

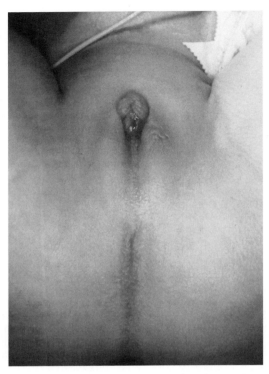

FIG. 38.6. Perineal anatomy of a female with persistence of the cloaca. The clitoris is surrounded by a hood and rudimentary labia minora, which are bunched up in front. The remaining structures of the vulva and the anus are absent. The single opening in the perineum is the distal end of the cloacal channel.

reared as females, anatomic definition is essential before to surgical reconstruction.

Persistent Cloaca

Girls with persistent cloaca have the typical appearance of a closed perineum with a single orifice for the cloaca usually located immediately behind the clitoris (Fig. 38.6), but a wide range of variations has been described.[14] In some cases the skin folds around the clitoris may be prominent, leading to a mistaken diagnosis of intersex. Less severe cases may present with a persistent urogenital sinus with an anterior ectopic anus or a perineal fistula. A duplicated uterus and septate or duplicated vagina is seen in approximately half of these cases.[12] Rarely, the vagina may be absent but the uterus present.[14] Usually the duplex vaginas lie side by side and have a common communication with the cloaca, but they may enter the cloaca separately. Associated urinary tract anomalies, including vesicoureteral reflux, neurogenic bladder dysfunction, solitary kidney, and anomalies of position of the kidney are present in 90% of the cases.[15, 16] In addition, persistence of the cloaca can be associated with esophageal atresia, duodenal atresia, and cardiac anomalies. Persistence of the cloaca can be seen in the VATER association, which may include

agenesis radius, tracheoesophageal fistula, and vertebral and renal anomalies.

A detailed anatomic evaluation is often conducted after the initial colostomy has been performed. If the condition of the newborn allows it, endoscopy may be performed at the time of the colostomy, but it is usually necessary to repeat it later to define the anatomy precisely.[14]

In addition to the steps described to evaluate simple cases, girls with persistent cloaca should undergo spine radiographs (or spinal ultrasound if the child is younger than 3 months old) to rule out vertebral malformations. Those with abnormal spine radiographs should be further evaluated with magnetic resonance imaging (MRI) to rule out cord abnormalities[17] In the newborn, spinal ultrasonography may be used to screen for cord abnormalities but the MRI provides for better anatomic definition. Overall, the incidence of spinal cord abnormalities in girls with persistent cloaca is 46%.[18] These anomalies include low placed or dysplastic conus medullaris and tethered cord with lipoma or myelolipoma, and they may have an adverse effect on future bladder, rectal, and pelvic floor function. Some authors also recommend evaluating the pelvic floor with MRI.

MANAGEMENT

Simple Urogenital Sinus

In newborns with hydrometrocolpos, prompt evaluation and decompression are necessary. Ultrasonography should be the initial study.[11] Stabilization of the general condition of the infant may require temporary, immediate tube drainage of a dilated bladder or vagina. When

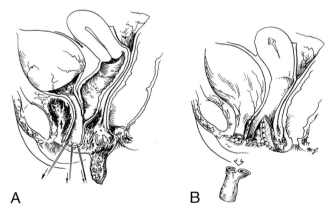

A   B

FIG. 38.7. A, To mobilize and advance the urogenital sinus when it is shorter than 3 cm. A posterior inverted-U flap is prepared from the perineal skin with the apex at the level of the opening of the sinus (see Fig. 38.8B). An incision is made around the meatus of the sinus and it is dissected circumferentially. The dissection should reach the prevesical space anteriorly and the peritoneal reflection posteriorly. **B,** The sinus is pulled down and excised. The posterior vagina wall is incised to accommodate the perineal U flap. Separate vaginal and urethral openings are created in the vestibule.

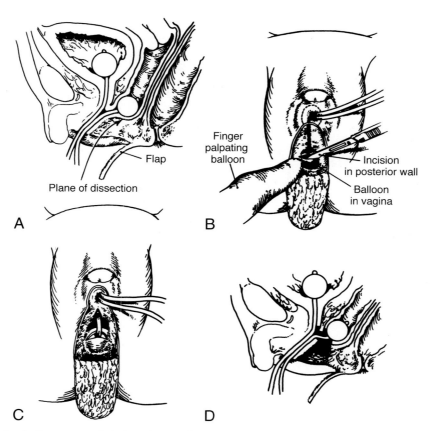

FIG. 38.8. A, To a urogenital sinus longer than 3 cm, two catheters—one in the vagina and one in the bladder—are inserted over guide wires under endoscopic guidance. **B,** An inverted U flap is prepared. It is preferable to make the skin base of this flap narrower than the apex to create a narrower posterior fourchette without compromising vaginal caliber. The vascularity of the flap is preserved by maintaining a broad base of subcutaneous tissue. The flap is elevated and the urogenital sinus is dissected posteriorly without opening it. Care is taken to dissect away the rectum, which usually occupies the space vacated by the absent distal vagina. When the distal end of the vagina is reached and the vaginal balloon can be palpated unequivocally, the vagina is opened transversely. **C and D,** Visualization of the junction of the vagina and the sinus, which is now divided. The anterior vaginal wall is dissected from the posterior urethral wall for an extension of 5 mm or more. **E and F,** The opening in the urogenital sinus is closed over the catheter in two layers. After traction sutures are placed in the edges of the vagina, the posterior vaginal wall is incised and the posterior skin flap is sutured to it. **G and H,** If there is clitoromegaly, the clitoris is reduced; then a flap is prepared from its hood and shaft skin to bridge the gap between the distal vagina and the vestibule. Windows are created in the flap at the appropriate places to accommodate the urethra and the glans clitoris. **I,** The completed reconstruction of the vulva. If the anterior flap is wide enough, it will fold longitudinally to resemble labia minora.

the newborn is stable, endoscopic evaluation should be undertaken. The endoscopic examination will help define the anatomy and establish if there is a persistent urogenital sinus responsible for the hydrometrocolpos. In the differential diagnosis of hydrometrocolpos, urogenital sinus anomalies must be distinguished from distal vaginal atresia and transverse vaginal septum with an intact urethra.

If the communication between the sinus and the vagina is patent and can be dilated, this may be sufficient treatment until the child is old enough for definitive repair. Intermittent catheterization of the sinus is often needed to maintain patency. Frequent renal ultrasonography is necessary to insure proper urinary tract drain-

age. Vesicostomy or vaginostomy may be needed to establish bladder emptying.[19] We reserve vesicostomy for instances when intermittent catheterization of the sinus to the bladder or vagina does not decompress the system. Tube vaginostomy has the disadvantages of all long-term catheters in infants, namely infection, dislodgement, and difficult handling for the parents. In addition, the scarring between the vagina and the abdominal wall after vaginostomy may make vaginal mobilization during the reconstruction more difficult.

In the stable infant, perineal vaginoplasty with preservation of the sinus as the urethra may be necessary if temporizing measures to decompress the vagina fail. We prefer to do the vaginoplasty and pull through using

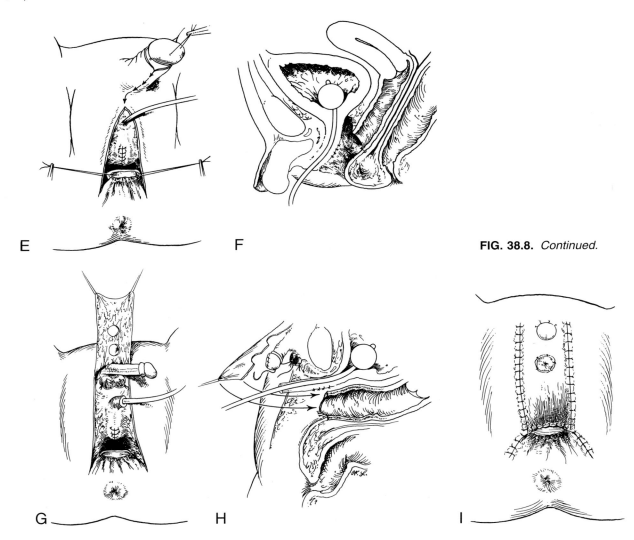

E

F

FIG. 38.8. *Continued.*

G H I

perineal sink flaps and perineal dissection under direct vision rather than in the manner described by Ramenofsky and Raffensperger,[20] which is done blindly and may impair future continence.

In the asymptomatic infant or if temporizing measures are successful, subsequent repair of the persistent urogenital sinus can be undertaken electively. We prefer early reconstruction in the first 2 years of life, but there is no evidence that waiting longer is detrimental other than for psychological reasons. Repair of the urogenital sinus with a common channel shorter than 3 cm can be done by a pull through technique.[21] This technique, originally described to repair cloacas, has been used by us and others to repair simple urogenital sinus malformations.[22] We do not hesitate to dissect circumferentially to the retropubic area ventrally and to the peritoneal reflection dorsally. A standard posterior inverted U flap is prepared at the time the incision is made and is then sutured to the longitudinally incised posterior wall of the descended vagina to prevent stenosis (Fig. 38.7). With this technique excellent cosmetic and func-

tional results are obtained with preservation or restoration of urinary continence.

When the sinus is longer, the principles of repair include preservation of the sinus as a distal extension of the urethra and the creation of skin flaps to bridge the gap between the vaginal edges and the skin. We are able to dissect behind the urogenital sinus to find the vagina and to divide it from its entrance to the sinus through a perineal approach in all cases not previously operated, even when the junction is as high as the bladder neck and the vagina is very short. This dissection is aided by first placing two balloon catheters, one in the urethra and one in the vagina under endoscopic control at the beginning of the procedure (Fig. 38.8A–F).[23] If the sinus is long, the segment that extends beyond the skin level is divided along the coronal plane and used to create a mucosal vestibule (Fig. 38.9). We have not had to use the transperitoneal, transvesical, or posterior sagittal approaches to separate the vagina from the sinus, but the surgeon should be familiar with these techniques, particularly for reoperative cases.[24, 25] Because

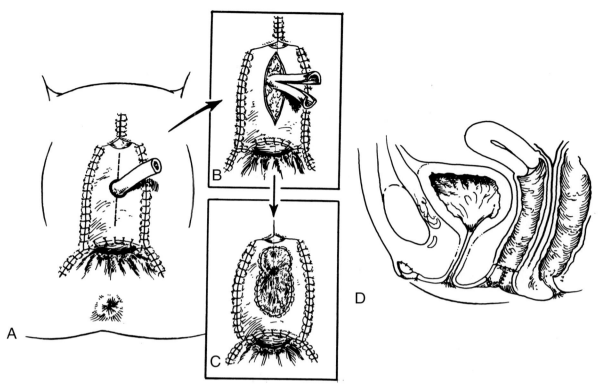

FIG. 38.9. When the length of the urogenital sinus exceeds the level of the vestibule, it can be incised in the coronal plane and interposed in a midline incision of the anterior flap to provide mucosal coverage of the vestibule. The anterior skin flap then forms the labia minora.

the condition is not usually associated with clitoromegaly, seldom is there enough skin to prepare anterior flaps, therefore, the use of labial flaps or flaps of the posteriorly incised distal urogenital sinus are more useful (Figs. 38.10 & 38.11). The use of tissue expanders in a preliminary surgical step is useful (Fig. 38.12)[26, 27] (see Chapter 32). An alternative for high or reoperative cases when the distal sinus is wide and serves well as a vagina but not as a urethra, is to extend the urethra distally by tubularizing a strip of the anterior vagina (or

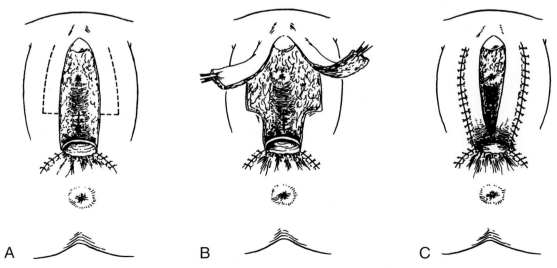

FIG. 38.10. Technique for creating the distal anterior vaginal wall from labial flaps when there is no clitoral skin available.

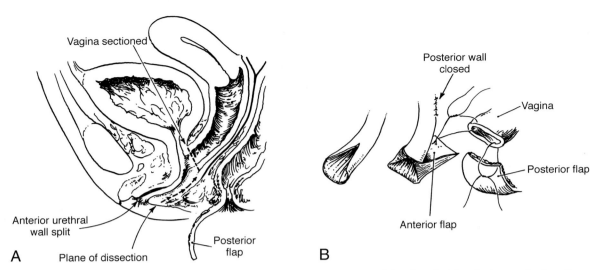

FIG. 38.11. The anteriorly incised and everted sinus can be used for the distal anterior vaginal wall when its length exceeds the level of the vestibule. This technique can be combined with the labial flaps shown in Figure 38.10. Modified from Passerini.

rather the wide sinus) and reconstructing the anterior vaginal wall with an anteriorly based buttocks flap as described by Hendren.[28, 29] This flap preserves vaginal caliber and prevents fistula formation. At a second surgical stage, the base of the flap, is divided and the labium, previously divided to bring in the flap, is reconstructed (Fig. 38.13). We have found this technique particularly

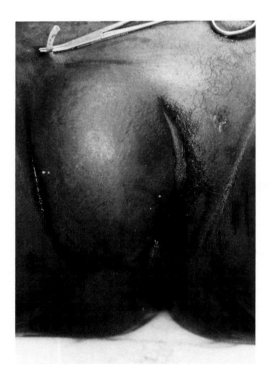

FIG. 38.12. Perineum of a female after implantation and expansion of a tissue expander to augment the labial skin and allow reconstruction of the distal vagina.

useful when the distal portion of the urogenital sinus is wide and the urethra is short, resulting from the congenital malformation or an ill advised "cut back" operation in a patient with a high urethrovaginal junction.

We have not had to resort to the posterior sagittal approach for the primary repair of urogenital sinus without anorectal malformation, an approach unnecessarily invasive because it not only requires the division of the normal anorectum but also requires a protective colostomy.[30] An intriguing compromise recently described involves the division of the anterior wall of the anus and rectum to gain additional exposure. The authors of this report claim colostomy may not be necessary.[31] We continue, though, to use the less invasive perineal approach, which in our hands yields satisfactory anatomic and cosmetic results.

In cases in which the proximal vagina is short, a segment of sigmoid colon is interposed between the proximal vagina and the skin flaps. This is accomplished through a combined abdominoperineal approach. The proximal vagina is dissected free from the urogenital sinus from below. The spaces between the vagina and the bladder anteriorly and the rectum posteriorly are dissected from below and above. The sigmoid segment is passed to a position distal to the vagina through the space dissected between the vagina and the rectum. It is usually necessary to perform the anastomosis between the vagina and the proximal end of the sigmoid segment anteriorly, through the space dissected between the vagina and the bladder. It is important not to bring the colon out to the skin surface to avoid the unsightly appearance of a perineal colostomy (Fig. 38.14). If there is insufficient introital skin to create distal flaps, we resort to the use of tissue expanders.

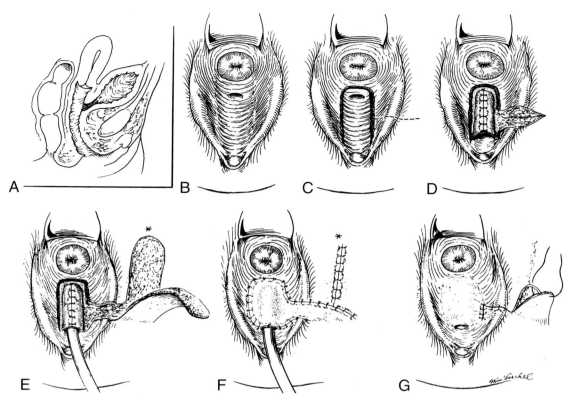

FIG. 38.13. Technique to construct the distal urethra with the anterior vaginal wall as described by Hendren.[28] We use this technique when the urethra is very high and the distal sinus which serves as vagina is wide. **A and B,** To construct the distal urethra, the patient is placed in the prone position with the thighs spread widely. **C,** Two parallel incisions are made on the anterior vaginal wall; the distance between the incisions determines the urethral circumference. **D,** The vaginal wall lateral to the incisions is mobilized, and a lateral episiotomy is made to increase exposure and allow the transposition of the buttocks flap. **E,** An anteriorly based generous flap of the skin, with subcutaneous tissue, is prepared. The base of this flap is lateral to the labium major, and the apex is in the vicinity of the ischial tuberosity (*star*). **F,** The flap is rotated and sutured to the vaginal edges; it prevents vaginal stenosis and the development of a urethrovaginal fistula. **G,** At the second stage, the base of the flap is divided, and the labia are reconstructed.

Intersex

The timing of reconstruction of children with intersex states requiring correction of a persistent urogenital sinus is controversial (see Chapter 32), but in general we recommend early repair in the first year of life. In cases with associated clitoromegaly, it is best to perform the correction of the urogenital sinus at the time of the clitoroplasty to take advantage of the redundant phallic skin and prepuce to create anterior vaginal flaps and labia minora. For cases with a high junction of the urethra and vagina, we prefer the technique described by González and Fernandes (Fig. 38.8)[23] with modifications to improve the cosmetic appearance of the vestibule by using the excess urogenital sinus tissue when available (Fig. 38.9). In our experience, techniques that do not use a posterior U flap of perineal skin to widen the posterior vaginal wall tend to lead to introital stenosis and are to be discouraged.[25, 32]

Cloaca

Repair of the persistent cloaca requires a team approach between the pediatric surgeon, the pediatric urologist, and, at times, the neurosurgeon. The surgeon or team of surgeons treating this rare and challenging malformation must be well-trained and experienced to have the flexibility necessary to solve difficult or unexpected situations. Errors caused by inexperience at the first operation compromise the long-term outcome.

Treatment starts in the newborn period with a colostomy and a radiologic and endoscopic evaluation. Peña makes a strong case in favor of a descending colon colostomy.[16] The advantages cited include a low incidence of prolapse and a reduced risk of the infant developing metabolic acidosis from absorption urine that may enter the colon through the urinary fistula. The disadvantage of this technique is that if construction of an intestinal vagina is required at the time of reconstruc-

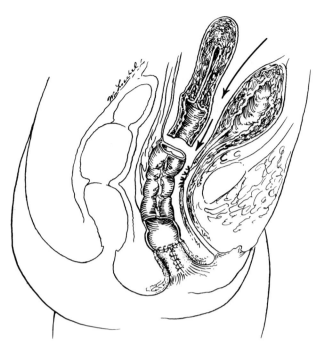

FIG. 38.14. Technique that uses the sigmoid colon to bridge the gap between a high short vagina (*arrows*) and the perineal skin flaps. The colonic segment is based on a distal vessel, usually the superior hemorrhoidal, and the marginal artery is carefully preserved. The rectovaginal and vesicovaginal spaces must be dissected. The sigmoid segment and its pedicle are brought down posteriorly, but the anastomosis between its upper portion and the distal vagina is best done from the front. To facilitate reaching the perineum, it is usually better to rotate the sigmoid segment 180° so that the proximal end of the color segment is positioned distal in the vaginal anastomosis.

tion, the colon distal to the colostomy is too short for this purpose. Others propose a transverse colostomy, which overcomes this objection and is preferred in cases of high confluence in which difficult vaginal reconstruction can be anticipated.[14] Whatever the location of the colostomy it should be a totally divided end colostomy and a mucus fistula to avoid passage of stool to the distal colon, common when a loop colostomy is done. Also, the marginal artery should be preserved to maintain the dual blood supply of the sigmoid colon and rectum from the superior and inferior mesenteric arteries. This is important when, at the time of the reconstruction, it becomes necessary to divide the inferior mesenteric artery to gain length of the rectum.

In many cases, a vagina distended with urine may cause urinary obstruction and, as in any case of hydrometrocolpos, this needs urgent management. Dilation or slight cutback of the sinus to facilitate intermittent catheterization of the vagina or the bladder usually suffices. When decompression cannot be achieved by this method, vesicostomy or rarely tube vaginostomy may be necessary.[14]

The repair is usually postponed until the child is 6 to 18 months of age, depending on the existence of associated malformations and the general health of the infant. Most surgeons agree that the posterior sagittal approach of DeVries and Peña[33] is the preferred method to repair these malformations.

When the sinus is shorter than 3 cm, the rectum is separated first from the vagina and mobilized (Fig. 38.7). The sinus need not be opened and no attempt is made to separate the vagina from the urethra. Instead, the intact urogenital sinus is mobilized and brought down. The common channel is excised and the separate openings of the urethra and vagina are placed in a normal anatomic perineal position.[21]

When the common channel is longer than 3 cm, the standard posterior approach is recommended (Fig. 38.15). However, this approach commonly needs to be combined with a laparotomy to better define the anatomy, particularly of the internal genitalia, and to help mobilize a high rectum and vagina. The child must be prepared and draped in such a way to allow for easy turning from prone to supine during the operation. The abdominal approach is also essential for the simultaneous correction of associated urologic anomalies such as refluxing or obstructed ureters.

Some important points of the technique include identifying the future site for the anus using a muscle stimulator to place the rectum at the center of the muscle complex, keeping the plane of incision strictly in the midline and marking with sutures the various muscle layers divided to facilitate their reapproximation during closure. In the original description of this operation the entire length of the cloaca was incised dorsally. However, this is unnecessary in many cases. Instead, the vagina is opened posteriorly to identify the point of confluence of the alimentary, genital, and urinary tracts but the sinus is preserved unopened to serve as the urethra. This is particularly important when the urethra above the confluence is short.

The most difficult part of the repair is usually the separation of the anterior vaginal wall from the urethra and bladder. The vaginal reconstruction is often challenging and can be made more difficult by a prior tube vaginostomy. The midline sagittal septum that divides the duplicated vaginas should be incised when present. When the vagina cannot be brought down by simple mobilization, the addition of a bowel segment to reach the skin may be necessary. A large vagina secondary to hydrocolpos may allow for the creation of vaginal wall flaps to reach the perineum.

Calibration or dilation of the anus and vagina is started after the 10th postoperative day and continued at intervals until the healing is complete and the colostomy is closed 10 to 12 weeks after the repair. Careful follow-up and periodic reevaluation of the digestive and urinary systems is necessary until adulthood. Genital

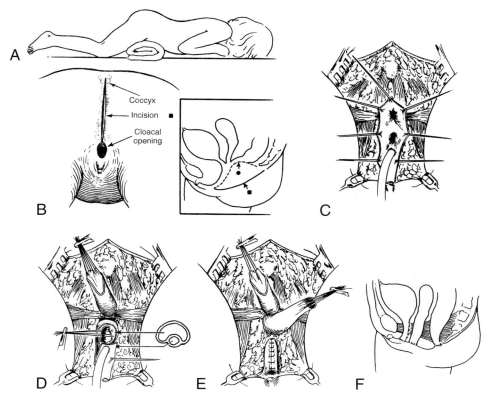

FIG. 38.15. A, For repair of a cloaca through the posterior sagittal approach, the patient is positioned prone with the thighs spread, but provisions are made to turn the patient and perform a laparotomy either before or after the posterior incision is made. The site for the future location of the anus is determined using a muscle stimulator to make the skin appropriately. **B,** A midline incision is made from the coccyx to the opening of the cloaca. **C,** Staying strictly in the midline, the muscular planes are tagged with sutures to facilitate their reapproximation during closure. **D,** The cloaca is opened in the midline. The rectum is first separated from the cloaca and mobilized superiorly; it often needs tapering, as shown. **E,** Next, the vagina is divided from the sinus and mobilized. The dissection of the vagina from the urethra can be difficult. At this point the surgeon must deal with possible problems presented by the associated vaginal anomalies such as septation, duplication, or short length. The addition of an intestinal segment to extend the vagina distally is sometimes necessary. Once the vagina is sufficiently mobilized, the cloaca is closed to serve as the distal urethra. **F,** The incision is closed, approximating all anatomical layers and positioning the anus, vaginal introitus, and urethral meatus in the appropriate locations.

evaluation under anesthesia is recommended around the onset of puberty.

Difficult vaginal or rectal mobilization may necessitate a combined abdominal and posterior sagittal approach. This possibility needs to be considered when positioning and preparing the patient for surgery.[14]

RESULTS

There are few published data that allow the surgeon to evaluate the long-term results of the techniques described. Bailez et al. reported on long-term data regarding vaginoplasties performed at an early age, suggesting that revisions may be necessary after puberty for introital stenosis in up to 78% of cases.[32] The authors of this report observed 28 females for a mean of 16 years who

underwent vaginoplasty for adrenal hyperplasia at a mean age of 22 months. The revisions done after puberty were successful in 72% of cases.

Although these data could be used to advance the argument of delaying vaginoplasty until after puberty, we continue to advocate early repair with careful follow-up.[23, 34] This attitude is in keeping with our general philosophy of early repair of genital malformations, but we recognize that only in the future, with long-term follow-up of patients operated early with current techniques, will the question of optimal timing for repair be answered. The high revision rate reported by Bailez et al. may be explained in part by the fact that many of their patients were operated on more than 20 years ago without the benefit of modern, sophisticated techniques that use a posterior flap for the vaginoplasty.[32] In any event, most of their patients required a minor revision after puberty to achieve an adequate introitus. We do not recommend routine dilations in prepubertal girls, but to examine them yearly in the clinic and if a stenosis is suspected, we perform an examination under anesthesia.

Reports on long-term results of cloacal reconstruction are few. Results of cloacal repairs must be evaluated from several angles, including rectal continence, urinary continence, ability to evacuate the rectum and the bladder spontaneously, preservation of renal integrity, adequacy of the vagina, sexual function, and general wellbeing of the individual. Because associated spinal cord anomalies are so common, many patients will have neurogenic dysfunction of the bladder and colon. For the bladder this often means the possibility of intermittent catheterization. Thus, the reconstructed urethral meatus should be readily accesible and the urethra easy to catheterize. Reconstructive surgery to correct reflux, enlarge the bladder, and enhance urethral resistance may be needed, and the results and complications must be taken into account when considering the overall success of a given procedure. In general, the principles and results of urologic management of these patients are similar to that of other patients with neurogenic bladder dysfunction, but with the aggravating feature that a reconstructed urethra may be inaccessible or difficult to catheterize.[35] Patients who do not achieve urinary or fecal control may require additional procedures to enhance bladder and bowel emptying, such as continent appendicovesicostomy,[36] or the Malone operation for antegrade enema administration.[37]

Peña reported the results of 26 cloaca abnormalities that had completed reconstrucion. Of the 19 patients with a normal sacrum, 18 had voluntary bowel movements, 14 exhibited some soiling, 3 had episodes of diarrhea, 2 had constipation, and 5 had urinary incontinence. In contrast, of seven patients with an abnormal sacrum, three had voluntary bowel movements, six soiled, two were constipated, and five had urinary incontinence.[16] These results highlight the importance of intact neural pathways to achieve good results.

Because extensive data on the long-term results of cloacal repairs are unavailable, we must rely on reports that address fecal continence and quality of life in patients with high imperforate anus. A group from the Netherlands observed 58 patients with a median age of 26 years who had repair of high anorectal malformations in childhood. No patient had normal fecal control, but 84% had socially acceptable defecation. Twelve percent felt socially handicapped by their condition, 24% never had a lasting relationship and of those who had, 48% felt that their problem interfered with the relationship.[38] Similar findings were reported by a group in Finland. Of 33 patients, including 8 females, only 18% had normal bowel movements and the quality

of life of the group was estimated to be poor.[39] These studies suggest that parental education and life-long counseling is an important part of the management of these patients.

CONCLUSION

The evaluation and treatment of patients with anomalies of the urogenital sinus and cloaca presents one of the greatest challenges of reconstructive pediatric urology and surgery. With precise diagnosis, evaluation of the anatomy and identification of potential functional disorders, the surgical treatment of these children is generally satisfactory. Cases of isolated persistence of the urogenital sinus can be usually reconstructed successfully, although the achievement of urinary continence and long-term adequacy of the vagina may require reoperation and long-term follow-up.

The long-term results of children with urogenital sinus anomalies associated with intersex is described in detail in Chapter 32. Cases of persistent cloaca are the most challenging of all. A team approach, early counseling of the family and later of the patient as well as life-long follow-up are essential to insure the greatest degree of patient satisfaction and psychosocial adjustment. Preservation of renal integrity, the attainment of urinary and fecal control and the reconstruction of an adequate vagina remain challenging goals for the treatment team.

REFERENCES

1. Patten BM. Human Embryology, 2nd ed. NY: McGraw-Hill, 1947;585.
2. Stephens FD. Congenital malformations of the urinary tract. In: Normal Embryology of the Cloaca. NY: Praeger Publishers, 1983;3–14.
3. O'Rahilly R. The development of the vagina in the human. In: Blandau RJ, Bergsma D, eds. Morphogenesis and Malformations of the Genital System. Birth Defects: Original article series 13. New York: Alan R Liss Inc. 1997;123–136.
4. Carlson B. Embryology of the urogenital sinus. In: Patten's Foundations of Embryology. New York: McGraw-Hill, 1981.
5. Witschi E. Development and differentiation of the uterus. In: HC Mack, ed. Prenatal Life. Detroit: Wayne University Press, 1970;11–35.
6. Bok G, Drews U. The role of the Wolffian ducts in the development of the vagina: an organ culture study. J Embryol Exper Morphol 1983;73:275–95.
7. Mauch RB, Thiedemann KU, Drews U. The vagina is formed by downgrowth of Wolffian and Müllerian ducts. Graphical reconstructions from normal and Tfm mouse embryos. Anat Embryol 1985;172:75–87.
8. Ufelder H, Robboy SJ. The embryologic development of the human vagina. Am J Obstet Gynecol 1976;126:769–776.
9. Cunha GR. The dual origin of the vaginal epithelium. Am J Anat 1975;143:387–392.
10. Peña A, Filmer B. Urogenital sinus surgery in pediatric patients. Infect Urol 1993, May/June.
11. Blask AR, Sanders RC, Gearhart JP. Obstructed uterovaginal anomalies: demonstration with sonography. Part I. Neonates and infants. Radiology 1991;179:79–83.
12. Peña A. The surgical management of persistent cloaca: results in

54 patients treated with a posterior sagittal approach. J Pediatr Surg 1989;24:590–598.

13. Tröger J, Greinacher I. The radiologic diagnosis of the sinus urogenitalis. Prog Pediatr Surg 1985;17:11–20.

14. Hendren WH. Cloacal malformations. In: Walsh PC, Retik AB, Stamey TA, Vaughan ED, eds. Campbell's Urology. Philadelphia: WB Saunders, 1992;1822–1850.

15. Sheldon CA, Gilbert A, Lewis AG, Aiken J, Ziegler MM. Surgical implications of genitourinary tract anomalies in patients with imperforate anus. J Urol 1994;152:196–199.

16. Peña A. Anorectal anomalies. In: Spitz L, Coran AC, eds. Rob & Smith's Operative Surgery. Pediatric Surgery. 5th ed. London: Chapman & Hall. 1995;423–451.

17. Beek FJA, Boemers TD, Witkamp MS, vanLeeuwen MS, Mali WPTM, Bax NMA. Spine evaluation in children with anorectal malformations. Pediatr Radiol 1995;25 (suppl 1):S28–32.

18. Appignani BA, Jaramillo D, Barnes PD, Poussaint TY. Dysraphic myelodysplasias associated with urogenital and anorectal anomalies: prevalence and types seen with MRI imaging. AJR 1994;163:1199–1203.

19. Alexander F, Kay R. Cloacal anomalies: role of vesicostomy. J Pediatr Surg 1994;29:74–76.

20. Ramenofsky MC, Raffensperger JG. An abdominal-perineal-vaginal pull through for the definitive treatment of hydrometrocolpos. J Pediatr Surg 1971;6:381–387.

21. Peña A. Total urogenital mobilization. An easier approach to repair cloacas. J Pediatr Surg 1997;32:263–268.

22. Ludwikowski B, Oesch Hayward I, González R. Total urogenital mobilization. Expand applications. BJU Int (In press).

23. González R, Fernandes E. Feminization genitoplasty. J Urol 1989;43:776.

24. Monfort G. Transvesical approach to utricular cysts. J Pediatr Surg 1982;17:406.

25. Passerini-Glazel G. A new 1-stage procedure for clitorovaginoplasty in severely masculinized female pseudohermaphrodites. J Urol 1989;142:565.

26. Patil U, Hixson FP. The role of tissue expanders in vaginoplasty for congenital malformations of the vagina. Br J Urol 1992;70:554–557.

27. Belloli G, Campobasso P, Musi L. Labial flap vaginoplasty using tissue expanders. Pediatr Surg Int 1997;12:168–171.

28. Hendren WH. Construction of female urethra from vaginal wall and perineal flap. J Urol 1980;123:657.

29. González R. Reconstruction of the female urethra to allow intermittent catheterization for neurogenic bladders and urogenital sinus anomalies. J Urol 1985;133:478.

30. Peña A, Filmer B, Bonilla E, Mendez M, Stolar C. Transanorectal approach for the treatment of urogenital sinus without anorectal malformation. J Pediatr Surg 1992;27:681–685.

31. Dòmini R, Rossi F, Ceccarelli PL, de Castro R. Anterior sagittal transanorectal approach to the urogenital sinus in adrenogenital syndrome. Preliminary report. J Pediatr Surg 1997;32:823.

32. Bailez MM, Gearhart JP, Migeon C, Rock J. J Urol 1992;148:680–682.

33. DeVries P, Peña A. Posterior sagittal anorectoplasty. J Pediatr Surg 1982;17:638–643.

34. de Jong TPVM, Boemers TML. Neonatal management of female intersex by clitorovaginoplasty. J Urol 1995;154:830.

35. Fernandes E, Reinberg Y, Vernier R, González R. Neurogenic bladder in children. Review of pathophysiology and current treatment. J Pediatr 1994;124:1–7.

36. Süser O, Vates TS, Freedman AL, Smith CA, González R. Results of the Mitrofanoff procedure in urinary tract reconstruction in children. Br J Urol 1997;79:279–282.

37. Malone PS, Ransley PG, Kiely EM. Preliminary report: the antegrade continence enema. Lancet 1990;336:1217–1218.

38. Hassnik EAM, Rieu PNMA, Brugman ATM, Festen C. Quality of life after operatively corrected high anorectal malformation: A long-term follow-up study of patients aged 18 years and older. J Pediatr Surg 1994;29:773–776.

39. Rintala R, Mildh H, Lindahl H. Fecal continence and quality of life for adult patients with an operated high or intermediate anorectal malformation. J Pediatr Surg 1994;29:777–779.

CHAPTER 39

The Role of Urinary Diversion in Childhood: Temporary, Continent, or Otherwise

Byron D. Joyner and Antoine E. Khoury

INTRODUCTION

The ideal urinary neobladder should provide for continent, low-pressure, non-refluxing storage of sterile urine which can be completely and conveniently emptied at the will of the patient. It should approximate normal bladder function, preserve renal tissue, and be psychologically and socially acceptable to the patient. The prerequisites for the ideal urinary diversion appear intuitive today only because so many historical contributions have led to the distillation of these concepts.

The concept of *cutaneous* urinary diversions began in the mid-1800s with Rayer's[1] correlation of renal failure with hydronephrosis. This association provided the rationale for surgical intervention in such cases. Aspiration of the hydronephrotic kidney involved percutaneous insertion of a bore needle to decompress the distended renal pelvis. In 1878, Robert Weir performed the first open drainage of a hydronephrotic kidney. Twenty years later, a nephrotomy was recommended by Henry Morris for a patient whose solitary hydronephrotic kidney drained for six years post-operatively.[2] The *continent* urinary diversion first appeared in 1851, when Simon[3] performed the first ureterosigmoidostomy in a patient with bladder exstrophy. After one year, the patient died of overwhelming urosepsis. Ten years later, Mikulicz performed the first successful human ileocystoplasty.[4]

For nearly the next century, advancement of urinary diversion was hindered by complications of the ureteral anastomosis, the most common of which were postoperative leakage and infection. It was not until Coffey's[5] anti-reflux "value" that the idea of protecting the upper urinary tracts became possible. Such a valve was created by tunneling the distal ureter through the submucosa of the large intestine. This technique prevented urinary reflux, ascending infection, and renal damage.

Despite the odd success story of the operation, mortality remained high, with death typically secondary to enteric soilage and inevitable urosepsis.

Solutions for these problems became apparent in the 1950s. Bricker's[6] popularization of the ileal conduit was one of them. Initially described in 1911 by Zaaijer,[7] the ileal conduit is still arguably the gold standard of urinary diversions. Born out of frustration with attempts at constructing an intra-abdominal receptacle for collection and storage of urine, the ileal conduit (ureterointestinal diversion) seemed to be a tacit admission of failure. Quite to the contrary: in 1950, the ileal loop was praised for its simplicity and low rate of complications. In the same year, Gilchrist and associates[8] revisited the continent urinary diversion previously set forth as the ureterosigmoidostomy. Their new technique, clearly the forerunner of most of the contemporary continent diversions, was largely ignored because of inconsistent results of continence, as well as skepticism regarding intermittent catheterization. Besides, Bricker's simple solution was the obvious choice for supravesical urinary diversion, so much so that for the next 30 years (1950 to 1980), enthusiasm for the continent urinary diversion waned almost to the point of extinction.

During this time, however, reasonable solutions to many recurring problems were described. Previous techniques of ureterointestinal anastomosis often led to urinary obstruction or leakage of urine. However, these serious complications were significantly lessened after the description of a careful mucosa-to-mucosa anastomosis by several investigators.[9–13] This new technique led to a significant reduction in the incidence of both obstruction and infection.[14, 15] Concurrently, the explosion of broad-spectrum antibiotics acted synergistically to improve success by providing greater protection from infection after enteric soilage. Furthermore, they provided the impetus to safely try innovative surgical techniques, which previously had been prohibitive. The role of antibiotics in the progress of urinary diversion should not be underestimated.

Another significant problem was solved with Lapides' landmark article on clean intermittent self-catheterization (CIC).[16] Prior to this, augmentation cystoplasty in children with neurogenic bladder dysfunction was contraindicated because most could not empty their bladder even before the augmentation. CIC allowed convenient and complete emptying of the bladder at regular, socially acceptable intervals. The technique was simple and convincing. The timing was impeccable. Lapides' contribution actually revolutionized the concept of continent urinary diversion.

In 1979, Camey and LeDuc,[17] realizing that there might be a better solution, devised an operation in which urethral voiding was maintained by utilizing a tubularized loop of ileum that could be attached to a urethral stump. Urinary continence was maintained by the individual's own external sphincter. The procedure was plagued by a high rate of both diurnal and nocturnal incontinence. But it was popular because, like Lapides' CIC, it rekindled enthusiasm in the search for the ideal continent diversion. The popularity of this concept has continued, especially following such landmark descriptions as the Koch detubularized reservoir[18] and the Mitrofanoff principle.[19]

The ingenuity of reconstructive surgeons continues to refine techniques for urinary diversion. In fact, in the last 10 years, over 40 operations for continent urinary diversion have been described. Although most of the operations differ from one another in only small details, each has made a contribution toward the construction of the ideal continent urinary reservoir. Another reason that continent urinary diversion has been so widely accepted is that indications for urinary diversion have been better defined and temporary urinary diversion is less frequently performed now compared to 20 years ago.[20, 21] Ironically, interest in the century-old ureterosigmoidostomy has resurfaced.[22, 23] Applying new techniques to old ideas has re-established the modified ureterosigmoidostomy, in selected patients, as yet another option for continent urinary diversion.

This historical perspective provides just some of the landmark advancements in the search for the perfect bladder substitute. It is by no means complete. The perfect bladder substitute continues to be elusive while the need for the ideal urinary diversion is becoming increasingly important owing to the greater number of operations performed for intrapelvic cancers, genitourinary anomalies, and neurogenic bladder diseases.[24]

TEMPORARY URINARY DIVERSIONS

Temporary urinary diversions may be classified variously as intubated or nonintubated, percutaneously or surgically placed, single or multi-staged, and continent or incontinent.[25] The fact that there are so many categories and even more types suggests that none of the categories would satisfy every situation in which a urinary diversion might be necessary. Any child who might require a urinary diversion should be evaluated individually, keeping in mind the child's needs as well as the limitations of each diversion. Despite new technical advances and earlier reconstructive surgery, temporary urinary diversions are still occasionally indicated.

Infravesical Intubated Diversion (Urethral Catheter)

Only certain conditions require transient, intubated urethral drainage. Common examples are children who require monitoring of their urine output, neonates who are being evaluated for posterior urethral valves, boys who have a urethral catheter placed after a hypospadias repair or urethral reconstruction, and children who receive a catheter after dilatation of a urethral stricture. Prolonged use of indwelling urethral catheters introduces infection, bladder inflammation, and stone formation.[26]

Intubated Cystostomy (Suprapubic Catheter)

Intubated cystostomies can be inserted either percutaneously or surgically. Percutaneous insertion of a suprapubic catheter is typically performed with one of the wide range of commercially available percutaneous cystostomy kits (Fig. 39.1). The procedure is generally easy and safe. Consequently, it has largely replaced the open cystostomy techniques.

An intubated cystostomy is indicated for patients who

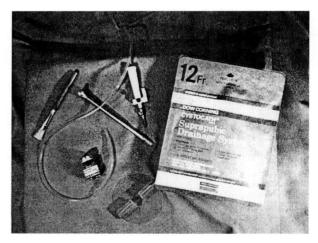

FIG. 39.1. CYSTOCATH Suprapubic Drainage System Set (Medical Products, Bulletin 51-009b, Dow Corning Corporation, Midland, Michigan). (From Ring KS, Hensle TW: Urinary Diversion. In: Kelalis PP, King LR, Belman AB, eds. Clinical Pediatric Urology, Vol 2, 3rd ed. Philadelphia: W.B. Saunders Co. 1992;866.)

require temporary urinary diversion, such as boys undergoing hypospadias repair, children suffering from urethral stricture disease, or those with severe lower urinary tract infections (urethritis or prostatitis). Open surgical placement of a suprapubic tube is preferable when the patient has had previous abdominopelvic surgery. Adhesions and scar tissue distort the normal anatomical landmarks, making percutaneous placement unpredictable.

Intubated cystostomies are not intended for long-term diversion. They should not be used in cases of secondary ureteral dilation and tortuosity, because bladder decompression would not address the primary problem and might actually exacerbate obstruction at the ureterovesical junction.[27] Complications of intubated cystostomies include infection, stone formation, and contraction of the anterior bladder wall.[28] Percutaneously placed intubated cystostomies have the additional complications of iatrogenic internal organ or vascular injury. Such problems can be minimized if ultrasound guidance is utilized during the procedure.

Cutaneous Vesicostomy

Since long-term indwelling catheters were known to cause a Pandora's box of problems, it became imperative to develop a tubeless diversion that would provide unobstructed flow of urine at the bladder level. The cutaneous vesicostomy was initially performed in 1956 in an elderly man with urethral carcinoma.[29] However, it was not accepted as an important method of temporary urinary diversion in children until the 1970s.[30]

Cutaneous vesicostomy is a tubeless, temporary urinary diversion that decompresses the entire urinary tract.[26] It is readily reversible, easy to perform with minimal operating time, and drains directly into a diaper (Fig. 39.2). A cutaneous vesicostomy might be indicated in a variety of situations.[26] These include posterior urethral valves, neuropathic bladder (secondary to myelomeningocele, sacral tumor removal, or sacral pull-through), Prune Belly syndrome, high-grade vesicoureteral reflux with tortuous megaureters, urethral stricture disease, ureteroceles, dysfunctional voiding (Hinman) syndrome, and urogenital-cloacal anomalies. It also might be indicated in children for whom clean intermittent self-catheterization is an unrealistic option.

Cutaneous vesicostomy is commonly employed in the neonate with posterior urethral valves when cystoscopic evaluation and primary valve ablation are inadvisable due to either a small urethral caliber or a sick neonate. In these situations, (until the child is old enough for

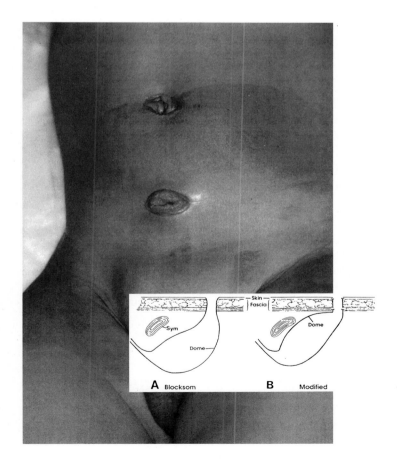

FIG. 39.2 Standard cutaneous vesicostomy. (Photograph courtesy of Antoine E. Khoury, The Hospital for Sick Children.) (Krahn CG, Johnson HW. Cutaneous vesicostomy in the young child: indications and results. Urology 1993;41(6):562.)

definitive reconstructive surgery) cutaneous vesicostomy is an effective temporizing solution.

The technique is simple and efficacious, providing at least a 60% improvement in upper urinary tract dilatation and a decreased rate of pyelonephritis.[26] Babies who do not improve, in spite of a cutaneous vesicostomy, may benefit from a supravesical urinary diversion and renal biopsy.

Babies who are candidates for a vesicostomy should have a voiding cystourethrogram (VCUG) in order to determine bladder capacity and configuration, as well as to establish the presence and grade of reflux. Prior to surgery, the parents should be informed that vesicostomy reversal and definitive reconstruction will be delayed until the child is between 1 and 3 years of age. Close follow-up, including serial blood work and imaging studies, is imperative to determine the child's progress.

Prolonged vesicostomy drainage can result in chronic bacterial colonization, vesical stone formation,[28, 30] bladder wall prolapse. Persistent upper tract deterioration might result from stomal stenosis which can be avoided by meticulous attention to surgical detail.

Intubated Nephrostomy (Nephrostomy Tube)

A nephrostomy tube may be placed as an open surgical or percutaneous procedure. Nephrostomy tubes are used to temporarily decompress an acutely obstructed upper urinary tract. Indications for nephrostomy tube insertion include relief of a congenital or acquired obstruction, especially in the presence of infection or acute renal deterioration. It is the first step in gaining antegrade renal access, which permits a wide range of diagnostic and therapeutic options. Percutaneous nephrostomies can be difficult because of the great mobility of the pediatric kidney.[31] Therefore, a certain amount of expertise is required.

Recently, we have developed a pyeloureteral tube which can be placed intraoperatively to divert the urine and stent the anastomosis following a dismembered pyeloplasty[32] (Fig. 39.3). The advantage of the new percutaneous pyeloureteral stent over the standard double J ureteral stent is that it can be removed easily in an outpatient setting without a general anesthetic.

As much as possible, prior to intracorporeal manipulation (nephrostomy tube) the patient should have sterile urine. Patients should have any bleeding diathesis and hypertension corrected initially to avoid renal hemorrhage, the most common complication of nephrostomy tube placement. Special consideration should be given to any child who might be a candidate for a nephrostomy tube. Majid and associates point out that in children with asymmetry of body structures, positioning for percutaneous placement and understanding individ-

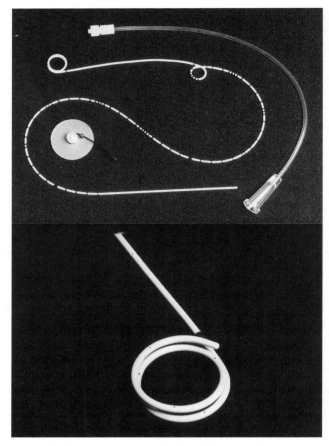

FIG. 39.3. Salle pyeloureteral stent. (Photograph courtesy of Cook Urological, Inc., A Cook Group Company, Spencer, Indiana.)

ual anatomical variations become exceedingly important when trying to avoid unnecessary morbidity.[33]

Incontinent Urointestinal Diversion (Ileal Loop Conduit)

Incontinent urinary conduits were at one time the standard method of urinary diversion in children with obstructive uropathy and neurogenic bladder dysfunction[34] (Fig. 39.4). But by the mid-1970s, a series of review articles had dismantled their foundation.[35-38] In the developing child, conduit urinary diversions have been associated with an unacceptable number of long-term complications, including metabolic acidosis, stomal stenosis, chronic low-grade bacilliuria, renal and bladder calculi, upper urinary tract deterioration, and unavoidable life-style problems.[20, 39]

Today, incontinent diversions are rarely indicated in the pediatric population.[40] They may be viable options for children with reduced renal function who are not capable of performing clean intermittent self-catheterization of a continent intestinocystoplasty and for those

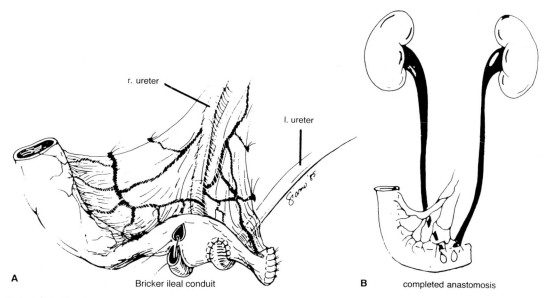

FIG. 39.4. Ileal conduit urinary diversion. (Adapted from Hampel N, Bodner DR, Persky L, eds.: Ileal and jejunal conduit diversion. Urologic Clinics of North America, 1986;13:207.)

children who have a poor life expectancy. Despite earlier enthusiasm, both the ileal conduit[37, 41] and the nonrefluxing colon conduit[42] are associated with considerable upper tract deterioration, especially when associated with functional or mechanical obstruction.[43] However, recently Stein et al. concluded that when a child does require an incontinent diversion, an isoperistaltic, anti-refluxing colonic conduit is preferable because it minimizes upper urinary tract deterioration.[23]

The cosmetically-acceptable continent urinary diversion has been a significant factor in making the ileal conduit obsolete in children. The continent diversion has led to an improved self-image and enhanced sexuality. Boyd and associates surveyed the psychological impact of continent and ileal conduit diversion on a large group of patients.[44] Those with external appliances had the poorest self-images, as defined by a decrease in libido and avoidance of all forms of social and physical contact. A subset of index patients who had undergone undiversion were the most physically and sexually active of all of the groups studied. Many children who in the past were once appliance-dependent are now kept dry and infection-free with a combination of medications and intermittent catheterization.[45] Measures that confront issues of bowel and bladder continence enhance the sexual appeal and improve socialization and sexual function.

End Cutaneous Ureterostomies

Coaptation is the method by which a bolus of urine is formed and carried distally into the bladder.[46, 47] Dilated ureters do not coapt, and urine transport primarily de-

pends on gravity and the hydrostatic forces generated by the kidney.[48] This method of drainage is ineffective, resulting in pooling of urine, stasis, and eventual dilation of the ureter (Fig. 39.5). Bacterial toxins released during a urinary tract infection further impair the already poorly functioning ureter, thus complicating the problem.[46, 49, 50]

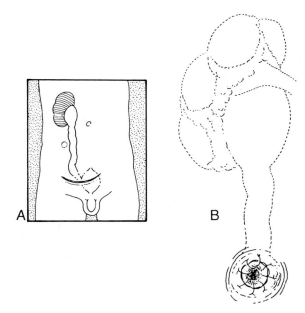

FIG. 39.5. End cutaneous ureterostomy. **A,** Incision for end cutaneous ureterostomy. **B,** Completed end cutaneous ureterostomy. (Adapted from Ring, KS and Hensle, TW: Urinary Diversion. In: Kelalis PP, King LR, Belman AB, eds. Clinical Pediatric Urology, Vol 2, 3rd ed. Philadelphia WB Saunders Co. 1992;874.)

Despite the fact that end cutaneous ureterostomy is easy to construct and has a low incidence of stomal stenosis,[51] there are two concerns with this form of diversion. The first is that this procedure does not allow the kidneys to be biopsied. This is merely a nuisance as a biopsy might be of prognostic value. The second concern arises at the time of closure and is more germane. The distal ureter, having been disconnected from the bladder at the original procedure, depends on its proximal blood supply. In order to reestablish vesicoureteral continuity, it must be mobilized again, further compromising its vascular supply. This is not an ideal situation for reimplantation of the ureters because it places them at an unnecessarily high risk for ischemia and ureteral stenosis.

Candidates for end cutaneous ureterostomy might be 1) a child with obstructed megaureters whose distal portions must be excised at reconstruction or 2) a child who has a poor life expectancy and for whom the urinary diversion is performed for palliation. But, in general, indications for end cutaneous ureterostomy are limited.

Cutaneous Pyelostomy and High Cutaneous Ureterostomy

Conditions which require immediate proximal temporary supravesical drainage are rare, indeed. They are typically restricted to newborns who have progressive hydroureteronephrosis, poor urinary drainage, renal compromise, and persistent infections despite initial urethral intubation. In this situation, the most common diagnoses are either posterior urethral valves (associated with a thickened, stiff bladder) or high-grade vesicoureteral reflux. Babies with these conditions often require stabilization in an intensive care unit where their fluid and electrolyte status can be optimized, acid-base problems can be corrected, and sepsis can be addressed.

A supravesical diversion allows the urine to bypass the long, tortuous ureter and the intramural tunnel, both of which could delay, if not substantially impede, urinary drainage. Theoretically, a more proximal diversion should provide for better drainage. Therefore, a supravesical diversion is occasionally useful in the management of vesical and urethral anomalies when persistence of severe upper urinary tract dilatation is unrelieved by either valve ablation or vesicostomy. Additionally, the stable child with massively dilated ureters may be decompressed with a supravesical ureteral diversion, making ureteral tapering unnecessary and allowing interval improvement of the renal function. Therefore, high loop cutaneous ureterostomies or pyelostomies continue to have clinical application in limited circumstances.

The cutaneous pyelostomy (Fig. 39.6) is preferred only when the renal pelvis is of sufficient size to reach the skin without tension or distortion of the ureteropelvic junction. A pyelostomy has the additional advantage of

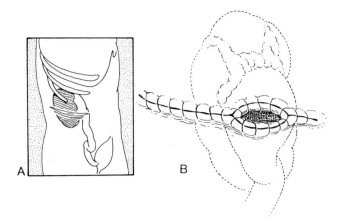

FIG. 39.6. Cutaneous pyelostomy. **A,** Incision for cutaneous pyelostomy. **B,** Completed cutaneous pyelostomy. (Adapted from Ring KS, Hensle TW: Urinary Diversion. In: Kelalis PP, King LR, Belman AB, eds. Clinical Pediatric Urology, Vol 2, 3rd ed. Philadelphia: W.B. Saunders Co. 1992;876.)

maintaining ureteral integrity. This makes subsequent closure and ureteral reimplantation easier by avoiding devascularization of the ureter. Pyelostomies or loop ureterostomies are the urinary diversions of choice for the child for whom vesical or infravesical diversion has failed and who consequently has a chronically dilated, obstructed, redundant ureter.[25]

Duckett[21] claims that infants with ipsilateral renal function less than 15% benefit from a supravesical diversion because this maneuver may allow the kidney to regain some of its function. In this setting, supravesical diversion has a threefold benefit. First, a biopsy of the kidney can be obtained during the procedure. A renal biopsy may have prognostic value in that the degree of renal dysplasia may be assessed. Additionally, a renal biopsy might be helpful in sorting out whether the baby whose creatinine continues to rise, despite adequate infravesical diversion, has poorly functioning kidneys or inadequate drainage. Second supravesical diversions allows the affected kidney to be monitored by sequential radiography in a retrograde or an antegrade fashion.[25] Third, in the interim, the surgeon can decide upon the most appropriate, definitive surgical management.

Supravesical diversion is rarely the initial procedure and is often performed only after a cutaneous vesicostomy does not improve progressive hydroureteronephrosis associated with azotemia, urosepsis, high-grade reflux, and/or incomplete bladder emptying. Some urologists utilize high diversion selectively, in the sickest children with progressive uropathy and severe hydroureteronephrosis. Others claim that there are no indications for supravesical diversions whatsoever, citing that they are prone to ureteral stricturing, difficult to reconstruct, and detrimental to the bladder.[26] The debate regarding the last claim has existed for many years and is unlikely to be resolved soon.

Some authors criticize bilateral proximal urinary diversion because it prevents bladder storage and expulsion of urine, which may result in defunctionalization of the bladder. This is an attractive but controversial theory. Some clinicians believe that postdiversion bladder defunctionalization is related to issues that are intrinsic to the bladder, such as posterior urethral valves or neurogenic bladder dysfunction. Others believe that postdiversion bladder contraction occurs as a result of either severe, chronic infections, of fibrosis secondary to multiple surgical procedures.[52] But, Jayanthi et al. concluded in a retrospective review of temporary vesical diversions that most patients can undergo primary reversal of the temporary cutaneous diversion with preservation of ultimate bladder function.[53]

ALGORITHM FOR TEMPORARY URINARY DIVERSION

The most effective management of the neonate with progressive renal failure and hydroureteronephrosis is to progress through a logical algorithm in order to establish adequate urinary drainage. Posterior urethral valves (PUV) are a common cause of infravesical obstruction in the male neonate. Patients with PUV offer some insight into the variability involved in deciding on the timing and the technique of urinary diversion. Therefore, PUV will be used as a model to illustrate several points.

When a neonate with suspected PUV has been identified, a 5-French pediatric feeding tube is inserted into the urethra to provide adequate urinary drainage. The response to catheter drainage will be determined by following the level of the serum creatinine. If the urethral catheter causes the creatinine to decrease daily by 10% to a nadir of less that 80 μmol/L by day 5,[54] then transurethral resection of the posterior urethral valves is performed. Primary valve ablation is the preferred treatment of choice, but temporary urinary diversion may be necessary if the creatinine continues to rise following valve ablation. Children who may be too small (<2.5 kg) or too sick for a technically satisfactory endoscopic procedure may require a cutaneous vesicostomy. Then, when the urethra is larger, endoscopic valve ablation can be performed simultaneously with vesicostomy closure.

Sometimes, an indwelling foley catheter can exacerbate detrusor irritability, leading to inflammation and bladder instability. In these cases, when drainage is not adequate, the creatinine level is not falling, and primary valve ablation is not prudent, the foley catheter should be removed and a cutaneous vesicostomy should be performed. Ureteral drainage will improve after resolution of vesical edema and muscle hypertrophy. Monitoring the response of the creatinine, in association with

sequential physical examinations and radiographic findings, is extremely important.

Review of the radiographic studies can direct further management. All babies with PUV should have a voiding cystourethrogram (VCUG) in order to determine the bladder capacity and configuration, as well as to establish the presence and grade of reflux. In the infant whose voiding cystourethrogram (VCUG) demonstrates massive bilateral reflux, for example, a cutaneous vesicostomy may be beneficial to decompress the upper urinary tracts and to provide better drainage. For babies who do not improve clinically in spite of a cutaneous vesicostomy, a temporizing supravesical urinary diversion and a renal biopsy may be appropriate. Likewise, the baby with Posterior urethral and ipsilateral renal *valves* (VURD syndrome) may benefit from a higher diversion. In these situations, higher urinary diversions may serve to decompress the bladder and protect the normal kidney. When the renal ultrasound reveals hyperechoic renal parenchyma consistent with renal dysplasia, a supravesical diversion might provide not only the best decompression, but it might also be the best method of monitoring the urine output from each renal unit.

A voiding cystourethrogram may provide further insight into the quality of the bladder, as well. A "good" bladder has a normal capacity for age and a normal bladder wall. In contrast, a "bad" bladder is abnormally small, thick-walled, and noncompliant. The detrusor muscle hypertrophies in response to infravesical obstruction, with consequent trabeculation and sacculation. These distinctive radiographic findings are extremely useful in managing the infant who may need some form of urinary diversion.

CONTINENT URINARY DIVERSIONS

Until the 1970s, an incontinent urinary diversion was the standard therapy used to treat children with various forms of obstructive and neurogenic uropathies.[20] In the middle part of that decade however, pediatric urologists recognized that long-term results of conduit diversions were not extremely encouraging.[38, 56] They resulted in late complication rates of 87% in certain pediatric cohorts.[37]

For a variety of reasons, there are fewer pediatric diversions being performed today compared to 20 years ago. The complications witnessed in the 1970s were clear reminders that cautious reserve should balance every innovation. These complications forced many clinicians to re-examine their therapeutic approach to obstructive and neurogenic uropathies. Hendren was one of those clinicians. In that same decade, he demonstrated that virtually everyone with a retained defunctionalized bladder could be successfully undiverted.[57] Hendren's concept of *urinary undiversion* was contingent upon the use of nonsterile clean intermittent catheterization, introduced by Lapides in 1972.[16] It was the combination of these two concepts that led to the current mode of therapy: preservation of the bladder and the upper tracts by clean, intermittent self-catheterization with or without anticholinergic medications. Urinary diversions in the pediatric population are the final recourse, performed only in selected cases where no alternative treatment is available. Thus, many patients who, in the past, would have been candidates for a urinary diversion are currently being managed by this conservative regimen, which has been shown to be safe and reliable.[59]

Another, perhaps less obvious, factor that has had an impact on limiting the number of children requiring urinary diversions is ultrasonography. The excellent resolution of dynamic ultrasonography has allowed physicians to diagnose a number of congenital problems *in utero*. For example, the sonographic images of a myelomeningocele are sensitive. Some of the prenatal findings have such a poor prognosis or predict such a poor quality-of-life that an increasing number of parents are opting for termination of pregnancy.

Surgical Management

Those patients who do not benefit from an exhaustive trial of conservative treatment may become candidates for surgical management, of which there are two broad categories. Surgical procedures that serve to divert the urine (*urinary diversion*) have previously been reviewed (see "Temporary Urinary Diversion"). The second category of surgical procedures is continent diversion, which can be subcategorized into *stomal reservoir* and *orthotopic neobladder*. The mechanisms of continence are similar in both categories in that the principle techniques for achieving continence rely on increasing resistance to flow.[60] In the cutaneous stomal reservoir, also referred to as *continent cutaneous diversion,* a surgically constructed cutaneous stoma must be catheterized to overcome this resistance. Representations of a cutaneous stomal reservoir include the nipple valve (e.g., Kock pouch)[61] and the tapered segment of bowel (e.g., Indiana pouch).[62] An orthotopic neobladder, also called a *bladder substitute,* is attached directly to the urethra and relies on the external urinary sphincter for continence.[63] The patients with an orthotopic neobladder empties by coordinate pelvic floor relaxation and abdominal straining (Credé or Valsalva) or, alternatively, by intermittent catheterization. Representations of an orthotopic neobladder include Le Bag[64] or the Mainz pouch.[65]

There is a third category of continent urinary reservoir which will be mentioned for completeness. The *enteric diversion*[66] uses the intact anal sphincter as its continence mechanism. The ureterosigmoidostomy is the only example in this category. It was, in fact, the first continent urinary diversion.[3] In spite of its recent

"rediscovery"[22, 23] and intelligent modifications,[67] its acceptance has been modest.

Definitions of a continent diversion are blurred sometimes because the names are used interchangeably. And, as if these names are not confusing enough, many of the innumerable continent techniques have been immortalized by using the city of origin as eponyms (e.g., Indiana, Bellevue, Charleston, Mainz).

Candidates for Continent Urinary Diversion

Sheldon and Snyder listed four components to balanced urinary tract function that are essential in achieving long-term success with urinary tract reconstruction.[70] Each component should be evaluated in every candidate being considered for a continent urinary diversion. The first component is a reservoir capacity large enough to allow a 4-hour catheterization (or voiding) interval during the day and an 8-hour interval at night. As the reservoir fills, it should maintain a low storage pressure. The second component is a continent bladder outlet (see "Mechanisms of Continence in Continent Urinary Diversion"). The third component involves a consistent and convenient method of emptying the reservoir. If the urethra is not an acceptable conduit, then catheterization of the native urethra or a cutaneous stoma should be considered. The fourth component of achieving balanced urinary tract function is maintaining sterile, unobstructed drainage of urine from the kidneys and preventing reflux in order to assure protection of the upper urinary tracts.

Candidates for continent urinary diversion include children with obstructive uropathy, exstrophy (classic or cloacal), neoplasms, neurogenic voiding dysfunction secondary to myelomeningocele, or failed first operations requiring "salvage procedures." Also, many of the patients who underwent ileal conduit diversion in the 1970s are candidates for urinary undiversion and an improved quality of life, free from all external appliances.[66] Newer technical advances have allowed the treatment of these candidates to be directed more toward the primary pathology. Efficient antireflux surgery, improved bowel preparations, more broad-spectrum antibiotics, and the development of newer absorbable staples[68] have all minimized.[69]

Complications of Continent Urinary Diversion

Continent urinary diversion has enjoyed a recent trend of success; however, potentially serious complications can occur. Recent articles have reviewed both medical and surgical complications of bladder augmentation.[70–74] Medical complications of bladder reconstruction using bowel include electrolyte disturbances, chronic pyelonephritis, secondary hypertension, altered pharmacokinetics, mucus production, calculi, B_{12} deficiency, tumor formation, and possible defective linear growth (the single-most critical consequence in children undergoing urointestinal diversion). Surgical complications include stomal stenosis, bowel obstruction, urinary leaks, spontaneous bladder rupture, and bladder stones.

Sometimes, a metabolic problem can manifest itself as a surgical issue. For example, the incidence of bladder stones in patients with a urointestinal diversion is dramatically increased, with a frequency as high as 50%.[75, 76] Urolithiasis occurs most commonly in children without dependent urinary drainage. This problem might occur, for example, in the Mitrofanoff construction to the abdominal wall.[70] Struvite stones are the most common type of stone formed in these situations, suggesting, in part, an infectious process.[75] However, the composition of the calculi in these children is variable, perhaps implicating a metabolic process. As of yet, there is no definitive cause of stone formation in these patients, but the process seems to be multifactorial.

The majority of stones occurring in patients with augmentations develop in the bladder, not in the kidneys— the most common site for urolithiasis in North America. This fact led Khoury[77] to be circumspect of the proposal by Cher and associates[43] that metabolic changes make precipitation of stones more likely. Khoury concluded that intestinal mucus acts as a nidus for urolithiasis and as a biofilm to protect pathogenic bacteria. In a study of 79 bladder augmentations performed between 1990 and 1994, 24 stones formed. Of these, only two stones formed in the kidney. In the same study, Khoury did not find a significant difference in the mean urinary excretion of the measured electrolytes (Ca, Mg, P, Na, K, and oxalate) between stone-formers and non–stone-

formers ($p < 0.05$) in a 24-hour urine collection. The only common finding between the two groups was hypocitraturia. Given this data, metabolic factors could not be solely responsible for urolithogenesis in this patient population.

Pre-Operative Evaluation of Children for Continent Urinary Diversion

Available Anatomy

Children being considered for a continent urinary diversion should have their anatomy defined by a serial review of their radiographic studies. Such studies include, but are not limited to, renal ultrasonography, contrast voiding cystourethrography, and intravenous urography. Retrograde ureterography offers complementary radiographic assessment when appropriate. Finally, a urodynamic evaluation should be performed to evaluate the bladder and sphincter function. After the anatomy and pathophysiology have been defined, the next objective is to decide which segment and length of bowel would be best to use in the reconstructive effort.

Stomach,[78] ileum,[79] right colon,[80] and sigmoid colon have all been used, alone and in various combinations,[62, 65] and in many different configurations to achieve a low-pressure, non-refluxing reservoir which can be completely and conveniently emptied by a predetermined schedule. Despite this, controversy continues to exist concerning the best segment of bowel to use.[81] In a recent article, Grune and Taylor listed criteria that they deemed applicable for the ideal urinary diversion[66] (see Table 39.1). Each available urinary diversion was

TABLE 39.1. *Criteria for an ideal urinary diversion—comparison to currently available options*

Criteria	Ileal conduit	Orthotopic	Kock	Indiana	Ureterosigmoid	Ureterostomy
Metabolic stability	4	3	3	3	2	5
Easy to construct/minimal morbidity	4	3	2	3	3	4
Preserve upper tract	3	3	3	3	3	3
Non-refluxing	1	4	4	4	4	1
Continent at all times	1	4	4	4	4	1
"Natural" cycling	1	3	1	1	3	1
No malignant changes	4	3	3	3	2	4
Sterile urine	2	4	2	2	2	2
Easy endoscopic access	3	2	3	2	2	4
Applicable to both genders	5	2	5	5	5	5
Catheterless	5	4	1	1	5	3
Stomaless	1	5	1	1	4	5
Valveless (continence)	5	5	1	1	5	5
Psychologically acceptable	3	4	4	4	3	2
Raw score	42	49	37	37	47	45
% Max score	60	70	53	53	67	64

(From Grune MT, Taylor RJ. Aspects of Urinary Diversion: The Current Role of Conduits. AUA Update Series Vol. 15, lesson 21, 1997, p. 167.)

Score: 1) criteria never met, 2) criteria seldom met, 3) criteria met at least half the time, 4) criteria met often, 5) criteria met always.

scored according to the specific criteria. Even the most popular diversions met only about half of their criteria, emphasizing that there is no one answer as to which form of urinary diversion is best. Once all of the information has been evaluated, the surgeon should summarize the goals of surgery in order to choose the appropriate operation to meet the needs of the child. Even in spite of this approach, special considerations need to be made in every case.

Certain axioms should be observed when considering a patient for a continent diversion. As much as possible, even small portions of the native bladder and outflow should be incorporated into the reconstruction. As a general rule, since genitourinary reconstruction attempts to achieve continence, a permanent, low-pressure continent reservoir should be the goal.

There are only a few relative contraindications to continent diversion in the pediatric population. First, ureterosigmoidostomy is not an appropriate urinary diversion for children with neurogenic bladder dysfunction. Continence would unlikely be attainable in these children, who almost always have some associated bowel or anal sphincter dysfunction. Second, the ileocecal valve is not recommended in reconstruction of the bladder because its absence may cause contumacious diarrhea.[82] Absence of an ileocecal junction may alter ileal function, both by allowing high concentrations of bacteria into the ileum and by interfering with the absorption process by decreasing bowel transit time.[70, 72] Additionally, malabsorption from ileal resection is directly related to the length of bowel resected. Because the ileum is the sole site of vitamin B_{12} absorption, megaloblastic anemia and spinocerebellar degeneration may occur.[81] Lastly, children with myelomeningocele have a redundant sigmoid colon which, for all intents and purposes, may maintain their fecal continence.

Another consideration worth mentioning is that bladder augmentation using stomach can be a double-edged sword. Its advantages are that it is ideal in those patients with short bowel syndrome and it is usually protected in patients who have received preoperative radiation therapy to the pelvis.[78, 83] The stomach is non-absorptive, decreases infection, and does not produce much mucus. Furthermore, in the patient with chronic acidosis and renal compromise, a wedge gastrocystoplasty serves as a route for acid excretion.[84] At the same time, however, acid excretion has the negative effect of causing severe dysuria and skin irritation, which outweighs its positive effects. Therefore, the interposition of stomach in the urinary tract has largely been abandoned owing to the unacceptably high number of patients who have what developed as the *dysuria-hematuria syndrome*.[85] Sheldon summarized the three factors contributing to this complex: acid hypersecretion, profound oliguria, and bladder neck incompetency.[70]

Vitamin B_{12} deficiency is yet another problem that may arise when stomach is used to augment the bladder.[72] A decreased parietal cell mass creates an interference with intrinsic factor (IF) production As mentioned previously, resection of long segments of ileum, as with the Kock pouch, may cause similar problems related to deficiency of this vitamin.[81] Typically, though, generous segments of small and large bowel can be resected in infants because of the great adaptation of their bowel in a relatively short period of time.[81]

Principles of Detubularization and Reconfiguration

Volume is a significant consideration when creating a reservoir for bladder augmentation, substitution, or continent diversion. Opening an isolated bowel segment along its antimesenteric border results in detubularization. In the case of a bladder substitution or a continent diversion, the flattened surface area can then be reconfigured into a sphere. The sphere's new volume is proportional to the cube of its radius as opposed to the square of the radius, as it is with a cylinder.[86] The sphere holds a larger volume than its original cylindrical shape[87] (Fig. 39.7). In the case of a bladder augmentation, the

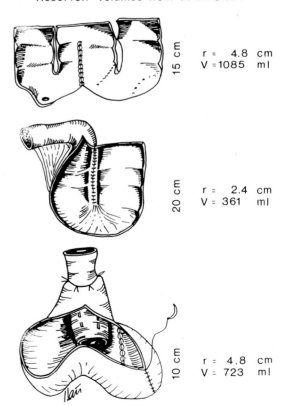

Reservoir Volumes from 60 cm Ileum

15 cm

r = 4.8 cm
V = 1085 ml

20 cm

r = 2.4 cm
V = 361 ml

10 cm

r = 4.8 cm
V = 723 ml

FIG. 39.7. Volume of a 60 cm segment of ileum detubularized and reconfigured into W- or U-shaped neobladders. (From Hautmann RE: Bladder Replacement Surgery. In: Krane RJ, Siroky MB, Fitzpatrick JM, eds. Clinical Urology. Philadelphia: JB Lippincott Co., 1994;727.)

flattened surface area can be anastomosed to the bi-valved bladder to create a larger spherical shape.

Clinically, this is important. As Rink[71] points out, the patient with a concentrating defect and consequent high urine output may need a much longer segment of bowel for augmentation than a child with normal renal tubular function. So important is this issue of detubularization and volume in cystoplasties that Koff[88, 89] established guidelines to determine the size and shape of intestinal segments used for bladder reconstruction. Despite the fact that the tables tend to be cumbersome, Koff's guidelines are a thoughtful approach to creating the largest reservoir possible with the smallest amount of bowel.

Urodynamic studies by Goldwasser et al. demonstrated that clinically significant contractions (>40 cm H_2O pressure at less than 200 mL) were seen in 10% of detubularized right colocystoplasties, compared to 0 percent of detubularized ileocystoplasties.[90] In a follow-up study, Hautmann confirmed Goldwasser's work in neobladders composed of small bowel and large bowel.[81] These findings are significant for at least two specific reasons. First, the importance of a low-pressure system was demonstrated by McGuire's 1981 landmark article in which he correlated resting bladder pressures of greater than 40 cm H_2O with significant upper urinary tract deterioration.[91] Along the same lines, in a continent neobladder, lower filling pressures are less likely to be associated with pouch-to-renal reflux, thus, maintaining renal integrity. Second, a low pouch pressure is a desirable feature in the maintenance of good sphincteric control.[81] Since lower pressures are generated with small bowel segments, they are less often associated with episodic incontinence.

Incontinence is much less of a concern ever since Hinman's description of physical and physiological properties involved in reconstructive bladder surgery.[87] Hinman's ideas embraced the essence of LaPlace's law: T = Pr where (T) is mural tension or stretch resistance, (P) is intravesical pressure, and (r) is the radius of a cylinder.[92] With filling, the wall tension (T) increases leading to an expansion of the reservoir (r) without a rise in pressure (P). Consequently, from a clinical standpoint, incontinence is less of a problem. Additionally, detubularized bowel segments have a blunted contractile ability since the strong circular muscle fibers have been divided. As a result of all of these physical properties, detubularized and reconfigured small bowel segments store more urine at lower pressures, rarely exceeding 40 cm H_2O at high volumes.[93]

Metabolic Consequences of Urointestinal Diversion

Metabolic complications resulting from interposition of bowel in the urinary tract were initially identified following the popularization of ureterosigmoidostomy in the 1950s. These complications were manifested by fatigue, weakness, anorexia, and polydypsia.[94] It was well known, even then, that more severe electrolyte abnormalities were evident in the presence of renal insufficiency. For this reason, patients who are being considered for an enterocystoplasty or a continent diversion should have a creatinine clearance greater than 35 mL/min.[72] In some cases, temporary diversion of a hydronephrotic upper tract might allow for satisfactory improvement in renal function, permitting ultimate reconstruction of the lower urinary tract with bowel.[21] Also, patients who are being considered for undiversion and subsequent renal transplantation are exceptions to the rule regarding the level of renal function. Undiversion would improve their quality of life, and transplantation of a kidney into an intact lower urinary tract is better than transplantation into an ileal conduit.[66] If the renal transplant is delayed, it is essential that the continent pouch be managed carefully and that serum electrolytes be monitored frequently.

Interposition of bowel into the urinary tract has variable metabolic consequences, the character and severity of which depend on the segment employed, the absorptive surface area, the dwell time, and the metabolic reserve of the patient.[70, 72] Basically, *metabolic acidosis* results when jejunum, ileum, or colon are incorporated into the urinary tract, with hyperchloremia being specific to the latter two. *Metabolic alkalosis* is a consequence of incorporating stomach into the urinary tract. As many as 14% of children who have an ileocystoplasty may develop some degree of metabolic acidosis.

The treatment for acute absorptive acidosis as a consequence of urointestinal diversion has been recently reviewed.[70] Initial therapy consists of proper drainage of the urinary neobladder or continent pouch, rehydration with sodium lactate, avoidance of chloride, and replacement of potassium with potassium citrate. Chronic metabolic acidosis may be treated with oral alkali such as Shohl's solution or polycitra. Nicotinic acid[95] and chlorpromazine[96] have had some experimental success in treating metabolic acidosis.

At one time, medical therapy for *metabolic alkalosis* consisted of vigorous rehydration and sodium chloride. However, this condition was generally unresponsive to standard acid-inhibiting or neutralizing therapies. Treatment for metabolic alkalosis and aciduria associated with gastrocystoplasty became available in the early part of this decade when omeprazole, a proton-pump inhibitor, was discovered to be successful.[97] Given the potential metabolic consequences, serum electrolytes should be monitored regularly in all patients with a urointestinal reconstruction.

Current Options in Nonbowel Augmentation Cystoplasty

The metabolic consequences of urinary diversion can be reduced in certain groups of children when nonab-

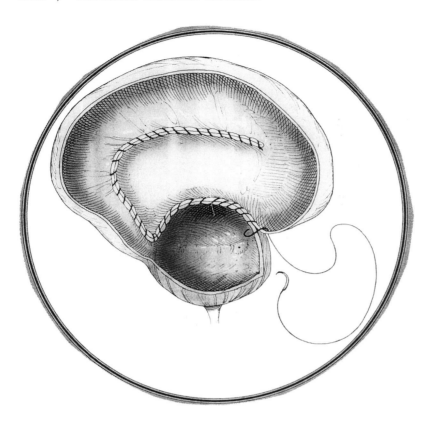

FIG. 39.8. Ureterocystoplasty. (From Bellinger MF: Ureterocystoplasty. In: Olsson CA, ed. Current Surgical Techniques in Urology. 1995;8:2.)

sorbing, impermeable tissue is used. Such tissue is available in selected patients. For example, megaureters subtending poorly functioning or non-functioning kidneys provide an ideal source of augmentation material (Fig. 39.8). This tissue is free of electrolyte and acid-base disturbances and mucus production. It is capable of sensing and tolerating distension without perforation. Furthermore, the megaureter has an extraperitoneal location that prevents complications associated with intra-abdominal surgery.

Churchill and colleagues[98] performed bladder augmentation in 16 patients with a dysfunctional bladder of inadequate capacity using detubularized, reconfigured megaureter. Renal function remained stable or improved in all patients. Complete postoperative urodynamic studies demonstrated a good capacity, low-pressure bladder without instability in 75% of the patients. Continence was reported in 63%. In a follow-up study, the same investigators concluded that ureteral augmentation improved storage function of the dysfunctional bladders to the same extent as that achieved with ileum, but without the complications inherent in ileocystoplasty.[99]

Other options that have been described to increase bladder capacity and reduce intravesical pressures include bladder autoaugmentation[100] and tissue engineering techniques.[101–103] Autoaugmentation has been performed as an open surgical procedure and also laparoscopically,[104] but the long-term efficacy of either technique is unsatisfactory. Autologous sheets of transitional epithelium grown on absorbable scaffolding have been proposed by Atala et al.[102] using tissue engineering techniques. This option is currently in the developmental phase, but may have exciting future potential.

Physical and Psychosocial Issues

Children being considered for a continent urinary reservoir should be evaluated using standard criteria. They should have a life expectancy of greater than one year. There should be no history of bowel disease (inflammatory bowel disease) or significant compromise of the bowel.[82] These children should be strongly motivated to be "bag free." The continent stomal reservoir requires a good deal of manual dexterity. Therefore, patients should be evaluated for their ability to perform clean intermittent self-catheterization. If the child is too young or for another reason unable to perform the catheterizations, then the family should be counseled to this end. The family is an integral part in the evaluation of these children, and each family should be evaluated with regard to their intelligence, motivation, compliance, and understanding of the patient's problems. Additionally, social, financial, and psychological support systems should not be neglected.

In those cases where bladder reconstruction is unavoidable, there has been a tremendous effort, especially in the last 10 years, to improve the quality-of-life issues.[23] For example, we prefer an umbilical stoma for the continent urinary reservoir in children who do not have a useable urethra. A recessed umbilical stoma is barely distinguishable from a normal umbilical dimple

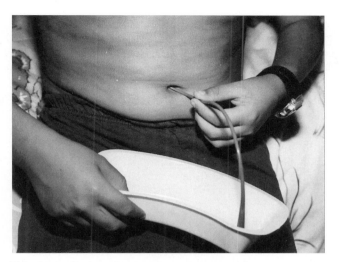

FIG. 39.9. Catheterization through the umbilical stoma of a urinary reservoir. (Photograph courtesy of The Hospital for Sick Children, 1996.)

(Fig. 39.9). This type of surgical cosmesis improves patient acceptance and builds self-esteem.

Certainly, prevention of acute and chronic postoperative complications and protection of the upper urinary tracts are still of paramount importance. In general, these goals have been achieved, as indicated by the excellent prognosis for longevity in these children.[20] Although there is still room for improvement, more emphasis is now being placed now on living as nearly a normal existence as possible, with a healthy body image and full sexual function.

Mechanisms of Continence in Continent Urinary Diversion

The nemesis of any continent urinary diversion is a poorly constructed continence mechanism. It is the single most demanding technical feature. In fact, it is the success or failure of this mechanism that determines the outcome of the entire procedure.[107] A continent urinary reservoir approximates normal bladder function inasmuch as it efficiently stores urine to be emptied at conveniently timed intervals. Just like a normal bladder, continence in the urinary neobladder depends on the relationship between the pressure generated in the reservoir and the resistance of the outlet. This is common to all continent neobladders. Differences are based on minor modifications of the *type of access* and the *mechanism of continence* (Fig. 39.10).

Continence in Cutaneous Stomal Reservoir

Sagalowsky has identified four methods by which continence is achieved in a stomal reservoir[108] (Fig. 39.11).

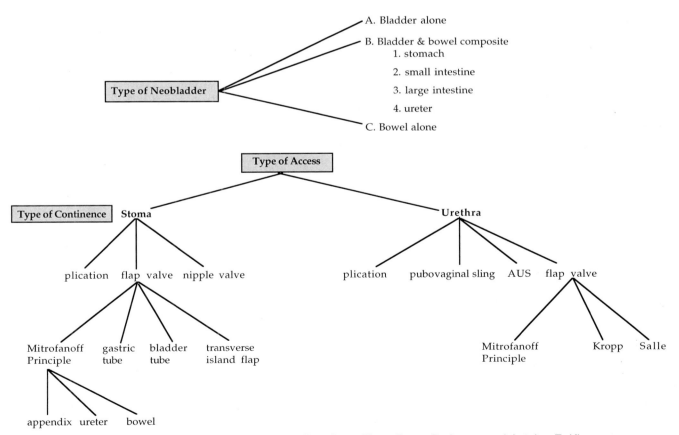

FIG. 39.10. Algorithm for continent urinary diversions. (From Byron D. Joyner and Antoine E. Khoury, The Hospital for Sick Children, 1997.)

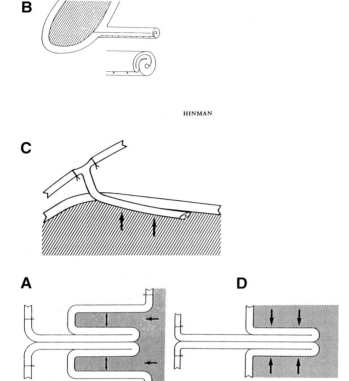

HINMAN

FIG. 39.11. Four methods of surgical continence in stomal reservoir **A,** Intussusception nipple valve. **B,** Terminal ileal plication. **C,** Mitrofanoff principle and **D,** Pressure equilibration principle. (Adapted from Sagalowsky AI: Mechanisms of continence in continent urinary diversions. AUA Update Series Vol. 11, lesson 5, 1992, p. 35.)

The common idea that unites each of the designs is an increase in the resistance to flow. In the first method, the *intussusception nipple valve,* the outlet is thickened by invaginating a segment of bowel to effectively create a partially compressive flap-valve. In the second method, referred to as the *terminal ileal plication,* the length of the narrowed lumen may be increased. The *Mitrofanoff principle* is the third design. It utilizes intraluminal fluid to compress an efferent flap valve. The *pressure equilibration principle* is the last method and it combines any of the first three techniques with an hydraulic catheterizable channel.

The Intussusception Nipple Valve

Initially, the nipple valve was plagued with complications. Inadequate stabilization of the nipple base to the abdominal wall caused significant problems with catheterization, especially with distension of the ileal reservoir. This efferent limb was eventually modified by intussuscepting the terminal ileum into the cecal lumen. Stabilization was achieved by suturing a rectus fascial sling to the cecum and the ileum.[109] Unfortunately, in-

continence also became a problem. Ultimately, Thüroff and associates[65] from Mainz, Germany, reported on a series of ileocecal reservoirs referred to as the Mainz (Mixed Augmentation with Ileum 'n' Zecum) pouch in which they, too, used a nipple valve for continence. The nipple valve good in principle, but it has its share of problems. Now, however, with newer modifications[110, 111,] these problems have been largely overcome. In fact, Skinner's most recent clinical experience with the modified, stapled intussuscepted nipple valve has demonstrated a reliable continence rate of 95%.

The Terminal Plication Principle

Plication procedures are familiar to most urologists.[112–114] Lengthening and plicating the bladder outlet to prevent urine leak has been a continence mechanism which has been adapted to several stomal reservoirs. Rowland and coworkers adapted this mechanism to the Gilchrist ileocecal reservoir to create the Indiana pouch,[62] and Lockhart applied *two* plicated rows to provide continence for the Florida Pouch.[115] There are distinct advantages to this technique. Suture plication avoids the use of staples and their inherent problems. Additionally, continence rates have been reported to be above 90%.[60, 116]

The Mitrofanoff Principle

The Mitrofanoff appendicovesicostomy[19] is an ingenious idea which applies an old technique (submucosal tunneled reimplantation) to solve the problems of incontinence. The appendix was the tubular structure originally used by Mitrofanoff and, at present, is the tissue of choice. But, if it is congenitally absent or has been surgically removed, a variety of tissues can be used as a substitute to construct a catheterizable channel including ureter[117–120,] bladder and gastric tubes,[121–124] tapered colon,[125] or ileum,[117, 119, 127] preputial skin,[126] and fallopian tubes[117, 124] (Fig. 39.12). But, when deciding which tissue to use, the most important criterion is, of course, tissue availability. Regardless of the tissue used, the principle is the same. Submucosal tunneling of any tubularized structure creates a flap-valve which provides continence.

The Mitrofanoff principle may be beneficial to those children who are plagued with either urinary incontinence owing to congenital, traumatic, or neoplastic bladder dysfunction or who have failed multiple continence procedures. These children might be good candidates for bladder neck closure and a catheterizable permanent, continent urinary diversion (e.g., an augmentation cystoplasty and a Mitrofanoff appendicovesicostomy). Counseling issues with this procedure include (1) the need for mandatory catheterization (2) the possibility of slow drainage, and (3) the risk of spontaneous rup-

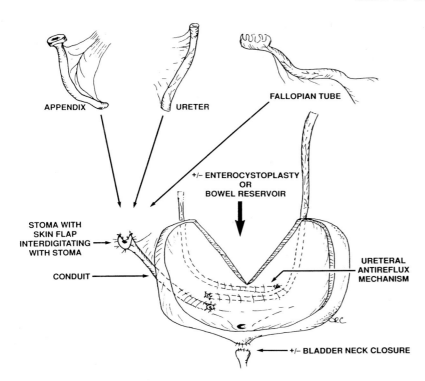

FIG. 39.12. Illustration of the Mitrofanoff principle—appendicovesicostomy. Alternatives are ureterostomy, fallopian tube conduit, tapered ileal conduit, bladder and gastric tubes, and preputial skin conduits. (From Cendron M, Gearhart JP: The Mitrofanoff principle: Technique and applications in continent urinary diversion. In: Marshall FF, ed. WB Saunders Co 1991;18:618.)

ture, of the bladder.[128, 129] Slow drainage is common through the small caliber catheter which must be used through the narrow channel, and this small catheter is also prone to muccus plugging.[60] Therefore, it is important that the continent diversions be irrigated regularly to reduce the copious amounts of mucus that can be produced by the intestinal components. Rink's[71] recommendations are to irrigate the neobladder with saline (or water) three times a day immediately post-operatively. At 2 to 4 weeks, saline irrigations are decreased to twice a day. Subsequently, saline irrigations should be performed every morning, regardless of the segment of bowel used for augmentation.

Mucus may not be troublesome for many patients, but it may interfere with bladder emptying in some. Mucus plugging could lead to incomplete pouch emptying with subsequent distension and spontaneous rupture. Also, attempts at catheterization during bladder overdistension can be a problem due to angulation of the catheterizing channel. In these situations, insertion of an 18-G needle through the anterior abdominal wall into the palpable neobladder would decompress the pouch sufficiently to allow for easy passage of the catheter. The safest site for percutaneous access is through the old suprapubic tube site—because this represents a cylinder of scar tissue where no bowel is present.

The Pressure Equilibration Principle

The last method incorporates the pressure equilibration principle to maintain urinary continence. Stomal resistance to leakage increases when the reservoir pressure or volume increases. The surrounding fluid neutralizes any net force toward the stoma to reinforce continence.[108] One example of this principle is the "ink-well" continence mechanism, first described by Benchekroun[130] in 1978. Koff's technique[131] is similar to that described by Benchekroun in that it is an hydraulic catheterizable channel. The complex design of the "ink-well" belies its consistent reproducibility.[132]

Continence in Urethral Neobladder

The orthotopic neobladder provides a low-pressure, high-capacity system which allows micturition through the urethra by straining (Valsalva technique). It represents a further refinement in the continuous evolution of lower urinary tract reconstruction. This type of construction avoids a cutaneous abdominal stoma while at the same time allows urethral micturition.[133] There are a variety of operative procedures that have been developed from each of the different segments of bowel.

One continent surgical procedure which utilizes the patient's native urethra while reinforcing the outlet resistance with an anterior bladder wall flap valve is the Salle procedure.[134] This procedure mandates catheterization, a consideration which should not be taken lightly when evaluating and counseling patients for a continent urinary neobladder.

If additional urethral resistance is necessary because of either functional or anatomic damage, urinary continence can be achieved through either surgical or nonsurgical mechanical compression. In selected patients, surgical techniques to improve urethral resistance include the pubovaginal sling procedure[135] and the artificial urinary sphincter.[136] Non-surgical techniques include endoscopic periurethral injectable substances such as collagen.[137]

SUMMARY

There is a tremendous foundation upon which the progress and philosophy of urinary diversion in the 1980s and 1990s has based its successes. The field of urinary diversion requires an appreciation of the contributions of our predecessors, as well as a thorough knowledge of the methods and surgical maneuvers of current experts. There is no substitute for this knowledge when treating a child who requires urinary diversion. The benefits can be extraordinary and include resolution of reflux, acquisition of continence, and preservation of the upper tracts. Unfortunately, the extraordinary benefits are matched by consequences which include chronic bacteriuria, metabolic disturbances, stone formation, risk of perforation, and malignancy.

In this chapter, the various aspects of urinary diversion in children have been reviewed. Urinary diversions have been classified as (1) those designed to be temporary and to use external appliances (including an intestinal conduit or a ureterostomy) and (2) those diversions designed to be permanent and continent.[66] Each classification has its own history, indications, benefits, and complications. None of the urinary diversions is appropriate for every child, nor is any diversion ideal in every setting. Each diversion should be tailored to the individual child through a discriminating selection process, careful and comprehensive counseling, and appropriate follow-up on the part of the surgical team, as well as the patient.

REFERENCES

1. Rayer. Traite Des Maladies Des Reins. Paris, 1837–1841.
2. Morris H. The origin and progress of renal surgery. London: Cassell 1893.
3. Simon J. Ectopica vesica: operation for directing the orifices of the ureters into the rectum. Lancet 1852;2:568.
4. Mikulicz J. Zur operation der Augerborener Blalsenspalte. Zentralb Chir 1899;26:641.
5. Coffey RC. Physiologic implantation of the severed ureter or common bile-duct into the intestine. JAMA 1911;56:397.
6. Bricker EM. Bladder substitution after pelvic evisceration. Surg Clin North Am 1950;30:1511.
7. Zaaijer JH. Discussion. Intra-abdominale plastieken. Med Tijdschr Geneesk 1911;65:836.
8. Gilchrist RK, Merricks JW, Hamlin HH, Rieger IT. Construction of a substitute bladder and urethra. Surg Gynec & Obst 1950;90:752.
9. Nesbit RM. Ureterosigmoid anastomosis by direct elliptical connection. University Hospital Bulletin, University of Michigan, Ann Arbor. 1948;14:14.
10. Cordonnier JJ. Ureterosigmoid anastomosis. Surg Gynec Obst 1949;88:441.
11. Leadbetter WF. Consideration of problems incident to the performance of ureteroenterostomy. Report of a technique. J Urol 1951;65:818
12. Gil-Vernet JM, Escarpenter JM, Perex-Trujillo G. A functioning artificial bladder: results of 41 consecutive cases. J Urol 1962;87:825.
13. Mogg RA. The treatment of neurogenic urinary incontinence using the colonic conduit. Br J Urol 1965;37:681.
14. Weyrauch HM, Young BW. Evaluation of common methods of uretero-intestinal anastomosis: an experimental study. J Urol 1952;67:880.
15. Weyrauch HM. Landmarks in the development of uretero-intestinal anastomosis. Annals of the Royal College of Surgeons, England, 1952;18:343.
16. Lapides J, Diokno AC, Gould FR. Clean intermittent self catheterization in the treatment of urinary tract disease. J Urol 1972;107:458.
17. Camey M, LeDuc A. L'Enterocystoplastie avec cystoprostatectomie pour cancer de la vessie. Ann Urol 1979;13:114.
18. Kock NG. Intraabdominal reservoir in patinets with permanent ileostomy. Arch Surg 1969;99:223.
19. Mitrofanoff P. Cystostomie continent transappendiculaire dans le traitement des vessies neurologiques. Chir Pediatr 1980;21:297.
20. Hensle TW, Nagler HM, Goldstein, HR. Long-term functional results of urinary tract reconstruction in childhood. J Urol 1982;128:1262.
21. Cendron M. Discussion: Temporary cutaneous urinary diversion in children. Dialogues in Pediatric Urology 1995;18:1.
22. Atta MA. Detubularized isolated ureterosigmoidostomy: Description of a new technique and preliminary results. J Urol 1996;156:915.
23. Stein R, Fisch M, Stockle M, Demirkesen O, Hohenfellner R. Colonic conduit in children: protection of the upper urinary tract 16 years later? J Urol 1996;156:1146.
24. Kock NG, Nilson AE, Norlen LJ, et al. Urinary diversion via a continent ilieum reservoir: Clinical experience. Scand J Urol Nephrol 1978;49:5.
25. Spring DB, Deshon GE Jr. Radiology of vesical and supravesical urinary diversions. In: Pollack HM, ed. Clinical Urography: An Atlas and Textbook of Urological Imaging. Philadelphia: W.B. Saunders, 1990;1:296.
26. Duckett JW. Uses and abuses of vesicostomy. AUA Update Series 1995;14:130.
27. Retik AB, Perlmutter AD. Temporary urinary diversion in infants and young children. In: Walsh PC, Gittes RF, Perlmutter AD, eds. Campbell's Urology. Philadelphia: W.B. Saunders Co. 1986;2:2116.
28. Ring KS, Hensle TW. Urinary Diversion. In: Kelalis PP, King LR, Belman AB, eds. Clinical Pediatric Urology. Philadelphia: W.B. Saunders Co. 1992;2:865.
29. Blocksom B. Bladder pouch for prolonged tubeless cystostomy. J Urol 1957;78:398.
30. Hurwitz RS, Ehrlich RM. Complications of cutaneous vesicostomy in children. Urol Clin North Am 1983;10:503.
31. Wammack R, Fisch M, Hohenfellner, R. Pediatric urinary diversion: review and own experience. Eur Urol 1992;22:177.
32. Salle JP. Salle Intraoperative Pyeloplasty Stent Set 1995.
33. Majid E, Reda EF, Franco I. Endoscopic surgery of the upper tract in children. In: Kelalis PP, King LR, Belman AB, eds. Clinical Pediatric Urology. Philadelphia: W.B. Saunders Co. 1992;2:726.
34. Stevens PS, Eckstein HB. Ileal conduit urinary diversion in children. Br J Urol 1977;49:379.
35. Smith ED. Follow-up studies on 150 ileal conduits in children. J Pediatr Surg 1972;7:1.
36. Schwarz GR, Jeffs RD. Conduit urinary diversion in children: computer analysis of follow-up from 2 to 16 years. J Urol 1975;114:285.
37. Shapiro SR, Lebowitz R, Colodny AH. Fate of 90 children with ileal conduit urinary diversion a decade later: analysis of complications, pyelography, renal function and bacteriology. J Urol 1975;114:300.
38. Middleton AW Jr., Hendren WH. Ileal conduits in children at

the Massachusetts General Hospital from 1955 to 1970. J Urol 1976;115:591.

39. Dunn M, Roberts JB, Smith PJ, Slade N. The long-term results of ileal conduit urinary diversion in children. Br J Urol 1979;51:458.

40. Hensle TW, Connor JP, Burbige KA. Continent urinary diversion in childhood. J Urol 1990;143:981.

41. Shandera KC, Thompson IM, Wong RW, Cossi AF. Delayed development of mid-ileal conduit stenosis: the importance of life-long urologic follow-up. South Med J 1995;88:1118.

42. Elder DD, Moisey CU, Rees RW. A long-term follow-up of the colonic conduit operation in children. Br J Urol 1979;51:462.

43. Cher ML, Roehrborn CG. Incorporation of intestinal segments into the urinary tract. In: Hohenfellner A, Wammack R, eds. Continent Urinary Diversion. Edinburgh: Churchill Livingstone, 1992.

44. Boyd SD, Feinberg SM, Skinner DG, Lieskovsky G, Baron D, Richardson J. Quality of life survey of urinary diversion patients: comparison of ileal conduits versus continent Kock ileal reservoirs. Journal of Urology 1987;138:1386–1389.

45. Stone AR, MacDermott JP. Sexual dysfunction in the neurologically impaired patient. In: Pauson DF, ed. Problems in Urology. JB Lippincott Co. 1989;147.

46. Weiss RM. Obstructive uropathy. In: Kelalis PP, King LR, Belman AB, eds. Clinical Pediatric Urology. Philadelphia: W.B. Saunders, 1992;2:674.

47. Woodburne RT, Lapides J. The ureteral lumen during peristalsis. American Journal of Anatomy 1972;133:255.

48. Rose JG, Gillenwater JY. Effects of obstruction upon ureteral function. Urology 1973;12:139.

49. Hellstrom M, Jodal U, Marild S, Wettergren B. Ureteral dilation in children with febrile urinary tract infection or bacteriuria. AJR 1987;148:483.

50. Boyarsky S, Labay P. Ureteral dynamics. Baltimore: The Williams & Wilkins Co. 1972.

51. Filmer RB, Honesty H. Problems with urinary conduit stomas in children. Urol Clin North Am 1974;1:531.

52. Burstein JD, Firlit CF. Complications of cutaneous ureterostomy and other cutaneous diversion. Urol Clin North Am 1983;10:433.

53. Jayanthi VR, McLorie GA, Khoury AE, Churchill BM. The effect of temporary cutaneous diversion on ultimate bladder function. J Urol 1995;154:889.

54. Claesson G, Josephson S, Robertson B. Experimental partial ureteric obstruction in newborn rats. IV. Do the morphological effects progress continuously? J Urol 1983;130:1217.

55. Deleted.

56. Hendren WH. Nonrefluxing colon conduit for temporary or permanent urinary diversion in children. J Pediatr Surg 1975;10:381.

57. Hendren WH. Tapered bowel segment for ureteral replacement. Urol Clin North Am 1978;5:607.

58. Bauer SB. Neurogenic bladder dysfunction. Pediatr Clin North Am 1987;34:1121.

59. Dionko AC, Sonda LP. Compatibility of genitourinary prostheses and intermittent self-catheterization. J Urol 1981;125:659.

60. Sagalowsky AI. Continent urinary diversion excluding the Kock pouch, part I. AUA Update Series 1987a;6:1.

61. Kock NG, Nilson AE, Nilsson LO. Urinary diversion via a continent ileal reservoir: Clinical results in 12 patients. J Urol 1982;128:469.

62. Rowland RG, Mitchell ME, RB. Indiana continent urinary reservoir. J Urol 1986;137:1136.

63. Carroll PR, Presti JC Jr. Comparison of plicated and stapled continent ileocecal stoma. Urology 1992;40:107.

64. Hautmann RE, Egghart G, Frohneberg D. The ileal neobladder. J Urol 1988;139:39.

65. Thuroff JW, Alken P, Riedmiller H, Engelmann U, Jacobi GW, Hohenfellner R. The Mainz pouch (mixed augmentation with ileum and cecum) for bladder augmentation and continent diversion. J Urol 1986;136:17.

66. Grune MT. Aspects of urinary diversion: the current role of conduits. AUA Update Series 1996;15(Lesson 21):166.

67. Fisch M, Wammack R, Steinbach F, Muller SC, Hohenfellner R. Sigma-rectum pouch (Mainz pouch II). Urol Clin North Am 1993;20:561.

68. Kirsch AJ, Olsson CA, Hensle TW. Pediatric continent reservoirs

and colocystoplasty created with absorbable staples. J Urol 1996;156:614.

69. Fisch M, Wammack R, Muller S, Hohenfellner R. The Mainz Pouch II (Sigma Rectum Pouch). J Urol 1993;149:258.

70. Sheldon CA, Snyder HM. Principles of urinary tract reconstruction. In: Gillenwater JY, Grayhack JT, Howards SS, Duckett JW, eds. Adult and Pediatric Urology. St. Louis: Mosby, 1997;3:2317.

71. Rink RC, Hollensbe D, Adams MC. Complications of bladder augmentation in children and comparison of gastrointestinal segments. AUA Update Series 1995;14:122.

72. McDougal WS. Use of intestinal segments in the urinary tract: Basic principles. In: Walsh PC, Retik AB, Stamey TA, Vaughan ED, eds. Campbell's Urology. Philadelphia: WB Saunders, 1992;3:2595.

73. Pompino HJ. Urinary diversion in children. Eur J Pediatr Surg 1992;2:67.

74. Hill JT, Ransley PG. The colonic conduit: a better method of urinary diversion? Br J Urol 1983;55:629.

75. Blyth B, Ewalt DH, Duckett JW, Snyder HMI. Lithogenic properties of enterocystoplasty. J Urol 1992;148:575.

76. Palmer L, Franco I, Kogan S, Reda E, Gill B, Levitt S. Urolithiasis in children following augmentation cystoplasty. J Urol 1993;150:726.

77. Khoury AE. Stone formation following augmentation cystoplasty: the role of intestinal mucous. J Urol 1997: in press.

78. Nguyen DH, Mitchell ME. Gastric bladder reconstruction. In: The Urologic Clinics of North America. Marshall FF, ed. Philadelphia: W. B. Saunders Co. 1991;18:649.

79. Skinner DG, Boyd SD, Lieskovsky G. Clinical experience with the Kock continent urinary reservoir for urinary diversion. J Urol 1984;132:1101.

80. Zinman L, Libertino JA. Right colocystoplasty for bladder replacement. In: Urologic Clinics of North America. Edited by W.B. Saunders Co. 1986;13:321.

81. Hautmann RE. Bladder replacement surgery. In: Krane RJ, Siroky MB, Fitzpatrick JM, eds. Clinical Urology. J.B. Lippincott. 1994;725.

82. Randall GR, Rink RC. Instructional Course #9683: Continent Urinary Diversion. 1996;1.

83. Adams MC, Mitchell ME, Rink RC. Gastrocystoplasty: an alternative solution to the problem of urological reconstruction in the serverly compromised patient. J Urol 1988;140:1152.

84. Rink RC, Mitchell ME. Gastrocystoplasty. Problems in Urology 1991;213.

85. Nguyen DH, Bain MA, Salmonson KL, Ganesan GS, Burns MW, Mitchell ME. The syndrome of dysuria and hematuria in pediatric urinary reconstruction with stomach. J Urol 1993;150:707.

86. Jurgensen RC, Brown RG, Jurgensen JW. In: Geomtry. Edited by Houghton Mifflin Co. 1985;437.

87. Hinman F, Jr. Selection of intestinal segments for bladder substitution: physical and physiological characteristics. J Urol 1988;139:519.

88. Koff SA. The shape of intestinal segments used for reconstruction. Journal d Urologie 1988;94:201.

89. Koff SA. Guidelines to determine the size and shape of intestinal segments used for reconstruction. J Urol 1988;140:1150.

90. Goldwasser B, Barrett DM, Webster GD. Cystometric properties of ileum and right colon after bladder augmentation, substitution or replacement. J Urol 1987;138:1007.

91. McGuire EJ, Woodside, JR, Borden TA, Weiss, RM. Prognostic value of urodynamic testing in myelodysplastic patients. J Urol 1981;126:205.

92. Hinman FJ, Miller ER. Mural tension in vesical disorders and ureteral reflux. J Urol 1964;91:33.

93. Fowler JE. Continent urinary reservoirs, bladder substitute in the adult: Part I. Monograms of Urology 1987;8.

94. Ferris DO, Odel HM. Electrolyte pattern of blood after urterosigmoidostomy. JAMA 1950;142:634.

95. Kock MO, McDougal WS. Nicotinic acid: treatment for the hyperchloremic acidosis following urinary diversion through intestinal segments. J Urol 1985;134:162.

96. Kock NG, Norlen LJ, Philipson BM. The continent ileal reservoir

(Koch pouch) for urinary diversion. World J Urol 1985;3:152.

97. Kinahan TJ, Khoury AE, McLorie GA, Churchill, BM. Omeprazole in post-gastrocystoplasty metabolic alkalosis and aciduria. J Urol 1992;147:435.

98. Churchill BM, Aliabadi H, Landau EH, McLorie GA, Steckler RE, McKenna PH, Khoury AE. Ureteral bladder augmentation. J Urol 1993;150:716.

99. Landau EH, Jayanthi VR, Khoury AE, Churchill BM, Gilmour, RF, Steckler RE, McLorie GA. Bladder augmentation: ureterocystoplasty versus ileocystoplasty. J Urol 1994;152:716.

100. Cartwright PC, Snow BW. Bladder autoaugmentation: early clinical experience. J Urol 1989;142:505.

101. Atala A. Current, future options in nonbowel augmentation cystoplasty. Dialogues in Pediatric Urology 1995;18:1.

102. Atala A, Freeman MR, Vacati JP. Implantation in vivo and retrieval of artificial structures consisting of rabbit and human urothelium and human bladder muscle. J Urol 1993;150:601.

103. Atala A, Vacanti JP, Peters CA. Formation of urothelial structures from dissociated cells attached to biodegradable polymer scaffolds in vitro. J Urol 1992;148:658.

104. Ehrlich RM, Gershman A. Laparoscopic seromyotomy (autoaugmentation) for non-neurogenic neurogenic bladder in a child: initial case report. Urology 1993;42:175.

105. Goldwasser B, Webster GD. Continent urinary diversion. [Review]. J Urol 1985;134:227.

106. Mansson W. Editorial. Continent urinary reconstruction—method-to-patient matching. J Urol 1996;156:936.

107. Benson MC, Olsson CA. Urinary Diversion. In: Walsh PC, Retik AB, Stamey TA, Vaughan ED Jr., eds. Campbell's Urology. W.B. Saunders Co. 1992;3:2654.

108. Sagalowsky AI. Mechanisms of continence in continent urinary diversions. AUA Update Series 1992;11:34.

109. Mansson W, Colleen S, Sudin T. The continent cecal reservoir in urinary diversion. World J Urol 1985;3:173.

110. Skinner DG, Lieskovsky G, Boyd S. Continent urinary diversion. J Urol 1989;141:1323.

111. King LR. Protection of the upper tracts in undiversion. In: King LR, Stone AR, Webster GD, eds. Year Book Medical Publishers, Inc. 1987;10:127.

112. Leadbetter GW Jr. Surgical correction of total urinary incontinence. J Urol 1964;91:261.

113. Dees JE, Durham NC. Epispadias with incontinence in the male. Surgery 1942;12:621.

114. Young HH. Exstrophy of the bladder. The first case in which a normal bladder and urinary control have been obtained by plastic operations. Surg Gynecol Obstet 1942;74:729.

115. Lockhart JL. Remodeled right colon: An alternative urinary reservoir. J Urol 1987;138:730.

116. Lockhart JL, Pow-Sang JM, Perky L, Kahn P, Helal M, Sanford E. A continent colonic urinary reservoir: The Florida pouch. J Urol 1990;144:864.

117. Woodhouse CRJ, Malone PR, Cumming J, Reilly TM. The Mitrofanoff principle for continent urinary diversion. Br J Urol 1989;63:53.

118. Hollowell JG, Ransley PG. Surgical management of incontinence in bladder exstrophy. Br J Urol 1991;68:543.

119. Duckett JW, Lotfi AH. Appendicovesicostomy (and variations) in bladder reconstruction. J Urol 1993;149:567.

120. Peters CA. Bladder reconstruction in children. Curr Opin Pediatr 1994;6:183.

121. Pope J, Koch MO. Ureteral replacement with reconfigured colon substitute. J Urol 1996;155:1693.

122. Kristic ZD. Preputial continent vesicostomy: preliminary report of a new technique. J Urol 1995;154:1160.

123. Adams MC, Bihrle R, Foster RS, Britto CG. Conversion of an ileal conduit to a continent catheterizable urinary diversion. J Urol 1992;147:126.

124. Woodhouse CR, MacNeily AE. The Mitrofanoff principle: expanding upon a versatile technique. Br J Urol 1994;74:447.

125. Sheiner JR, Kaplan GW. Spontaneous bladder rupture following enterocystoplasty. J Urol 1988;140:1157.

126. Elder JS, Snyder HM, Hulbert WC, Duckett JW. Perforation of the augmented bladder in patients undergoing clean intermittent catheterization. J Urol 1988;140:1159.

127. Benchekroun A. Continent caecal bladder. Eur J Urol 1978;3:248.

128. Koff SA, Cirulli C, Wise HA. Clinical and urodynamic features of a new intestinal urinary sphincter for continent urinary diversion. J Urol 1989;142:293.

129. Quinlan DM, Leonard MP, Brendler CB, Gearhart JP, Jeffs RD. Use of Benchekroun hydraulic valve as a catheterizable continence mechanism. J Urol 1991;145:1151.

130. Light JK, Marks JL. Total bladder replacement in the male and female using the ileocolonic segment (LeBag). Br J Urol 1990;65:467.

131. Salle JL, de Fraga JC, Amarante A, Silveira, ML, Lambertz M, Schmidt M, Rosito NC. Urethral lengthening with anterior bladder wall flap for urinary incontinence: a new approach. J Urol 1994;152:803.

132. Blaivas JG. Treatment of female incontinence secondary to urethral damage or loss. In: Leach GE, ed. The Urologic Clinics of North America. W.B. Saunders Co. 1991;18;355.

133. Kreder KJ, Webster GD. Evaluation and management of incontinence after implantation of the artificial urinary sphincter. In: Leach GE, ed. Urologic Clinics of North America. W.B. Saunders Co. 1991;18:375.

134. Monga AK, Robinson D, Stanton SL. Periurethral collagen injections for genuine stress incontinence: a 2 year follow-up. Br Urol 1995;76:156.

CHAPTER 40

Indications for Laparoscopic Procedures in Pediatric Urology

Harry P. Koo, J. Stuart Wolf, Jr., and David A. Bloom

Laparoscopic surgery is a rapidly developing technique in minimally invasive surgery that began at the turn of the century when Kelling[1] and Jacobaeus[2] developed techniques for peritoneoscopy in animals and cadavers and then applied the methods to living patients. The primary application of peritoneoscopy throughout most of this century has been gynecologic.[3] Outside gynecologic practice, diagnostic peritoneoscopy grew slowly, despite the efforts of its early pioneers. The use of laparoscopy in the pediatric age group was virtually unkown until Gans and Berci[4] and Cognat and associates[5] independently reported their successful application using prototype instruments. The first major genitourinary application of laparoscopy was described by Cortesi in 1976, for diagnosis of intraabdominal testes in an 18-year-old man.[6]

Aided by the development of miniature television cameras, high-resolution color monitors, and instruments specific to various endosurgical procedures, there has been a tremendous expansion of interest in laparoscopic surgery. Today, laparoscopy has been used directly in pediatric urology for: (a) localization and evaluation of nonpalpable testis; (b) orchiectomy for undescended testis; (c) two-stage orchidiopexy; (d) single-stage orchidopexy; (e) gonadal examination and biopsy in patients with intersex disorders; (f) as an adjunct in diagnosis and directly in the treatment of pediatric indirect inguinal hernias; (g) nephrectomy; (h) pyeloplasty; (i) ureteral and bladder surgery.

SPECIAL CONSIDERATIONS FOR PEDIATRIC LAPAROSCOPIC SURGERY

Just as pediatric urology is a specialty unto itself, pediatric laparoscopic surgery is an extended subspecialty. As such, surgical considerations in children must be the central focus of procedural planning. There are unique anatomic, physiologic, and pathologic conditions

that must be understood to prevent laparoscopic complications in children.

The margin for error in pediatric laparoscopic surgery is inversely proportional to the age and size of the patient. The smaller the abdominal cavity, the relatively larger the instruments, the decreased distance between the anterior abdominal wall and major retroperitoneal structures, and the intraperitoneal position of the bladder presents inherent difficulties in children.[7] The aorta and inferior vena cava may be found only 1 to 2 cm below the anterior abdominal wall and are at great risk for injury when using blind Veress needle and trocar insertion techniques.[8] Children are also at risk for gastric distension. The child often undergoes anesthesia while crying with concomitant air swallowing. Gastric distension predisposes to injury during insufflation needle placement or primary access cannula placement.[9]

There are benefits to children's dimensions. Landmarks are readily palpable; the bifurcation of the great vessels and the sacral promontory are usually easily felt. In addition, abdominal or pelvic masses are easily detected in most children. Children also tend to have less preperitoneal fat, making the depth of the abdominal wall thinner with less of a chance of inappropriate preperitoneal insufflation.[9]

Children are especially susceptible to emphysematous complications during insufflation. Not uncommonly, one will see extraperitoneal emphysema, omental emphysema, or emphysema en flax. Emphysematous complications arise more frequently in children because of their looser attachments of the peritoneum to the extraperitoneal structures.[9]

In initial experience with children's laparoscopy, hypercarbia was thought to be related to the development of emphysema. It was therefore presumed that children were at an increased risk and required more intensive monitoring than adults. Recent experience has disproved this fear. Children tolerate pneumoperitoneum well with little hypercarbia.[10] With diligent monitoring of end tidal carbon dioxide and with minimal hyperventilation, children can have end tidal CO_2 levels kept well within acceptable ranges.

There are certain pediatric patients with special congenital medical conditions who may not be suitable for laparoscopy. The patients include those with large ventricular septal defects, ventriculoperitoneal shunts, or prune belly syndrome. There is an increased risk of morbidity if a gas embolus occurs in a patient with a ventricular septal defect. The gas bubble can cross the septal defect and enter the systemic circulation. Massive strokes have occurred in patients with carbon dioxide embolus and a concurrent ventricular septal defect.[11] In patients with ventriculoperitoneal shunts or intracranial lesions, the pneumoperitoneum pressures must be kept low, the tilt of the Trendelenburg position should be kept to a minimum, and intracranial pressure monitoring used to ensure that adequate cerebral perfusion is being maintained. Antibiotic prophylaxis must be administered to decrease the chance of shunt infection and care must also be taken to avoid damaging the shunt with instruments during surgery.[12] In patients with prune belly syndrome, inadequate development of the anterior abdominal wall makes trocar insertion difficult. In addition, the location of the testes is known to be intraabdominal and extensive dissection is necessary to bring the testes down to a scrotal position in these patients.

ANATOMY

Normal Anatomy

A review of the embryologic development of the umbilical cord and pelvic structures is pertinent to understanding the normal laparoscopic anatomic landmarks. Several vestigial structures, particularly those related to the umbilicus, are important in the endoscopic examination of the pelvis. At birth, two umbilical arteries and the single umbilical vein are present in the umbilical cord (Fig. 40.1). The umbilical vein and the ductus venosus atrophy to become the ligamentum teres and the ligamentum venosum, respectively, of the liver. The umbilical arteries persist in the deep pelvis as the internal iliac and proximal superior vesical artery, whereas the more anterior aspects remain as the solid medial umbilical ligament on each side. The medial umbilical ligament is perhaps the most visually obvious structure in the pelvis and it permits quick identification of the internal inguinal ring, which lies lateral to it.[13]

Normal laparoscopic anatomy at the internal ring consists of a substantial leash of spermatic vessels proceeding into a closed ring lateral to the vas deferens. Endoscopically the spermatic vessel leash and vas are configured like an upside-down V. Another fairly consistent finding in boys is the transverse vesical fold that

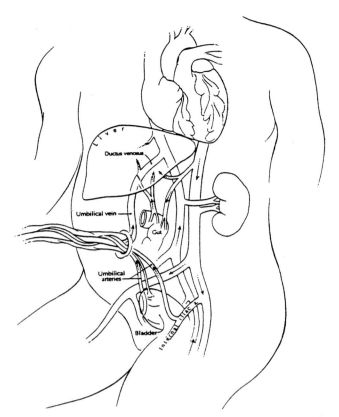

FIG. 40.1. The fetal umbilical circulation. [From Bloom DA, et al., Urology 1994;44:905.]

blends into the anterior margin of the ring or fans out and disappears just above it. The transverse vesical fold is readily seen in prepubertal boys and adolescents, but the fold is less obvious later in life (Fig. 40.2).

It is useful for laparoscopic surgeons to identify the precise location of the distal ureter so that it can be spared injury or be used surgically. The ureter passes from a point medial to the distal spermatic vessels, deviating from them toward the midline across the iliac vessels to pass underneath the vas deferens. Sometimes, a wave of peristalsis is observed in the distal ureter during laparoscopic examination. On occasions when the distal ureter is obscured by fat or bowel, a sense of the appropriate location of the ureter will facilitate its identification. Geometrically, the ureter forms a triangular space with the vas caudally and the medial umbilical ligament laterally (Fig. 40.2). Three fluids (blood, semen, and urine) in three tubes of intersecting axes define the space, which has been defined as the vasal triangle.[13]

Abnormal Anatomy

The spermatic vessels are the critical anatomic landmark for locating a nonpalpable testis or declaring its absence. The vessels should be identified and followed to their termination or point of entry into the internal

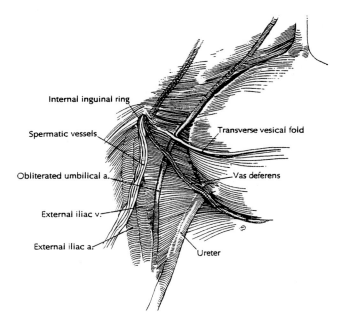

FIG. 40.2. Laparoscopic pelvic anatomy and the left vasal triangle. [From Bloom DA, et al., Urology 1994;44:905.]

inguinal ring. The important characteristics of the spermatic vessel leash are direction, caliber, and termination. A leash of spermatic vessels that terminates blindly and proximal to the internal ring is proof that there is no distal gonad. A hypoplastic spermatic vessel leash implies a similar situation. The presence of spermatic vessels indicates that a testis was present at some point during fetal development, but disappeared subsequently, presumably because of vascular accident. This phenomenon occurs more often on the left side, suggesting a specific vulnerability of that set of spermatic vessels.[14]

Complete absence of the spermatic vessels or of visible remnants above the internal inguinal ring is an uncommon situation and is indicative of an ectopic testis or complete agenesis. In transverse testicular ectopia, one spermatic vessel leash crosses the midline to join its contralateral mate at its internal inguinal ring.[15] In testicular agenesis, there is absence of the ipsilateral kidney.[13]

A patent processus vaginalis is a common abnormality at the internal ring. Weiss and Seashore[16] have shown that the presence of a patent processus vaginalis predicts a distal (canalicular or lower) testis. Such testes can be brought into the scrotum by conventional orchidopexy.

TECHNIQUE OF PEDIATRIC LAPAROSCOPY

Laparoscopy is performed with the patient under general anesthesia with the abdomen, groin, scrotum, and upper thigh regions prepped to facilitate laparotomy, if necessary. The bladder is emptied before laparoscopy to prevent inadvertent bladder injury. An orogastric tube decompresses the stomach before the needle placement and peritoneal insufflation. The arms are tucked at the side to prevent brachial plexus injury. The child is secured to the table to prevent inadvertent shifting during movement of the table.

Before a pneumoperitoneum is obtained, the proper equipment should be prepared and inspected. With the table in a slight (15°) Trendelenburg position, a small semilunar incision is made along the inferior or superior border of the umbilicus and the fascia scored. The periumbilical skin is grasped and held upward while the Veress needle is advanced at a 45° angle caudad. With proper placement of the needle, there is a slight "pop" as the needle pierces the fascia and then another less pronounced one as the peritoneum is entered. Correct intraperitoneal placement of the needle tip is essential and must be verified before insufflation. Easy instillation of saline through the needle and no return on aspiration indicates proper placement (Fig. 40.3). Another effective method of verifying proper position is placing a drop of saline solution in the hub of the Veress needle. When the stopcock is opened or the abdominal wall lifted upward, the drop should flow into the abdominal cavity. Several early warning signs of improper needle placement include the return of air or succus, which may indicate intravisceral placement; urine, which indicates intravesical placement; and frank blood, which suggests placement in a large vessel and should prompt immediate exploration. An alternative to using the Veress needle is the open Hasson technique[17] whereby a small peritonotomy is made, and under direct vision, the trocar is introduced into the abdominal cavity.

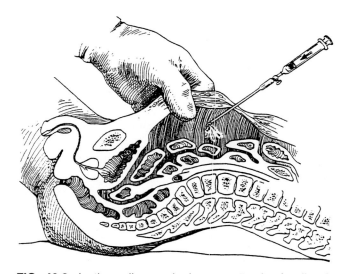

FIG. 40.3. In the saline aspiration test, 5 mL of saline is injected. One should not be able to aspirate if the needle is in the appropriate position. [From Elder JS. Urol Clin North Am 1989;16:399.]

Opening pressure must be noted and be less than 5 mm Hg. Maintenance of low intraabdominal pressure during the early moments of insufflation is the best indicator of intraperitoneal placement. As the pneumoperitoneum progresses, tympany noted on percussion should be equal in all abdominal quadrants. Insufflation with CO_2 is continued until the intraabdominal pressure is 15 to 20 mm Hg, at which time the Veress needle is removed and the appropriate sized trocar and laparoscope is inserted. A 5-mm laparoscope is usually sufficient for diagnostic laparoscopy; however, a larger trocar and scope and additional ports are necessary if more complicated procedures are anticipated. If working ports are necessary, they are placed under direct vision.

At the completion of diagnostic or operative laparoscopy, the intraabdominal pressure is lowered and the surgical sites and port sites inspected carefully for bleeding. Trocar sheaths are removed sequentially under vision and fascial defects closed with absorbable interrupted sutures. The skin is closed with subcuticular sutures.[18]

LAPAROSCOPIC MANAGEMENT OF NONPALPABLE UNDESCENDED TESTIS

Although it is unclear whether the cause of an undescended testicle is mechanical or hormonal or a combination of these factors, it is known that gross and microscopic abnormalities exist in the undescended testis and genital ducts. The goal of treatment is permanent fixation of the testis in the scrotum. Although this may be achieved in some instances by hormonal therapy, it is most consistently accomplished by one of several surgical techniques. Orchidopexy allows for (1) potential improvement of fertility; (2) relocation of the testis to a site amenable to examination (given the higher incidence of malignancy of an undescended testis); (3) correction of an associated hernia; (4) prevention of testicular torsion; and (5) alleviation of the psychological trauma resulting from an empty scrotum.[19]

Diagnostic Evaluation of Nonpalpable Testis

Approximately 20% of undescended testes are truly nonpalpable.[20] A nonpalpable testis may be intraabdominal (normal or dysgenetic), inguinal, or absent. Laparoscopy has gained acceptance as the most accurate diagnostic procedure to identify the exact anatomy of the nonpalpable testis and its adnexae.[6, 21, 22]

Testes should not be declared nonpalpable until a deliberate set of maneuvers does not elicit either a gonad or a remnant of one. Good physical examination requires placing the child at ease. A warm room, warm hands, and attempting to ease the child's anxiety help to achieve an accurate physical examination. An attempt is made to milk the testis down from the internal ring through the inguinal canal into the scrotum. Lubricating jelly sometimes helps one feel the gonad by decreasing the tactile friction. Placing the child in a cross-leg posture may further help deliver the testis. If a testis is still not palpable, examination should be repeated with the child under anesthesia at the time of operation. If the testis remains unequivocally nonpalpable, laparoscopy is performed.

The main area of interest is the internal inguinal ring. A spermatic vessel leash that ends blindly proximal to the internal ring proves absence of the testis; there is no distal gonad, and further exploration is unnecessary (Fig. 40.4). In other instances laparoscopy reveals attenuated or hypoplastic vessels still present at the internal inguinal ring. When we have explored the canal in instances of considerable hypoplasia, the gonadal remnants have generally been nonviable, but the persistent instances with discernible germ cells argue for remnant orchiectomy.[23]

Laparoscopic observation of an inguinal hernia is predictive of a distal gonad, which may be seen by passing the scope into the hernia sac. Alternatively, squeezing the scrotum or milking back the pubic and lower inguinal areas may cause the testes to peek through the internal ring, confirming its presence. Normal spermatic vessels at the internal ring mandate distal exploration (Fig. 40.5).

Laparoscopic Orchiectomy

An atrophic abdominal testis, particularly given a normal contralateral testis, should be removed. Laparoscopy offers several advantages. The simplest approach is to illuminate the abdominal wall adjacent to the abdominal testis and then make a small direct incision over the testis and remove it conventionally. Another option is placement of two additional ports and performance of laparoscopic orchiectomy.[24] The peritoneum over the spermatic vessels is incised. The vessels are doubly clipped and divided in between. The vas is similarly clipped and divided. The testis is mobilized and brought directly out a port site with the aid of an endobag.

When a diagnosis of unilateral testicular absence is made, we follow the advice of Harris, Kogan, and their coworkers to pex the contralateral solitary testis.[25, 26] Although the remaining solitary gonad may not have an increased risk of torsion, its loss, however unlikely, would be catastrophic. At the time of laparoscopy, we carefully place a few extraparenchymal sutures for fixation within a dartos pouch to minimize the risk of subsequent intravaginal spermatic cord torsion. It is important to secure the testis without injury to the gonad.[27]

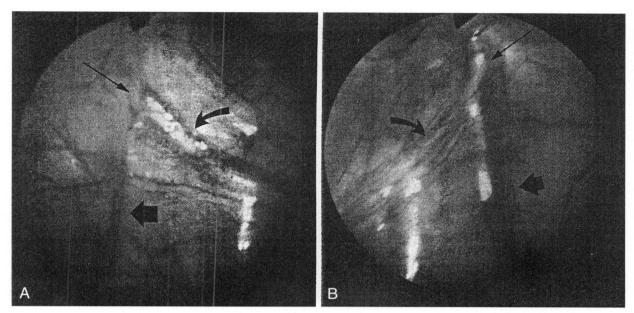

FIG. 40.4. Blind-ending spermatic vessels on the left side in a boy with a nonpalpable left testis and normal right testis. **A,** Left side: spermatic vessels (*short thick arrow*) end above the closed internal inguinal ring (*thin arrow*). Normal vas deferens (*curved arrow*). **B,** Right side: normal spermatic vessels (*short thick arrow*) cross into internal ring (*thin arrow*) adjacent to vas deferens (*curved arrow*). [From Bloom DA, et al., Pediatric Endoscopic Surgery, Norwalk: Appleton and Lange, 1994;41–50.]

Bilateral blind-ending spermatic vessels are uncommon. When this diagnosis is made, careful and compassionate counseling is mandatory. Given normal penile morphology, these boys will be completely normal until puberty, but will then need hormonal replacement for puberty and maintenance of secondary sexual character-

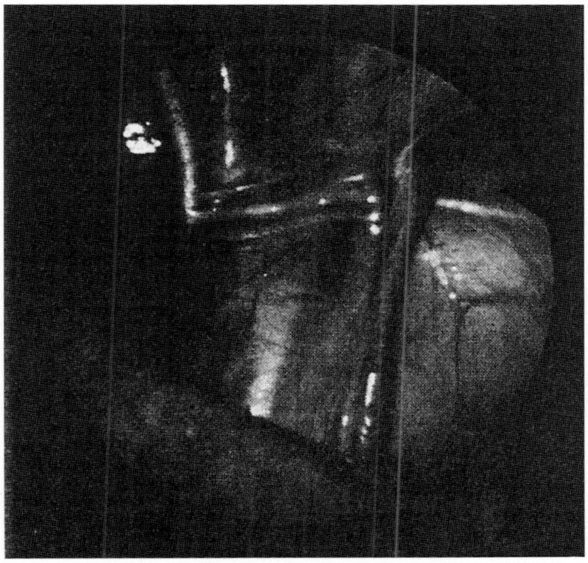

FIG. 40.5. Right hernia sac containing a distal testis in the inguinal canal. [From Bloom DA, et al., Clinical Pediatrics Feb 1993;100.]

istics. Early pediatric endocrinologic consultation is necessary. Anorchid adults will be infertile but should have normal sexual desires and function normally if maintained on appropriate exogenous hormonal support. Because the completely empty scrotum is flat and small, we favor early placement of small testicular prostheses and replacement with adult sizes after puberty. The anxiety over risks from silicon gel prostheses has raised concerns among patients and their families.[28]

Intraabdominal Testis

In approximately a third of the patients with a nonpalpable testis, the gonad will be situated above the internal inguinal ring. Laparoscopy is reliable in locating these organs. A true abdominal testis in our opinion is a gonad that lies consistently within the abdominal cavity, 1 cm or more above the internal inguinal ring. Some testes lie just within or at the internal ring and we describe them as "peeping" testes (Fig. 40.6). Traditional surgical exploration from the external ring craniad tends to chase these testes into the peritoneal cavity and thereby mislabel them as abdominal organs.[29]

The management of an intraabdominal testis remains controversial. Hinman advised that, given a normal contralateral gonad, most abdominal testes are best removed because of their doubtful fertility value and substantial malignancy risk.[30] In some instances, salvage of an abdominal testis is warranted. This is true in small

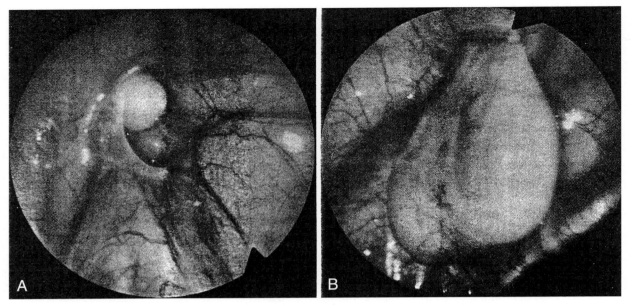

FIG. 40.6. **A,** A "peeping testis" at the internal ring. **B,** Laparoscopic view of a true intraabdominal testis. [From Bloom DA, et al., Pediatric Endoscopy Surgery, Norwalk: Appleton and Lange, 1994;41–50.]

children with a fairly normal-looking intraabdominal testis or in patients with bilateral abdominal testes. Laparoscopy provides the advantage of precise localization and inspection.

A variety of techniques are applicable for intraabdominal testis including conventional orchidopexy, staged orchidopexy, microsurgical autotransplantation, and Fowler-Stephens orchidopexy.[31–34] We have found that staged orchidopexy with endoscopic clip occlusion of the spermatic vessel leash with a Fowler-Stephens type of orchidopexy 6 months later is reliable and suc-

cessful even in children without long vasal loops (Fig. 40.7).[14, 35] Some authors have voiced concern regarding the high number of spermatic vessel divisions performed during laparoscopic surgery and the tendency to move away from the standard orchidopexy as a valid option for the intraabdominal testis.[36, 37] With more extensive use of pediatric laparoscopy, we should strive toward establishing accurate criteria for determining laparoscopically the testes that are descended sufficiently to allow for a single stage laparoscopic or open orchidopexy, or a staged repair.

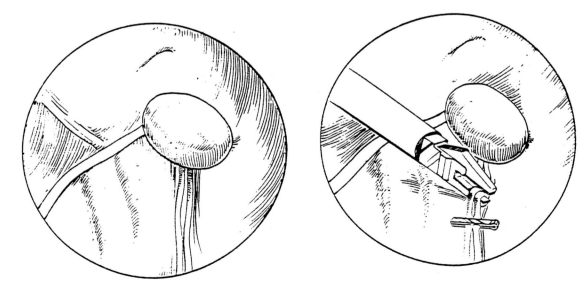

FIG. 40.7. An intraabdominal right testis with laparoscopic ligation of the spermatic vessels. [From Bloom DA, et al., Pediatric Endoscopic Surgery, Norwalk: Appleton and Lange, 1994;41–50.]

Primary Laparoscopic Orchidopexy

With increasing improvements in techniques and instrumentation, primary laparoscopic orchidopexy offers a viable alternative to the open technique. For an impalpable testicle that is emerging or peeping (high inguinal) or is immediately proximate to the internal ring (intraabdominal), single-stage laparoscopic orchidopexy have shown successful results.

The procedure can be performed endoscopically using two lateral 5-mm accessory cannulas and a midline 10/11-mm trocar. The testis, spermatic vessels, and vas deferens are mobilized by keeping a triangular flap of peritoneum attached between the distal vasculature and vas deferens. By including the peritoneum between the vessels and vas, fallback maneuvers including primary Fowler-Stephens after orchidopexy or a staged orchidopexy are possible if there is insufficient length adequate vascular dissection. After creation of a subdartos pouch in the scrotum, a 5-mm blunt rod with a threaded dilator is guided up through the canal and into the peritoneal cavity under direct vision. The testis is then delivered into the scrotum with grasping forceps and secured to the dartos pouch.[38]

In 1992, Jordan and associates[39] were the first to perform a laparoscopic single stage orchidopexy in a 10-year-old boy. Since this report, Jordan has completed 24 laparoscopic orchidopexies.[38] Others have shown successful results with the primary laparoscopic orchidopexy.[40, 41]

INTERSEX EVALUATION

Genital ambiguity at birth requires urgent evaluation to avoid the consequences of a social stigma. Physical examination, gestational history, and family history should be obtained. Phallic measurement is made according to the stretched length from pubic symphysis to tip of glans. Gonads should also be sought and measured if found. Rectal examination is performed to palpate for a cervix and uterus. Pelvic ultrasound may also help delineate the presence of a uterus. Critical laboratory studies include karyotype and electrolytes. The karyotype can be obtained from leukocyte tissue culture within 48 hours and has largely supplanted the buccal smear. Electrolytes are important in children with congenital adrenal hyperplasia (CAH), at the time of initial evaluation and over the ensuing 2 weeks, because maternal adrenocortical steroids may still be active in maintaining neonatal homeostasis.

Laparoscopic techniques have variable applications in diagnostic and reconstructive management of intersex conditions. Particularly appealing is inspection, biopsy, and removal of internal gonads and ductal structures. Few intersex patients will require laparoscopic management, and laparoscopy should be used only when it can be of real value. The neonatal applications remain of questionable value, but if used, laparoscopy essentially is an alternative to laparotomy for gonadal biopsy. However, laparoscopy for intersex management in older children and young adults has proven value. Yu et al.[42] reported on their 5-year laparoscopic experience in six intersex patients. Laparoscopy was valuable in defining internal ductal anatomy, in performing gonadectomy, and in removing inappropriate wolffian and Müllerian structures.

INDIRECT INGUINAL HERNIAS/ EXAMINATION OF CONTRALATERAL INGUINAL RING

Laparoscopic inguinal herniorrhaphy in the adult has some advantages over conventional open herniorrhaphy, especially in the case of bilateral or recurrent inguinal hernia. However, pediatric hernia repair holds little reason for laparoscopy. The open pediatric herniorrhaphy is practically a minimally invasive procedure that can be performed quickly, safely, and with absolute certainty of success. Nonetheless, laparoscopy may be performed in patients with hernia for another indication (i.e., hernia associated with an undescended testicle or a contralateral hernia discovered at the time of laparoscopy for an undescended testis).

One of the great dilemmas with the pediatric hernia has been whether to explore the asymptomatic contralateral side. Lobe and Schropp[43] were the first to report laparoscopic evaluation for contralateral inguinal hernia in children and reported an accuracy of 96% in diagnosing hernia. The incidence of contralateral inguinal hernia diagnosed by laparoscopy or open exploration is similar at 50 to 57%.[43–45] Other investigators have reported great satisfaction of inspection of the contralateral side through the patent processus vaginalis of the operated side.[46–49] However, it should be noted that the patency of the processus vaginalis is not equivalent to a clinical hernia. The major drawback to this method is that the small or friable patent processus tissue may not permit passage of the 5-mm optical sleeve. In addition, the increased cost of laparoscopic equipment and the extended time are considerations. Recently, Kaufman et al.[44] have reported a cost-effective way in examining the contralateral ring using a nondisposable cystoscope with 110° side-viewing lens.

RENAL PROCEDURES

While laparoscopic evaluation of genital structures in children has become an accepted technique, the laparoscopic approach to urinary tract structures (i.e., kidney, ureter, and bladder) in the child remains controversial. When evaluating a nonpalpable testicle, laparoscopy offers some important technical advantages over open surgery, including better access to the deep pelvis and a higher degree of magnification. Laparoscopic surgery of the urinary tract offers no such technical advantage; these procedures are generally considered more difficult than their open counterparts. The general advantages of laparoscopy over open surgery in the adult population are shortened hospital stay, decreased postoperative pain, more rapid return of normal pulmonary function, shortened duration of ileus, and more rapid return to normal activity. Compared to adults undergoing the same surgical procedure, children tend to require a shorter hospital stay, have less pain, more quickly resume normal pulmonary and bowel function, and return to normal activity sooner. Thus, the marginal benefit of laparoscopy would appear to be less in the child; therefore, the technical difficulties of urinary tract laparoscopy must be considered more carefully.

Nephrectomy

Laparoscopic nephrectomy in a child may be performed for any benign disease of the kidney requiring nephrectomy. Such conditions would include multicystic kidneys, poorly functioning or nonfunctioning kidneys associated with ureteropelvic junction obstruction, dysplastic kidneys causing hypertension, end-stage renal failure associated with excessive urinary protein loss or nephrogenic diabetes insipidus, or other symptomatic atrophic or dysplastic kidneys. Most experiences to date have been with a transperitoneal approach to the kidney. A retroperitoneal approach to pediatric nephrectomy has been described as well. Although the retroperitoneal technique suffers from a smaller working space and less distinct anatomic landmarks, it has some potential advantages, including a decreased risk of injury to bowel and intraabdominal viscera and possibly decreased postoperative discomfort.

Several investigators have reported individual cases or small series of pediatric laparoscopic nephrectomies.[50–53] The largest reported experience appears to be that of Ehrlich and associates,[54] who have reported performing 15 nephrectomies over a 2.5-year period. In all but two instances, the procedure was performed through a transperitoneal route. A retroperitoneal approach has been described by other authors as well. The largest pediatric retroperitoneoscopic nephrectomy series has been reported by Grune and associates,[55] who have described nine retroperitoneal pediatric nephrectomies. Their experience is summarized in Table 40.1. The average age of the patients was 8.8 years. The mean operative time was 263 minutes. All patients resumed oral intake the same day of the operation and the average hospital stay was 1.1 days, with an overnight admission in eight patients, and a 2-day admission in one patient. There were no complications reported. These results are compared in Table 40.1 to our experience at

the University of Michigan with nine consecutive, open, simple nephrectomies performed over the past year. The average age in these patients was 4.5 years. The mean operative time was 146 minutes. Patients resumed a normal diet in an average of 2.1 days after the procedure, and were discharged from the hospital an average of 2.9 days after the procedure. There were no complications in this group.

From a rough comparison of these data, it seems that the same advantages of laparoscopic surgery noted in adults occur in children, albeit of somewhat lesser magnitude in comparison to the open procedure. At the expense of almost 2 hours longer in the operating room, the patients resumed oral intake a day sooner and left the hospital almost 2 days earlier. Unfortunately, no data are available for postoperative convalescence at home, but it may be reasonable to assume that the improvements in morbidity from the laparoscopic procedure persisted during this time. The question then becomes: Is the increase in operative time justified by the decreased postoperative morbidity experienced by the patient? There is scant cost data available for these procedures in the pediatric population, but extrapolation from the adult experience would suggest that the laparoscopic procedure is at least $1,000 more expensive than the open procedure when all operative and in-hospital postoperative costs are included. It is apparent that a decrease in operating time would render the laparoscopic procedure more cost-effective. Given the modest improvements in postoperative morbidity in the younger pediatric population, it would seem most reasonable to consider laparoscopic nephrectomy in two situations. The first would be that of the older child in whom the marginal difference in morbidity between the laparoscopic and open procedures may be greater (as it is in the adult patient). The second would be a simple nephrectomy for a noninflammatory condition, such as multicystic dysplastic kidney or renal hypertension. The laparoscopic dissection is usually more difficult for a kidney that has suffered infection. For a noninfected kidney in a thin child, it would be expected that the operative time would be less than 2 or 3 hours. Although this appears to be a reasonable plan to use, the true usefulness of laparoscopic pediatric nephrectomy cannot be ascertained until a randomized trial between open and laparoscopic nephrectomy in the appropriate population is undertaken.

Other Renal Procedures

Other laparoscopic renal procedures have been reported occasionally in the literature. Ehrlich and associates[54] reported the excision of a giant renal cyst in two patients, nephroureterectomy in four patients, and a heminephrectomy for upper or lower pole hydronephrosis in four patients. Peer-reviewed reports of

TABLE 40.1. *Comparison of laparoscopic and open pediatric nephrectomy*

	Grune, 1996 Laparoscopic (retroperitoneal)	University of Michigan, past year Open (extraperitoneal)
No. of patients	9	9
Age, years	8.8 (7–14)*	4.5 (0.5–14)
Operative time, minutes	263 (70–300)	146 (80–176)
Time to resume diet, days	same day in all	2.1 (1–3)
Hospital stay, days	1.1 (1–2)	2.9 (2–4)

*Mean (range)

nephroureterectomy has been offered by other groups as well.[56, 57] All procedures were reported to be uneventful and followed by a rapid convalescence. Of all these procedures, the laparoscopic approach to nephroureterectomy would seem to hold the most potential advantage because the larger incisions necessary for open nephroureterectomy can be replaced by only four or five laparoscopic trocars for the laparoscopic procedure.

URETERAL AND BLADDER PROCEDURES

Pyeloplasty

Several authors have reported laparoscopic pyeloplasty for ureteropelvic junction obstruction in adults. The experience in children appears to be limited, with the only published report being that of Peters and associates.[58] The technical difficulty of this procedure and the high success rates of traditional open dismembered pyeloplasty raise questions about the advisability of this laparoscopic procedure in the pediatric population on a routine basis.

Repair of Vesicoureteral Reflux

In the United States, high-grade reflux is most commonly addressed with an operative procedure. Intravesical and extravesical techniques have been reported with high success rates, exceeding 95 to 97%. With the increased popularity of the extravesical approach, a laparoscopic technique of extravesical repair of vesicoureteral reflux has been considered by many urologists. After promising results with extravesical repairs in animal models,[59–61] small clinical series have been reported.[62, 63] With short-term follow-up, the results have been favorable. The benefits of the extravesical approach, with the shortened period or no catheter drainage and less potential for bladder pain and hematuria, combined with the minimally invasive nature of laparoscopy, may make this an important addition to pediatric surgery if these promising initial results are corroborated by future investigators. An alternative laparoscopic technique, endoscopic trigonoplasty, has been described by two groups.[64, 65] In this procedure, the trigone is drawn together by a series of midline sutures

that are placed using laparoscopic intravesical access. This intriguing technique deserves further study.

Ureterolysis

The first report of laparoscopic ureterolysis in 1992 by Kavoussi and associates[66] was in a 15-year-old girl with unilateral retroperitoneal fibrosis. The ureter was intraperitonealized without omental wrapping. Although an uncommon procedure, laparoscopic ureterolysis in adults has been shown to be an effective procedure and to have minimal morbidity compared to the open surgical approach. This would appear to be a reasonable option for the rare child who requires ureterolysis.

Bladder Autoaugmentation

Introduced by Cartwright and Snow in 1989,[67] this procedure has been performed laparoscopically in children. The initial reports appeared favorable,[68, 69] but subsequent experience has been disappointing.[70] The long-term results of autoaugmentation by the open technique recently have come into question. The future of laparoscopic bladder autoaugmentation remains in doubt.

Appendicovesicostomy

Jordan and Winslow,[71] reported the laparoscopic approach to appendicovesicostomy in a 15-year-old girl with a history of multiple failed bladder neck reconstructions. The recovery was uneventful, and at 18 months follow-up she was doing well. This case exemplifies the creative laparoscopic procedures that can be devised by a team of motivated surgeons.

COMPLICATIONS

The incidence of complications in pediatric laparoscopy is low with the overall estimates ranging from 0 to 5%.[72] Laparoscopy with gas insufflation introduces a unique set of physiologic complications, including: tension pneumoperitoneum, cardiac dysrhythmia, venous stasis and thrombosis, cerebral edema, cerebral ischemia, ocular hypertension, oliguria and fluid overload, hypothermia, hypercarbia, acidosis, acute respiratory insufficiency, hypoxia, subcutaneous emphysema, pneumomediastinum, pneumopericardium, pneumothorax, gas embolism, and intraabdominal explosion.[48]

Of greater concern during laparoscopy in children are potential technical errors. The most frequent technical complications are minor and are associated with the passage of the Veress needle, Hasson cannula, or secondary trocars; these include abdominal wall bleeding, preperitoneal and retroperitoneal insufflation, or minor lacerations of the omentum, mesentery, or bowel surface. Abdominal wall bleeding can often be controlled with direct pressure or a figure-of-eight suture (which can be placed under laparoscopic guidance). Damaged abdominal wall vessels often do not bleed significantly until after the tamponading laparoscopic port has been removed; port sites must always be inspected externally and internally (with the laparoscope) after removal of the port. Depending on their severity, minor omental, mesenteric, or bowel lacerations may be observed or may be managed with laparoscopic suturing. More serious complications include visceral or vascular punctures and these may require open surgical intervention for management.

The concern regarding injury by the Veress needle, given the minimal margin for error in the small abdominal cavity of the child, is part of the reason why many pediatric urologic laparoscopists use "open" placement of a Hasson cannula to gain laparoscopic access. In addition the preperitoneal space is "looser" in the child than in the adult,[9] which predisposes to preperitoneal insufflation or emphysema, and the technical consequences of preperitoneal gas (i.e., the hindered discernment of extraperitoneal structures) may be more significant in the child than in the adult. Thus, the proponents of the "open" laparoscopic access have some good arguments for the use of this technique, although we use the Veress needle in most patients who do not have a history of abdominal surgery because of its speed and effectiveness when used carefully.

Visceral or vascular injuries may also occur during the operative manipulation. The most common causes are inadequate identification of structures during dissection and electrocautery injury. With regards to the latter, all instruments should be inspected for defects in the insulation before insertion into the operative field. If electrocautery is applied and effects are not seen immediately at the tip of the instrument, attention should be directed along the shaft of the instrument to detect inadvertent conduction of energy to another instrument or a visceral structure.

Delayed complications of pediatric laparoscopy include infection, omental or bowel evisceration, bowel obstruction, and adhesion formation. As opposed to the usual recommendations in adults, even 5-mm port sites should be closed in children because of the potential for herniation.[73] The findings of Moore and associates[74] suggest that postoperative adhesion formation is minimal after pediatric laparoscopy; these authors noted an adhesion rate of only 9.8% at the time of "second-look" laparoscopy in 41 pediatric patients

FUTURE PERSPECTIVES

Laparoscopy for the diagnostic evaluation of undescended testes is one of the few laparoscopic procedures that is a "treatment of choice" for most pediatric urologists. The other laparoscopic procedures described in this chapter are: more expensive than their open counterparts (because of increased operative time and instrumentation), more difficult than their open counterparts because of absolute technical issues or because of the additional training required to perform the laparoscopic procedure, or too infrequently performed for a reasonable assessment to be made. There is no doubt that laparoscopic procedures benefit adult patients in terms of lessened postoperative morbidity. The marginal benefit of the decreased postoperative morbidity in the pediatric patient is more open to debate. All of these issues need to be addressed before the future role of laparoscopy in the practice of pediatric urology can be clarified. We need to compare directly the morbidity of open and laparoscopic surgery in similar groups of children, preferably in a prospective, randomized fashion. We need to decrease the costs of laparoscopic procedures by using fewer disposable devices and by simplifying procedures to decrease operative time. Finally, great improvements need to be made in laparoscopic instrumentation and techniques so that advanced laparoscopic procedures such as nephrectomy can be practiced more widely outside of large referral centers.

REFERENCES

1. Kelling G. Zur colioskopie. Arch Klin Chir 1923;126:226.
2. Jacobaeus HC. Kurze ubersicht uber meine erfahrungen mit der laparoskopie. Munch Med Wochenschr 1911;58:2017.
3. Palmer R. La celioscopie gynecologique. Rapport du Professeur Mocquet. Acad de Chir 1946;72:363.
4. Gans SL, Berci G. Peritoneoscopy in infants and children. J Pediatr Surg 1973;8:399.
5. Cognat M, Rosenberg D, David L, Papathanassious Z. Laparoscopy in infants and adolescents. Obstet Gynecol 1973;42:515.
6. Cortesi N, Ferrari P, Zambarda E, Manenti A, Baldini A, Pignatti Morano F. Diagnosis of bilateral abdominal cryptorchidism by laparoscopy. Endoscopy 1976;8:33.
7. Lobe TM. Basic laparoscopy. In: Holcomb GW, ed. Pediatric Endoscopic Surgery, Norwalk: Appleton & Lange 1993:83.
8. Capeluto CC, Kavoussi LR. Complications of laparoscopic surgery. Urology 1993;42:2.
9. Jordan GH, Bloom DA. Laparoendoscopic genitourinary surgery in children. In: Gomella LG, Kozminski M, Winfield HN, eds. Laparoscopic Urologic Surgery, NY: Raven Press, 1994;223.
10. McCammon KA, Jordan GH. Complications and changes in pediatric laparoscopic surgery. Dialogues Pediatr Urol 1995;18(9):3.
11. Naitoh J, Shichman SJ. Urological laparoscopic complications. In: Sosa RE, Jenkins AD, Albala DM, Perlmutter AP, eds. Textbook of Endourology, Philadelphia: WB Saunders, 1997;523.

12. Borten M. Contraindications. In: Friedman ED, ed. Laparoscopic Complications, Prevention and Management. Toronto: BC Decker 1986;139.

13. Bloom DA, Guiney EJ, Richey ML. Normal and abnormal pelviscopic anatomy at the internal inguinal ring in boys and the vasal triangle. Urology 1994;44:905.

14. Bloom DA, Semm K. Advances in genitourinary laparoscopy. Adv Urol 1991;4:167.

15. Golladay ES, Redman JF. Transverse testicular ectopia. Urology 1982;19:181.

16. Weiss RM, Seashore JH. Laparoscopy in the management of the nonpalpable testis. J Urol 1987;138:382.

17. Hasson HM. Open laparoscopy: a report of 150 cases. J Reprod Med 1974;12:234.

18. Faerber GJ, Bloom DA. Pediatric endourology. In: Gillenwater JY, Grayhack JT, Howards SS, Duckett JW, eds. Adult and Pediatric Urology, St. Louis: Mosby-Year Book, Inc., vol. 3, 1996;2739.

19. Kogan SJ. Cryptorchidism. In: Kelalis PP, King LR, Belman B, eds. Clinical Pediatric Urology, Philadelphia: WB Saunders, 1985;864.

20. Levitt SB, Kogan SJ, Engel RM, Weiss RM, Martin DC, Ehrlich RM. The impalpable testis: a rational approach to management. J Urol 1978;120:515.

21. Castilho LN. Laparoscopy for the nonpalpable testis: how to interpret the endoscopic findings. J Urol 1990;144:1215.

22. Naslund MJ, Gearhart JP, Jeffs RD. Laparoscopy: its selected use in patients with unilateral nonpalpable testis after human chorionic gonadotropin stimulation. J Urol 1988;142:108.

23. Rozanski TA, Wojno KJ, Bloom DA. The remnant orchiectomy. J Urol 1966;155:712.

24. Castilho LN, Ferreira U, Netto NR Jr, et al. Laparoscopic pediatric orchiectomy. J Endourol 1992;6:155.

25. Harris BH, Webb HW, Wilkinson AH, Steven PS. Protection of the solitary testis. J Pediatr Surg 1982;17:950.

26. Kogan SJ, Gill B, Bennett B, Smey P, Reda EF, Levitt SB. Human monorchism: a clinicopathological study of unilateral absent testes in 65 boys. J Urol 1986;135:758.

27. Bellinger MF, Abramowitz HB, Brantley S, Marshall G. Orchidopexy: an experimental study of the effect of surgical techniques on testicular histology. J Urol 1989;142:553,

28. Ehrlich RM. Silicon testicular prosthesis. Soc Pediatr Urol Newslett 1992;Oct:31–32.

30. Hinman F, Jr. Survey: localization and operation for nonpalpable testes. Urology 1987;30:193.

31. Youngson GG, Jones PF. Management of the impalpable testis: long-term results of the preperitoneal approach. J Pediatr Surg 1992;26:618.

32. Steinhardt GF, Kroovand RL, Perlmutter AD. Orchiopexy: planned 2-stage technique. J Urol 1985;133:534.

33. Stephens FD. Fowler-Stephens orchiopexy. Semin Urol 1988;6:103.

34. Silber SJ, Kelly J. Successful autotransplantation of an intra-abdominal testis to the scrotum by microvascular technique. J Urol 1976;115:452.

35. Elder JS. Two-stage Fowler-Stephens orchidopexy in the management of intra-abdominal testes. J Urol 1992;148:1239.

36. Heiss KF, Shandling B. Laparoscopy for the impalpable testes: experience with 53 testes. J Pediatr Surg 1992;27:175.

37. Ferro F, Lais A, Gonzalez-Serva L. Benefits and afterthoughts of laparoscopy for the nonpalpable testis. J Urol 1996;156:795.

38. Jordan GH, Bloom DA. Laparoscopic treatment of the impalpable undescended testicle. In: Smith AD, Bagley DH, Badlani GH, et al., eds. Smith's Textbook of Endourology, St. Louis: Quality Medical Publishing, 1996;2:1486.

39. Jordan GH, Robey EL, Winslow BH. Laparoendoscopic surgical management of the abdomina/transinguinal undescended testicle. J Endourol 1992;6:157.

40. Peters CA, Kavoussi LR, Retik AB. Laparoscopic management of intraabdominal testes. J Endourol 1993;7(suppl): S170.

41. Bogaert GA, Kogan BA, Mevorach RA. Therapeutic laparoscopy for intra-abdominal testes. Urology 1993;42:182.

42. Yu TJ, Shu K, Kung T, Eng HL, Chen HY. Use of laparoscopy in intersex patients. J Urol 1995;154:1193.

43. Lobe TE, Schropp KP. Inguinal hernias in pediatrics: initial experience with laparoscopic inguinal exploration of the asymptomatic contralateral side. J Laparoendosc Surg 1992;2:135.

44. Kaufman A, Ritchey ML, Black CT. Cost-effective endoscopic examination of the contralateral inguinal ring. Urology 1996;47:566.

45. Sparkman RS. Bilateral exploration in inguinal hernia in juvenile patients. Surgery 1962;51:393.

46. Chu C, Chou C, Hsu T, et al. Intraoperative laparoscopy in unilateral hernia repair to detect a contralateral patent processus vaginalis. Pediatr Surg Int 1993;8:385.

47. Holcomb GW. Diagnostic laparoscopy: equipment, technique, and special concerns in children. In: Lobe TE, Schropp KP, eds: Pediatric Laparoscopy and Thoracoscopy, Philadelphia: WB Saunders, 1994;19.

48. Wolf JS Jr, Stoller ML. The physiology of laparoscopy: basic principles, complications, and other considerations. J Urol 1994;152:294.

49. Wolf SA, Hopkins JW. Laparoscopic incidence of contralateral patent processus vaginalis in boys with clinical unilateral inguinal hernias. J Pediatr Surg 1994;29:1118.

50. Ehrlich RM, Gershman A, Mee S, Fuchs G. Laparoscopic nephrectomy in a child: expanding horizons for laparoscopy in pediatric urology. J Endourol 1992;6:463.

51. Koyle MA, Woo HH, Kavoussi LR. Laparoscopic nephrectomy in the first year of life. J Pediatr Surg 1993;28:696.

52. Suzuki K, Ihara H, Kurita Y, et al. Laparoscopic nephrectomy for atrophic kidney associated with ectopic ureter in a child. Eur Urol 1993;23:463.

53. Diamond DA, Price HM, McDougall EM, Bloom DA. Retroperitoneal laparoscopic nephrectomy in children. J Urol 1995;153:1966.

54. Ehrlich RM, Gershman A, Fuchs GJ. Laparoscopic renal surgery. In: Smith AD, Bagley DH, Badlani GH, et al., eds. Smith's Textbook of Endourology, St. Louis: Quality Medical Publishing, 1996;2:1496.

55. Grune MT, Donovan JM, Gill IS. Pediatric retroperitoneoscopic nephrectomy (abstract #P15-441). J Endourol 1996; 10(Suppl):S170.

56. Das S, Keizur JJ, Tashima M. Laparoscopic nephroureterectomy for end-stage reflux nephropathy in a child. Surg Laparosc Endoscop 1993;3:462.

57. Figenshau RS, Clayman RV, Kerbl K, McDougall EM, Colberg JW. Laparoscopic nephroureterectomy in the child: initial case report. J Urol 1994;151:740.

58. Peters CA, Schussel RN, Retik AB. Pediatric laparoscopic dismembered pyeloplasty. J Urol 1995;153:1962.

59. Atala A, Kavoussi LR, Goldstein DS, Retik AB, Peters CA. Laparoscopic correction of vesicoureteral reflux. J Urol 1993; 150:748.

60. Shimberg W, Wacksman J, Rudd R, Lewis AG, Sheldon CA. Laparoscopic correction of vesicoureteral reflux in the pig. J Urol 1994;151:1664.

61. McDougall EM, Urban DA, Kerbl K, et al. Laproscopic repair of vesicoureteral reflux utilizing the Lich-Gregoir technique in the pig model. J Urol 1995;153:497.

62. Ehrlich RM, Gershman A, Fuchs G. Laparoscopic vesicoureteroplasty in children: initial case reports. Urology 1994;43:255.

63. Janetschek G, Radmayr C, Bartsch G. Laparoscopic ureteral antireflux plasty reimplantation. First clinical experience. Ann Urol 1995;29:101.

64. Okamura K, Ono Y, Yamada Y, et al. Endoscopic trigonplasty for primary vesico-ureteric reflux. Br J Urol 1995;75:390.

65. Cartwright PC, Snow BW, Mansfield JC, Hamilton BD. Percutaneous endoscopic trigonplasty: a minimally invasive approach to correct vesicoureteral reflux. J Urol 1996;156:661.

66. Kavoussi LR, Clayman RV, Brunt M, Soper NJ. Laparoscopic ureterolysis. J Urol 1992;147:426.

67. Cartwright PC, Snow BW. Bladder augmentation: partial detrusor excision to augment the bladder without use of bowel. J Urol 1989;142:1050.

68. Ehrlich RM, Gershman A. Laparoscopic seromyotomy (auto-augmentation) for non-neurogenic neurogenic bladder in a child: initial case report. Urology 1993;42:175.

69. Braren V. Laparoscopic bladder autoaugmentation. Dial Pediatr Urol 1994;Feb:3.

70. Poppas DP, Uzzo RG, Britanisky RG, Miniberg DT. Laparoscopic laser assisted auto-augmentation of the pediatric neurogenic bladder: early experience with urodynamic followup. J Urol 1996;155:1057.

71. Jordan GH, Winslow BH. Laparoscopically assisted continent cutaneous appendicovesicostomy. J Endourol 1993;7:517.

72. Holcomb GW III, Brock JW III, Morgan WM III. Laparoscopic evaluation for a contralateral patent processus vaginalis. J Pediatr Surg 1994;29:970.

73. Bloom DA, Ehrlich RM. Omental evisceration through small laparotomy ports sites. J Endourol 1993;7:31.

74. Moore RG, Kavoussi LR, Bloom DA, Bogaert GA, Jordan GH, Kogan BA, Peters CA. Postoperative adhesion formation after urological laparoscopy in the pediatric population. J Urol 1995;153:792.

Bloom DA. Two-step orchiopexy with pelviscopic clip ligation of the spermatic vessels. J Urol 1991;145:1030.

Subject Index

717